Anatomy and Physiology of Speech and Hearing

Bernard Rousseau, PhD, MMHC, CCC-SLP, ASHA Fellow
Associate Vice Chair for Research, Department of Otolaryngology
Chancellor Faculty Fellow
Associate Professor of Otolaryngology, Hearing and Speech Sciences, and
    Mechanical Engineering
Director, Laryngeal Biology Laboratory
Vanderbilt University Bill Wilkerson Center
Nashville, Tennessee, USA

Ryan C. Branski, PhD, ASHA Fellow
Associate Director
NYU Voice Center
Associate Professor
Otolaryngology–Head and Neck Surgery and Communicative Sciences and
    Disorders
New York University School of Medicine
New York, New York, USA

460 illustrations

Thieme
New York • Stuttgart • Delhi • Rio de Janeiro

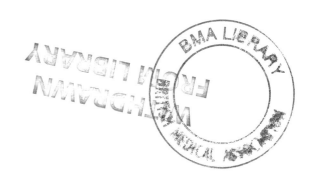

Acquisition Editor: Delia K. DeTurris
Managing Editor: Kenneth Schubach
Editorial Assistant: Rina Mody
Director, Editorial Services: Mary Jo Casey
Production Editor: Kenny Chumbley
In-House Production Editor: Torsten Scheihagen
International Production Director: Andreas Schabert
Editorial Director: Sue Hodgson
International Marketing Director: Fiona Henderson
International Sales Director: Louisa Turrell
Director of Institutional Sales: Adam Bernacki
Senior Vice President and Chief Operating Officer: Sarah Vanderbilt
President: Brian D. Scanlan

Library of Congress Cataloging-in-Publication Data

Names: Rousseau, Bernard, editor. | Branski, Ryan C., editor.
Title: Anatomy and physiology of speech and hearing / [edited by] Bernard
Rousseau, Ryan C. Branski.
Description: New York : Thieme, [2018]
Identifiers: LCCN 2017051277| ISBN 9781626233379 (softcover) |
ISBN 9781626233386 (ebook)
Subjects: | MESH: Speech--physiology | Hearing--physiology |
Respiratory System--anatomy & histology
Classification: LCC QP399 | NLM WV 501 | DDC 612.7/8--dc23
LC record available at https://lccn.loc.gov/2017051277

Important note: Medicine is an ever-changing science undergoing continual development. Research and clinical experience are continually expanding our knowledge, in particular our knowledge of proper treatment and drug therapy. Insofar as this book mentions any dosage or application, readers may rest assured that the authors, editors, and publishers have made every effort to ensure that such references are in accordance with **the state of knowledge at the time of production of the book**.

Nevertheless, this does not involve, imply, or express any guarantee or responsibility on the part of the publishers in respect to any dosage instructions and forms of applications stated in the book. **Every user is requested to examine carefully** the manufacturers' leaflets accompanying each drug and to check, if necessary in consultation with a physician or specialist, whether the dosage schedules mentioned therein or the contraindications stated by the manufacturers differ from the statements made in the present book. Such examination is particularly important with drugs that are either rarely used or have been newly released on the market. Every dosage schedule or every form of application used is entirely at the user's own risk and responsibility. The authors and publishers request every user to report to the publishers any discrepancies or inaccuracies noticed. If errors in this work are found after publication, errata will be posted at www.thieme.com on the product description page.

Some of the product names, patents, and registered designs referred to in this book are in fact registered trademarks or proprietary names even though specific reference to this fact is not always made in the text. Therefore, the appearance of a name without designation as proprietary is not to be construed as a representation by the publisher that it is in the public domain.

© 2018 Thieme Medical Publishers, Inc.
Thieme Publishers New York
333 Seventh Avenue, New York, NY 10001 USA
+1 800 782 3488, customerservice@thieme.com

Thieme Publishers Stuttgart
Rüdigerstrasse 14, 70469 Stuttgart, Germany
+49 [0]711 8931 421, customerservice@thieme.de

Thieme Publishers Delhi
A-12, Second Floor, Sector-2, Noida-201301
Uttar Pradesh, India
+91 120 45 566 00, customerservice@thieme.in

Thieme Publishers Rio de Janeiro, Thieme Publicações Ltda.
Edifício Rodolpho de Paoli, 25º andar
Av. Nilo Peçanha, 50 – Sala 2508
Rio de Janeiro 20020-906, Brasil
+55 21 3172 2297

Cover design: Thieme Publishing Group
Typesetting by Prairie Papers

Printed in India by Replika Press Pvt. Ltd.

ISBN 978-1-62623-337-9

Also available as an e-book:
eISBN 978-1-62623-338-6

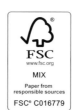

FSC
www.fsc.org
MIX
Paper from
responsible sources
FSC® C016779

To Dr. Diane Bless, for teaching me to embrace science and find happiness in the promise of discovery; to Mom and Dad for teaching me about sacrifice and perseverance; and to Alicia, Clara, and Camille for allowing me to pursue my life passion every day.

—*Bernard Rousseau*

To Drs. Sam Brown and Christine Sapienza, who taught me anatomy and physiology as an undergraduate student and helped shape my career; Dr. Zemlin's tattered text will remain on my bookshelf forever. And to Sarah and TR for simply being awesome.

—*Ryan Branski*

Contents

Preface...ix
Acknowledgments...xi
Contributors xiii

Part I: Foundations of Human Anatomy and Physiology 1

1   Framework for Anatomy and Physiology...3
    Samuel R. Atcherson, Melanie L. Meeker, and Bonnie K. Slavych

2   Composition of the Body: Cells, Tissues, Organs...31
    Elizabeth Erickson-DiRenzo and Daniel DiRenzo

3   Genetics..73
    Barbara A. Lewis, Sudha K. Iyengar, and Catherine M. Stein

4   Embryology and Development of the Speech and Hearing Mechanism 103
    Steven L. Goudy and Christen Lennon

Part II: Foundations of the Nervous System 135

5   Neuroanatomy...137
    Torrey Loucks and Li-Hsin Ning

6   Neurophysiology...171
    Michelle R. Ciucci, Erwin B. Montgomery Jr., and Lyn S. Turkstra

7   Suprasegmental Motor Control 191
    Erwin B. Montgomery Jr., Michelle R. Ciucci, and Lyn S. Turkstra

8   Peripheral Motor Control..233
    Mary J. Sandage and David D. Pascoe

9   Sensory Systems...263
    Richard D. Andreatta and Nicole M. Etter

Part III: The Anatomy and Physiology of Speech and Language, Swallowing, Hearing, and Balance 309

10 Respiration 311
    Erin P. Silverman and Bari Hoffman Ruddy

11 Phonation 351
    Christopher R. Watts

12 Articulation and Resonance..391
    Kate Bunton and Jessica E. Huber

13 Hearing...443
    Jason Tait Sanchez and Tina M. Grieco-Calub

14 Swallowing 483
    Michelle S. Troche and Alexandra E. Brandimore

15 Balance 523
    Elizabeth Meztista Adams

Glossary...557
Index...611

Preface

Anatomy and Physiology of Speech and Hearing serves an important need in the training of students in the field of communication sciences and disorders. The Council for Clinical Certification in Audiology and Speech-Language Pathology (CFCC) is a semi-autonomous credentialing body of the American-Speech-Language-Hearing Association. The CFCC establishes standards for obtaining the Certificate of Clinical Competence (CCC) in Audiology and Speech-Language Pathology. CFCC certification standards require that applicants for the CCC have knowledge of the biological and physical sciences. This includes biology, human anatomy and physiology, neuroanatomy, neurophysiology, human genetics, physics, and chemistry. Students should also have knowledge of basic human communication and swallowing, including the underlying biological, neurological, and developmental bases of speech, language, swallowing, hearing and balance disorders. *Anatomy and Physiology of Speech and Hearing* is the most contemporary title on the market, unrivaled in its coverage of anatomy and physiology, including recent advances in the understanding of basic cell functions, biological control systems, and coordinated body functions.

Careful attention is given to detail and in the consistency and presentation of information throughout the title to maximize learning. *Anatomy and Physiology of Speech and Hearing* contains expertly written chapters that make anatomical and physiological concepts readily accessible to even the novice reader. Illustrations are beautifully prepared, and each contributor ensures that the subject matter is accessible, straightforward, and easy to understand. This book incorporates the latest developments in the biological underpinnings of respiration, phonation, articulation, hearing, swallowing, and balance function and dismisses many common misconceptions that have permeated the field of communication sciences and disorders over the years, replacing them with the most accurate and contemporary account available in the literature. This book sets the standard for what future titles that teach communication sciences and disorders students will look like.

FEATURES: The following features make the content of each chapter readily accessible to students.

1. Detailed and modern anatomical drawings in a style that students have enthusiastically endorsed. A few examples are shown below.

2. Recent developments in cellular biology and physiology; providing a contemporary understanding of the biological foundations of speech, language, swallowing, hearing and balance, and new concepts that are not found in any other title available on the market.

3. In all chapters, textboxes and sidebars are used to provide meaningful examples of clinical disorders and a context for applying newly learned concepts. This connection between basic and clinical science provides students with additional opportunities to maximize learning and apply this new knowledge in clinical practicum settings.

4. Didactic features to assist educators and students in consolidation of learning, including learning objectives at the start of every chapter, the highlighting of key terms and concepts throughout the book, review questions, and chapter ending summaries.

5. Online access to illustrations for use in presentations and lecture notes.

6. Online access to review questions and answers for interactive study and review.

Bernard Rousseau, PhD, MMHC, CCC-SLP, ASHA Fellow
Ryan C. Branski, PhD, ASHA Fellow

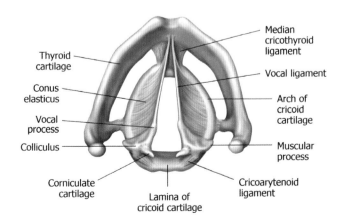

Structures of larynx (superior view)

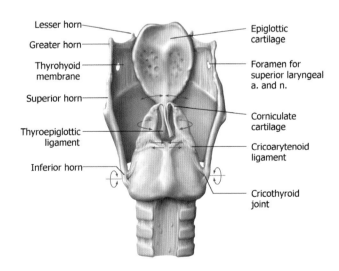

Structures of larynx (posterior view)

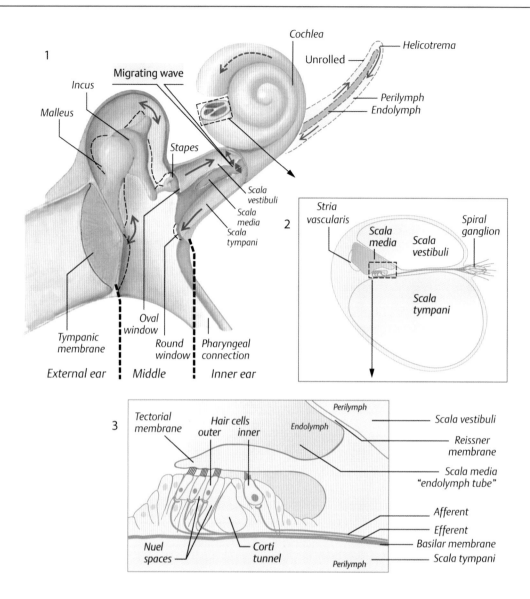

Acknowledgments

The authors of each chapter are owed a debt of gratitude. Not simply for creating an invaluable resource for the field, but also for displaying collegiality and an esprit de corps throughout all stages of manuscript preparation. The editors also wish to thank Thieme Medical Publishers, Inc. for believing in this project from the beginning, and allowing us to create a one-of-a-kind resource that will be used to prepare communication sciences and disorders trainees for many years to come.

Contributors

Elizabeth Meztista Adams, PhD
Department Chair and Associate Professor
Department of Speech Pathology and Audiology
University of South Alabama
Mobile, Alabama, USA

Richard D. Andreatta, PhD
Associate Professor
Department of Rehabilitation Sciences
University of Kentucky
Lexington, Kentucky, USA

Samuel R. Atcherson, PhD
Professor and Director of Audiology
Department of Audiology and Speech Pathology
Clinical Adjunct Associate Professor
Department of Otolarynology–Head and Neck Surgery
University of Arkansas at Little Rock
University of Arkansas for Medical Sciences
Little Rock, Arkansas, USA

Alexandra E. Brandimore, PhD, CCC-SLP
Assistant Professor
Department of Communication Sciences and Disorders
University of South Florida
Tampa, Florida, USA

Ryan C. Branski, PhD, ASHA Fellow
Associate Director
NYU Voice Center
Associate Professor
Otolaryngology–Head and Neck Surgery and
   Communicative Sciences and Disorders
New York University School of Medicine
New York, New York, USA

Kate Bunton, PhD
Associate Professor
Department of Speech, Language, and Hearing Sciences
University of Arizona
Tucson, Arizona, USA

Michelle R. Ciucci, PhD, CCC-SLP
Associate Professor
Department of Communication Sciences and Disorders
Department of Surgery–Otolaryngology Head and Neck Surgery
Neuroscience Training Program
University of Wisconsin–Madison
Madison, Wisconsin, USA

Daniel DiRenzo, PhD
Division of Vascular Surgery
Stanford University School of Medicine
Stanford, California, USA

Elizabeth Erickson-DiRenzo, PhD, CCC-SLP
Assistant Professor
Department of Otolaryngology–Head and Neck Surgery
Stanford University School of Medicine
Stanford, California, USA

Nicole M. Etter, PhD, CCC-SLP
Assistant Professor
Department of Communication Sciences and Disorders
The Pennsylvania State University
University Park, Pennsylvania, USA

Steven L. Goudy, MD
Associate Professor
Director of Pediatric Otolaryngology
Department of Otolaryngology
Emory University
Atlanta, Georgia, USA

Tina M. Grieco-Calub, PhD, CCC-A
Assistant Professor
The Roxelyn and Richard Pepper Department of
   Communication Sciences and Disorders
Northwestern University
Evanston, Illinois, USA

Jessica E. Huber, PhD
Professor
Speech, Language, and Hearing Sciences
Purdue University
West Lafayette, Indiana, USA

Sudha K. Iyengar, PhD
Professor and Vice Chair for Research
Department of Population and Quantitative Health Sciences
School of Medicine
Case Western Reserve University
Cleveland, Ohio, USA

Christen Lennon, MD
Department of Otolaryngology–Head and Neck Surgery
Vanderbilt University Medical Center
Nashville, Tennessee, USA

Barbara A. Lewis, PhD
Professor
Psychological Sciences
Case Western Reserve University
Cleveland, Ohio, USA

Torrey Loucks, PhD
Research Chair in Stuttering
Associate Professor
Department of Communication Sciences and Disorders
Institute for Stuttering Treatment and Research
University of Alberta
Edmonton, Alberta, Canada

Melanie L. Meeker, PhD, CCC-SLP
Assistant Professor
Communication Sciences & Disorders
Harding University
Searcy, Arkansas, USA

Erwin B. Montgomery Jr., MD
Professor
Division of Neurology
Department of Medicine
The Michael De Groote School of Medicine
McMaster University
Hamilton, Ontario, Canada
Medical Director
Greenville Neuromodulation Center
Greenville, Pennsylvania, USA

Li-Hsin Ning, PhD
Assistant Professor
Department of English (Linguistics Track)
National Taiwan Normal University
Taipei, Taiwan

David D. Pascoe, PhD
Humana Germany Sherman Distinguished Professor
Director of the Thermal and Infrared Labs
School of Kinesiology
Auburn University
Auburn, Alabama, USA

Bernard Rousseau, PhD, MMHC, CCC-SLP, ASHA Fellow
Associate Vice Chair for Research, Department of
    Otolaryngology
Chancellor Faculty Fellow and Associate Professor of
    Otolaryngology, Hearing and Speech Sciences and
    Mechanical Engineering
Director, Laryngeal Biology Laboratory
Vanderbilt University Bill Wilkerson Center
Nashville, Tennessee, USA

Bari Hoffman Ruddy, PhD
Professor
Department of Communication Sciences and Disorders
Professor of Internal Medicine
College of Medicine
University of Central Florida
Orlando, Florida, USA
Director
The Center for Voice Care and Swallowing Disorders
The Ear, Nose, Throat, and Plastic Surgery Associates
Winter Park, Florida, USA

Jason Tait Sanchez, PhD, CCC-A
Assistant Professor
The Roxelyn and Richard Pepper Department of
    Communication Sciences and Disorders
Northwestern University
Evanston, Illinois, USA

Mary J. Sandage, PhD, CCC-SLP
Assistant Professor
Department of Communication Disorders
Auburn University
Auburn, Alabama, USA

Erin P. Silverman, PhD, CCC-SLP, CCRC
Research Coordinator III and Adjunct Assistant Professor
Department of Medicine
University of Florida
Gainesville, Florida, USA

Bonnie K. Slavych, PhD
Speech Language Pathologist
Adjunct Instructor
Audiology and Speech Language Pathology
University of Arkansas for Medical Sciences
North Little Rock, Arkansas, USA

Catherine M. Stein, PhD
Associate Professor
Department of Population and Quantitative Health
    Sciences
Case Western Reserve University
Cleveland, Ohio, USA

Michelle S. Troche, PhD, CCC-SLP
Assistant Professor, Speech–Language Pathology Program
Director, Laboratory for the Study of Upper Airway
    Dysfunction
Department of Biobehavioral Sciences
Teachers College, Columbia University
New York, New York, USA

Lyn S. Turkstra, PhD, CCC-SLP, BC-ANCDS
Assistant Dean
Speech-Language Pathology Program
Professor
School of Rehabilitation Science
McMaster University
Institute for Applied Health Sciences
Hamilton, Ontario, Canada

Christopher R. Watts, PhD, ASHA Fellow
Director
Davies School of Communication Sciences & Disorders
Texas Christian University
Fort Worth, Texas, USA

Part I

Foundations of Human Anatomy and Physiology

1

Framework for Anatomy and Physiology

Samuel R. Atcherson, Melanie L. Meeker, and Bonnie K. Slavych

■ Chapter Summary

The human body is undeniably complex, yet it works in ways that can be understood in functional "bite-size" units, from micro (biochemical and cellular) to macro (system and body) levels. The study of anatomy and physiology is essential to the understanding of the human body. To fully appreciate a disorder, speech-language pathologists and audiologists must have a working knowledge of how various parts of the body function and how they work together toward a meaningful goal. The purpose of this chapter is to set the stage for the study of anatomy and physiology for speech, language, swallowing, hearing, balance, and related disorders. Specifically, we introduce terminology commonly used in the study of anatomy and physiology; provide an overview of the various body systems, including those used for speech, language, swallowing, hearing, balance, and related functions; and relate these concepts to disorders managed by speech-language pathologists and audiologists.

■ Learning Objectives

- Define and differentiate common terms used in the study of anatomy and physiology
- Understand the functions of the basic tissue and joint types in the human body
- Describe the general functions of the body systems supporting speech, language, swallowing, hearing, balance, and related functions

■ Putting It Into Practice

- Speech-language pathologists and audiologists are the professionals involved in the treatment of speech, language, swallowing, hearing, balance, and related disorders.
- The assessment and management of disorders related to speech, language, swallowing, hearing, and balance require a basic understanding of normal structure and function.
- The study of anatomy and physiology provides an essential framework in the practice of speech-language pathology and audiology.

■ Introduction

The study of human anatomy and physiology provides an important foundation for the speech-language pathologist and audiologist. The basic concepts of anatomy and physiology serve as the essential framework upon which to build an understanding of a variety of human activities. Students approaching the study of anatomy and physiology for the first time are often overwhelmed by the new terminology. Students will encounter many prefixes and suffixes that are used throughout the practice of medicine and related healthcare fields. Many of these roots are Latin or Greek in origin. For example, the prefix "a-" or "an-" is from a Greek word meaning "not" or "without." You may have encountered this prefix in the words *atypical* (meaning *not typical*) or *anaerobic* (meaning *with-*

3

out oxygen). An understanding of prefixes and suffixes will facilitate your learning of the material and increase the relevance of these terms to the practice of speech-language pathology and audiology.

A strong foundation in anatomy also provides important information about how the body works. Take the stylohyoid muscle as an example. Its name can be broken down into its component parts: *stylo-* (referencing the styloid process of the temporal bone) and *hyoid* (referencing the **U**-shaped bone above the larynx). The stylohyoid muscle spans the distance between the two structures. Knowing that striated skeletal muscles contract when stimulated, you can deduce that stimulation of this muscle draws the hyoid bone closer to the styloid process. An understanding of where the structures are located then provides information about function, which is to move the hyoid backward (posteriorly) toward the styloid. Although some exceptions to this general rule exist, a basic understanding of the general principles that underlie physiological function will provide a solid foundation upon which to build a conceptual framework.

To facilitate learning, students are encouraged to read assigned materials prior to class and to make purposeful notes in the margins of this text or on study cards. This preparation will allow you to more fully engage in lectures and acquire a deeper understanding of the concepts discussed during class. Consider incorporating a variety of cognitive and physical modalities in your learning. Practice drawing and labeling structures or manipulating them mentally to visualize them from different angles. Recite unfamiliar words aloud and practice their pronunciation. Explore topics of interest by accessing the supplemental materials referenced at the end of each chapter. Use the study questions at the end of each chapter to prepare for exams. These techniques will actively involve and engage aspects of your working memory and help you to organize and store information in your long-term memory for later retrieval (e.g., on an exam or when working with a patient). Mnemonic memory aids (e.g., acronyms or clever phrases) may also be helpful.

This text utilizes a variety of techniques to teach students keys to anatomical exploration and related physiology. The major anatomical systems are presented to familiarize students with the entire body. Glossary terms are bolded throughout the text, and definitions can be found within each chapter and at the end of the book. In addition, each chapter includes clinically relevant text boxes to increase the relevance of key concepts to clinical practice. Finally, a list of suggested readings in each chapter will guide the interested student to more information on the topics in the chapter.

Now that we have set the stage for your exploration of anatomy and physiology, let's begin. Simply stated, **anatomy** is the study of the structure of an organism. Gross anatomy consists of what can be inspected with the naked eye, such as what might occur in a cadaver lab. **Physiology** explores the functions of structures in a living organism. Together, the study of anatomy and physiology explores the structure and function of a living organism in terms of its parts and the organism as a whole. **Pathology** is the study of diseases and the structural and functional changes that affect an organism. This text provides a solid foundation in anatomy and physiology relevant to the practice of speech-language pathology and audiology.

■ Basic Elements of Anatomy

General Anatomical Terms and Anatomical Position

Early anatomists named structures based on what they resembled. As an example, a structure deep within the brain has a curly shape that, upon discovery, was thought to resemble a seahorse, so it was named the hippocampus from the Greek word for that animal. Hippos, "horse," is also found in hippotherapy, which makes use of the rhythmic movements of the horse.

Once you learn to deconstruct the vocabulary of anatomy, you will be on your way to mastery of the material. **Table 1.1** provides roots, their meanings, and an example of each root in the context of some commonly used terms in speech-language pathology and audiology.

Terms of Orientation

Used as a reference to describe various body parts relative to one another, the standard posture when in the anatomic position is with your full body standing straight, with the face directed forward, the arms hanging down at your sides with your palms facing forward, fingers pointing straight down, and the knees facing forward with the feet slightly apart and pointed forward. Anatomic position is important as it is the assumed position of reference when using directional terms to describe position or direction of body structures. Anatomic position is shown in **Fig. 1.1**.

Just as the directional terms north, east, south, and west serve as a reference on a compass (or GPS system), directional terms are commonly used to

Table 1.1 Meanings and examples of some common medical root words

Root	Meaning	Example	Definition
a-	without	aphonia	without voice
ab-	away from	abduction	draw away from midline (as in vocal folds)
ad-	toward	adduction	draw toward midline
-algia	pain	neuralgia	nerve-related pain
an-	without	anoxia	without oxygen
angio-	related to blood vessels	angiography	method of imaging vasculature
ante-/ antero-	before	antepartum	related to the time before birth
arth-	related to joint	arthritis	joint inflammation
bi-	two	bisect	divide into two portions
brachy-	short	brachydactyly	shortness of the fingers or toes
brady-	slow	bradykinesia	slow movement
capit-	toward the head	capital	the "head" location of government
cephalo-	the head or toward the head	cephalohematoma	a hemorrhage under the periosteum of the newborn skull
contra-	opposite	contralateral	the opposite side
-culum/ -culus	diminutive form for a noun	homunculus	"little man"
de-	away from; cessation	denervation	loss of nerve supply
di-	two	diplophonia	perception of two pitches simultaneously
dys-	disordered	dysphonia	disordered phonation
ecto-	outer	ectoderm	outermost layer of tissue in the embryo
-ectomy	excision	appendectomy	removal of the appendix
-emia	blood	septicemia	serious infection of the blood
endo-	inner	endoscopy	a procedure that looks inside the body using a scope
ep-/ epi-	upon or above something else	epidural hematoma	bleeding above (superficial to) the dura mater
extra-	outside	extraocular muscles	muscles outside of the eye that control its movement
-gen/-genic	producing; pertaining to	neurogenic	arising from the nervous system
hemi-	half	hemispherectomy	removal of a hemisphere of the brain
hyper-	above, or increased, or too much	hypertonic	containing more dissolved material than blood does
hypo-	below, decreased, or too little	hyporeflexia	reduced reflexive action
infra-	below	infrahyoid musculature	muscles that are situated below the hyoid bone
inter-	between	intercostals	muscles that are between the ribs
intra-	within; inside	intracranial	within the cranium
ipsi-	same	ipsilateral	referencing the same side
-itis	inflammation or irritation	pericarditis	inflammation of the sac around the heart
kine-	movement	kinesiology	the scientific study of human movement
latero-	side	lateral sulcus	the primary cerebral fissure situated on the side of the cortex
leuco- / leuko-	white	leukoplakia	thickened, white patches sometimes found on the vocal folds
macro-	large	macrocephaly	an abnormally large head

(Continued on page 6)

Table 1.1 *(Continued)*   Meanings and examples of some common medical root words

Root	Meaning	Example	Definition
medio-	middle	medial compression	the force pressing the vocal folds toward each other and toward the midline during phonation
micro-	small	microcephaly	an abnormally small head
mono-	single	monaural	referring to one ear
morph-	form	morphology	the study of the form of something
my-/myo-	muscle	myalgia	muscular pain
naso-	nose	nasopharynx	the upper part of the pharynx behind the nose
neo-	new	neoplasm	new growth (as in tumor)
neuro-	nerve	neuropathology	disorders of the nervous system
oculo-	eye	oculomotor nerve	cranial nerve that controls eye movement
-oma	tumor	vestibular schwannoma	benign tumor of myelin covering the vestibulocochlear nerve
oro-	mouth	oropharynx	the part of the pharynx behind the mouth
-osis	a state or condition	osteoporosis	lack of bone density
osteo-	bone	osteophyte	bone spur
ot-	related to the ear	otology	the study of the ear
palato-	referencing the palate	palatine tonsils	masses of lymphatic tissue situated on either side of the back of the palate
para-	beside	paraprofessional	individual who is trained to assist or "work alongside" other professionals
patho-	abnormal	pathophysiology	the disordered physiology associated with diseases or injuries
-pathy	disease state	myopathy	muscle disease
ped-/paed-	child	pediatrics	specialty of medicine dealing with care of children
ped-/pod-	foot	podiatry	specialty of medicine dealing with care of feet
peri-	around	periventricular	the area around the cerebral ventricles
-phage/-phagia	eating	dysphagia	a disorder of feeding/swallowing
pharyngo-	related to the pharynx	pharyngitis	inflammation of the pharynx
-plasia	growth	hyperplasia	excessive growth
-plasty	molding or forming	tympanoplasty	surgical repair of structures related to the ear drum
poly-	many; multiple	polycystic	characterized by many cysts
post-	after; behind	postpartum	after childbirth
pre-/pro-	before; in front of	prefix	an affix placed at the beginning of a root word
quadra-/quadri-	four	quadriparesis	partial paralysis of all four extremities
re-	repeating; turned back	recurrent laryngeal nerve	a branch of the vagus nerve (CN X) that descends into the chest before running back upward (recurring) to innervate structures of the larynx
retro-	toward the rear; backward	retrograde amnesia	loss of memory of events before an injury
-rrhea	flow	logorrhea	extreme verbosity

Table 1.1 *(Continued)* Meanings and examples of some common medical root words

Root	Meaning	Example	Definition
sclero-	hard	scleroderma	disease characterized by hardening of the skin and connective tissues
sclerosis-	hardening	arteriosclerosis	thickening or hardening of the arterial wall
scolio-	curved	scoliosis	sideways curvature of the spine
semi-	half	semicircular canals	half-circle structures in the inner ear that help with equilibrium and balance
soma-/somato-	referencing the body	somatosensory	part of the nervous system that tells us about the environment around us using touch, temperature, taste, and other sensory information
steno-	narrowing	tracheostenosis	narrowing of the tracheal lumen
-stomy	to create an opening	tracheostomy	a surgically created opening in the trachea
sub-	under	subglottic	below the glottis (vocal folds)
super-	above	superficial	area above (skin is superficial to bones)
supra-	above	suprasegmentals	features of speech (e.g., rate, stress, rhythm) that "lie over" the speech sound or segments; also known as prosody
sym-/syn-	with; together	synthesis	to pull together; combine
tachy-	fast	tachycardia	rapid heart rate
tetra-	four	tetraplegia	paresis or paralysis of all four limbs (also known as quadriplegia)
-tomy	cutting	tracheotomy	a surgical incision in the trachea
trans-	on the other side	transfusion	giving blood or blood products from one individual to another
tri-	three	tricuspid	upper third molar with three cusps/points
-trophic	nourishment	hypertrophy	increase in size due to growth
-trophy	growth; expansion	atrophy	tissue wasting
uni-	one	unilateral	on one side

orient to a specific area of the body. Perhaps the most commonly used terms are *superior*, *inferior*, *anterior*, and *posterior*. These terms tell you the position of a point of interest in the body relative to some other body part. When something is superior, it is above or higher than another structure; when inferior, it is below or under; when anterior, it is in front; and when posterior, it is behind or in back of another structure (see **Fig. 1.1**). For example, the head is superior to the neck, the ankle is inferior to the knee, the spine is posterior to the heart, and the sternum (breastbone) is anterior to the spine.

Other commonly used directional terms include *dorsal*, *ventral*, *rostral*, *caudal*, *superficial*, and *deep*. **Dorsal** refers to the posterior surface (as in a dolphin's dorsal fin) and **ventral** refers to the anterior surface (toward the belly). **Rostral** means toward the nose, while **caudal** indicates toward the tail. (A speaker's platform is called a *rostrum* after the Ros-

tra in the ancient Roman Forum, which was decorated with the rams from the bow ends of captured warships.) The term **superficial** indicates toward the surface, while **deep** references away from a surface. Putting it into practice, you could say that the heart is deep to the rib cage and your skin is superficial to your bones.

The terms *proximal*, *distal*, *medial*, and *lateral* are used to describe the position of a structure relative to the central part of the body (**Fig. 1.1**). When something is **proximal** to another structure, it is nearer to the trunk (the shoulder is proximal to the elbow). Conversely, **distal** indicates that something is further from the trunk (the elbow is distal to the shoulder). The term **medial** indicates that a structure is toward the middle, whereas **lateral** is used to indicate toward the side. For example, the lungs are lateral to the heart and the heart is medial to the lungs.

You should also become familiar with the terms *ipsilateral* and *contralateral*. You just learned that *lateral* (the root word in both terms) means side. Considering that *ipsi-* means same, **ipsilateral** means "on the same side." For example, the left arm and left leg are ipsilateral to one another; they are on the same side of the body. The prefix *contra-* means against or in opposition to. When *contra-* is paired with *lateral*, they give the meaning *opposite side* for the word **contralateral**. Your ears are on contralateral sides of your head. Combining these ideas and putting them into practice, we might say that the right arm is ipsilateral to the right leg and contralateral to the left arm. See **Table 1.2** for a summary of directional terms.

Anatomic Planes

A body part, such as the brain, may be imaged or dissected for many reasons, including the need to make a diagnosis (e.g., stroke), to observe changes during and/or after treatment, or to increase our knowledge of its internal structure. When referring to the sectioned body part, medical professionals use terms to orient observers to the surface or **plane** being viewed (**Fig. 1.2**). In human anatomy, the three basic planes are sagittal, coronal, and transverse. A **sagittal plane** divides the body or structure into left and right parts. If it divides the body *equally* into left and right parts, it may be called a **midsagittal plane**; else it is **parasagittal**. A **coronal** (or **frontal**) **plane** divides the body into front and back (anterior and posterior) parts. A **transverse** (also called **horizontal**, **axial**, or **transaxial**) **plane** divides the body into top and bottom (superior and inferior) parts.

■ Building Blocks: Tissues and Systems

The structures that make up the human body are composed of cells: living units that contain a nucleus and supporting cellular structures. The body's cells serve specialized functions that are critical to normal tissue and organ function. Four basic tissue types make up all of the structures in the human body. The tissue types are epithelial, connective, muscular, and nervous tissue. The tissues combine to form the structures that are explored deeply in this text. These essential building blocks are covered in more detail in Chapter 2.

Epithelial tissue makes up the outer layer of mucous membrane and the cells of your skin. Epi-

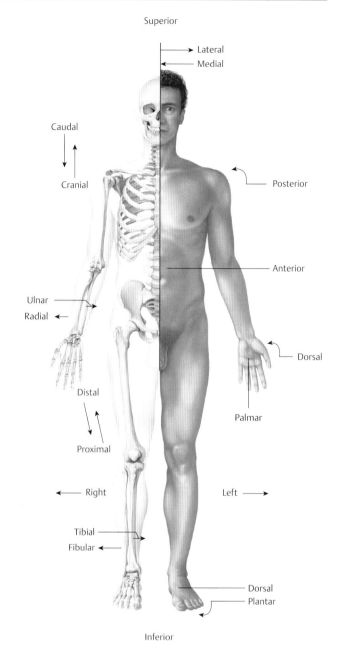

Fig. 1.1   Anatomic position. Anterior view.

thelial cells are found in the linings of body cavities, including your mouth, nose, trachea, esophagus, and digestive tract. Epithelial cells are tightly packed together and form a protective membranous sheet that serves as a barrier to infectious agents. In addition, epithelial cells of your skin help keep your body from losing moisture. Some epithelial cells contain cilia, or hairlike structures, such as those found lining the passageways of the respiratory system and middle ear. The cilia trap pollutants, and their beating motion serves to move the contaminants out of the body.

Table 1.2 General terms of location and direction

Upper body (head, neck, and trunk)	
Term	**Explanation**
Cranial	Pertaining to, or located toward, the head
Caudal	Pertaining to, or located toward, the tail
Anterior	Pertaining to, or located toward, the front; "ventral" usually a synonym (used for all animals)
Posterior	Pertaining to, or located toward, the back; "dorsal" usually a synonym (used for all animals)
Superior	Upper or above
Inferior	Lower or below
Axial	Pertaining to the axis of a structure
Transverse	Situated at right angles to the long axis of a structure
Longitudinal	Parallel to the long axis of a structure
Horizontal	Parallel to the plane of the horizon
Vertical	Perpendicular to the plane of the horizon
Medial	Toward the median plane
Lateral	Away from the median plane (toward the side)
Median	Situated in the median plane or midline
Peripheral	Situated away from the center
Superficial	Situated near the surface
Deep	Situated deep beneath the surface
External	Outer, superficial, or lateral
Internal	Inner, deep, or medial
Apical	Pertaining to the top or apex
Basal	Pertaining to the bottom or base
Sagittal	Situated parallel to the sagittal suture
Coronal	Situated parallel to the coronal suture (pertaining to the crown of the head)
Limbs	
Term	**Explanation**
Proximal	Close to, or toward, the trunk, or toward the point of origin
Distal	Away from the trunk (toward the end of the limb), or away from the point of origin
Radial	Pertaining to the radius or the lateral side of the forearm
Ulnar	Pertaining to the ulna or the medial side of the forearm
Tibial	Pertaining to the tibia or the medial side of the leg
Fibular	Pertaining to the fibula or the lateral side of the leg
Palmar (volar)	Pertaining to the palm of the hand
Plantar	Pertaining to the sole of the foot
Dorsal	Pertaining to the back of the hand or the top of the foot

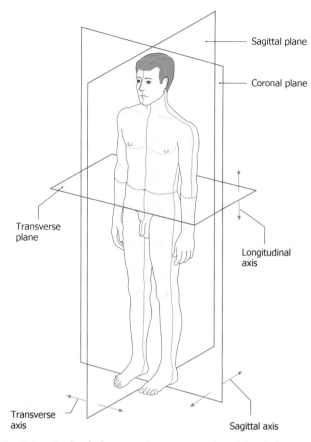

Fig. 1.2 Cardinal planes and axes: neutral position, left anterolateral view.

The body contains many types of connective tissue, including blood, cartilage, and bone. **Cartilage** is a strong and elastic tissue that provides a smooth articulating surface where the bones of your body meet. Cartilage absorbs shock, which is crucial in joints like the knees. Disks of cartilage can be found between the vertebrae and serve to cushion the joints. Cartilage provides structure to familiar facial features, such as the nose and ears, and also forms structures you cannot see, such as the larynx. Rings of cartilage hold the trachea open so it does not collapse during inhalation. The elastic and flexible nature of the cartilage in the rib cage supports the expansion of your ribs for inhalation and the return of these structures to "resting position" with exhalation.

Bone is the hardest of the connective tissues and forms the skeleton, to which muscles attach, allowing movement of the various body parts. The average adult human skeleton contains 206 bones of varying sizes and shapes. In addition to providing

a framework for the body, the skeletal system also provides protection for underlying organs.

■ Skeletal and Muscular System

When referencing the skeletal system, you may hear and see the terms *axial* and *appendicular*. The axial skeleton supports the central portion of the body and is composed of the 80 bones that form the skull, vertebral column, and thoracic cage (chest region). The axial skeleton provides support and protection for the brain, spinal cord, and organs in the thorax. The appendicular skeleton (or system) supports the extremities (arms and legs) and is composed of 126 bones that form the upper and lower limbs. The appendicular skeleton is joined to the axial skeleton through sets of bones and joints called *girdles*. The pectoral girdle joins the upper extremities to the thorax, and the pelvic girdle provides the attachment for the lower extremities. Movement of the appendicular skeleton supports mobility and physical interaction with the environment.

Skull

Composed of 22 bones, the human skull serves several important purposes, including housing and protecting the brain and organs of equilibrium, hearing, vision, smell, and taste, as well as providing points of attachment for muscles that allow head movement and facial expression. The human skull may be divided into two parts: the **neurocranium** and the **viscerocranium**. The neurocranium (or simply *cranium*) is the part of the skull that surrounds the brain. It is composed of eight **cranial bones**: the frontal, two parietal, two temporal, occipital, sphenoid, and ethmoid bones. The parietal and temporal bones are paired (**Fig. 1.3** and **Fig. 1.4**), meaning they have symmetrical and distinct contralateral counterparts.

The cranial vault (or cranial cavity) is the space within the cranium occupied by the brain; the calvaria (or skullcap) is the top portion of the cranium and covers the cranial vault. **Fig. 1.5** shows the cranial vault with the calvaria removed. At the base of the cranium (in the occipital bone) there is a very large opening called the **foramen magnum**. The foramen magnum is the space through which the spinal cord exits the skull at the base of the brain (**Fig. 1.6**). The viscerocranium is also known as the

Box 1.1   Otitis Media

Otitis media (ear infection) is acute inflammation or chronic fluid in the middle ear that can lead to conductive hearing impairment and balance problems and has been linked to speech and language delays in young children. The prefix *oto-* refers to the ear, the suffix *-itis* refers to inflammation, and *media* refers to the "middle of things." The peripheral hearing apparatus resides *deep* within the petrous portion of the temporal bone and includes the ear canal, the middle ear (air-filled space with three small transmission bones), and the inner ear (receptor organ for hearing). With otitis media, the middle ear (**Box Fig. 1.1**) is subjected to abnormal negative pressure (vacuum) and/or fluid buildup (infected or not). Otitis media is typically secondary to a temporary or permanent malfunction of the **Eustachian tube**. The middle ear space is lined with tissues that can absorb gases. When gases are absorbed, the middle ear space develops negative pressure. Whenever we swallow or yawn, the eustachian tube opens and a small amount of air is delivered from the back of the throat to the middle ear space, reestablishing equilibrium of air pressure on both sides of the tympanic membrane (eardrum). The eustachian tube is angled in a lateral-posterior to medial-anterior manner from the middle ear to the back of the throat. With otitis media, conductive hearing loss can occur. In severe cases, the significant negative pressure can pull fluid back out of the surrounding tissues, and overaccumulation of fluid in the middle ear can cause the tympanic membrane to rupture.

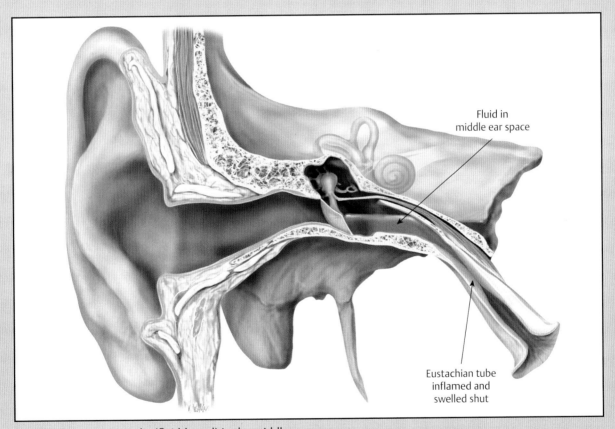

Fluid in middle ear space

Eustachian tube inflamed and swelled shut

Box Fig. 1.1   Otitis media (fluid-based) in the middle ear space.

Box 1.2 Tracheoesophageal Fistulas

Tracheoesophageal fistulas (TEFs) are openings that connect the trachea to the esophagus (**Box Fig. 1.2**). In healthy individuals, there is no connection between these passageways. Swallowed material stays in the esophagus (food tube) on its way to the digestive system, while respiration occurs via the **trachea** (windpipe). The word *fistula*, from a Latin word for pipe, means an abnormal opening. TEFs provide the opportunity for swallowed material to enter the respiratory system, resulting in aspiration and potentially life-threatening complications. Air may also enter the esophagus via a TEF, although the resulting complications are not generally as serious.

TEFs can be congenital (present from birth) or acquired. For example, tracheostomy tubes that put pressure on the posterior wall of the trachea can cause the tissue to wear away, resulting in a hole or passageway between the two structures. TEFs can also develop as a complication of surgical procedures, such as laryngectomy. Congenital TEF may also occur with esophageal atresia (EA), where the esophagus does not properly connect to the stomach. Both TEF (whether congenital or acquired) and EA have life-threatening implications and are treated surgically.

Interestingly, a connection between the esophagus and trachea can be useful for communication in certain situations. A laryngectomee (i.e., an individual whose larynx has been removed surgically) may have a tracheo-esophageal puncture (TEP), which is a surgically created passageway between the esophagus and trachea. Using a prosthesis inserted into the TEP, the laryngectomee can produce sound by shunting air from the lungs to the esophagus. The vibratory source for speech becomes the esophageal tissue rather than the vocal folds, which were removed with the larynx. Aspiration of swallowed material that "leaks" through the TEP remains a concern for individuals using TEP for speech; candidates for this method of communication are carefully selected and closely followed by the healthcare team.

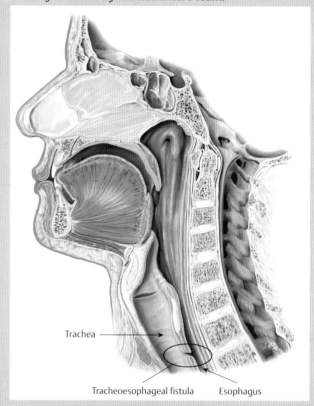

Box Fig. 1.2 Tracheoesophageal fistula.

facial skeleton and is composed of 14 facial bones: the mandible, maxilla, palatine bone (not pictured), zygomatic bone, nasal bone, lacrimal bone, vomer (not pictured), and inferior nasal conchae, all of which are paired except the mandible and vomer (**Fig. 1.3** and **Fig. 1.4**).

At birth, the human skull consists of about 44 bones. Upon birth and for the first 18 to 24 months afterward, the infant's cranial bones are not firmly articulated (joined together). For example, in the adult skull, there is only one frontal bone. However, in the infant skull, there are two frontal bones that fuse during postnatal development. The presence of many smaller bones at birth that later fuse together is necessary for the newborn's passage through the birth canal and the subsequent rapid brain and skull growth over the following years. Sutures, bands of fibrous material that allow rapid expansion during growth, hold the infant's cranial bones together until they fuse or ossify, forming the 22 bones in the adult skull. The infant skull has four sutures: frontal, coronal, sagittal, and lambdoid (**Fig. 1.7** and **Fig. 1.8**).

The frontal suture, also called the metopic suture, extends down the middle of the forehead toward the nose and is the site where the two frontal bones fuse. The coronal suture extends over the head from ear to ear and is the site where the frontal bone fuses with the two parietal bones. The sagittal suture extends length-

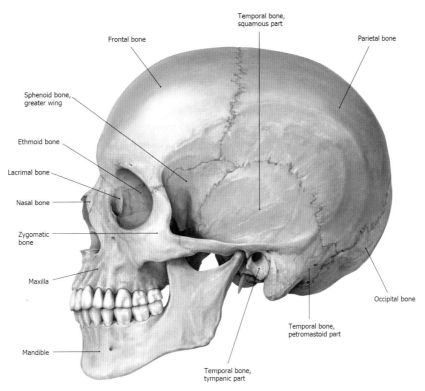

Fig. 1.3 Cranial and facial bones.

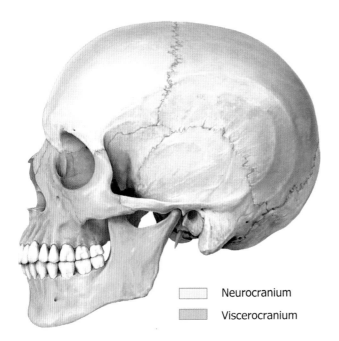

Neurocranium

Viscerocranium

Fig. 1.4 Bones of the neurocranium and viscerocranium.

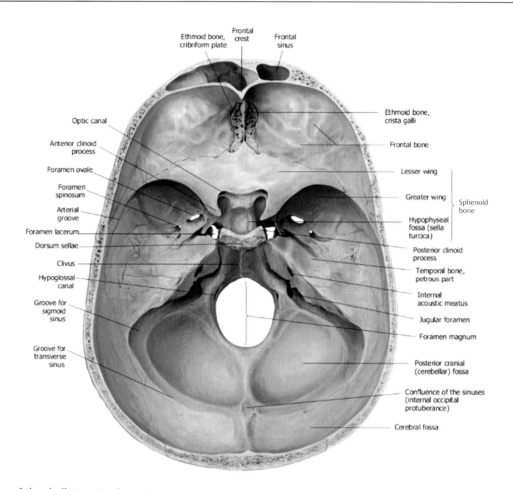

Fig. 1.5 Base of the skull: interior. Superior view.

wise down the top of the head, from anterior to posterior, and is the site where the two parietal bones fuse. The lambdoid suture extends across the posterior portion of the head and is the site where each parietal bone fuses with the occipital bone.

Fontanelles, colloquially referred to as soft spots, are the spaces between the cranial bones where the sutures eventually meet (**Fig. 1.7** and **Fig. 1.8**). They are covered by tough membranes to protect the brain. The anterior fontanelle is found at the junction of the two frontal and two parietal bones and typically closes between 18 and 24 months of age. The posterior fontanelle is found at the junction of the two parietal bones and the single occipital bone and usually closes within the first several months of life.

Vertebral Column

Composed of 33 bones called vertebrae, the vertebral column (commonly referred to as the backbone or spine) houses and protects the spinal nerve roots and spinal cord (**Fig. 1.9**). Starting at the base of the skull, it extends in a single column down the back, ending at the pelvis. The vertebral column is divided into five groups of vertebrae, called spinal regions. From superior to inferior (top to bottom), the regions are termed *cervical, thoracic, lumbar, sacral,* and *coccygeal*. Each vertebra is labeled according to its spinal region and serial placement within that region (e.g., the fifth cervical vertebra is labeled C5). Each vertebra (except for C1) is separated from the one that follows by an intervertebral disk made of cartilage, which helps cushion or absorb shock during movement.

Fig. 1.6 Foramen magnum.

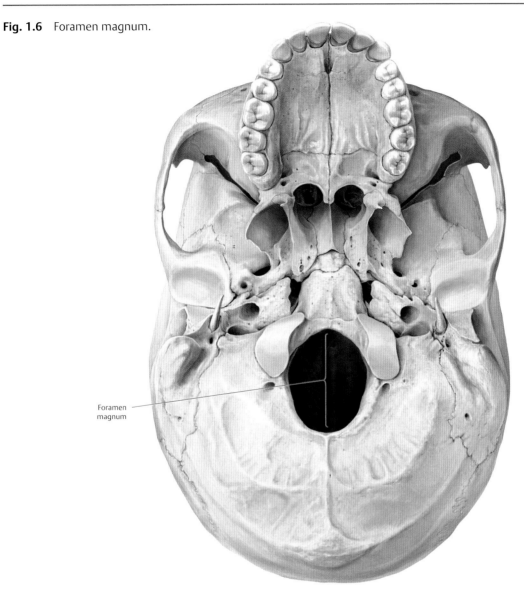

Foramen
magnum

Fig. 1.7 Cranial sutures and fontanelles. Superior view.

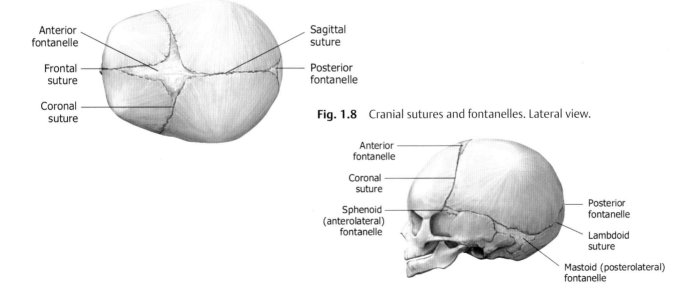

Anterior
fontanelle

Frontal
suture

Coronal
suture

Sagittal
suture

Posterior
fontanelle

Fig. 1.8 Cranial sutures and fontanelles. Lateral view.

Anterior
fontanelle

Coronal
suture

Sphenoid
(anterolateral)
fontanelle

Posterior
fontanelle

Lambdoid
suture

Mastoid (posterolateral)
fontanelle

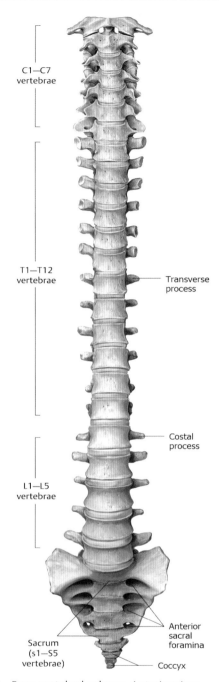

C1—C7
vertebrae

T1—T12
vertebrae

Transverse
process

Costal
process

L1—L5
vertebrae

Sacrum
(s1—S5
vertebrae)

Anterior
sacral
foramina

Coccyx

Fig. 1.9 Bony vertebral column. Anterior view.

Consisting of seven vertebrae, the cervical spine (C1–C7) is the most superior spinal region. It is designed for flexibility and is located in the neck. Highly specialized and given unique names (atlas and axis), the first two vertebrae within this region differ from the other vertebrae in that they are designed specifically for rotation. The *atlas* (C1) is located at the base of the skull and sits atop the *axis* (C2). The axis has a bony prominence (odontoid process or dens) that juts upward and articulates with the atlas, allowing rotational movement of the head.

Consisting of 12 vertebrae, the thoracic spine (T1–T12) is inferior to the cervical spine and is located in the upper and middle back. The thoracic spine is distinguished from the other spinal regions by the articulation of a rib on the right and left side of each thoracic vertebra. Built for stability, the thoracic spine is important for holding the body upright and for providing protection for the vital organs in the chest.

Consisting of five vertebrae, the lumbar spine (L1–L5) is inferior to the thoracic spine and is located in the lower back. The lumbar spine is distinguished from the other spinal regions in that the lumbar vertebrae are the largest of all unfused vertebrae. Built for power and flexibility, the lumbar spine is important for lifting, twisting, and bending.

Consisting of five vertebrae, the sacral spine (S1–S5) is inferior to the lumbar spine and is located posterior to the pelvic cavity. The sacral spine is composed of vertebral segments that begin to fuse during late adolescence and early adulthood to form a single triangular bone by around 30 years of age. This strong bone, the sacrum, supports the weight of the upper body and, in part, surrounds and protects the spinal nerves of the lower back. Last, the coccygeal vertebrae, which usually consist of five fused vertebrae forming the coccyx, are the most inferior of the spinal regions.

Torso

The torso, or trunk, refers to the portion of the axial skeleton that includes the thorax and abdomen; it excludes the head, arms, and legs. Located within the torso, the thoracic, abdominal, and pelvic cavities contain visceral organs, nerves, and blood vessels. Commonly referred to as the chest, the thorax is the region between the neck and diaphragm (**Fig. 1.10**). Its shell is referred to as the thoracic wall or cage (you've probably heard the term *rib cage*). The thoracic cage is made up of the 12 thoracic vertebrae aligned vertically along the upper and middle back and 12 pairs of ribs that extend from either side of each thoracic vertebra, curving outward from the back before turning inward toward the front of the body. There ten rib pairs attach to costal cartilage, which then attaches to the sternum or breastbone (**Fig. 1.11**). As the second largest hollow space within the body, the thoracic cavity houses the heart and great vessels,

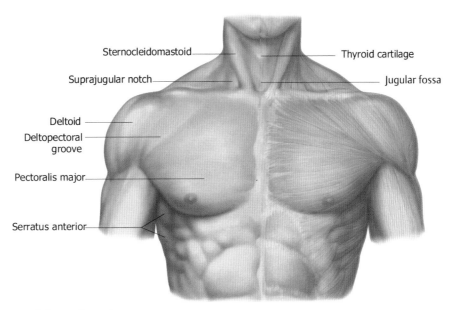

Fig. 1.10   Anterior view of thorax (torso).

the lungs, and other important structures, such as the trachea (windpipe) and esophagus. Specifically, the heart and other structures of the thorax, except the lungs, are contained within the mediastinum, the middle portion of the thoracic cavity.

The abdominal and pelvic cavities are both located within a larger, single cavity called the abdominopelvic cavity, which is inferior to the thoracic cavity. The abdominal and pelvic cavities are continuous with one another, distinguished only by the bony boundaries of the pelvis. The abdominal cavity is located superior to the pelvic cavity and houses the bulk of the visceral organs, including the stomach, intestines, pancreas, kidneys, and liver. The pelvic cavity, located immediately inferior to the abdominal cavity, contains the reproductive

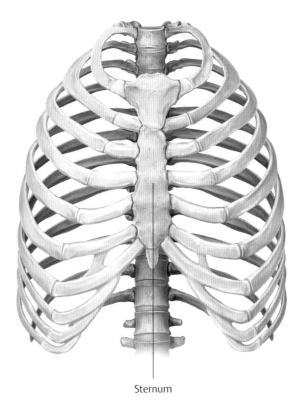

Fig. 1.11   Thoracic wall.

Sternum

organs, urinary bladder, portions of the colon, and the rectum.

Extremities

Composed of 30 bones on each side, the upper extremities consist of arms, forearms, wrists, hands, and fingers. Bones forming the pectoral girdle (commonly called the shoulder or shoulder girdle) provide a point of articulation for the clavicle (collarbone). The clavicle is located on either side of the body, superficial to the first rib, and connects the pectoral girdle to the thorax through its articulation with the sternum (anteriorly) and the scapula (or shoulder blade) posteriorly (**Fig. 1.12**). Extending distally from the shoulder to the elbow, the humerus forms the upper arm and articulates with the radius and ulna of the forearm. The forearm articulates distally with the carpal bones of the wrist, which, in turn, articulate with the metacarpals that form the palm of the hand. The bones of the fingers are known as proximal, middle, and distal phalanges. The thumb, however, has only proximal and distal phalanges.

The lower extremities are composed of 32 bones (on each side) that comprise the thighs, legs, ankle, and feet. As the pectoral girdle does for the upper extremities, the pelvic girdle connects the trunk to the lower extremities. The femur, commonly referred to as the thighbone, is the longest, heaviest, and strongest bone in the body. The femur forms the upper leg and extends distally from the coxa (hip bone) to the tibia and fibula of the lower leg. The tibia and fibula articulate with the tarsal bones, which articulate with the metatarsals forming the foot. The metatarsals articulate with the bones of the toes, which are also called phalanges and are similar in number and arrangement to the phalanges in the hand.

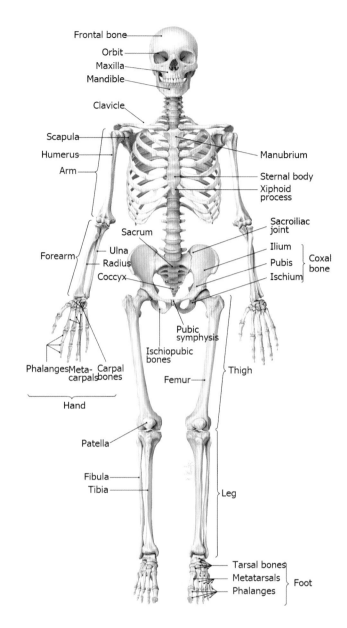

Fig. 1.12   Extremities.

Joints

A **joint** is the union of two or more bones. Most joints, such as the elbow, are movable. For example, the elbow is where the humerus of the upper arm articulates with the ulna and radius of the lower arm, as just described. The body employs several types of joints to allow various levels of range of motion. The most common type of joint is the freely moving **synovial joint**. The knee (a hinge joint), the hip and shoulder (ball and socket joints), and the

gliding costovertebral joints (articulations of ribs and vertebrae) are all examples of synovial joints.

Other joint types afford less movement. The articulation of the bony portion of the ribs with the sternum occurs via cartilage (costal portion of the rib). This type of joint, a **cartilaginous** joint, provides the flexibility needed to support respiration, which is explored in more detail in Chapter 10. **Fibrous** joints are generally immovable and join structures with fibrous connective tissue. The cranial sutures that join the bones of the skull are examples of fibrous joints. With more than 200 joints, the body can move not only in very obvious ways (e.g., for balancing, bending, jumping, and twisting) but also in ways that you may not have considered (e.g., for chewing, changing vocal pitch, hearing, and writing).

Muscular System

Muscles make it possible for us to breathe, to maintain balance, and, in general, to move. Your muscles enable you to read this page and then turn to the next. Muscular tissue contracts and relaxes. These simple actions form the basis for all muscle movement. Some muscles are not under direct control (involuntary muscle movement), such as those that contract when you get goose bumps. You do have control over other muscles (voluntary muscle movement), such as those used when you put on a jacket. The muscular system is described in greater detail in Chapter 8.

The body contains three kinds of muscles: cardiac, smooth, and skeletal. **Cardiac muscle** is found only in the heart, and its contraction is involuntary. This muscle regulates and provides rhythmic contraction and relaxation so that blood is pumped throughout the body via the circulatory system. **Smooth muscle** is located in the walls of the blood vessels and in the hollow internal organs, such as the stomach and intestines. Smooth muscle is typically under involuntary control. **Skeletal muscle**, which includes most muscles discussed in this text, is generally attached (at least at one end) to a bone and, unlike cardiac and smooth muscles, is under voluntary control. Skeletal and cardiac muscle fibers are striated, giving them a striped microscopic appearance. Contraction of muscle fibers provides the primary mechanism for movement. Two terms are critical to understand both the anatomy and physiology of muscles: **origin** and **insertion**. The origin of a muscle is generally the point of attachment that is least mobile. The insertion is the point of attachment that is more mobile. In the earlier example of the stylohyoid muscle, the origin of the muscle is the styloid process of the temporal bone in the skull—definitely the less mobile point of attachment. At the inferior end of the muscle is the insertion, or the attachment to the hyoid bone, which is a very mobile structure.

■ Nervous System

The fourth type of tissue introduced in this chapter is **nervous tissue** (also called neural tissue). This tissue consists of nerve cells (**neurons**) and supporting cells (**glial cells**). Neurons transmit information through both electrical and chemical mechanisms, and this communication is responsible for directing all voluntary and involuntary muscle contractions, such as those responsible for maintaining homeostasis, postural support, and voluntary movements. The nervous system is also responsible for higher-order cognitive skills, such as language, learning, and thinking. Highly complex and interactive, the nervous system consists of the brain, spinal cord, and a network of nerves, and it is organized both functionally and anatomically. Functionally, the nervous system may be divided into the **autonomic nervous system (ANS)** and the **somatic nervous system (SNS)**. Anatomically, it is divided into the **central nervous system (CNS)** and the **peripheral nervous system (PNS)**. The nervous system communicates within itself and with outlying regions through an array of afferent and efferent nerve fibers. **Efferent** nerve fibers deliver commands from the CNS to the muscle for a particular type of movement, while **afferent** nerve fibers deliver sensory information to the CNS, where its meaning is processed.

Autonomic and Somatic Nervous Systems

The ANS functions largely on a subconscious level, mostly making minor but important adjustments to the body's function. The ANS triggers the fight or flight responses (some argue that "fright" and "freeze" should also be included) whenever you feel fear or stress. The ANS also supports functions of "rest and digest" when you feel calm and relaxed in an effort to return the body to homeostasis. The ANS influences the function of your internal organs when it increases your heart rate as you sprint to class, responds to the chill you feel by producing goosebumps, or constricts the eye's pupil size in response to sudden bright light. All of these actions occur automatically and without your voluntary control. The SNS is associated with voluntary control of muscle movement as well as the processing of sensory information received from the external environment. In addition to voluntary control of muscle movement, the SNS is also associated with involuntary movements, such as reflex arcs, as is demonstrated when your knee jerks in response to a tap below your kneecap.

Central Nervous System

Consisting of the brain and spinal cord, the CNS is responsible for processing information received from sensory receptors located all over the body and transmitting motor commands to muscles in response to the sensory information received (**Fig. 1.13**). For example, imagine you are having a bowl of soup. You have just spooned a bit of soup to take your first bite. You see the steam rising from the spoon. Instinctively, you gently blow across the spoon to cool the soup before taking the bite. Do you see the involvement of your CNS in this scenario? The sensory information transmitted to your CNS involved what you saw with your eyes: the steam. After analyzing and interpreting its meaning (i.e., steam equals "hot"), your CNS responded to this potential threat by transmitting motor signals to the muscles involved in the act of blowing air toward the food.

The brain is the body's central processing unit where all voluntary and involuntary activities of the body are controlled (**Fig. 1.14** and **Fig. 1.15**). The brain as a whole comprises numerous structures, performing a variety of functions, and the structures are classified in various ways. To begin with, brain tissue may be classified loosely into **gray matter** and **white matter** (**Fig. 1.16**), which differ not only in their superficial and deep locations within the tissue, but also by which part of the neurons (brain cells) is present in that area to impart the color observed (i.e., gray = cell bodies and white = connections between cells).

The brain can also be divided based on location within the skull. Much of the brain can be divided into the **cerebrum** and the **cerebellum**, and each of these components is further divided into left and right halves called hemispheres. The cerebrum makes up the largest portion of the brain, whereas the cerebellum is smaller and is located caudal to the posterior end of the cerebrum. The outer surface of the cerebrum (cerebral cortex), with its **gyri** (ridges) and **sulci** (valleys), is the most recognizable part of the brain. Some fissures (large sulci) run deep and long, forming clear boundaries defining the lobes of the brain. For example, the longitudinal fissure is the deep sulcus that divides the cerebrum into hemispheres. Other fissures divide the hemispheres into lobes named after the skull bones superficial to them (the temporal lobe lies deep to the temporal bone). Each major lobe of the brain can be assigned an overall task, although many tasks, such as emotion or formulating an

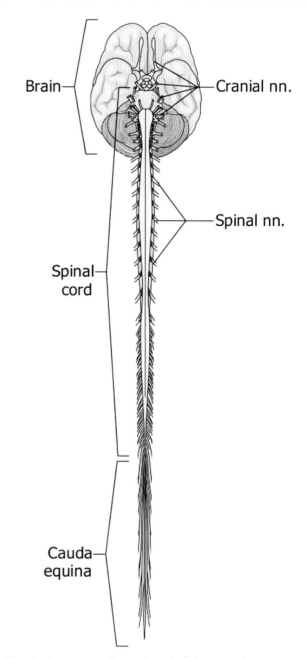

Fig. 1.13 Brain and spinal cord of the central nervous system with cranial and spinal nerve roots.

overall opinion about food, are integrated across the brain and are quite complex. In general, the **frontal lobe** is associated with motor movement, the **parietal lobe** interprets most sensory stimuli, the **temporal lobe** is responsible for evaluating sound, and the **occipital lobe** enables vision. Much more information on the structure and function of the CNS is presented in Chapter 5.

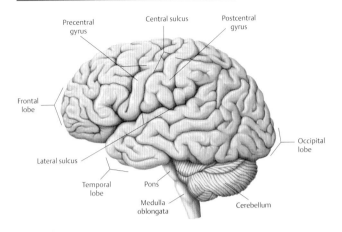

Fig. 1.14 Left lateral surface of the adult brain.

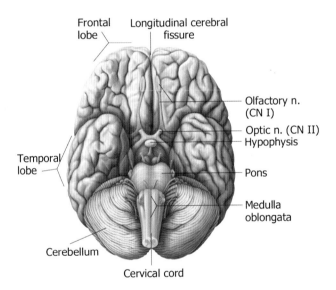

Fig. 1.15 Inferior surface of the adult brain.

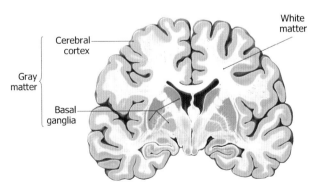

Fig. 1.16 Gray and white matter of the brain.

Peripheral Nervous System

The PNS is composed of 12 pairs of cranial nerves and 31 pairs of spinal nerves. These nerves serve the critical function of transmitting sensory information from the body to the brain and sending motor commands from the brain to the muscles. Cranial nerves, as their name suggests, arise, in part, from neurons in the brain. Similarly, the spinal nerves arise from the nervous tissue in the spinal cord. Cranial nerves relay information between the sense organs of the head and neck (e.g., eyes, nose) and the brain. They also provide the pathway for motor control of the muscles of speech and swallowing, as well as many other motor functions. The 12 cranial nerves (CN) are identified by Roman numerals, and primarily follow the rostral to caudal axis of the brain (**Fig. 1.17**). The cranial nerves are: olfactory (CN I, sensory), optic (CN II, sensory), oculomotor (CN III, motor), trochlear (CN IV, motor), trigeminal (CN V, sensory and motor), abducens (CN VI, motor), facial (CN VII, sensory and motor), vestibulocochlear (CN VIII, sensory), glossopharyngeal (CN IX, sensory and motor), vagus (CN X, sensory and motor), accessory (CN XI, motor), and hypoglossal (CN XII, motor). Spinal nerves are numbered according to the segment of the spinal cord where they exit the CNS and are generally divided into cervical (neck), thoracic (trunk), lumbar (lower back), and sacral segments. Spinal nerves transmit sensory input to the brain (afferent tracts) and motor output from the brain and spinal cord (efferent tracts) to regulate limb and organ function throughout the body.

■ Cardiovascular System

Consisting of the heart, blood vessels, and blood, the cardiovascular system serves to transport nutrients throughout the body. A muscle roughly the size of a large fist, your heart pumps blood throughout the body via two pathways: the systemic circuit and the pulmonary circuit. In systemic circulation, oxygen-rich blood travels away from your heart through arteries to deliver nutrients to your body's organs and tissues. Once the oxygen and nutrients are delivered, deoxygenated blood and waste products travel back to the heart through the veins. In the pulmonary circulation, deoxygenated blood returning through the veins moves from the heart to the lungs, in order to be reoxygenated, and then moves back to the heart to be sent out to tissues.

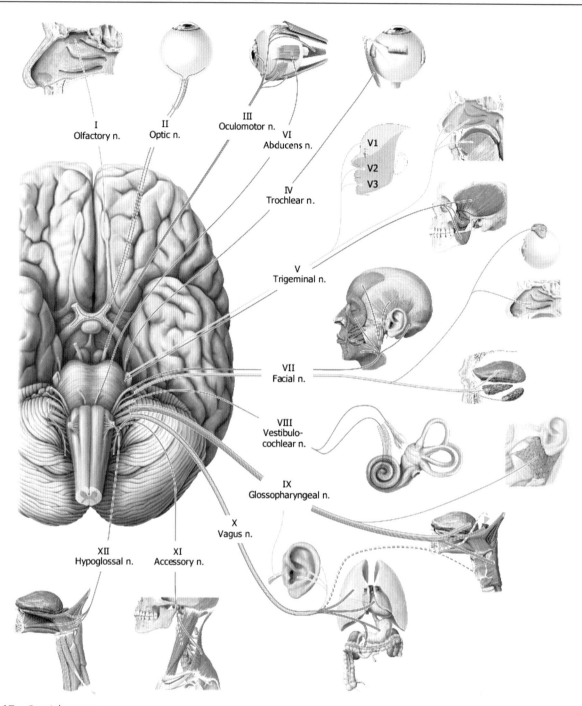

Fig. 1.17 Cranial nerves.

Box 1.3   Benign Paroxysmal Positional Vertigo

Benign paroxysmal positional vertigo (BPPV) is a disorder arising in the inner ear. Its symptoms are repeated episodes of positional vertigo, that is, a spinning sensation caused by changes in the position of the head. BPPV is the most common cause of the symptoms of vertigo ("spinning sensation"). The two otolithic organs in the inner ear, the utricle and saccule, house tiny calcium carbonate crystals (otoliths or otoconia) in a gelatinous mass. (The term *otolith* is derived from the roots *oto-*, which refers to the ear, and *-lith*, which means "stone.") When the head moves in a linear direction (e.g., forward), the otoliths in the utricle lag slightly behind the head movement and tiny receptor cells inside the utricle detect that particular motion. When otoliths become dislodged (e.g., by head injury or aging) from the utricle and enter into the nearby semicircular canals, vertigo is common with any sudden head movement or change in head position. Unless the free-floating otoliths make their way back into the utricle to be disposed of (i.e., absorbed by the body), patients with BPPV will be compelled to minimize head movement in order not to feel sick and dizzy. Like the utricle and saccule, the semicircular canals also have tiny receptor cells. Whenever we rotate our heads, our semicircular canals send signals to the brain to cause an equal and opposite reaction of the eyes. Otoliths in the semicircular canals, where they do not belong, result in prolonged stimulation of the receptor cells, and our eyes move for a brief period even though our head is completely still. Various head maneuvers can be used by qualified health professionals to help patients place the otoliths back into the utricle. **Box Fig. 1.3** shows the physical relationship between the utricle, saccule, and semicircular canals.

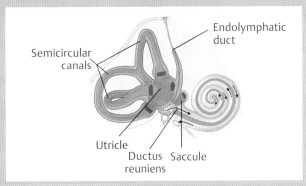

Box Fig. 1.3   Vestibular structure of the inner ear. Benign paroxysmal positional vertigo (BPPV) occurs when otoliths break loose from the utricle and float freely or become lodged within the semicircular canals.

Respiratory System

The respiratory system is composed of the organs and muscles that function in breathing (e.g., nose, mouth, lungs, diaphragm). During inhalation, oxygen (O_2), along with other atmospheric gases, enters the mouth and/or nose, travels down the pharynx, through the larynx, into the trachea, through the bronchi, and finally to the lungs. This process is reversed during exhalation. The process of breathing, then, may be divided into two phases: **inspiration** and **expiration**.

Inspiration occurs when air is inhaled. When you inspire, your body takes in O_2 (along with several other gases). The process of respiration occurs at the cellular level. This process enables the body to use the O_2 from the inhaled air to support the work of the cells in your body. Inhalation does not occur just by opening the mouth; rather, inspiration relies on muscular effort and expansion of the thoracic cavity. The primary muscles of inspiration include the **diaphragm** (often referred to as the principal muscle of inspiration) and the **external intercostal muscles**. The diaphragm, a large, single, dome-shaped muscle, lies inferior to the lungs and separates the thorax from the abdomen. The external intercostal muscles are located between the ribs; their contraction expands the rib cage and contributes to inhalation.

Expiration occurs when air is exhaled. Expiration removes carbon dioxide (CO_2), a waste product of cellular respiration. Like inspiration, expiration requires more than opening the mouth. Expiration relies on the elastic recoil of the lungs and compression of the thoracic cavity. The primary muscles of expiration include the internal intercostal muscles and the abdominal muscles. Like the external intercostal muscles, the internal intercostal muscles are located between the ribs; however, their course is perpendicular to that of the external intercostals. This arrangement allows the action of the internal intercostals to be in direct opposition to that of the external intercostals, allowing for the distinct contribution of each muscle group to the expansion (external intercostals) and compression (internal intercostals) of the rib cage. The group of six abdominal muscles that lies between the thorax and the pelvis contributes to exhalation through compression of the abdominal cavity. The anatomy and physiology of the respiratory system are examined in much greater detail in Chapter 10.

■ Digestive System

The digestive system consists of the gastrointestinal (GI) tract (also called the digestive tract), gallbladder, pancreas, liver, and salivary glands. The digestive system extracts nutrients from consumed food and drink to feed cells, organs, and tissues of the body. The process of digestion begins at the lips, with food and/or drink traveling through a series of cavities (e.g., oral cavity) and hollow organs (e.g., stomach, small intestine) that contribute to the mechanical and chemical processes of converting a mass of food, or **bolus**, into nutrients to be absorbed into the bloodstream. It is primarily in the digestive system that smooth muscles are found.

■ Speech Systems

Speech is the product of several systems working together. The systems supporting speech production include the respiratory, phonatory, resonatory, and articulatory systems. The respiratory system provides the airflow to support voicing (phonation). The sound wave produced by the vocal folds and shaped by the resonators is formed into speech sounds by the articulatory system. A thorough understanding of the structures and functions of each of these systems is important to the practice of speech-language pathology and audiology. Each of these subsystems is described in greater detail in Chapters 10, 11, and 12.

Box 1.4   Respiration and Phonation

As is discussed in Chapters 10 and 11, the respiratory system provides the driving force for phonation (voicing). Simply, air in the lungs serves as the "gas in the tank" for producing voice. Using that analogy, if there's insufficient gas in the tank, the car won't go very far. With inadequate respiratory driving pressure for phonation, the quality of the resulting voice diminishes. A number of conditions result in reduced respiratory driving pressure. Cystic fibrosis is a genetic disorder without a cure. One feature of this disease is the production of thick mucus in the lungs, with resulting breathing difficulties and frequent respiratory infections. The reduction in lung elasticity and capacity that results from the disease will often have a negative impact on voice, possibly resulting in low volume, shortened phrase length, and reduced variability in pitch and loudness.

Neurological diseases can also affect the respiratory system. Parkinson's disease results from a decrease in dopamine-producing neurons in the midbrain. The impact of reduced dopamine is manifested in rigidity that affects many muscle groups, including those of the phonatory and respiratory systems. The rigidity limits the speed and extent of rib cage expansion, resulting in less "gas in the tank" and less control in managing exhalation for phonation. The rigidity also limits flexibility and range of movement in the phonatory system, yielding a voice that lacks inflection. Taken together, rigidity in the skeletal muscles results in a voice that is classically low in volume (hypophonia), and lacks intonation (monotone). Phrase length may be short, because the speaker needs to take frequent "refueling" breaks. The speech disorder common in Parkinson's disease is hypokinetic dysarthria.

The relationship between the respiratory and phonatory systems is important for the speech-language pathologist who treats patients with voice disorders. Poor coordination between breathing and speaking can result in dysphonia. An understanding of the relationship between the systems is critical to establish an effective treatment plan to facilitate healthy, efficient voice use.

Box 1.5 Cleft Lip and Cleft Palate

Clefts of the lip and/or palate are one of the most common birth defects and belong to a group of features called craniofacial anomalies. Clefting occurs during early fetal development (between 6 and 12 weeks), when tissues that form the lip and roof of the oral cavity (palate) fail to fuse. Clefts can vary in degree and severity, and their impacts on speech and swallowing vary accordingly. Clefts may be complete, incomplete, unilateral, or bilateral. **Box Fig. 1.4** illustrates various types and degrees of oral clefting. Clefting is a recognized feature of over 400 syndromes (e.g., Down's syndrome, Pierre Robin sequence, and 22q deletion, among many others). Clefting can also occur in isolation, without any other anomalies or as part of an identified syndrome. A submucosal cleft occurs in the palate but is covered by the oral mucosa, which obscures the cleft. Submucosal clefts can be more difficult to identify than the obvious clefts of the lip and palate. Clefts are treated surgically, often during the first weeks of life, with ongoing management usually continuing for years afterward. Speech-language pathologists and audiologists are part of a multidisciplinary team involved in the treatment of patients with clefting of the lip and/or palate. The craniofacial team also includes surgeons, dentists, pediatricians, dietitians, and social workers.

Clefts of the lip and palate can impact an infant's ability to latch on to a nipple and to generate sufficient intraoral pressure for feeding. Later in development, speech sound acquisition and language development may be delayed. Speech-language pathologists work with the infant and family to facilitate feeding, speech, and language development. Frequent ear infections (chronic otitis media) and the resulting hearing loss are often a complication of clefting. When hearing loss is present, audiologists and ear, nose, and throat physicians work together with the cleft and craniofacial team to recommend and fit an appropriate hearing aid or implantable device.

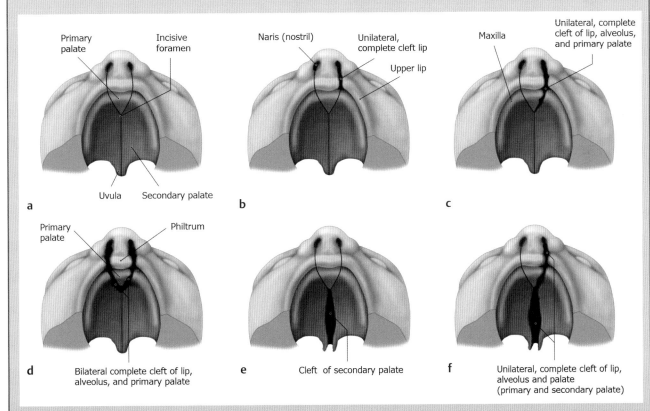

Box Fig. 1.4 Examples of cleft lip and/or palate. **(a)** An anatomically normal palate and the primary (anterior) and secondary (posterior) palates, where clefting occurs. **(b)** Unilateral and complete cleft of the lip without palatal involvement. **(c)** Unilateral and complete cleft of the lip and alveolus and cleft of the primary palate. **(d)** Bilateral complete cleft of the lip, alveolus, and primary palate. **(e)** Cleft of the secondary palate without clefting of the lip. **(f)** A complete cleft of both the primary and the secondary palate, with unilateral complete cleft of the lip.

Box 1.6 Chiari Malformation

In conjunction with several other structures, the cerebellum ("little brain") is important for motor control and regulation of muscle activities. The cerebellum is located inferior to the occipital lobes and dorsal to the brainstem. Together, the cerebellum and brainstem are located at the base of the skull just above the foramen magnum. When part of the cerebellum (known as the cerebellar tonsils) descends below the foramen magnum, it is called a Chiari malformation (**Box Fig. 1.5**). Although Chiari malformation is not a syndrome, it can be caused by exposure to toxins during fetal development or by genetic mutations. Four types of Chiari malfor-

mation have been described. Type I (which is the most common) is the only acquired type and may not cause symptoms. Types II, III, and IV, however, are congenital (present from birth) and are associated frequently with symptoms. Although the three congenital types vary in presentation, in each type, the cerebellar tonsils (and possibly other nearby tissue) push through the foramen magnum, causing displacement of other tissues. This displacement causes a disruption in the flow of cerebrospinal fluid and a variety of other problems, depending on the type and severity. Symptoms of Chiari malformation may include headache, numbness, weakness, disequilibrium, and/or hearing loss.

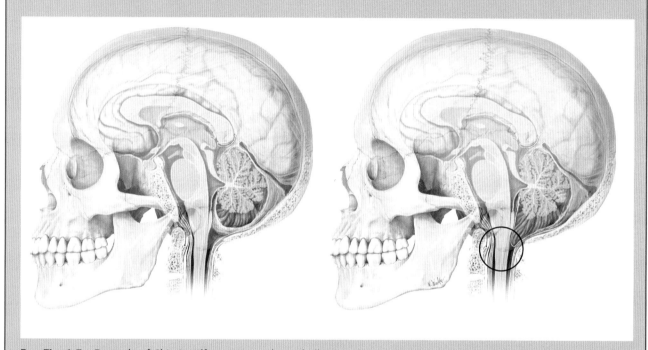

Box Fig. 1.5 Example of Chiari malformation with cerebellar tonsils exiting the foramen magnum (*right*). Contrast Chiari malformation with the normal cerebellum (*left*).

Box 1.7 Labyrinthine Artery

The labyrinthine artery provides the blood supply to the inner ear, which houses the structures responsible for hearing and balance. The labyrinthine artery gets its name because the inner ear is likened to a maze (Latin: *labyrinthus*) of channels within the temporal bone of the skull. The labyrinthine artery can have one of two origins and provides blood to many areas of the brain. For a large portion of the population (> 85%), the labyrinthine artery arises from the an-

terior inferior cerebellar artery (AICA), and the AICA arises from the large basilar artery. For 10% to 15% of the population, the labyrinthine artery arises directly from the basilar artery. Even rarer (< 5% of the population), the labyrinthine artery may arise from other nearby arteries, such as the vertebral artery and the superior cerebellar artery (SCA). These variations (and others) help to explain why a disruption somewhere in the blood supply may cause different functional deficits among patients.

■ Suggested Readings

Arvedson JC, Brodsky L. Pediatric Swallowing and Feeding: Assessment and Management. 2nd ed. Clifton Park, NY: Delmar Cengage Learning; 2002

Cohen BJ. Memmler's Structure and Function of the Human Body. 8th ed. Baltimore, MD: Lippincott Williams & Wilkins; 2005

Desmond AL. Vestibular Function: Clinical and Practice Management. New York, NY: Thieme; 2011

Gazzaniga M. Tales from Both Sides of the Brain: A Life in Neuroscience. New York, NY: Harper Collins; 2015

Møller AR. Hearing: Anatomy, Physiology, and Disorders of the Auditory System. San Diego, CA: Plural; 2013

■ Study Questions

Choose the correct term to describe the relationship between the structures.

1. Your fingers are _____ to your elbow.

A. medial
B. distal
C. lateral
D. inferior
E. dorsal

2. Your scalp is _____ to your skull.

A. deep
B. medial
C. lateral
D. superior
E. superficial

3. Your lungs are _____ to your rib cage.

A. inferior
B. deep
C. lateral
D. caudal
E. superficial

4. The lumbar spine is _____ to the cervical spine.

A. inferior
B. distal
C. rostral

D. superior
E. dorsal

5. The ears are _____ to the eyes.

A. medial
B. distal
C. superficial
D. lateral
E. dorsal

6. The sternum (breastbone) is _____ to the spinal column

A. anterior
B. posterior
C. lateral
D. superficial
E. dorsal

7. The abdominal cavity is _____ to the thoracic cavity.

A. ventral
B. dorsal
C. superior
D. inferior
E. anterior

8. Choose the plane that divides the brain into equal halves (left and right).

A. Transverse
B. Midsagittal
C. Coronal
D. Frontal
E. Horizontal

9. Choose the plane that divides the brain into anterior and posterior sections.

A. Frontal
B. Sagittal
C. Horizontal
D. Vertical
E. Midsagittal

10. Choose the plane that divides the spinal column between the thoracic and lumbar sections.

A. Sagittal
B. Transverse
C. Coronal
D. Dorsal
E. Frontal

11. Which statement about the appendicular skeleton is true?

A. It is composed of the upper and lower limbs.
B. It is medial to the axial skeleton.
C. It contains only afferent nerve fibers.
D. It contains the ribs and sternum.
E. None of these statements is true.

12. Which statement describes the cerebral cortex?

A. It is superficial to the brainstem.
B. It features gyri and sulci.
C. It is part of the peripheral nervous system.
D. It contains only efferent nerve fibers.
E. It is deep to the spinal cord.

13. Which statement best describes the cranial nerves?

A. They exit the nervous system between the vertebrae.
B. They are part of the central nervous system.
C. They are superficial to the cerebral cortex.
D. They have both afferent and efferent functions.
E. They are the primary pathway for sensory information traveling from the appendicular skeleton to the cerebral cortex.

14. The nervous system can be classified in a variety of ways. Which of the following is the system that functions largely out of conscious control to maintain homeostasis?

A. Central nervous system
B. Peripheral nervous system
C. Somatic nervous system
D. Autonomic nervous system
E. All of these

15. Which type of muscle is striated, is controlled voluntarily, and will be the primary type of muscle explored in this text?

A. Cardiac
B. Smooth
C. Skeletal
D. All of these
E. None of these

16. Which of the following does *not* describe anatomic position?

A. Standing
B. Palms facing forward
C. Fingers pointed down
D. Arms hanging at side
E. Arms extended at the side

17. The root *a-* means

A. within
B. between
C. outside of
D. without
E. related to the eyes

18. The root *myo-* references

A. bones
B. nerves
C. muscles
D. red
E. blood

19. The root *contra-* indicates

A. opposite
B. without
C. same
D. inflammation
E. within

20. The root *oto-* references

A. the eye
B. the ear
C. the oral cavity
D. the nose
E. the larynx

■ Answers to Study Questions

1. The correct answer is *distal* (B). The term *distal* refers to a body part that is farther from the point of origin than another part. The fingers are further away from the elbow.

If (A) were correct, the fingers would be between the shoulder and the elbow. If (C) were correct, the fingers would be on the side of the elbow. Answer choice (D) indicates that the fingers are below the elbow, which is true in anatomic position; however, common usage dictates that the terms *distal* and *proximal* are used in discussion of extremities. The term *dorsal* (E) indicates that the fingers are on the back surface of the elbow.

2. The correct answer is *superficial* (E). The term *superficial* indicates that something is closer to the surface than something else. The scalp is closer to the surface of the body compared to the skull.

Answer (A) is incorrect for the same reason—the skull does not lie over the scalp. The terms *medial* and *lateral* refer to a side-by-side relationship, so (B) and (C) are incorrect. Answer (D) might seem to be correct, as the scalp is above the skull, but common usage of the terms *superficial* and *deep* indicates that (E) is the correct answer.

3. The correct answer is *deep* (B). The term *deep* indicates that something is farther from the surface compared to something else. The lungs are further from the surface of the body when compared to the ribs.

   Answer (E) is incorrect because the ribs are superficial to the lungs, not the other way around. The term *inferior* (A) would indicate that the lungs are below the rib cage when the body is in anatomic position (standing) and is therefore incorrect. The term *lateral* refers to a side-by-side relationship and is not correct in this context. One could say that the lungs are medial to the rib cage, as they are closer to the center of the body (the axis). The term *caudal* indicates that the lungs are "toward the tail" and is incorrect.

4. The correct answer is *inferior* (A). The term *inferior* indicates that something is farther from the top than/below something else.

   Answer (A) is incorrect because the ears are to the side of the eyes. The term *distal* (B) refers to a point away from the point of origin and is incorrect in this context. *Superficial* (C) refers to a plane closer to the surface than another plane and is incorrect here. *Dorsal* (E) refers to "the back side" (as in a dolphin's dorsal fin) and is also incorrect.

5. The correct answer is *lateral* (D). The term *lateral* indicates that something is more to the side than something else.

   Answer choice (A) is incorrect because the ears are to the side of the eyes. The term distal (B) refers to a point away from the point of origin and is incorrect in this context. Superficial (C) refers to a plane closer to the surface than another plane and is incorrect here. Dorsal (E) refers to "the back side" (as in a dolphin's dorsal fin) and is also incorrect.

6. The correct answer is *anterior* (A). The term *anterior* indicates that something is in front of something else. In anatomical position, the sternum is in front of the spinal column. Answers (B) and (E) would indicate that the sternum is behind the spinal cord. Choice (C) indicates that the sternum is to the side of the spinal column, and answer (D) indicates that the sternum is closer to the surface of the body than the spinal column—both of these are incorrect.

7. The correct answer is (D). The term *inferior* indicates that something is situated below something else. The abdominal cavity is below the thoracic cavity, and the two are separated by the diaphragm.

   Choice (C) is incorrect because its use in this statement would indicate that the abdominal cavity (containing the visceral organs) is above the thoracic cavity containing the heart and lungs. *Ventral* (A) and *dorsal* (B) indicate front and back surfaces of the body, respectively, and are incorrect. *Anterior* (E) indicates the front side of something. The abdomen and thorax have an above–below rather than a side-by-side arrangement. Thus choice (E) is incorrect.

8. The correct answer is *midsagittal* (B). A midsagittal plane divides a structure into two equal left and right halves.

   A transverse (A) or horizontal plane (E) would create top and bottom sections. Coronal (C) and frontal (D) planes would divide the brain into front and back sections.

9. The correct answer is *frontal* (A). A frontal plane divides a structure into two sections, yielding front and back portions. The coronal plane would also be a correct answer here.

   The correct answer is *frontal* (A). A frontal plane divides a structure into two sections, yielding front and back portions. The coronal plane would also be a correct answer here.

10. The correct answer is *transverse* (B). A transverse plane divides a structure into top and bottom sections. Because the thoracic vertebrae are above the lumbar vertebrae, a transverse plane would separate the divisions.

    Sagittal sections (A) divide structures into left and right portions. Frontal (E) and coronal (C) planes would create front and back sections. The term *dorsal* (D) refers to a surface of the body and not a plane, so it is incorrect.

11. The correct answer is (A). The appendicular skeleton is composed of the appendages or extremities.

    The axial skeleton (B) is composed of the trunk of the body and the appendicular skeleton is distal to the trunk of the body. The appendages contain afferent and efferent fibers, so answer (C) is not correct. The ribs and sternum are part of the axial skeleton, so D is not true.

12. The correct answer is (B); *gyri* and *sulci* are distinguishing characteristics of the cerebral cortex.

    The cortex is superior to (not superficial) to the brainstem and spinal cord, so (E) and (A) are incorrect. The cortex is part of the central (not peripheral) nervous system, which eliminates choice (C), and it contains cell bodies rather than either afferent or efferent nerve fibers, which eliminates choice (D).

13. The correct answer is (D). The cranial nerves exit the central nervous system at the level of the brainstem and contain both sensory (afferent) and motor (efferent) fibers.

The cranial nerves exit the nervous system at the brainstem, so (A) is incorrect, and are part of the peripheral nervous system, so choice (B) is incorrect. They are not superficial to the cortex, which eliminates answer (C), but they do contain sensory (afferent) and motor (efferent) fibers. The spinal cord and spinal nerves would be the pathway for motor and sensory information between the cortex and the muscles/tissues of the appendicular skeleton, which eliminates choice (E). After the other choices are eliminated, the correct answer, (D), remains.

14. The correct answer is (D). The autonomic nervous system functions largely out of conscious control to maintain homeostasis and to return the body to equilibrium following a "fight or flight" response.

The somatic nervous system (C) involves voluntary control of skeletal muscles and is part of the peripheral nervous system (B). The central nervous system (A) is not the correct answer because it does not primarily act to maintain homeostasis.

15. The correct answer is (C). Skeletal muscles are striated and controlled voluntarily via the cranial and spinal nerves. Cardiac (A) and smooth muscles (B) function largely outside of conscious control and are not explored in depth in this text.

16. The correct answer is (E). Anatomic position is described as the body standing erect (A), with arms at the sides (D), fingers pointed down (C), and palms facing forward (B). All of these answer choices are part of the definition of anatomic position, with the exception of choice (E).

17. The correct answer is *without* (D); the root *a-* means without.

The root *oculo-* refers to the eyes (E), the root *extra-* means outside of (C), *intra-* means within (A), and *inter-* means between (B).

18. The correct answer is *muscles* (C); the root *myo-* means related to muscles.

The root *osseo-* refers to bones (A), *neuro-* refers to nerves (B), and *hem-* refers to blood (E). The root *rubr-* or *erythr-* indicates the color red (D).

19. The correct answer is *opposite* (A); the root *contra-* indicates opposite.

The root *a-* means without (B), *ipsi-* refers to same (C), *-itis* indicates an inflammation (D), and *intra-* means within (E).

20. The correct answer is *the ear* (B); the root *oto-* refers to the ear.

The root *oculo-* refers to the eye (A); *oro-* refers to the oral cavity (C); *naso-* indicates the nose (D); and *laryngo-* references the larynx (E).

2

Composition of the Body: Cells, Tissues, Organs

Elizabeth Erickson-DiRenzo and Daniel DiRenzo

■ Chapter Summary

The human body has a complex hierarchical organization. This hierarchy is a framework for understanding human anatomy and physiology. Cells are the basic units of life and have remarkable diversity in terms of structure and function. Unique types of cells are organized into collective entities called tissues. The four main tissue types of the human body are epithelial, connective, nervous, and muscle tissue. Multiple tissue types form organs and groups of organs, called organ systems. These systems work in concert to fulfill all functions necessary for our existence, including processes essential for speech, language, swallowing, hearing, and balance. The purpose of this chapter is to provide the basic understanding of the levels of organization of the human body necessary for speech, language, swallowing, hearing, and balance. Specifically, the chapter provides an overview of cell structure and reviews the cellular processes essential to survival, discusses how cells form the specialized tissues of the body and the functions of these tissues, explains how tissues are further organized into organs and organ systems, and relates these concepts to disorders managed by speech-language pathologists and audiologists.

■ Learning Objectives

- Describe the structure and function of the components of the eukaryotic cell
- Explain the processes that support cell health and survival
- Identify the four major tissue types of the body and discuss their unique structure and function
- Explain how tissues form organs and organ systems

■ Putting It Into Practice

- Disorders of speech, language, swallowing, hearing, and balance are often the consequence of structural and/or functional changes within the various cells, tissues, and organ systems of the human body.
- An understanding of the biological organization of structures of the human body, including the oral and nasal cavities, larynx, auditory and vestibular systems, and the central and peripheral nervous systems, is necessary to understand the etiology of speech, language, swallowing, hearing, and balance disorders.
- Speech-language pathologists and audiologists use information about the human body to understand the pathophysiology of disorders and to make informed, evidence-based treatment decisions.

◼ Introduction

The human body has multiple levels of hierarchical biological organization. Increased complexity is observed at each higher level of organization. The **cell** is the smallest living unit of the body. Individual cells vary widely in shape and size, and each cell type plays a specific role within the body. **Tissues** are groups of connected cells that share a similar function. The four basic tissue types in humans are epithelial tissue, connective tissue, nervous tissue, and muscle tissue. Each tissue has a characteristic role in processes related to communication. An **organ** is a structure composed of at least two different tissue types that work synergistically. Examples of organs include the brain, heart, and lungs. As expected, functions that are more complex emerge at this level. Finally, an organ system is a group of organs that work together to carry out complex bodily functions essential to human survival.

Knowledge of human biological composition is fundamental to health-related professions, including speech-language pathology and audiology. In this chapter, levels of hierarchical organization are introduced, beginning with the cell and ending with organ systems. At the core of many communication disorders are abnormalities at the cell, tissue, or organ level. Thus, familiarity with our biological makeup is necessary to understand the etiology of these disorders and their associated symptoms and to make evidence-based treatment decisions. Over the past decade, there has been a remarkable increase in research in the biology of communication disorders. The breadth of currently available information requires speech-language pathologists and audiologists to have a basic understanding of the composition of the body and the biological approaches used to understand the function of organ systems.

◼ The Cell

Cells are the most basic structural and functional unit of all living organisms. Some forms of life, such as many species of bacteria, are **unicellular**—composed of a single cell. Other highly complex organisms, such as humans, are **multicellular** and are composed of trillions of cells. Whether in a unicellular organism or as part of a multicellular organism, cells contain the machinery (organelles) and knowledge (deoxyribonucleic acid—DNA)

necessary to carry out basic functions of life, which they perform throughout their existence. Cells have a multitude of common features, yet they can look different and vary dramatically in their function. For example, epithelial cells protect the outside surface of the body as well as cover the outermost surface of internal organs. Blood cells carry important nutrients and oxygen throughout the body while removing carbon dioxide waste, whereas bone cells provide essential structural support to the body. Despite their diversity, cells share certain fundamental processes and features.

Defining a Cell

All cells, from simple to complex, must fulfill three basic requirements. First, cells must be distinct entities. Second, cells must be able to interact with the surrounding environment and acquire energy in order to support maintenance and growth. Third, a cell must be able to replicate itself. Each of these requirements is discussed further throughout this chapter, except for replication, which is addressed in detail in Chapters 3 and 4.

Cells are considered the most basic units of living organisms, due, in part, to the fact that they come in distinct identifiable packages. Furthermore, all cells have a common set of four key components: a plasma membrane, cytoplasm, DNA, and ribosomes. Cells are surrounded by a structure called the **plasma membrane**, which allows them to be identified as separate or distinct entities. Also called the cell membrane, this structure is composed primarily of fat molecules called phospholipids, with proteins interspersed throughout. Enclosed within the plasma membrane is the water-based inside environment called the **cytoplasm**. Suspended within the cytoplasm are significant structural and functional elements essential to cell survival.

◼ Prokaryotes and Eukaryotes

Cells have striking diversity in terms of structure (e.g., shape, size, form) and function. It is somewhat surprising, however, that cells can be divided into only two types: prokaryotic and eukaryotic cells. Key characteristics of prokaryotic and eukaryotic cells are displayed in **Table 2.1** and **Fig. 2.1**. Prokaryote simply means

Table 2.1 Comparison of prokaryotic and eukaryotic cells

Characteristic	Prokaryotes	Eukaryotes
Size of cell	Small (< 5 μm)	Large (> 10 μm)
Level of organization	Always unicellular	Often multicellular
Nucleus	Absent	Present
Genetic material	Singular, circular DNA	Multiple strands of linear DNA
Organelles	Absent	Present
Cytoplasm	No cytoskeleton	Cytoskeleton
Cell wall	Yes	No (animals), Yes (plants)
Ribosomes	Smaller (70S)	Larger (80S)
Reproductive strategy	Asexual	Asexual or sexual
Oxygen requirement	Anaerobic (does not require oxygen)	Aerobic (requires oxygen)

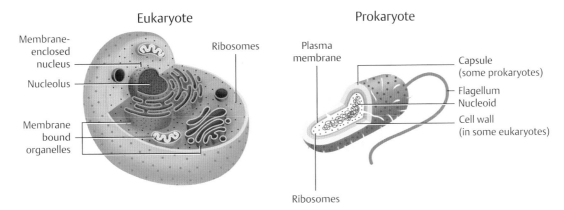

Fig. 2.1 A eukaryotic cell (*left*) has a membrane-enclosed nucleus containing DNA and other specialized membrane-bound organelles. In contrast, a prokaryotic cell (*right*) has no nucleus or any other organelles. Other distinct features of prokaryotic cells include a cell wall, capsule, and flagellum.

"before nucleus"; therefore, **prokaryotic cells** do not have a cell nucleus or other organelles. Most prokaryotes are unicellular and generally are extremely small, ranging from 0.1 to 2 μm. Bacteria are an example of prokaryotes. Prokaryotic cells also exhibit some unique features, such as a rigid, protective **cell wall** covering the plasma membrane, and certain subtypes of prokaryotes have a sticky, outermost layer called the **capsule**. Furthermore, prokaryotic DNA consists of a single chromosomal loop found in the **nucleoid** region of the cytoplasm. Finally, many of these cells use a specialized whiplike protein, the **flagellum**, for locomotion.

All other forms of life are typically multicellular and eukaryotic. Eukaryote means "true nucleus." **Eukaryotic cells** are often more complicated than prokaryotic cells. Animals and plants are perhaps the most familiar multicellular eukaryotic organisms. Other eukaryotes, such as fungi or protists (e.g., unicellular algae), may be unicellular. Eukaryotic cells are substantially larger than prokaryotic cells, ranging in size from 10 to 100 μm. **Fig. 2.2** displays the sizes of prokaryotic and eukaryotic cells, as well as other molecules and organisms, in a logarithmic scale, with each unit in the scale representing a tenfold increase in size. As the name describes, the primary defining feature of eukaryotic cells is a membrane-bounded **nucleus**, where multiple DNA-containing, linear chromosomes are stored. In addition, eukaryotic cells contain a number of highly specialized membrane-bound organelles, such as mitochondria. Both prokaryotes and eukaryotes contain **ribosomes**, the protein-synthesizing machinery of the cell. Ribosomes are RNA and protein complexes made up of a large subunit and small subunit. Overall, eukaryotes'

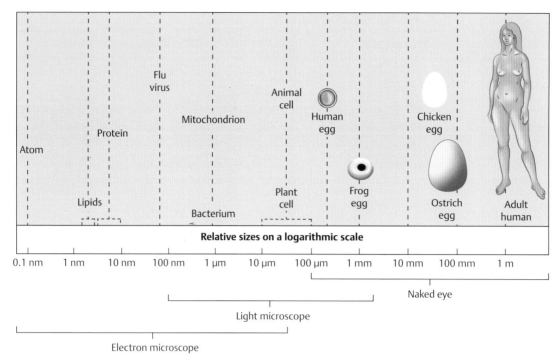

Fig. 2.2 The relative sizes of molecules and biological structures. Cells can vary between 1 micrometer (μm) and hundreds of micrometers in diameter.

ribosomal unit is referred to as 80S and is larger than the 70S unit of the prokaryote. The structure and function of animal (eukaryotic) cells are the primary focus of this chapter.

■ Tools of Cell Biology

An understanding of the biology of prokaryotic or eukaryotic organisms depends heavily on laboratory methods used to investigate the structure and function of cells. **Microscopes** are essential tools of cell biology, because the cells of uni- and multicellular organisms usually cannot be observed with the naked eye. Simply stated, microscopes make small objects appear larger. However, this is not the only function of a microscope. A microscope must be able to separate details in the image (this ability is referred to as its resolving power), and then render the details visible to the human eye or a camera. Microscopy is important because it enables close examination of cell structure and leads to improved understanding of cell function. Two common microscopy techniques are **light microscopy** and **electron microscopy**. Examples of molecules and structures that can be observed with light and electron microscopy are shown in **Fig. 2.2**.

■ Cell Structure

The term *cell* comes from the Latin word *cellula*, meaning a small compartment. Cells in turn contain numerous smaller compartments, termed **organelles**, each with a specialized function (**Fig. 2.3**). In this section, the structure of animal (eukaryotic) cells is presented in detail, because they are the cell types that make up the human body. Specifically, we introduce the various cellular organelles, describe the cytoplasm, and characterize the extracellular matrix.

The Plasma Membrane

A semipermeable plasma membrane, also called the cell membrane, surrounds the cell. The plasma membrane has both barrier and gatekeeper functions in the cell. As a barrier, the membrane defines the cell boundaries, effectively dividing the living insides of the cell from the nonliving outside of the cell (extracellular space). As a gatekeeper, the plasma membrane helps determine which molecules may enter or exit the cell and facilitates signaling between cells. The basic structure of the plasma membrane is shown in **Fig. 2.4**. Approximately 20% to 79% of the plasma membrane is composed of phospholipids,

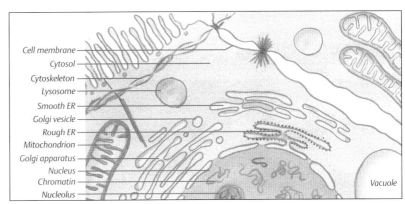

Fig. 2.3 Cell structure. A cell and some of its organelles. ER, endoplasmic reticulum.

which are modified lipid molecules containing two fatty acids. Each phospholipid molecule contains two "water-repelling," or **hydrophobic** tails and a "water-loving," or **hydrophilic**, head. Phospholipids are organized into two layers that form a **phospholipid bilayer**. Phospholipids are oriented so that the tails of each molecule face inward, keeping both the hydrophobic surfaces together on the inside of the membrane bilayer, and the hydrophilic heads contact water on

Box 2.1   Electron Microscopy of Inner Ear Hair Cells

Hair cells are the sensory receptors in the inner ear that detect sound and head motion. In humans, hair cell loss caused by acoustic overstimulation, ototoxic drugs, aging, or genetic defects is irreversible, leading to permanent loss of function. Electron microscopy can be used to study hair cell structure and function. Specifically, electron microscopy can be used to assist in the identification of factors associated with hearing loss, in testing and development of new drugs, and in evaluating the regeneration or repair of damaged hair cells. Here we display electron microscopic images of the hair cells of the mouse inner ear. **Box Fig. 2.1a** was acquired using **transmission electron microscopy (TEM)**, while **Box Fig. 2.1b** was acquired using **scanning electron microscopy (SEM)**. There are obvious differences in the appearance of the images. SEM produces a three-dimensional image of the hair cells, while TEM creates a flat, two-dimensional image. The three-dimensional image captured by SEM provides more detailed information about the shape and location of the hair cells relative to each other. On the other hand, the TEM image provides higher magnification and greater resolution than SEM. Often it is useful to acquire both TEM and SEM images of cells such as hair cells in order to examine these structures in three dimensions and at high resolutions.

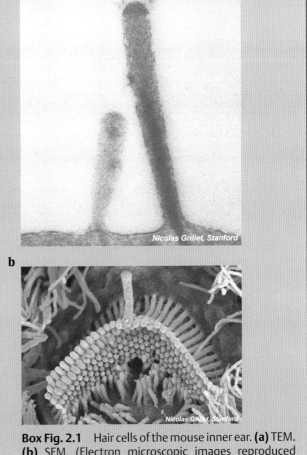

Box Fig. 2.1   Hair cells of the mouse inner ear. **(a)** TEM. **(b)** SEM. (Electron microscopic images reproduced courtesy of Nicolas Grillet, PhD, Stanford University.)

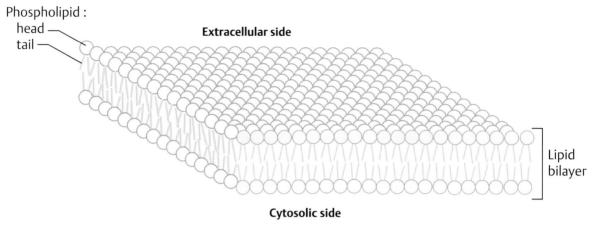

Phospholipid :
head
tail

Extracellular side

Lipid bilayer

Cytosolic side

Fig. 2.4 Plasma membrane. Biological membranes are bilayers composed of amphipathic phospholipids. The polar heads (blue) of the phospholipid form the outer surface (extracellular side) and inner surface (cytosolic side) of the membrane, whereas the nonpolar hydrophobic tails (yellow) form the interior.

the interior and exterior of the cell. Since the membrane has both hydrophobic and hydrophilic regions, it is referred to as **amphipathic**. Proteins are also embedded throughout the plasma membrane, and the membrane may consist of approximately 30% to 50% proteins. These membrane proteins act as carriers for transport of molecules into and out of the cell, provide specialized sites for attachment and communication with neighboring cells, and serve as receptors for chemical messengers. Depending on their particular type of association with the membrane, the proteins can be characterized as peripheral or integral (**Fig. 2.5**). **Peripheral proteins** are hydrophilic and are bound only to the interior or exterior surface of the plasma membrane or to other membrane proteins. Conversely, **integral proteins**, also called transmembrane proteins, are amphipathic and pass through the entire plasma membrane, thereby connecting the interior and exterior of the cell. The hydrophobic region of these proteins

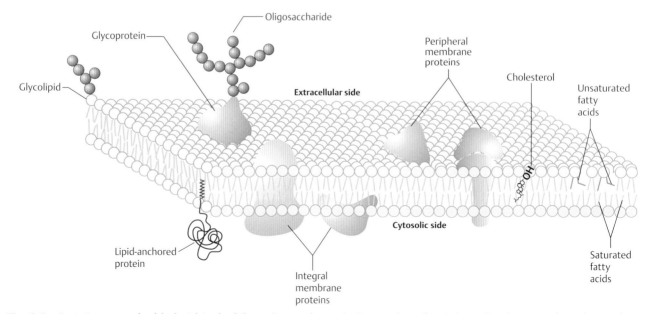

Oligosaccharide

Glycoprotein

Glycolipid

Peripheral membrane proteins

Cholesterol

Unsaturated fatty acids

Extracellular side

Lipid-anchored protein

Cytosolic side

Integral membrane proteins

Saturated fatty acids

Fig. 2.5 Proteins are embedded within the bilayer (integral proteins) or anchored to it (peripheral proteins). Both membrane lipids and membrane proteins are frequently glycosylated (attached to carbohydrate molecules) on the extracellular side of the lipid bilayer.

passes through the interior of the membrane, and the hydrophilic regions are exposed to the membrane surface. Additionally, proteins and lipids found in the plasma membrane can be covalently linked to carbohydrates (i.e., glycosylated) to form advanced glycoprotein and glycolipid molecules. These components form the general structure of the cellular plasma membrane. Of note, the membrane structure is highly dynamic, and the protein, phospholipid, and carbohydrate composition of the plasma membrane may change rapidly in response to a variety of environmental stimuli.

The Nucleus

The **nucleus** is the largest and arguably most critical organelle in eukaryotes. The nucleus serves as the cellular control center and has two major functions: to store genetic material (DNA), and to coordinate cell activities, including growth, protein production, and replication. Generally, the nucleus is spherical and occupies about 10% of the total cell volume (**Fig. 2.6**). The nucleus can be broken down into substructures with specific and important functions. The **nucleolus** is a subregion within the nucleus that is responsible for the manufacture and assembly of ribosomes. The **nuclear envelope** is also a critical substructure and is responsible for separating the contents of the nucleus from the cytoplasm and other organelles. The nuclear envelope is composed of a double-layered (inner and outer) membrane that is perforated with pores to selectively regulate the passage of certain molecules between the nucleus and the cytoplasm. Additionally, the outer membrane of the nuclear envelope is attached to a network of tubules and sacs, called the rough endoplasmic reticulum, which is discussed shortly.

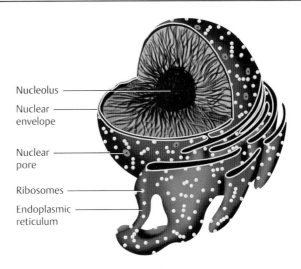

Nucleolus

Nuclear envelope

Nuclear pore

Ribosomes

Endoplasmic reticulum

Fig. 2.6 Cell nucleus. The nucleus is the control center of the cell. The nuclear envelope surrounds the nucleus and all of its contents. Within the envelope, there are pores and spaces for molecules to pass through. Within the nucleus is a dense structure composed of RNA and proteins called the nucleolus.

Mitochondria

Mitochondria are considered the "power plants" of the eukaryotic cell. Most cells contain hundreds of rod-shaped mitochondria; however, the exact number depends upon the metabolic requirements of the cell (**Fig. 2.7**). Mitochondria use oxygen to extract energy from sugar, fat, and other "fuel" molecules to produce **adenosine triphosphate (ATP)** in much greater amounts than could be obtained without mitochondria to use oxygen. This process is called **cellular respiration**, and ATP is the essential fuel source for powering a host of cellular reactions and mechanisms. (Cellular respiration is discussed in detail later in this chapter.) Mitochondria have two membranes: an outer membrane, which separates the mitochondrion from the cytoplasm, and an inner

Box 2.2 Mitochondrial DNA and Alzheimer's Disease

Alzheimer's disease is an irreversible, progressive type of dementia in which there is slow deterioration of memory and thinking skills and, eventually, of the ability to carry out daily tasks. The pathological changes that underlie Alzheimer's disease often begin decades prior to the manifestation of dementia symptoms. A promising area of research in improving early diagnosis is the analysis of biomarkers. Biomarkers are early biological signs of disease found in brain images, cerebrospinal fluid, and blood in persons who may be at risk for development of a specific disease. Biomarkers for Alzheimer's disease may be detected in the preclinical state, or prior to the appearance of dementia symptoms. Scientists believe that reduced levels of mitochondrial DNA in cerebrospinal fluid may be a biomarker of preclinical Alzheimer's disease (Podlesniy et al 2013). Specifically, in asymptomatic, at-risk individuals and in symptomatic patients with the disease, mitochondrial DNA levels were significantly lower than in age-matched controls.

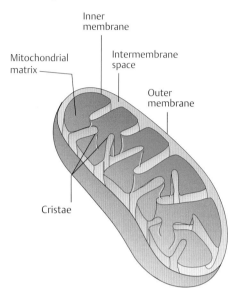

Membranes and compartments

Inner
membrane

Mitochondrial
matrix

Intermembrane
space

Outer
membrane

Cristae

Fig. 2.7 Structure of mitochondria. Mitochondria are cellular organelles composed of a central mitochondrial matrix enclosed by an inner membrane that is bent into folds (cristae). The inner membrane is surrounded by an outer membrane, and the space separating the membranes is called the intermembrane space.

membrane that is bent into folds called **cristae.** Mitochondria are unique organelles because they can divide independently of the cell and contain their own circular form of DNA, which is similar to that observed in prokaryotic cells (**Box 2.2**).

Endomembrane System

The endomembrane system is a group of closely related cell membranes and organelles that serve a variety of functions within the cell. Organelles that belong to this system include the endoplasmic reticulum, Golgi apparatus, and lysosomes. The vesicles that facilitate movement of molecules between these organelles are also part of the endomembrane system. The central role of this system is the production, modification, and transport of proteins, either to the plasma membrane or for secretion out of the cell. Other functions include production and transport of lipids, storage of nutrients, and breakdown of unwanted molecules.

The **endoplasmic reticulum** (ER) is a continuous series of flattened sacs and branching tubules that extend throughout the cytoplasm. The ER is bound by a single membrane to form a highly convoluted lumen, or internal space, that is continuous with the outer membrane of the nuclear envelope. Consequently, there is close communication between the nucleus and ER.

The ER can be divided into two distinct regions: the rough and smooth ER. The **smooth ER** has a variety of functions within the cell, including the synthesis of lipids (such as cholesterol and phospholipids), detoxification of substances such as drugs and toxic byproducts of metabolism, and the storage of ions that regulate cell signaling. In contrast, the **rough ER** is named for its "rough" appearance on electron micrographs, where it appears bumpy due to the many ribosomes attached to the outer, cytoplasmic surface of the membrane (**Fig. 2.8**). The rough ER is primarily involved in the assembly of amino acid subunits into proteins and the transfer of these proteins to

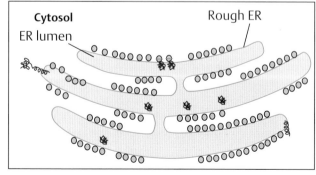

Cytosol   Rough ER

ER lumen

Fig. 2.8 Structure of the endoplasmic reticulum. The rough ER is an organelle composed of a continuous series of flattened sacs and branching tubes. Ribosomes are attached to the outer surface of the rough ER.

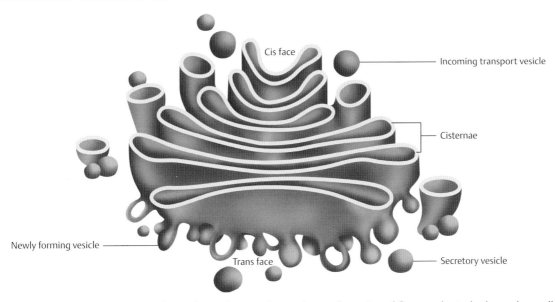

Fig. 2.9 The Golgi apparatus is a membrane-bound organelle made up of a series of flattened, stacked pouches called cisternae. Molecules packaged in vesicles from the ER fuse with the *cis* face of the apparatus. Modified molecules then exit from the *trans* face.

other regions of the cell or into the Golgi apparatus for further processing. Most proteins produced in the rough ER are packed into **vesicles** that pinch off from a transitional zone between the rough and smooth ER, devoid of ribosomes.

The **Golgi apparatus** (**Fig. 2.9**) is composed of stacks of flattened, membrane-covered sacs called **cisternae.** Animal cells typically contain between ten and twenty cisternae in the Golgi apparatus. The Golgi apparatus, also referred to as the Golgi body or Golgi complex, is often described as the distribution and shipping department of the cell. Vesicle-packaged proteins and lipids arrive at the Golgi apparatus and fuse with the *cis* face of this organelle, the surface of the Golgi nearest to the ER. As proteins and lipids progress through the Golgi apparatus, they undergo a series of modifications. The modified molecules that are ready for shipping out of the Golg apparatus are found at its *trans* face, the surface of the Golgi furthest from the ER. The molecules are then extruded from the Golgi in secretory vesicles and are directed to their final destination within the cell or to the extracellular space. For example, vesicles containing membrane proteins are delivered to the plasma membrane, whereas other vesicles may fuse with the plasma membrane and discharge their contents to the cell's exterior. Some vesicles may be directed to other organelles within the cells, such as lysosomes.

Lysosomes have been referred to as "cell stomachs" or the "recycling centers" of the cell. The interior of the lysosomes is highly acidic and is packed with powerful digestive enzymes that are specifically designed to work in acidic environments. Therefore, lysosomes are capable of degrading materials that have exceeded their lifetime or are no longer useful to the cell. Cellular waste products, fats, carbohydrates, and proteins are broken down by the lysosome into simple compounds that are then moved back to the cytoplasm for use in other cellular processes.

Cytoplasm

In general terms, the **cytoplasm** is the interior portion of the cell that is not occupied by the nucleus. In a typical animal cell, the cytoplasm occupies most of the cellular volume and includes organelles (i.e., mitochondria, Golgi apparatus, etc.) as well as important cellular machinery for the synthesis of proteins, lipids, and energy (ATP). These organelles are suspended within a viscous fluid called the **cytosol**. However, the cytosol is not simply a structureless fluid. Instead, it contains an intricate system of interconnected fibers and tubules that make up the cell's structural framework. This system is called the **cytoskeleton**, meaning "cell skeleton" (**Fig. 2.10**). The cytoskeleton helps shape and support the plasma membrane as well as the cell's interior. Unlike the permanence and rigidity that characterize the human skeletal system, the cellular cytoskeleton exhibits extreme plasticity and can be rapidly remodeled in response to internal and external

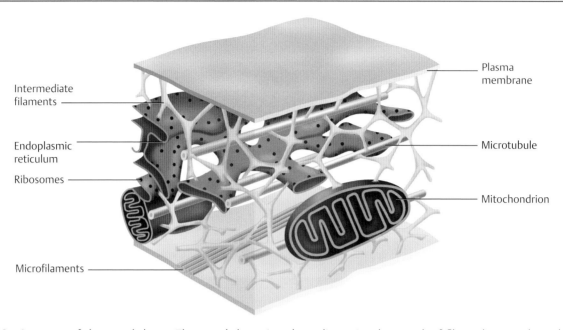

Intermediate filaments

Endoplasmic reticulum

Ribosomes

Microfilaments

Plasma membrane

Microtubule

Mitochondrion

Fig. 2.10 Structure of the cytoskeleton. The cytoskeleton is a three-dimensional network of fibers that run throughout the cytoplasm of living cells. Three main protein structures constitute the cytoskeleton: microfilaments, microtubules, and intermediate filaments.

stimuli. Due to this plasticity, the cytoskeleton is able to accomplish major functions within the cell, including the positioning of organelles, providing a system for the transport of vesicles, and facilitating cellular locomotion.

The cytoskeleton is composed of three major structural elements: microtubules, microfilaments, and intermediate filaments. **Microtubules** are the largest of the cytoskeletal fibers, with a diameter of about 25 nm, and are formed from the smaller protein **tubulin**. In these fibers, tubulins, specifically α-tubulin and β-tubulin, are arranged to form a hollow, strawlike tube (**Fig. 2.11**). Microtubules resist compression, support cell structure, participate in cell division, and are major contributors to cytoplasmic organization and transport. **Microfilaments** are found in almost all eukaryotic cells and are the thinnest component of the cytoskeleton, with a diameter of only 6 nm. These fibers are formed from links of individual subunits called

---

Box 2.3   Dystrophin and Duchenne Muscular Dystrophy

Duchenne muscular dystrophy (DMD) is a genetic disorder characterized by progressive muscle degeneration and weakness. Onset of symptoms typically occurs in boys during early childhood. Muscles first affected include those in the hips, pelvic area, thighs, and shoulders; later, the disease affects muscles in the arms, legs, and trunk. In advanced stages of DMD, the heart and respiratory muscles are affected. Dysphagia (difficulty swallowing) is reported in the advanced stages of DMD. Specifically, the oral phase of the swallow is primarily affected, as evidenced by reduced strength of oral muscles, including the tongue, which influences deglutition of solid foods. Individuals with DMD often require treatment from a speech-language pathologist to develop compensatory strategies for safe swallowing.

DMD is caused by mutations in the gene that encodes the cytoskeletal protein dystrophin. Dystrophin has a major structural role in muscles because it connects the internal cytoskeleton of the cell to the extracellular matrix. In other words, dystrophin is essential for keeping muscle cells intact. The majority of patients with DMD lack dystrophin, causing their muscle cells to be fragile and easily damaged. Increased knowledge of the structure and function of dystrophin and its role in the muscle has led scientists to a better understanding of DMD. Further advances in the understanding of the cytoskeleton and its function in DMD and other diseases may lead to new diagnostic and therapeutic applications for dysphagia and other features of these disorders.

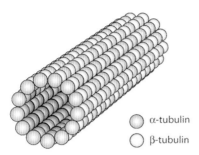

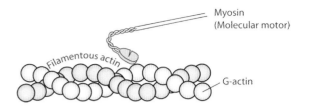

Fig. 2.11 Structure of a microtubule. A microtubule is made of α-tubulin and β-tubulin. Thirteen of these subunits form rings that stack up to form a hollow tubule.

Fig. 2.12 Structure of a microfilament. A microfilament is made of subunits of actin. These subunits create a structure resembling a double helix. The molecular motor myosin pulls the actin to make the cytoskeleton contract.

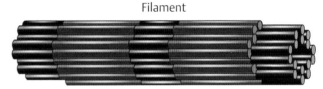

Fig. 2.13 Structure of an intermediate filament. An intermediate filament has variable composition. Structurally, most intermediate filaments contain rodlike segments.

actin, creating a structure that resembles a double helix (**Fig. 2.12**). Microfilaments are best known for their role in cellular events requiring motion and are particularly evident under the surface of the plasma membrane. Microfilaments were first discovered in skeletal muscle, where myosin pulls actin filaments to make the cytoskeleton contract. However, microfilaments have other important functions, including playing a role in cell division, supporting vesicle movement throughout the cell, and determining cell shape. **Intermediate filaments** are considered the most stable structure of the cytoskeleton; consequently, they play an essential structural role in the cell. They are termed intermediate because, with a diameter of about 10 nm, they are smaller than microtubules and larger than microfilaments. Unlike microtubules and microfilaments, intermediate filaments are not found in all animal cells and have variable composition depending on cell type. However, intermediate filaments do have structural similarities, including a central rodlike segment that is similar from one protein to another (**Fig. 2.13**).

Aberrations in cytoskeletal or cytoskeleton-associated proteins are implicated in a variety of disease states.

Extracellular Matrix

Thus far, we have focused on the structural composition of individual cells. However, the external environment, or extracellular space, is also critical. Most cells secrete a variety of macromolecules, the essential functional elements of cells, into the extracellular space, and this complex meshwork of proteins and carbohydrates forms the **extracellular matrix** (ECM; **Fig. 2.14**).

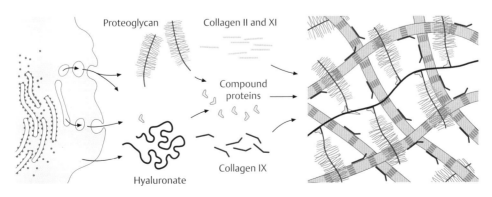

Fig. 2.14 Structure of the extracellular matrix. Cells secrete macromolecules into the extracellular space to form the extracellular matrix. The extracellular matrix is a meshwork composed of fibrous proteins (e.g., collagen) and carbohydrates (e.g., proteoglycans and hyaluronate).

The ECM is closely associated with the cells that produced it by surrounding and supporting these cells as well as regulating their progression from individual cells into tissues during development.

The composition of the ECM can vary widely. The macromolecules that make up the ECM are mostly dependent upon the specific type of nearby cells. Largely, cells called **fibroblasts** produce matrix macromolecules, and, generally two main classes of macromolecules constitute the ECM. The first class is a specific type of polysaccharide chain (i.e., carbohydrate chain) called a **glycosaminoglycan** (GAG). Hyaluronan is a simple GAG and major component of the ECM. When GAGs are linked to proteins, they are called proteoglycans. Proteoglycans fill the majority of the extracellular space in the form of a ground substance or hydrated gel. The second classes of ECM macromolecules are fibrous proteins, which include collagen, elastin, fibronectin, and laminin. When these classes of molecules are together, the proteoglycans form a hydrated gel ground substance in which fibrous proteins are embedded.

Of the fibrous proteins of the ECM, collagen is the most abundant and primary structural element of the ECM. In fact, collagen constitutes up to 30% of the total protein mass of a multicellular organism. Collagen fibers contribute to both the strength and organization of the matrix. Elastin, another fibrous ECM protein, often associates with collagen and is often described as "rubber-like," giving the matrix its elasticity and resilience. A third fibrous protein, fibronectin, is important for mediating cell attachment to the ECM. Integral membrane proteins on the cell surface called **integrins** attach to both the fibrous proteins of the ECM and the cytoskeleton.

■ Cellular Processes

The complex and diverse cell machinery described in the previous section is critical for a variety of cellular processes. These processes are essential to cell survival and adaptation to the constantly changing environment. In the next section, two major cellular processes, cellular respiration and cellular transport, are presented.

Cellular Respiration

Cells require energy in order to accomplish the tasks of life and, like humans, cells need to locate a source of energy from their environment. The sun is the ultimate source of energy for almost all cells. Photosynthetic prokaryotes, algae, and plant cells utilize solar energy to make the complex organic food molecules on which cells rely for energy as well as oxygen gas. Common cellular foods include carbohydrates (i.e., sugars), lipids, and even proteins. The large nutrient-rich macromolecules are composed of subunits, and energy is stored within the molecules as chemical bonds holding the subunits together. Consequently, the chemical bonds must be broken to harness the energy contained within. Cells release energy from food molecules through controlled **oxidation** reactions, multistep reactions during which electrons are transferred from one molecule to another. At the start of the reaction, food molecules act as the electron donor. As food molecules are broken down, electron acceptor molecules capture some of that energy and store it for later use. Once a food molecule is completely broken down, or oxidized, what remains is carbon dioxide (CO_2), which is released as waste.

Cells do not immediately use the energy released from oxidation reactions. Instead, it is converted into energy-rich molecules, such as adenosine triphosphate (ATP) and nicotinamide adenine dinucleotide (NAD). ATP is the primary cellular molecule used for storage and transfer of energy and is composed of three main parts (**Fig. 2.15**). In the center of ATP, a ribose (sugar) molecule is bound on one side to a nucleobase, adenine, and bound on the other side to a series of three connected phosphate molecules, a triphosphate group. High-energy bonds connect the phosphate molecules, and when the bond between the second

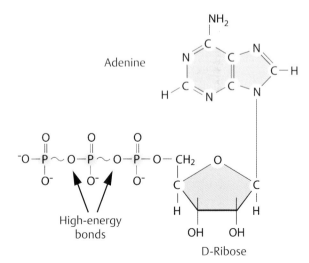

Fig. 2.15 Structure of ATP. ATP is composed of three main parts: ribose, adenine, and phosphate molecules. High-energy bonds connect the three phosphate molecules.

and third phosphate molecule is broken, energy is released and is available for the cell to use. This molecule is adenosine diphosphate (ADP). The reaction is reversible, and when energy is available for storage, ADP is converted back to ATP through the addition of a third phosphate group.

The process by which cells convert cellular foods into ATP is called **cellular respiration**. There are two types of cellular respiration: aerobic respiration and anaerobic respiration. During **aerobic respiration**, cells produce energy using oxygen to help power the process. This long, multistep process takes place in both the cytoplasm and mitochondria of the cell and produces approximately 38 ATP molecules. The basic formula for aerobic respiration is as follows. In this formula, $C_6H_{12}O_6$ is the

carbohydrate glucose, O_2 is oxygen, CO_2 is carbon dioxide, and H_2O is water.

$$C_6H_{12}O_6 + 6O_2 \rightarrow 6CO_2 + 6H_2O + \sim 38 \text{ ATP}$$

To summarize, during aerobic respiration, glucose is oxidized into CO_2 and H_2O, thereby releasing energy in the form of ATP. With modification, aerobic respiration can occur with other molecules beside glucose, such as lipids and proteins. However, we will focus on glucose as the primary fuel source for this process. This eukaryotic energy pathway can be broken down into four stages (**Fig. 2.16**). The first stage occurs in the cytoplasm of the cell and is **glycolysis**. Glycolysis means "sugar splitting" and does not require oxygen. During gly-

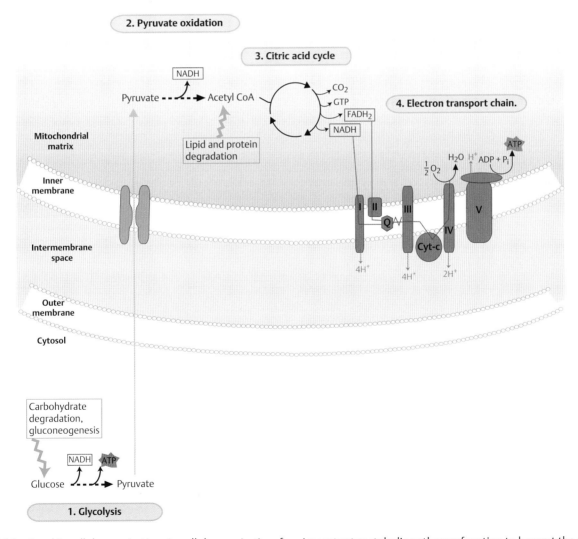

Fig. 2.16 Aerobic cellular respiration. In cellular respiration, four important metabolic pathways function to harvest the energy contained within the bonds of carbohydrates, proteins, and lipids and convert it to ATP. These metabolic pathways are (1) glycolysis, (2) pyruvate oxidation, (3) the citric acid cycle, and (4) the electron transport chain.

colysis, a single glucose molecule is split into two molecules of pyruvate and produces only two molecules of ATP. The next stage is pyruvate oxidation, also referred to as the transition reaction. Pyruvate is transferred into the innermost compartment of mitochondria, where it is converted into acetyl CoA, a two-carbon energy carrier, for further breakdown. Acetyl CoA then enters the third stage of aerobic respiration called the citric acid cycle, or Krebs cycle. In the presence of O_2, all hydrogen atoms are stripped from acetyl CoA to extract the electrons needed to make ATP. When this process is complete, all that is left of glucose is CO_2, a waste product, and H_2O. The citric acid cycle produces only four ATPs; however, it does create ample amounts of NADH that is used in the fourth and final stage of aerobic respiration. The final stage is called the electron transport chain and occurs in the cristae of the mitochondria, resulting in a large ATP yield. The electrons acquired during the citric acid cycle are carried by NADH and passed down an electron transport chain, resulting in the production of about 32 ATPs for every glucose molecule. Any excess energy from aerobic respiration is stored in large, energy-rich molecules, such as the carbohydrates called glycogens and lipids.

Anaerobic respiration, also called fermentation, is the breakdown of cellular food that does not require oxygen. This process occurs much faster than aerobic respiration, but during anaerobic respiration, only a partial breakdown of sugar occurs, and typically this process only reaches the stage of glycolysis. Therefore, it produces only two ATPs per glucose, much less than the 38 produced during aerobic respiration. During strenuous exercise, human muscle cells undergo a type of anaerobic respiration that produces lactic acid, which builds up in the tissue, causing fatigue and soreness.

■ Cellular Transport

Cellular transport is the movement of substances (e.g., atoms, ions, or molecules) across the plasma membrane into or out of the cell. Cellular transport is a critical cellular process for a variety of reasons. To begin with, the process allows molecules manufactured within the cell (e.g., carbohydrates, proteins, lipids) to be transported outside of the cell and to the rest of the body. Cellular transport also permits essential molecules such as glucose and amino acids to enter the cell, while allowing the removal of cellular waste products. Before the processes in cellular transport can be understood, it is necessary to understand why the processes are required. As discussed previously, the plasma membrane of the cell is a semipermeable barrier composed of an amphipathic bilayer of phospholipids and proteins. Semipermeability means that only certain substances can pass through the barrier. The ease with which substances move through the plasma membrane is usually a function of molecular polarity and size. Polarity is the arrangement of electrons on a molecule that can create either a positive or a negative charge. The phospholipids that make up the cellular membrane have hydrophobic (uncharged) interiors, which prevent charged particles from crossing the cell membrane, even small ions such as sodium, potassium, calcium, and chloride. Polar molecules also have difficulty passing through the hydrophobic interior of the membrane. For example, water molecules can pass

---

Box 2.4 Aerobic and Anaerobic Respiration During Exercise

Exercise requires the release of energy from ATP in order for our muscles to contract. During aerobic exercise, large amounts of oxygen are shuttled to our working muscles to serve as an energy substrate in the metabolism of cellular food, such as glucose, to ATP. Aerobic respiration is the only source of ATP during sustained exercise of moderate intensity. However, in some instances, such as sprinting or lifting heavy weights, we require energy production faster than our bodies can adequately deliver oxygen to the exercising muscles. This is when our bodies may begin to obtain energy anaerobically. During anaerobic exer-

cise, ATP is produced from glucose without the need for oxygen, and lactic acid is produced as a byproduct. A healthy person can perform aerobic exercise for several hours. On the other hand, the magnitude of energy from anaerobic sources depends on a person's capacity and tolerance for lactic acid accumulation. Typically, anaerobic exercise can be sustained at a high rate for only 1 to 3 minutes, during which time lactic acid can accumulate to high levels. Lactic acid accumulation causes the burning sensation often experienced in active muscles during intense exercise. This often-painful sensation also gets us to stop overworking our muscles, thus forcing a recovery period in which the body clears the lactic acid.

through the membrane only at a very slow rate. On the other hand, molecules that are electrically neutral (nonpolar) and small, including such gases as O_2 and CO_2, can typically move uninterrupted through the plasma membrane. Consequently, transmembrane proteins are needed to assist in the movement of charged molecules and large, uncharged particles across the plasma membrane. The two primary types of transport by which substances move across the plasma membrane are passive transport and active transport.

Passive Transport

Passive transport is the simplest form of transport across the plasma membrane. During passive transport, no energy is expended, because passive transport involves diffusion of a substance down a concentration gradient. The concentration gradient is simply a space where the concentration of a substance is not equal. Substances naturally move down their concentration gradient, from areas of high concentration to areas of low concentration. Types of passive transport include diffusion, facilitated diffusion, and osmosis.

Diffusion is the movement of particles from an area of high concentration to an area of low concentration, until equilibrium is reached or the concentration becomes uniform throughout (**Fig. 2.17**). Movement of substances does not stop at equilibrium; constant, minor movements of substances back and forth across the membrane continue. Substances may move throughout the cytosol by diffusion. This process is also used to

move small, uncharged molecules through the plasma membrane. The rate of diffusion is variable and depends on temperature as well as size and type of molecule. As described in Chapter 10, an example of diffusion is respiratory gas exchange, where oxygen diffuses from the blood, where it is at a higher concentration, into a tissue with respiring cells low in oxygen. In contrast, carbon dioxide diffuses in the opposite direction, from the tissue into the blood and back to the lungs for exhalation.

Facilitated diffusion is the movement of specific molecules down a concentration gradient and passage through the plasma membrane using membrane proteins. In this type of passive transport, membrane proteins allow larger and polar molecules to pass across the hydrophobic core of the plasma membrane (**Fig. 2.18**). Transport proteins used in facilitated diffusion are very selective and permit transport of only one substance or a few closely related substances. Two major classes of transport proteins are channel

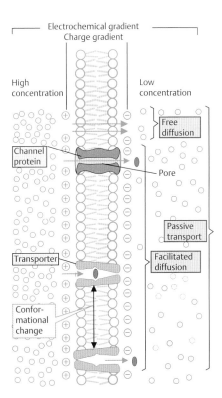

Fig. 2.18 Facilitated diffusion is the movement of specific molecules down a concentration gradient and passage through the plasma membrane using membrane proteins. This type of diffusion can occur using channel proteins and carrier proteins. Channel proteins make a tunnel across the membrane, allowing molecules to pass through by diffusion. Carrier proteins change shape when they encounter the target molecule, allowing the material to cross the membrane.

A Simple diffusion
(movement from high to low concentration; energy-independent)

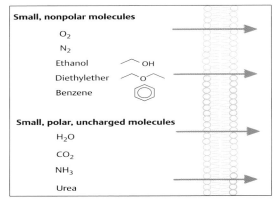

Fig. 2.17 Diffusion. Passive transport is the energy-independent movement of molecules from an area of high concentration to one of lower concentration. During diffusion, only nonpolar and some small, uncharged polar molecules pass through the lipid bilayer without help.

and carrier proteins. **Channel proteins** span the plasma membrane and make tunnels across it, allowing specific substances to pass through via diffusion. A common channel protein is aquaporin, which is always open and allows water to cross the membrane easily. On the other hand, some channels are "gated" and selectively open and close to regulate the movement of materials across cellular membranes. In contrast to channel proteins, which create membrane tunnels, **carrier proteins** change shape when they encounter their target substance, thereby allowing the desired materials to pass across the membrane—their action is similar to a one-way revolving door. Glucose is a common example of a molecule moved through the plasma membrane by a carrier protein.

Osmosis is the movement of water across a semipermeable membrane from a region of high concentration to a region of low concentration. In other words, it is simply the diffusion of water. To understand how osmosis works in cells, you first have to understand the concept of solutions. Solutions have two parts—the solute, which is being dissolved, and the solvent, which does the dissolving. Water is the primary solvent in cells, and if the total amount of dissolved solutes is not equal inside and outside of the cell, there will be net movement of water into or out the cell. For instance, when the environment inside and outside of the cell is **isotonic**, the concentrations of dissolved solutes are equal and there will be no net water movement across the cellular membrane. In general, animal cells perform best in isotonic environments. A **hypertonic solution** has a higher concentration of dissolved solutes than another solution. Therefore, in a hypertonic environment, for example, the concentration of water is lower outside the cell and water from the cytoplasm flows out of the cell, causing it to shrink (**Fig. 2.19**). On the other hand, a **hypotonic** extracellular environment would have very little dissolved solute and lots of water compared to the cytoplasm. A cell in a hypotonic environment will swell, due to the flow of water across the membrane and into the cell (**Fig. 2.19**).

Active Transport

Active transport is the process that takes place when the movement of substances across the plasma membrane requires the expenditure of cellular energy, such as ATP. Active transport can involve the movement of substances against a concentration gradient, from an area of low concentration to an area of high concentration. Additionally, ions carry a positive or negative electrical charge and may form an electrical gradient across the cell membrane, referred to as a **membrane potential**. In this case, active transport and the use of cellular energy are required to move charged particles across the membrane. A common example of active transport across a membrane potential is the **sodium-potassium pump** (e.g., Na^+,K^+-ATPase; **Fig. 2.20**). The sodium-potassium pump is one of the most important pumps in

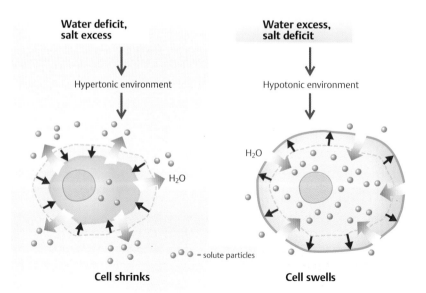

Fig. 2.19 Water output and intake from the cell by osmosis. In a hypertonic environment, there is a higher concentration of solutes outside the cell than inside, so water moves out of the cell by osmosis. In a hypotonic environment, there is a higher concentration of solutes inside the cell, so extracellular water moves into the cell by osmosis.

Box 2.5   Cellular Transport in the Vocal Folds

A thin layer of fluid covers the surface of the vocal folds. This layer, called vocal fold surface fluid (VFSF), has numerous important functions. VFSF acts as a barrier that helps protect the underlying tissue from damage by inhaled irritants such as pollutants and cigarette smoke. It also helps lubricate the vocal folds while they are vibrating and helps support a healthy sounding voice. Over the past decade, vocal fold researchers have discovered that the cellular transport of ions is the primary mechanism for regulating the amount and composition of VFSF. Specifically, the active transport of small, electrically charged molecules through vocal fold cells creates a gradient for osmosis that causes water movement in and out of the VFSF.

A model of the pathways for ion and water movement through vocal folds is displayed in **Box Fig. 2.2**. The epithelial cells, or the outermost cell layer of the vocal folds, support this cellular transport. Transmembrane ion and water transport proteins are located on the apical (i.e., outer) and basolateral (i.e., inner) epithelial cell membranes. In this model, Na^+,K^+-ATPase is the primary driving force behind the active ion transport and is located on the basolateral cell membrane. The Na^+,K^+-ATPase creates an electrical gradient by transporting three sodium (Na^+) ions out of the cell in exchange for two potassium (K^+) ions into the cell. This electrical gradient is used to help move Na^+ and chloride (Cl^-) ions through separate transmembrane proteins located on the apical cell membrane. Specifically, Na^+ is absorbed into the epithelium through the epithelial sodium channel (ENaC), and Cl^- is secreted out of the epithelium through the cystic fibrosis transmembrane regulator (CFTR). The transport of the Na^+ and Cl^- ions creates the osmotic gradient that drives water movement across the vocal fold epithelium. Specifically,

water movement into the epithelium is associated with Na^+ absorption, while water movement into the VFSF is associated with Cl^- secretion. Water movement occurs through water-specific transmembrane proteins called aquaporins. Understanding of these pathways may lead to the development of clinical treatments directed toward facilitating vocal fold epithelial ion and fluid transport. These treatments have the potential to benefit healthy speakers, those with voice disorders, and those at risk for developing voice problems.

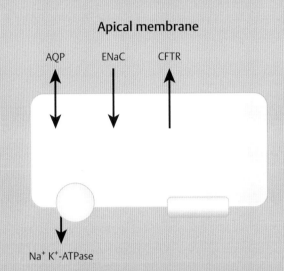

Box Fig. 2.2   Model illustrating ion and water transport across vocal fold epithelial cells. The Na^+,K^+-ATPase, localized to the basolateral cell membrane, provides the primary driving force behind active ion transport. The Na^+,K^+-ATPase creates an electrochemical gradient that supports Na^+ absorption (through ENaC) and Cl^- secretion (through CFTR). Both ENaC and CFTR have been localized to the apical cell membrane. Bidirectional water fluxes, driven primarily by Na^+ absorption and Cl^- secretion, occur through aquaporin channels (AQP) located on the apical membrane.

animal cells and is found in particularly high concentrations in nerve cells, where it moves three Na^+ molecules out of the cell and two K^+ into the cell. Consequently, the exterior of the cell becomes positively charged relative to the interior of the cell, creating an electrical gradient. If given the chance, positive charges move across the membrane to neutralize this difference; consequently, the pump must act continuously to maintain the membrane potential. In nerve cells, these electrical gradients are used to propagate electrical signals. (The physiology of neurotransmission is discussed in detail in Chapter 6.)

The movement of very large molecules across the plasma membrane is called bulk transport. Bulk transport processes, including endocytosis and exocytosis, require the expenditure of ATP and are forms of active transport. **Endocytosis** is the process of capturing substances from outside of the cell and bringing them into the cell's interior (**Fig. 2.21**). Briefly, the cell membrane engulfs the target substance and invaginates to form a pouchlike, membrane-bound vesicle that is then pinched off and moved into the cytoplasm. In contrast, **exocytosis** describes the process of already formed vesicles fusing with the plasma membrane and

2 Active Na$^+$-K$^+$-pump

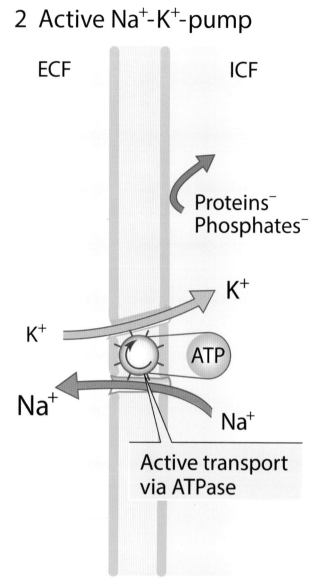

ECF   ICF

Proteins$^-$
Phosphates$^-$

K$^+$

K$^+$

ATP

Na$^+$

Na$^+$

Active transport via ATPase

Fig. 2.20 Sodium-potassium pump. The sodium-potassium pump uses energy from the hydrolysis of ATP to move sodium and potassium ions across the cell membrane against their concentration gradients. For each ATP broken down, two potassium ions are transported into the cell and three sodium ions out of the cell. ECF: extracellular fluid, ICF: intracellular fluid.

releasing their contents outside of the cell (**Fig. 2.21**). Both of these processes are critical for regulating cellular homeostasis by moving very large molecules across the cell membrane.

In sum, cellular respiration and transport are processes essential to cell survival. Cellular respiration is the process by which cells acquire energy in order to accomplish the tasks of life. Aerobic respiration is the primary eukaryotic energy pathway and uses oxygen to create the energy-yielding substance ATP. Anaerobic respiration occurs in the

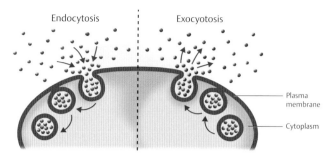

Endocytosis   Exocyotosis

Plasma membrane

Cytoplasm

Fig. 2.21 Endocytosis and exocytosis. Endocytosis (left) is a process by which cells take in molecules that are too large to pass through the plasma membrane. Exocytosis (right) is a process by which a cell expels molecules that are too large to pass through the plasma membrane. Both processes require energy and make use of vesicles for transport.

absence of oxygen and, although a faster reaction, its ATP output is dramatically less. Cellular transport is the movement of substances across the plasma membrane, either to enter or to exit the cell. Cellular transport is divided into two general types: passive and active. Passive transport moves substances down their concentration gradient without the use of energy and occurs through diffusion, facilitated diffusion, and osmosis. Conversely, active transport uses energy in the form of ATP to move substances against their concentration or electrical gradient.

◼ Cellular Communication

Survival of cells in a multicellular organism depends on the ability of the cell to monitor the environment and to communicate effectively using a variety of chemical messengers. The nucleus is the "control center" of the cell and it is essential for information from the extracellular environment to be efficiently and accurately relayed to the nucleus. This information can be conveyed mechanically, such as by stretching and pulling, or it may come from other cells in the form of chemical messengers. The signals are received by the cell using specialized **receptors** that transmit the information to the nucleus, allowing the cell to respond appropriately. Cells are constantly surrounded by hundreds of different signals, but if a cell lacks the receptor for a particular signal, that information will not be received and there will be no response. The ability of cells to respond only to certain signals allows for specialization of groups of cells within the body. These specialized cells can join with other specialized groups to form tissues that can then coordinate to accomplish tasks a single cell type could not perform on its own. In the next section, the cellular interactions within multicellular organisms are presented, as well as the types of cell signaling molecules and their cognate receptors.

Types of Cell Signaling

In general, cells communicate with one another through four types of signals: juxtacrine, paracrine, autocrine, and endocrine signals. The type of signal is determined by the nature of the signal (chemical, protein), the type of responding cell, and the distance traveled to reach the intended target. The first type of signaling is **juxtacrine** signaling, which requires direct contact between communicating cells. A type of juxtacrine signaling is when the signaling molecule stays attached to the signaling cell and binds to a membrane-bound protein receptor on the target cell (**Fig. 2.22**). This type of signaling is important for cells to identify the adjacent cell and to determine their position in three-dimensional space. Another type of juxtacrine signaling is when cells cooperate to open a communication channel or **gap junction** between their plasma membranes (**Fig. 2.23**). Gap junctions, which are made up of proteins called connexins, are unique because they directly connect the cytoplasm of adjacent cells and allow small molecules, such as calcium (Ca^{2+}), to pass directly between them. However, larger molecules, such as DNA and proteins, cannot fit through gap junctions. Additionally, gap junctions serve an important physiological function, because it is essential for cells to synchronize their response to a stimulus. For example, cardiac cells of the heart pass the signal to beat through their gap junctions, allowing the cells to contract in unison. Therefore, juxtacrine signaling is an important method for neighboring cells to communicate and serves an essential physiological function.

    Paracrine signaling allows cellular communication when cells are not in direct contact and involves the secretion of molecules into the extracellular space, where they can then diffuse to target cells in close proximity (**Fig. 2.24**). It is important to note that nearby cells will respond to a paracrine signal only if they have the appropriate or cognate receptor. Interestingly, the diffusible signaling molecules can bind to receptors on the cell from which they were secreted and signal back to the original cell or another cell of the same type, which is referred to as **autocrine** signaling (**Fig. 2.25**). An example of paracrine signaling is the secretion of growth

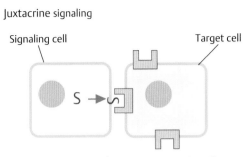

Juxtacrine signaling

Signaling cell   Target cell

Fig. 2.22 Juxtacrine signaling. Juxtacrine signaling requires direct contact between communicating cells. In this example, the signaling molecule stays attached to the secreting cell and binds to a receptor on the adjacent target cell.

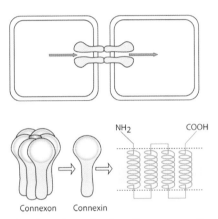

Connexon   Connexin

Fig. 2.23 Gap junctions. Gap junctions connecting adjacent cells are designed to permit free communication through them. A gap junction is made up of two connexons, one in the membrane of each of the adjacent cells (top). Each connexon is made up of six connexins (bottom left). Each connexin (bottom middle) is made up of a long peptide chain that traverses the membrane four times (bottom right).

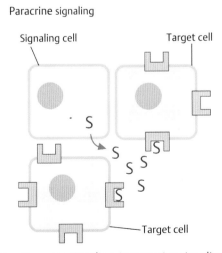

Paracrine signaling

Signaling cell   Target cell

Target cell

Fig. 2.24 Paracrine signaling. In paracrine signaling, the signaling molecule is released by one cell type and diffuses to a neighboring target cell that has a receptor for that molecule.

Autocrine signaling

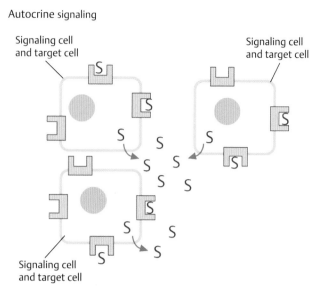

Fig. 2.25 Autocrine signaling. In autocrine signaling, the signaling molecule acts on secreting cell itself or a cell of the same type.

Endocrine signaling

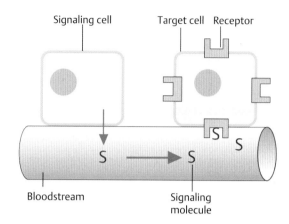

Fig. 2.26 Endocrine signaling. In endocrine signaling, the signaling molecule is released by a cell distant from the target cell and is transported via the bloodstream to the target cell.

factors during embryonic development. Certain growth factors are secreted by individual cell types at specific times and places to coordinate cell division and extracellular matrix deposition, as well as to specify tissue organization. In this way, growth factors and paracrine signaling are critical to the coordination of growth and development of the organism.

In humans and many other multicellular organisms, cells in distant regions of the body must communicate to maintain homeostasis. The bloodstream is an excellent conduit for transmitting these signals, as it is already delivering oxygen and nutrients to all cells and tissues of the body. The process by which cells transmit chemical signals, called hormones, through the bloodstream to cells in other areas of the body is **endocrine signaling** (**Fig. 2.26**). An example of endocrine signaling is the release of the hormone insulin from pancreatic cells when blood glucose levels increase after a meal. Insulin travels through the bloodstream and stimulates all cells of the body to take up glucose from the blood and to turn it into cellular fuel. In this way, cells of the pancreas signal to distant tissues of the body to regulate blood glucose levels and cellular energy stores.

The nervous system is composed of several specialized cell types involved in transmitting signals throughout the body. One particular cell type in this system, neurons, uses a special type of cellular communication called **synaptic signaling** (**Fig. 2.27**). In synaptic signaling, two neurons bring their plasma membranes in close proximity to form a unique structure called a **synapse**. When a neuron is stimulated, chemical messengers called **neurotransmitters** are released into the synaptic cleft (the narrow space between the cell membranes), where they signal to the adjacent cell. This type of signaling is distinct from paracrine signaling in that the messengers travel a very short distance, signal only to the other cell in the synaptic cleft, and have a very narrow range of influence. In this way, the nervous system regulates signals through essential organs, such as the brain and spinal cord, to ensure the accurate and efficient transmission of information.

Receptors

Cellular signals are sent through a variety of means, and cells will recognize a signal only if they have the receptor for that particular message. Cellular receptors are responsible for binding to a specific molecule, called a **ligand**, and then transmitting the information the ligand represents to the nucleus, where the cell will interpret and respond to the signal. Cellular receptors are found throughout the cell, including the plasma membrane, cytoplasm, and nucleus. **Cell surface receptors** are integral membrane proteins that bind to diverse ligands in the extracellular environment that cannot pass through the plasma membrane, such as nutrients, growth factors, or hormones. Upon binding, the receptors are said to be activated. In contrast, **intracellular receptors** are found in the cytoplasm and nucleus

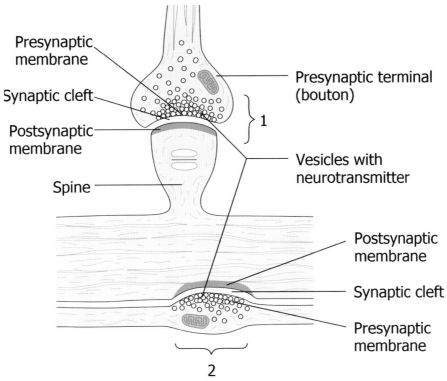

Fig. 2.27 Synaptic signaling. In synaptic signaling, the signaling molecules, or neurotransmitters, are released into the synaptic cleft, where they signal to the adjacent cell via the postsynaptic membrane, where the receptors are located.

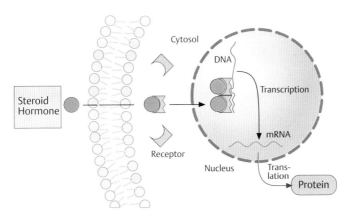

Fig. 2.28 Intracellular receptor. Steroid hormones diffuse through the plasma membrane and interact with receptors in the cytoplasm or nucleus. The resulting hormone–receptor complex alters gene transcription and causes the synthesis of proteins.

of the cell. Some signaling molecules, such as steroid hormones, are hydrophobic and can cross the plasma membrane into the interior of the cell, where they bind to intracellular receptors (**Fig. 2.28**). Intracellular receptors also bind a group of molecules produced when cell surface receptors are activated.

In order for a cell to respond appropriately to the environment, information must be received and transmitted to the nucleus. However, since many signals are received at the cell surface by membrane-bound receptors, cells use a process called **signal transduction** to pass information throughout the cell. In some cases, the receptor itself can act as an **enzyme** and can modify other proteins near the plasma membrane, often by adding or removing phosphate groups. These receptors are called **enzyme-linked receptors** and they have an extracellular portion that binds to the ligand in the environment and an intracellular, enzyme portion that catalyzes the modifications of nearby proteins (**Fig. 2.29**).

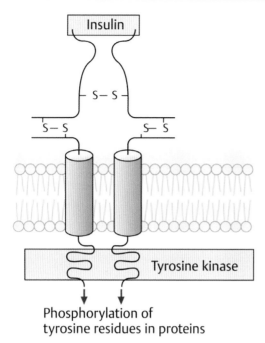

Fig. 2.29 Enzyme-linked receptor. In this example, insulin is the ligand that binds to an extracellular receptor. This causes the enzyme tyrosine kinase to phosphorylate tyrosine residues in proteins. These proteins can then signal other proteins to form, thus exerting a physiologic effect.

Another category of membrane receptors is **G-protein-coupled receptors (GPCRs),** which, as their name suggests, are bound in a complex to a signaling molecule called a G-protein (**Fig. 2.30**). When the GPCR binds to its ligand, a change occurs in the structure of the complex that causes the G-protein to separate from the receptor and to signal to other regions of the cell. While activated and signaling, G-proteins may participate in the production of **second messengers**, which are nonprotein molecules, such as Ca^{2+} or cyclic adenosine monophosphate (AMP). These messengers relay information from membrane-bound receptors and activated G-proteins to the rest of the cell and are often the chemical "trigger" for intracellular signaling cascades. A signaling cascade is a series of chemical reactions that occur one after another that serve to amplify a signal and elicit a cellular response, such as cell growth, locomotion, or death. Second messengers are also the ligands for several intracellular receptors that are activated upon binding and move to the nucleus to alter the production of proteins in the cell.

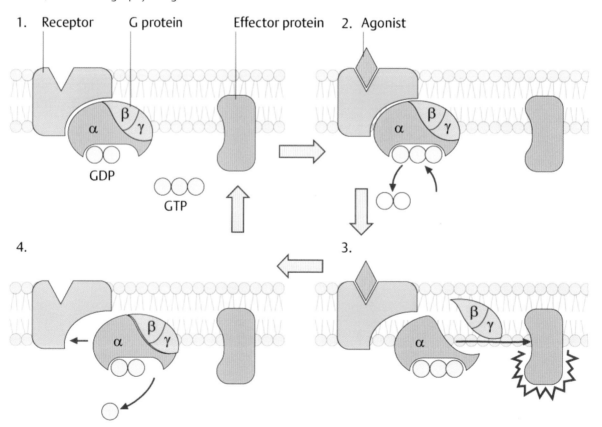

Fig. 2.30 G-protein-coupled receptors. (1) The G-protein-coupled receptor (GPCR) in the resting state. (2–3) When a ligand or agonist binds to the GPCR, it causes the receptor and G-protein to change conformation. The α-subunit exchanges GTP for GDP and dissociates from the other subunits, where it interacts with an effector protein. The effector protein then stimulates or inhibits second messengers to produce a physiological effect. (4) The α-subunit then hydrolyzes the bound GTP to GDP and reassociates with the other subunits.

Box 2.6   Parkinson's Disease and Cell Signaling

Parkinson's disease (PD) is one of the most common progressive neurodegenerative disorders. Specifically, PD is a "movement disorder," meaning it primarily affects the nerve cells in the brain responsible for body movement. Typical symptoms include shuffling gait, tremor of the arms and legs, muscle stiffness, slowed movement, and stooped posture. Movement disturbances related to speech and swallowing are also prevalent in PD. Dysarthria, the disruption of muscular control for speech, and dysphagia, the inefficient or unsafe transfer of food, liquid, or saliva from the mouth into the stomach, are also observed in PD.

Many of the symptoms of PD are associated with the loss of nerve cells that contain the neurotransmitter dopamine (**Box Fig. 2.3**). Dopamine enables messages to be transmitted to other parts of the brain that coordinate movement. Dopamine, like all neurotransmitters, is a chemical released by nerve cells to communicate with other nerve cells. In the normal state, release of dopamine in the presynaptic neuron results in signaling in the postsynaptic neuron through dopamine receptors, a class of G-protein-coupled receptors. Presynaptic neuron terminals release a neurotransmitter in response to an action potential. A postsynaptic neuron receives the electrical impulse that is transmitted. In the case of PD, the dopamine-producing neurons of the substantia nigra, a hub of nerve cells in the brainstem, slowly die. The resulting reduction in dopamine levels causes an imbalance with other neurotransmitters, leading to the common movement disturbances of PD.

No known treatments can stop or reverse the breakdown of nerve cells that causes PD. However, pharmacologic treatments are available that rely on principles of cell signaling to relieve symptoms of the disease. Two common treatment options include levodopa (L-dopa) and dopamine receptor agonist therapy. L-dopa is considered the most effective treatment for PD. L-dopa is a chemical precursor of dopamine. When L-dopa is administered, it is absorbed by the gastrointestinal tract and then is transported to brain cells and is converted into dopamine by brain enzymes. It is then released by brain cells and activates dopamine receptors. Dopamine receptor agonists, a class of drugs used to treat PD symptoms, mimic the action of naturally occurring dopamine. Specifically, they stimulate dopamine receptors directly. Unlike L-dopa, these medications do not have to be modified by brain enzymes in order to activate dopamine receptors.

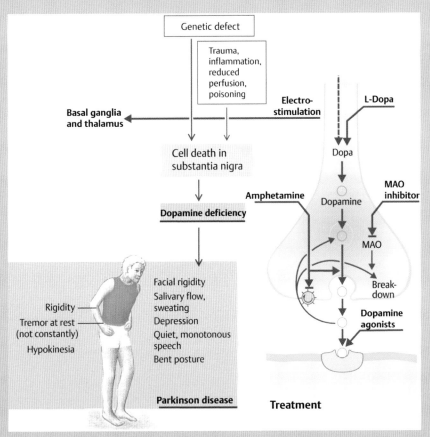

Box Fig. 2.3   In Parkinson's disease, the death of dopaminergic neurons in the substantia nigra results in less dopamine available to neurons in the striatum. Treatment aims to increase dopamine in neurons.

■ Tissues and Organs

The human body is composed of approximately 200 different types of cells organized into collective entities called **tissues**, in which groups of cells work together to carry out a common function. There are four main tissue types: epithelial tissue, connective tissue, nervous tissue, and muscle tissue. The tissue types are classified based upon their embryonic development, structure, and function within the body. In a developing embryo, cells occur in three major layers from which all body tissues later develop: the ectoderm, mesoderm, and endoderm. In general, the ectoderm, or outer layer, forms the skin and nervous system of the developing embryo, whereas the mesoderm, or middle layer, develops into connective tissue, muscle, and circulating blood cells. The endoderm, or inner layer, forms the two main tubes of the body the respiratory and digestive systems. In this chapter, the main tissue types that arise from the embryonic layers are presented, along with information regarding their structural organization and functional properties. In addition, the formation of **organs** to carry out complex physiologic functions is discussed. Finally, organ systems, or groups of organs that cooperate to perform critical processes in the body (many of which are related to speech, language, swallowing, hearing, and balance) are presented.

Epithelial Tissue

Epithelial tissue embryonically derives from all three germ layers (ectoderm, mesoderm, and endoderm) and primarily covers the body surface and lines the internal body cavity. Also known as the epithelium, epithelial tissue is formed by one or more sheets of epithelial cells closely packed to form a protective barrier. Other functions of the epithelium include absorption, excretion, secretion, filtration, and sensory reception. Epithelial tissues have five main characteristics. The first is polarity, which, in this context, means that the epithelium has one free surface (apical), with no additional cellular or extracellular structures, and one surface that is firmly attached to the ECM (basal). The second characteristic of epithelial tissue is the presence of specialized cell–cell contacts. Given that the primary function of epithelial tissue is to form a barrier, individual cells are densely packed together in single, or sometimes multiple, sheets. Individual cells are held together in the sheets by specialized contacts called cell junctions. The third characteristic of epithelium is that the cells are supported by connective tissue. The basal surface of the epithelium is attached to connective tissue through a type of ECM called the **basement membrane**. Macromolecular secretions from both the epithelium and connective tissue form the basement membrane. The fourth characteristic of epithelial tissue is that it is avascular. A tissue is described as avascular if there are no blood vessels interspersed throughout its cells. In this case, cells must rely on diffusion of nutrients and oxygen from nearby tissues, rather than direct delivery. The final and perhaps most important characteristic of epithelial tissues is their ability to regenerate. In certain tissues, such as the intestinal mucosa, epithelial cells survive only three to five days before they are replaced by new epithelium.

Epithelial tissues are classified based on the number of cell layers or by the arrangement and shape of the cells. In short, four common epithelial tissue arrangements have been described: simple, stratified, pseudostratified, and transitional (examples of these arrangements are described in **Table 2.2**). Epithelial cell shape is important for the cell to function properly, because the cell shape helps establish polarity, a hallmark of the epithelium. **Table 2.3** explains the

Table 2.2 Arrangements of epithelial cells

Cell Arrangement	Description
Simple	Single layer of cells attached to a basement membrane
Stratified	Two or more layers of cells found on top of each other
Pseudostratified	Single layer of cells that appears to be multiple layers due to varying cell height and location of nuclei
Transitional	Cells are rounded and slide around each other, allowing stretching

Table 2.3 Shapes of epithelial cells

Cell Shape	Description
Squamous	Flattened cells
Cuboidal	Cube-shaped cells, with equal cell height and width
Columnar	Tall, rectangular or column-shaped cells, with greater height than width

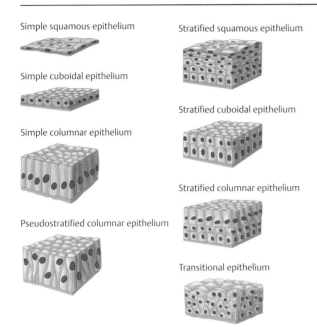

Simple squamous epithelium

Simple cuboidal epithelium

Simple columnar epithelium

Pseudostratified columnar epithelium

Stratified squamous epithelium

Stratified cuboidal epithelium

Stratified columnar epithelium

Transitional epithelium

Fig. 2.31 Epithelial tissues are characterized by the number of cell layers and cell shape. Various types of epithelial tissues are found throughout the body.

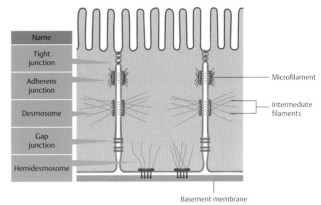

Fig. 2.32 Epithelial cells are joined by specialized contacts called cell junctions. Tight junctions are the most apically located cell junctions and tightly seal the space between epithelial cells. Adherens junctions, desmosomes, and hemidesmosomes form bonds between the cytoskeletal components of adjacent cells.

typical shapes of epithelial cells, including squamous, cuboidal, and columnar. The middle ear is lined with simple squamous epithelium. Stratified squamous epithelium covers both the surface of the esophagus and the vocal folds. Finally, the trachea is lined with pseudostratified columnar, or respiratory, epithelium. Schematics of common types of epithelial tissue are depicted in **Fig. 2.31**.

An important feature of epithelial tissues is specialized contacts called **cell junctions.** The cell junctions seal the space between adjacent cells, effectively creating a barrier (**Fig. 2.32**). Cell junctions are a hallmark of epithelial tissue and are necessary for the mechanical stability of the epithelium. In epithelial tissue, the various types of cell junctions have several overlapping and unique functions. **Tight junctions** are the most apically located cell junctions. They are located where plasma membranes of adjacent epithelial cells come together and form a tight, waterproof seal. Other types of junctions include adherens junctions, desmosomes, and hemidesmosomes. These junctions provide strong adhesive bonds between the cytoskeletal components of adjacent epithelial cells and are important for providing mechanical stability to epithelial tissue. **Adherens junctions** join the microfilaments of neighboring cells together. Even stronger connections are formed between neighboring cells at **desmosomes,** which connect intermediate filaments of adjacent cells, and **hemidesmosomes,** which join the intermediate filaments of cells to the basement membrane.

Epithelial cells are highly specialized and often have a variety of special features and machinery to accomplish specific functions. For example, many types of epithelial cells contain cilia, which are hair-like structures composed of microtubules and are found on the epithelial cell surface. As described in Chapter 10, cilia are important sensory organelles that respond to a variety of mechanical and chemical stimuli. Although nearly all human cells have non-motile, primary cilia, some cells, such as respiratory epithelial cells, have specialized motile cilia that are critical for clearing trapped irritants from the lungs (**Box 2.7**). Furthermore, certain types of epithelial cells are responsible for the synthesis and secretion of specific chemical substances, such as secretion of mucus onto the respiratory epithelial surface. These secretory, or glandular, cells are incorporated into multicellular glands made up of multiple secretory cells or they can form unicellular glands in the epithelium, called goblet cells (**Fig. 2.33**).

Connective Tissue

Connective tissue is embryonically derived from the mesoderm and is among the most abundant and widely distributed tissue in the body. It is incredibly diverse in composition and vascularity, and it provides structural support for the body by binding together cells and tissues. Generally speaking, connective tissue consists of ECM macromolecules, including a hydrated gel ground substance and protein fibers, with a sparse amount of cells embedded within. Ground substance is an amorphous gel consisting mainly of GAGs and proteoglycans. Common connective tissue protein fibers include collagen, elastin, and reticular fibers. Unlike in epithelial tissue,

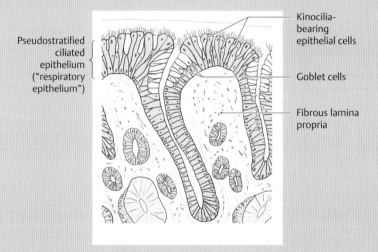
where cells are tightly packed, in connective tissue cells are widely distributed throughout the ECM. A variety of cell types are found in connective tissue, and they can be divided into two general categories:

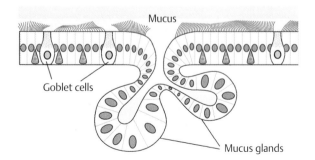

Mucus

Goblet cells

Mucus glands

Fig. 2.33 Glandular cells. Epithelium may contain glands that are unicellular (i.e., goblet cells) or multicellular (i.e., mucus glands). Both types of glands are responsible for secreting mucus and other substances onto the epithelial surface.

resident, or fixed cells, and nonresident, or wandering cells. As the name implies, fixed cells are permanent residents of the connective tissue. Fibroblasts are the principal fixed cells of connective tissues and are responsible for synthesis of ECM components, including the complex ground substance (e.g., proteoglycans and hyaluronic acid) and protein fibers (e.g., collagen and elastin). Other fixed cells, such as adipocytes, have the unique function of storing fat molecules, while tissue-resident macrophages are responsible for engulfment and digestion of cellular debris. Nonresident cells enter the connective tissue via the bloodstream, usually in response to a specific stimulus. These wandering cells include lymphocytes, plasma cells, and eosinophils, which have important immune functions in the connective tissue.

The classification and function of connective tissue is largely dependent on the quantity and composition of cells, fibers, and ground substance. Prominent types of connective include connective tissue proper and specialized connective tissue. Connective tissue proper includes dense irregular tissue, dense regular connective tissue, and loose connective tissue (**Table 2.4**). Examples of dense regular and dense irregular connective tissue are shown in **Fig. 2.34**. Specialized connective tissues include adipose tissue, reticular tissue, and elastic tissue (**Table 2.5**). Some of these specific connective tissues, as well as other unique types of connective tissue, including bone and cartilage, are discussed later in the chapter.

Nervous Tissue

Nervous tissue is embryonically derived from the ectoderm and functions to initiate and conduct electrochemical impulses to coordinate all body functions. Nervous tissue is composed mainly of two cell types: neurons and neuroglia, which are found throughout the nervous system, including the brain, spinal cord, and peripheral nerves. Nervous tissues also interact with other cells and tissues, either directly or indirectly, to coordinate

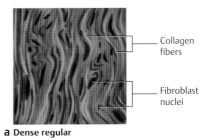

a **Dense regular**

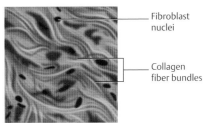

b **Dense irregular**

Fig. 2.34   Connective tissue. **(a)** Dense regular connective tissue consists of fibers packed in parallel bundles. **(b)** Dense irregular connective tissue consists of collagenous fibers interwoven into a meshlike network.

Table 2.4   Characteristics of connective tissue proper

Tissue Type	Cells	Fibers	Tissue Characteristics	Function	Locations
Dense irregular	Mostly fibroblasts	Collagen, elastin, reticular	Fewer cells; more fibers arranged in meshwork without definite orientation	Resist stress, protect organs	Skin, capsules of organs
Dense regular	Mostly fibroblasts	Collagen, elastin, reticular	Fewer cells; more fibers arranged in uniform orientation	Resistance to traction forces	Tendons, ligaments
Loose	Fibroblasts, macrophages, adipocytes, mast cells, leukocytes	Mostly collagen	More cells; fewer randomly distributed fibers	Protection, suspension, support	Gastro-intestinal tract

Table 2.5   Characteristics of specialized connective tissues

Tissue Type	Cells	Fibers	Tissue Characteristics	Function	Locations
Adipose	Mostly adipocytes	Collagen, reticular	Fibers form network that separates adipocytes	Cushioning for organs, energy storage	Hypodermis of skin, mammary glands
Reticular	Fibroblasts, reticular cells, hepatocytes, smooth muscle cells	Reticular fibers	Fibers form delicate meshlike network; cells attach to network with cell processes	Supportive framework for hematopoietic and solid organs	Liver, pancreas
Elastic	Mostly fibroblasts or smooth muscle cells	Mostly elastic fibers	Fibers form parallel, wavy bundles	Support; accommodates pressure changes in arteries	Large arteries; Vertebral ligaments

complex body functions. **Neurons** are specialized cells that quickly conduct impulses, called **action potentials**, to other neurons or onto tissues, such as muscles and glands. Using action potentials, neurons communicate information from the environment to the brain or spinal cord and between the various components of the sensory and nervous systems. Interestingly, neurons have a unique structure that greatly supports their function and consists of three basic parts: the dendrites, cell body, and the axon (**Fig. 2.35**). **Dendrites** are the input portion of the neuron, and their branched structure enables the neuron to receive information from a large surface area. This information is passed on to the cell body and is then conducted along the axon as an action potential. The elongated **axon** enables the neuron to communicate with distant neurons or cells from other tissues and organs. For example, the axon of a motor neuron originating in the spine can extend over three feet to reach muscle tissue in the leg. Due to the highly specialized function of neurons, they require numerous types of supportive cells, called neuroglia or **glial cells**. More abundant than neurons, glial cells support neurons by assisting in the propagation of nerve impulses, transfer of nutrients, and removal of waste. Types of glial cells in the nervous system include astrocytes, oligodendrocytes, microglial cells, and Schwann cells. For example, oligodendrocytes and Schwann cells make up the myelin sheath that covers some axons. These cells promote rapid impulse transmission along the axon and enable action potentials to be stronger and to travel farther (**Fig. 2.36**). Not surprisingly, nervous tissue is extremely important for several processes related to speech, language, swallowing, hearing, and balance. The anatomy and physiology of tissues in the nervous system are discussed in greater detail in Chapters 5 and 6.

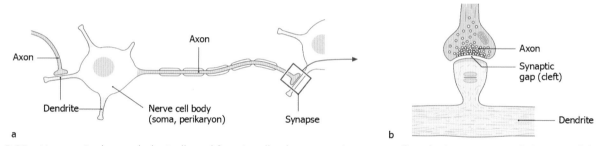

Fig. 2.35 Neuron. Both morphologically and functionally, the neuron (or nerve cell) is the basic structural element of the nervous system. Nerve cells generate electrical signals (action potentials) and pass them on to other nerve or muscle cells. **(a)** Attached to the cell body are at least two projections of different lengths. The dendrite is typically short and highly branched. The axon is typically longer. **(b)** At synapses, the axon of one nerve cell comes into very close contact with other cells. There is a gap between the axon and the receptor cell where the electrical signal is converted to a chemical signal or transmitter.

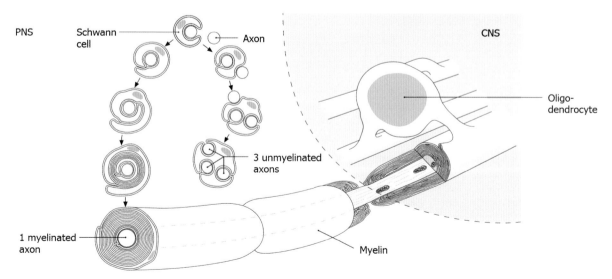

Fig. 2.36 Glial cells. The other distinctive cell type of the nervous system is the glial cell (neuroglia). Glial cells do not carry nerve impulses, but they are crucial in determining the speed with which impulses travel through the nervous system. Glial cells, including Schwann cells and oligodendrocytes, accomplish this by forming sheaths of myelin around the axons of nerve cells.

Muscle Tissue

Muscle tissue is embryonically derived from the mesoderm and is characterized based on its most basic functional property: the ability to contract. Consequently, muscle tissue is composed of specialized cells that contract, or shorten, in order to produce movement of body parts. Without muscle tissue, body movement would not occur; however, muscle tissue has other important functions, including maintaining posture, providing body support, and heat production. Common characteristics of all muscle tissue include specialized cells, irritability, contractility, extendibility, and elasticity. For example, specialized muscle cells called myocytes exhibit irritability, meaning they are able to receive and respond to impulses from nervous tissue. Responses to stimuli typically come in the form of contraction, or shortening of the muscle tissue. Once the stimulus has subsided, the tissue then demonstrates its extendibility by passively stretching back to its precontractile shape, or it may be actively pulled by the contracting fibers of an opposing muscle. Finally, muscle tissue has an innate tension, or elasticity, that causes it to assume a unique shape after relaxation.

Three main types of muscle tissue are found in the body: skeletal, smooth, and cardiac muscle. Each type has a distinctive structure and function and is found in different parts of the body. An overview of each muscle type is provided in **Table 2.6**. The muscle types are distinguishable based on the arrangement of the contractile proteins actin and myosin within the cell, the cellular shape, and the mechanism for contractile control. A brief introduction to the three types of muscle tissue is provided in the next section of this chapter. Additional details regarding the anatomy and physiology of muscle tissue are available in Chapter 8.

Skeletal muscle is the only muscle tissue that is voluntary, or under conscious control, and it is primarily responsible for the movement of the bones of our skeleton. Specifically, most skeletal muscle is connected to bones through fibrous attachments called tendons. The contraction of skeletal muscles

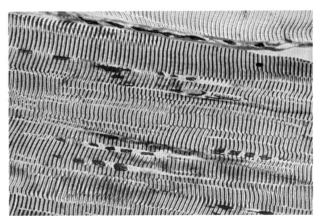

Fig. 2.37 Skeletal muscle fibers. Skeletal muscles are striated and occur in slender bundles with multiple nuclei.

pulls on the skeleton and produces the movements necessary for walking, breathing, and speaking. Of the three types of muscle tissue, skeletal muscle constitutes the greatest portion of the body's total weight, on average comprising approximately 40% of body mass. Skeletal muscle tissue is organized into basic units called muscle fibers, which are thick bundles of cylindrical, multinuclear cells (**Fig. 2.37**). Actin and myosin proteins of skeletal muscle cells are precisely arranged and parallel to each other along the long axis of the cells, giving the fibers a striated appearance. The bundles of skeletal muscle fibers are then surrounded by sheaths of connective tissue referred to as muscle fascia.

In contrast to skeletal muscle, **smooth muscle** contraction is involuntary and under intrinsic, autonomic, or hormonal control. Smooth muscle is responsible for the contractility of hollow organs, such as the gastrointestinal tract, the bladder, the uterus, and blood vessels. Specifically, the slow contraction of smooth muscles produces body movements primarily associated with digestion and the flow of fluids (**Box 2.8**). On a cellular level, smooth muscle cells are spindle-shaped and have a single nucleus (**Fig. 2.38**). Furthermore, their actin fila-

Table 2.6 Characteristics of muscle tissue

Tissue Type	Structural Features	Function	Location
Skeletal	Striated, cylindrical muscle fibers occurring in slender bundles with multiple nuclei	Rapid, voluntary movement of joints of skeleton	Attached to bony skeleton via tendons
Smooth	Elongated, spindle-shaped muscle fibers with a single nucleus	Slow, involuntary movements of internal organs	Walls of hollow internal organs
Cardiac	Branched, striated muscle fibers with single nucleus and intercalated disks	Rapid, involuntary, rhythmic contractions	Wall of heart

Box 2.8   Esophageal Peristalsis

The esophagus is a hollow muscular tube, closed proximally and distally by muscular sphincters (**Box Fig. 2.5**). The upper esophageal sphincter and proximal one-third of the esophagus are composed of skeletal muscle. The lower esophageal sphincter and distal one-half to two-thirds of the esophagus are composed of smooth muscle. The primary function of the esophagus is to propel swallowed food and liquid into the stomach. This occurs secondary to sequential, or peristaltic, contraction of the muscles of the esophagus. Esophageal motility disorders involve dysfunction of the esophagus and cause symptoms such as dysphagia, heartburn, and chest pain. Dysphagia can occur at different stages in the swallowing process, including the oral phase, pharyngeal phase, and esophageal phase. One of the most well-known esophageal motility disorders is diffuse esophageal spasm. Diffuse esophageal spasm is characterized by high-pressure, repetitive, simultaneous (rather than peristaltic) contractions in the smooth muscle portion of the esophagus, resulting in pain and spasm as well as dysphagia. Regurgitation may occur because of the swallowing dysfunction. Diagnosis is typically by esophageal manometry, a diagnostic test that examines pressure in the esophagus, or by a barium swallow study.

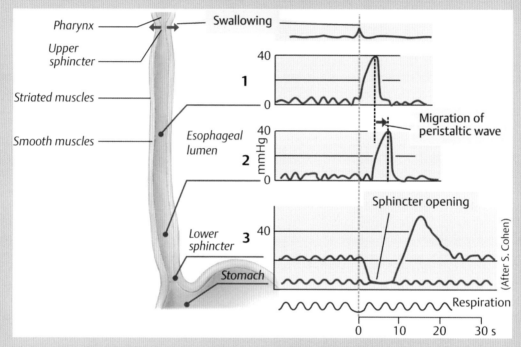

Box Fig. 2.5   Esophageal motility. Esophageal motility is usually examined by measuring the pressure in the lumen during a peristaltic wave (1,2). The resting pressure within the lower esophageal sphincter (LES) is normally 20 to 25 mm Hg. During reflex relaxation, esophageal pressure drops to match the lower pressure in the proximal stomach (3), indicating opening of the LES. Vagal pathways are involved in reflex relaxation of the LES.

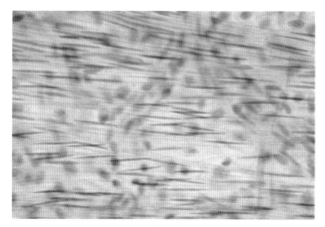

Fig. 2.38   Smooth muscle fibers. Smooth muscles are nonstriated and spindle-shaped, with a single nucleus.

ments are oriented in slightly different directions within cytoplasm; consequently, there are no visible striations.

Cardiac muscle, found only in the heart, is specialized to perform the essential function of pumping blood powerfully and efficiently throughout the body. This process is under involuntary control, meaning cardiac muscle contracts in its own intrinsic rhythms without external stimuli. Cells of cardiac muscle are called cardiomyocytes and have a branched appearance and a single central nucleus (**Fig. 2.39**). As in skeletal muscle, their actin and myosin are precisely arranged, giving cardiomyocytes a striated appearance.

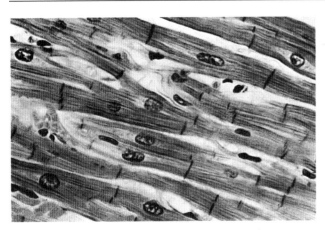

Fig. 2.39 Cardiac muscle fibers. Cardiac muscles are striated and branched with a single nucleus.

■ Stem Cells

Stem cells have three general properties. The first is self-renewal, or the ability to divide and renew through cell division over long periods of time. Second, stem cells are unspecialized, meaning that, unlike epithelial cells, muscle cells, or neurons, stem cells have no specialized functions within the body. Finally, stem cells have the potential to differentiate or develop into many different cell types with specialized functions in the body. In many tissues, stem cells contribute to regeneration by acting as internal repair systems and dividing to replenish lost or damaged cells.

The major classes of stem cells are embryonic stem cells, adult stem cells, and induced pluripotent stem cells. **Embryonic stem cells** occur in early-stage embryos. (When used in studies or treatments, these cells are obtained from embryos that develop from eggs that have been fertilized in vitro, or outside of the body. They are not derived from eggs fertilized within women's bodies.) Embryonic stem cells are pluripotent, meaning they can develop into each of the more than 200 cell types in the adult body and into all three primary germ layers. These cells can be cultured; however, culturing of embryonic stem cells is challenging and requires careful attention and observation. As long as embryonic stem cells are cultured under appropriate conditions, they remain undifferentiated. To obtain different types of specialized cells in culture, scientists change the chemical composition of the culture medium or modify the cells by inserting specific genes to force the cells to differentiate.

Adult stem cells are undifferentiated cells found among differentiated cells in a specific tissue. Adult stem cells have a lesser ability than embryonic stem cells to give rise to the various cell types and tissues of the body. However, these cells have the capacity to regenerate the cell types of the tissue in which they reside. Adult stem cells are responsible for tissue maintenance and repair and can be found in small numbers in most adult tissues, including blood, blood vessels, skeletal muscle, skin, teeth, heart, gut, liver, and epithelium. The area of the tissue in which the adult stem cells reside is called the stem cell niche. Once removed from the body, adult stem cells are even more challenging than embryonic stem cells to grow in culture, due to their small numbers and limited capacity to divide.

The third class of stem cells are called **induced pluripotent stem cells,** or iPS cells. These are adult cells, such as blood or skin cells, that have been genetically reprogrammed to a pluripotent, embryonic-like stem cell state. This reprogramming earned its discoverers the 2012 Nobel Prize in Physiology or Medicine. This reprogramming is accomplished by forcing the cells to express a cassette of genes typically found only during embryogenesis.

Scientists believe that stem cells will increase our understanding of disease development and lead to tissue-regeneration techniques capable of replacing injured or diseased cells with healthy tissue. Currently, scientists are exploring the use of stem cells to grow inner ear hair cells. This work may lead to stem cell–based therapies to cure hearing loss.

■ Organs and Organ Systems

Organs are structures made up of two or more kinds of tissues organized into a recognizable structure that performs a more complex function than any tissue alone. Organs group together to form organ systems, which can perform more complex functions than any single organ alone. Organ systems perform specialized functions necessary for the survival of an organism. If a single organ is not functioning, an organism may still survive. However, if an entire organ system shuts down, the life of that organism will be compromised. It is important to remember that organ systems are not independent of one another. In fact, organ systems must work together to ensure continued viability. Eleven organ systems are described in the body: integumentary, skeletal, muscular, nervous, endocrine, circulatory, lymphatic, respiratory, digestive, urinary, and reproductive. The organ components and general function of each of these systems are described in **Table 2.7.** Many organ systems are intimately involved in processes related to speech, language, swallowing, hearing, and balance.

Table 2.7　Organ systems

Organ System	Organ Components	Functions
Integumentary	Hair, nails, glands, skin	Protective barrier for the human body; regulates body temperature
Skeletal	Bones, cartilage, tendons, ligaments	Structural framework providing support, shape, and protection for the body; attachment site for organs
Muscular	Skeletal muscle, smooth muscle, cardiac muscle	Provides movement to the body; maintains posture; produces heat
Nervous	Brain, spinal cord, nerves	Conducts information in the form of electrical impulses throughout the body and regulates and controls physiologic processes of other organ systems
Endocrine	Pituitary gland, pineal gland, hypothalamus, thyroid gland, parathyroid gland, thymus, adrenal glands, pancreas, ovaries, testes	Regulates and controls physiologic processes of the body; accomplishes processes by sending hormones into the blood
Circulatory	Heart, blood vessels, blood	Circulates blood throughout the body and transports gases, nutrients, and wastes to and from tissues
Lymphatic (Immune)	Lymph, lymph nodes, lymph vessels, thymus, spleen, tonsils	Defends body against microorganisms and other foreign bodies; transports fluids from body's tissues to the blood
Respiratory	Nose, pharynx, larynx, trachea, bronchi, lungs	Exchanges gases between the body's tissues and the external environment
Digestive	Mouth, pharynx, esophagus	Digests and absorbs nutrients from the food ingested in the body; transports foods through the gastrointestinal tract
Urinary	Kidney, ureters, urinary bladder, urethra	Removes excess water and nutrients and filters waste from the circulatory system
Reproductive	Female: Ovaries, fallopian tubes, vagina, vulva, mammary glands Male: Testes, vas deferens, urethra, penis, scrotum, prostate	Structural and physiologic network to create new life

Musculoskeletal System

One of the essential systems critical for speech, language, swallowing, hearing, and balance is the musculoskeletal system, which, as the name implies, is a combination of the muscular and skeletal systems. The primary function of the musculoskeletal system is to provide support to the body and give us the ability to move body parts. This organ system uses a variety of organs and tissues, including muscles, bones of the skeleton, cartilage, joints, tendons, ligaments, and other connective tissues. Bones and cartilage are the supportive connective tissues of the skeletal system that provide structural framework as well as protection of the internal organs. Muscles are attached to bones via tendons and, through contraction, produce a diverse range of body movements. A joint is the location at which bones connect, and joints are specially constructed to allow specific ranges of motion. Other connective tissues, like tendons and ligaments, are critical for connections between bone, cartilage, and muscles. For example, ligaments help connect and stabilize bones. Tendons, on the other hand, primarily attach muscle to bone. The makeup

and function of these unique structures are described in the following section.

Supportive Connective Tissues

Bone and cartilage are the two types of supportive connective tissues and are the strongest and most durable tissues in the body. The principal components of connective tissues are cells and ECM. The ECM, in turn, contains protein fibers embedded in a specialized ground substance. Bones and cartilage both contain unique cell types and ECM components that are essential for providing these tissues with their unique supportive function.

Bones, or osseous tissue, is the framework that supports the body and forms the majority of the adult skeleton. The most obvious functions of bone are clear upon observation. First, bones provide protection to the vital organs in the body by surrounding or covering them. For example, your ribs protect your heart and lungs, and the bones of your skull enclose your brain. In addition, by providing an attachment point for skeletal muscles, bones facilitate movement. The other critical functions of bones are less obvious. Bones are reservoirs for minerals, particularly calcium and phosphorus, which are important for essential body functions. Finally, the bone marrow, or substance in the cavities of bones, is important for metabolic processes, including fat storage and production of blood cells. The adult skeleton contains over 200 bones, which are classified into five general categories based upon their shapes and functions. The categories include long, short, flat, irregular, and sesamoid, and are described in **Table 2.8**.

Bone tissue contains relatively few cells, which are widely separated in a hardened ECM. Osteoblasts are one type of bone cell. Osteoblasts are "bone-building" cells that synthesize the matrix of bone tissue. On the other hand, osteoclasts are cells that release enzymes that break down bone tissue. A third cell type, osteocytes, are mature cells of the bone tissue that no longer secrete ECM. However, osteocytes are important for other functions within bone, including nutrient and waste exchange with the blood. The matrix of bones is unlike any other type of connective tissue. The matrix consists of collagen fibers embedded in a ground substance containing mineral salts, mostly calcium phosphate and some calcium carbonate. These salts are crystallized, which confers a unique hardness to bone tissue. Collagen fibers, on the other hand, provide bone with its flexibility.

There are two textures of mature bone tissue: compact and spongy (**Fig. 2.40**). Most bones contain both textures, but the distribution and concentration of compact and spongy bone vary based upon location and function. As the name suggests, **compact bone** is the denser and stronger type of bone and is typically found in the hard outer layer. Structurally, compact bone is arranged in units called osteons, also called haversian systems. Osteons are cylindrical structures that consist of layers of compact matrix that surround a central canal, which contains blood vessels and nerve fibers. **Spongy bone**, or cancellous bone, is the porous and vascular inner portion of bone tissue. Spongy bone does not contain osteons but instead consists of a lattice of thin columns called trabeculae. Bone marrow is found between the trabeculae, and blood vessels are located within the spongy bone, where they deliver important nutrients to osteocytes and remove waste. Two important coverings are also found in bones. The outer surface of bone is covered with a dense connective tissue called the periosteum. The periosteum contains blood vessels and nerves and is the point where tendons and ligaments attach to bone. The endosteum is a thin layer of connective tissue that lines the inside of the marrow cavity of spongy bone and any canals of compact bone and is where bone growth, repair, and remodeling occur.

Cartilage is a strong, flexible, semirigid form of supportive connective tissue that can bend and withstand compression forces. Like bone, cartilage forms a supportive and protective framework for many organs. For example, the cartilage found in the walls of the airway (nose, larynx, trachea, and bronchi) is essential for preventing airway collapse. Cartilage is also found where some bones articulate, or come together. By providing a surface for free movement, cartilage helps to minimize the friction between bones. Finally, cartilage forms the template for the growth and development of long bones and makes up most of the fetal skeleton.

The two types of cartilage cells are chondroblasts and chondrocytes. The ECM of cartilage is secreted by chondroblasts, which are found in the perichondrium, the outer covering layer of the cartilage. As chondroblasts secrete ECM, they become trapped inside and mature to form advanced cartilage cells called chondrocytes. The ground substance and fibers of cartilage form a unique matrix that is very flexible but also resistant to compressive forces. There are three types of

Table 2.8 Bone classification

Bone Classification	Structural Features	Functions	Example Locations
Long	Cylindrical	Levers that move when muscles contract	Arms, fingers, toes
Short	Cubelike	Stability and support; some limited motion	Wrists, ankles
Flat	Thin and curved	Point of attachment for muscles; protect internal organs	Skull, scapulae, sternum, ribs
Irregular	No characteristic shape; irregular	Protect internal organs	Vertebrae, facial bones
Sesamoid	Small and round	Protect tendons from compressive forces	Patellae

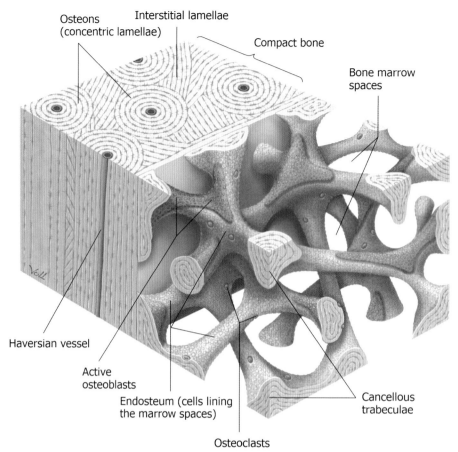

Fig. 2.40 Bone structure. Two textures of mature bone include compact bone and spongy or cancellous bone. Compact bone is the hard outer layer of bones. It is permeated by an elaborate system of interconnecting canals, the haversian systems, which contain the blood supply for bone cells. The bone is arranged in concentric layers around the canals, forming structural units called osteons. Spongy bone is a light, porous bone with a spongelike appearance. It is organized into a three-dimensional latticework of bony processes called trabeculae. These spaces are often filled with bone marrow and blood vessels.

cartilage: hyaline, fibrous, and elastic cartilage, which differ mostly in the type of fibers they contain. The features of each type of cartilage are displayed in **Table 2.9**. The most abundant type of cartilage in the body is hyaline. Fibrous and elastic cartilages are also critical supporting structures found throughout the body. Unlike bone and other connective tissues, cartilage is avascular, meaning that it lacks blood vessels. Consequently, cartilage is nourished with nutrients and oxygen by long-range diffusion into the perichondrium.

Joints

Joints, also referred to as articulations, are the sites where two bones come together, or articulate with one other. Joints are important for providing stability and mobility to the skeletal system. In joints, stability and mobility are closely related. For example, very stable joints allow minimal movements between two bones. On the hand, joints that allow for ample movement between bones are highly unstable. Joints are classified both structurally (**Table**

Table 2.9 Types of cartilage

Type of Cartilage	Structural Features	Functions	Example Locations
Hyaline	Predominantly collagen, glassy appearance, covered by perichondrium	Provides stiff but flexible support, covers bone surfaces at synovial joints	Ribs, nose, larynx, trachea
Fibrous cartilage	Alternating layers of hyaline cartilage and thick collagen fibers, not covered by perichondrium	Resists compression, prevents bone-to-bone contact, limits relative movement	Intervertebral disks, joint capsules, ligaments
Elastic cartilage	Predominantly elastin, covered by perichondrium	Provides strength and elasticity, maintains shape	External ear, epiglottis

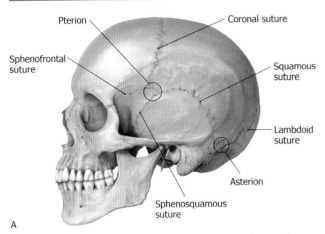

Pterion
Sphenofrontal suture
Coronal suture
Squamous suture
Lambdoid suture
Asterion
Sphenosquamous suture

A

Fig. 2.41 Skull sutures are junctions between adjacent bones of the skull. Sutures are an example of a synarthrosis type of fibrous joint. They help protect the brain by forming a tight union that prevents most movement between the bones.

2.10) and functionally (**Table 2.11**). Structural classifications are based on the kind of materials that are present in the joint. Fibrous joints are composed of dense connective tissue containing high amounts of collagen. Cartilaginous joints are made of a band of cartilage that binds bones together. Finally, at a synovial joint, articulating bones are not directly connected, but instead are separated by a joint capsule filled with lubricating fluid called synovial fluid. These are the most common joints of the body.

Functional joint classifications are determined by the degree of mobility found at each joint. An immobile joint, or synarthrosis, is highly stable and provides strong connections between articulating bones. Depending upon location, fibrous and cartilaginous joints may be classified as synarthroses. For example, a suture of the skull is an example of a fibrous synarthrosis (**Fig. 2.41**). An amphiarthrosis is a joint that permits a slight amount of mobility. Like a synarthrosis, an amphiarthrosis may be both fibrous

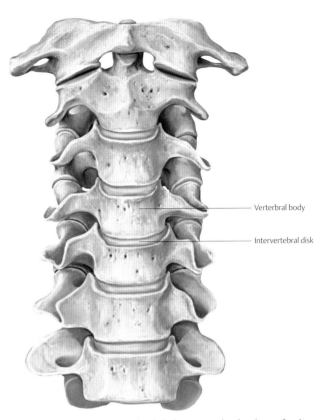

Verterbral body
Intervertebral disk

Fig. 2.42 An intervertebral disk unites the bodies of adjacent vertebrae within the vertebral column. Each disk forms an amphiarthrosis type of cartilaginous joint. This joint permits limited movement between the vertebrae.

and cartilaginous. Intervertebral disks of the spine are an example of cartilaginous amphiarthroses (**Fig. 2.42**). The third functional class of joints is the freely movable diarthrosis. All synovial joints are diarthroses. The structure of a synovial joint is displayed in **Fig. 2.43**. These joints are primarily found in the limbs, permitting a wide range of movement in, for example, the elbow, knee, shoulder, and wrist.

Table 2.10 Structural joint classification

Type of Joint	Description
Fibrous	Bone articular surfaces are held together by fibrous connective tissue
Cartilaginous	Bone articular surfaces are held together by hyaline cartilage of fibrocartilage
Synovial	Bone articular surfaces are not directly connected, surfaces come in contact within a joint cavity that is filled with synovial fluid

Table 2.11 Functional joint classification

Type of Joint	Description	Example Location
Synarthrosis	Immobile joint	Sutures of skull, gomphosis joints that anchor the root of the tooth into its bony socket of the jaw
Amphiarthrosis	Slightly movable joint	Intervertebral disks of the spine, pubic symphysis of the pelvis
Diarthrosis	Freely movable joint	Knee, elbows, shoulders

Tendons, Ligaments, and Fascia

The term *musculoskeletal system* clearly suggests that muscles and bones are the key components. However, without supporting structures, such as tendons, ligaments, and fascia, the critical functions of the musculoskeletal system could not be accomplished. Tendons, ligaments, and fascia are all types of dense, regular connective tissue characterized by an abundance of closely packed fibers and a predominance of collagen content. Their composition makes these tissues ideal for support and resistance to the excessive traction forces that occur during movement.

Tendons are fibrous tissues that attach muscle to other body parts, usually bone. A common example is the Achilles tendon, which attaches the calf muscle to the heel bone (**Fig. 2.44**). However, tendons may also attach muscle to cartilage, and in some instances to other muscles, such as in the omohyoid muscle of the neck (**Fig. 2.45**). Tendons are composed of parallel arrangements of collagen, with few elastin fibers, and their shape and size vary widely depending upon location. Tendons are

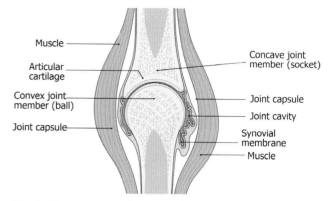

Fig. 2.43 Structure of a synovial joint. Synovial joints allow for smooth movements between adjacent bones. The joint is surrounded by a tough capsule lined with synovial membrane. This forms a joint cavity filled with synovial fluid, which lubricates the joint and reduces friction and wear. A thin layer of articular cartilage covers articulating surfaces of the bone.

remarkably strong, which is necessary for them to withstand the stress of muscle contraction and to transmit mechanical forces to bone.

Ligaments connect bone to bone, but may also join bone to cartilage or attach cartilage to carti-

Box 2.9   Traumatic Brain Injury and Sutures

Traumatic brain injury (TBI) is caused by external forces resulting in sudden damage to the brain. Depending on the source of the force, TBIs can be due to open or closed head injuries. Consequences of TBI are widespread and include physical, sensory, cognitive, communication, swallowing, and behavioral symptoms. Speech-language pathologists play an important role as members of the rehabilitation team for patients with TBI.

TBI is prevalent across the life span. It is the leading cause of disability and death in children and adolescents in the United States. A group at greatest risk for TBI is young children, from birth to age 4. Specifically, children in this age group are particularly susceptible to skull fractures. Skull fractures, or a break in the skull bone, are a type of open head injury. A specific type of open head injury that commonly occurs in children is called a diastic skull fracture. Diastic skull fractures occur along the suture joints in the skull. The sutures are the areas between the bones in the head that fuse as the child grows (**Box Fig. 2.6**). In this type of fracture, the normal suture lines are widened. These fractures are more often seen in newborns and older infants.

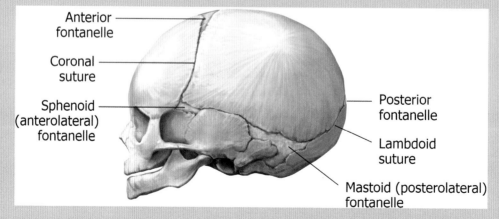

Box Fig. 2.6 Cranial sutures of the neonatal skull. The flat cranial bones grow as the brain expands; thus, the sutures between them remain open after birth. In the neonate, there are areas (fontanelles) between the still-growing cranial bones that are occupied by unossified fibrous membrane.

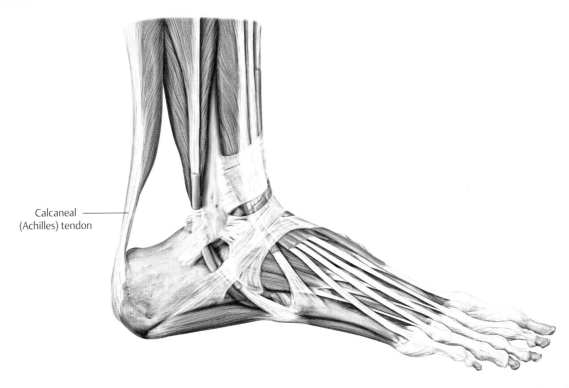

Calcaneal (Achilles) tendon

Fig. 2.44 Achilles tendon. The Achilles tendon attaches the calf muscle to the heel bone, or calcaneus. It is also referred to as the calcaneal tendon.

lage. In general, ligaments are less organized than tendons and contain more elastin fibers and slightly fewer collagen fibers. Ligaments are found in every joint in the body, and the many ligaments of the hand are displayed in **Fig. 2.46**. Ligaments primarily function to stabilize joints, but they also define

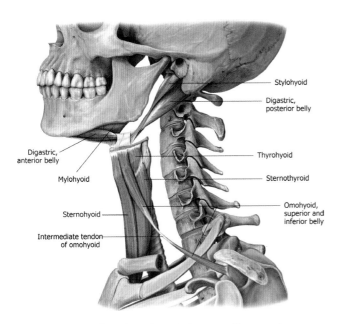

Stylohyoid

Digastric, posterior belly

Digastric, anterior belly

Thyrohyoid

Mylohyoid

Sternothyroid

Sternohyoid

Omohyoid, superior and inferior belly

Intermediate tendon of omohyoid

Fig. 2.45 Omohyoid tendon. An intermediate tendon separates the two bellies of the omohyoid muscle.

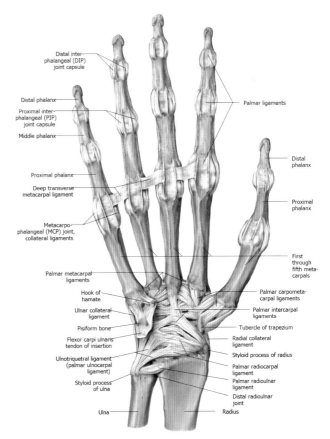

Distal interphalangeal (DIP) joint capsule

Distal phalanx

Proximal interphalangeal (PIP) joint capsule

Middle phalanx

Proximal phalanx

Deep transverse metacarpal ligament

Metacarpophalangeal (MCP) joint, collateral ligaments

Palmar metacarpal ligaments

Hook of hamate

Ulnar collateral ligament

Pisiform bone

Flexor carpi ulnaris tendon of insertion

Ulnotriquetral ligament (palmar ulnocarpal ligament)

Styloid process of ulna

Ulna

Palmar ligaments

Distal phalanx

Proximal phalanx

First through fifth metacarpals

Palmar carpometacarpal ligaments

Palmar intercarpal ligaments

Tubercle of trapezium

Radial collateral ligament

Styloid process of radius

Palmar radiocarpal ligament

Palmar radioulnar ligament

Distal radioulnar joint

Radius

Fig. 2.46 Ligaments. The ligaments of the hand. Ligaments typically connect bone to bone.

their range of motion and serve to protect bones and joints. Due to their composition, ligaments can stretch and contract when necessary, which allows them to act as shock absorbers.

Fascia is a fibrous tissue that holds the body together by surrounding muscle and other organs to keep them in place. The fascia is arranged into sheets of collagen interspersed with elastin fibers and fibroblasts, which allow it to be both supportive and flexible. In addition to its connective function, the fascia separates muscles, allowing them to contract independently. There are three main types of fascia: superficial, visceral, and deep fascia. Superficial fascia is primarily found under the skin in all areas of the body but can also surround glands, where it supports the tissues and allows for the storage of water and fat. Visceral fascia surrounds internal organs and is critical to supporting the organs and holding them in place. Finally, deep fascia is a dense tissue that surrounds major muscle groups and contains a higher presence of elastin fibers. The three types of fascia are critical for supporting the major organs and tissues of the body and maintaining their functional capacity.

In summary, the musculoskeletal system allows for the movement of body parts in a coordinated fashion. To accomplish this very difficult task, a variety of tissues and organs must work together. Muscle groups are the energy source of the system and, through their contractions, drive the movement of bones, the major structural components of the body. In support of this system, the tendons and ligaments bind bones and muscles, allowing them to function as a single unit. Various types of joints permit more advanced body movements by allowing two bones to come together and to move without causing damage. Finally, cartilage and fascia support the organs and tissues by providing structural and shock-absorbing functions.

■ Suggested Readings

Allen T, Cowling G. The Cell: A Very Short Introduction. New York, NY: Oxford University Press; 2011

Betts JG, Desaix P, Johnson E, et al. Anatomy & Physiology. Houston, TX: Rice University; 2017. https://openstax.org/details/books/anatomy-and-physiology

Bray D. Cell macromolecules. http://www.els.net/WileyCDA/ElsArticle/refId-a0001269.html

Cooper GM. The Cell: A Molecular Approach. Sunderland, MA: Singulair Associates; 2000

Frantz C, Stewart KM, Weaver VM. The extracellular matrix at a glance. *The Journal of Cell Science, 123,* 4195–4200; 2010

Lodish H, Berk A, Zipursky SL, Matsudaira P, Baltimore D, Darnel J. Molecular Cell Biology. 4th ed. New York: W. H. Freeman; 2000

O'Connor CM, Adams JU. Essentials of Cell Biology. www.nature.com/scitable/ebooks/essentials-of-cell-biology-14749010

■ Reference

Podlesniy P, Figueiro-Silva J, Llado A, et al. Low cerebrospinal fluid concentration of mitochondrial DNA in preclinical Alzheimer disease. *Annals of Neurology, 74*(5), 655–668; 2013. doi:10.1002/ana.23955

■ Study Questions

1. Which of the following is a characteristic of prokaryotes?

A. Nucleus
B. Membrane-bound organelles
C. Nucleoid
D. Typically multicellular
E. Large cell size

2. Which of the following techniques uses electrons to produce a three-dimensional image of the sample of interest?

A. Scanning electron microscopy
B. Cell culture
C. Light microscopy
D. Phase-contrast microscopy
E. Transmission electron microscopy

3. Which of the following describes the plasma membrane?

A. Control center of the cell
B. Phospholipid bilayer
C. Site of protein synthesis
D. Occupies most of the cellular volume
E. Power plant of the cell

4. Which of the following is the largest cellular organelle?

A. Mitochondria
B. Endoplasmic reticulum
C. Nucleus
D. Plasma membrane
E. Golgi apparatus

5. Which of the following organelles is *not* part of the endomembrane system?

A. Golgi apparatus
B. Rough endoplasmic reticulum
C. Lysosomes
D. Nucleus
E. Smooth endoplasmic reticulum

6. Where is energy packaged into usable units for the rest of the cell?

A. Mitochondria
B. Nucleus
C. Plasma membrane
D. Endoplasmic reticulum
E. Lysosomes

7. Which of the following statements is true of the extracellular matrix?

A. The primary cell type is the fibroblast.
B. It is primarily responsible for movement of the skeleton.
C. It contains neurons and glial cells.
D. It forms a protective barrier.
E. Its three major structural elements are microtubules, microfilaments, and intermediate filaments.

8. The four stages of aerobic respiration occur in which order?

A. Glycolysis, citric acid cycle, pyruvate oxidation, electron transport chain
B. Glycolysis, pyruvate oxidation, citric acid cycle, electron transport chain
C. Electron transport chain, pyruvate oxidation, citric acid cycle, glycolysis
D. Pyruvate oxidation, citric acid cycle, glycolysis, electron transport chain
E. Citric acid cycle, glycolysis, pyruvate oxidation, electron transport chain

9. Which of the following is true for anaerobic cellular respiration?

A. Occurs during strenuous exercise
B. Produces minimal ATP
C. Does not require oxygen
D. Occurs at faster rate than aerobic cellular respiration
E. All of the above

10. Which of the following statements below is *not* true of cellular transport?

A. Small, nonpolar molecules move easily into and out of the cell.
B. Movement of material depends on size and polarity of the molecule.
C. Cell transport allows all substances to pass in and out of the cell.
D. Cell transport involves moving materials in and out of the cell.
E. Cells need to transport to maintain the stability of the cell.

11. Which of the following statements best describes facilitated diffusion?

A. Movement of particles from an area of high concentration to an area of low concentration
B. Movement of water across a semipermeable membrane from a region of high concentration to lower concentration
C. The process of capturing substances from the outside of the cell and bringing them into the cell's interior
D. Movement of particles against a concentration gradient
E. Movement of specific molecules down a concentration gradient while passing through the plasma membrane using membrane proteins

12. Which type of cell signaling requires direct contact between communicating cells?

A. Paracrine
B. Juxtacrine
C. Autocrine
D. Endocrine
E. Synaptic

13. The presence of a basement membrane is most characteristic of what type of tissue?

A. Epithelial tissues
B. Connective tissues
C. Nervous tissues
D. Muscle tissues
E. Cartilage

14. Which type of cell junction joins the actin filaments of neighboring epithelial cells?

A. Hemidesmosome
B. Tight junction
C. Gap junction
D. Adherens junction
E. Desmosome

15. Connective tissue is primarily made up of what three components?

A. Cell junctions, protein fibers, ground substance
B. Cells, protein fibers, ground substance
C. Cells, carbohydrate fibers, ground substance
D. Cilia, protein fibers, cell junctions
E. Cells, basement membrane, protein fibers

16. Striations, cylindrical cells, and multiple nuclei are observed in what type of tissue?

A. Nervous tissue
B. Smooth muscle
C. Cardiac muscle
D. Connective tissue
E. Skeletal muscle

17. Which of the following best describes adult stem cells?

A. Pluripotent
B. Genetically reprogrammed to an embryonic stem cell–like fate
C. Reside in a "stem cell niche"
D. Derived from early-stage embryos
E. Found in adult tissue in large numbers

18. Which of the following choices denotes the correct order of the structural organization of the body (from smallest to largest)?

A. Cells, organs, tissues, organ systems
B. Cells, tissues, organs, organ systems
C. Tissues, organ systems, cells, organs
D. Organ systems, organs, tissues, cells
E. Organs, tissues, organ systems, cells

19. Which of the following structures are components of the musculoskeletal system?

A. Bones
B. Ligaments
C. Joints
D. Cartilage
E. All of the above

20. Which of the following is a functional class of joints?

A. Fibrous joint
B. Synovial joint
C. Amphiarthrosis
D. Cartilaginous joint
E. None of the above

■ Answers to Study Questions

1. The answer is (C) because the DNA of prokaryotes consists of a single chromosomal loop found in an area called the nucleoid. The answer is not (A), (B), (D), or (E) because these are all characteristics of eukaryotes, not prokaryotes.

2. The answer is (A) because scanning electron microscopy uses electron beams to scan the surface of a sample in order to form an image depicting the three-dimensional, external shape of a sample. The answer is not (C), (D), or (E) because these types of microscopy produce two-dimensional images. The answer is not (B) because cell culture involves growth of cells in an artificial environment, not cellular and tissue imaging.

3. The answer is (B) because a phospholipid bilayer forms 20% to 79% of the plasma membrane of the cell. The answer is not (A) because the nucleus is the control center of the cell. The answer is not (C) because the primary site for protein synthesis is the rough ER. The answer is not (D) because the cytoplasm occupies most of the cellular volume. The answer is not (E) because mitochondria are the power plants of the cell.

4. The answer is (C) because the nucleus, or the control center of the cell, is the largest cellular organelle. The answer is not (A), (B), (D), or (E) because, while they are all cellular organelles, each of them is smaller than the nucleus.

5. The answer is (D) because the nucleus is not part of the endomembrane system and its primary function is to coordinate cell activities, including growth, protein production, and replication. The answer is not (A), (B), (C), or (E) because these organelles are all part of the endomembrane system, where the primary goals include production, modification, and transport of proteins.

6. The answer is (A) because mitochondria extract energy from sugar, fat, and other cellular fuel molecules to produce ATP. The answer is not (B) because the nucleus is the control center of the cell. The answer is not (C) because the plasma membrane is the organelle that surrounds the cell and acts as a barrier and gatekeeper. The answer is not (D) or (E) because these organelles are part of the endomembrane system and are involved in protein synthesis and degradation.

7. The answer is (A) because fibroblasts are the primary cell type that produces the macromolecules that make up the extracellular matrix. The answer is not (B) because muscle tissue is primarily responsible for movement of the skeleton. The answer is not (C) because nervous tissue contains neurons and glial cells. The answer is not (D) because epithelial tissue forms a protective barrier. The answer is not (E) because microtubules, microfilaments, and intermediate filaments are the major structural elements of the cytoskeleton.

8. The answer is (B) because aerobic respiration, or the process by which cells convert cellular food into ATP, is broken into four stages that occur in the following order: glycolysis, pyruvate oxidation, citric acid cycle, and electron transport chain. The answer is not (A), (C), (D), or (E) because, while the listed stages are part of aerobic respiration, they are not in the correct order.

9. The answer is (E) because all of the statements describe anaerobic cellular respiration.

10. The answer is (C) because cellular transport is a selective process and does not allow all substances to pass freely in and out of the cell. Specifically, cellular transport is the selective movement of materials across the plasma membrane into or out of the cell. The plasma membrane is semipermeable, meaning only certain materials can pass through the barrier. The answer is not (A), (B), (D), or (E) because these statements are all true of cellular transport.

11. The answer is (E) because facilitated diffusion is a type of diffusion that involves the movement of specific molecules down a concentration gradient while passing through the plasma membrane via the use of specialized membrane proteins. The answer is not (A) because it describes (nonfacilitated) diffusion. The answer is not (B) because it describes osmosis. The answer is not (C) because it describes endocytosis. The answer is not (D) because it describes active transport.

12. The answer is (B) because juxtacrine signaling requires direct contact between communicating cells. A type of juxtacrine signaling involves the use of gap junctions. The answer is not (A) because paracrine signaling allows for cell communication when the cells are not in contact and involves the secretion of molecules into the extracellular space, where they then diffuse to target cells in close proximity. The answer is not (C) because autocrine signaling involves signaling molecules binding to the receptors on the cell from which they were secreted or another cell of the sample type. The answer is not (D) because endocrine signaling involves the transmission of hormones through the bloodstream to other areas of the body. The answer is not (E) because synaptic signaling involves the communication between a neuron and another cell bring their plasma membranes in close proximity to form a unique structure called a synapse.

13. The answer is (A) because the basal surface of epithelial tissue is attached to a type of ECM called the basement membrane. The answer is not (B), (C), (D), or (E) because these tissues are not typically directly associated with a basement membrane.

14. The answer is (D) because adherens junctions are a type of cell junction that provides strong adhesive bonds between the actin filaments of adjacent epithelial cells. The answer is not (A) or (E) because hemidesmosomes and desmosomes connect intermediate filaments of adjacent cells. The answer is not (B) because tight junctions are the most apically located cell junctions, where plasma membranes of adjacent epithelial cells come together to form a tight, waterproof seal. The answer is not (C) because gap junctions are communication channels between neighboring cells.

15. The answer is (B) because, while connective tissue is incredibly diverse in terms of composition, its three primary components are cells, protein fibers, and ground substance. The answer is not (A) because cell junctions are a component of epithelial tissue. The answer is not (C) because protein, not carbohydrate fibers, is a component of connective tissue. The answer is not (D) because cilia are a feature of epithelial tissue. The answer is not (E) because the basement membrane is a type of extracellular matrix closely associated with epithelial tissue.

16. The answer is (E) because skeletal muscle is a type of tissue under voluntary control that is organized into basic units called muscle fibers, which are thick, cylindrical cell bundles with multiple nuclei. Because of the arrangement of actin and myosin, skeletal muscle also has a striated appearance. The answer is not (A) or (D) because these are not types of muscle tissue. The answer is not (B) because smooth muscle cells have a single nucleus and no visible striations. The answer is not (C) because cardiac muscle cells have a branched appearance and a single, central nucleus.

17. The answer is (C) because the area of tissue where adult stem cells reside is called the stem cell niche. The answer is not (A) because embryonic, not adult, stem cells are pluripotent. The answer is not (B) because induced pluripotent stem cells are genetically reprogrammed to an embryonic stem cell–like fate. The answer is not (D) because embryonic stem cells are derived from early-state embryos. The answer is not (E) because adult stem cells are found in tissues in only small, not large, numbers.

18. The answer is (B) because cells are the smallest living unit of an organism. Cells are organized into tissues. An organ is an anatomically distinct structure of the body composed of two or more types of tissue. Finally, organs are organized into organ systems, which work together to perform a major function. The answer is not (A), (C), (D), or (E) because the structural units of the body are not in the correct order of smallest to largest.

19. The correct answer is (E) because all of the listed structures are part of the musculoskeletal system. These structures all assist in providing form, support, stability, and movement to the body.

20. The answer is (C) because amphiarthrosis joints are classified based upon their specific function of permitting a slight amount of mobility. The answer is not (A), (B), or (D) because these are structural classes of joints, which are classified based upon what kind of material is present in the joint, not function.

3

Genetics

Barbara A. Lewis, Sudha K. Iyengar, and Catherine M. Stein

■ Chapter Summary

Genes, in combination with the environment, may contribute to the development of speech, language, swallowing, hearing, and balance disorders. Some disorders may result from a single chromosomal abnormality, some from a single gene variant, and others from a combination of many different genes. For some disorders, the genetic basis may be unknown, or the disorder may be predominantly environmental. In the last decade, technological advances enabled for sequencing of an individual's genome relatively inexpensively, making personalized medicine a reality. Targeted treatments based on an individual's genome may soon be feasible. The study of genetics will aid the speech-language pathologist and audiologist in clinical decision making, facilitate the selection of intervention strategies and educational placements, and assist with making appropriate referrals to geneticists and genetic counselors to help guide families to achieve optimal outcomes for their children. The purpose of this chapter is to examine the structural and functional coding of genes and their potential impact on speech, language, swallowing, hearing, and balance disorders. Specifically, the chapter covers (1) what genes are made of and how they code for proteins, (2) syndromes that illustrate different means of genetic transmission of disorders, and (3) recent discoveries in **epigenetics** (heritable changes in gene activity that do not involve mutation of genes) and the potential ties to clinical practice.

■ Learning Objectives

- Describe the human genome and its implications for speech, language, swallowing, hearing, and balance disorders
- Understand the differences between genotype and phenotype
- Describe the features of inheritance, such as imprinting, copy number variants, and epigenetics
- Understand the relationship between the environment and genetics

■ Putting It Into Practice

- Speech-language pathologists and audiologists are an important resource for families and individuals with speech, language, swallowing, hearing, and balance disorders.
- Knowledge of how genetic information is transcribed and translated is important in the understanding of how genes and environmental influences contribute to speech, language, swallowing, hearing, and balance disorders.
- Speech-language pathologists and audiologists should be familiar with the impact of genetic syndromes on typical human development in order to make referrals, when appropriate, to professionals for genetic testing and counseling.

■ Introduction

Genetics is the study of how common **traits** are passed along from previous generations. A trait is a distinguishing quality or characteristic of a specific part of a person. Traits can be physical, such as height, eye color, and hair color. Traits may also be behavioral. For example, a golden retriever's instinct to fetch is a behavioral trait. Traits can also predispose us to medical conditions, such as cystic fibrosis and heart disease. These traits are usually described by the genetic information carried by **deoxyribonucleic acid (DNA)**. All of the instructions for constructing and operating an organism are contained in DNA. Genetics may inform clinical practice by improving early identification and treatment of children at risk for speech, language, swallowing, hearing, and balance disorders. In addition, the discovery of key genetic pathways may improve our understanding of the neurobiological basis of these disorders. Discoveries in genetics may result in new diagnostic categories based on shared underlying deficits and the validation of current diagnostic categories based on behavioral observations. From an evolutionary perspective, the study of genetics may provide insight into the origins of speech and language. The emergence of speech and language is one of the most important developments in the evolution of man.

Genetics is essential to the clinical practice of speech-language pathology and audiology. Genetic testing is frequently performed on children with developmental delays, including speech and language disorders or hearing impairment. Clinicians require a working knowledge of genetics to understand and interpret the results of such testing. In fact, speech-language pathologists and audiologists are often the first professionals to treat a child with developmental delay and serve as an important resource for families during referral for genetic testing and counseling (**Box 3.1**). Familiarity with the features of genetic conditions enables targeted interventions, informed prognoses, and appropriate educational plans. Technologies for testing specific genetic variants are described in **Box 3.4**.

Genetic studies of speech, language, swallowing, hearing, and balance disorders have uncovered candidate genes for these disorders (**Box 3.2**).

Box 3.1   Should I Refer This Patient for Genetic Counseling?

Genetic counselors are professionals trained to help individuals or families understand a genetic condition, interpret genetic tests and findings, make decisions about treatments, and understand the risk of having a child with a genetic condition. In essence, genetic counselors provide support to parents and families. Genetic counselors hold a master's degree and are board certified by the National Society of Genetic Counselors. Genetic counselors often work with a clinical geneticist, who is a medical doctor trained in genetics. Genetic counseling may be performed both before and after genetic testing to ensure that patients understand the test and its implications for healthcare. Often genetic counseling is performed during prenatal counseling.

Who should be referred for genetic counseling?
Often, speech-language pathologists and audiologists are the first professionals to assess a child with speech, language, swallowing, hearing, and balance deficits. If the child presents with other developmental delays (e.g. motor, cognitive, or social) or health problems, a referral for genetic testing may be warranted to determine whether there is a genetic basis for the disorder. Children may also be referred for genetic testing if there is a family history for a genetic condition. Parents may also seek genetic testing to learn the recurrence risk before attempting future pregnancies. If a genetic condition is apparent at birth, such as Down's syndrome, or detected through newborn screenings, the parents may seek genetic counseling to learn more about their child's condition so that they may plan for the child's future.

What happens during genetic counseling?
The genetic counselor will compile a detailed family history for speech, language, swallowing, hearing, and balance disorders and other medical conditions and construct a pedigree. The genetic counselor will provide information on the child's genetic condition, explain how the condition may be transmitted within the family, and offer emotional support to family members. The genetic counselor may recommend additional tests that may aid in diagnosing the condition and will explain the test results. Recurrence risk of the disorder in future pregnancies may also be discussed. The genetic counselor, along with other team members, will assist the family in choosing treatment options, in managing their child's care, and in long-term planning.

(See also National Society for Genetic Counselors, http://www.nsgc.org.)

> **Box 3.2 A Gene for Speech and Language: The Story of the KE Family**
>
> Over a decade ago, a gene for speech sound disorder, the *FOXP2* gene located on chromosome 7q31, was discovered in a large British family referred to as the "KE family." Affected family members, spanning three generations, presented with orofacial apraxia. The causative gene was identified as a brain-expressed transcription factor called FOXP2. The mode of transmission of the *FOXP2* gene in the KE family was autosomal dominance. Individuals who carried the mutant *FOXP2* allele had persistent speech sound disorders, as well as impairments in IQ, language, and reading. Findings from neuroimaging studies of the KE family suggested that the *FOXP2* gene had pleiotropic effects on multiple aspects of brain development related to speech and language. Since the original report, other mutations in *FOXP2*, encompassing a spectrum from rare point mutations to translocations and several deletions of varying length, have been identified in patients with verbal dyspraxia of speech. *FOXP2* has also been implicated in sex differences in vocal communication in mammals. See also Morgan et al (2017).

Although many genes are associated with hearing loss (**Box 3.3**), only a few have been identified for speech and language impairments. To date, no gene responsible for the majority of disorders has been identified. It is likely that, in a few cases, a single gene variant may be responsible for a disorder. However, in most cases, many genes and environmental influences likely contribute to a disorder. This chapter reviews basic genetic principles and how they relate to speech, language, swallowing, hearing, and balance disorders.

■ Ethical, Legal, and Social Issues

Before proceeding with the discussion of genetics, it is important to note the ethical, legal, and social issues surrounding genetic testing. As our knowledge of the genetics underlying speech, language, swallowing, hearing, and balance disorders increases, genetic testing has become more routine in clinical practice for screening, diagnosis, and treatment. This results in ethical, legal, and social challenges.

A major concern involves the protection of an individual's genetic information. Insurance companies and employers could potentially use personal genetic data to deny insurance coverage or employment to individuals with known genetic conditions or genetic risk factors. The Genetic Information Nondiscrimination Act of 2008 (GINA) was passed to prohibit health insurers or employers from using genetic information to determine coverage, rates, hiring, firing, or promotion decisions. Although GINA was a first step to protect genetic information, there are some exceptions to the law. Employers with fewer than 15 employees are exempt. GINA does not extend to life insurance, disability insurance, or long-term-care insurance. Related to this issue is identification of nonparentage. If family members all conduct genetic testing, and if the results are not consistent with familial inheritance, the test may reveal nonpaternity, for example. Such situations must be handled delicately, and confidentiality must be maintained.

Another issue is whether or not family members of an individual with a genetic condition or predisposition should be informed of their risk for the disease. Do individuals have the right to know their genetic information? What responsibility does an individual have to inform family members? These decisions should be discussed with a genetic counselor both before and after genetic testing.

Advancing technologies in the field of genetics enable the detection of hundreds or even thousands of genetic variants, but the medical implications of many of these variants are not yet known. Furthermore, questions arise about whether the result is clinically actionable and whether it has implications for family planning. Knowledge of a genetic condition or predisposition to a condition may cause psychological distress. Informed consent is essential prior to genetic testing. Patients should be informed of the risk that they may have a condition, how predictive or definitive the genetic test may be, whether or not the condition is treatable, and the likelihood that, given a genetic predisposition, a disorder will evolve. These issues are particularly important in prenatal testing, because genetic conditions often have variable expression and the severity of the disorder may be modified by the environment as well as other protective factors.

Finally, the individual's cultural background and religious and moral beliefs must be respected. Ultimately, the individual has the right to choose whether or not to know his/her personal and genetic information and how to use that information should he/she acquire it.

Box 3.3 Genetics of Deafness

Recently, the genetics underlying hearing loss and deafness have been described. The following are highlights of relevant research.

- *Fifty to sixty percent of congenital moderate to profound hearing loss has a genetic etiology.* Other causes of congenital deafness may be environmental; for example, cytomegalovirus infections. One in every 1,000 children has some form of hearing impairment, and one in 2,000 is genetic in origin. The human genome houses about 20,000 to 30,000 genes, and about 10% of them are related to hearing loss. Genetic deafness is heterogeneous, with many genes across the genome involved. Many different genes may give rise to similar phenotypes, and, conversely, a single gene variant may result in multiple phenotypes.

- *Genetic bases for hearing loss may be syndromic or nonsyndromic.* Sixty to seventy percent of hearing loss is nonsyndromic, meaning that other medical or physical conditions are not present, while 30% to 40% of hearing loss is syndromic, meaning that the genetic mutation affected multiple body systems and organs. About 60% to 75% of the mutated genes are autosomal recessive, 20% to 30% are autosomal dominant, and about 2% are X-linked or mitochondrial. Deafness that is due to an autosomal recessive gene tends to be more severe and across more frequencies than deafness due to an autosomal dominant gene.

  Nonsyndromic Hearing Loss
  Most genes for hearing loss have a role in cochlear structures and function. Three autosomal recessive genes (*GJB2*, *GJB6*, and *SLC26A4*) account for more than one-third of nonsyndromic hearing loss. Connexin 26/connexin 30 mutations (*GJB2/GJB6* genes) are the most common cause of congenital sensorineural hearing loss. A mutation in the *GJB2* gene results in a disruption in the coding of the protein connexin, which regulates potassium flow in the inner ear. The *GJB6* gene codes for connexin 30, which interacts with connexin 26 mutation to cause deafness. Individuals with connexin 26 mutations do well with cochlear implants. These patients are cognitively normal

and have normal inner ear gross anatomy. Some patients may present with both hearing and vestibular dysfunction. Only a small percentage of hearing loss can be attributed to mitochondrial genes. An example is a mutation in the mitochondrial gene *MT-RNR1* that increases aminoglycoside-induced ototoxicity. Profound hearing loss may result from taking an aminoglycoside antibiotic.

Syndromic Hearing Loss
  - Waardenburg's syndrome, a pigmentary syndrome, is the most common autosomal dominant syndrome associated with sensorineural hearing loss and accounts for 2% of congenital deafness. It has been mapped to *PAX3* on chromosome 2q37. The prevalence of Waardenburg's syndrome is 1 in 42,000 births. Clinical features of Waardenburg's syndrome include a white forelock, pale blue or different-colored eyes, widely spaced eyes, and, in some cases, a cleft lip and/or palate.

  - Usher's syndrome is a common autosomal recessive syndrome associated with deafness and accounts for half of individuals who are deaf and blind. Usher's syndrome has several subtypes located in different chromosome regions. Its prevalence is 3 or 4 in 100,000 births, with a higher prevalence in the Louisiana Acadian population and the Ashkenazi Jewish population.

  - Alport's syndrome is an example of an X-linked syndrome in which approximately 80% of patients have sensorineural hearing loss. Other features include kidney disease and eye abnormalities.

- *Clinical relevance of genetic testing for hearing loss*

  Knowledge of the underlying cause for the hearing loss can help predict whether the loss will remain the same or change. By understanding how the gene has impacted the auditory system, decisions about treatment can be made; for example, to determine whether a cochlear implant is appropriate. Identification of the genetic basis for the hearing loss may indicate other potential medical issues, as in the case of syndromes. Genetic information may also be useful in family planning.

■ Genes

There are ~ 20,000 genes in the human genome, many of which are actively transcribed into **ribo-nucleic acid (RNA)** (transcription and translation are discussed below). The process whereby DNA is read and leads to the creation of a product is called gene expression. Gene expression is used to make proteins, such as hormones and receptors, that perform essential functions in the body, but not all genes code for proteins. Sometimes, RNA itself is the final product. The latter molecules also have very important functions in the cellular machinery. Furthermore, genes do not express the same amount of product in all cells (e.g., a liver cell expresses different genes than a heart cell does), although the expression of genes may be shared. These differences lead to natural alterations in protein synthesis, giving tissues and organs their own identity. Molecular technologies are available

Box 3.4   Molecular Technologies and Diagnostic Testing Used in Speech, Language, Swallowing, Hearing, and Balance Disorders

A variety of molecular tests are used for diagnosis, prevention, or treatment of disease. Also known as molecular diagnostics, this area of personalized medicine employs a range of molecular biological techniques to analyze an individual's genetic code. Technologies can examine a single variant (e.g., SNP or mutation) or perform high-dimensional whole-genome or whole-proteome analyses. Samples for testing are typically obtained from cells in blood or saliva, as a surrogate for the tissue or cell type predominantly involved in the disease or condition. Because of technological advancements, many assays can also be performed prenatally with samples obtained from maternal blood (which has fetal DNA or proteins circulating in it) or from chorionic villus sampling of the placenta.

The technologies vary in their degrees of reliability and range of detection (i.e., sensitivity and specificity), and the results can be interpreted using simple processes or fairly complex algorithms. Prior to releasing results to the patient, consultation with a licensed medical expert, such as a board-certified molecular pathologist, medical geneticist, or genetic counselor, is recommended because of the complexity of the testing paradigms. In the United States, release of molecular or genetic testing results to patients is federally regulated through the Clinical Laboratory Improvement Act (CLIA'88), which requires laboratories to adhere to specific quality control standards (42 CFR 493); other countries generally have similar regulations in place.

Knowledge of genetic or molecular testing results provides insight into the clinical phenotype expressed by an individual. Identification of the precise genetic cause of a disease, syndrome, or condition also enable medical teams to understand the natural disease course, based on similar profiles in other individuals, and to prescribe an appropriate program of additional clinical testing, along with therapy or medication. This is known as personalized medicine or precision medicine. For example, a recent review of the literature on genetic testing for speech and language conditions (Barnett and Van Bon 2015) noted that optimal management of patients with 22q11.2 deletions should include audiometric evaluations for hearing loss, whereas lifelong evaluation of cardiovascular function should be performed in patients with duplications of 7q11.23.

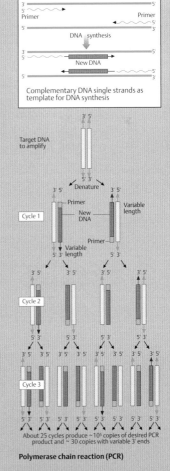

Box Fig. 3.1   A polymerase chain reaction (PCR), one of the molecular biological techniques used to analyze an individual's genetic code.

to study gene expression one gene at a time, or to examine all genes in a cell; the latter is called the transcriptome. Gene expression varies with developmental stage (e.g., birth, puberty, and aging), time, tissue, and even cell type. Many genes show noncharacteristic expression patterns with disease. The field of transcriptomics is attempting to determine whether such differences can be used as biomarkers for disease.

Human beings are highly complex, with over 200 cell types in the body, yet each cell has the same DNA. Specifically, the nucleus of each cell contains 22 pairs of autosomal **chromosomes** and one pair of sex chromosomes, all of which contain the genetic code in DNA (**Fig. 3.1**). Chromosomes

are inherited from parents, normally one set from the mother and the other from the father. The chromosomes contain ~ 20,000 genes. Each gene has a defined location on a chromosome, referred to as a gene locus, and the sequence of **nucleic acids** is structured into coding regions (**exons**) and noncoding regions (**introns**). Only the exons are spliced together to code for a protein after **transcription** (**Fig. 3.2**). In genetic nomenclature, human genes are referred to in all capital letters, usually italicized. Gene names are usually related to their cellular function, although some have been named by the scientist who discovered them.

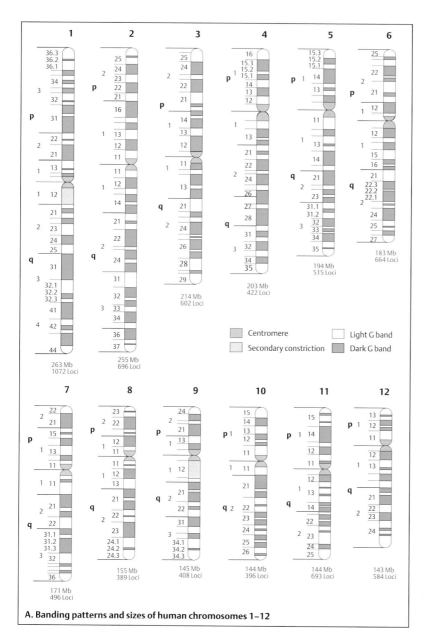

Fig. 3.1 Banding patterns, and sizes, of chromosomes 1 through 12. Each chromosome is made up of a short arm (p arm) and a long arm (q arm) joined by the centromere. The banding patterns are created by the different staining of regions on the chromosome. Regions on each arm of the chromosome are numbered starting at the centromere.

A. Banding patterns and sizes of human chromosomes 1–12

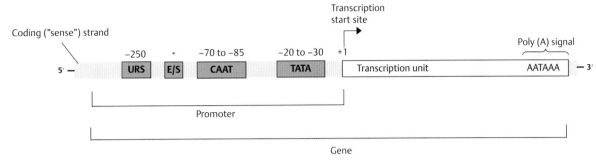

Fig. 3.2 Coding regions, or exons, and noncoding regions, or introns, occur along a gene. Exons are transcribed and joined together to form the code for a protein

It is important to note that not all of the 3 billion base pairs in the human **genome** code for genes. As molecular geneticists further characterize DNA variation and function, it is clear that regions of the genome that were previously considered "junk" may actually have critical functions for gene expression and cellular function.

Nucleic Acids

Genetic information is stored in a chain of **nucleotides**, which in sequence determine the function of the gene. Chemically, each nucleotide is composed of three parts: a five-sided sugar molecule called deoxyribose, a phosphate group, and a nitrogenous base. In human DNA, there are four nitrogenous bases: adenine (A), guanine (G), thymine (T), and cytosine (C), as shown in **Fig. 3.3**. Adenine and guanine are purine bases, and cytosine and thymine are pyrimidine bases. The phosphate of one nucleotide bonds to the sugar of the next in an offset manner, so DNA forms a helix, and is double-stranded, with the sides of the helix parallel, and the strands linked by hydrogen bonds between the bases. The biochemical structure of the nucleotide bases determines that a purine always pairs with a pyrimidine; adenine always pairs with thymine, and cytosine always pairs with guanine, thus forming complementary pairs A-T and G-C. Other pairings are not possible in humans. Furthermore, three hydrogen bonds link guanine and cytosine, but only two hydrogen bonds link thymine and adenine. This specificity of base pairing determines the helical and double-stranded structure of DNA.

RNA differs from DNA in that the sugar moiety is ribose; one of the bases, thymine, is replaced with another base, uracil (U); and RNA is usually single stranded.

Polymorphisms

Each individual genome differs from others by differences in DNA nucleotide sequences. On average, one out of every 300 nucleotides is polymorphic, meaning that differences in the human genome typically occur with at least a 1% frequency. Variants with frequencies less than 1% are called rare variants. Many general types of polymorphisms (**Fig. 3.4**) exist: single-nucleotide polymorphisms, small insertions and deletions (indels), and repeating changes, such as copy number variants, microsatellites, and minisatellites. Single-nucleotide polymorphisms (SNPs) can occur at any single nucleotide among the 3 billion base pairs. If a change (mutation) occurs on one part of the double helix, a complementary change occurs on the other part, so that the pairing of A-T and G-C remains intact.

As mentioned, humans have two copies of each autosome (chromosomes 1 to 22). The location, order, and sequential arrangement of the bases on each human chromosome have been systematically identified, recorded into a database, and codified into a nucleotide coordinate system. For example, chromosome 1, which is the largest human chromosome, has ~ 249 million base pairs arranged from 1 to 249,000,000. Other chromosomes follow similar coordinate assemblies. Since all humans show variation from others at many locations in the genome, this universal coordinate system makes it possible to compare genetic differences among two or more individuals using whole-genome or whole-exome sequencing or genotyping technology.

At a particular nucleotide location on a specific chromosome (generally called a **locus,** but also specified using the human genome coordinates), there may exist generally two, but possibly more than two, nucleotide alternatives that can occur naturally in the population. This naturally occur-

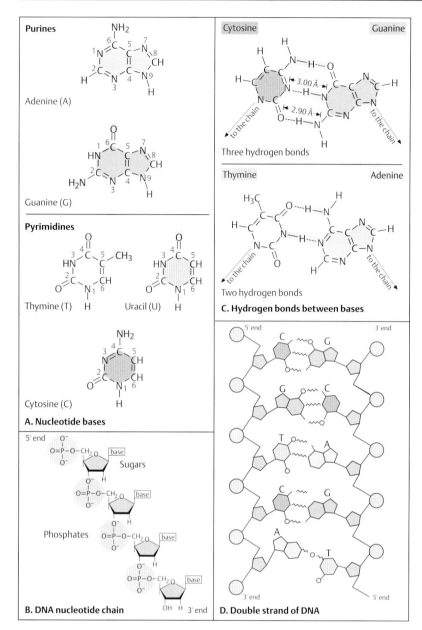

Fig. 3.3 DNA components include the purine bases adenine and guanine and the pyrimidine bases cytosine and thymine. The sugars and phosphates join to form a nucleotide chain. Cytosine is linked with guanine and thymine with adenine by hydrogen bonds to keep the double strand of DNA together.

ring variation due to different DNA forms (**alleles**) is called polymorphism. For a single-nucleotide variant, only one base is different (e.g., either the A nucleotide or the G nucleotide at that locus). Because each individual has two copies of every chromosome (one inherited from the mother, the other inherited from the father), using the allele A and G notation described above, only three possible **genotypes**—AA, AG, or GG—can be present at a particular locus in an individual. In the population, it is possible for other allelic forms besides A and G (e.g., T or C) to exist, but generally two alleles dominate. A deletion or addition of one or more base pairs may also occur. The latter variants are also called single-nucleotide polymor-

phisms but are sometimes called small indels. Indels can range in size from 1 to 100,000 bases and have recently been treated as their own category of polymorphism if more than one base pair is involved.

Microsatellites are variable numbers of short tandem repeats in sequence. For example, there may be regions where two nucleotides C and A repeat sequentially, so one possible allele might be CACACACA—labeled $(CA)_4$—and another allele might be CACACACACA—$(CA)_5$. Generally, the repeats are di-, tri- or tetranucleotide repeats. Minisatellites, also known as variable-number or tandem repeats, consist of a variable number of longer repeat units that are 20 to 500 nucleotides

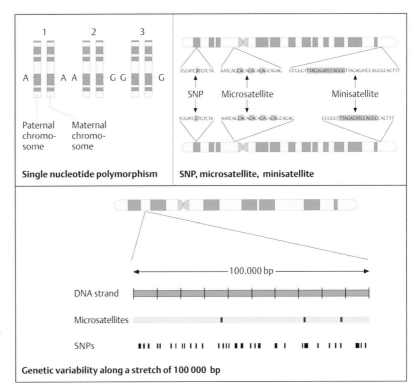

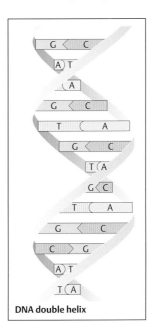

Fig. 3.4 A single-nucleotide polymorphism (SNP) has two alleles, one inherited from the mother and one inherited from the father. As shown in the single nucleotide polymorphism box, there are three possible combinations of the alleles. SNPs, microsatellites, and minisatellites contribute to genetic variability and are useful as markers for gene mapping.

(or base pairs) long. Allelic variant forms have their own nomenclature system, which, together with the chromosomal coordinate system of nucleotides, allow us to fully describe the variation that is present in humans from all populations. These genetic polymorphisms, also referred to as **markers**, are used for gene mapping, which is discussed later in the chapter.

■ DNA and RNA

In 1953, James Watson and Francis Crick discovered that DNA was structured as a double helix (**Fig. 3.5**). Because of the pairing that occurs between purines and pyrimidines, two complementary strands of nucleic acids bond together. This complementary arrangement of base pairs allows one strand to serve as a template to generate another strand of DNA in replication. This arrangement also implies that the strands run opposite to each other. The direction of the strands is determined by their biochemical structure. In replication, the DNA sequence is read from the 5′ end to the 3′ end, and the complementary strand is read from 3′ to 5′. In order to replicate DNA, it is first necessary to break the hydrogen bonds between the bases and unzip the double helix, after which new complementary strands of DNA

can be generated using the old strands of DNA as a template. The cellular machinery for DNA replication is fairly complex, involving many enzymes and proteins, and many stages. Enzymes called

Fig. 3.5 DNA consists of two polynucleotide chains wrapped around each other to form a double helix. The nucleotide bases form pairs, guanine with cytosine and adenine with thymine. During replication, the chains separate and serve as a template, so that a copy of the strands of DNA is created. Through transcription and translation, proteins are produced.

DNA polymerases can replicate about 50 bases per second. Since the average chromosome is about ~ 150,000,000 base pairs long, replication would take a very long time if the process occurred from end to end (i.e., only a single replication fork were created). Instead, replication occurs in multiple forks along the chromosome where topoisomerases relax the DNA, and DNA helicases break open the hydrogen bonds between bases to separate the double helix and initiate the process, allowing DNA polymerases to start replicating small segments of DNA. DNA replication is generally completed within an hour.

Replication is critical to create daughter cells that replenish aging cells throughout an individual's lifetime, and also for encoding nearly identical information in germ cells (ova or sperm) passed down from parent to offspring. Thus, replication is critical for inheritance of DNA from one generation to the next.

RNA is created through **transcription**, which is described in more detail below (**Fig. 3.6**). The type of RNA that is translated into a protein is called messenger RNA (mRNA) and consists of a long single strand. DNA encodes detailed instructions to create RNA, similar copying written text, with letters (bases), paragraphs (exons), and volumes (RNA molecules), complete with punctuation and formatting (splicing of exons in mRNA, when and how much mRNA should be expressed, and tissue specificity). Each cell type within a tissue has

instructions to turn only certain genes on or off (i.e., transcribe certain genes). As previously mentioned, the segments of DNA sequence that code for proteins are called exons, and the regions in between exons are called introns. DNA bases on a chromosome form a continuous sequence. The vast majority of human DNA is noncoding (~ 98%). Originally, the noncoding DNA was thought to be junk, but it is now understood that noncoding DNA has complex regulatory functions.

Although every exon is generally faithfully copied between the DNA and mRNA, a molecular editing process involving cellular machinery later clips out some exons in a process called alternative splicing. Some exons are skipped in the mature mRNA, giving rise to splice isoforms. Some genes can repurpose the same transcript to create a large number of isoforms to diversify function from the same gene across tissues. Similar flexibility is also encoded in a promoter region of DNA typically upstream from the gene, which helps the gene start transcription of mRNA. Proteins called transcription factors bind in clusters to DNA signatures of promoters, setting the stage for mRNA transcription. Some genes may have alternative promoters, with differential transcription-factor binding capacity, allowing the cell to choose when a gene is expressed and how much mRNA is expressed. Cells in close proximity to each other or in particular areas of tissue may synchronize gene expression (transcription).

Like DNA replication, transcription occurs in multiple steps, but the actual process of transcription varies by the length of the gene across the DNA strand. Elongation of RNA by RNA polymerase takes place at between 30 and 50 nucleotides per second. However, the largest gene is not necessarily the one for the biggest protein. *CNTNAP2*, a gene associated with speech and language and autism (OMIM 604569), is the biggest gene across the DNA segment, at 2.3 Mb, but the smaller gene for Duchenne muscular dystrophy (OMIM 300377), *dystrophin*, at 2.22 Mb, has a larger RNA size, 14.1 versus 9.9 kb.

Messenger RNA (mRNA) is single-stranded. Again, RNA bases are all the same as DNA bases except that uracil (U) substitutes for thymine (T). The genes that are transcribed within each cell depend on that cell's function, which is how cells can contain the same DNA but have very different functions from other cells.

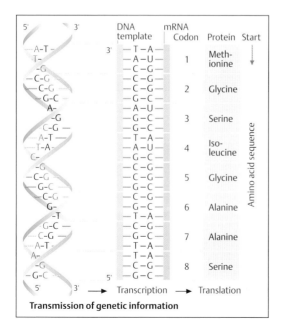

Fig. 3.6 Genetic information is transmitted through transcription and translation.

■ Proteins

mRNA is **translated** into amino acids, and the amino acids are then assembled into **proteins**. The proteins are the outward product of the genetic code. It should be noted that one gene may code for more than one protein, depending on alternative splicing, which is when particular exons of a gene are included or excluded from the final mRNA produced from that gene. The total complement of proteins in a given cell is called its **proteome**.

■ Transcription (mRNA synthesis) and Translation (Polypeptide Synthesis)

The entire process from the DNA sequence to protein synthesis is referred to as the central dogma of genetics (**Fig. 3.7**). In other words, the central dogma is that DNA is transcribed into RNA and RNA is then translated into protein. First, DNA is unwound to expose the sequence of bases (**Fig. 3.8**). The DNA helix is opened and one strand of DNA serves as a template in the 3′ to 5′ direction. RNA polymerase reads the sequence of nucleotides and generates a complementary strand of RNA in the 5′ to 3′ direction. Another proofreading enzyme proofreads the sequence, and the DNA molecule zips back together.

Once a single-stranded mRNA molecule has been transcribed, it provides the information to produce a protein through the process of translation. The RNA strand can be read as a series of **codons**, which are triplets of RNA nucleotides (**Fig. 3.9**). That is, once the mRNA molecule is in the cytoplasm, it attaches to a **ribosome**, and the ribosome moves along the mRNA molecule reading the codons. Translation does not start until a start codon, AUG, is found (**Fig. 3.8** and **Fig. 3.9**). Amino acids are the building blocks for proteins. Note that some redundancy is present in the genetic code, and different triplets of nucleotides may code for the same amino acid; thus, the genetic code is degenerate. This redundancy is important when considering the impact of nucleotide changes in DNA and RNA; if there is a change in one nucleotide base that does not result in a

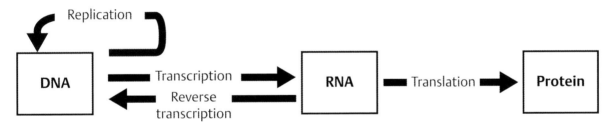

Fig. 3.7 The central dogma of genetics refers to the entire process that begins with the DNA sequence and ends with the protein product. In this process, DNA is transcribed into RNA and RNA is translated into a protein.

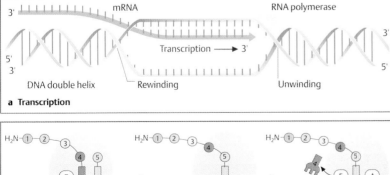

Fig. 3.8 **(a)** During transcription, the double helix of DNA is opened and serves as a template for RNA. **(b)** Translation occurs when the mRNA is read to form amino acids, which are the building blocks of proteins.

Box 3.5 Technologies for Analysis of Gene Expression

Gene expression analysis is a quickly evolving field. Every few years, a new technology to measure the amount of RNA transcripts from each gene in different cell types is created. Currently, the main technologies available differ in the type of result produced, and the number of genes that can be measured at a given time.

Real-time polymerase chain reaction (RT-PCR) is used to detect gene expression qualitatively through creation of complementary DNA (cDNA) transcripts from RNA. Primer sequences are designed to target

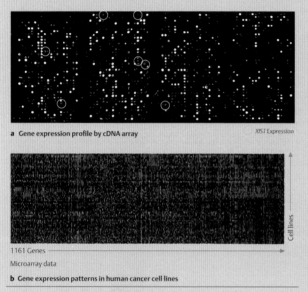

a Gene expression profile by cDNA array *XIST Expression*

1161 Genes
Microarray data

b Gene expression patterns in human cancer cell lines

Box Fig. 3.2 **(a)** Gene expression profile by cDNA array. **(b)** Gene expression patters in human cancer cell lines.

a specific gene's transcript. RT-PCR is used to clone expressed genes by reverse transcribing the RNA of interest into its DNA complement through the use of reverse transcriptase. Although this method is considered "low throughput" because it can assess only one gene product at a time, it is also considered the most sensitive and quantitative, and it is often used to validate higher-throughput methods (**Box Fig. 3.2**).

In microarray technology, the gene transcript (RNA sequence) is broken up into smaller bits, or primer sequences. The primer sequences are overlapping, so there are multiple primers per gene. All possible genes that could be transcribed are referred to as the transcriptome. All primers from the transcriptome are put onto a small chip with RNA. The primers are so specific that the matching RNA anneals to only the primer. A solution is used that includes a marker that lights up when RNA attaches to the primer. The chips are then read by a special machine that translates the image into quantities of each RNA transcript.

RNA-sequencing (RNA-Seq) technology also captures the entire transcriptome, but it does so using sequencing technology similar to that described in **Box 3.4**. The technology also has the ability to detect smaller RNAs that do not necessarily get translated into protein as well as transcripts that are alternatively spliced. Because the method captures sequence, special methods are required to align the RNA-Seq with a reference sequence. Coverage (the number of copies of a specific transcript) is also important, because it determines the reliability of the result. This technology returns the number of sequences of a particular transcript, so it is only semiquantitative, compared to microarray technology.

different amino acid, this change is referred to as synonymous, but if the nucleotide change results in an amino acid change, it is referred to as nonsynonymous. Since a synonymous variant does not result in an amino acid change, the final protein will not be different; however, an amino acid change resulting from a nonsynonymous variant could cause the protein to change either in structure or function. As each triplet is read, another molecule, **transfer RNA (tRNA)**, which is specific to the triplet, carries the requested amino acid to the ribosome, where the acids are linked together to form a protein. This process continues until the ribosome reaches a stop codon (UAA, UAG, or UGA). The entire process of the ribosome moving along the mRNA strand with the growing polypeptide chain is depicted in **Fig. 3.8**. Technologies for analyzing the amount of RNA in a sample are summarized in **Box 3.5**.

■ Regulation of Protein Synthesis

Proteins are the building blocks of all parts of the body, and they are active players in many cellular processes. Translation is the essential process by which proteins are synthesized. Protein synthesis requires all three classes of RNA (mRNA, tRNA, and **ribosomal RNA** or **rRNA**), and is used in gene regulation (transcription). The amount, location, and timing of protein production and degradation are carefully controlled by cells and are maintained in equilibrium in a process called **homeostasis**. Because transcription of a gene determines how much mRNA is available to make proteins, transcription and translation are highly coordinated. The presence of certain molecules inside the cell (e.g., glucose) determines which protein is made, how much protein is made, and how much is destroyed.

Fig. 3.9 The genetic code is a set of biological rules by which nucleotide base pairs code amino acids. Each code word consists of three nucleotides. The genetic code also specifies the beginning (start codon) and end (stop codon) of the coding region. An abbreviated code is used consisting of the first letter of each nucleotide.

First	Nucleotide base				Third
	Second				
	Uracil (U)	Cytosine (C)	Adenine (A)	Guanine (G)	
Uracil (U)	F Phenylalanine (Phe)	S Serine (Ser)	Y Tyrosine (Tyr)	C Cysteine (Cys)	U
	F Phenylalanine (Phe)	S Serine (Ser)	Y Tyrosine (Tyr)	C Cysteine (Cys)	C
	L Leucine (Leu)	S Serine (Ser)	Stop Codon	Stop Codon	A
	L Leucine (Leu)	S Serine (Ser)	Stop Codon	W Tryptophan (Trp)	G
Cytosine (C)	L Leucine (Leu)	P Proline (Pro)	H Histidine (His)	R Arginine (Arg)	U
	L Leucine (Leu)	P Proline (Pro)	H Histidine (His)	R Arginine (Arg)	C
	L Leucine (Leu)	P Proline (Pro)	Q Glutamine (Gln)	R Arginine (Arg)	A
	L Leucine (Leu)	P Proline (Pro)	Q Glutamine (Gln)	R Arginine (Arg)	G
Adenine (A)	I Isoleucine (Ile)	T Threonine (Thr)	N Asparagine (Asn)	S Serine (Ser)	U
	I Isoleucine (Ile)	T Threonine (Thr)	N Asparagine (Asn)	S Serine (Ser)	C
	I Isoleucine (Ile)	T Threonine (Thr)	K Lysine (Lys)	R Arginine (Arg)	A
	Start (Methionine)	T Threonine (Thr)	K Lysine (Lys)	R Arginine (Arg)	G
Guanine (G)	V Valine (Val)	A Alanine (Ala)	D Aspartic acid (Asp)	G Glycine (Gly)	U
	V Valine (Val)	A Alanine (Ala)	D Aspartic acid (Asp)	G Glycine (Gly)	C
	V Valine (Val)	A Alanine (Ala)	E Glutamic acid (Glu)	G Glycine (Gly)	A
	V Valine (Val)	A Alanine (Ala)	E Glutamic acid (Glu)	G Glycine (Gly)	G

A. Genetic code for all amino acids in mRNA

Start	AUG	F (Phe)	UUU	L (Leu)	CUU	R (Arg)	CGU	V	GUU
Stop	UAA		UUC		CUC		CGC		GUC
	UAG				CUG		CGG		GUG
	UGA	G (Gly)	GGU		CUA		CAA		GUA
A (Ala)	GCU		GGC		UUG		AGG		
	GCC		GGG		UUA		AGA	W (Trp)	UGG
	GCG		GGA	M (Met)	AUG	S (Ser)	UCU	Y (Tyr)	UAU
	GCA	H (His)	CAU	N (Asn)	AAU		UCC		UAC
C (Cys)	UGU		CAC		AAC		UCG		
	UGC						UCA	B (Asx)	Asn
		I (Ile)	AUU	P (Pro)	CCU		AGU		or
D (Asp)	GAU		AUC		CCC		AGC		Asp
	GAC		AUA		CCG	T (Thr)	ACU		
					CCA		ACC	Z (Glx)	Gln
E (Glu)	GAG	K (Lys)	AAG	Q (Gln)	CAG		ACG		or
	GAA		AAA		CAA		ACA		Glu

B. Abbreviated code

Cells are capable of responding to extracellular stimuli via signaling cascades, which then signal DNA within the cell nucleus to increase or decrease protein production, maintenance, and destruction.

In humans and other eukaryotes, protein synthesis can extend from hours to days, because mRNA is present in eukaryotic cells for a longer period of time than in prokaryotic cells. Blocking prokaryotic protein synthesis is often the mechanism of action for antibiotics, but, because RNA can be produced anew, the medications require continuous administration over time to keep blocking protein synthesis.

■ Protein Degradation

Protein degradation is the cellular process in which misfolded and damaged proteins are removed from circulation. Animal cells have two fundamental means of degrading proteins: via compartments inside the cell called lysosomes, or via a protein complex called the proteasome. Both processes use specialized enzymes (e.g., proteases) and other specialized cell machinery to earmark proteins scheduled for destruction. Protein degradation serves to regulate cellular metabolism, to recycle amino acids (building blocks of proteins), and to keep the production of new proteins active. The rate of protein degradation varies widely from protein to protein. Some proteins are degraded quickly, while others persist in the cell. Because of the variation in protein turnover, some proteins have longer half-lives. The half-life of a protein is the time it takes for half of the protein to be degraded, and degradation continues at an exponential rate after that. Half-life also refers to the amount of time it takes for a protein to lose half its physiologic activity.

■ Replication of Genetic Material, the Processes of Mitosis and Meiosis, and Cell Division

In eukaryotic cells, the genetic material (DNA) resides inside the nucleus. The length of the DNA strands is greater than what would ordinarily fit in the nuclear compartment without additional packaging. As described earlier, DNA is bundled into structures called chromosomes. Humans have 23 pairs of chromosomes: a matched pair (two copies) of 22 autosomes numbered in size from chromosome 1, the largest, to chromosome 22, the smallest, and a pair of sex chromosomes, XY in males and XX in females (**Fig. 3.1**).

DNA is replicated via processes called **mitosis** and **meiosis**. Mitosis is the process of formation of new cells during the lifetime of an individual (**Fig. 3.10**). Mitosis occurs in almost all cells of the body. Meiosis is a specialized case of formation of new cells that occurs only in reproductive cells, and leads to the formation of ova in females and sperm in males (**Fig. 3.11**). Ova and sperm contain

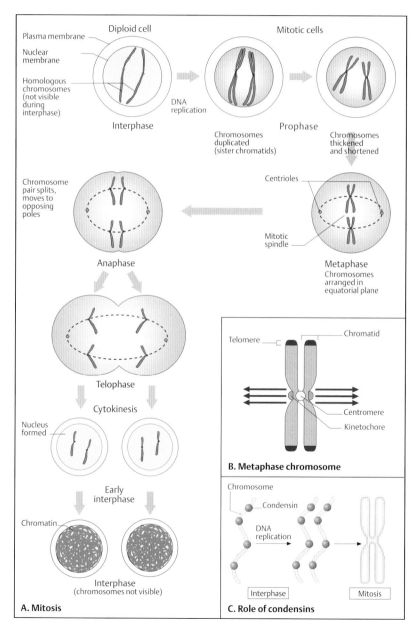

Fig. 3.10 Cell division occurs through a process known as mitosis. Nuclear division consists of prophase, metaphase, anaphase, and telophase. Mitosis results in two genetically identical cells.

only one copy of each chromosome, as opposed to the normal two; at fertilization, ova and sperm fuse to form the zygote (fertilized egg), which will then contain a normal complement of 23 pairs of chromosomes: a total of 44 autosomes and 2 sex chromosomes, either XX (female) or XY (male; **Fig. 3.12**). Because DNA contains the instructions for making RNA and subsequently protein, replication of DNA is vital to survival of an organism. The process of replication can be divided into stages and is dependent on the cell cycle (**Fig. 3.10** and **Fig. 3.11**).

■ Features of Inheritance

Mendelian Traits

As stated earlier, a trait is a distinguishing quality or characteristic of a specific part of a person. A simple example of a trait is blue eyes. Some traits are transmitted by a single gene, while other traits are polygenic or influenced by the interaction of several or more genes. Traits transmitted by single genes are often referred to as Mendelian traits. Gregor Mendel (1822–1884) was an Austrian monk

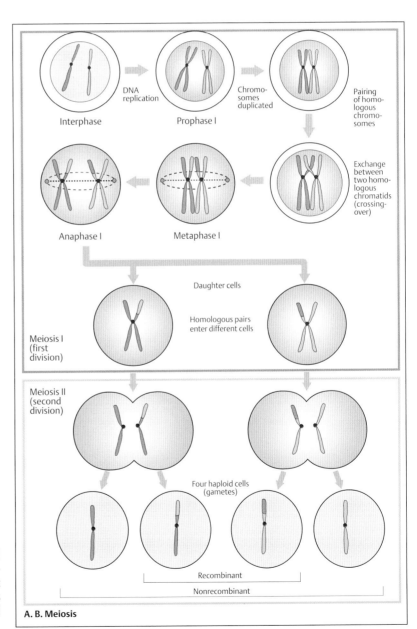

Fig. 3.11 Meiosis is a special type of cell division that results in the formation of gametes (haploid cells). Recombination of genetic material may occur during meiosis. Meiosis leads to the formation of sperm in males and ova in females.

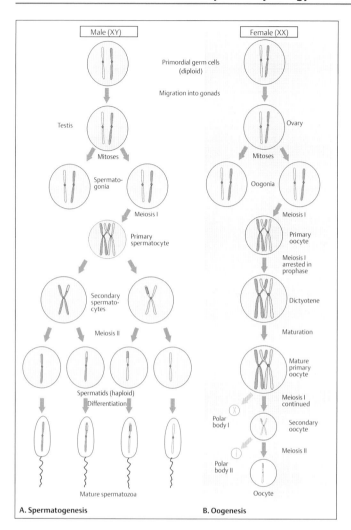

Fig. 3.12 The formation of germ cells is called spermatogenesis in males and oogenesis in females. The formation of germ cells begins with meiosis, and the process differs in males and females.

Table 3.1 Patterns of inheritance

Mode	Pattern	Characteristics	Examples
Autosomal dominant	Vertical transmission. Does not skip a generation. Males and females equally affected.	Affected individuals have an affected parent. Child of an affected parent has a 50% chance of inheriting the causal variant.	Apert's syndrome, Beckwith-Wiedemann syndrome, Crouzon's syndrome, neurofibromatosis
Autosomal recessive	Horizontal transmission. Skips generations. Males and females equally affected.	Parents are usually not affected. Siblings of an affected child have a 25% chance of inheriting the causal variant.	Dysautonomia, Goldberg-Shprintzen syndrome, Hurler's syndrome
X-linked dominant	Vertical transmission. Does not skip a generation. Males and females may be affected.	All daughters of an affected father are affected.	Rhett's syndrome, fragile X syndrome, Alport's syndrome
X-linked recessive	Never transmitted father to son. Uncles may be affected. Males are affected, females are carriers.	Parents are usually not affected. Brothers of an affected boy have a 50% chance of inheriting the causal variant.	Hunter's syndrome, red–green color blindness, hemophilia, Duchenne muscular dystrophy
Y-linked	Vertical transmission. Does not skip a generation. Only males are affected.	All sons of an affected father are affected.	
Mitochondrial	Vertical transmission. All children of an affected mother may be affected. Highly variable within a family.	All children of an affected father are unaffected.	Exercise intolerance, Kearns-Sayre syndrome

who discovered the phenomenon of dominant and recessive traits while breeding pea plants. A simple example in humans is attached versus unattached earlobes: attached earlobes are dominant over unattached earlobes. When Mendel bred yellow and green plants, the hybrid offspring were green rather than yellow and green. He concluded that green was a dominant trait and yellow was recessive. Some human traits, including those that influence speech and language disorders, follow these patterns of inheritance. Traits may be carried on the autosomes or on the X chromosome. As shown in **Table 3.1**, Mendelian traits may be autosomal dominant, autosomal recessive, or X-linked. Each has a unique pattern of transmission and rate of affecting offspring.

For an autosomal recessive trait to be expressed, the offspring must inherit a copy of the gene or allele carrying the trait from each parent. The allele combination is said to be homozygous, because both alleles for the trait are the same. The chance of offspring inheriting the causal variant from both parents is 25%. Parents are usually not affected; therefore, the trait is said to "skip a generation."

Autosomal dominant traits are expressed if the offspring inherits the allele for the trait from one or both parents. The combination of alleles from the parents may be homozygous (alleles from both parents carry the trait) or heterozygous (one allele carries the trait and one allele does not carry the trait). Affected offspring typically have one or both parents affected. Transmission is said to be vertical because the trait seldom skips a generation. Children with one affected parent have a 50% chance of inheriting the trait. Males and females are equally affected.

X-linked traits are carried on the X chromosome. They are never transmitted father to son because the father contributes the Y chromosome in male offspring. X-linked traits are typically inherited by males and are neither dominant nor recessive, because males have only a single X chromosome. If an X-linked trait is recessive and is carried by the mother, sons may be affected. If an X-linked trait is recessive, a daughter who inherits the variant will not demonstrate the trait but will be a carrier of the trait, because females have two X chromosomes. However, if an X-linked trait is dominant and the father has the trait, all daughters will be affected.

Y-linked traits are rare, and only males will be affected. All sons of an affected father will be affected. The Y chromosome carries only about 50 genes, none of which is essential to life.

■ Mitochondrial Inheritance

Mitochondria are unique cellular organelles that possess their own DNA. Mitochondria serve as the powerhouse for the cell, producing the energy needed for cellular function. A mutation in a mitochondrial gene can result in defective energy production. Disorders with mitochondrial inheritance may result in muscle weakness, exercise intolerance, blindness, or deafness. There is great variability in mitochondrial inheritance, since not every cell in an individual will carry a given mitochondrial mutation. The expression of mitochondrial inheritance is highly variable within a family.

■ Penetrance and Expressivity

Genotype can be the specific alleles at a specific location in a gene, or it may be the combination of all genetic variation in a person's genome. **Phenotype** is the outward manifestation of genotype, or, in other words, a trait. The expression of a particular genotype may vary among individuals with the same genotype due to **penetrance** and variable expressivity. Penetrance is the probability that a particular phenotype will be expressed. A combination of other genes and the environment may determine whether the individual manifests a particular genetic trait. A gene may show very high penetrance (e.g., it is almost always expressed) or low penetrance, as in the case of multifactorial inheritance; also, it may appear that a genetic condition skips generations, when in fact the gene was not fully penetrant and was not expressed. Genetic conditions also demonstrate **variable expressivity**. Some individuals may present with all the features of a particular condition, while other individuals may express only some of the features. An example is neurofibromatosis, where patients with the same genetic mutation show different signs and symptoms of the disease. The pedigree of the family shown in **Box 3.6** contains some family members who present with only a speech and language disorder, while other family members demonstrate speech, language, reading, and learning disabilities. The unique background of an individual's genotype and environment is responsible for the variable expressivity of a gene.

■ Recombination

One mechanism causing genetic variability occurs via recombination during meiosis and how this pattern can be seen within families (**Fig. 3.12**). As the corresponding chromosomes line up next to each other, some genetic material crosses over to the other chromosome and is exchanged. This swapping of genetic material between the two chromosomes creates novel combinations of genes. **Fig. 3.13** shows the formation of new combinations of genes as a result of crossing-over of homologous chromosomes during meiosis. The newly combined DNA must retain the original structure without losing or adding a base pair in order to function properly.

■ Copy Number Variation

About 12% of the human genome has **copy number variation (CNV)**, which is more or less than the usual two copies of a gene (one each from both parents). CNV may be responsible for the diversity we see in humans and the variability in complex human behavioral traits, such as speech and language. Approximately 0.4% of genomes of unrelated people differ in CNV. CNVs have been observed in identical twins, who have otherwise identical genomes. CNVs are widespread in humans: about 2,000 CNVs have been identified in humans. CNVs can be duplications, deletions, inversions, or translocations. Not all CNVs are benign. CNVs have been associated with susceptibility to disease, including developmental disorders, such as autism, schizophrenia, and learning disabilities.

■ Chromosomal Abnormalities

Genetic disorders may also result from chromosomal abnormalities, as described in **Table 3.2**. Chromosomal abnormalities occur during cell division and include errors in chromosome number (deletion or additions of entire chromosomes), deletion of a segment of a chromosome, translocation (rearrangements of chromosomes in which a segment of a chromosome breaks and attaches to another), or inversion (a chromosome breaks and a segment is reattached opposite its original alignment). Many chromosomal abnormalities result in syndromes, such as Down's syndrome (**Box 3.7**), and have associated features, including speech, lan-

Table 3.2 Some types of chromosomal abnormalities

Errors in chromosome number	
Monosomy	Deletion of an entire chromosome, usually due to nondisjunction
Trisomy	An entire extra chromosome, also due to nondisjunction, such as trisomy 21 (Down's syndrome)
Polyploidy	Presence of an entire extra set of chromosomes
Deletions: Absence of a segment of a chromosome	
Terminal	Deletion from the end of the chromosome
Interstitial	Deletion from the interior of the chromosome
Translocations: Rearrangements of chromosomes in which a segment of one chromosome breaks and attaches to another	
Balanced	No genes are lost; phenotype is normal
Unbalanced	Genetic material is lost
Dicentric chromosomes: Chromosomes that have two centromeres because they are made up of two broken segments of other chromosomes	
Inversions: Interstitial break and segment reattaches opposite its original alignment	
Ring chromosome: Two breaks in chromosome and ends join to form a ring	

guage, and hearing difficulties (**Box 3.8**, **Box 3.9**, **Box 3.10**).

■ Multifactorial Inheritance

Many traits, such as speech, language, and hearing, are determined by multiple genes (they are **polygenic**) and environmental factors. As described in **Box 3.11**, speech and language are complex human traits, with many genes likely contributing to individual function. Environmental factors may also influence gene expression. **Table 3.3** provides a list

of the **candidate genes** for speech, language, and reading disorders, their function, and the phenotypes that have been associated with each gene. Many of these genes affect neural development, structures, and functions. Most speech and language disorders result from multifactorial inheritance.

■ Epigenetics

Epigenetics is the study of heritable changes in gene activity that do not involve alterations to the genetic code. Epigenetic marks inform genes to

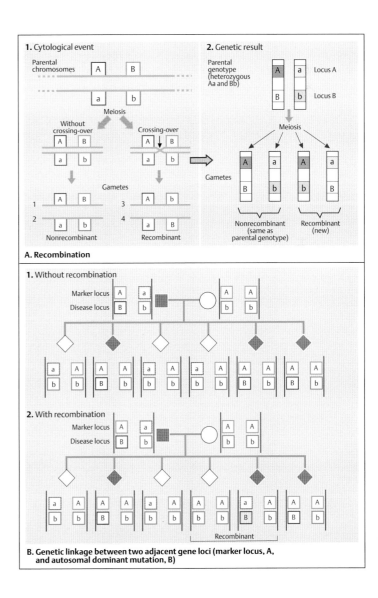

Fig. 3.13 Meiosis, with and without recombination. The gametes formed without recombination are the same as the parental genotype. The gametes formed with recombination differ from the parental genotype, creating new genetic combinations.

Table 3.3   Candidate genes for speech-language disorders and dyslexia

Gene(s)	Chromosome location	Function(s)	Phenotype
FOXP2	7	A brain-expressed transcription factor that affects brain development	Apraxia Developmental delays Language impairment
ROBO1 and *ROBO2*	3	Guide axons and influence neuronal axon growth	Dyslexia
KIAA0319, TTRAP, and *DCDC2*	6	Disrupt neuronal migration	Dyslexia Speech sound disorders Phonological awareness
BDNF	11	Brain-derived neurotrophic factor related to nerve growth and differentiation in the brain	Language impairment Articulation
DRD2	11	Dopamine receptor; involved in motor control, endocrine function, cognition, language learning, procedural learning, and working memory, as well as motor region of the brain	ADHD Stuttering Vocabulary
AVPR1a	11	Arginine-vasopressin (AVP) affects social behavior and vocalization	Autism Memory Vocabulary Reading decoding
ASPM	11	Involved in mitotic spindle formation, neurogenesis, and cognition, and is associated with intracranial volume	Word reading Speech sound disorder Microcephaly
DYX1C1	15	Mediates protein-to-protein interactions	Dyslexia
CYP19A1	15	Controls cell differentiation in specific brain areas	Dyslexia Speech sound disorder
CNTNAP2	7	A gene that is regulated by the *FOXP2* gene	Language impairment Autism spectrum disorder Nonword repetition
GNPTAB, GNPTG, and *NAGPA*	12	Regulate the development of pathways to the lysosomes of the cell	Stuttering

Box 3.6 Drawing a Family Pedigree

Family history can be valuable in identifying children at risk for speech and language disorders, screening children for early intervention programs, and predicting educational and social outcomes for children. Taking an accurate family history is an important part of speech, language, and hearing assessments. Constructing a family pedigree allows the clinician to obtain family history systematically and provides a pictorial summary of the history information. Begin with the individual who was referred for the assessment (the **proband**) using the symbols shown below. Note the proband's name, date of birth, and clinical features, such as hearing impairment, language and/or speech disorder, learning disabilities, stuttering, etc. Some disorders are seemingly unrelated, such as ADHD, autism, and other cognitive disorders, but are noted on the pedigree. Next, draw the nuclear family of the proband, including parents, siblings, spouses, and children, and record the clinical features as you did for the proband. Ask about siblings' spouses and children. Draw in the paternal and maternal aunts and uncles and cousins. Finally, add both paternal and maternal grandparents, again noting any pertinent history information. Review the pedigree with the parents to check for accuracy and update the pedigree on subsequent visits.

The example pedigree in **Box Fig. 3.3** shows the proband, a 4-year-old boy, with a phonology disorder. (Males are indicated by squares and females by circles. Affected individuals are indicated by shaded squares and circles.) The proband's brother was a late talker, although he never received speech-language therapy. The parents report never having had speech disorders; however, the maternal aunt had speech, language, and reading difficulties. A male cousin also had a speech and language disorder. A paternal uncle reportedly had reading and learning disabilities as well as being a late talker. Grandparents are reported as unaffected (although history information on grandparents is often unknown or inaccurate).

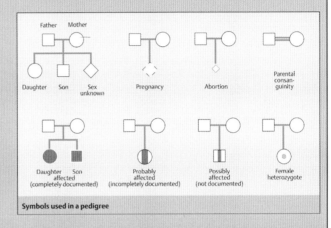

Symbols used in a pedigree

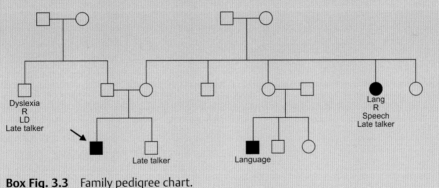

Box Fig. 3.3 Family pedigree chart.

Box 3.7   Down's Syndrome: Nondisjunction of Chromosome 21

Nondisjunction occurs when both copies of a chromosome end up in the same cell during cell division (meiosis); one cell receives 24 chromosomes and the other only 22 chromosomes. The cell (sperm or egg) with 24 chromosomes may go on to be fertilized, and the resulting embryo contains three copies (instead of two) of the chromosome. Down's syndrome is the most common condition resulting from nondisjunction, in this case nondisjunction of chromosome 21, with a prevalence ranging from 1 in 700 to 1 in 1,000 births. In 95% of children, the condition is sporadic (nonfamilial). Children born with Down's syndrome usually present with multiple medical conditions and cognitive impairments. Although individuals with Down's syndrome vary greatly in the features they demonstrate, common physical findings are hypotonia, small head, macroglossia (large tongue), flat nasal bridge, epicanthal folds, upward slant to the eyes, small ears, broad neck, and small stature. About 75% of individuals with Down's syndrome present with hearing loss. Cognitive impairments may be mild (IQ = 50–70), moderate (IQ = 35–50), or severe (IQ = 20–35). Social skills are a relative strength for individuals with Down's syndrome compared to their cognitive abilities. Individuals with Down's syndrome may have limitations in adaptive skills.

Children with Down's syndrome have speech and language impairments due to structural and functional abnormalities of the articulators as well as due to reduced cognitive abilities. Speech sound errors are similar to those in other children with speech delays, such as consonant cluster reduction, final consonant deletion, and reduced intelligibility in conversation (Kent and Vorperian 2013). Notable speech characteristics include lack of articulatory precision, lack of appropriate pausing and phrasing, and vowel errors (Bunton and Leddy 2011). If the child has a hearing loss, speech perception may also be impaired. Language abilities often are below expectations for the child's nonverbal skills. Language may be telegraphic, omitting grammatical markers, articles, pronouns, and prepositions. Syntax and morphology usually show the greatest deficits. Mean length of utterance (MLU) is reduced. Receptive language is generally better than expressive language.

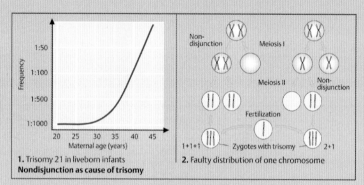

1. Trisomy 21 in liveborn infants
Nondisjunction as cause of trisomy

2. Faulty distribution of one chromosome

Box Fig. 3.4   Nondisjunction as cause of trisomy.

Box 3.8 Parent-of-Origin Effects

Does it matter which gene comes from your father and which comes from your mother? Maybe. Parent-of-origin effects (or imprinting) occur when the same trait has different phenotypic outcomes depending on whether it's inherited from the mother or the father. Imprinted genes often occur in clusters along a chromosome. Some imprinted genes affect cognitive and neurodevelopmental processes. Specific genetic syndromes may result from mutated genes that are imprinted. Examples of such syndromes are Angelman's syndrome and Prader-Willi syndrome.

Angelman's syndrome results when the mother's segment of the chromosome is missing (a deletion in the 15q11–q13 region of chromosome 15 known as the PWS/AS region) or both copies of the region are the father's copy. Angelman's syndrome is characterized by severe to profound mental retardation, with little speech or language development. Other characteristics of Angelman's syndrome are failure to thrive as an infant, progressive ataxia, hypotonia, seizures, cortical atrophy, outbursts of laughter, and arm flapping.

Prader-Willi syndrome results from an abnormality in the father's segment of chromosome 15 in the 15q11–13 region. Prader-Willi syndrome may be due to a deletion of the paternally contributed chromosome 15 PWS/AS region (70% of cases), maternal uniparental disomy (UPD; 29% of cases), or a translocation or other structural abnormality of the PWS/AS region (< 1% of cases). Individuals with Prader-Willi syndrome present with an IQ of 70 and typically have speech and language delays. Speech and language characteristics include poor speech sound development, reduced oral motor skills, abnormal pitch, hypernasality, receptive/expressive language delays, and poor pragmatic skills. Other characteristics of Prader-Willi syndrome include hyperphagia (excessive hunger) and food seeking (leading to obesity), neonatal and infantile hypotonia, feeding problems in infancy, and developmental delays. Males and females are equally affected, with an incidence of 1:10,000.

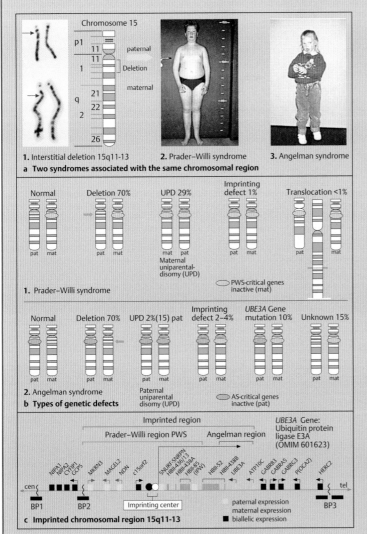

Box Fig. 3.5 (a) Two syndromes associated with the same chromosomal region. **(b)** Types of genetic defects. **(c)** Imprinted chromosomal region 15q11-13.

Box 3.9 Fragile X Syndrome: A Case of X-Linked Mental Retardation

Fragile X syndrome is the most common cause of inherited mental retardation, with about 30% of individuals with fragile X also presenting with autism. Fragile X is caused by a mutation of a gene on the X chromosome called *FMR1*, for Fragile X Mental Retardation-1. A region of DNA at the start of this gene (a CGG trinucleotide) expands beyond the normal range (more than 200 repeats) and turns off the gene. The neural synaptic protein coded by this gene is not produced, and thus does not perform its function during brain development. A woman is a carrier of the gene if the DNA region is somewhat longer than is typical. Fragile X is more common in males (1 in 4,000 males) than in females (1 in 6,000 females), because males inherit only one X chromosome, whereas females inherit two. Boys are more severely affected than girls, with only about 30% to 50% of girls demonstrating mental retar-

dation. However, girls often demonstrate a nonverbal learning disability (e.g., math difficulties). Physical features of individuals with fragile X syndrome include a long face, large prominent ears, flat feet, hyperextensible joints, low muscle tone, seizures, and chronic ear infections. Males may have large testes after puberty.

Cognitive/behavioral characteristics include intellectual disabilities (ranging from mild to severe), ADHD, anxiety, autistic behaviors, sensory integration problems (hypersensitivity to touch), hand flapping and hand biting, and speech delay, with expressive language more severely affected than receptive language. Speech and language difficulties include perseveration and echolalia in speech, auditory memory deficits, poor syntax and semantics, articulation and phonological errors, stuttering and cluttering, and a hoarse breathy voice. Relative strengths include sequential processing, good long-term and visual memory, and adaptive skills in males.

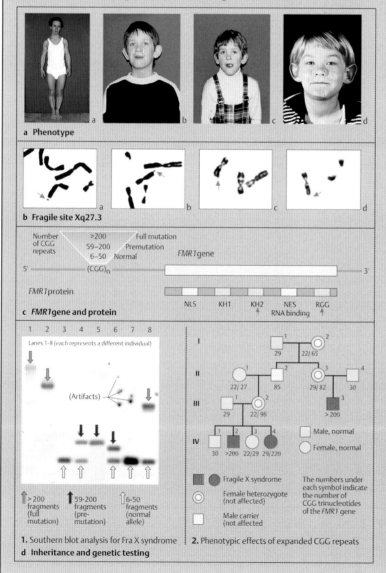

Box Fig. 3.6 **(a)** Phenotype. **(b)** Fragile site Xq27.3. **(c)** FMR1 gene and protein. **(d)** Inheritance and genetic testing.

Box 3.10   Genetics of Cleft Lip and Palate

The genetics of cleft lip and palate is often multifactorial, involving both genetic bases and environmental risk factors (smoking, alcohol and diet, steroids, lack of folic acid and multivitamins in early pregnancy, and use of steroids and anticonvulsants during pregnancy). Cleft lip and palate may be either syndromic (appearing with other malformations in a recognizable pattern) or nonsyndromic (appearing in isolation). Syndromic and nonsyndromic cleft lip and palate may have common genetic bases. Genes for cleft lip and palate have variable expressivity, meaning that their expression may vary from very severe in some children to less severe in others.

- The following are some genes in which some variations lead to syndromic cleft lip and palate.
    - **T-box transcription factor-22** (*TBX22*) is X-linked and semidominant and may result in cleft palate and tongue tie. It may contribute to both syndromic and nonsyndromic forms of cleft palate. The clinical expression is highly variable, with milder cases in males presenting with high arched palate, bifid uvula, and tongue tie. Female carriers may be asymptomatic.
    - **Poliovirus receptor-like-1** (*OVRK1*) is related to cleft lip and palate and ectodermal dysplasia syndrome. It demonstrates an autosomal recessive pattern of inheritance.
    - **Interferon regulatory factor-6** (*IRF-6*) may result in van der Woude's syndrome and accounts for 2% of all cleft lip and palate. Individuals with the gene may present with a cleft lip with or without cleft palate, an isolated cleft palate, pits or cysts on the lower lip, and hypodontia. *IRF-6* expression is highly variable in family members. The gene is located on chromosome 1 (1q32–q41).
- Nonsyndromic cleft lip and palate may result from the following mutations.
    - ***TGFA* mutation** combined with maternal smoking increases risk of a cleft palate six to eight times.
    - ***MSX1* mutation** is related to tooth agenesis and cleft lip with or without cleft palate and contributes to 2% of nonsyndromic clefts.
    - ***MTHFR C677T***, a single-nucleotide polymorphism, is related to folic acid deficiency and increases the risk of cleft lip and palate ten times.
- Orofacial cleft lip and palate syndromes may result from genes that affect bone development. Examples include:
    - **Apert's syndrome** results from mutation of the *FGFR2* gene, which produces a fibroblast growth factor receptor that signals cells to become bone cells during development. The gene causes prolonged signaling that results in premature fusion of bones in the skull, hands, and feet. It is autosomal dominant, and most cases are due to new mutations in the gene.
    - **Crouzon's syndrome** is also caused by a mutation in *FGFR2* gene that results in premature fusion of the skull bones. It demonstrates an autosomal dominant mode of inheritance.
    - **Hemifacial macrosomia** is a condition in which the lower half of one side of the face is underdeveloped and does not grow normally.
    - **Pierre Robin sequence** results from changes in the DNA near the *SOX9* gene that regulates genes important for the development of the skeleton, including the mandible. Changes in the DNA near the *SOX9* gene disrupt enhancers that regulate the gene. Most cases are due to new mutations and may occur as part of a syndrome that affects other organs.
    - **Treacher Collins syndrome** results from mutations in the *TCOF1, POLRIC,* or *POLRID* gene that code for proteins responsible for early development of bones and tissues of the face. Mutations in the genes cause reduction in the production of rRNA, which causes cell death. The syndrome demonstrates an autosomal dominant mode of inheritance, and 60% of cases are due to new mutations.

Box 3.11 Speech and Language Disorders: A Complex Trait

The biological underpinnings of speech and language are complex. In genetic terminology, speech and language disorders are complex traits, in that no single gene is responsible for the majority of cases or deficits of any particular developmental disorder. Heterogeneous effects of risk genes may act alone or together to give rise to multiple profiles of speech and language skills that may culminate in the same diagnosis and general impairment on the surface. Further, a single genetic defect may result in multiple problems if it is present early in development. Different components of this complex phenotype can be linked to distinct genetic loci. The nature and severity of the disorder might vary at different developmental stages; genes may be turned on and off during the life span. Environmental effects may be unique to individuals (nonshared environment). **Box Fig. 3.7** illustrates the genetic architecture of a complex trait. Multiple genes and environmental factors give rise to proteins that influence underlying skills or traits, called **endophenotypes**, such as phonological awareness skills, memory, vocabulary, and cognitive abilities. These endophenotypes contribute to disorders such as speech sound disorders, language impairment (LI), or reading disability (RD). Environmental factors (such as early intervention or speech-language therapy) might modify the resulting phenotype.

The hunt for genes that influence speech-language disorders and dyslexia has uncovered many candidate genes distributed across the genome. Some of these genes broadly influence brain development by guiding axons to specific areas of the brain or controlling neuronal growth. Component skills or endophenotypes, such as memory, phonological and linguistic processing, and cognition, may be disrupted by abnormalities in brain growth and development. These skills may affect both spoken and written language, resulting in speech, language, or reading disorders, and may explain high rates of comorbidity among the disorders. Clinically, children with early speech and language disorders are at higher risk for literacy difficulties at school age than their peers, even if early speech-language problems have resolved.

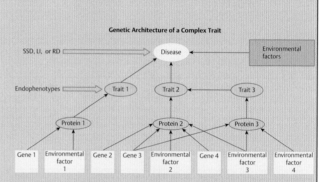

Box Fig. 3.7 As shown in the figure, multiple genes code for proteins that influence cognitive traits. The combination of these traits and environmental influences may give rise to a disorder.

switch on or off based on several factors. Two types of epigenetic marks have been described: chemical (e.g., methylation) and protein (e.g., histones). Through epigenetic marks on the genome, environmental factors, such as diet, stress, and prenatal nutrition, can make an imprint on genes passed from one generation to the next. These marks do not change the DNA, but rather change the DNA's instructions to cells. Epigenetic changes can be inherited (nature) or accumulated (nurture). Tissues have specific patterns of epigenetic modification. The Human Epigenome Project will eventually yield a detailed map of the human epigenome. Discovery of the location and marks will make personalized medicine a possibility. Sometimes, diseases appear to follow a recessive mode of inheritance, in that they skip a generation, but in fact the transmission patterns are due to epigenetic marks on the DNA and are referred to as "transgenerational inheritance" or "horizontal inheritance."

■ Suggested Readings

Angeli S, Lin X, Liu XZ. Genetics of hearing and deafness. *The Anatomical Record, 295,* 1812–1829; 2012

Barnett CP, van Bon BW. Monogenic and chromosomal causes of isolated speech and language impairment. *J Med Genet.* 2015 Nov;52(11):719-29. doi: 10.1136/jmedgenet-2015-103161

Cloud J. Why your DNA isn't your destiny. *Time,* Jan. 6, 2010

HereditaryHearingLoss.www.hereditaryhearingloss.org

HumanGenomeProjectInformation.www.genomics.energy.gov

Keats B. Genetics and hearing loss. *The ASHA Leader, 10,* 6–18; 2006

Mercer D, Tsien F. Genetics of Auditory Disorders. www.asha.org/Articles/Genetics-of-Auditory-Disorders/

National Human Genome Institute. Talking Glossary of Genetic Terms. www.genome.gov/glossary/

On-line Mendelian Inheritance in Man. www.ncbi
.nlm.nih.gov/omim

Peter B. The future of genetics at our doorstep. *The
ASHA Leader, 17,* 16–19; 2012

Raskind WH, Peter B, Richards T, Eckert, Barninger
VW. The genetics of reading disabilities: from
phenotypes to candidate genes. *Frontiers in
Psychology, 3,* Article 601; 2013

Read A, Donnai D. New Clinical Genetics. 3rd ed.
Banbury, UK: Scion Publishing Limited; 2015

Shprintzen R. Syndrome Identification for Speech-
Language Pathologists. San Diego, CA: Singular
Publishing; 2000

■ References

Bunton K, Leddy M. An evaluation of articulatory
working space area in vowel production of
adults with Down syndrome. *Clinical Linguistics
& Phonetics, 25,* 321–334; 2011

Kent RD, Vorperian HK. Speech impairment in
Down syndrome: A review. *Journal of Speech,
Language, and Hearing Research, 56*(1), 178–
210; 2013

Morgan A, Fisher SE, Scheffer I, Hildebrand M.
FOXP2-related speech and language disorders.
GeneReviews; 2017. https://www.ncbi.nlm.nih.
gov/books/NBK368474/

■ Study Questions

1. Which of the following statements is true about
the autosomal dominant mode of inheritance?

A. It skips a generation.
B. It affects only males.
C. It demonstrates vertical transmission.
D. A child of an affected parent has a 1 in 4
chance of being affected.
E. None of these choices is correct.

2. Which of the following statements is true about
an X-linked dominant trait?

A. Vertical transmission.
B. All sons of an affected father will be affected.
C. All daughters of an affected mother will be
affected.
D. Horizontal transmission.
E. All of these choices are correct.

3. A complex human trait implies that

A. A single gene is responsible for the majority of
disorders.
B. No single gene is responsible for the majority
of disorders.
C. There are no environmental contributions to
the disorder.
D. Genes that influence the trait are difficult to find.
E. None of these choices is correct.

4. All of the following statements are true
concerning parent-of-origin effects, *except*:

A. Parent-of-origin effects are also called imprinting.
B. The phenotype differs depending on whether
the gene comes from the father or the mother.
C. Down's syndrome is an example of a disorder
with parent-of-origin effects.
D. Imprinted genes may affect cognitive and
neurodevelopmental processes.
E. Some genetic syndromes result from mutated
imprinted genes.

5. The central dogma of genetics states:

A. DNA is transcribed into RNA and RNA is then
translated into protein.
B. DNA is translated into RNA and RNA is then
transcribed into protein.
C. RNA is transcribed into DNA and DNA is then
translated into protein.
D. RNA is translated into DNA and DNA is then
transcribed into protein.
E. All heritable changes in gene activity involve
changes in the genetic code.

6. Which statement is *not* true about the process
of translation?

A. The ribosomes move along the mRNA
molecule reading codons.
B. Different triplets of nucleotides may code for
the same amino acid.
C. Changes in one nucleotide base may result in
the coding of a different amino acid.
D. As the ribosome moves along the mRNA, it
creates a polypeptide chain.
E. Translation takes place in the nucleus of the cell.

7. A genetic counselor's role is to:

A. Interpret genetic tests and findings.
B. Make decisions about treatments.
C. Identify risk factors within a family for having
a child with a genetic condition.
D. Provide support to the family.
E. All of these choices are correct.

8. The process of protein degradation is significant because:

A. Misfolded and damaged proteins are removed from circulation.
B. It serves to regulate cellular metabolism.
C. Amino acids are recycled.
D. It keeps the production of proteins active.
E. All of these choices are correct.

9. Which of the following statements is *not* true about gene expression?

A. Gene expression involves transcription and translation.
B. RNA is a product of gene expression.
C. The same amount of gene product is found in all cells of the body.
D. Different tissues and organs result from differences in gene expression.
E. Some genes may produce only RNA when expressed.

10. Which is *not* true about the process of recombination?

A. Recombination occurs during meiosis.
B. Recombination results in different genetic combinations from the parents.
C. Nonhomologous regions of the chromosome may cross over without the risk of losing function.
D. Recombination is a frequent occurrence during gamete production.
E. Recombination may occur without loss of function.

11. Suppose a family with apraxia of speech undergoes genetic testing, including the child and his two parents. The child has a novel mutation (one allele) in a gene, and neither parent carries that mutation. Which of the following are possible explanations?

A. It is a mutation that arose in this child "de novo."
B. The child is adopted; therefore, we should not expect to see inheritance.
C. The father is not related to the child (nonpaternity).
D. All of the above.
E. None of the above.

12. What is *not* true about drawing a pedigree diagram?

A. Squares represent boys; circles represent girls.
B. As many people as possible should be included.
C. Shading indicates the individual is not affected by a disorder.
D. Arrows point to the proband.
E. Disorders presenting in the proband are noted on the pedigree even if they appear unrelated to the trait of interest.

13. Which of the following is *not* true about penetrance and expressivity?

A. Variable expressivity means that people with the same genotype may have different severity of the disease.
B. Penetrance means that there is a probability of having disease associated with each genotype.
C. If a disease is incompletely penetrant, it may appear to skip a generation.
D. In variable expressivity, the gene expression patterns (RNA levels) may differ between subjects.
E. An individual's genotype and environment are both responsible for variable expressivity.

14. What is a generic term for "disorder" when discussing genetics?

A. Trait
B. Genotype
C. Phenotype
D. (A) and (C)
E. None of the above

15. On which of the following chromosomes are sex-linked traits carried?

A. Chromosome 2
B. Chromosome 6
C. Chromosome 15
D. Chromosome 21
E. X chromosome

16. A person who has two copies of the same allele is:

A. Hemizygous
B. Homozygous
C. Heterozygous
D. Homologous
E. None of the above

17. Which statement is *not* true about the GINA laws:

A. GINA stands for Genetic Information Nondiscrimination Act.

B. GINA prohibits health insurers or employers from denying insurance or employment based on genetic information.

C. Employers with fewer than 15 employees are exempt from the GINA laws.

D. GINA does not apply to life insurance.

E. None of the above.

18. The discovery of the *FOXP2* gene mutation in the KE family is important because:

A. The *FOXP2* mutation is found in most individuals with speech and language disorders.

B. It demonstrates how a rare mutation in a family may cause speech delay.

C. FOXP2 is a brain-expressed transcription factor that affects brain development.

D. (A) and (B)

E. (B) and (C)

19. What statement(s) is (are) true about polymorphisms?

A. Polymorphisms are naturally occurring variations in the DNA.

B. Rare variants are polymorphisms that occur in < 1% of the population.

C. An SNP is a single-nucleotide polymorphism.

D. All of the above.

E. None of the above.

20. What is *not* an ethical concern about genetic testing?

A. An individual's genetic information may not be kept confidential.

B. An individual may be discriminated against if he/she carries a genetic disease.

C. Genetic testing may reveal nonpaternity.

D. A parent may decide to have a child tested for genetic disease before the age of 18.

E. None of the above.

■ Answers to Study Questions

1. The correct answer is (C). An autosomal dominant mode of transmission means that the trait will be expressed each time it is transmitted and therefore it does not skip a generation (A). Since it is autosomal (not X- or Y-linked), males and females are equally affected (B). A child of an affected parent has a 1 in 2 chance of being affected (D), since the affected parent has at least one allele with the dominant gene.

2. The correct answer is (A). An X-linked dominant trait demonstrates vertical transmission similar to an autosomal dominant trait. If the father is affected, he will transmit the trait to daughters and not sons (B), since the father contributes an X chromosome to his daughters but a Y chromosome to his sons. Daughters of an affected mother have a 1 in 2 chance of being affected if the mother is heterozygous (C). There is no such thing as horizontal transmission (D).

3. The correct answer is (B). A complex human trait means that no single gene is responsible for the disorder (A). Environmental factors may influence the expression of the gene (C). Genes have been identified for many complex human traits, such as speech and language disorders (D).

4. The correct answer is (C). Down's syndrome results from nondisjunction of chromosome 21. All other answer choices are true statements.

5. The correct answer is (A). DNA is transcribed into RNA; it is not translated into RNA (B), translated into protein (C), or transcribed into protein (D). Similarly, RNA is translated into protein; it is not transcribed into protein (B) or into DNA (C) or translated into DNA (D). Therefore, the central dogma of genetics states that DNA is transcribed into RNA and RNA is then translated into protein. Finally, epigenetics demonstrates that not all heritable changes in gene activity involve changes in the genetic code (E).

6. The correct answer is (E). Translation takes place in the cytoplasm of the cell. The other four statements accurately describe the process of translation.

7. The correct answer is (E). All of these activities are within the genetic counselor's scope of practice.

8. The correct answer is (E). Protein degradation performs all of the above functions.

9. The correct answer is (C). Various types of cells differ in the amount of gene product. All of the other answer choices are true statements.

10. The correct answer is (C). Only homologous regions of the chromosome can cross over without base pairs being lost or added, preserving function. All of the other answer choices are true statements.

11. The correct answer is (D). If the child has only one copy of an allele, he inherited it from one parent. In some family studies, nonpaternity and adoption are not reported. If the child is not biologically related to the parents, he could carry alleles that neither parent carries. Said another way, inheritance of alleles from parent to child would not be observed. However, sometimes mutations occur during DNA synthesis, which is another possible explanation. These situations must be handled carefully and with a genetic counselor.

12. The correct answer is (C). Shading indicates that the individual *is* affected by the disorder. The other answer choices are true statements.

13. The correct answer is (D). Variable expressivity is a concept that refers to the relationship between genotype (at the DNA level) and phenotype. It means that individuals with the same genotype may have different manifestations of the phenotype, whether it be in severity or clinical symptoms. It has nothing to do with RNA expression. The other answer choices are true statements.

14. The correct answer is (D). Trait (A) and phenotype (C) are used interchangeably in genetics, and disorders are specific examples of traits. Traits and phenotypes may include other things that are not disorders, such as hair color. The other answer choices are not correct.

15. The correct answer is (E). Sex-linked traits are carried on the X chromosome. Numbered chromosomes (A through D) are called autosomes.

16. The correct answer is (B). None of the other answer choices is correct.

17. The correct answer is (E). All are true.

18. The correct answer is (E). Answer (A) is not a true statement.

19. The correct answer is (D). Statements (A), (B), and (C) are all true.

20. The correct answer is (E). All of the statements are ethical concerns about genetic testing.

4

Embryology and Development of the Speech and Hearing Mechanism

Steven L. Goudy and Christen Lennon

■ Chapter Summary

Language and communication separate humans from other species on our planet. From fertilization to birth, to the first word, to the first public speech, the ability to communicate using speech and language makes us uniquely human. The study of embryology is essential to the understanding of the embryonic development of the brain, spinal cord, face, nose, mouth, teeth, tongue, larynx, respiratory system, and inner and outer ears and development of the speech and hearing mechanism. This chapter explores the initiation of life through mitosis and meiosis, fertilization, and early embryonic development. The purpose of this chapter is to set the stage for the study of embryology and development of the structures supporting speech, language, swallowing, hearing, and balance. Specifically, the chapter (1) describes the stages of development that support structure and function of the mechanisms involved in speech, language, swallowing, hearing, balance, and related functions, (2) introduces anatomic variants of development in addition to syndromes relevant to aspects of the development of speech, language, swallowing, hearing, and balance, and (3) provides an overview of clinical disorders and anatomic variants relevant to the practice of speech-language pathology and audiology, including branchial cleft anomalies, facial and orofacial clefts, choanal atresia, cleft palate, lingual and labial ties, and aural atresia.

■ Learning Objectives

- Understand the general stages of embryologic development
- Describe development of the laryngeal and respiratory systems, tongue, teeth, and inner and outer ear
- Understand the development of the nervous system and how its various components interact to produce speech and language
- Describe lip and palate development and understand how facial clefts form

■ Putting It Into Practice

- Speech-language pathologists and audiologists should be familiar with normal development of the speech and hearing mechanism.
- The study of embryology is critically important to provide an understanding of typical and atypical development of the anatomical structures involved in speech, language, swallowing, hearing, and balance.
- Speech-language pathologists and audiologists often work on multidisciplinary teams of specialists involved in the assessment and treatment of individuals with congenital abnormalities, such as cleft lip and palate and aural atresia.

■ Introduction

An understanding of embryology and the development of the mechanisms involved in speech, language, swallowing, hearing, and balance is critical to fully appreciating the complex anatomical and physiologic relationships among structures of the head and neck. In order to comprehend development, production, processing, and comprehension of speech, it is necessary to understand not only the pathways underlying speech production, but also how auditory stimuli are transmitted and processed. In that regard, speech-language pathologists and audiologists must be able to synthesize the study of embryology with the overall understanding of human body function, or physiology. This chapter discusses the processes involved in fertilization, gastrulation, and development of the structures supporting speech, language, swallowing, hearing, and balance.

■ Mitosis and Cell Division

Mammalian cells divide through a process called **mitosis,** a form of asexual reproduction where the parent cell divides into two equal parts. For successful reproduction, mitosis must meet the challenge of maintaining the same amounts of genetic material in the daughter cells as in the parent cells.

Replication of genetic material is manageable for the cell due to structures called **chromosomes,** which package DNA molecules. Every species has a characteristic number of chromosomes in each cell nucleus of parent cells. In humans, this number is 23. Therefore, the nuclei of human somatic cells (all body cells except the reproductive cells) each contain 46 chromosomes, with one set of 23 chromosomes from each parent. As the cells mature and die, they must be replaced in order for the entire organism to continue to thrive. A more comprehensive overview of genetics is provided in **Chapter 3**.

Duplication of genes and chromosomes is the first step in the division of the cell (cell cycle). Once this is accomplished, division of the cytoplasm and reconstruction of the nuclei can take place. The result is two cells, each identical in genetic characteristics. The stages of the cell cycle are divided into interphase, prophase, metaphase, anaphase, and telophase, as shown in **Fig. 4.1.**

Interphase accounts for about 90% of the cell cycle. During this phase, the cell grows and copies its chromosomes in preparation for cell division. The chromosomes cannot be seen individually because they have not yet condensed. They are contained within the nucleus and are bound by the nuclear envelope. In the cytoplasm, two centrosomes are present. Centrosomes are organelles that serve as the main microtubule organizing center of the cell. They also play a role in cell-cycle progression. Cen-

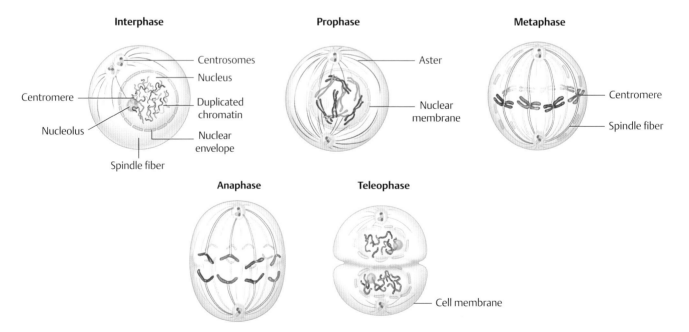

Fig. 4.1 Schematic representation of the five phases of mitotic cell division. Interphase is a resting phase where chromosomes are copied in preparation for cell division. Prophase is the first stage of mitosis, when the nucleoli disappear and chromosomes condense. In metaphase, the nuclear envelope breaks down, the chromosomes attach to the microtubules of the mitotic spindle, and the microtubules align the chromosomes on the metaphase plate. Anaphase is characterized by the splitting of chromosomes and migration of sister chromatids to opposite poles of the cell. Finally, in telophase, the nuclear envelopes form and cytokinesis occurs.

trosomes each contain a pair of centrioles, which are sets of microtubules arranged in a cylinder.

Prophase is the first phase of mitosis. The chromosomes begin to condense; each duplicated chromosome appears as two long, thin threads joined together. These threads are called sister chromatids. In addition, the nucleoli, which are concentrations of DNA within the nucleus, diminish in size and eventually disappear. The mitotic spindle, composed of two centrosomes and microtubules extending between them, begins to form. This apparatus forms scaffolding over which chromosomes are pulled throughout mitosis.

Metaphase is the longest stage of mitosis. It begins with fragmentation of the nuclear envelope, which exposes the sister chromatids to the microtubules of the spindle. Each of the two chromatids of a chromosome has a kinetochore, a specialized protein structure located at the region joining the two sister chromatids, called the centromere, which enables attachment to a microtubule. Once attached, the microtubules align the chromosomes on the metaphase plate, which is an imaginary plane that is equidistant between the two poles at either end of the cell.

Anaphase is the shortest phase of mitosis, during which the sister chromatids of each pair are pulled apart. Each chromatid then becomes a chromosome once unpaired from its sister chromatid. Chromosomes are pulled by microtubules toward opposite ends of the cell. The cell elongates. At the end of anaphase, the two ends of the cell have equivalent collections of chromosomes.

In **telophase,** a nuclear envelope begins to form around each group of chromosomes. The chromosomes begin to uncoil and become less condensed. Cytokinesis begins, with the division of the cytoplasm by formation of the cleavage furrow, which pinches the cell in two. The result is two cells ready to enter resting phase before the next division is initiated.

■ Early Embryonic Development

Gametogenesis

Survival depends upon the ability to reproduce. In fact, this quality sets living things apart from nonliving matter. All animals reproduce, from single-celled protozoans to complex mammals. To ensure genetic diversity, complex life forms, such as humans, have developed **sexual reproduction**, which involves the union of two sexual germ cells (**gametes**). Two gametes (one male and one female) combine genetic material to form a new cell (**zygote**), which gives rise to a new individual

organism. The new cell is made up of the genetic material from the two parent cells.

In humans, the female germ cell is called an **ovum**, or egg, and the male germ cell is called a **sperm**. The sperm and ovum are the only cells in the human body not produced by mitosis. If they replicated via mitosis, the zygote would have 92 chromosomes, or twice as many chromosomes as needed. To avoid this scenario, the process of **meiosis** reduces the number of sets of chromosomes from the **diploid** number (2n) which is the number found in all body cells, to the **haploid** number (n), the number found in the germ cells. Simply put, this process consists of two nuclear divisions during maturation of the sex cell, with only one division of chromosomes. Before any germ cell is capable of reproduction, the number of chromosomes must be reduced by half.

The process of meiosis differs between **spermatogenesis** for sperm and **oogenesis** for eggs. These processes are outlined in **Fig. 4.2**. Both processes begin with a diploid parent cell. In spermatogenesis, chromosomes replicate and are divided between two separate cells in meiosis I. The two cells each are haploid cells with replicated chromosomes. In the second division, meiosis II, the sister chromatids separate and each cell then divides again, creating haploid cells with unreplicated chromosomes. This process is similar in oogenesis. However, during the first division, the primary oogonium divides

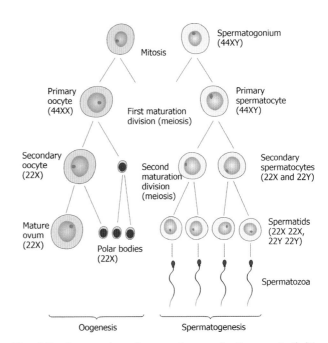

Fig. 4.2 Oogenesis and spermatogenesis. Oogenesis (left) and spermatogenesis (right) are similar processes with important distinctions. Two rounds of meiotic division each produce haploid gametes; however, in spermatogenesis, four gametes are produced, but in oogenesis one gamete and three polar bodies are produced.

meiotically (meiosis I) into a secondary oocyte and a **polar body**, which is a small haploid cell without adequate cytoplasm to support a zygote if fertilized. The cells often die (apoptosis), but the first polar body may divide again to form two polar bodies. During the second division, the secondary oocyte again divides meiotically to form both a second polar body as well as the mature ovum. Thus, for every one parent cell that undergoes meiosis, one egg and three polar bodies are formed. In the case of spermatogenesis, four sperm are produced for each parent cell that undergoes meiosis.

The mature germ cell contains 22 ordinary chromosomes plus one sex chromosome, either the **X chromosome** or the **Y chromosome**. An egg contains 22 chromosomes and an X chromosome. However, sperm may contain 22 chromosomes and either an X chromosome or a Y chromosome. Fertilization of an egg by a sperm with an X chromosome creates the combination XX, which results in a female zygote. Fertilization of an egg by a sperm with a Y chromosome results in the combination XY, creating a male zygote. Thus, the type of sperm that fertilizes the egg determines the sex of the offspring.

Fertilization

During reproduction, millions of sperm are deposited within the female reproductive tract. The sperm travel toward the ovum, but no more than one sperm will successfully fertilize the egg. Secretions in the female reproductive tract increase sperm motility. In humans, this enhancement of sperm function requires about 6 hours of exposure to the female reproductive tract.

The process of fertilization is shown in **Fig. 4.3**. The mammalian egg has an extracellular matrix called the **zona pellucida**, which has receptor molecules that bind to the sperm. This binding induces the acrosomal reaction, in which sperm release hydrolytic enzymes into the zona pellucida to break it down. The binding also triggers a release of enzymes from the egg in cortical granules that alter and harden the zona pellucida in order to prevent the fertilization of an egg by multiple sperm. Once the sperm reaches the plasma membrane of the egg, the sperm membrane fuses with that of the egg, and the nucleus and other components of the sperm cell enter the egg. With fertilization complete, the zygote is formed.

Cleavage

Initial cell division occurs 12 to 36 hours after sperm binding to the oocyte in mammals. This process is shown in **Fig. 4.4**. These divisions parti-

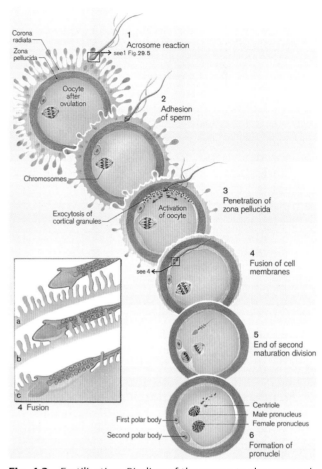

Fig. 4.3 Fertilization. Binding of the sperm to the zona pellucida induces an acrosomal reaction (1) to break down this barrier. Once the sperm adheres (2) and penetrates the zona pellucida (3), it reaches the plasma membrane of the egg. The sperm membrane fuses with that of the egg (4), and the nucleus and other components of the sperm cell enter the egg. As the second meiotic division of the oocyte has ended (5), the pronuclei are then able to form (6).

tion the cytoplasm of the initial zygote into many smaller cells, called **blastomeres**, each with its own nucleus. This process continues until a round mass of about 12 to 16 cells is formed, known as a **morula**. With continued cell division, a fluid-filled cavity called the blastocoele begins to form, creating the **blastocyst**, which is a hollow ball of cells.

A cross-section of a blastocyst, shown in **Fig. 4.5,** reveals an outer layer of cells called a **trophoblast,** which surrounds a cluster of cells called the **inner cell mass**. The inner cell mass will later develop into the embryo and form, or contribute to, all of the extraembryonic membranes.

The trophoblast secretes enzymes that break down the endometrium, or the lining of the uterine cavity. This process allows the blastocyst to invade the endometrium, implanting itself so that the inner cell mass is deepest in the uterine lining.

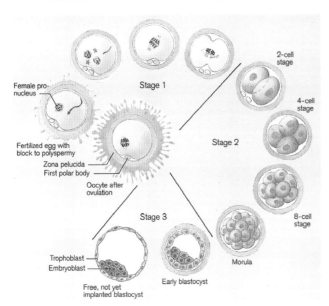

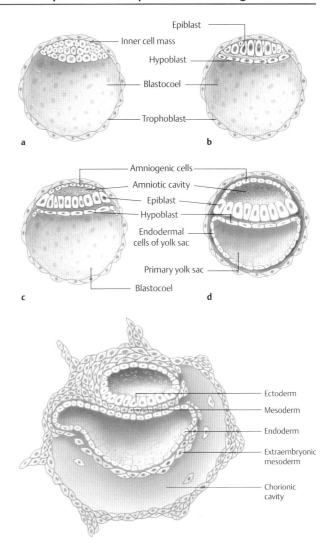

Fig. 4.4   Development of oocyte to blastocyst. The first cell division takes place anywhere from 12 to 36 hours after fertilization (Stage 1). Division of blastomeres (Stage 2) continues until there is a morula, which consists of about 12 to 16 cells. Finally, a blastocoele forms within the cell mass, creating a blastocyst (Stage 3).

Development of the Yolk Sac

Around the time of implantation, the inner cell mass of the blastocyst forms a flat disk with an upper layer of cells, called the **epiblast**, and a lower layer of cells, called the **hypoblast,** as shown in **Fig. 4.6.** The epiblast proliferates and begins to secrete fluid, which creates the **amniotic cavity** covered by the **amniotic membrane**, or **amnion**. Concurrently, the hypoblast proliferates and in part gives rise to the **yolk sac**.

The cells of the inner cell mass begin to move inward from the epiblast through a **primitive streak**, a structure that forms on the surface of the blastula and establishes bilateral symmetry (**Fig. 4.5**). The primitive streak is a temporary structure that gives rise to the mesoderm. Migration of cells of the inner cell mass initiates the process of **gastrulation**, or the creation of three germ layers. The **ectoderm** forms the outer germ layer of the gastrula, the **endoderm** lines the embryonic digestive tract, and the **mesoderm** partly fills the space between the ectoderm and endoderm. These three cell layers will eventually form all of the tissues within the human body.

While the amniotic sac and yolk sac are being formed, cells from the inner surface of the trophoblast proliferate to form a loose network of **extraembryonic mesoderm**, which gives rise to structures supporting embryonic growth but does not contribute to the formation of the embryo. The **chorion**, which completely surrounds the embryo

Fig. 4.5   **(a)** The early amnion and its relation to the inner cell mass and yolk. **(b)** The inner cell mass proliferates and forms the epiblast and hypoblast, shown in. **(c)** A secretion of fluid inside the epiblast is derived from the inner cell mass to create the amniotic cavity. **(d)** At the same time, cells move inward from the epiblast to form mesoderm and endoderm. **(e)** The chorionic cavity develops encircles the extraembryonic mesoderm.

and the other extraembryonic membranes, functions in gas exchange. The **allantois** forms blood vessels that transport oxygen and nutrients from the placenta to the embryo and rid the embryo of carbon dioxide and nitrogenous wastes.

Establishment of Maternal/ Fetal Communication

The endometrium responds to implantation by growing over the blastocyst. During the first two to four weeks of development, the embryo obtains

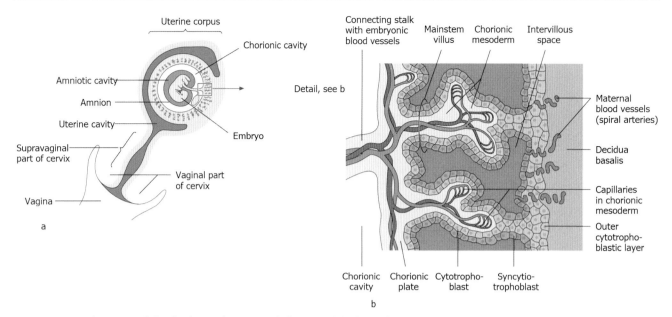

Detail, see b

Fig. 4.6 Development of the fetal membranes and placenta. **(a)** The embryo is immediately surrounded by the amniotic cavity. The chorionic cavity separates the amnion from the chorion. **(b)** The chorionic villi grow into the endometrium. These are separated from the maternal uterine tissue by the cytotrophoblast, which penetrates the maternal spiral arteries. The syncytiotrophoblast conducts maternal-fetal gas and nutrient exchange.

nutrients from the endometrium. As proliferation of the trophoblast continues after implantation, fingerlike processes (**trophoblastic villi**) begin to extend out in all directions from the blastocyst into the endometrium. These villi grow into **chorionic villi** and join with the extraembryonic mesoderm (**Fig. 4.6**).

The villi use two major cell layers in order to facilitate effective implantation in the endometrium. The **cytotrophoblast** is a layer of cells that serves both to anchor the growing fetus to the maternal uterine tissue as well as to penetrate the maternal spiral arteries and route the blood flow through the placenta for the growing embryo to use. The **syncytiotrophoblast** layer plays an important role in maternal–fetal gas exchange, nutrient exchange, and immunologic and metabolic functions.

Villi first develop all over the surface of the blastocyst, but later degenerate, except at the region of the inner cell mass. This restricted area where villi continue to develop is known as the **chorion frondosum**. The extraembryonic mesoderm extends between this area, which remains implanted in the endometrial lining, and the embryonic disc by means of a **body stalk**.

The Primitive Streak and Notochord

While the yolk sac and amnion are being formed, the embryonic disc is beginning to ingress at the primitive streak, as described above. The primi-

tive streak is formed by rapid proliferation of the columnar ectodermal cells in the floor of the amniotic cavity. The ingression of mesoderm progenitors gives rise to both endodermal cells as well as **intraembryonic mesoderm**.

A layer of mesodermal cells begins to grow out laterally from the primitive streak between the ectoderm and endoderm, forming a trilaminar embryonic disc. At one end of the primitive streak (away from body stalk), the mesenchyme condenses and forms an area known as the **notochord**. It defines the primitive axis of the embryo (**Fig. 4.7**). The notochord has a key role in signaling and coordinating development. A postembryonic vestige of the notochord is found in the nucleus pulposus of the intervertebral disks.

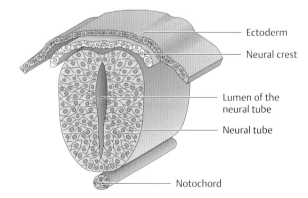

Fig. 4.7 Cross section of the neural tube, neural crest, and notochord during the third week. The notochord is a primitive structure required for signaling to, and patterning, surrounding tissues, including the neural tube.

The intraembryonic mesoderm (notochord) continues its growth cephalically, but it is limited because the ectoderm and endoderm are in such intimate contact at the very cephalad portion that the notochord is unable to separate them. This small area of tightly bound ectoderm and endoderm, called the **prechordal plate**, forms the **buccopharyngeal membrane** (discussed later in this chapter). Below this area of the primitive streak, the intraembryonic mesoderm continues to proliferate and forms an intermediate layer between ectoderm and endoderm. This layer is present everywhere in the body except for the procardiac area, where it is found only at the midline.

Development of the Neural Tube

The notochord signals to the overlying ectoderm, inducing this region of ectoderm to become the **neural plate**. The lateral margins of the neural plate grow upward to form the paraxial **neural folds.** The neural folds develop just behind the rostral end of the embryonic disc, where they are continuous with one another and extend inferiorly (**Fig. 4.8**). Between the neural folds lies the **neural groove**, which deepens as the folds become elevated. Eventually, the neural folds meet at the midline, fuse, and form the neural tube, which is the precursor to the central nervous system (**Fig. 4.9**).

Formation of the Somites

At the beginning of the third week, the mesoderm on either side of the neural tube and notochord, called the paraxial mesoderm, begins to form transversely segmented structures called **somites**. Somites occupy the entire length of the trunk of the embryo and are below the ectoderm. Even in a very early embryo, somites bear a resemblance to the vertebral column in humans, and the vertebrae are adult derivatives of the somites. However, human somites give rise to virtually all connective, muscular, and dermal tissue (except in the head), in addition to the vertebrae. Somite derivatives during weeks 4 to 8 are shown in **Fig. 4.10**.

The first pair of somites appears around the sixteenth day after fertilization; there are 3 occipital, 8 cervical, 12 thoracic, 5 lumbar, and about 5 coccygeal somites. The occipital and coccygeal somites dedifferentiate and disappear, so they seem to have a transitory role. The remaining somites differentiate into three cell groups: **sclerotomes**, **myotomes**, and **dermatomes**.

Sclerotomes are formed from the most medial region of a somite. The cells migrate to surround the notochord and neural tube. Their migration dorsally around the neural tube forms the vertebral arch, and the lower half of one sclerotome fuses with the upper half of the adjacent sclerotome to form each vertebral body. Eventually, sclerotomes give rise to the individual vertebral bodies, the intervertebral disks, the ribs, and part of the occipital bone.

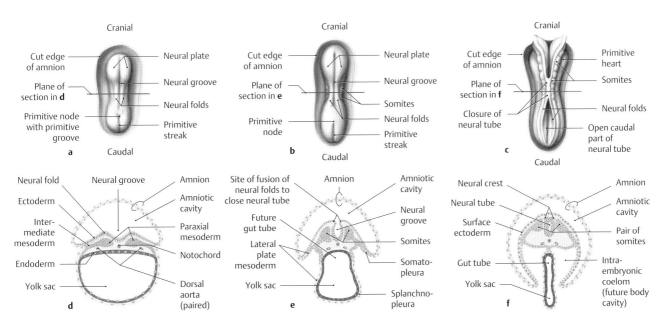

Fig. 4.8 Neurulation. Embryonic disc at 19 days, dorsal view after removal of the amnion **(a)** and schematic cross section **(d)** of plane of section in **(a)**. Embryonic disc at 20 days, dorsal view after removal of the amnion **(b)** and schematic cross section **(e)** of plane of section in **(a)**. Embryonic disc at 22 days, dorsal view after removal of the amnion **(c)**, and schematic cross section **(f)** of plane of section in **(c)**.

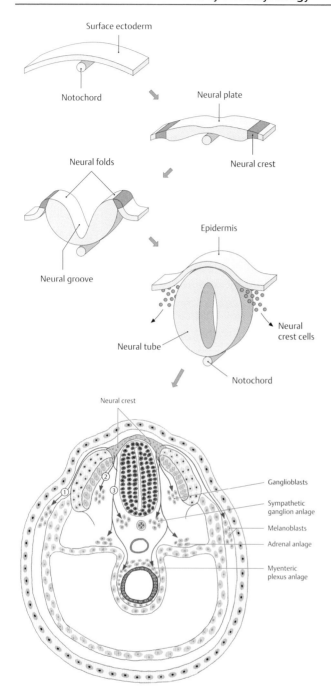

Fig. 4.9 Neural tube formation and neural crest migration. The infolding of the neural plate to create the neural groove and neural tube enable neural crest cells to begin their migration. These cells migrate to multiple levels of the body and give rise to a diverse cell lineage.

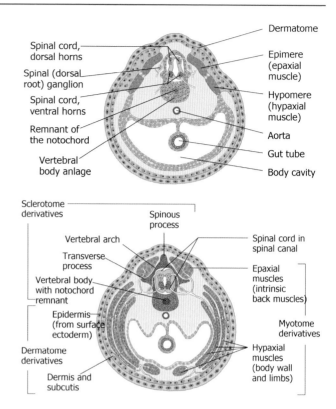

Fig. 4.10 Formation of the somites and sclerotome, myotome, and dermatome derivatives. Sclerotomes form the vertebral arch, myotomes the muscles of the trunk, and dermatomes the skin, fat, and connective tissue of the neck and trunk.

Myotomes are located immediately lateral to the sclerotome. These cells become elongated and spindle-shaped, and they will eventually give rise to the muscles of the trunk. Each myotome is divided into an epaxial region dorsal to the vertebrae and a hypaxial region ventral to the vertebrae. Myoblasts from the hypaxial division form the muscles of the thoracic and anterior abdominal walls. The epaxial

muscles form the extensor muscles of the neck and trunk.

The anatomical innervation path of each muscle indicates that the muscle has a similar embryonic origin and migratory path. For example, the phrenic nerve supplies the diaphragm with motor fibers and emerges from the fourth and fifth cervical nerves of the embryo. In a flexed embryo, this course is rather straightforward. However, as the embryo grows, the course is extended, yielding a much longer course from the neck to the diaphragm in an adult. Facial muscles, which are branchiomeric in origin, exhibit similar migratory trends.

Furthermore, an original single primordial muscle mass may split longitudinally into two or more muscle masses. The sternocleidomastoid and trapezius muscles provide examples of such a split. These muscles stem from the same primordial muscle mass, which explains why they are innervated by the same nerve: the accessory nerve (CN XI).

Conversely, certain portions of successive myotomes may fuse to form a single muscle. An example of fusion is the digastric muscle, which has both an anterior and a posterior belly. The posterior belly is innervated by the digastric branch of the facial nerve (CN VII), and the anterior belly is innervated by the mylohyoid branch of the trigeminal nerve (CN V). Innervation differs due to the varying embryologic origin of each belly, although they are fused to form a single muscle.

Finally, degeneration of portions of muscle or an entire muscle segment may occur. In this case, the muscle tends to convert into connective tissue. Many aponeurotic sheets in the body can be attributed to muscle degeneration. Examples are the abdominal aponeuroses as well as the galea aponeurotica that connects the occipitalis and frontalis muscles.

Dermatomes are formed from the most lateral portion of a somite and develop into skin, fat, and connective tissues of the neck and trunk. Most of the skin, however, is derived from a specific portion of the mesoderm: the lateral plate mesoderm.

Division of Intraembryonic Mesoderm

During the latter part of the third week, the embryo begins flexing as intraembryonic structures begin growing too rapidly to be maintained in a straight position. This brings both the buccopharyngeal membrane and the developing heart ventral to the neural plate. In order to accommodate this flexion, the intraembryonic mesoderm divides into three parts: the paraxial mesoderm alongside the notochord (which divides into the somites), the intermediate mesoderm, and the lateral plate mesoderm.

The lateral plate mesoderm divides into two layers. The upper layer of the lateral plate mesoderm, called the somatopleuric intraembryonic mesoderm, is in contact with the ectoderm of the dorsum of the embryo and forms the body wall. The lower layer of the lateral plate mesoderm, called the splanchnopleuric intraembryonic mesoderm, is in contact with the endoderm and forms the circulatory system. This division, in turn, produces a cavity called the intraembryonic coelom, which subsequently divides into the pericardial, pleural, and peritoneal cavities in the developing embryo.

■ Development of the Nervous System

Introduction

The development of the nervous system spans the embryonic period and completes after birth. The nervous system is the most complex system in the human body. For these reasons, insults during gestation can have consequences for development, and understanding the origins of the nervous system as well as its complex functions in the context of speech and hearing is critical.

The early central nervous system begins as an invagination from the primitive streak, and the neural folds join to form the neural tube. Within the neural tube, stem cells generate two major classes of cells that contribute to the nervous system: neurons and glia. Differentiation of cells of the nervous system, as well as the establishment of cellular populations and networks establishing the layered structure seen in the brain and spinal cord, are complex and interdependent, and any alteration to the process can lead to significant neural dysfunction.

Fusion of the Neural Folds

Fusion of the neural folds is a complex process that begins rostrally in the region of the future hindbrain and extends both rostrally and caudally. As the embryo grows in the caudal direction, the neural groove and folds grow concurrently. The rostral opening of the neural tube, the **anterior neuropore**, seals off at about the 20-somite stage. The open caudal end of the neural tube, the **posterior neuropore**, closes off at about the 25-somite stage (**Fig. 4.8**).

Prior to fusion of the neural folds, a ridge of ectodermal cells, which gives rise to neural crest cells, appears just lateral to each fold. Neural crest cells give rise to spinal and cranial nerve ganglia and the ganglia of the sympathetic trunk of the autonomic nervous system. Migration of neural crest cells between the ectoderm and mesoderm in the head region begins before the neural tube closes. Neural crest cells migrate between the ectoderm and mesoderm. The cells that migrate the most ventrally contribute to the pharyngeal arches. The remaining head and neck neural crest cells are associated primarily with mid- and hindbrain development. Midbrain neural crest cells move around the developing eye into the region around the forebrain and behind the eye, into the first pharyngeal arch. Hindbrain neural crest cells contribute to the remainder of the pharyngeal arches. Other contributions of the neural crest cells include the meninges, ganglia, and the nasal placode and nose. The migratory pathways of the neural crest cells are shown in **Fig. 4.9**.

The cephalic neural crest cells that contribute to the third, fourth, and sixth pharyngeal arches may also migrate beyond their respective arches into the area of the developing heart. These cells contribute to the initial development of the truncoconal septum, which is responsible for the separation of arterial outflow. In fact, since the cephalic, and not truncal, neural crest has the ability to form mesenchyme (embryonic connective tissue), these cells are imperative for the development of the truncoconal septum. Therefore, failure of migration of cephalic neural crest cells may result in problems affecting both structures derived from pharyngeal arches as well as the heart. Many syndromes have combinations of craniofacial and cardiac malformations; this connection is due to the commonality of neural crest cells (e.g., DiGeorge's syndrome).

Differentiation of Primitive Medullary Cells

At the time of formation, the wall of the neural tube is composed of a single layer of columnar ectodermal cells with the nuclei located toward the lumen end of the cell. These cells are known as the primitive medullary epithelial cells, from which most of the cells in the nervous system are derived.

Medulloblast formation within the neural tube is characterized by clustering of the cytoplasm and nuclei toward the lumen side of the neural tube. These cells form either the neuroepithelial lining of the neural tube or **glioblasts**. Glioblasts differentiate into astrocytes and **oligodendrocytes**, the glia of the central nervous system. Glia connect throughout development to form a network of supportive fibers throughout the spinal cord and brain, providing metabolic and structural support to the neurons of the central nervous system.

Oligodendrocytes are unique in that they are responsible for the formation of **myelin** around the nerve fibers of cells in the brain and spinal cord. Myelin is a white, fatty substance that surrounds nerve fibers (**axons**) and insulates and therefore promotes conduction of neuronal signal. It does not appear until the nerve processes are well developed.

Differentiation of the Neural Tube

The central canal of the neural tube takes on an oblong shape, with a small concavity in the central region, and effectively divides the lateral walls of the neural tube into ventral and dorsal zones (basal and alar laminae, respectively). Cells of the basal lamina become involved in motor function (efferent), and cells of the alar lamina become sensory (afferent). Neuroblasts in the basal lamina send out extensions that course toward the periphery as motor nerve fibers and eventually form the ventral (motor) roots of the spinal nerves. The division of

the spinal cord as well as projection of spinal nerves are shown in **Fig. 4.10**.

Zones of the Neural Tube

Due to proliferation and differentiation of the cells of the lateral walls of the neural tube, three layers or zones are defined: an internal (ependymal) zone, an intermediate (mantle) zone, and an external (marginal) zone. The ependymal zone gives rise to epithelial-like lining of the central canal of the spinal cord and ventricular system of the brain. The mantle zone is composed of neuroglia and neuroblasts, and this area eventually makes up the gray matter (i.e., cell bodies) of the spinal cord. The marginal zone is outside the mantle zone and is relatively free of developing nerve cells. However, processes from the mantle zone eventually extend into this zone and become the white matter (i.e., axons and myelin) of the spinal cord.

As proliferation continues within the neural tube, the central canal narrows. Furthermore, local proliferation in the mantle zone results in four clusters of cell bodies, or gray matter, on each side that run the length of the spinal cord. Dorsally, there are two columns of somatic and visceral afferent (sensory) nerve bodies. Ventrally, there is a somatic efferent column as well as a visceral efferent column. The somatic nervous system is the part of the nervous system associated with voluntary skeletal muscle. The visceral nervous system is the part of the nervous system associated with involuntary control of internal organs.

Development of the Spinal Cord

The differential arrangement of neuroblasts in the spinal cord leads to the general organization of the spinal cord nerves in the adult. The cells of the ventral columns become the somatic motor neurons of the spinal cord and innervate somatic motor structures, such as the voluntary (striated) muscles of the extremities. The cells of the dorsal columns develop into association neurons, which receive synapses from afferent fibers from the sensory neurons of the dorsal root ganglia. The efferent motor neuron fibers exit via the ventral roots. As a rule, the dorsal spinal root is involved in sensory function and the ventral spinal root is involved in motor function. This basic division, often called Bell's law, is restricted to the spinal cord and part of the brainstem and does not apply to the cephalic portion of the neural tube, which develops into the brain.

The embryonic spinal cord develops periodic regions of intensified proliferation. Each segment is called a **neuromere** and is located at intervals that correspond with somites. Each neuromere supplies a defined segment of the body, with the ventral root ganglion supplying muscles from the somatic myomeres that lie in close proximity to the developing neuromeres. The spinal cord is covered in greater detail in **Chapter 5.**

Development of the Brain

The rostral portion of the neural tube begins to enlarge and differentiate before the neuropores close. Three dilations of the neural tube develop: **prosencephalon**, **mesencephalon**, and **rhombencephalon**. These dilations are known as the primary brain vesicles. Shortly after these initial dilations appear, the prosencephalon develops diverticula on either side at its cephalic extreme to form the **telencephalon**. The remainder of the prosencephalon is known as the **diencephalon**.

Due to unequal growth of these various segments, the developing brain begins folding and forming flexures (**Fig. 4.11**). The first flexure, the **cephalic flexure**, occurs in the midbrain region. A sharp U-shaped bend forms ventrally, causing the midbrain to protrude dorsally. At about the same time, the **cervical flexure** appears at the junction of the brain and the spinal cord, so that the hindbrain and spinal cord are located at a right angle

to one another. However, as the entire head flexes ventrally and the body grows, this flexion gradually disappears. Finally, the **pontine flexure** also forms, although this structure also straightens with body growth.

During the flexure stage, the mesencephalon remains relatively unchanged; however, the rhombencephalon differentiates into the metencephalon (cephalic portion) and the myelencephalon (caudal portion). The myelencephalon gives rise to the medulla oblongata, which is the most caudal portion of the brainstem. The early medulla oblongata is characterized by a roofplate and floorplate. The roofplate is nonnervous in its structure, and a vascular mesenchyme (the pia mater) known as the tela choroidea is located on the ependymal roof. The tela choroidea forms the **choroid plexus** of the fourth ventricle, which is responsible for the formation of cerebrospinal fluid. Localized resorption of the roofplate results in paired lateral apertures (foramina of Luschka) and a medial aperture (foramen of Magendie) that permit communication with the subarachnoid space.

Sensory fibers from the facial (CN VII), glossopharyngeal (CN IX), and vagus (CN X) nerves grow from their respective neural crest ganglia into the alar lamina of the medulla to form the **solitary tract** in the marginal zone. This tract contains primary visceral afferent (sensory) fibers. The olivary nuclei are also derivatives of the alar lamina of the

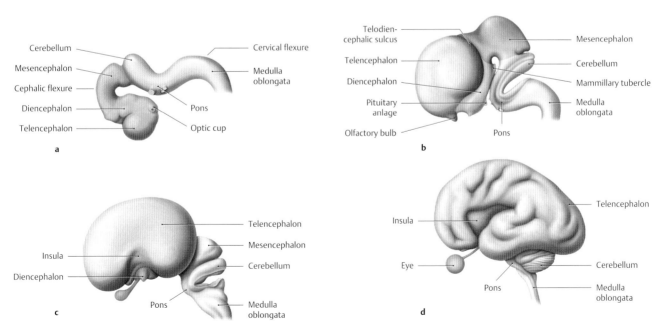

Fig. 4.11 Development of the brain. **(a)** The neural tube differentiates into the telencephalon (red), diencephalon (yellow), mesencephalon (dark blue), cerebellum (light blue), and pons and medulla oblongata (gray) at the beginning of the second month of development. **(b)** At the end of the second month, the cephalic and cervical flexures become more pronounced and the telencephalon grows over the diencephalon. **(c)** The fetal brain during the third month of development. **(d)** In the seventh month of development, the fetal brain greatly resembles the developed brain.

medulla. They arise from cells that migrate from the alar lamina into the basal lamina.

The basal lamina of the myelencephalon differentiates slightly earlier than does the alar lamina. Basal lamina neuroblasts give rise to the motor nuclei of origin for certain cranial nerves. Laterally, the nucleus ambiguus forms, from which the glossopharyngeal (CN IX), vagus (CN X), and accessory (CN XI) nerves acquire their special visceral efferent (motor) fibers that supply muscles of the branchial arch derivatives.

The **metencephalon** is a part of the hindbrain and is located superior to the myelencephalon and inferior to the mesencephalon. The cephalic border is the isthmus and the caudal border is the pontine flexure. The metencephalon gives rise to the **pons** and **cerebellum**. The function of the cerebellum is to coordinate and regulate muscle activity. The pons is part of the brainstem and lies between the midbrain (superior) and the medulla oblongata (inferior) and anterior to the cerebellum. It contains white matter tracts as well as nuclei that relay signals from the forebrain to the cerebellum, along with nuclei that deal primarily with sleep, respiration, swallowing, bladder control, hearing, equilibrium, taste, eye movement, facial expressions, facial sensation, and posture.

The alar lamina of the metencephalon develops sensory relay nuclei for the trigeminal (CN V), facial (CN VII), and vestibulocochlear (CN VIII) nerves. It also contributes to the development of the cerebellum and cerebellar peduncles. The peduncles are three pairs of stalks that connect the cerebellum with other parts of the brain. The basal lamina of the metencephalon differentiates into motor nuclei of origin for the trigeminal (CN V), abducens (CN VI), and facial (CN VII) nerves.

The mesencephalon, or midbrain, is associated with vision, hearing, motor control, sleep/wake, arousal (alertness), and temperature regulation. The cavity of the mesencephalon constricts to form the **cerebral aqueduct**, which establishes a communication between the third and fourth ventricles. Neuroblasts near the aqueduct (from the basal lamina) develop into motor nuclei for the oculomotor (CN III) and trochlear (CN IV) nerves. The region dorsal to the cerebral aqueduct forms the tectum, and the region ventral to the aqueduct forms the tegmentum. The tegmentum develops two prominent nuclei: the red nucleus (nucleus ruber) and the black nucleus (**substantia nigra**). The red nucleus is involved in motor coordination, and the substantia nigra plays an important role in reward, addiction, and movement.

Thickening of the tectum on either side of the midline creates the **superior** and **inferior colliculi**.

The superior colliculus is associated with vision, and the inferior colliculus constitutes the principal midbrain nucleus of the auditory pathway. The inferior colliculus receives input from several peripheral brainstem nuclei in the auditory pathway as well as input from the auditory cortex in the temporal lobe. Auditory fibers course from the inferior to the superior colliculus, paving the way for auditory-visual reflexive responses.

The prosencephalon is divided into the diencephalon and the telencephalon. The diencephalon is the most caudal part of the forebrain and develops into the epithalamus, the thalamus, the hypothalamus, and the third ventricle. The cavity of the diencephalon forms the third ventricle, with its roofplate also forming a choroid plexus.

The remainder of the diencephalon derives from the alar lamina. The **epithalamus** is the most dorsal structure. Its function includes regulation of the secretion of metatonin (a hormone similar to melatonin) by the pineal body and regulation of motor pathways and emotions. The pineal body is a small endocrine gland in the brain that produces melatonin and thus affects modulation of sleep patterns in both seasonal and circadian rhythms.

The **thalamus** is a symmetrical structure made up of gray matter, with its medial surfaces constituting the upper part of the lateral walls of the third ventricle. The two halves of the thalamus are connected across the third ventricle by a band of gray matter called the interthalamic adhesion. The thalamus is the principal avenue by which all impulses from cutaneous, visual, and auditory senses are relayed to the cerebral cortex.

The **hypothalamus** is located below the thalamus, just above the midbrain, and is part of the limbic system. It forms the ventral aspect of the diencephalon. This brain structure is made up of nuclei, many of which communicate with the pituitary gland.

The axons of the paraventricular nucleus and the supraoptic nucleus of the hypothalmus contain oxytocin and vasopressin and project into the posterior pituitary gland. Other cells in the paraventricular nucleus release corticotropin-releasing hormone as well as other hormones of the hypophyseal portal system, through which the hormones diffuse to the anterior pituitary gland.

The telencephalon gives rise to the mature cerebrum and basal ganglia. Initially, the walls of the hemispheres remain the primitive neural tube, with ependymal, mantle, and marginal zones. However, during the third month of development, neuroblasts migrate to the periphery from the mantle and ependymal zones. These cells collect in the deeper layer of the marginal zone, forming the outer layer or **gray matter** of the cerebral cortex. The processes of the cells project toward the depths of the brain to form the **white matter**, which appears white due to myelination.

Cerebral hemispheres grow rapidly until, by the fifth month of development, they overgrow the diencephalon, mesencephalon, and part of the cerebellum. The rostral border of the neural tube does not expand, and remains relatively stable in its position. This portion forms the **lamina terminalis**, and as the hemispheres expand forward on either side, the lamina terminalis is eventually positioned at the bottom of the deep longitudinal fissure.

The cerebral hemispheres are divided into three functionally distinct parts, known as the **rhinencephalon**, the **corpus striatum**, and the white matter. The rhinencephalon is the part of the brain involved with olfaction and includes the olfactory bulb, olfactory tract, anterior olfactory nucleus, anterior perforated substance, medial olfactory stria, lateral olfactory stria, parts of the amygdala, and prepiriform area. The **archipallium,** a component of the primitive cortex, is included in the rhinencephalon. Part of the archipallium enlarges to form the olfactory lobes. This enlargement occurs initially as a longitudinal ridge on the ventral surface of each hemisphere. The remainder of the archipallium comprises the **hippocampus**, so named due to its resemblance to a seahorse.

The corpus striatum is anatomically continuous with the thalamus and is also functionally similar to the thalamus, because it is a high-order relay center. It is part of the basal ganglia. The dorsal striatum is called the internal capsule and is divided into the caudate and lenticular nuclei. The internal capsule emerges from the base of the cerebral hemispheres as one of the cerebral peduncles. The corpus striatum elongates in concert with the growth of the cerebral hemispheres, conforming somewhat to the shape of the lateral ventricle, so that its caudal portion curves around to the tip of the inferior horn of the lateral ventricle.

White matter forms by nerve processes extending up into the cerebral hemispheres. Due to the sheer volume of cortical substance, multiple gyri form, which are separated by sulci. The deepest sulci are called fissures and begin to form by the fourth month. The smaller sulci do not appear until the very end of fetal development. This mechanism explains the prominent **lateral fissure** (lateral sulcus) as well as the **insular cortex**. The insular cortex is a region of the cerebral cortex that is buried in the folds of the lateral fissure. The folds overlying this area are the opercula, which are formed from parts of the enclosing frontal, temporal, and parietal lobes. The lateral fissure separates the temporal lobe from the parietal and frontal lobes. The insu-

lar cortex is thought to be involved in consciousness and to play a role in diverse functions linked to emotion or regulation of homeostasis. Furthermore, it is located in close proximity to the **claustrum**, which is a small strip of gray matter that is separated from the cortex during rapid expansion.

Finally, the two hemispheres of the telencephalon are connected by bundles of fibers known as commissures. The three commissures in the telencephalon are the corpus callosum, the fornix, and the anterior commissure. All three arise from the lamina terminalis. Around the fourth month of development, a thickening forms on the lamina terminalis. The lower part of this thickening becomes the anterior commissure, and the upper part of the thickening continues to grow caudally and is invaded by both transverse (connecting hemispheres) and longitudinal fibers. Transverse fibers pass through the dorsal aspect, effectively creating the **corpus callosum**. Longitudinal fibers originate in the hippocampus, arch over the thalamus, and course toward the mamillary bodies, creating the **fornix**.

Language development, of course, does not occur during embryonic development. However, the structures necessary for neural processing begin to form. Language-processing centers are located in the cerebral cortex, with the two well-described areas vital for human communication being the Wernicke and Broca areas. These areas are typically located in the dominant hemisphere (which is the left hemisphere in most people).

The **Wernicke area** is classically located in the posterior section of the superior temporal gyrus. This area is traditionally associated with receptive speech, including the comprehension of language and the communication of coherent ideas, whether the language is vocal, written, or signed. The **Broca area** is typically formed by the pars triangularis and the pars opercularis of the inferior frontal gyrus. It is involved in the production of speech and signals to the larynx, tongue, and mouth motor areas in the motor cortex. The arcuate fasciculus is a bundle of fibers that connects the Broca and Wernicke areas.

Speech production and processing centers develop as children learn language. Cortical plasticity allows the brain to store linguistic information, not only for the nuances of one language, but also multiple language acquisition if necessary. The development of neuronal connections for speaking and language comprehension develop during the first years of life by a process that is thought to be innate or inherent and biologically determined. This complex developmental process is beyond the scope of this chapter; however, the structures relevant to communication are described in the following sections.

■ Development of the Structures for Speech and Hearing

Development of the Branchial Arches

The ectoderm, mesoderm, and endoderm are intimately involved in the development of the complex head and neck anatomy of the human body. During the fourth week of development, they organize into the pharyngeal apparatus, which is formed by six pairs of **branchial/pharyngeal arches** as well as a set of **branchial/pharyngeal pouches** and **grooves** (**Fig. 4.12**).

The derivatives of each arch are illustrated in **Fig. 4.13**. Each arch consists of ectodermal tissue covering mesenchymal tissue, with epithelium of endodermal origin lining the inside body cavity. The muscular components of each arch have corresponding cranial nerve innervation. Furthermore, each arch has its own arterial component as well.

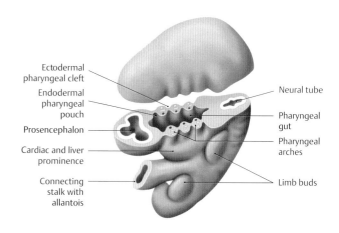

Fig 4.12 Pharyngeal (branchial) arches in a 5-week-old embryo. Although they appear in succession, this cross-sectional view represents a snapshot of a developing embryo and its pharyngeal arches and grooves. Each pharyngeal arch contains an artery, vein, and nerve, in addition to its skeletal and muscular components.

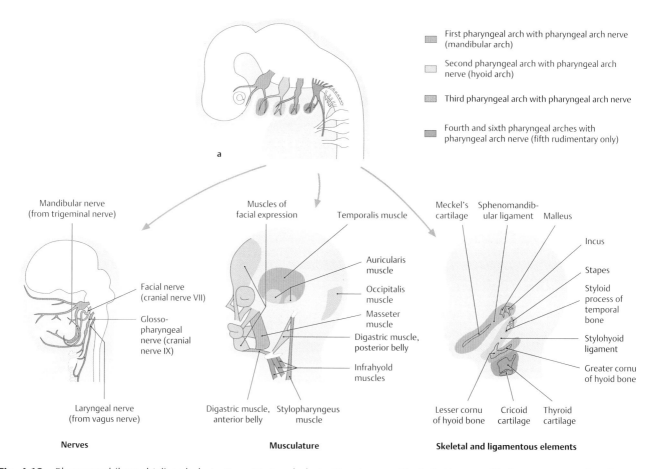

Fig. 4.13 Pharyngeal (branchial) arch derivatives. First arch derivatives (orange) include the mandibular nerve, muscles of mastication, mandible, malleus, and incus. Second arch derivatives (green) include the facial nerve (CN VII), muscles of facial expression, and upper hyoid bone. Third arch derivatives (blue) include the glossopharyngeal nerve (CN IX), the stylopharyngeus, and the lower hyoid bone. Fourth and sixth arch derivatives (purple) include the vagus nerve (CN X), the pharyngeal and laryngeal muscles, and the thyroid and cricoid cartilages.

The nerves lie anterior to their respective arteries, except in the sixth arch, where the nerve is posterior to the artery. Finally, a cartilaginous component is contained within each arch. Although six branchial arches are present, only the first four are externally visible. Furthermore, the fifth arch does not appear to have any contribution to adult anatomy and disappears (**Table 4.1**).

The first branchial arch is also known as the mandibular arch. It gives rise to the lower lip, the muscles of mastication (temporalis, masseter, medial and lateral pterygoids, tensor palatini, and tensor tympani), the mandible proper, the anterior portion of the tongue, and some of the structures of the middle ear. It also gives rise to the maxilla and palate, which effectively divide the first arch into maxillary and mandibular portions. It is innervated by the trigeminal nerve (CN V) to provide efferent information to the muscles of mastication, the anterior belly of the digastric, the mylohyoid, the tensor tympani, and the tensor veli palatini. Its cartilaginous components derive from Meckel's

cartilage. This cartilage forms the malleus, incus, sphenomandibular ligament, and mandible. The arteries of this arch include the maxillary artery and the external carotid artery.

The second branchial arch is often referred to as the hyoid arch. It is innervated by the facial nerve (CN VII) and gives rise to the platysma, stapedius muscle and tendon, muscles of facial expression, the posterior belly of the digastric, the stylohyoid, and auricular muscles. Its skeletal derivatives form from Reichert's cartilage and include the lesser horn and upper part of the hyoid body, the temporal styloid process, and the stylohyoid ligament. Its arteries are the stapedial and hyoid arteries.

The third branchial arch is innervated by the glossopharyngeal nerve (CN IX) and gives rise to the stylopharyngeus muscle as well as the greater horn and lower part of the body of the hyoid, the thymus, and inferior parathyroid glands. The arteries of this arch are the common carotid and the internal carotid branch.

Box 4.1 Branchial Cleft Anomalies

Branchial cleft anomalies are abnormalities of the pharyngeal (branchial) arches and can arise in various areas of the neck due to failure of obliteration of one of the pharyngeal grooves. A branchial cleft cyst occurs when the structure is lined with squamous epithelium and does not communicate with the skin or digestive tract. A sinus, however, has a single opening to the skin or digestive tract, and a fistula has both an opening to the skin and an opening to the digestive tract. Branchial cleft anomalies also include cartilaginous remnants appearing as neck masses.

First branchial cleft cysts typically present as a mass in the preauricular region (type I) or at the angle of the mandible (type II). A type I first branchial cleft cyst includes ectodermal elements only, presents as a mass periauricularly, courses lateral to the facial nerve (CN VII), and typically terminates as a blind sac near the mesotympanum. A type II first branchial cleft cyst occurs more commonly than a type I cyst and contains both ectodermal and mesodermal elements. It presents as a duplicated membranous external auditory canal, with cartilaginous elements, near the angle of the mandible. The tract can pass lateral or medial to the facial nerve and ends near or in the external auditory canal, and may also be associated with the parotid gland.

Second branchial cleft cysts account for 95% of all branchial cleft abnormalities. They present as cysts along the anterior border of the sternocleidomastoid muscle. Fistulas are an external opening at the anterior neck. The tract extends along the carotid sheath and between the external and internal carotid arteries. The tract passes deep to the facial nerve (CN VII) and superficial to the glossopharyngeal (CN IX) and hypoglossal (CN XII) nerves. The internal opening is usually within the tonsillar fossa.

Third branchial cleft cysts can present as neck masses and are often associated with dysphagia, stridor, recurrent acute suppurative thyroiditis, and/or neck abscesses. A fistula can open at the lower anterior neck and track superficial to the common carotid artery as well as vagus (CN X) and hypoglossal (CN XII) nerves and pass deep to the glossopharyngeal nerve (CN IX) into the thyrohyoid membrane above the superior laryngeal nerve. The internal opening is at the base of the piriform recess. Excision of a third branchial cleft cyst includes excision of the superior pole of the ipsilateral thyroid lobe.

Fourth branchial cleft cysts are extremely rare. They have an external opening at the lower anterior neck, similar to third branchial cleft cysts, but they track deep to the hypoglossal nerve (CN XII) and posterior to the common carotid artery. They also have a thoracic component, with a loop inferior to the aorta on the left and the subclavian artery on the right. The tract passes posterior to the thyroid gland, along the tracheoesophageal groove, and into the cricothyroid membrane beneath the superior laryngeal nerve. The internal opening is at the apex of the piriform recess.

The fourth branchial arch is innervated by the vagus nerve (CN X). The cricothyroid muscle as well as all intrinsic muscles of the soft palate, except for the tensor veli palatini, are derived from this arch. Intrinsic muscles of the soft palate include the tensor veli palatini, palatoglossus, palatopharyngeus, levator veli palatini, and musculus uvulae. The cartilaginous structures derived from this arch include the thyroid cartilage and the epiglottic cartilage. The superior parathyroid glands are also derived from the mesenchymal portion of this arch. The fourth right arch forms the right subclavian artery, while the fourth left arch forms the arch of the aorta between the origin of the left carotid artery and the termination of the ductus arteriosus.

The sixth branchial arch is innervated by the vagus nerve (CN X) as well. The intrinsic muscles of the larynx, except the cricothyroid muscle, derive from this arch. The cartilaginous contributions include the cricoid, arytenoid, corniculate, and cuneiform cartilages. The sixth right arch forms the pulmonary artery, and the sixth left arch forms the pulmonary artery and the ductus arteriosus.

The pharyngeal pouches penetrate the mesenchyme and are endodermal in nature. However, they do not connect with the ectodermal grooves. During development, they appear simultaneously with the arches. The first pharyngeal pouch gives rise to the eustachian tube. The second pharyngeal pouch mostly disappears, but its very medial segment gives rise to the tonsillar fossae. The third pharyngeal pouch gives rise to the inferior parathyroid gland and the thymus. The fourth pharyngeal pouch gives rise to the superior parathyroids and parafollicular cells of the thyroid gland. These cells secrete calcitonin, a hormone involved in the regulation of calcium in the blood.

The branchial grooves are ectodermal structures separating the arches and are visible on the outside of the developing embryo. They are essentially obliterated except for the first branchial groove, which forms the concha of the auricle and external auditory meatus.

Development of the Face

When the embryo is about three weeks old, the primitive facial region begins to form. By 24 days, a series of smooth, relatively undifferentiated bulges evolve (**Fig. 4.14**). Five swellings make up the

Table 4.1 Branchial (pharyngeal) arch derivatives

Branchial Arch	Muscular & Glandular Derivatives	Skeletal Derivatives	Nerve	Artery
First (mandibular) arch	Muscles of mastication, anterior belly of the digastric, mylohyoid, tensor tympani, tensor veli palatini	Mandible, premaxilla, maxilla, zygomatic bone, part of temporal bone, incus, malleus, sphenomandibular ligament	Trigeminal nerve (CN V)	Maxillary artery, external carotid artery
Second (hyoid) arch	Muscles of facial expression, buccinators, platysma, stapedius, stylohyoid, posterior belly of the digastric, auricular	Stapes, temporal styloid process, lesser horn and upper part of body of the hyoid bone, stylohyoid ligament	Facial nerve (CN VII)	Stapedial artery, hyoid artery
Third arch	Stylopharyngeus, thymus, inferior parathyroids	Hyoid (greater horn and lower part of body)	Glossopharyngeal nerve (CN IX)	Common carotid, internal carotid
Fourth arch	Cricothyroid muscle, all intrinsic muscles of the soft palate except the tensor veli palatini, superior parathyroids	Thyroid cartilage, epiglottic cartilage	Vagus nerve (CN X), superior laryngeal nerve	Right fourth arch—subclavian artery; left fourth arch—aortic arch
Sixth arch	All intrinsic muscles of the larynx except cricothyroid muscle	Cricoid cartilage, arytenoid cartilages, corniculate cartilage, cuneiform cartilages	Vagus nerve (CN X), recurrent laryngeal nerve	Right sixth arch—pulmonary artery; left sixth arch—pulmonary artery and ductus arteriosus

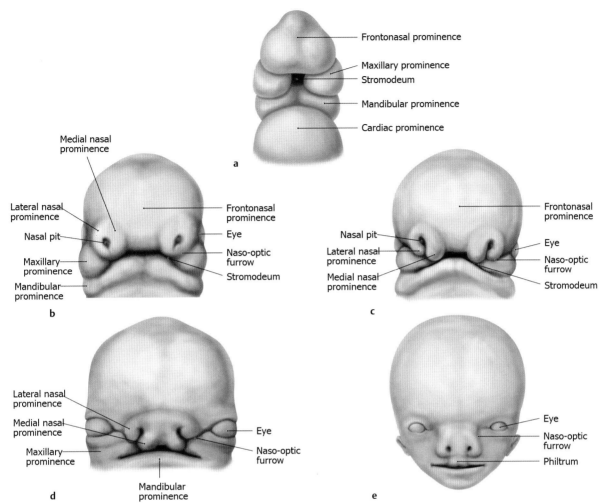

Fig. 4.14 Development of the face (after Sadler) **(a)** Anterior view at 24 days. The surface ectoderm of the 1st pharyngeal arch invaginates to form the stromodeum, which is a depression between the forebrain and the pericarlium in the embryo. It is the precursor of the mouth, oral cavity, and the anterior pituitary gland. At this stage, the stromodeum is separated from the primitive pharynx by the buccepharyngeal (erepharyngeal) membrane. This membrane later breaks down and the stromodeum become continuous with the pharynx. The stromodeum is surrounded by five neural-crest-cell-derived mesenchymal swellings, known as prominences, which contribute to the development of the face. **(b)** Anterior view at 5 weeks. Nasal placodes, ectodermal thickenings, form on each side of the frontonasal prominence. Invagination of the nasal placodes into the frontonasal prominence leads to the formation of the lateral and medial nasal prominences. The placodes now lie in the floor of a depression knowns as the nasal pit. The maxillary prominences continue to increase in size and merge laterally with the mandibular prominences to form the cheek. Medially, the maxillary prominences compress the medial nasal passage prominences toward the midline. A furrow (the naso-optic furrow) separates the nasal processes from the maxillary process. Ectoderm from the floor of the nasolacrimal groove (nasoptic furrow) will give rise to the nasolacimal duct that connects the orbit with the nasal cavity; the two prominences will join to close the groove and create the nasolacrimal canal. **(c)** Anterior view at 6 weeks. The medial nasal swellings enlarge, grow medially, and merge with each other to form the inter maxillary segment. **(d)** Anterior view at 7 weeks. The medial nasal processes have fused with each other along the midline and with their lateral margins. **(e)** Anterior view at 10 weeks. Cell migration is complete.

primitive face: the frontonasal prominence, two maxillary prominences, and two mandibular prominences. These facial prominences derive from the first and second branchial arch mesenchyme, but they originate from neural crest cells, which have an ectodermal origin.

The **frontonasal prominence** begins to form from the ventral aspect of the forebrain and is derived from neural crest cells that migrate from the ectoderm as the forebrain closes and that invade the frontonasal prominence area. The stomodeum is a depression between the forebrain and the pericardium in an embryo. It is lined by ectoderm and is separated from the anterior end of the foregut by the buccopharyngeal membrane.

The **mandibular prominences** form from the first branchial arch and are located immediately caudal to the stomodeum/oral groove. These prominences fuse together into a ventral bar early in development. At this time, the **maxillary prominences** also begin to form from the first branchial arch, with each prominence located superior and lateral to the stomodeum.

The maxillary processes fuse laterally and rostrally with the mandibular prominences to form the early cheeks. During the later part of the third week and the beginning of the fourth, neural crest–derived areas on either side of the frontonasal process begin to proliferate. These areas thicken to form **nasal placodes**, and the centers then sink to form **nasal pits**. This area gives rise to the olfactory epithelium of the nose. As shown in **Fig. 4.14**, the nasal pits divide the frontonasal process into a **medial** and two **lateral nasal processes**. The lateral nasal process is separated from the maxillary prominence by the nasolacrimal groove.

During the fifth week, a fusion of the frontonasal and the maxillary processes constricts the opening of the nasal pits. Around the sixth week of development, the most medial edge of the medial nasal process, known as the **globular process**, projects posteriorly into the nasal cavity and forms two plates known as the **nasal laminae**. As the nasal pits are pushed closer together by the maxillary processes, these laminae fuse to form the **nasal septum**. Meanwhile, the lateral nasal prominence gives rise to the alae of the nose and fuses with the maxillary prominence, which forms the nasolacrimal duct.

Development of the Lip and Palate

Beginning at the end of the sixth week and completing around the tenth of embryonic development, growth of the maxillary prominences compresses the medial nasal prominences and causes them to fuse. This intermaxillary segment yields the bridge of the nose, the upper lip containing the **philtrum**, the upper jaw with four incisors, and the **primary palate**. Upper lip morphogenesis results from contact and fusion between the maxillary and medial nasal processes (**Fig. 4.14**).

Due to the posterior projection of the globular process, the nasal pits are pushed deep into the nose, and the posterior aspect of the pits becomes closed off posteriorly by the **bucconasal membrane**. In the seventh week, this membrane disappears, and the communication between the nasal cavities and the future pharynx is established. These communications on either side of the septum are the primitive **choanae.** In order for these tracts to mature and to represent the openings of the nasal cavities to the nasopharynx, the secondary palate must form to separate them from the oral cavity.

The development of the **secondary palate** begins during the sixth week of development. In the early stages of secondary palatal development, the tongue nearly completely fills the oral cavity and is in contact with the nasal laminae. The oral cavity is open to the nasal cavity (**Fig. 4.15**). Two **palatal shelves** form on the maxillary prominences. These shelves are also known as the palatine processes of the maxillae, and their growth, at this stage, is directed inferiorly from the maxillary prominences

---

Box 4.2 Choanal Atresia

Since newborns are preferential nasal breathers for about the first six to twenty weeks of life, newborn nasal obstruction must be evaluated and treated promptly. Nasal obstruction will often present with cyclical cyanosis (worse with feeding, improves with crying), increased difficulty breathing, failure to thrive, rhinorrhea, and inability to pass flexible suction catheters through the nose.

Choanal atresia is a common cause of nasal obstruction in newborns and occurs when the bucconasal membrane persists or with abnormal migration of neural crest cells into the nasal vault, resulting in a complete bony, mixed bony-membranous, or membranous (rare) defect of the posterior nasal cavity. The obstruction can be unilateral or bilateral, with about 65% being unilateral. Unilateral choanal atresia usually presents with rhinorrhea within the first few months of life, although it can go undiagnosed until later in childhood. Bilateral choanal atresia presents within the first few days of life with cyclical cyanosis.

Diagnosis of choanal atresia is confirmed with nasal endoscopy. As it is often associated with CHARGE, Apert's syndrome, Treacher Collins syndrome, Crouzon's syndrome, trisomy 21, and 22q11 deletion syndrome, further workup may be warranted. A CT scan is often performed to assess the nature of the defect prior to surgical correction. Early interventions include establishing an oral airway (e.g., with use of a McGovern nipple, which can also be used for feeding). Transnasal surgical opening of the choana is the treatment of choice and should be performed at birth for bilateral atresia, whereas unilateral atresia can be addressed when the child is older if he or she is breathing and eating well.

Box 4.3 Facial and Orofacial Clefts

Facial clefts are openings or gaps in the face that can be caused by failure of fusion of bony structures, soft tissue, and/or skin. Clefts are extremely rare congenital abnormalities, but they have a significant aerodigestive and psychosocial impact on those affected. Many hypotheses have been proposed about the etiology of facial clefts, including failure of mesoderm fusion and amniotic bands. In 1976, Paul Tessier created a classification of facial clefts based on the anatomical location of the cleft. Tessier clefts are numbered 0 to 14, but can be grouped based on position into midline clefts, paramedian clefts, orbital clefts, and lateral clefts. Due to the large variation in types of facial clefts, there is not a one-size-fits-all approach to treatment. Furthermore, the timing of reconstruction is controversial. Early reconstruction poses the risk of recurrence of the deformity and damage to the tooth germs located in the maxilla. Functional repair is more urgent than cosmetic repair and should be performed at an earlier age. That decision is weighed against the potential psychological impact of the cleft on the individual.

Orofacial clefts are a group of conditions that include cleft lip (CL), cleft palate (CP), and cleft lip and palate together (CLP). Cleft lip is caused by failure of fusion of the frontonasal prominence and the maxillary prominence. These clefts are classified as unilateral or bilateral, as well as complete (involving the nasal floor) or incomplete. Cleft lip can also present as a microform cleft (forme fruste), which may appear as a small indentation on the vermilion of the upper lip with or without what appears as a scar extending to the nostril.

Orofacial cleft formation is illustrated in **Box Fig. 4.1**. In a unilateral cleft lip, the orbicularis oris muscle is directed superiorly in a complete cleft or is hypoplastic at the area of the defect in an incomplete cleft. The maxilla is hypoplastic on the affected side, and the alar base is displaced inferolaterally. The nasal dome is flattened and rotated downward. The nostril on the cleft side is horizontally positioned, with a shortened columella. In bilateral cleft lip, the floor of the nose communicates with the oral opening on both sides. The central aspect of the alveolus protrudes anteriorly and superiorly, with underdeveloped prolabium skin. The columella is short, and the nasal tip is widened. These defects may or may not involve clefting of the alveolar ridge.

Children with orofacial clefting require close management. Feeding presents significant challenges, including poor suction, prolonged feeds, inadequate intake, excessive air intake, and poor airway protection. Special nipples have been developed to help with difficulty obtaining a seal. Preoperative nasoalveolar molding (PNAM) may also be utilized in order to reduce the overall width of the cleft and make subsequent surgical procedures less technically challenging. Genetic evaluation and syndromic screening are useful to obtain thorough evaluation for potential heart, genitourinary, limb, or other anomalies. Following repair, speech and swallowing therapy is needed to improve function after correction of the cleft. Cleft lip is ideally repaired within the first 3 months of life, with surgical planning depending on the size of the defect and indications for PNAM or taping of the defect in order to optimize surgical repair.

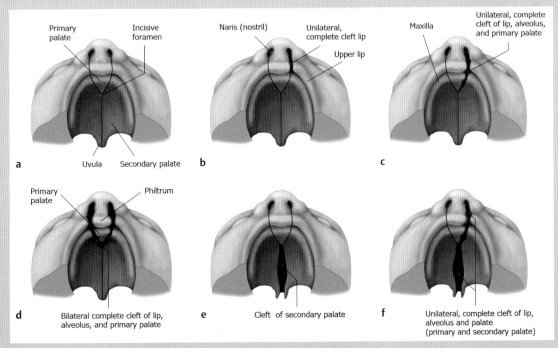

Box Fig. 4.1 Formation of facial clefts. (After Sadler.) Inferior view. (*Continued on page 122*)

Box 4.4   Cleft Palate

Cleft palate is caused by failure of apoptosis of opposed epithelial surfaces during palatal closure. Because closure progresses in an anterior to posterior direction, failure of fusion will be present posteriorly in mild defects but will extend anteriorly in severe clefts. Cleft palate is classified as complete (extending anteriorly to the incisive foramen) or incomplete, unilateral or bilateral (with laterality being applicable if it does extend anterior to the incisive foramen), and involving the secondary (posterior to the incisive foramen) or primary (anterior to the incisive foramen) palate. These various classifications are shown in **Box Fig. 4.1**. Submucosal clefts are a minor form of secondary cleft palate that causes a midline diastasis of the levator muscles, with the mucosa remaining intact. This causes a blue streak (zona pellucida) associated with a bifid uvula and notching at the posterior aspect of the bony hard palate.

Cleft palate is often associated with cleft lip, but it brings with it a unique set of challenges that must be managed in addition to those already described for cleft lip. For example, additional feeding difficulties are caused by velopharyngeal insufficiency (VPI), which arises due to failure of closure between the posterior palate and posterior pharyngeal wall during swallowing. This can cause both inadequate suction as well as nasal regurgitation. Even after repair, children with cleft palate are at risk for VPI, leading to hypernasal speech. These children may require extensive speech therapy and/or surgical repair of the VPI (pharyngoplasty) later on in their development. Finally, due to abnormal attachment of the tensor palatini, the children are at increased risk for eustachian tube dysfunction and often require multiple sets of pressure equalization (PE) tubes throughout their childhood. While a palatoplasty will usually improve eustachian tube dysfunction, it is imperative to monitor the patients closely for otitis media with effusion in order to prevent hearing loss. Cleft palate is ideally repaired between 9 and 12 months of age, which allows adequate palatal growth for optimal surgical repair but closure of the defect prior to the development of speech.

A unique presentation of cleft palate occurs with Pierre Robin sequence (PRS), where micrognathia leads to glossoptosis, with tongue-based airway obstruction caused by the tongue's obstructing palate elevation, resulting in cleft palate. The cleft palate observed in PRS is actually **U**-shaped rather than the classic **V**-shape. PRS may be due to autosomal recessive or sporadic causes and may be syndromic or nonsyndromic. Syndromic PRS can be associated with Stickler's syndrome, 22q11, Treacher Collins syndrome, Goldenhar's syndrome, and Nager's syndrome. It is important to note that PRS is not in itself a syndrome—it is a sequence of abnormalities caused by one abnormality (micrognathia).

---

so that the palatine processes are growing on either side of the tongue and extend posteriorly to the lateral walls of the pharynx. The incisive foramen marks the boundary between the primary and secondary palates.

Between the seventh and eighth week, the mandibular arch elongates, allowing the tongue to descend. Descent of the tongue allows the palatal shelves to elongate and elevate. The shelves begin to elevate to a horizontal position (**Fig. 4.16**), due to rapid proliferation of mesodermal cells on the lat-

---

Box Fig. 4.1   (*Continued*) Formation of facial clefts. (After Sadler.) Inferior view.
Clefts (fissures or openings) can involve the lips and/or the palate. Clefts are classified as isolated (cleft lip or cleft palate), unilateral or bilateral, and as complete (when they cross the nasal philtrum)
(a) Normal lips and palate, in which the maxillary prominences and medial nasal prominences have merged to form the upper lip and primary palate. The primary palate has also fused with the palatine processes of the maxillary prominences (secondary palate) to form the complete, unified, hard palate. The posterior portion of the secondary palate is unossified and forms the soft palate and uvula. **(b)** Unilateral, complete cleft lip results from failure of fusion of the maxillary prominence with the medial nasal prominence on the affected side. **(c)** Unilateral, complete cleft lip, alveolus, and primary palate (part of palate anterior to the incisive foramen) results from failure of fusion of the maxillary prominence with the medial nasal prominence on the affected side. **(d)** Bilateral, complete cleft lip, alveolus, and primary palate result from failure of the maxillary prominence to fuse with the medial nasal prominences on both sides. **(e)** Cleft of secondary palate (part of palate posterior to the incisive foramen) results from incomplete fusion of the two lateral palatine processes.
(f) Unilateral, complete cleft lip and complete cleft palate (involving both primary and secondary palate) result from failure of fusion of the maxillary prominence with the medial nasal prominence and failure of fusion of the two lateral palatine processes on the affected side. Cleft lip and palate can cause difficulty in eating and speaking, and result in failure to thrive in infants. Treatment by a multidisciplinary team of healthcare professionals principally involves corrective surgery, which is usually performed between 6 and 12 months of age, often followed by surgical revisions, speech therapy, and orthodontic therapy.

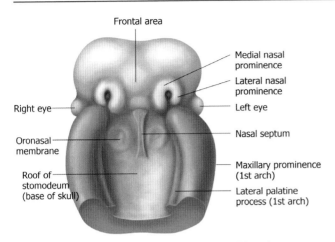

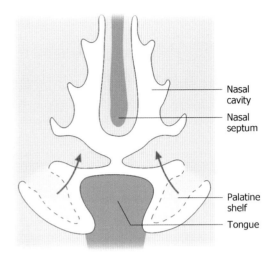

Fig. 4.15   Palate formation; 7- to 8-week-old embryo.

Fig. 4.16   Elevation of the palatine shelves. The palatine shelves, which form the secondary palate, are seen at around 6 weeks and are directed obliquely downward on each side of the tongue. At around 7 weeks, the palatine shelves ascend to a horizontal position above the tongue and fuse.shelves, which form the secondary palate, are seen at around 6 weeks and are directed obliquely downward on each side of the tongue. At around 7 weeks, the palatine shelves ascend to a horizontal position above the tongue and fuse.

eral (oral) surface of the palatine processes, causing a change in growth from the vertical to the horizontal plane. The palatine processes fuse in an anterior to posterior direction via apoptosis of the opposed epithelial surfaces (**Fig. 4.17**). The palatine processes form both the soft palate and part of the hard palate. The nasal septum grows inferiorly from the merged nasal laminae and fuses with the palatine processes between the ninth and the eleventh week.

The roof of the mouth is bound laterally and anteriorly by the **tectal ridge** following palate fusion. The tectal ridge is essentially an inward projection of the globular process and is the equivalent

of the premaxillary process. Later, the alveolar ridge will arise from a layer of mesodermal tissue that is located in the sulcus between the palate and the lip.

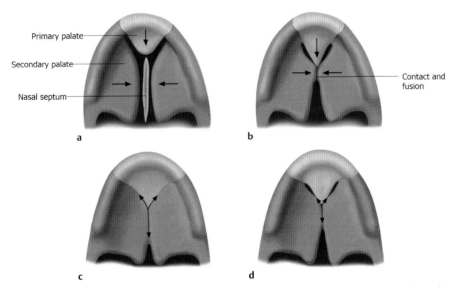

Fig. 4.17   Fusion and merging of the palatine shelves. Fusion of the palate begins at around 9 weeks and is completed posteriorly by week 12. **(a)** The primary palate and both halves of the secondary palate migrate toward each other as indicated by the arrows. **(b)** They contact and fuse at a point (marked by the incisive foramen) and merge anteriorly and posteriorly, as shown in **(c)** and **(d)**. The primary and secondary palates ossify, forming the hard palate. The posterior portions of the palatine shelves do not become ossified but extend beyond the nasal septum to form the soft palate and uvula.

Development of the Tongue

The tongue has contributions from all of the branchial arches. Embryos in the fifth week develop paired lateral thickenings (**lateral lingual swellings**) on the internal surface of the mandibular arch (**Fig. 4.18**) that consist of rapidly proliferating mesenchyme covered by epithelium. Small elevations called the **tuberculum impar** are located between these swellings. Just inferior to the tuberculum impar, another midline swelling, the **copula**, forms from the second and third branchial arches. This structure forms a transverse groove that shapes the epiglottis. Ventrally, the copula spreads in a **V**, and forms the posterior or pharyngeal part of the tongue.

In adults, the union of the anterior (first arch) and posterior (second, third, and fourth arches) parts of the tongue is marked by the **sulcus ter-minalis**, the apex of which is the **foramen cecum**. The primitive thyroid gland appears in this area and later descends through the body of the tongue into the neck along a tract known as the thyroglossal duct, passing through the hyoid bone.

By the seventh week, a distinct tonguelike structure is evident. The foramen cecum separates paired symmetric tongue primordia. The cephalic pair are the **anterior lingual primordia**, located at the level of the first branchial arch, and the caudal pair are the **root primordia**, located at the level of the second branchial arch.

The muscles of the tongue derive from occipital somites. Migrating muscle cells follow the path of the hypoglossal nerve (CN XII), and all intrinsic, as well as most of the extrinsic, muscles of the tongue are innervated by this nerve (CN XII). The extrinsic muscles of the tongue include the genioglossus, sty-

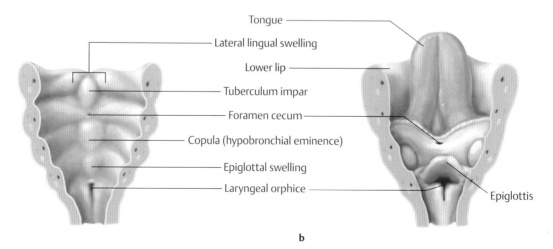

Tongue
Lateral lingual swelling
Lower lip
Tuberculum impar
Foramen cecum
Copula (hypobronchial eminence)
Epiglottal swelling
Laryngeal orphice
Epiglottis

a   b

Fig. 4.18 Tongue Development. **(a)** The tuberculum impar appears at 4 weeks. The anterior two-thirds of the tongue is formed from the two lateral lingual swellings (one on each side of the tuberculum impar). The posterior one-third of the tongue arises from the copula/hypobranchial eminence. An epiglottal swelling appears in the midline. Immediately behind this swelling is the laryngeal orfice, which is flanked by arytenoid swellings. **(b)** Anterior two-thirds of the tongue develops from the lateral lingual swellings and the tuberculum impar. The base of tongue develops from the copula/hypobranchial eminence and is divided from the anterior two-thirds of the tongue by the foramen cecum. The epiglottis and laryngeal orfices develop accordingly.

loglossus, and the hypoglossus; all are innervated by the hypoglossal nerve. The palatoglossus is also an extrinsic muscle of the tongue; however, it is innervated by the vagus nerve (CN X). Intrinsic muscles of the tongue include the superior longitudinal, inferior longitudinal, verticalis, and transverse muscles; all are innervated by the hypoglossal nerve (CN XII).

Development of the Respiratory System

The **median laryngotracheal groove** appears on the floor of the foregut in the fourth week of development (**Fig. 4.19**). This groove deepens and, with further development, becomes a diverticulum referred to as the tubular lung bud. The diverticulum continues to grow and becomes separated from the pharynx by the tracheoesophageal septum, which divides the foregut into the laryngotracheal tube and the esophagus. The tube is lined with endoderm, and from this, the epithelial lining of the entire respiratory tract develops. The cranial part of the tube becomes the laryngeal epithelium; the caudal part forms the epithelium of the lower respiratory system.

At the caudal aspect of the tube, two lateral outgrowths form. These primitive right and left **lung buds** will grow to form the main bronchi, and all branching of the bronchi within the lungs takes place from these two primitive structures. The lung buds divide into lobules, with three on the right and two on the left.

Four phases of lung tissue differentiation have been described: pseudoglandular, canalicular, saccular, and alveolar. The pseudoglandular phase takes place between weeks 5 and 17 and is critical for the formation of all conducting airways. In this phase, the conducting epithelial tubes are surrounded by mesenchyme, and extensive airway branching occurs. By two months, all segmental bronchi are present. The epithelial tissue resembles glandular tissue before it differentiates to tall columnar epithelium proximally, with the more distal structures lined with cuboidal epithelium.

The canalicular phase takes place between weeks 16 and 24. In this phase, the delineated respiratory segments form and establish a relationship with the vascular system. Bronchioles are produced, and their cuboidal epithelium comes in close contact with capillaries. The lungs begin producing surfactant, which decreases the surface tension of the alveoli and is critical to pulmonary function.

The saccular phase is the final stage of lung development within the womb and begins at 6 months. During this phase, most peripheral airways form widened airspaces called saccules. New bronchi and alveoli continue to form even after birth in the alveolar stage.

The alveolar stage begins close to term and continues 1 to 3 years postnatally. Alveoli form through septation, a process that increases the gas exchange surface area. During development, the lungs migrate caudally, and at birth, the bifurcation

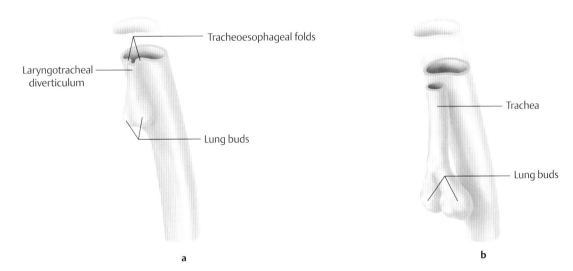

Fig. 4.19 **(a)** The laryngotracheal groove develops at the ventral aspect of the foregut in the 4th week. The laryngotracheal diverticulum becomes separated from the foregut by the tracheoesophageal folds. The right and left lung buds appear before the laryngotracheal groove has been converted into a tube. **(b)** The tracheoesophageal folds fuse to become the tracheoesophageal septum. The lung buds divide into lobules, with three on the right and two on the left.

of the trachea (carina) is located at the level of the fourth thoracic vertebra.

Development of the Larynx

The cranial end of the laryngotracheal tube develops into the larynx. Rudiments formed here are bound ventrally by the hypobranchial eminence, a derivative of branchial arches III and IV, and laterally by the ventral ends of the sixth arch. The laryngeal cartilages are produced from the fourth and sixth arches. Two arytenoid swellings develop on either side of the groove, meet the hypobranchial eminence, and approximate one another. Initially, the opening to the larynx is a slit, but the arytenoid swellings eventually develop a **T**-shaped cleft (**Fig. 4.20**). The horizontal aspect lies anteriorly and separates the arytenoid swellings from the hypobranchial eminence, which will eventually form the epiglottis.

Soon after the appearance of the cleft, however, the two walls adhere together, effectively closing off the entrance to the trachea until the third month of development, when the lumen is established by the resorption of tissue. Should this process be inter-

rupted, congenital laryngeal webs may form. Following the establishment of the glottis, a pair of lateral recesses, the laryngeal ventricles, form; they are bound cranially and caudally by the future vestibular (false) and vocal (true) folds, respectively.

The arytenoid swellings form both the **arytenoid** and **corniculate cartilages** of the larynx. The folds joining the arytenoids to the epiglottis (the aryepiglottic folds) are also formed from the arytenoid swellings. The **cuneiform cartilages,** however, are derived from the hypobranchial eminence. These cartilages all form from the sixth arch.

The thyroid cartilage is developed from the fourth arch. It appears as two lateral plates joined at the midline by a fibrous membrane that give rise to the constrictor muscles of the pharynx. The cricoid cartilage is a derivative of the sixth arch.

The laryngeal muscles develop from muscle elements in branchial arches IV and VI and are innervated by laryngeal branches of the vagus nerve (CN X). The bilateral recurrent laryngeal nerves innervate all intrinsic muscles of the larynx except the cricothyroid muscle and also supply sensation to the subglottis. The course of the recurrent laryngeal nerves

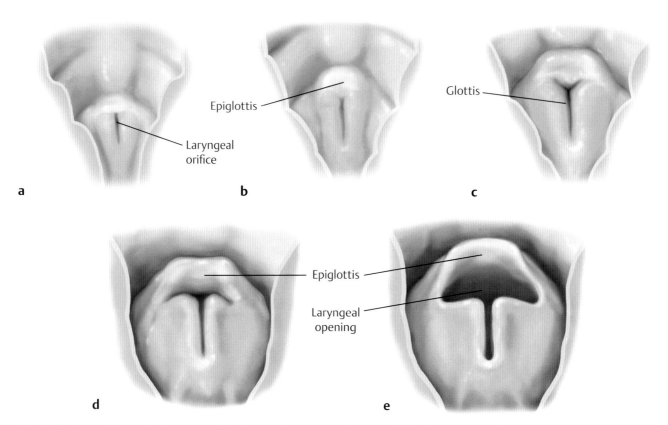

Fig. 4.20 Stages in the development of the human larynx, viewed posteriorly. **(a)** The arytenoid swellings enlarge and meet the hypobranchial eminence. **(b)** The initial laryngeal opening is a verticle slit, but it is converted to a T-shaped cleft **(c)** due to the enlargement of the arytenoid swellings. **(d)** The epiglottis and arytenoids continue to develop, shown at 9 weeks and **(e)** 10 weeks.

illustrates a unique embryological relationship. The recurrent laryngeal nerves on either side are produced from the nerve of the sixth pharyngeal arch. On the right side, the artery of the sixth pharyngeal arch is obliterated, while on the left, the artery persists as the ductus arteriosus, which is a vital structure for human embryonic circulation. After birth, this artery closes and becomes the ligamentum arteriosum. The left recurrent laryngeal nerve has an elongated recurrent path around the aortic arch inferior to the ductus arteriosus, because it is not allowed to migrate superiorly, due to the persistence of the ductus arteriosus on the left. On the right, the recurrent laryngeal nerve passes around the subclavian artery, unless there is an anomalous origin of the subclavian, in which case the nerve directly innervates the larynx.

Development of the Teeth

Development of the teeth, also known as odontogenesis, is a complex and staged process by which teeth form, grow, and erupt into the mouth. Primary (baby) teeth start to form between the sixth and eighth week of prenatal development. Permanent teeth begin to develop during the twentieth week.

The growth of the tooth spans many different stages and includes the beginning formation of the tooth bud, specialization and arrangement of cells in the form of the future tooth, and deposition of the enamel and dentin matrix (**Fig. 4.21**).

The initial stage of tooth growth is the initiation of the tooth germ, an aggregation of cells that eventually form a tooth. These cells are derived from the ectoderm of the first pharyngeal arch. During the sixth week, the oral epithelium is separated from the underlying connective tissue by a thin basement membrane. Dental epithelium begins to proliferate and extends into the mesoderm to form a thin strand of tissue called the **dental lamina**.

During the seventh week of development, swellings begin to develop in the dental lamina. These swellings are known as **tooth buds**. Once they are formed, tooth development has entered the bud stage. The dental lamina connects the developing tooth bud to the epithelial layer of the mouth for a significant time. A grouping of cells, called the **dental papilla**, underneath the tooth bud begins to aggregate, forcing the proliferating cells within the tooth bud to grow in a differential manner, so that it takes on the appearance of a cap, marking the cap stage of tooth development. At this stage, the dental cap is surrounded by mesoderm, which ultimately forms the **cementum**

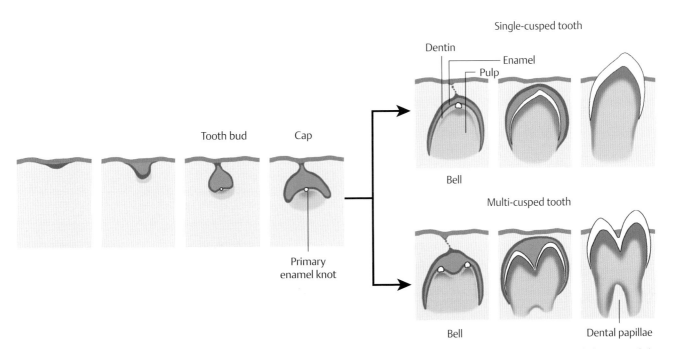

Fig. 4.21   Tooth development. The first stage of tooth development is the initiation of the bud from the epithelial tissue of the alveolar ridge. Its cells begin to proliferate at unequal rates, resulting in the invagination of the deeper surface of the tooth bud, which marks the cap stage. As proliferation continues, the dental cap is surrounded by mesoderm. In the Bell stage, cells begin to differentiate into three distinct layers—those in contact with the very inside of the tooth are enamel cells (ameloblasts). Those on the outer layer are called external enamel epithelium. The cells located in the intermediate layer between these two give rise to the dental pulp and contributes to the formation of dentin.

of the tooth as well as the periodontal tissue. The cap itself also surrounds mesoderm contained within it, and this mesoderm gives rise to the dental pulp and contributes to the formation of **dentin**.

The bell stage is known for the differentiation of the histology and morphogenesis of the cells within the tooth. Layers begin to form within the tooth. The cells in contact with the papillae undergo modifications and acquire the ability to form enamel and form the inner enamel epithelium. Cells in the outer layer of the cap are called the external enamel epithelium. These cells, plus the cells in the stratum intermedium (between the inner enamel epithelium and the dental organ), become modified to form the **enamel organ**.

At the same time, a condensation of ectomesenchymal cells called the dental sac surrounds the enamel organ. The enamel organ eventually produces enamel, the dental papilla produces dentin and pulp, and the dental sac produces all the supporting structures of the tooth, called the periodontum. The enamel organ and its dental papilla, plus the dental sac, constitute the formative tissues for the tooth and periodontal tissue. These structures are collectively called the **tooth germ**.

Dentin formation, known as dentinogenesis, is the first identifiable feature in the crown stage of tooth development. Dentin, a calcified tissue of the body, is less mineralized and less brittle than enamel. Formation of dentin must always occur before the formation of enamel. Dentinogenesis is initiated by the odontoblasts of the enamel pulp and is derived from the dental papilla of the tooth germ. Unlike enamel, dentin continues to form throughout life and can be initiated in response to stimuli, such as tooth decay or attrition.

Enamel formation or amelogenesis also occurs in the crown stage of tooth development. Enamel makes up the normally visible part of the tooth, covering the crown, and is the hardest substance in the human body. Generally, enamel formation occurs in two stages: the secretory and maturation stages. Proteins and an organic matrix form partially mineralized enamel in the secretory stage, and in the maturation stage, the enamel completes mineralization.

Development of the Outer Ear

During the sixth week of development, several small buds begin to appear at the hyoid-mandibular arch area. These six buds are the beginnings of the margins of the **auricle** and are termed the **auricular hillocks** (**Fig. 4.22**). Three auricular hillocks derive from both the first and second arches. At the same time, an elongated elevation develops caudal to the three

---

Box 4.6   Aural Atresia

Aural atresia is a spectrum of ear deformities that involve absence or abnormal narrowing of the external auditory canal associated with underdevelopment of the middle ear. These abnormalities occur as a result of abnormal development of the first and second branchial arches. They are often associated with microtia, or underdevelopment of the pinna (external ear). In fact, both microtia and atresia imply an arrest in ear development at any stage. Atresia is also associated with malformed semicircular canals, stapes fixation, malformed cochlea, and cholesteatoma. Fusion of the malleus and incus with sparing of the footplate is the most common middle ear anomaly.

Atresia is often associated with craniofacial syndromes. For example, Treacher Collins syndrome, or mandibulofacial dysostosis, involves first and second arch abnormalities, including downward-slanting eyes, micrognathia (a small lower jaw), conductive hearing loss, underdeveloped zygoma, drooping of the lateral lower eyelids, and malformed or absent ears. These patients have normal intelligence but may have a developmental delay due to hearing loss. Although many benefit from bone conduction hearing aids, surgical repair of the atresia using rib cartilage usually offers definitive correction of this deformity. Other syndromes with which aural atresia is associated include Nager's syndrome (acrofacial dysostosis), Crouzon's syndrome (craniofacial dysostosis), and Goldenhar's syndrome (oculoauriculovertebral syndrome or hemifacial microsomia).

In the treatment of children with unilateral atresia, it is particularly important to preserve hearing in the contralateral ear, which typically involves aggressive treatment of otitis media in the normal hearing ear throughout childhood. Should initial newborn screening fail in the contralateral ear, an auditory brainstem response (ABR) and a CT scan of the temporal bones are indicated. The treatment of bilateral aural atresia is aimed at aiding hearing immediately at birth with bone conduction hearing aids and possible surgical repair around the age of 6 to 7 years after microtia repair. The prognosis for aiding with a bone-anchored hearing aid (BAHA) is good; 85% of patients experience air–bone gap closure. Furthermore, patients experience improvement in hearing of 30 dB hearing loss or better with surgery in 50 to 75% of cases.

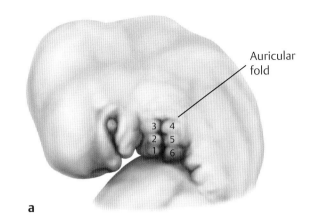

Auricular fold

a

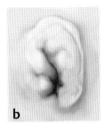

b

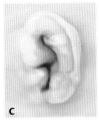

c

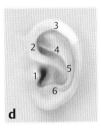

d

Fig.4.22 Embryonic development of the auricle. **(a)** The external ear develops from the first and second arches and the first branchial groove. At about 6 weeks, six small elevations called hillocks appear around the first branchial groove – three on the caudal border of the first arch and three on the cephalad border of the second arch. Furthermore, cephalad to the three hillocks on the second arch, there is an elongated elevation called the auricular fold. **(b,c,d)** These elevations migrate to become 1- tragus, 2,3- helix, 4,5- antihelix, and 6- antitragus.

hillocks on the second arch called the **auricular fold**. Although the auricular hillocks and the auricular fold are originally on the neck, the apparatus moves cranially during mandibular development.

The first branchial groove eventually develops into the concha of the auricle and the external auditory meatus. The ectodermal floor of the groove is in contact with the endoderm of the first pharyngeal pouch, but this contact is lost with growth. Toward the end of the second month, the first branchial groove deepens to form a funnel-shaped pit. The medial aspect of this pit develops an ectodermal plate that continues to grow medially until it reaches the wall of the tympanic cavity. During the seventh month of development, this plate splits. The resultant cleft constitutes the most medial aspect of the external auditory meatus. The tympanic membrane develops in this area, abutting the wall of the tympanic cavity. The tympanic membrane is formed from ectodermal endothelium externally and from endodermal epithelium internally.

Development of the Inner Ear

Although reception and transmission of sound energy are the functions of the external and middle ears, the function of the inner ear involves conversion of that energy into neural signals as well as regulation of the equilibrium of the body. The inner ear is derived from a pair of sensory placodes, called **otic placodes**, that appear posterior to the second branchial arch during the fourth week of development. The otic placode is initially a thickening of ectoderm that develops into a pit. It invaginates and pinches off from the surface to form epithelium surrounding a fluid-filled **auditory vesicle** embedded in mesoderm, which lies close to the early developing hindbrain and the developing vestibulocochlear-facial ganglion complex.

The epithelium of the auditory vesicle then begins to form the primitive membranous labyrinth around the fifth week of development (**Fig. 4.23**). The **endolymphatic sac** extends medially and continues to dilate. The epithelium further varies in thickness and begins to distort, and vestibular (dorsal) and cochlear (ventral) regions form. The intermediate region subdivides into the **utricle** and **saccule**. They are both otolithic organs located in the vestibule of the inner ear. The saccule collects information primarily from the vertical planes, and the utricle collects information about head tilt. Together, these organs use mechanoreceptors to transmit information about orientation of the head in space to the brain.

By the sixth week, two flattened pouches that give rise to the semicircular canals begin to form on the auditory vesicle. A single pouch forms at the dorsal limit of the vesicle, giving rise to both the posterior and superior canals. The lateral canal emerges from a horizontal outpouching. Meanwhile, the cochlear area begins to form its first turn. By the end of the seventh week, the auditory vesicle has begun to take the shape of the membranous labyrinth, with semicircular canals and a cochlea with one turn.

By the eighth week, the endolymphatic duct and the three semicircular canals are well defined. The utricle and saccule are also now distinct. The cochlear duct begins to coil and now resembles a snail shell. The superior and posterior semicircular canals have a common crus, which converges onto the utricle, where the ampulla is now located.

Further development results in complete separation of the utricle and saccule, each of which remains attached to the endolymphatic duct by a short, slender canal. By the third month, the adult form of the inner ear is nearly complete. The membranous labyrinth is lodged within the bony labyrinth and has the same general form, although it

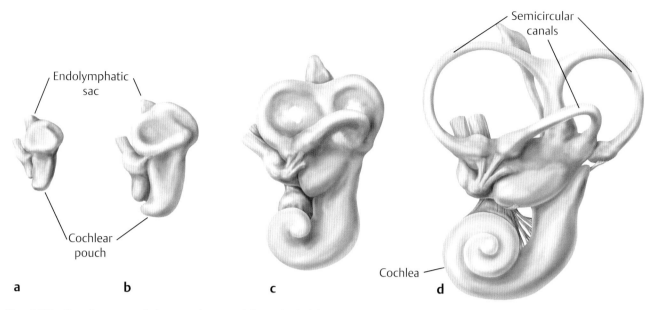

Fig. 4.23 Development of the membranous labyrinth. **(a,b)** Diverticula of the auditory vesicle give off the endolymphatic sac, the cochlear pouch, and the semicircular ducts. **(c)** The semicircular canals become defined, with the superior semicircular canal as the first to be completed and the lateral the last. **(d)** The membranous vestibule separates into the saccule and utricle.

is smaller. It contains endolymph and is lined with distributions of the vestibulocochlear nerve (CN VIII). The epithelium of the membranous labyrinth is initially a single layer of columnar cells. Early in development, fibers of the auditory nerve grow between the cells in regions where subsequent thickening results in the development of the special sense organs. These include the **cristae ampullaris** in the ampullae of the semicircular canals, the **macula** in the utricle and saccule, and the **spiral organ** in the cochlear duct.

The cristae ampullaris forms in each ampulla of the semicircular canals from a curved ridge, called the crista, in the epithelium and underlying tissue of the ampullae at the end of each semicircular canal. These cells differentiate into supportive and sensory cells. The supportive cells secrete the **cupula**, a jellylike substance that covers sensory cells. Sensory cells develop **kinocilia**, which project out into the cupula. Deposits of minerals, or **otoconia,** also cover the kinocilia to provide mass over the top of the cupula, so that movements of the head result in an inertial lag that bends the kinocilia of the sensory cells. This movement results in stimulation of the sensory cells, which transmit a signal to the brain in order to provide orientation awareness. The development of the macula is very similar to that of the cristae described previously.

The epithelium of the spiral organ divides into an inner and outer ridge. Cells of the inner ridge become the **spiral limbus**, and the outer ridge is the primordium of the spiral organ. Supportive and sensory cells are again differentiated. Both ridges are covered by a tectorial membrane that is secreted by the epithelium of the spiral limbus.

In the ninth week, chondrification of the mesenchyme around the membranous labyrinth is induced by the otic vesicle. The newly formed cartilaginous otic capsule undergoes vacuolization around the tenth week of development to produce the perilymphatic cavity surrounding the membranous labyrinth. The otic capsule eventually ossifies by 23 weeks, forming the bony labyrinth of the petrous portion of the temporal bone.

The cochlear duct coils to about 2.5 spirals and elongates in the fifth week. It is triangular in cross section, and its inner angle is attached to the axis (modiolus) of the cochlea. Perilymphatic spaces (periotic) develop above and below the cochlear duct. The upper space is the scala vestibuli and the lower is the scala tympani; each is lined with squamous mesodermal cells. The thin partition separating the scala vestibuli from the cochlear duct (scala media) is known as the vestibular membrane. It is composed of a single layer of mesoderm on the side of the scala vestibuli, and a single layer of epithelium on the cochlear duct side. The organ of Corti is innervated by the spiral ganglion of the modiolus, whose fibers form the cochlear branch of the vestibulocochlear nerve (CN VIII). The organ of Corti is fully differentiated by the seventh week. By the middle of fetal life, the inner ear has reached its final size.

■ Suggested Readings

Gilbert SF. Developmental Biology. 9th ed. Sunderland, MA: Sinauer Associates, Inc.; 2010

Kandel ER, Schwartz JH, Jessell TM. Principles of Neural Science. 4th ed. New York: McGraw-Hill; 2000

Moss-Salentijn L. Pharyngeal Arches. www.columbia.edu/itc/hs/medical/humandev/2004/Chapt9-PharyngealArches.pdf

Pasha R, Golub JS. Otolaryngology—Head and Neck Surgery: Clinical Reference Guide. San Diego, CA: Plural Publishing; 2013

Schoenwolf GC, Bleyl SB, Brauer PR, Francis-West PH. Larsen's Human Embryology, 4th ed. New York, NY: Churchill Livingstone; 2009

Standring S. Gray's Anatomy, 40th ed. New York, NY: Churchill Livingstone; 2008

Schoenwolf GC, Bleyl SB, Brauer PR, Francis-West PH. Larsen's Human Embryology, 4th ed. New York, NY: Churchill Livingstone; 2009

Standring S. Gray's Anatomy, 40th ed. New York, NY: Churchill Livingstone; 2008

Zemlin WR. Speech and Hearing Science: Anatomy and Physiology, 4th ed. Columbus, OH: Pearson; 1997

■ References

Bear MF, Connors BW, Paradiso MA. Neuroscience: Exploring the Brain, 2d ed. Baltimore, MD: Lippincott Williams & Wilkins; 2001

Bischof P, Irminger-Finger I. The human cytotrophoblastic cell, a mononuclear chameleon. *International Journal of Biochemistry & Cell Biology*, 37(1), 1–16; 2005

Campbell NA, Reece JB. Biology, 2d ed. San Francisco, CA: Pearson Benjamin Cummings; 2005

Gilbert SF. Developmental Biology, 9th ed. Sunderland, MA: Sinauer Associates, Inc.; 2010

Hill MA. Embryology: Tongue Development. embryology.med.unsw.edu.au/embryology/index.php/Tongue_Development.

Kandel ER, Schwartz JH, Jessell TM. Principles of Neural Science, 4th ed. New York: McGraw-Hill; 2000

Moss-Salentijn L. Pharyngeal Arches. www.columbia.edu/itc/hs/medical/humandev/2004/Chapt9-PharyngealArches.pdf

Nanci A. Ten Cate's Oral Histology, 8th ed. New York, NY: Elsevier Health Sciences; 2013

Pasha R, Golub JS. Otolaryngology—Head and Neck Surgery: Clinical Reference Guide. San Diego, CA: Plural Publishing; 2013

Posnick JC. Treacher Collins syndrome: perspectives in evaluation and treatment. *Journal of Oral and Maxillofacial Surgery, 55*(10), 1120–1133; 1997

■ Study Questions

1. What is the defining characteristic of metaphase?

A. Sister chromatids of each pair are pulled to opposite poles of the cell.

B. Kinetochores attach to microtubules, which align the chromosomes along the central axis of the cell.

C. DNA condenses into discrete chromosomes observable with a light microscope.

D. The cell grows and copies its chromosomes in preparation for cell division.

E. The organelles and DNA line up in the center of the cell.

2. How many chromosomes does a human haploid mature germ cell contain?

A. 22

B. 23

C. 24

D. 44

E. 46

3. Which of the following structures gives rise to the embryo?

A. Yolk sac

B. Amniotic sac

C. Trophoblast

D. Inner cell mass

E. Allantois

4. Which of the following is *not* a derivative of the somites?

A. Dermatome

B. Neurotome

C. Sclerotome

D. Myotome

E. None of the above

5. Which of the following cell types gives rise to the nasal placodes?

A. Neural crest
B. Endoderm
C. Neuroectoderm
D. Mesenchyme
E. Mesoderm

6. Which of the following is a correct pairing between neural tube zone and derived structure?

A. Ependymal zone—gray matter
B. Mantle zone—white matter
C. Mantle zone—somatic efferent cell bodies
D. Marginal zone—visceral afferent cell bodies
E. Marginal zone—central canal

7. Which area of the neural tube does the Broca's area derive from?

A. Anterior neuropore
B. Prosencephalon
C. Mesencephalon
D. Rhombencephalon
E. Posterior neuropore

8. Which of the following serves as the principal midbrain nucleus of the auditory pathway?

A. Mammillary bodies
B. Substantia nigra
C. Superior colliculus
D. Inferior colliculus
E. None of the above

9. Which pharyngeal (branchial) arch do most of the intrinsic muscles of the soft palate derive from?

A. First
B. Second
C. Third
D. Fourth
E. Sixth

10. What is the most common type of branchial cleft cyst?

A. First
B. Second
C. Third
D. Fourth
E. Sixth

11. Cleft lip results from failure of fusion of which two structures?

A. The frontonasal prominence and the maxillary prominence
B. The nasal laminae and the maxillary prominence
C. The nasal pit and the maxillary prominence
D. The nasal laminae and the mandibular prominence
E. The maxillary prominence and the mandibular prominence

12. Which of the following is an incorrect classification of a cleft lip and/or palate?

A. Complete bilateral cleft lip, alveolus, and palate
B. Complete unilateral cleft lip, alveolus, and primary palate
C. Incomplete cleft of the secondary palate
D. Complete cleft of the secondary palate
E. Incomplete cleft of the primary palate without cleft lip

13. Choanal atresia is associated with which of the following syndromes?

A. CHARGE
B. Treacher Collins syndrome
C. Crouzon's syndrome
D. 22q11 deletion syndrome
E. All of the above

14. Which of the following muscles is *not* innervated by the hypoglossal nerve (CN XII)?

A. Genioglossus
B. Styloglossus
C. Hypoglossus
D. Palatoglossus
E. Intrinsic muscles of the tongue

15. The bilateral recurrent laryngeal nerves innervate all intrinsic muscles of the larynx except the:

A. Thyroarytenoid
B. Cricothyroid
C. Posterior cricoarytenoid
D. Lateral cricoarytenoid
E. Interarytenoid

16. Which of the following branchial arches are involved in aural atresia?

A. First arch
B. Second arch
C. Third arch
D. Both A and B
E. Both B and C

■ Answers to Study Questions

1. The correct answer is (B). Metaphase is the longest stage of mitosis, during which the nuclear envelope fragments, the chromosomes attach at their kinetochores to the microtubules of the mitotic spindle, and the microtubules align the chromosomes on the metaphase plate. Answer choice (A) refers to anaphase, (C) refers to prophase, and (D) refers to interphase. (E) is not a part of cell division (organelles do not align along the metaphase plate).

2. The correct answer is (B). The mature germ cell contains 23 chromosomes.

3. The correct answer is (D). The inner cell mass will develop into the embryo and form, or contribute to, all of the extraembryonic membranes. The yolk sac (A) is a membranous sac attached to the embryo, formed by cells of the hypoblast adjacent to the embryonic disc. The amniotic sac (B) is the closed sac between the embryo and the amnion, containing amniotic fluid. The trophoblast (C) forms the outer layer of a blastocyst, which develops into a large part of the placenta. The allantois (E) is a saclike structure that helps the embryo exchange gases and handle liquid waste.

4. The correct answer is (B). The cervical, thoracic, and lumbar somites differentiate into three cell groups: sclerotomes (C), myotomes (D), and dermatomes (A). Sclerotomes form from the most medial region of a somite and give rise to the individual vertebral bodies, the intervertebral disks, the ribs, and part of the occipital bone. Myotomes are located immediately lateral to the sclerotome and are the group of muscles that a single spinal nerve root innervates. Dermatomes are formed from the most lateral portion of a somite. They develop into the skin, fat, and connective tissue of the neck and trunk.

5. The correct answer is (A). Neural crest cells from the forebrain region are involved in the development of the nasal placode and the nose.

6. The correct answer is (C). The mantle (intermediate) zone gives rise to four clusters of cell bodies on each side of the central canal, including somatic and visceral afferent, as well as somatic and visceral efferent, nerve bodies. The ependymal (internal) zone gives rise to epithelial-like lining of the central canal of the spinal cord. The marginal (external) zone is relatively free of developing nerve cells and contains axons and myelin of the spinal cord (white matter).

7. The correct answer is (C). Broca's area is in the cerebral cortex and is involved in the production of speech. The prosencephalon gives rise to the telencephalon and diencephalon. The telencephalon forms the cerebral cortex.

8. The correct answer is (D). The inferior colliculi serve as the principal midbrain nuclei of the auditory pathway, located on the tectal region of the midbrain.

9. The correct answer is (D). The fourth branchial arch is innervated by the vagus nerve (CN X). The cricothyroid muscle as well as all intrinsic muscles of the soft palate *except* for the tensor veli palatini are derived from this arch. Intrinsic muscles of the soft palate include the tensor veli palatini, palatoglossus, palatopharyngeus, levator veli palatini, and musculus uvulae

10. The correct answer is (B). Second branchial cleft cysts account for 95% of all branchial cleft abnormalities. They present as cysts, sinuses, or fistulas along the anterior border of the sternocleidomastoid muscle. Fistulas will have an external opening at the anterior neck. The tract of a sinus or fistula extends along the carotid sheath and between the external and internal carotid arteries. It passes deep to the facial nerve and superficial to the glossopharyngeal and hypoglossal nerves. The internal opening is usually within the tonsillar fossa.

11. The correct answer is (A). Cleft lip is caused by failure of fusion of the frontonasal prominence and the maxillary prominence. It is classified as unilateral or bilateral as well as complete (involving the nasal floor) or incomplete. Cleft lip can also present as a microform cleft (forme fruste), which may appear as a small indentation on the vermilion of the upper lip, with or without what appears as a scar extending to the nostril.

12. The correct answer is (E). Cleft palate is classified as unilateral or bilateral, complete (involving the incisive foramen) or incomplete, and of the primary or secondary palate. Since the palatal shelf elevation is a separate process from fusion of the frontonasal process with the maxillary process, a cleft of the primary palate needs to be accompanied by either a cleft lip or a complete cleft of the secondary palate (passing the incisive foramen).

13. The correct answer is (E). Choanal atresia is often associated with CHARGE, Apert's syndrome, Treacher Collins syndrome, Crouzon's syndrome, trisomy 21, and 22q11 deletion syndrome.

14. The correct answer is (D). All of the intrinsic, as well as most of the extrinsic, muscles of the tongue are innervated by the hypoglossal nerve (CN XII). The extrinsic muscles of the tongue include the genioglossus, the styloglossus, and the hypoglossus, which are all innervated by the hypoglossal nerve. The palatoglossus is also an extrinsic muscle of the tongue; however, it is innervated by the vagus nerve (CN X). Intrinsic muscles of the tongue include the superior longitudinal, the inferior longitudinal, verticalis, and transverse muscles, which are all innervated by the hypoglossal nerve.

15. The correct answer is (B). The laryngeal muscles develop from muscle elements in branchial arches IV and VI. The bilateral recurrent laryngeal nerves, which are branches of the vagus nerve (CN X), innervate all intrinsic muscles of the larynx except the cricothyroid muscle and also supply sensation to the subglottis.

16. The correct answer is (D). Aural atresia is a spectrum of ear deformities that involve absence or abnormal narrowing of the external auditory canal associated with underdevelopment of the middle ear. It occurs as a result of abnormal development of the first (A) and second (B) branchial arches.

Part II
Foundations of the Nervous System

5

Neuroanatomy

Torrey Loucks and Li-Hsin Ning

■ Chapter Summary

The study of neuroanatomy is necessary to provide an understanding of the building blocks of the nervous system and how behaviors ultimately arise from integrated networks of neurons. This chapter provides an introduction to the nervous system and focuses on its major subdivisions and building blocks. Specifically, chapter (1) discusses the division of the nervous system into the central nervous system and peripheral nervous system, followed by a description of neural tissue and neurons; (2) describes the cerebral cortex and its organization, with a focus on the lobes and gyrus/sulcus system, together with structure–function associations; (3) provides an overview of the major subcortical structures, including the basal ganglia, hippocampus, thalamus, limbic system, and hypothalamus, with emphasis on anatomical position and relationships; (4) introduces the two circulation systems of the brain, starting with the arterial supply of the brain and brainstem, followed by the ventricular system and cerebrospinal fluid; (5) describes the cerebellum in terms of a straightforward anatomical organization that encompasses functional connections with the rest of the nervous system; (6) discusses the anatomical organization of the brainstem and spinal cord in detail to emphasize continuity with the cerebrum and to show distinctions in these essential structures; and (7) describes several disorders that affect speech, language, swallowing, hearing, balance, or related functions to illustrate how neuroanatomy and function are related and critical to the practice of speech-language pathology and audiology.

■ Learning Objectives

- Describe the divisions of the nervous system and their major functions
- Identify the major gyri and sulci and the functions of selected gyri of the cerebral cortex
- Describe the anatomy and functions of the subcortical systems, including the thalamus, basal ganglia, and cerebellum
- Understand the anatomy of neurons and the composition of white matter and gray matter
- Explain the functions of the 12 cranial nerves

■ Putting It Into Practice

- The brainstem is the major superhighway that connects the brain with the body, but it also contains many of the cranial nerves that make speech, language, swallowing, hearing, and balance possible.
- The cerebral cortex is the source of consciousness, volition, executive function, and language. Subcortical structures are vital for modulating the activity of the cerebral cortex, particularly the basal ganglia, cerebellum, and thalamus.
- Speech-language pathologists and audiologists should be familiar with how sensory information related to speech, language, swallowing, hearing, and balance are received and how motor commands are used to control movement.

■ Introduction

Neuroanatomy is the oldest branch of neuroscience, just as gross anatomy is the oldest branch of medicine. Early theories of brain function followed from observations of how different parts of the brain were arranged. The history of how the study of neuroanatomy led to modern neuroscience is tightly linked to advances in knowledge of speech and language production. In the late 19th century, physician-scientists, including Paul Broca and Carl Wernicke, discovered that stroke-induced lesions in specific parts of the left hemisphere led to different deficits in language and speech. These discoveries were part of the fundamental revolution in neurology and psychology that brain function and structure displayed close connections—now commonly referred to as structure–function associations.

This chapter introduces the parts of the brain, from the neurons that serve as the essential building blocks to the different anatomical systems, including the cerebral hemispheres, brainstem, cerebellum, and spinal cord. Although with modern neuroscience methods certain parts of the brain seem to be studied in isolation, a more comprehensive framework is needed to put emerging knowledge within the right context. An appropriate analogy for neuroanatomy is a classic Victorian mansion. The external features of the mansion suggest the importance of the building, but one needs to enter the building to understand what is behind the elegant architecture. Inside, there is an elaborate system of rooms that have specific functions. Yet none of the rooms functions in isolation. An elaborate system connects the rooms and serves a higher function. Extending this analogy to the brain and nervous system, imagine exploring the grand mansion from the outside and the inside. Understand how the different parts of the nervous system are like the rooms of the mansion while remembering that they function together to achieve speech, language, memory, and executive function.

■ Divisions of the Nervous System

The nervous system has two divisions: the **central nervous system** (**CNS**) and the **peripheral nervous system** (**PNS**; **Fig. 5.1**). The CNS consists of the **spinal cord** and the brain and is the site of all central operations that interpret sensory information, generate motor responses, store information, provide consciousness and volition, and produce and comprehend language. The PNS, consisting of 31 pairs

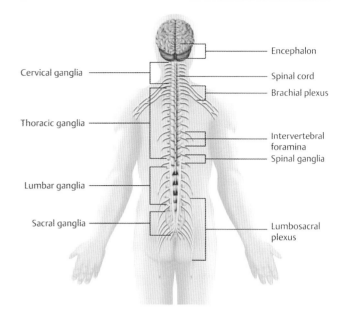

Fig. 5.1 The nervous system. Central nervous system (brain and spinal cord), pink; peripheral nervous system (nerves and ganglia), yellow.

of spinal nerves, 12 pairs of cranial nerves, and peripheral autonomic and sensory ganglia, implements sensory and motor functions and carries information to and from the central nervous system. All sensory information received by the CNS is conveyed through the PNS, while descending motor commands generated by the CNS rely on the PNS for transmission to muscles and glands.

Central Nervous System (CNS)

The CNS consists of the brain and spinal cord. The spinal cord begins at the base of the brain (at the foramen magnum) and extends caudally to the first lumbar vertebra. The spinal cord is entirely enclosed and protected within the vertebral column, which is longer than the spinal cord. The spinal cord is the major structure for information transfer between the brain and the PNS. It involves sensory processing and contains neurons responsible for implementing voluntary movements and generating reflexes.

The brain proper is rostral to the spinal cord and is divided into four regions: the **cerebral hemispheres** (or **telencephalon**), **diencephalon** (**thalamus, hypothalamus,** subthalamus), the brainstem (**midbrain, pons,** and **medulla**), and **cerebellum** (**Fig. 5.2**, right hemisphere). The major divisions of the brain and their functions are shown in **Table 5.1**. Each of these divisions is paired, but differs slightly across hemispheres.

The cerebral hemispheres are the largest regions of the human brain. They include the **cerebral cortex** (including the heavily folded cortical surface), **basal ganglia**, and **limbic system**. The cerebral cortex is responsible for the planning and execution of actions, including speech and language, and the interpretation and moderation of all sensations. The basal ganglia are associated with the control of desired actions and thoughts and the inhibition of unwanted movements and thoughts. The limbic system in particular is thought to be involved in the regulation of emotion and memory formation. As a result, the importance of the cerebral hemispheres as the center of our ability to learn, understand, and respond in a volitional and personal way cannot be understated.

The diencephalon includes two major structures: the thalamus and hypothalamus. The thalamus resides between the cerebral cortex and the midbrain and is an essential pathway for all afferent (or sensory) information traveling to the cerebral cortex, such as hearing, vision, pain, temperature, touch, and limb position. The hypothalamus, below the thalamus, regulates the hormonal secretions of the **pituitary gland** (or **hypophysis**). The hypothalamus plays an important role in regulating basic life functions, such as body temperature, circadian rhythms, sleep, hunger, stress and arousal, and reproductive behaviors.

The midbrain, pons, and medulla are collectively known as the **brainstem**. The brainstem is situated below the diencephalon and above the spinal cord. All major pathways that send information

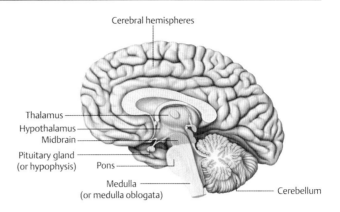

Fig. 5.2 Medial view of the major regions in the brain.

to and from the brain pass through, or terminate in, the brainstem. The brainstem gives rise to 10 of the 12 cranial nerves and houses their cell bodies. These 10 nerves determine eye movements, facial sensation and control, oral movements, oral sensation, and many other sensory and motor functions essential to eye gaze, speech, and swallowing. There are also critical centers in the midbrain that regulate wakefulness, stages of sleep, levels of arousal, taste, breathing, swallowing, and even vomiting. The midbrain is most rostral, and the pons is caudal to the midbrain and connects to the medulla, which transitions into the spinal cord.

Finally, the cerebellum, located posterior to the brainstem and connected to the pons, is the essential brain area for motor learning. Therefore, the

Table 5.1 Major divisions of the brain

Major divisions*	Related structure	Subdivision	Function
Forebrain	Telencephalon (end brain)	Cerebral hemispheres	Cerebral cortex	Executive function, voluntary movement control
			Basal ganglia	Modulation of movement commands Memory, emotion
			Limbic system	
	Diencephalon (interbrain)		Thalamus	Relay station for afferents before they reach cerebral cortex Controlling homeostasis
			Hypothalamus	
Midbrain	Mesencephalon (midbrain)	Brainstem	Midbrain	Visual and auditory reflexes, dopamine generation, sensory and motor pathways
Hindbrain	Metencephalon (after brain)		Pons	Sensory and motor pathways, cerebello-cortical pathways, nuclei for oral sensation and jaw movement control
	Myelencephalon (marrow brain)		Medulla	Nuclei for taste, hearing, facial pain sensation, breathing, speech, and balance
	Cerebellum			Motor learning, coordination, cognition

* One common categorization system uses the base form *encephalon* (meaning brain) modified by a prefix.

cerebellum plays an important role in the learning and coordination of movements of the head, eye, and body. It is also involved in the learning of new motor skills (e.g., dart throwing) and maintaining posture. Although the cerebellum has previously been considered a purely motor structure, recent research has shown that the cerebellum contributes to cognitive functions, including language.

Peripheral Nervous System (PNS)

The PNS consists of **afferent** nerves (meaning "carrying toward"), which collect information about both the internal and the external environment and deliver that information as messages to the

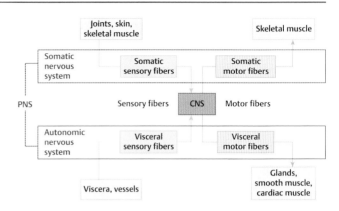

Fig. 5.3   Information flow in the nervous system. Fibers that carry information to the central nervous system (CNS) are called sensory or afferent fibers (teal); fibers that carry information away from the CNS are called motor or efferent fibers (pink).

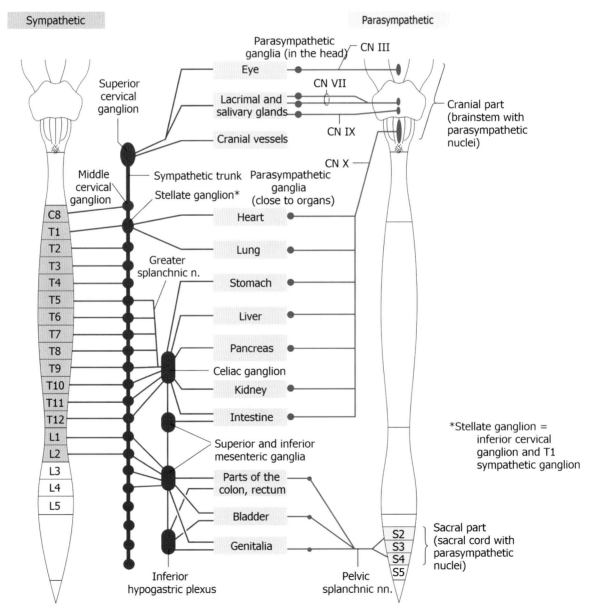

Fig. 5.4   Autonomic nervous system. The autonomic nervous system is subdivided into the sympathetic (red) and parasympathetic (blue) systems, which often act in antagonistic fashion to regulate blood flow, secretions, and organ function.

CNS, and also **efferent** nerves (meaning "carrying away from"), which deliver messages from the CNS to control muscle contraction and gland secretion. The PNS can be subdivided into the **somatic nervous system** and the **autonomic nervous system**.

The somatic nervous system is associated with voluntary control of body movements and perception of somatic sensory information. It includes **somatic sensory fibers** (afferent fibers) and **somatic motor fibers** (efferent fibers) (**Fig. 5.3,** upper half). The somatic sensory fibers receive information from the skin, skeletal muscles, and joints to relay information about limb position, touch, and pressure at the body surface to the CNS. The somatic motor fibers receive commands from the CNS and are responsible for stimulating muscle contraction.

The autonomic nervous system mediates visceral sensation and regulates involuntary efferent functions, such as heart rate, respiration, urine production, digestion, and motor control of the vascular system and exocrine glands. The autonomic nervous system innervates smooth and cardiac muscle and glands and contains afferent (**visceral sensory fibers**) and efferent (**visceral motor fibers**) nerves (**Fig. 5.3,** lower half). The autonomic nervous system has two subdivisions: the **sympathetic system** and the **parasympathetic system** (**Fig. 5.4**). The sympathetic system contains neurons in the lateral gray column from the thoracic to the lumbar spinal cord as well as in the paravertebral ganglia in paired trunks outside the spinal cord, while the parasympathetic system contains neurons in the brainstem and sacral spinal cord. The sympathetic system participates in stimulating the body's **fight or flight response**, a physical and quick reaction to stress, attack, or threat. The parasympathetic system, complementary to the sympathetic system, restores homeostasis in the body. The parasympathetic system is often considered the rest-and-digest or feed-and-breed system, because it calms the body and controls the body's responses while at rest, including digestion, defecation, urination, salivation, lacrimation, and sexual arousal.

■ Neurons and Neural Tissue

Neural tissue (also called **nervous tissue**) is the cells of the nervous system that in turn make up each aspect of the nervous system, including the CNS and PNS. Neural tissue includes **neurons** (also called nerve cells) and **glial cells** (also called neuroglia or glia). The neuron is the primary unit of the nervous system: it receives incoming (or afferent) signals,

integrates the signals, and possibly generates the characteristic output signal—the action potential. The genetic and metabolic machinery of the neurons share many common attributes with other cells in the body. However, unlike other cells, neurons generate bioelectrical signals that contribute to intercellular communication (action potentials). The glial cells are nonneuronal cells that form myelin and support the metabolic requirements of neurons.

Anatomy of Neurons

The structure of a typical neuron includes a **soma** (or cell body), one or more **dendrites**, an **axon**, and one or more **terminal boutons**, illustrated in **Fig. 5.5**. The soma and dendrites are the **receptor segment** (or input zone) that receives input signals from other neurons (**Fig. 5.6**). The axon is the **transmission segment** (or conducting zone) that propagates the bioelectrical action potential. The terminal bouton is the **terminal segment** (or output zone) of chemical synapses that contains organelles, pro-

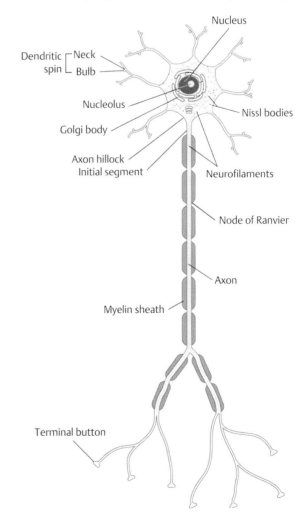

Fig. 5.5 Structure of a neuron.

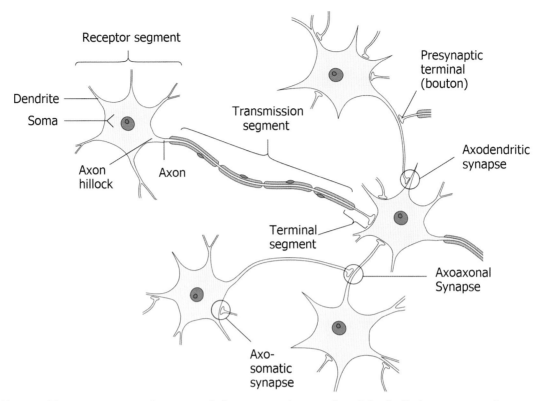

Fig. 5.6 Neurons. The nervous system is composed of neurons and supporting glial cells. Each neuron contains a soma with one axon (transmission segment) and one or more dendrites (receptor segments). The release of neurotransmitters at synapses creates an excitatory or inhibitory postsynaptic potential at the target neuron.

Box 5.1   Multiple Sclerosis

Multiple sclerosis is a degenerative disease of the central nervous system in which demyelination decreases or even terminates neural signal transmissions. The term *sclerosis* refers to the plaque along the axon created during recovery. The term *multiple* indicates that demyelination can happen simultaneously in various parts of the central nervous system. Multiple sclerosis is not a contagious or fatal disease, but an autoimmune disease. The immune system mistakes the myelin for a foreign substance invader and thus attacks and eventually destroys the myelin covering.

Symptoms
Multiple sclerosis has a variety of symptoms depending on the location of the sclerotic plaques and whether the plaques have resolved. Patients may have visual symptoms (blurred vision, blind spots, loss of sight, or twitching eyes) or somatic symptoms (muscle spasms, loss of coordination, dizziness, vertigo, fatigue, or frequent urination). Slow speech, poor articulation, and swallowing difficulty are usually seen only in more advanced cases. Multiple sclerosis may lead to cognitive problems in advanced stages, including loss of short-term memory and impaired executive function.

Symptoms often appear between the ages of 20 and 40 years. The disease is two to three times more common in females than in males. While multiple sclerosis is not considered a hereditary disease, the risk increases if relatives are affected.

Diagnosis
Multiple sclerosis can be diagnosed by magnetic resonance imaging (MRI), lumbar puncture, and evoked potentials. For 70 to 95% of individuals with multiple sclerosis, the axonal damage can be detected on MRI. Lumbar puncture is used to collect cerebrospinal fluid. The number of immune cells in cerebrospinal fluid tends to increase in patients with multiple sclerosis. An evoked potential is a record of how the brain responds to a sensory stimulus, such as light, sound, or touch. Because of the demyelinated axons in multiple sclerosis, the electrical impulses in neurons are reduced compared to those in undamaged neurons.

teins, and chemicals for the synthesis/release of neurotransmitters that affect downstream effectors (other neurons, muscles, or glands).

The soma contains a nucleus, nucleolus, and organelles that function to produce proteins (**Fig. 5.5**). The thin plasma membrane forms the neuronal "skin" that encases the cytoskeleton, made from filamentous proteins that give structure to the neuron. Protein synthesis, which requires energy (obtained from mitochondria), takes place at Nissl bodies, which contain rough endoplasmic reticulum and ribosomes.

The dendrites are branching projections that extend from the soma and are the primary locations of contact with presynaptic neurons. More specifically, the point of synaptic contact between the cells occurs at short projections (about 100 μm) called **dendritic spines** that are found on the dendrites. The dendritic spines have a bulb (the head, like a mushroom cap) that is in close proximity to the presynaptic terminal bouton (presynaptic axon terminal) and a neck that connects the bulb to the dendrite. Dendrites that receive excitatory signals typically have spines, while dendrites without spines (called smooth) are usually associated with inhibitory signals.

The axon is a long extension from the soma. Axons can be very short (< 100 μm) or very long (> 1 meter). Their primary function is to conduct the action potential to other neurons, muscles, or glands. There are two types of axons in the nervous system: **myelinated** and **unmyelinated axons**. **Myelin**, formed by glial cells, is a fatty coating (or a fatty layer, **myelin sheath**) that insulates axons. Unmyelinated gaps called **nodes of Ranvier** occur along the myelin sheaths and primarily function to increase the speed of action potential propagation. Demyelination of axons leads to impaired functions of the nervous system and is a primary symptom of the neurological disease **multiple sclerosis** (**Box 5.1**).

The terminal bouton found at the end of axons is the input structure for synapses, the tiny gaps between two neurons. Communication between most neurons is managed by the release of neurotransmitters from the terminal bouton into the synapse, which alters the membrane properties of the downstream dendrite. Axon terminals can contact a dendrite of another neuron (**axodendritic synapse**, most common), the soma of another neuron (**axosomatic synapse**), or another axon (**axoaxonal synapse**) (**Fig. 5.6**). Therefore, a neuron can receive information from hundreds or up to thousands of other neurons. The human brain has an average of 100 billion neurons and many more glial cells. As each neuron may contact up to 10,000 synapses, the number of synapses is estimated to exceed one trillion.

Classification of Neurons

Neurons are the specialized cells that receive and transmit information in the nervous system. Certain neurons can be classified by their structure, as illustrated in **Fig. 5.7**. The **multipolar neuron** (**Fig. 5.7a, b**) has many dendrites projecting from the soma. The axon of a multipolar neuron is usually long relative to the rest of the cell. The multipolar neuron is a typical neuron in the CNS and is similar to motor neurons that innervate muscles. The **pyramidal cell** (**Fig. 5.7c**) and **Purkinje cell** (**Fig. 5.7d**) are examples of multipolar neurons. The pyramidal cell is a type of neuron found particularly in the cerebral cortex. It has a conical soma, multiple short basal dendrites, and a single long axon. The Purkinje cell is a neuron located in the cerebellum and is characterized by a flasklike soma, an elaborate dendritic tree, and a single long axon. The **bipolar neuron** (**Fig. 5.7e**) has a single dendrite extending in one direction from the soma and an axon extending in the opposite direction. It is the typical neuron that is associated with special

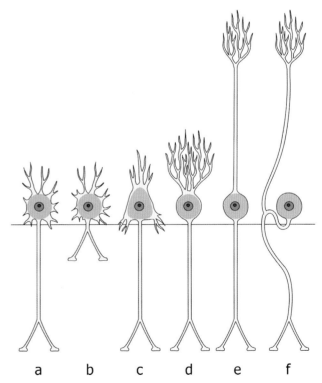

Fig. 5.7 Structural classification of neurons. **(a)** Multipolar neuron with a long axon. **(b)** Multipolar neuron with a short axon. **(c)** Pyramidal cell—dendrites are present only at the apex and base of the tridentate cell body and the axon is long. **(d)** Purkinje cell—an elaborately branched dendritic tree arises from a circumscribed site on the cell body. **(e)** Bipolar neuron—the dendrite branches in the periphery. **(f)** Unipolar or pseudounipolar neuron—the dendrite and axon are not separated by a cell body.

senses, including vision, audition, and olfaction. The **unipolar neuron** or pseudounipolar neuron (**Fig. 5.7f**) has only one projection from the soma, where the dendrite and axon are not separated. It is the typical neuron in the PNS that carries somatosensory impulses.

Neurons can also be classified by their function and projection distance, including **projection neurons** and **interneurons**. Projection neurons have a long axon that projects far from the soma, sending signals to a distant target neuron. Projection neurons can be afferent or efferent. The sensory afferent neurons receive information from the periphery via sensory receptors and send the sensory impulses to the CNS (see the blue lines in **Fig. 5.8**). Motor efferent projection neurons carry neural instructions from the cortex throughout the brainstem (see **Fig. 5.8** for a representation of projection neurons). Interneurons are usually smaller than other neurons and often function locally, with projections to proximal neurons. Interneurons serve as a processing connection between the afferent and efferent pathways or other neuronal circuits. Interneurons are the most abundant neuron type, easily outnumbering the sensory and motor neurons.

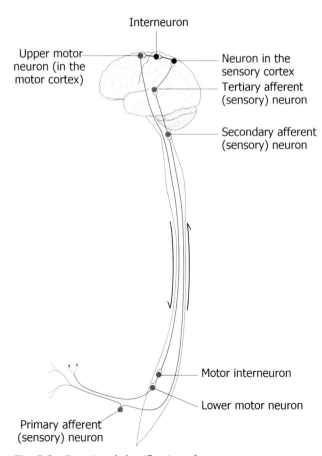

Fig. 5.8 Functional classification of neurons.

Glial Cells

The glial cells or glia (Greek for "glue") provide nutrients and essential metabolic support to neurons in the CNS and PNS. The principal glial cells include **astrocytes**, **oligodendrocytes**, and **microglia** in the CNS, and **Schwann cells** in the PNS (**Fig. 5.9**).

Astrocytes have numerous projections extending from the soma. Astrocytes are commonly found close to neuronal cell bodies, dendrites, and synapses. They have multiple roles, including passing nutrients and oxygen to neurons, removing waste products from neurons, recycling neurotransmitters from synaptic clefts, contributing to the **blood–brain barrier**, regulating local blood flow, and forming scars in damaged neural tissues.

Oligodendrocytes form myelin in the CNS and facilitate the propagation of action potentials along myelinated axons. Myelination in the PNS, however, is formed by a different cell type, the Schwann cell. Individual oligodendrocytes can have branches that myelinate different axons, but a Schwann cell myelinates a single axon. For unmyelinated axons, Schwann cells provide multiple indentations to encase them. Microglia are a special type of phagocyte that are the primary immune defense in the CNS. They recognize neural tissue damage and foreign bodies, surround/absorb them, and modulate local inflammatory responses.

Neural Tissue

Neurons and glial cells, taken together, constitute neural tissue. Neural tissue can be categorized into four types, including **gray matter** and **white matter** in the CNS (**Fig. 5.10**), and **nerves** and **ganglia** in the PNS (**Fig. 5.11**).

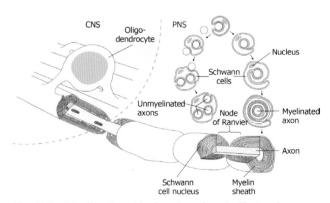

Fig. 5.9 Myelination. Myelination electrically insulates axons, thereby increasing impulse conduction speed. In the CNS, one oligodendrocyte myelinates one internode on multiple axons; in the PNS, one Schwann cell myelinates one internode on a single axon.

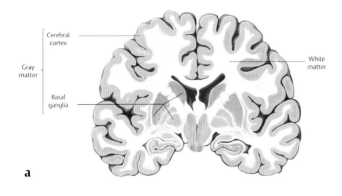

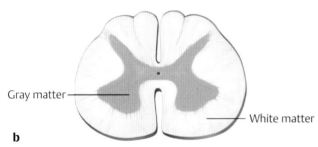

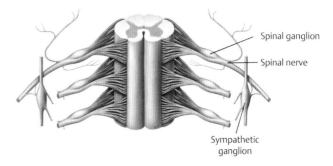

Fig. 5.11 Neural tissue in the PNS: nerves and ganglia.

Fig. 5.10 Gray and white matter in the CNS. Nerve cell bodies appear darker or gray upon gross inspection, whereas nerve cell processes (axons) and their insulating myelin sheaths appear lighter. **(a)** Coronal section through the brain illustrating cortical gray matter and underlying gray matter along with adjacent white matter. **(b)** Transverse section through the spinal cord illustrating central gray matter and surrounding white matter.

Gray matter, which is darker in unstained dissections and in certain other staining preparations, contains cell bodies, dendrites, unmyelinated axons, axon terminals (synapses), and glial cells of the CNS. The cerebral cortex and basal ganglia are examples of gray matter (see below). White matter is named for its lighter color (unstained dissections and certain preparations) due to the high density of myelinated axons and glial cells that form myelin. In general, gray matter corresponds to the input zone and output zone of neurons, while the white matter constitutes the conduction zone of neurons.

In the PNS, ganglia (singular, ganglion) are clusters of neuron cell bodies. Nerves have a bundle-like structure containing numerous axons and glial cells. Nerves can be classified into two types, based on where they are connected. **Cranial nerves** emerge from the brainstem and brain, while spinal nerves emerge from the spinal cord. Both types of nerves serve sensory and motor functions.

■ Cerebrum

The **cerebrum** is the largest portion of the CNS in terms of surface area, weight, and volume. It involves the cerebral cortex and subcortical struc-

tures, including the basal ganglia, thalamus, hypothalamus, hippocampus, and amygdala, along with subcortical white matter.

Cerebral Cortex

The cerebral cortex is a thin (2–3 mm) covering of neuronal tissue that is deeply folded and entirely encloses the two hemispheres. The cerebral cortex is formed by gray matter (**Fig. 5.10**), as it is mainly composed of neuronal cell bodies and dendrites. The surface of the cortical folds are termed **gyri** (singular, **gyrus**), while the grooves or valleys between the gyri are termed **fissures** or **sulci** (singular, **sulcus**). Approximately two-thirds of the cerebral cortex is buried in the sulci. If the cerebral cortex were unfolded, its flattened surface area would approximate 2,500 cm^2. This massive wrinkling or infolding of the gyri and sulci surface, which is referred to as gyrification, is a significant mammalian adaptation that increases the total surface area of the brain that the skull can accommodate. This means that there is a greatly expanded cortical volume that can accommodate more input, more processing, and more complex output. The human brain is generally far more folded than the brains of other mammals, although some other mammals, such as dolphins, also show extensive gyrification.

The gyri and sulci are the most striking features of the surface of the human brain when it is visually inspected. However, differences in the function of the multiple cortical regions are determined by their connections with other parts of the brain and the particular arrangement of cortical neurons, referred to as cytoarchitecture. During the early 20th century, Korbinian Brodmann became famous for his description of 52 distinct areas of the cerebral cortex, known as Brodmann areas. A sample map of **Brodmann areas** is presented in **Fig. 5.12**. Certain evidence has shown that the Brodmann areas are correlated with distinct cortical functions. For example, areas 41 and 42 in the temporal lobe are related to hearing; areas 44 and 45 are related to motor speech; and areas 1, 2, and 3 are the primary

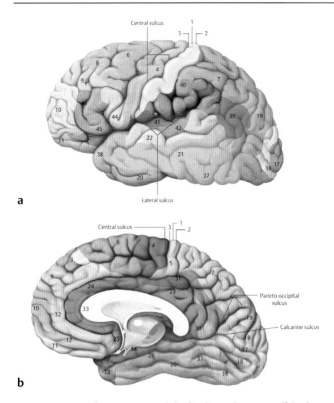

Fig. 5.12   Brodmann areas. **(a)** The lateral aspect. **(b)** The medial aspect.

somatosensory cortex. This relationship between anatomy and behavior is referred to as **functional localization**. Although the Brodmann system is not the only approach to classifying cortical functions, it offers an example that helps us to understand the complicated nature of the cerebral cortex.

Although the appearance of the gyri and sulci varies widely across individuals, there are prominent gyri and sulci that have been used as landmarks for anatomical localization. The cerebral cortex is divided into the left and right sides by the **longitudinal fissure** (**Fig. 5.13c**). However, the two hemispheres are closely connected by the massive bundle of white matter fibers known as the **corpus callosum** (**Fig. 5.13b**). There are two other deep fissures in the brain: the **central sulcus** (also called central fissure, Rolandic fissure, or the fissure of Rolando) that generally separates each hemisphere into anterior and posterior parts, and the **lateral fissure** (also called lateral sulcus, Sylvian fissure, or the fissure of Sylvius) that divides the cerebrum into the upper and lower portions (see below and **Fig. 5.13a, b**).

The sulci are important boundaries that have been used to classify the cortex into distinct **lobes** (**Fig. 5.13a**). The central sulcus separates the **frontal lobe** from the **parietal lobe**, while the lateral sulcus separates the **temporal lobe** from other lobes. Near the back of the brain and above the cerebellum is a small groove in the gyral structure called the **preoc-**

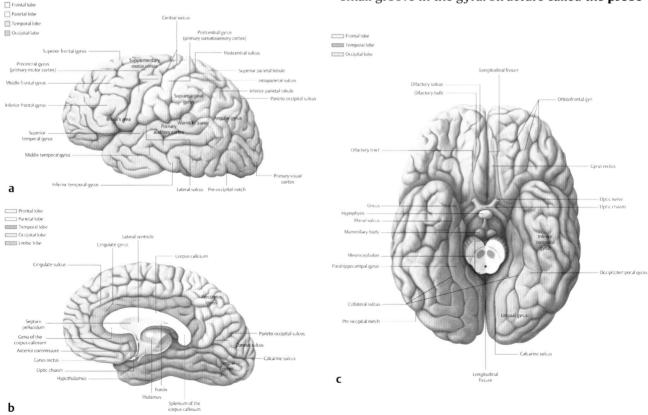

Fig. 5.13   Lobes and major sulci in the cerebral hemispheres. **(a)** The lateral aspect. **(b)** The medial aspect. **(c)** The ventral aspect.

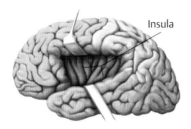

Fig. 5.14 Insula.

cipital notch. An imaginary projection between the **parietooccipital sulcus** and the preoccipital notch separates the **occipital lobe** from the parietal lobe.

An internal lobe that is not visible from the lateral surface but that is recognized by anatomists is the **limbic lobe**. It is a C-shaped structure comprised of cortical tissue that originates with the **cingulate gyrus** on the medial aspect of the brain inferior to the **cingulate sulcus** (**Fig. 5.13b**). The cingulate gyrus extends into the brain to eventually form the hippocampus. Another cortical area that is not visible from the lateral surface but that is recognized by some anatomists as a distinct lobe is the **insula** (**Fig. 5.14**). Despite its name, the insula is not an isolated structure; rather, it is a continuous volume of cortical tissue buried deeply within the lateral sulcus, and extends beneath the frontal, temporal, and parietal lobes. It can be seen if the temporal lobe is gently pulled apart from the frontal lobe and parietal lobe.

Lateral View of the Cerebral Hemispheres

Fig. 5.13a depicts the primary gyri that are visible from the lateral surface. Starting from the frontal lobe, an important gyrus anterior to the central sulcus is the **precentral gyrus**. The precentral gyrus is primarily occupied by **primary motor cortex** (Brodmann area 4) and is known to be associated with the generation of motor commands that are sent directly to cranial nerves and spinal nerves through long axons of pyramidal cells. The primary motor cortex has a characteristic somatotopic organization (**Fig. 5.15**). This means that each subregion of the cortex corresponds to the motor control of specific muscles, but the size of the subregions is associated with the complexity of the actions that an effector can produce. Effectors such as the lips, tongue, and hand, in particular, occupy much larger subregions of the primary motor cortex. This confirms the importance that these effectors have in speech production. Anterior to the primary motor cortex is the **premotor cortex** (Brodmann area 6), which is responsible for the planning of move-

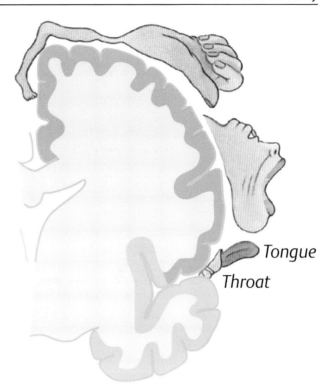

Fig. 5.15 Somatotopic organization of the primary motor cortex. The primary motor cortex exhibits somatotopic organization with respect to the target muscles it controls.

ment production and influences the motor signals generated by the primary motor cortex. Three obvious gyri in the anterolateral frontal lobe are the superior frontal gyrus adjacent to the longitudinal fissure, the middle frontal gyrus inferior to the superior frontal gyrus, and the inferior frontal gyrus inferior to the middle frontal gyrus. These gyri participate in higher cognitive functions, with the inferior frontal gyrus being particularly known for its importance to language and speech because it contains **Broca's area** (Brodmann area 44).

Broca's area is named after Pierre Paul Broca, a 19th-century French neurologist and anthropologist. Broca's observations revealed that patients who had lesions in the posterior inferior frontal gyrus lost their ability to speak, despite intact comprehension and mental function. The disorder thus identified was named **Broca's aphasia** (**Box 5.2**). Broca's work was the first to provide evidence for functional localization within the cortex.

Moving ventrally to the temporal lobe, the gyrus immediately adjacent to the lateral sulcus is the **superior temporal gyrus** (**STG**). It extends from the most anterior portion of the temporal lobe superiorly to the parietal lobe. The STG plays an important role in language. It is associated more closely with language input than with language output. In the two-thirds posterior to the superior temporal gyrus and on its dorsal

Box 5.2 Aphasia

Aphasia is a language disorder following a stroke, tumor, or head injury that is caused by cell death within portions of the brain that are responsible for language. Most often aphasia follows from damage to the left hemisphere. Aphasia is relevant for the study of language because clusters of symptoms are associated with different lesion locations. Aphasias are classified according to relative deficits in expression or comprehension ability. The five major types of aphasia are Broca's aphasia, Wernicke's aphasia, conduction aphasia, global aphasia, and anomic aphasia. The symptoms are summarized in **Table 5.2**.

Broca's Aphasia
Broca's aphasia is also called expressive aphasia. The site of lesion is typically the gray matter and white matter linked to function of Broca's area, a region of the left, posterior inferior frontal gyrus (although the location of this region varies across individuals). Individuals with Broca's aphasia have difficulty in expressing their thoughts, naming objects, reading aloud, repeating words, or writing. Often they can produce short meaningful phrases, but typically with great effort and frequent pauses. Adjectives, adverbs, and articles (such as *the*) are often omitted, making the sentences agrammatic. An extreme case is the patient whom Broca examined in 1861 who lost his ability to speak any word other than the syllable *tan*. Individuals with Broca's aphasia do not lose the ability to understand speech, but a certain level of impairment is often present. Patients are aware of their difficulties in speech and express frustration.

Wernicke's Aphasia
Wernicke's aphasia is also called receptive aphasia. The site of the lesion is often within the superior posterior temporal lobe. Patients are known to pro-

duce abundant fluent utterances, but in semantically meaningless sentences, essentially a string of intelligible words randomly strung together. Patients use unnecessary words or even create new words in sentences. They have difficulty comprehending speech, repeating words, and naming objects, along with reading and writing deficits. Typically, individuals with Wernicke's aphasia are not aware that their speech lacks meaning, at least in the acute stage.

Conduction Aphasia
Conduction aphasia may be caused by damage to white matter tracts, primarily the arcuate fasciculus, or temporoparietal cortex within the left hemisphere. The arcuate fasciculus is the white matter fiber bundle that includes direct connections between Broca's area and Wernicke's area. The junction of the temporal and parietal cortex in close proximity to Wernicke's area has also been identified as another vulnerable region. Conduction aphasia is characterized by a specific difficulty in repeating words, but there can be difficulties in naming objects and in reading aloud as well. Individuals with conduction aphasia display relative sparing of auditory comprehension and reading comprehension. They are able to write, but certain words are sometimes skipped, repeated, or substituted. In some ways, this aphasia can manifest as an intermediate syndrome between receptive and expressive aphasia. Compared to other forms of aphasia, conduction aphasia can be a milder disorder.

Global Aphasia
Global aphasia involves damage to the widespread language area in the dominant (left) hemisphere through blockage near the origin of the MCA. Individuals with global aphasia lose almost all receptive and expressive language abilities. They have difficulty in understanding spoken and written language, writing, speaking, repeating words, and naming objects. Com-

Table 5.2 Symptoms of aphasia

Aphasia	Speaking	Auditory comprehension	Reading comprehension	Repeating	Naming	Writing
Broca's aphasia	Reduced speech output	Fair	Impaired	Impaired	Impaired	Impaired
Wernicke's aphasia	Fluent but full of jargon	Impaired	Impaired	Impaired	Impaired	Impaired
Conduction aphasia	Fluent	Close to normal	Close to normal	Impaired	Spared	Spared
Global aphasia	Severely reduced	Impaired	Impaired	Impaired	Impaired	Impaired
Anomic aphasia	Fluent	Normal	Normal	Normal	Impaired	Normal

surface is the **primary auditory cortex** (Brodmann area 41), consisting of **Heschl's gyrus** (also called the transverse gyrus). The primary auditory cortex is responsible for the reception of auditory stimuli, including frequency, location, and intensity. The primary auditory cortex is tonotopic, which means that distinct neurons respond to particular frequencies. The anterior area responds to higher frequencies, while the posterior portion responds to lower frequencies. Damage to this region of the cortex leads to a rare form of hearing loss called cortical deafness. Just posterior to the primary auditory cortex is **Wernicke's area** (Brodmann areas 22, 41, and 42), named after the German physician Carl Wernicke, who in the 19th century proposed a link between lesions in the left STG and impaired language comprehension. Subsequent validation of his proposal led to the naming of temporal lobe lesions that impair speech understanding as **Wernicke's aphasia** (**Box 5.2**).

In the parietal lobe, the prominent gyrus posterior to the central sulcus is the **postcentral gyrus**. This gyrus is known to receive somatic sensation (such as touch and position) from all over the body, and is accordingly termed the **primary somatosensory cortex**. Similar to the primary motor cortex, the primary somatosensory cortex is organized somatotopically, with particular regions also showing a magnified representation (**Fig. 5.16**). The size of the cortical area devoted to each part is determined by the density of its sensory receptors. For example, the fingers and lips are far more sensitive than the legs and torso, meaning that there are more neurons associated with the face and hands in the primary somatosensory cortex and hence a larger cortical surface. In other words, the amount of cortex is directly related to its sensitivity. Moving posteriorly, a discontinuous sulcus called the intraparietal sulcus separates the superior parietal lobule from the inferior parietal lobule. The inferior parietal lobule is significant for language because it includes two important gyral formations: the **supramarginal gyrus** and the **angular gyrus**. The supramarginal gyrus (Brodmann area 40) curves around the end of the lateral sulcus. It is associated with a broad range of language formulation operations, ranging from semantic to phonologic processing. The angular gyrus (Brodmann area 39) is located posterior to the supramarginal gyrus and is responsible for semantic processing (particularly understanding metaphors) and mathematics. Although language skills are left-brain dominant, semantic processing appears to involve both the left and right sides of the parietal lobe. Damage to this area is associated with aphasia, including conduction aphasia, which compromises word repetition (left hemisphere damage), metaphor comprehension (right hemisphere damage), and basic arithmetic ability.

In the occipital lobe, the cortex around the **calcarine sulcus** (located on the caudal part of the medial surface, **Fig. 5.13b**) is called the **primary visual cor-**

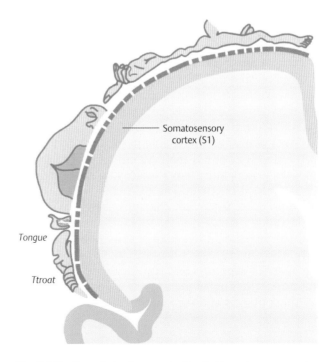

Somatosensory cortex (S1)

Tongue

Ttroat

Fig. 5.16 Somatotopic organization in the primary somatosensory cortex. The primary somatosensory cortex has somatotopic organization, meaning that each part of the body is represented in a particular cortical area.

tex (Brodmann area 17) because it is the first cortical area to receive information from the retinas. Due to its striped appearance under magnification, it is also called the striate cortex. Other areas in the occipital lobe proximal to the primary visual cortex are called extrastriate cortex (also called visual association cortex). Damage to the primary visual cortex can lead to cortical blindness for some portion of the visual field. Damage to the extrastriate cortex can result in the inability to recognize familiar faces.

Medial View of the Cerebral Hemispheres

Fig. 5.13b illustrates the primary gyri and structures that are visible from the medial surface. The cingulate gyrus is an arc-shaped structure extending across the medial surface of the frontal and parietal lobes and is separated from them by the cingulate sulcus. Below the cingulate gyrus is the corpus callosum and **lateral ventricle**. The corpus callosum is an enormous bundle of myelinated axons that enables the two hemispheres to communicate. The anterior portion of the corpus callosum is called the **genu**, while the posterior portion is called the **splenium**, with the body of the corpus callosum interposed between them. The bottom of the splenium connects to a large fiber bundle called the **fornix**, which communicates with the hippocampus of the temporal lobe (not visible from the medial surface, but see **Fig. 5.21**). The structures sitting beneath the fornix are the thalamus and hypothalamus. Another prominent but much smaller fiber bundle that connects the two hemispheres is the **anterior commissure**, which connects the ventral frontal lobe and anterior temporal lobe. The lateral ventricles are paired, with one in each hemisphere, and each has a medial membrane wall called the **septum pellucidum** that extends from the corpus callosum to the fornix.

The gyral structure visible in the medial surface of the parietal lobe is the **precuneus gyrus**, which engages in episodic memory, working memory, and visual-spatial function. The calcarine sulcus of the occipital lobe separates the gyri into two parts: the **cuneus** (wedgelike) **gyrus** in the superior part and the **lingual** (tonguelike) **gyrus** in the inferior part. The cuneus gyrus is associated with processing spatial awareness and recognizing objects from memory. The lingual gyrus is involved in encoding complex images and recognizing words.

Ventral View of the Cerebral Hemispheres

Fig. 5.13c illustrates the principal gyri and structures that are visible from the ventral or inferior surface. Near the midline of the frontal lobe are the

olfactory sulci in each hemisphere. The **olfactory tracts** and **olfactory bulbs** in the olfactory sulci process the incoming sensory information from the nose. The olfactory sulcus divides the ventral frontal lobe into the **gyrus rectus** at the medial region and the **orbitofrontal gyri** in the remaining portion of the ventral frontal lobe.

The ventral surface of the temporal lobe is occupied primarily by the inferior temporal gyrus. Additional gyri on the medial side of the ventral temporal lobe include the **occipitotemporal gyrus** and the **parahippocampal gyrus**, with a protuberance at the anterior extremity called the **uncus**. The two gyral structures are separated by two sulci: the **rhinal sulcus** at the anterior side and the **collateral sulcus** at the posterior side. The vital structure that resides inside the parahippocampal gyrus is the hippocampus. Its cross section has been likened to a seahorse in appearance, and it consists of cortical tissue folded into the temporal lobe that is central to forming new memories. The uncus sits on top of the large gray matter nucleus called the amygdala, which is commonly associated with fear processing.

Also along the midline on the ventral surface are the **optic chiasm**, pituitary gland (or hypophysis), and the **mammillary bodies** (part of the hypothalamus). The mammillary bodies connect to the hippocampus and thalamus and serve as an important support for the hypothalamus.

Subcortex

The subcortex is necessarily complex, because it supports the functions of the cortex. It is comprised of both characteristic gray matter and white matter. Several subcortical gray matter structures have already been discussed (hippocampus and amygdala), but there are other primary structures, including the basal ganglia and diencephalon (thalamus and hypothalamus). The vital function of these gray matter nuclei in regulating cortical activity cannot be overstated.

Basal Ganglia

The word *ganglia* typically refers to neuronal cell bodies in the PNS. However, the term *basal ganglia* is used to refer to a large network of embedded gray matter structures (an alternative term is basal nuclei). The nuclei of the basal ganglia include the **caudate nucleus**, **putamen**, and **globus pallidus** (**Fig. 5.17** and **Fig. 5.18**). The caudate nucleus has an odd C-shape, with a large head anteriorly, a smaller body close to the lateral ventricle, and a narrowing curved tail inferiorly that connects to the amygdala.

The putamen is a rounded mass that merges with the caudate nucleus anteriorly. The globus pallidus is closely connected to the putamen, with the putamen located at the lateral side and the globus pallidus at the medial side. The globus pallidus has two parts, the external segment (GPe) close to the putamen and the internal segment (GPi) that has white matter connections to the thalamus. The putamen and globus pallidus are collectively referred to as the lenticular nucleus because of their conelike structure (see the coronal section in **Fig. 5.18**). The caudate and the putamen, taken together, are called the **striatum** because of the striped appearance of the layered gray and white matter.

The basal ganglia are involved in complex network connections that modulate cortical output. The connections can be simplified as: cerebral cortex → striatum → GPi → thalamus → cerebral cortex. The striatum is the major input zone, collecting signals from throughout the cerebral cortex. The GPi is the major output structure that sends signals to the thalamus and then to cortical areas forming multiple parallel loops. The putamen receives signals from regions associated with somatomotor functions, while the caudate nucleus receives signals from higher association areas and cognitive areas, giving it a role in thought regulation, working memory, and perhaps language fluency. Generally, the basal ganglia are responsible for releasing desired movements and cognitive processes (thoughts and impulses) while inhibiting competing or undesired movements and thoughts. Damage to this area results in characteristic tremors and uncontrolled movements. Parkinson's disease (**Box 5.3**) and Huntington's disease (characterized by jerky uncontrollable movements), obsessive-compulsive disorder (OCD for short, characterized by uncontrollable behaviors, such as frequent hand washing), and Tourette's syndrome (characterized by motor and vocal tics) are associated with basal ganglia degeneration.

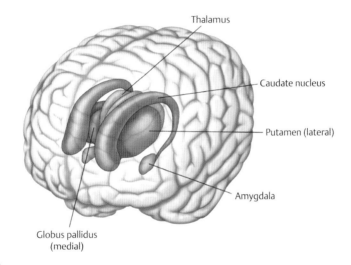

Fig. 5.17   The basal ganglia.

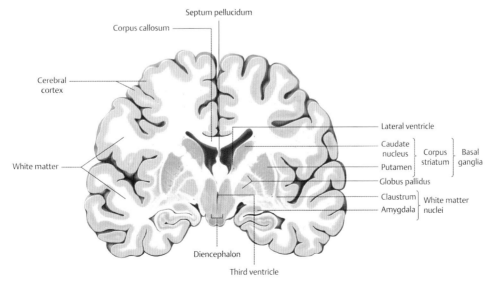

Fig. 5.18   Coronal section of the basal ganglia.

Box 5.3   Parkinson's Disease

Parkinson's disease is a progressive neurological disorder that affects movement-related behaviors. It usually appears between the ages of 55 and 60 years. The disease is caused by the death of dopamine-generating cells in the substantia nigra of the midbrain, which projects to the striatum. Degeneration of nigral dopaminergic neurons results in disruption of neural transmission through the basal ganglia, essentially causing movement control to become hypokinetic (there is slowness and paucity of movement). In the decline and eventual absence of basal ganglia modulation, an excitatory neurotransmitter (acetylcholine) becomes excessive, giving rise to resting tremor, shaking, and rigidity. Approximately 60 to 90% of individuals with Parkinson's disease have a breathy and hoarse voice, and slow and slurred speech. In later stages, dysarthria, dysphagia, and cognitive decline become clinically significant. Lee Silverman Voice Treatment is a therapy program designed for patients with Parkinson's diseases to improve laryngeal and articulatory function.

Diencephalon: Thalamus and Hypothalamus

The diencephalon refers to the thalamus, hypothalamus, and other proximal structures (shaded blue in **Fig. 5.19**). These structures are functionally important because they are involved in almost all operations of the nervous system, but they remain distinct in specific functions. The thalamus consists of twin bulb-shaped regions, symmetrical across the midline of the brain and occasionally connected by a gray band called **interthalamic adhesion**. The thalamus, near the center of the forebrain, is located generally posterior to the basal ganglia (**Fig. 5.17**). The medial surface of the thalamus encloses the **third ventricle** (**Fig. 5.18**), while its ventral surface forms the floor of the lateral ventricle. The **pineal gland** is posterior to the thalamus and secretes melatonin in response to seasonal changes in light.

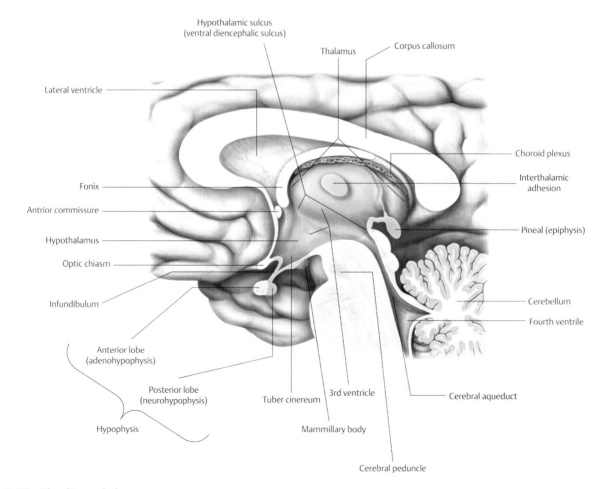

Fig. 5.19   The diencephalon.

The complexity of the thalamus is beyond the scope of this chapter, but it contains a large number of nuclei that send and receive projections from different regions of the cerebral cortex. A primary role of the thalamus is to serve as the relay station between the sensory signals originating in the PNS and their target regions in the cerebral cortex. For example, signals of somatic sensation from the spinal cord and brainstem pass the ventral posterior thalamic nuclei and then project to the postcentral gyrus. Comparable pathways have been identified for hearing and vision.

The hypothalamus is the cone-shaped structure located beneath the thalamus, and it is about the size of a sugar cube. As shown in **Fig. 5.19**, the hypothalamus is bounded by the optic chiasm at the anterior region and has structures known as the mammillary bodies at the posterior region. At the medial region, there is a small swelling called the tuber cinereum that narrows into the infundibulum, where the pituitary gland (or hypophysis) is attached. The hypothalamus is involved in all nonconscious regulation of bodily homeostasis and hormone secretion via the pituitary gland. Proper function of the hypothalamus is essential to health.

Limbic System

The limbic system, which is located in the medial region of the brain, is phylogenetically older than other brain regions, because it exists in nonmammalian species as well. It is sometimes referred to as the old brain. The primary structures of the limbic system include the hippocampus, the amygdala, and the cingulate gyrus, but there are other regions involved. The hippocampus arches anterosuperiorly over the thalamus and becomes the fornix (**Fig. 5.20a**). The amygdala is an almond-shaped nucleus found in the temporal lobe, anterior to the tail of the caudate nucleus and rostral to the hippocampus (**Fig. 5.20b**). The hippocampus complex is associated with memory formation, while the amygdala is involved in emotional responses (anger, happiness, fear, sadness, surprise, and disgust; **Box 5.4**).

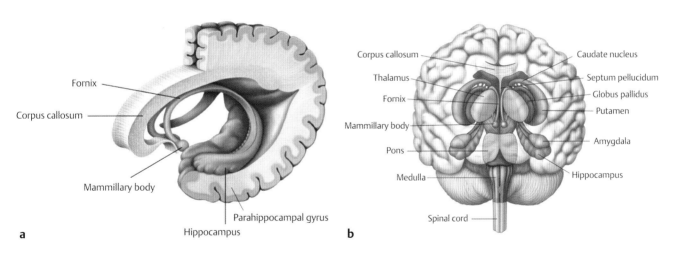

Fig. 5.20 The limbic system. **(a)** Left anterior oblique view. **(b)** Anterior view.

Box 5.4 Cerebellar Mutism

Cerebellar mutism is the loss of the ability to produce voluntary speech and is typically caused by the surgical removal of a tumor in the posterior fossa of the brain, where the cerebellum is located. This devastating complication of life-saving surgery occurs with disappointing regularity, particularly in the pediatric population. The most noticeable symptom is absent or reduced speech, almost always accompanied by impaired swallowing, visual impairment, and gross/fine movement discoordina-tion. It is not clear which are the most vulnerable structures, although removal of cerebellothalamic output connections or the vermis region appears to be implicated. Size of the tumor and whether bilateral resection is needed may also be related to this complication. Treatments are typically not successful, but a considerable number of cases show some improvement over time. The focus is on early identification so that tumors can be identified and removed with minimal collateral damage to surrounding healthy tissue.

Cerebrovascular System: Nourishment and Protection of the Brain

The brain requires a constant blood supply to maintain proper function. Because neurons cannot store glycogen (astrocytes supply glycogen), the supply of blood has to be sufficient and constant. A compromised blood supply to the brain quickly leads to unconsciousness, neuronal cell death, and loss of life. Localized interruption of the blood supply can lead to stroke and cause conditions like Broca's aphasia and Wernicke's aphasia. Although the brain comprises a mere 2% of body weight, it consumes approximately 20% of the blood flowing from the heart.

Divisions of Blood Supply

Blood vessels, including arteries, veins, and capillaries, are involved in transporting blood to and from the brain. The arterial systems that provide blood to the brain include the internal carotid system and the vertebrobasilar system, as illustrated in **Fig. 5.21** and **Fig. 5.22**.

The vertebrobasilar system forms from the right and left **vertebral arteries**, which follow the medulla and fuse near the pons to form the single **basilar artery**. A sequence of three (paired) major arteries arise from this system to supply the brainstem and cerebellum. These arteries, in a caudal to rostral sequence, are: the posterior inferior cerebellar artery, anterior inferior cerebellar artery, and the superior cerebellar artery. The vestibulocochlear artery supplying the inner ear often emerges from the anterior inferior cerebellar artery or is in close proximity. At the rostral head of the vertebrobasilar system, the artery splits into the (paired) **posterior cerebral artery** (**PCA**). The PCA supplies the occipital lobe, inferior surfaces of hemispheres, thalamus, and hypothalamus. Strokes that disrupt PCA flow result in **dyslexia** (trouble reading) and **dysarthria** (impaired articulation) if the thalamus and white matter projections are affected.

The **internal carotid arteries** have two major branches: the **anterior cerebral artery** (**ACA**) and **middle cerebral artery** (**MCA**). Together with the PCA, the ACA and MCA form the blood supply to the entire cerebrum. The ACA supplies the frontal lobes, corpus callosum, and medial surfaces of the hemispheres. The MCA supplies the lateral aspects of

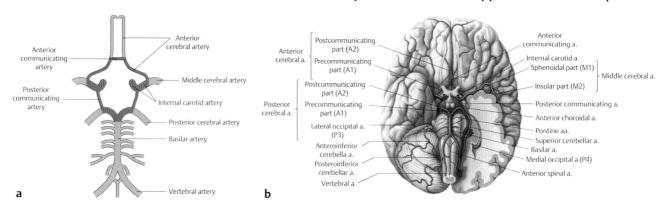

Fig. 5.21   Vertebrobasilar and internal carotid branches. **(a)** Schematic illustration of the cerebral blood supply. The circle of Willis is highlighted in dark red. **(b)** Ventral view.

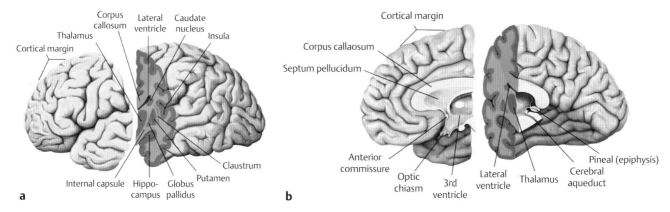

Fig. 5.22   The distribution of cerebral arteries. The central gray matter and white matter have a complex blood supply (yellow) that includes the anterior choroidal artery. **(a)** Lateral view of the left hemisphere. **(b)** Medial view of the right hemisphere.

hemispheres and the basal ganglia. The MCA is the largest cortical artery and is more directly continuous with the internal carotid artery than the ACA; however, this continuity may render it more susceptible to ischemic strokes that block arteries. Damage to the MCA can lead to weakness and paralysis of the limbs and face on the opposite side of the body. Furthermore, interruption of the MCA supply in the temporal or frontal lobe greatly impairs language formulation and production, depending on the site of damage (recall the examples of Broca's versus Wernicke's aphasia). Interestingly, the internal carotid and vertebrobasilar systems are connected at the base of the brain by communicating arteries

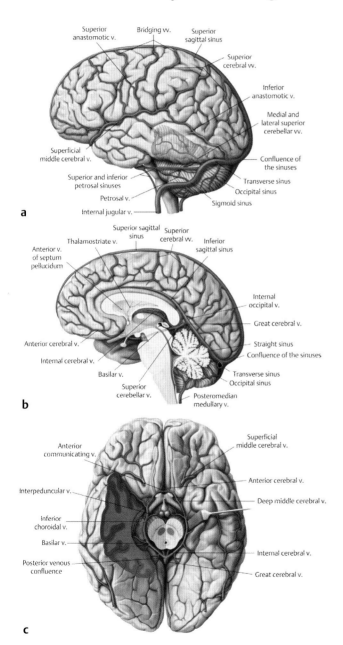

Fig. 5.23 Cerebral veins. **(a)** Lateral view. **(b)** Medial view. **(c)** Ventral view.

to form a continuous arterial ring called the **circle of Willis** (**Fig. 5.21a**). In some cases of damage or blockage, the circle of Willis can preserve sufficient blood flow to various parts of the brain.

The **superficial cerebral veins** on the medial and lateral surface of the cerebral hemispheres receive deoxygenated blood from the cortical surface and empty into the **superior sagittal sinus** on the dorsal brain surface. The **deep cerebral veins** drain the deep structures of the brain and converge on the **internal cerebral veins** above the third ventricle. The internal cerebral veins join to form the **great cerebral vein**, which continues into the **straight sinus**. The superficial and deep venous systems meet at the **confluence of sinuses** and then drain through to the transverse sinuses and sigmoid sinuses into the internal jugular veins and eventually to the heart for oxygenation (**Fig. 5.23**).

Meninges

The brain is protected by the cranial bones, the meninges, and the ventricular system. The meninges comprise three layers: the **dura mater** (outer layer), the **arachnoid mater** (middle layer), and the **pia mater** (inner layer), as shown in **Fig. 5.24**.

The dura mater is the toughest and most fibrous membrane, and it protects the inner meningeal layers. The arachnoid mater is deep to the dura and contains a layer of cells that are bound tightly to the dura mater. Tight junctions between cells of the arachnoid mater serve as a barrier (**arachnoid barrier**) to keep blood separate from the cerebral cortex. The innermost layer, the pia mater, closely adheres to the surface of the cerebral cortex. The **subarachnoid space** between the arachnoid mater and the pia mater contains the superficial arteries and veins. This space is traversed further by **arachnoid trabeculae** (spiderweblike extensions between the layers) and is filled with **cerebrospinal fluid (CSF)**.

Head trauma can lead to bleeding and tearing of the meninges. Bleeding occurring outside of the meninges (between the dura mater and the skull) is an **epidural hematoma**. Bleeding between the dura and the cortex is a **subdural hemorrhage** (or subdural hematoma; **Fig. 5.24**). The symptoms of an epidural hematoma include a loss of consciousness, bruising near the eyes and ears, nausea, vomiting, and seizures. The symptoms of subdural hemorrhage include a loss of consciousness, headache, confusion, impaired speech, blurred vision, difficulty walking, and personality changes. If untreated, these hematomas can lead to rapid deteriorations in brain function and eventually death.

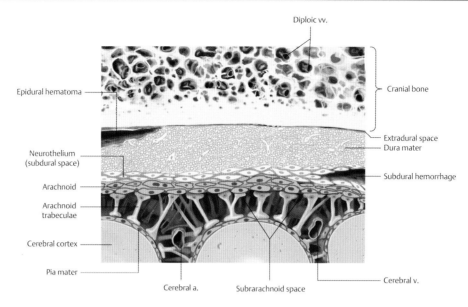

Fig. 5.24   Layers of the meninges.

Ventricular System of the Brain and Cerebrospinal Fluid

The brain has four interconnected ventricles that extend from the cerebrum to the medulla. The ventricles are the product of the expanding central canal of the neural tube in early human development. The ventricles are not empty cavities, but are filled with CSF. The four ventricles include the paired lateral ventricles in the telencephalon, the third ventricle in the midline of the diencephalon, and the **fourth ventricle** dorsal to the pons and medulla (**Fig. 5.25**). The right and left **interventricular foramina** connect the lateral ventricles and the third ventricle, and the midline **cerebral aqueduct** in the midbrain connects the third ventricle and the fourth ventricle.

The paired lateral ventricles are positioned in the middle of each cerebral hemisphere and are present in each major lobe (**Fig. 5.25**). The anterior horn of the lateral ventricle appears in the frontal lobe, the central part appears in the parietal lobe, the posterior horn penetrates the occipital lobe, and the inferior horn curves along the temporal lobe. The third ventricle sits in the midline, surrounded by the thalamus and hypothalamus. Extending from the cerebral aqueduct at the midbrain, the most caudal ventricle is the fourth ventricle.

CSF is produced by **choroid plexus** cells (**Fig. 5.26**) within each ventricle. CSF flows primarily from the lateral ventricles, through the interventricular foramina into the third ventricle, through the cerebral aqueduct into the fourth ventricle, and then through median and lateral apertures of the fourth ventricle into the subarachnoid space around the brain and spinal cord. After CSF flows into the subarachnoid space, it passes through the **arachnoid granulations** (or arachnoid villi) along

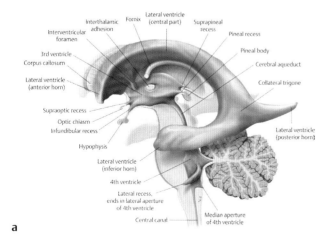

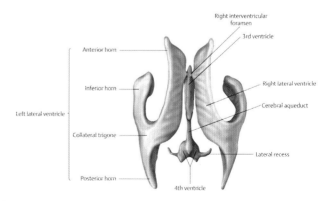

a   b

Fig. 5.25   The ventricular system. **(a)** Left lateral view. **(b)** Superior view.

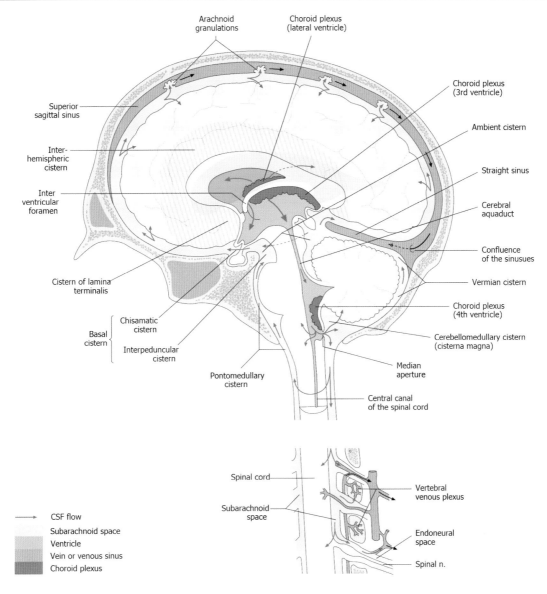

Fig. 5.26 Circulation of cerebrospinal fluid.

the dorsal midline of the brain and empties into the venous system at the superior sagittal sinus. Surprisingly, most CSF resides in the subarachnoid space instead of the ventricles, because the subarachnoid space is a much larger cavity overall.

Because the cranial bones fit tightly together, they do not allow much room for expansion. The amount of CSF produced by the choroid plexus is larger than the amount that can be placed in the brain. Therefore, the cerebrospinal fluid must empty continuously into the venous return system. Interruption of CSF circulation results in surplus fluid in the cavities, leading to **hydrocephalus** (water on the brain). The consequent increase in CSF pressure and abnormal enlargement of the ventricles interfere with cognitive development, learning ability, and motor control.

Blood–Brain Barrier

The blood–brain barrier is formed by the tight junctions between the endothelial cells of brain capillaries, which are surrounded by astrocyte endfeet (**Fig. 5.27**). The **endothelial cells** in the blood vessels of the brain also prevent the movement of material from the vessel lumen to the extracellular space of the CNS. This relatively impermeable barrier prevents large water-soluble molecules and many toxic substances from diffusing into the brain. Small fat-soluble components, such as alcohol, cocaine, and many hormones, can quickly travel through the endothelial cells and enter the brain, but large molecules such as glucose need to be transported across the capillary endothelium by transporter proteins in the vessel walls. Unfortunately, this

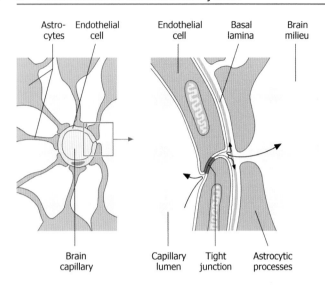

Fig. 5.27 Structure of the blood–brain barrier.

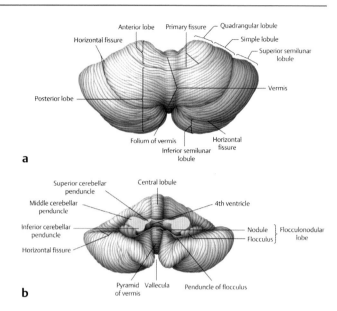

Fig. 5.28 Cerebellum. **(a)** Superior view. **(b)** Inferior view.

protective barrier may also hinder the delivery of potentially effective neurological treatments.

Cerebellum

Of all the brain structures introduced in this chapter, the cerebellum is the most interesting because it shows so many features of the entire brain itself, although it is separated from the cerebrum. The cerebellum features a proper cortex and distinct subcortical nuclei that mark its resemblance to the cortex and thereby earns it the name the "little brain." The cerebellum lies below the occipital cortex and posterior to the brainstem, placing it within the most inferior and posterior portion of the cranium. The cerebellum receives myriad afferent inputs from many areas of the cortex, brainstem, and spinal cord, and, accordingly, sends out a similar number of efferent outputs to cortical and brainstem regions.

The cerebellum's function was more difficult to understand than other parts of the brain because it was less accessible initially for neuroscientific study, and lesion effects were more subtle than those of most cortical lesions. Even more perplexing was the revelation, via improved anatomical descriptions, that the architectonics of the cerebellar cortex and subcortical nuclei are essentially identical throughout the entire structure, unlike the cerebral cortex, which shows wide variation. This suggests that, whatever the function of the cerebellum, it is replicated throughout the entire cerebellum.

There have been various attempts to organize the cerebellum in a systematic anatomical framework. While not exhaustive, a simple anatomical description with functional implications is provided here. The external cerebellum is crossed by narrow gyri and sulci that run in a general lateral-to-medial direction (**Fig. 5.28**). The sulci have a foliated or flowerlike appearance. A large fissure, the **primary fissure**, runs in the same direction and separates the cerebellum into anterior and posterior lobes. Coursing down the middle of the cerebellum is the phylogenetically oldest structure of the cerebellum, the **vermis** (Latin for "worm"). Its gyri and sulci are distinct from those of the two cerebellar hemispheres, which extend laterally from the vermis. Two other important fissures are the horizontal fissure and the **posterolateral fissure**. The horizontal fissure separates the cerebellum into superior and inferior sections and is continuous with the posterolateral fissure, which separates two adjoining cerebellar structures called the **nodulus** and **flocculus** from the main body. These two structures share similar properties with the vermis (also called the **flocculonodular lobe**).

The surface anatomy can be further classified into functional divisions related to the input and output relationships of the cerebellum with the cerebrum, brainstem, and spinal cord. These divisions are longitudinal zones that run perpendicular to the fissures and can be visualized as three bands. The medial functional zone, corresponding to the vermis and flocculonodular lobe, is called the vermal zone. Extending laterally onto the cerebellar hemisphere is the intermediate hemisphere functional zone. The most lateral portion of the hemispheres corresponds to the lateral functional zone. The vermal zone, intermediate zone, and lateral zone each project to distinct subcortical nuclei and then to different parts of the CNS.

Input–Output Connections

The input and output connections of these functional zones aid in understanding how cerebellar connectivity works. All input to the cerebellum, regardless of its origin within the CNS, travels to the cortex, but to different regions. All output from the cerebellum comes from the subcortical nuclei, regardless of its destination. The input and output pathways are located on the dorsal aspect of the brainstem. There are three prominent tracts, collectively called the **cerebellar peduncles**, that are fully visible only if the cerebellum is removed in a cadaver specimen or with a high-resolution MRI scan. The peduncles, the **superior**, **middle,** and **inferior cerebellar peduncles**, are the superhighways for cerebellar connections with the CNS (**Fig 5.28b** and **Fig. 5.29**). Most of the neurons traveling to the cerebellum enter through the middle and inferior peduncles, while most of the neuronal output is through the superior peduncle and a smaller tract from the vermal zone.

Input from the cerebral cortex that is related to complex actions and cognitive operations passes into the brainstem (pons subsection) and makes synaptic contact (corticopontine fibers; **Fig. 5.30**). From there , the pontocerebellar fibers arise, cross the midline, and project to the lateral zone of the hemispheres via the middle cerebellar peduncle. Cortical input related to coordinated movements follows an almost identical pathway, except the pontocerebellar fibers project to the intermediate functional zone. Proprioceptive information on body position (leg, arm, trunk, and jaw) from the spinal cord and brainstem also crosses the midline in the pons and projects to the intermediate zone. Vestibular information related to balance and head- and eye-orienting reflexes enter through the inferior cerebellar peduncle and project to the vermal zone. In this manner, the cerebellum receives selected input from throughout the CNS.

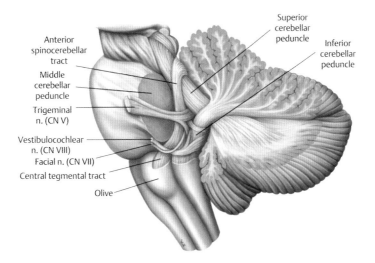

Fig. 5.29 Cerebellar peduncles.

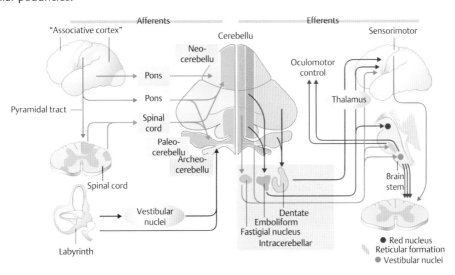

Fig. 5.30 Tracts and function of the cerebellum.

Output from the cerebellum originates in the subcortical nuclei and passes through the superior cerebellar peduncle, crosses the midline again, and then goes to specific targets. The three subcortical nuclei are the **dentate nucleus**, **interpositus nucleus**, and **fastigial nucleus** (**Fig. 5.30**). The three nuclei are arranged in a lateral-medial axis that corresponds to the functional zones mentioned earlier. The lateral zone of the cerebellar cortex projects to the dentate nucleus. Output from the dentate nucleus projects back to the cerebral cortex via the thalamus. The intermediate zone projects to the interpositus nucleus, which in turn projects to motor centers. The medial zone projects to the fastigial nucleus, which sends its output through a small tract to vestibular spinal cord regions. There are three principles to remember here: First, the cerebellum receives input from specific CNS regions and sends processed commands back to the same CNS regions, which acts to promote learning and refinement of activity in those regions. Second, inputs and outputs of the cerebellum preserve the somatotopy of the cerebral cortex and other regions. Third, the cerebellum influences CNS function contralaterally through its crossed input and output configuration. For example, operations on the left side of the brain are influenced by the right cerebellar hemisphere.

Cerebellar Neuronal Circuitry

Of all the interesting features of the cerebellum, described, it is important to emphasize that the gross anatomy is arranged around the most highly stereotypical neuronal circuitry within the nervous system. The cerebral cortex is fascinating because of its broad variation, while the cerebellar cortex and associated nuclei are equally as remarkable for their lack of variation. An approximate analogy is a circuit board in which all the features are replicated over and over in a highly precise manner to ensure speed and efficiency of operation. A brief review is provided here (**Fig. 5.31**).

There are two types of input neurons: **mossy fibers** and **climbing fibers**. The mossy fibers are the widespread projection neurons from the CNS. The climbing fibers are specific cells that originate in the contralateral brainstem (inferior olivary nucleus). Both the mossy fibers and the climbing fibers synapse in the cortex. The mossy fibers connect to cortical interneurons called **granule cells**, which have very long axons that make connections to the only cortical output neuron, the Purkinje cells. The climbing fibers connect directly to Purkinje cells. The climbing fibers make in excess of a trillion synaptic connections with the cerebellar cortex. The cortical Purkinje cells in turn project to deep cerebellar nuclei to terminate on the neurons that project back to the CNS. As already suggested, the number of cerebellar neurons and synaptic connections is vast, accounting for half of all the neurons and connections in the nervous system.

The pattern of excitatory and inhibitory connections of these neurons is also stereotyped, as would be predicted. The mossy and climbing fibers are both excitatory species. The granule cells contacted by mossy fibers are also excitatory. The Purkinje cells, in contrast, are exclusively inhibitory, while the cerebellar output projection neurons are excitatory. The inhibitory function of the Purkinje is the strongest modulatory effect on cerebellar function, enabling

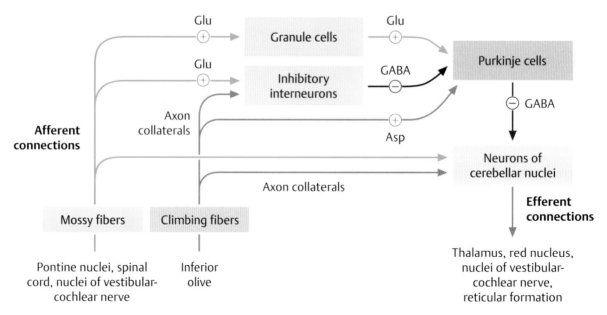

Fig. 5.31 Synaptic circuitry of the cerebellum.

highly selective and potent influences on the rest of the CNS. These influences have been highly studied in the context of motor learning, in which the cerebellum is more active during the learning phase, but less involved once the movement becomes routine.

■ Brainstem

The brainstem combines a vital highway with a vital processing center essential for life. As a highway, the brainstem connects the spinal cord with the cerebrum via numerous ascending and descending myelinated pathways that carry cortical impulses to the spinal cord and inform the brain of its environment. As a processing center, the brainstem contains gray matter nuclei essential to breathing, speech, swallowing, consciousness, pain processing, and the special senses. Given its fundamental role in connectivity and the maintenance of life, it is not surprising that the brainstem is also protected by the cranium. Upon observation, the organization of the brainstem is immediately different from the cerebrum and cerebellum, as the external tissue consists of white matter that encapsulates multiple gray matter nuclei.

Although the brainstem is continuous with the spinal cord and may appear similar, the cross-sectional organization differs from that of the spinal cord. Within the brainstem, sensory nerves enter laterally, while motor nerves exit anteromedially. Accordingly, sensory nuclei are positioned laterally and dorsally and motor nuclei are positioned medially and ventrally. Interposed among the sensory and motor nuclei are other gray matter nuclei that function as processing and relay centers.

The anatomical divisions of the brainstem are the midbrain, pons, and medulla oblongata (short form, medulla). The common feature of these divisions is that ascending and descending white matter tracts have a characteristic spatial organization that must cross the entire brainstem. Otherwise, the divisions are distinctive in overall morphology, internal organization, and relationship to the cranial nerves.

Midbrain

Rostrally, the midbrain merges with the diencephalon, with several thalamic nuclei in close proximity. The ventral (anterior) region is distinctive because it has large right and left columns of descending white matter called the **cerebral peduncles**. These are the continuation of the **corticospinal** and **cor-**

ticobulbar tracts that are distributed to brainstem centers and to the spinal cord. Internal and roughly parallel to the peduncle are large gray matter nuclei called the **substantia nigra**. On the dorsal aspect are two pairs of prominences, the **superior** and **inferior colliculi** (or "little hills"). The superior–inferior layout of the colliculi divides the midbrain into rostral and caudal divisions. In the center of the midbrain is a narrow channel, the cerebral aqueduct, which connects the third ventricle with the fourth ventricle. Surrounding the aqueduct is a complex processing center called the periaqueductal gray matter that is involved in generating nonvolitional vocalizations and processing of pain sensations. The prominent cranial nerves associated with the midbrain are the **oculomotor nerve** (**CN III**) and the **trochlear nerve** (**CN IV**), which are described later (**Fig. 5.32**).

Pons

The pons is distinctive for its bulging white matter that makes it larger than the other brainstem sections. The corticospinal tract and corticobulbar tracts contribute to the white matter of the pons, but it is also the region through which the massive white matter bundles traveling to and from the cerebellum are located. Corticopontine fibers that carry messages from the brain intended for the cerebellum make synaptic connections in the pons. From there, pontocerebellar fibers enter the cerebellum and synapse throughout that structure. On the dorsal aspect of the pons are the three prominent cerebellar peduncles, which connect the rest of the CNS with the cerebellum. In between the peduncles lies the origin of the fourth ventricle, which widens and extends into the rostral aspect of the dorsal medulla. The lateral margin of the pons is distinguished by the large root of the **trigeminal nerve** (**CN V**; **Fig. 5.32**). The internal structure of the pons is marked to a great extent by the white matter connections. The other major features are the gray matter nuclei of the cranial nerves. The largest set of nuclei is that of the trigeminal nerve, of which the largest is the chief or principal sensory nucleus.

Medulla

The medulla is perhaps the most complex region of the brainstem and most significant for speech production and deglutition because most of the motor and sensory nerves associated with these behaviors exit at the medulla. However, the trigeminal nerve from the pons is also fundamentally important for oral behaviors. The medulla also has dis-

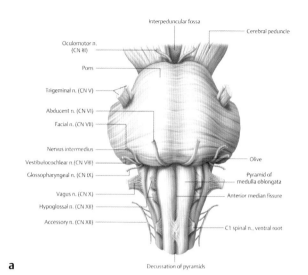

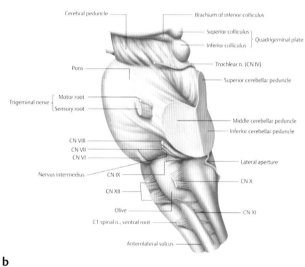

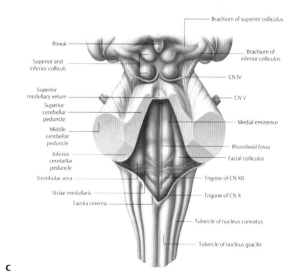

Fig. 5.32 Brainstem and associated cranial nerves. **(a)** Anterior view. **(b)** Lateral view. **(c)** Posterior view.

tinctive features on the dorsal, lateral, and ventral margins. The dorsal margin is dominated by the fourth ventricle rostrally. The ventricle narrows and ends approximately two-thirds of the way toward the caudal aspect. Along the caudal aspect are two large white matter columns on each side that carry almost all somatic sensation from the limbs, trunk, and legs. The medial column, called the **fasciculus gracilis**, conveys sensation from the legs to the brain. The lateral column, the **fasciculus cuneatus**, conveys sensation from the arms to the brain. On the lateral aspect is a large bulging rounded structure, the **olive**, that covers gray matter and has extensive connections with the cerebellum and other sensory centers. On the ventral aspect are the prominent and large white matter bundles called the **pyramids**. The pyramids are the continuation of the corticospinal tract on its way to the spinal cord.

The other distinctive external features of the medulla are the remaining cranial nerve roots present on the ventral and lateral aspects (**Fig. 5.32**). At the junction of the pons and medulla is the pontomedullary junction, at which the roots of the **abducens nerve** (**CN VI**), **facial nerve** (**CN VII**), and **vestibulocochlear nerve** (**CN VIII**) emerge. These three nerves exit along the motor-sensory distribution described above: the abducens nerve, a pure motor nerve, exits medially; the facial nerve, a mixed motor/sensory nerve, exits at an intermediate location; and the vestibulocochlear nerve, a pure sensory nerve, exits laterally. Moving in a rostral to caudal direction along the medulla are the roots of the glossopharyngeal to hypoglossal nerves. The smaller **glossopharyngeal nerve** (**CN IX**) and larger **vagus nerve** (**CN X**) exit as rootlets on the ventrolateral aspect of the medulla, indicating that these are mixed motor/sensory nerves. The **accessory nerve** (**CN XI**) actually originates in the upper spinal cord, where its cell bodies reside, but it exits medially from the brainstem. The last cranial nerve is the **hypoglossal nerve** (**CN XII**), which exits medially from the indentation between the pyramids and the olive.

The internal organization of the medulla is mostly arranged around the nuclei of the cranial nerves, where the cell bodies reside and the white matter tracts pass to and from the spinal cord. Properly viewed, these nuclei are arranged in a columnar structure placed in a lateral to medial organization depending on their function as sensory, mixed, or motor functions (**Fig. 5.33**). The other gray matter nuclei have very complicated functions that are not fully understood. They are thought to act as pattern-generating mechanisms for basic life

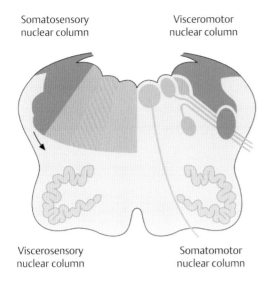

Somatosensory
nuclear column

Visceromotor
nuclear column

Viscerosensory
nuclear column

Somatomotor
nuclear column

Fig. 5.33 Location of the cranial nerve nuclei in the adult brain (medulla).

functions. One example is the **reticular system**, which has scattered gray matter nuclei within the medulla and extending up to the pons. These nuclei contribute to wakefulness. The pattern-generating neurons aid in chewing behavior, swallowing motions, respiratory cycles, vomiting, and balance. Motor neurons from these regions exit the brainstem to target the muscles involved in these cyclical patterns. Because so many nuclei are packed into the brainstem, it is particularly sensitive to small strokes, which damage multiple nuclei, impairing a range of basic behaviors and often compromising the motor control of speech. Damage to this area can lead to slurred and imprecise articulation (i.e., dysarthria).

■ Cranial Nerves

There are 12 cranial nerves in all mammals. Across species, only two of the cranial nerves have their origin outside of the brainstem. The cranial nerves vary from having highly specific functions as either pure sensory or pure motor nerves to mixed nerves that have broad functions. The highly specific nerves typically are associated with a single nucleus, while the mixed nerves receive contributions from multiple nuclei (**Fig. 5.34**). The following review summarizes the anatomy and function of the cranial nerves along with their organization in the CNS (for a summary, see **Table 5.3** and **Table 5.4**). It is a common convention to discuss sensory nerves as entering the CNS and motor nerves as exiting the CNS. With regard to the brainstem, motor nerves arise on the medial ventral surface (the trochlear nerve on the dorsal side is the sole exception), mixed nerves enter and exit the mediolateral surface, and pure sensory nerves enter on the most lateral position.

The first cranial nerve is the **olfactory nerve** (**CN I**), which is a specialized sensory nerve that carries odor information from the periphery into the CNS. The olfactory nerve terminates on the olfactory bulb, which, in turn, sends secondary afferent neurons directly to the cortex. Olfactory sensation is recognized as being the only sensation that is not relayed through the thalamus.

The second cranial nerve is the **optic nerve** (**CN II**), which is the specialized cranial nerve that conveys visual information from the retina. The optic nerves follow a complicated trajectory, in that half of the nerves cross over to the opposite side of the CNS before terminating in the thalamus. Second-order afferents project to the occipital lobe (pri-

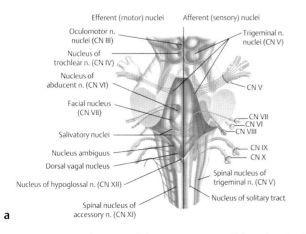
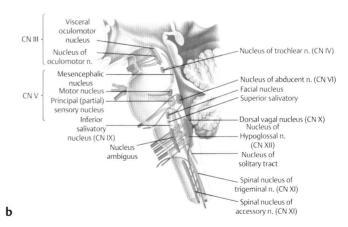

Fig. 5.34 Cranial nerves. **(a)** Posterior view. **(b)** Midsagittal section.

Table 5.3 Origin and function of cranial nerves

Cranial nerve	Origin	Functional fiber types
CN I: Olfactory n.	Telencephalon*	●
CN II: Optic n.	Diencephalon*	●
CN III: Oculomotor n.	Mesencephalon	● ●
CN IV: Trochlear n.	Mesencephalon	●
CN V: Trigeminal n.	Pons	● ●
CN VI: Abducent n.	Pons	●
CN VII: Facial n.	Pons	● ● ● ●
CN VIII: Vestibulocochlear n.	Pons	●
CN IX: Glossopharyngeal n.	Medulla oblongata	● ● ● ● ●
CN X: Vagus n.	Medulla oblongata	● ● ● ● ●
CN XI: Accessory n.	Medulla oblongata	● ●
CN XII: Hypoglossal n.	Medulla oblongata	●

* The olfactory and optic nerves are extensions of the brain rather than true nerves; they are therefore not associated with nuclei in the brainstem.

Table 5.4 Classification of cranial nerve fibers

Fiber Type		Function
General somatic motor	●	Innervate voluntary muscle
General visceral motor	●	Constitute the cranial component of the parasympathetic system, innervate involuntary muscles and glands
Special visceral motor (branchial motor)	●	Innervate muscles that developed from the primitive pharynx (pharyngeal arches)
General somatic sensory	●	Carry sensations such as touch, temperature, pain, and pressure
Special somatic sensory	●	Carry impulses from the eye for sight and from the ear for hearing and balance
General visceral sensory	●	Transmit information from viscera such as carotid bodies, the heart, esophagus, trachea, and gastrointestinal tract
Special visceral sensory	●	Transmit information regarding smell and taste

mary visual cortex), serving visual perception, or to brainstem regions to regulate visual reflexes.

The third cranial nerve, the oculomotor nerve, exits from the rostral, ventral midbrain in the midline because it is a pure motor nerve. The cell bodies of this nerve reside in the oculomotor nucleus located in the midline of the midbrain. The oculomotor nerve innervates four of the six extraocular muscles that control eye movements.

The fourth cranial nerve, the trochlear nerve, is also a pure motor nerve that innervates one of the extraocular muscles. This nerve is unique because it is the only one that emerges from the dorsal surface, at the level of the midbrain. The nerve circles all around the midbrain to exit the cranium and reach the muscle. Because it is a pure motor nerve, the cell bodies are within the medial midbrain and the nerve root exits medially.

The fifth cranial nerve, the trigeminal nerve, is the largest of all the cranial nerves. It arises from the lateral pons and is the only nerve arising from this structure. The nerve has a large sensory root entering the brainstem and a much smaller motor root that exits the brainstem. Each root connects to separate gray matter nuclei within the pons, illustrating how a single mixed nerve supports distinct functions. The sensory root has its ganglion of cell bodies outside the brainstem, and it splits into three branches (hence 'tri') that receive almost all sensory information from the face, oral cavity, nasal cavity, teeth, and parts of the pharynx. The first branch (**ophthalmic**, or V$_1$) innervates the upper face above the midline of the eyes up to the top of the forehead, carrying all forms of somatic sensation. The second branch (**maxillary**, or V$_2$) mediates all somatic sensation from the intermediate face, from the lower half of the eyes down to the upper lip, including the nasal cavity, upper teeth, and palate. The third branch (**mandibular**, or V$_3$) similarly carries all somatic innervation from the lower face, stretching from the lower lip around the jaw and chin to the upper neck. It also innervates the lower oral cavity, including the anterior two-thirds of the tongue, and provides jaw proprioception. The motor root travels with the mandibular branch to reach all the muscles controlling the jaw (muscles of mastication). Because the face and oral tract deliver abundant sensory information to the brainstem, the laterally positioned trigeminal nucleus is accordingly the largest nucleus of the cranial nerves, stretching from the brainstem up to the midbrain. The largest portion of the sensory nucleus, called the chief sensory nucleus, is contained within the pons. The motor branch of the trigeminal nerve has a small medially oriented nucleus within the pons. The trigeminal nerve is important for speech, as all of the oral somatosensations associated with articulatory motions are carried by this nerve.

The next set of cranial nerves exit the pontomedullary junction, as described above. The most medial is the abducens nerve, which is a small pure motor nerve that innervates one of the six external eye muscles. The motor nucleus is also at the midline. The nerve at the intermediate portion of the junction is the facial nerve, which is another mixed nerve. There is a large motor branch, which innervates all the muscles of the upper and lower face that control expressions and one of the small middle ear muscles (stapedius). The smaller somatic sensory branch innervates parts of the outer ear. The last important branch of the facial nerve is the

chorda tympani. This branch carries taste sensation to the gustatory nucleus in the brainstem. The sensory and motor nuclei serving the facial nerve are arrayed along a lateral-to-medial axis positioned proximal to the pontomedullary junction. The facial nerve has a critical role in speech production because it carries motor signals for the labial motions of many consonants and vowels.

The most lateral cranial nerve emerging at the pontomedullary junction is the vestibulocochlear nerve. This specialized sensory nerve has two roots from the inner ear: one that carries hearing sense and the other that carries vestibular sense (balance and head position). Separate groups of nuclei in the brainstem receive information from these nerves and are located at the most lateral portions of the brainstem proximal to the pontomedullary junction.

The rest of the cranial nerves have their roots on the medulla. The glossopharyngeal nerve is a mixed cranial nerve with a few small roots in the rostral medulla on the lateral side of the olive. It sends some somatic information to the CNS from the middle ear cavity and parts of the pharynx and visceral information from the carotid body and sinus. The final form of sensory information is taste sensation from the posterior third of the tongue. There is also a small motor root that innervates a single pharyngeal muscle called the stylopharyngeus. The nuclei serving this nerve are arranged in a complex manner because they are shared with the trigeminal, facial, and vagus nerves.

The vagus ("wandering") nerve is not the largest cranial nerve but carries afferent and efferent information from the most diverse set of organs. The numerous rootlets of the vagus resemble those of the glossopharyngeal nerve, but extend further caudally. The vagus carries afferent information throughout most of the larynx and pharynx up to two major sensory centers in the brainstem (solitary tract nucleus and trigeminal nucleus). The vagus nerve is also a motor nerve that sends motor innervation to many of the pharyngeal and laryngeal muscles. Therefore, the control of phonation and coordination of swallowing depends on intact function of the vagus. The vagus further carries visceral sensation from the thorax, heart, and abdomen that is essential for the brain in monitoring visceral health.

The accessory nerve is a motor nerve that originates from the caudal medulla and upper spinal cord. It is a pure motor nerve, so it exits medially. This nerve innervates two muscles that control head and shoulder movements.

The final cranial nerve, the hypoglossal nerve, is a pure motor nerve that exits from the lower medulla between the pyramid and olive. The multiple rootlets, which come from a large elongated midline nucleus, merge into a single motor nerve that innervates all of the tongue muscles. These muscles participate in most of the sounds of speech and allow for normal mastication and swallowing.

Understanding the organization of the brainstem is made easier by knowing both the cranial nerves and their nuclei. This perspective distinguishes the lateral-to-medial alignment of these structures because sensory nerves are lateral, mixed nerves are intermediate, and motor nerves are in the midline. If this lateral-to-medial axis is extended throughout the brainstem, one can visualize the nerves and nuclei as lying in a special sensory column (hearing and vestibular sense), a somatosensory column (the trigeminal nucleus), and a motor column (eye motor, facial motor, and tongue motor). In this way, the functions and general positions of the nerves can be recalled.

■ Spinal Cord

The brainstem is continuous with the spinal cord, and they are similar in two important ways. First, the gray matter for sensory and motor nuclei is arranged in a regular pattern. Second, many of the white matter pathways that pass through the brainstem are present in the spinal cord. The spinal cord is the part of the nervous system that carries all sensation and directs movement while regulating a large proportion of the sympathetic and parasympathetic drive for the body.

The spinal cord extends from the base of the skull down to the lower back. It is shorter than the vertebral column, but nerves from the spinal cord extend throughout the column. The sections of the spinal cord correspond to the sections of the vertebral column and have peripheral nerves that correspond to each vertebral level and exit at those levels. The sensory and motor nerves at each level arise separately but merge together before exiting the vertebral opening as a spinal nerve. There are 30 vertebral bones that make up the vertebral column, but there are 31 pairs of nerves because the first cervical nerve pair arises at the top of the vertebral column (i.e., there are eight cervical nerves, but only seven cervical vertebrae). At the termination of the spinal cord, the **conus medullaris**, the peripheral nerves continue their path toward their respective vertebral exits. The collection of nerves vaguely resembles a horse's tail and is called the

cauda equina. The inner core of the spinal cord is comprised of gray matter covered by external white matter. The three meningeal layers protect the spinal cord.

Gray Matter

The gray matter has a characteristic distribution throughout the length of the spinal cord that follows from the brainstem. The dorsal gray matter consists of neuronal cell bodies that receive afferent input from peripheral sensory nerves. These peripheral sensory neurons are called primary afferents, while the cell bodies within the dorsal gray matter and their afferents that project rostrally are called secondary afferents. This is exactly the same pattern as that of the brainstem, except that the sensory gray matter is shifted dorsally. The ventral gray matter consists of the cell bodies of **lower motor neurons**. The axons from these neurons project to target muscles. The somewhat prominent appearance of the gray matter in the spinal cord has been associated with horns, so that the dorsal gray is referred to as the dorsal horns and the ventral gray as ventral horns (**Fig. 5.35**). There is intermediate gray matter between the dorsal and ventral horns that houses the cell bodies of autonomic neurons (in thoracic regions), as well as interneurons, which modulate spinal cord activity.

The quantity of gray matter varies across the sections of the spinal cord. There are localized increases of gray matter within the cervical and lumber sections because these regions innervate the arms and legs, respectively. The thoracic and sacral sections have relatively less gray matter. Each section of gray matter, whether it is sensory or motor, innervates a distinct region of the body called a **dermatome**.

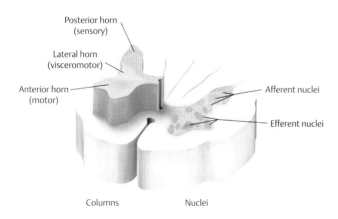

Fig. 5.35 Organization of gray matter in the spinal cord.

White Matter

Myelinated axons surround the midline gray matter and form the surface of the spinal cord. The number of axons (and volume of white matter) increases from the caudal extent to the most rostral portion simply because more axons are going to and coming from the brain. This means that the spinal cord narrows toward its caudal terminal point. The white matter is systematically compartmentalized into distinct afferent and efferent tracts. For the most part, these tracts traverse a considerable length of the spinal cord as they send or receive branches from the different sections. Anatomists have differentiated these tracts, but their distribution is complex. The largest tracts with sensory and motor significance are described next, but the list is far from exhaustive.

On the dorsomedial aspect are two separate columns of white matter (**Fig. 5.36**). The most medial is the fasciculus gracilis, which carries cutaneous information and limb position information from the lower extremities to the brain. The lateral column is the fasciculus cuneatus, which carries the same information, but from the upper extremities to the brain. Collectively, they are called the **dorsal column** system. These columns preserve a somatotopic organization of limb sensation. Pain and temperature information is relayed separately through a large tract on each side called the **spinothalamic tract**, which is located anteriorly and laterally within the spinal cord and is sometimes called the anterolateral pathway. Again, this tract has a somatotopic arrangement. There is also a specific decussation pattern for the tracts that is important to remember when assessing spinal cord injury. The dorsal column system remains ipsilateral until it reaches the brainstem and then crosses over. The spinothalamic system, in contrast, crosses over locally at the level where it enters the brainstem. This means that pain and somatosensory information from exactly the same part of the body ascend through the spinal cord on different sides.

The efferent tracts involve the all-important corticospinal tract, which provides voluntary movement control, and supplementary tracts, which support less volitional functions for balance (**Fig. 5.36**). The corticospinal tract descends from the primary motor cortex to synapse directly on the cell bodies of the lower motor neurons in the ventral horn. This tract is intriguing because 85% of the fibers cross over at the level of the pyramids in the brainstem. The remainder of the fibers remain ipsilateral until they reach the target level and either cross over locally or remain ipsilateral. The corticospinal fibers have the widest diameter and

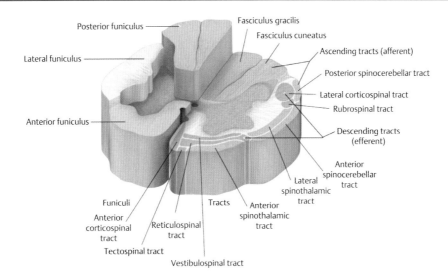

Fig. 5.36 White matter tracts within the spinal cord. The white matter of the spinal cord contains ascending tracts (afferent, in blue) and descending tracts (efferent, in red).

thickest myelin coat of all neurons in the CNS. As a result, action potential conduction is most rapid in this system. **Somatotopy** is preserved, as would be predicted, with the proximal muscles (torso, hip, and shoulder) represented most medially and the axial muscles (leg and arm) laterally.

The **vestibulospinal tract** descends from the vestibular nuclei to coordinate the body with the head in order to maintain balance. The signals, which terminate on cervical, thoracic, and lumbar gray matter, are heavily influenced by cerebellar efferents as well. The **reticulospinal** system descends from the reticular formation in the brainstem. It influences automatic posture- and gait-related movements. Interestingly, these ipsilateral tracts are found on both sides of the spinal cord.

Autonomic Nervous System

Typical peripheral efferent nerves have a direct connection between the spinal cord and the muscle. However, autonomic nerves project from gray matter to a synapse in a peripheral ganglion, from which another nerve arises and projects to the visceral muscle or gland. The sympathetic preganglionic neurons are in the thoracic and lumbar divisions of the spinal cord. These neurons project to the sympathetic trunk, which runs from the cervical to sacral levels, enabling the sympathetic system to reach the entire body and to regulate fight or flight responses. The parasympathetic preganglionic neurons arise from a much more limited set of regions (CN IX, CN X, and sacral levels) and project to a limited set of ganglia, but these ganglia in turn project to many organs to regulate rest/relax responses.

Upper and Lower Motor Neurons

There is a fundamental distinction between the two main types of neurons that excite muscles and result in volitional movement. **Upper motor neurons** arise from the cerebral cortex and descend to synapse on the motor nuclei of cranial motor nerves and spinal motor nerves. These neurons carry impulses that are analogous to commands from the brain for muscle to contract with a particular force and duration. However, these neurons remain exclusively within the CNS. The synaptic targets of upper motor neurons are the cell bodies of **lower motor neurons**, which also reside in the CNS. It is the axons of the lower motor neurons that leave the CNS and reach the actual muscle fibers and provide excitatory activation, resulting in muscle fiber contraction. The distinction of either being within the CNS or leaving the CNS is what separates the upper motor neuron from the lower motor neuron.

Yet, the influence of these neurons on movement differs, which is apparent when one of the neuron types is selectively damaged. Damage to upper motor neurons results in spasticity and heightened reflexes because the modulating influence of the corticospinal/corticobulbar tract is compromised. Damage to lower motor neurons results in muscle wasting and diminished reflexes because the muscle itself loses innervation. Damage to either neuron type results in selective weakness or broadly spread paresis, depending on the extent of involvement.

Reflexes

Reflexes are an extensive topic, and the afferent and efferent connections of the nervous system must be familiar before the neuroanatomy of a reflex can be understood. The most basic reflex is the tendon **stretch reflex** of the spinal cord. When a skeletal muscle is stretched rapidly, it activates a proprioceptive neuron that projects to the spinal cord through a peripheral afferent nerve. A branch of the neuron must ascend the spinal cord, but another branch extends to the cell body of the lower motor neuron of exactly the same muscle. This excitatory synapse causes contraction of the same muscle to counteract the stretch. There is only one synapse in this reflex chain, and hence it is called the monosynaptic stretch reflex. In the leg extensor muscles, this type of reflex functions to maintain balance.

Even a monosynaptic reflex is not simple. If an **extensor muscle** is stretched and the stretch reflex is activated, a third branch of the proprioceptive neuron projects to an inhibitory interneuron that projects to the corresponding **flexor muscle** of the joint, preventing it from contracting. This allows the extensor muscle to contract without interference from the flexor muscle. Consequently, even the simplest reflex in the nervous system has three synapses to coordinate contraction.

Other reflexes are more complex but follow the same general pattern. Most other reflexes in the body do not involve monosynaptic pathways. Instead, afferent fibers terminate on interneurons that project to the lower motor neurons of the target muscles. The interneurons can elicit variable patterns of excitation and inhibition, which accordingly render the reflex manifestation variable as well. Nonetheless, the reflexes can be quite rapid and elicit strong contractile effects in muscles.

■ Suggested Readings

Blumenfeld, H. Neuroanatomy through Clinical Cases. 2d ed. Sunderland, MA: Sinauer Associates ; 2011

Daneman R. The blood–brain barrier in health and disease. *Annals of Neurology, 72*, 648–672; 2012

Frings M, Maschke M, Timmann D. Cerebellum and cognition. *Cerebellum, 6*(4), 328–334; 2007

Gebhart AL, Petersen SE, Thach WT. Role of the posterolateral cerebellum in language. *Annals of the New York Academy of Sciences, 978*, 318–333; 2002

Jones EG, Peters A. Cerebral Cortex Series. Vol. 1–14. New York, NY: Plenum Press; 1984

Vanderagh TW, Gould DJ. Nolte's The Human Brain. 7th ed. New York, NY: Elsevier; 2015

Vecchio JL, Kearney CA. Selective mutism in children: Comparison to youths with and without anxiety disorders. *Journal of Psychopathology and Behavioral Assessment, 27*, 31–37; 2005

■ Study Questions

1. Which of the following structures is *not* in the CNS?

A. Visceral sensory fiber
B. Cerebellum
C. Hippocampus
D. Basal ganglia
E. Hypothalamus

2. What is the pathway of excitation and action potential transmission between neurons?

A. Axon → dendrite → synapse → soma → axon
B. Synapse → dendrite → axon → soma → synapse
C. Synapse → dendrite → soma → axon → synapse
D. Dendrite → synapse → soma → axon → dendrite
E. Axon → soma → synapse → dendrite → axon

3. Which of the following is *not* found in gray matter?

A. Synapse
B. Dendrite
C. Neuronal cell body
D. Astrocyte
E. Oligodendrocyte

4. The following structures can be seen from the inferior cortical surface, except for the:

A. Uncus
B. Mammillary bodies
C. Optic chiasm
D. Hippocampus
E. Pituitary gland

5. What is the primary symptom of Wernicke's aphasia?

A. Paucity of speech and preserved speech comprehension
B. Nonsensical but fluent speech and impaired speech comprehension
C. Paucity of speech and impaired speech comprehension
D. Impaired word repetition and preserved speech comprehension
E. Inability to read

6. The major source of input to the globus pallidus is the:

A. Striatum
B. Cerebral cortex
C. Thalamus
D. Corticospinal pathway
E. Cerebellum

7. With regard to the hippocampus, which of the following statements is *false*?

A. The hippocampus is located within the temporal lobe.
B. The hippocampus connects to the fornix anteriorly.
C. The hippocampus is associated with memory formation.
D. The hippocampus is involved in motor control.
E. The hippocampus is composed of highly folded cortical layers.

8. The middle cerebral artery supplies the:

A. Cingulate cortex
B. Occipitotemporal gyrus
C. Primary auditory cortex
D. Primary visual cortex
E. Corpus callosum

9. Which structure produces cerebrospinal fluid?

A. Superior sagittal sinus
B. Arachnoid granulations
C. Choroid plexus
D. Arachnoid mater
E. Pituitary gland

10. Cerebrospinal fluid circulates around the following locations, except for the:

A. Lateral ventricles
B. Subarachnoid space
C. Apertures in the fourth ventricle
D. Venous system
E. Fornix

11. The anatomy of the cerebellum has a functional organization that reflects how it connects to the rest of the brain. The most lateral portion of the cerebellar cortex is connected to the:

A. Spinal cord
B. Brainstem
C. Basal ganglia
D. Cerebral cortex

12. The midline section of the cerebellum, called the vermis, is concerned with:

A. Memory
B. Hearing
C. Balance

13. Which of the following is *not* part of the brainstem?

A. Midbrain
B. Putamen
C. Pons
D. Medulla

14. Which section of the brainstem contains the cell bodies that control tongue movements?

A. Substantia nigra
B. Midbrain
C. Pons
D. Medulla

15. Which cranial nerve carries sensation from the larynx?

A. Abducens nerve (CN VI)
B. Glossopharyngeal nerve (CN IX)
C. Vagus nerve (CN X)
D. Accessory nerve (CN XI)

16. Which branch of the trigeminal nerve carries motor commands to the jaw muscles?

A. V_1
B. V_2
C. V_3

17. Which section of the spinal cord contains the gray matter for the arm muscles?

A. Cervical
B. Thoracic
C. Lumbar
D. Sacral

18. The gray matter of the spinal cord is divided into two sections. Which of the sections represents sensory function of the body?

A. Corticospinal tract
B. Ventral horn
C. Dorsal horn
D. Sacrum

19. The simplest reflex in the body is called the:

A. Spinal reflex
B. Brainstem reflex
C. Stretch reflex
D. Contraction reflex

20. The simplest reflex is notable because it has ____ synaptic relay(s):

A. 1
B. 2
C. 3
D. 4

■ Answers to Study Questions

1. The correct answer is (A). Visceral sensory fibers innervate internal organs and are found in the peripheral nervous system. All the other answer choices are structures within the CNS.

2. The correct answer is (C). The dendrite and soma occupy the input zone of neural transmission. The conduction zone is the axon. The output zone is the synapse. Neural signals transmit from the synapse of the upstream neuron to the dendrite and soma of the downstream neuron, which in turn passes the information down to its respective axon and synapse(s).

3. The correct answer is (E). Oligodendrocytes form the myelin sheath around axons in white matter regions only.

4. The correct answer is (D). The hippocampus is not visible on the surface of the brain because it is located within the parahippocampal gyrus.

5. The correct answer is (B). Answer (A) describes symptoms of Broca's aphasia. Answer (C) describes symptoms of global aphasia. Answer (D) describes conduction aphasia. Answer (E) describes dyslexia. Answer (B) emphasizes the empty speech or jargon and difficulties with speech comprehension caused by damage to this critical auditory integration region in the posterior temporal lobe.

6. The correct answer is (A). The globus pallidus is the major output structure of the basal ganglia that primarily receives input from the striatum. (B) The cerebral cortex is the source of input to the striatum. (C) The globus pallidus sends information to the thalamus. (D) The corticospinal pathway does not connect with the basal ganglia directly, but its activity is modified by basal ganglia output. (E) The cerebellum has no direct connections with the basal ganglia.

7. The correct answer is (D). The hippocampus is not responsible for movement control.

8. The correct answer is (C). The MCA also supplies most of the lateral portion of the cerebral cortex. (A) The cingulate cortex is supplied by the ACA and PCA. (B) The occipitotemporal gyrus is supplied by the PCA. (D) The primary visual cortex is supplied by the PCA. (E) The corpus callosum is supplied by the ACA and PCA.

9. The correct answer is (C). CSF is produced by the choroid plexus within the ventricles.

10. The correct answer is (E). CSF flows from the ventricles into the venous system, not including the fornix (nerve fibers).

11. The correct answer is (D). The most lateral portions of the *cerebellar* cortex form a circuit that connects to the *cerebral* cortex through the dentate nucleus. The spinal cord and brainstem are influenced by the cerebellum directly, but those connections are primarily through the medial cerebellum.

12. The correct answer is (C). The cerebellum is a primary center for balance control.

13. The correct answer is (B). The putamen is part of the basal ganglia in the telencephalon.

14. The correct answer is (D). The hypoglossal nucleus, which contains the lower motor neurons for all the muscles of the tongue, is located in the medial medulla.

15. The correct answer is (C). All the sensory fibers of the larynx travel with the vagus nerve.

16. The correct answer is (C). It is the only branch of the trigeminal nerve that includes motor fibers.

17. The correct answer is (C). All of the lower motor neurons for the arms are located in medial motor nuclei within the cervical region of the spinal cord.

18. The correct answer is (C). All of the sensory nerves enter the spinal cord at the dorsal horn.

19. The correct answer is (C). The stretch reflex is a monosynaptic reflex that controls the level of tension in a muscle via connections between a single sensory fiber and a single motor fiber. Spinal and brainstem reflexes are real (A and C), but they do not necessarily refer to the monosynaptic reflex. There is no reflex called a contraction reflex (D).

20. The correct answer is (A). One sensory fiber connects to one motor fiber via a single synapse.

6

Neurophysiology

Michelle R. Ciucci, Erwin B. Montgomery Jr., and Lyn S. Turkstra

■ Chapter Summary

The function of the nervous system is to encode, process, and transmit information. The study of neurophysiology is essential to the understanding of how neurons function and form networks to mediate actions controlled by the nervous system. The purpose of this chapter is to provide information on how neurons use electrical and chemical signaling for processes such as sensation, movement, thought, language, and the regulation of body functions. Specifically, we will (1) discuss how neurotransmitters and structures within the cell membrane act as messengers that alter electrical activity in the nervous system; (2) explore how neurons function as circuits to process incoming stimuli, make decisions, and modulate communication functions such as hearing and speech production; and (3) discuss how drugs and disease can alter neuronal transmission and thus affect speech, language, swallowing, hearing, and balance function.

■ Learning Objectives

- Identify the structures of the neuron and describe their key functions
- Understand how neurons use chemicals called neurotransmitters to communicate with other neurons and cause the contraction of muscles
- Describe the effects of drugs and disease on synaptic transmission
- Describe the implications of rehabilitation after disease or injury for neuroplasticity.

■ Putting It Into Practice

- Speech-language pathologists and audiologists should be familiar with the normal functioning of the nervous system and how these critical functions are altered during disease.
- Knowledge of how synaptic transmission influences behavior is necessary to understand how diseases of the nervous system contribute to speech, language, swallowing, hearing, and balance disorders.
- The study of neurophysiology provides an essential framework for understanding how neurons communicate with other neurons, muscles, and glands.

■ Introduction

In Chapter 5, you learned about neuroanatomy, the *structure* of the nervous system. This chapter focuses on neurophysiology, or the *functions* of the nervous system. In this chapter, you will learn how structures at the anatomic, cellular, and molecular levels operate to perform speech, language, swallowing, hearing, and balance functions. We will begin by describing brain function as a complex electrical computational entity. We will then use this framework and relevant physiology to explain the normal functioning of neurons as circuits that underlie behaviors in typical speech, language, swallowing, hearing, and balance. We will also discuss how alterations to physiology at the level of the neuron can result in functional impairments.

The goal of this chapter is to introduce neuronal physiology in a way that is accessible to readers who may not have a strong background in cellular and molecular neurobiology or biophysics. We approach this topic by drawing parallels between neurons and examples of electrical circuits and computers to illustrate the vast computing power of the brain. We do so to present a framework for understanding how the brain works as a complex, dynamic system rather than a linear system. To achieve this, descriptions of terminology and philosophical principles are provided to assist with the understanding of recent research on complex systems. Fundamental principles important for understanding how neurons function are presented first, followed by the physiology underlying speech, language, swallowing, hearing, and balance functions.

■ Fundamental Operating Units and Logical Operators

Have you ever wondered how the brain can perform multiple complicated tasks at the same time and in a fraction of a second? For example, as you read this chapter, you might also be drinking coffee, and you might hear your phone ring and choose to direct it to voicemail—all without much thought. For centuries, humans have been studying the brain and its various functions, but how this living organ can perform such complex tasks almost simultaneously and seamlessly remains largely a mystery. The key to understanding how the brain works is by thinking about the nervous system as a dynamic and multilevel parallel processing system. Complex systems are often simplified to describe their critical functions as if they were linear, but this simplification can result in a somewhat limited understanding of actual function. Major advances in the understanding of how the brain works have been made possible through collaborative research efforts across the fields of neuroscience, physics, biomedical engineering, mathematics, and chemistry. We now have the conceptual and computational tools needed to think about the brain in complex, dynamic, parallel processing terms. In this chapter, we will introduce a few of these tools, particularly from the fields of engineering and computer science, to help you develop a comprehensive understanding of basic neurophysiology. We begin with the basic functional elements of the brain.

The nervous system consists primarily of two main cell types: **neurons** and **glial cells**. The neuron is the fundamental operating element in the ner-

vous system. Analogies may be helpful to illustrate this important concept. A modern digital computer consists primarily of a collection of transistors, and these transistors are considered the fundamental operating elements of the computer. However, a computer's function is not based on individual transistors, but rather groups of transistors that are connected in specific circuits called logic circuits. The logic circuits represent **fundamental logical operators**, meaning that they can perform functions at the smallest scale on the smallest amount of information possible. If you increase the number of logic circuits or fundamental logical operators, a computer increases its power to solve complex problems. Like the transistor, a neuron is the fundamental operating element in the nervous system, and neuronal physiology is part of the collective system of operating elements that work together to create or suppress movement, sensation, or thought. However, neurons also function as circuits, representing fundamental logical operators, outputting information based on combinations of signals from other neurons. By combining these operators, the brain displays tremendous computational power to perform exceptionally complex activities, such as speaking. Understanding the concept of logical operators is very important to avoid the misconception that neuronal signaling is a discrete, linear event and to form a modern framework for neurophysiology.

■ Structure and Function of Neurons and Glial Cells

Neurons

Recall that the neuron is the basic operating element in a complex system of circuits. Neurons come in many shapes and sizes, but share key structures (**Fig. 6.1**). The **soma**, or cell body, contains the cell nucleus and other organelles responsible for cell metabolism, transcription, synthesis of **neurotransmitters**, and other essential functions. The soma is the location where information from other neurons and glial cells is integrated. **Dendrites** are the structures where the neuron receives input from other neurons, primarily through the release of neurotransmitters, in addition to contact from neurons on other parts of the cell. The **axon** is a long, thin extension of the neuron that shuttles proteins and molecules such as neurotransmitters as well as the neuron's electrical output (an **action potential**) to the **axon terminal**. The axon terminal (**terminal bouton**) is where neurotransmitters are released to the next substrate

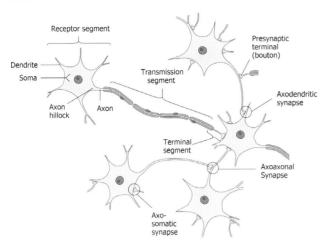

Fig. 6.1 The nervous system consists primarily of neurons (nerve cells) and supporting glial cells, which vastly outnumber neurons (10 to 1). Each neuron contains a cell body (soma) with one axon (projecting segment) and one or more dendrites (receptor segments). The release of neurotransmitters at synapses creates an excitatory or inhibitory postsynaptic potential at the receiving neuron. If the postsynaptic membrane potential exceeds the depolarization threshold of the postsynaptic neuron, the axon fires an action potential, initiating the release of a transmitter from its presynaptic terminal (bouton). Gilroy et al: Atlas of Anatomy. © 2008-2015 Thieme Medical Publishers, Inc. All rights reserved.

(e.g., another neuron, a muscle cell, or a gland cell) that receives the signal from the neuron.

The neuron has a resting electrical membrane potential that is negative relative to the surrounding cell medium. The electrical potential across the neuronal membrane is a function of the relative balance of positively and negatively charged ions between the outside and inside of the neuron. A typical electrical membrane potential is –70 millivolts, which means that there are relatively more negative charges or fewer positive charges inside the neuron compared to the outside. By altering this membrane potential, neurons can encode and process input from other neurons and convert them to an electrical output signal. The axon carries these electrical signals away from the cell body toward the axon terminal. These electrical signals can have one of two effects. First, they can stimulate neurotransmitter release at the axon terminal, where neurotransmitters are stored: neurotransmitters are released into the space between neurons, called the **synapse**. Second, alternatively, one neuron can directly stimulate another neuron or another tissue via **gap junctions**. Gap junctions are found throughout the body and brain, most notably in cardiac tissue. The main focus of this chapter will be on the action potential and how it causes the release of neurotransmitters onto adjacent neurons, muscles, visceral tissue, and glands.

Understanding the membrane that surrounds the neuron is key to understanding neuronal physiology. The neuronal cell membrane, like the membranes surrounding other types of cells, consists of a bilayered structure of phospholipids (**Fig. 6.2**). Within this bilayer are protein channels that allow ions to move in or out of the cell. An ion is an atom or molecule that does not have the same number of electrons and protons. If there are fewer electrons than protons, the atom will have a net positive electrical charge and be known as a **cation**. Conversely, if there are more electrons than protons, the atom will have a net negative electrical charge and be known as an **anion**. Ion channels allow specific ions to cross the cell membrane in response to various electrical or chemical stimuli. An ion channel that responds to changes in electrical potential across the cell membrane is a **voltage-gated ion channel**. An ion channel that responds to chemical **ligands**, or substances that can attach to receptors, is a **ligand-gated ion channel**. Opening and closing of these ion channels changes the electrical potential of the membrane and thus the probability of generating an action potential and releasing neurotransmitters or to communicate electrically through gap junctions. When a membrane ion channel opens to allow an ion to move into or out of the neuron, we say that the neuron changes its **permeability** for that ion. For example, opening of sodium channels makes the neuronal membrane more permeable to sodium.

Because the phospholipid bilayer is semipermeable to ions, fluids within the cell (intracellular), and outside of the cell (extracellular) can have very different compositions. Many ions and forces are at work, but for the sake of simplicity, only two ions are discussed here: potassium (K^+) and sodium (Na^+), both of which are positively charged ions, or cations. At rest, there is a higher concentration of K^+ inside the cell and a higher concentration of Na^+ outside the cell. This difference in ion concentration results in a **concentration gradient** (**Fig. 6.3**). Ions will flow from high to low concentrations if membrane permeability allows (i.e., if the ion channels for that particular ion are open). In addition to the concentration gradient, there is an electrostatic field generated by the difference in the voltage across the neuronal membrane, and that electrical gradient acts to move ions through the neuronal membrane. The flow of ions through ion channels depends on these concentration gradients, electrical potentials, and the membrane permeability to each ion.

In brief, neurons are specialized to use the opening and closing of ion channels and the resulting flows to respond to, create, and transmit signals representing information.

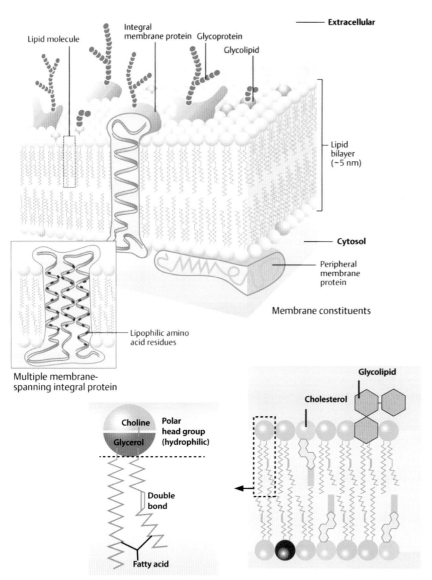

Fig. 6.2 Structure of the cell membrane. The cell membrane consists of a phospholipid bilayer. Each phospholipid molecule has a phosphatidyl head (such as phosphatidylcholine), which is hydrophilic, and two fatty acid tails, which are hydrophobic. When the phospholipid is surrounded by water, the molecules arrange themselves so that the heads face the water while the hydrophobic tails face each other inside the bilayer. Integral proteins and cholesterol are embedded within the bilayer. Other proteins may lie peripherally. Carbohydrate moieties may bind to lipids and proteins on the extracellular surface of the membrane, forming glycolipids and glycoproteins. From: *Physiology: An Illustrated Review.*

Glial Cells

The second major cell type in the nervous system are glial cells, which do not process information like neurons but provide essential supporting services to neurons. Glial cells are quite numerous. In fact, we have more glial cells than we do neurons. There are four different glial cell types in the central nervous system (**Fig. 6.4**). These glial cells serve many functions. **Astrocytes** provide structure and nutrients, influence neurotransmitter and ion levels, and form part of the blood–brain barrier. **Ependymal cells** generate cerebrospinal fluid by filtering it from the bloodstream. **Microglia** are macrophage-like and act as immune responders. **Oligodendrocytes** provide myelination (discussed in **Chapter 5** and later in this chapter under "Saltatory Conduction")

to neurons in the central nervous system, whereas **Schwann cells** provide myelination to neurons in the peripheral nervous system. Recent research suggests that glial cells serve other important roles in the nervous system (Gundersen et al 2015; De Zeeuw and Hoogland 2015).

Resting Membrane Potential

At rest, the membrane is negatively charged, meaning that the intracellular fluid has a more negative charge (more negative ions and fewer positive ions) than the extracellular fluid. Electrical charge across a cell membrane (membrane potential) is always stated as inside the cell relative to the outside, so a negative membrane potential indicates that the

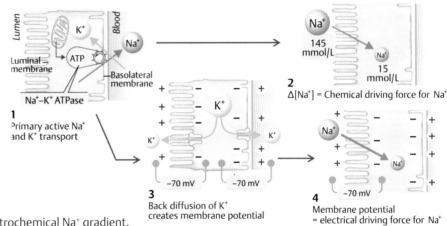

Fig. 6.3 Electrochemical Na+ gradient.

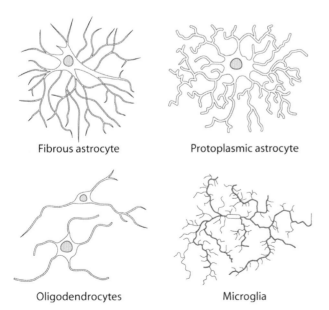

Fibrous astrocyte

Protoplasmic astrocyte

Oligodendrocytes

Microglia

Fig. 6.4 Four glial cell types in the central nervous system.

inside of the cell is more negative than the outside, and a positive potential indicates that the inside of the cell is more positive than the outside. A negative charge is present at rest because of two main features of the neuron. First, the neuronal cell membrane has "leaky" K+ ion channels, so the membrane allows small amounts of potassium ions to leave the cell. When positive ions leave, the inside of the cell becomes more negative. Second, the **sodium-potassium pump** in the cell membrane actively pumps more positive ions out than it pumps in. Specifically, it carries three Na+ ions out of the cell for every two K+ ions it carries into the cell. This exchange goes against both the ion concentration gradient and the membrane electrical potential, so it needs energy. Every exchange of three Na+ for two K+ uses one molecule of **adenosine triphosphate (ATP)**. Thus, this pump is also referred to as the Na+, K+-ATPase. As a result of the leaky K+ channels and the pumping action of Na+, K+-ATPase, most neuronal cells have a membrane potential of –70 millivolts at rest.

Action Potential

Changing their membrane potential is the major way in which neurons carry signals in the nervous system, while making the cell membrane potential more positive than the resting potential is called **depolarization**, while making the membrane potential more negative than the resting potential is called **hyperpolarization**. If the cell membrane becomes very positive, past a specific voltage threshold, then a rapid transition to a fast depolarization, followed by a hyperpolarization ensues. This is referred to as all-or-nothing depolarization–repolarization, or an action potential (**Fig. 6.5**).

Neurons change their resting membrane potential by the opening and closing of ion channels, especially Na^+ and K^+ channels. Depolarization is due to the opening of voltage-gated Na^+ channels, which allow Na^+ to enter the cell rapidly, following the Na^+ concentration gradient as well as the membrane potential. As the membrane potential becomes positive, these voltage-gated Na^+ channels close and become inactivated, and voltage-gated K^+ channels open. These allow K^+ to leave the cell rapidly, so the cell has a progressively more negative charge that triggers rapid hyperpolarization (below the resting membrane potential). Hyperpolarization is necessary to reactivate the Na^+ channels. After these two rapid changes the membrane returns to its resting potential through the sodium-potassium pump and leaky K^+ channels. The full cycle of depolarization, repolarization, hyperpolarization in an action potential takes ~ 2 milliseconds. Other cations such as calcium (Ca^{2+}) also cause depolarizations that can trigger action potentials. For a complex behavior, such as speech production or singing, tens of thousands of neurons generate millions of action potentials and communicate with thousands of other neurons. This complexity makes speech and vocalization especially vulnerable to nervous system injury.

After an action potential has been generated, there is a period in which additional stimulation cannot cause another action potential, referred to as the absolute **refractory period**, because inactivated Na^+ channels have not yet been reactivated. The absolute refractory period is followed by a relative refractory period, during which additional stimulation may indeed cause another action potential to occur (**Fig. 6.6**).

Depolarization or Hyperpolarization Caused by Postsynaptic Potentials

Neurons receive thousands of signals from other cells, which require integration. These signals often result in movement of positive and negative ions across the cell membrane and can shift the local cell membrane potential in a positive or negative direc-

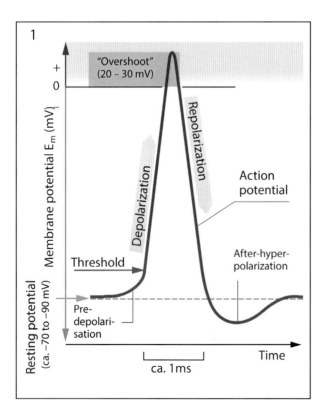

Fig. 6.5 Action potential ion conductivity. From: Color Atlas of Physiology, 6th ed.

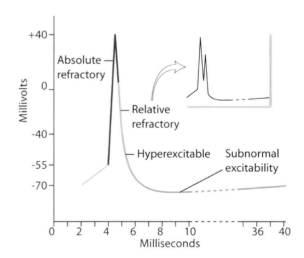

Fig. 6.6 Refractory periods of an action potential. Inset shows a second, smaller action potential triggered during the relative refractory period. From: Fundamentals of Medical Physiology.

Box 6.2 Tetrodotoxin

Drugs and toxins can disturb ion channels. Tetrodotoxin is one such toxin, found in puffer fish. The existence of this toxin became known to the West in 1774 when Captain James Cook and his crew ate puffer fish while at sea and experienced numbness and shortness of breath. Unfortunately, their livestock suffered a worse fate, because the crew threw them the entrails of the puffer fish, particularly the liver, where the toxin is found in high concentrations. The pigs were lifeless the next morning. Tetrodotoxin was first isolated and then named by Japanese scientist Yoshizumi Tahara in 1909. Tetrodotoxin is specific for voltage-gated Na$^+$ ion channels. It binds to the P-loop of the alpha (α) subunit of the receptor, which controls ion selectivity of the channel. These voltage-gated channels are important in generating the depolarizing events in action potentials, including action potentials in alpha lower motor neurons that travel to the neuromuscular junction and cause contraction of postsynaptic muscles. By blocking these channels, tetrodotoxin prevents activation of the muscle by the alpha lower motor neuron. If this happens in respiratory muscles, it can cause death (Lee and Ruben 2008).

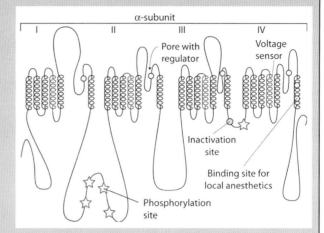

Box Fig. 6. 1 The ultrastructure of the α-subunit of the sodium channel showing its functionally important sites. (From *Fundamentals of Medical Physiology*)

tion. Signals that cause cell membrane depolarization increase the probability of an action potential; these potentials are often called excitatory postsynaptic potentials (EPSPs). Traditionally, it was believed that hyperpolarization decreased the probability of action potential generation, so inputs that led to hyperpolarization were called inhibitory postsynaptic potentials (IPSPs).

The term "excitatory" can be inaccurate, because in some circumstances there can be prolonged subthreshold depolarizations. Simply, the membrane potential is depolarized but not to the threshold necessary to cause an action potential. This partial depolarization will fail to activate Na$^+$ channels, and there will be no action potential. As such, EPSPs are more accurately termed depolarizing postsynaptic potentials (DPSPs). Similarly, hyperpolarization can lead to an *increased* probability of action potential generation at the end of the hyperpolarization phase. Activation of greater numbers of Na$^+$ channels during periods of more negative membrane potentials is one mechanism. Opening of these sodium channels primes the neuron for another action potential. Thus, what have been traditionally called IPSPs are more accurately termed hyperpolarizing postsynaptic potential (HPSPs). The term "HPSP" has not yet gained widespread popularity, but it is the most accurate term to describe these underlying physiological events.

Many different substrates (ligands), mainly neurotransmitters, cause small positive or negative shifts in polarization of the neuronal membrane when they bind to receptors, through several different mechanisms. Small positive or negative shifts in membrane potential are called **graded potentials**. The summed graded potentials received by a neuron leads to an action potential if depolarization is great enough to shift the membrane potential above its threshold for generating an action potential. That is, the sum of the graded potentials can lead to an increase or decrease in the probability of an action potential. The neuron sums these graded potentials over space (**spatial summation**) and time (**temporal summation**). The charge across any section of the cell membrane is determined by ion concentrations across that membrane. The ions will not only be in the fluid immediately next to one small section of membrane but also will diffuse into fluid adjacent to that area. The cell membrane responds to the concentrations in the area; summation of many different stimuli at different locations across a cell is called spatial summation. The neuron can also sum inputs delivered with high frequency over a short period of time; this process is called temporal summation. Both spatial and temporal summation can affect the membrane potential and cause action potentials to occur. The differences between graded and action potentials are shown in **Table 6.1**.

Table 6.1   Differences between graded potential and action potential

Graded potential	Action potential
Amplitude proportionate to stimulus strength and can be summed	Amplitude constant for all suprathreshold stimuli and cannot be summed
Can be a depolarization or hyperpolarization	Always a depolarization
Conduction is associated with reduction in magnitude	Conducted without reduction in magnitude
Can be generated spontaneously in response to physical or chemical stimuli	Generated only in response to membrane depolarization

---

Box 6.3   Channelopathies: Myasthenia Gravis and Episodic Ataxia Type 2

Ion channels are critical to the operation of neurons. These channels control the electrical operations of the neuron, just as electrical switches control the functions of electronic devices. Just as electrical devices act faulty when switches malfunction, ion channels can also malfunction. Diseases that affect ion channel functions are referred to as *channelopathies*.

Ionic conductance channels can be altered in many different ways. For example, myasthenia gravis is an autoimmune disorder characterized by extreme muscle fatigue, which can impair facial expression, speaking, walking, eating, and in severe cases breathing. In myasthenia gravis, antibodies block or alter postsyn-

aptic receptors for **acetylcholine**. Acetylcholine is the ligand for ligand-gated Na^+ channels on the muscle; thus, dysfunction of the acetylcholine receptor means that alpha lower motor neurons projecting to the muscle are unable to initiate a postsynaptic membrane depolarization that leads to muscle contraction.

Channelopathies can also be genetic. Abnormalities of the calcium channel Ca V 2.1 are associated with a syndrome called *episodic ataxia type 2* (EA2). EA2 syndrome is associated with episodes of vertigo and loss of coordination, or **ataxia**. At first, the episodes are brief, but over time, the symptoms persist. The Ca V 2.1 calcium channel is expressed primarily in the Purkinje cells of the cerebellum, a part of the brain involved in coordination of movements.

Saltatory Conduction

An action potential is generated at the **action potential–initiating segment** of the cell membrane, which is typically at the **axon hillock**, or the membrane segment where the axon joins to the soma. As mentioned previously, the action potential consists of rapid depolarization followed by hyperpolarization of the cell membrane. During depolarization, Na^+ enters the neuron's axon and diffuses along the length of the axon. Na^+ ions that diffuse under the neighboring axonal membrane depolarize that segment of the membrane (e.g., spatial summation) to produce an action potential in the next portion of the axon. This process proceeds down the length of the axon toward the axon terminal. The refractory period in the previous segment of the axon prevents the action potential from spreading backward. This process takes a relatively long time, and in long axons, K^+ and other ions can leak out of the cell membrane, causing a drop below the threshold for generating an action potential and thus ending propagation of the action potential along the length of the axon.

As a solution to the problem of action potentials dying out along the axon, many neurons have

myelin, which is a lipid-rich substance that wraps around axons in sheaths. As mentioned previously in **Chapter 5** and the discussion of glial cells in this chapter, Schwann cells in the peripheral nervous system and oligodendrocytes in the central nervous system provide these myelin sheaths. Myelin is hydrophobic, so it prevents ions from flowing across it; thus there is a decrease in Na^+ flow in through the cell membrane of a myelinated segment of an axon. By Kirchhoff's law, the net current flows in and out of an axon segment have to be equal. Therefore, with less flow of current into the segment through the membrane, the current flow into the axon through the end of the segment is increased. In between segments of myelin sheath are **nodes of Ranvier**. The cell membrane at these nodes is packed with ion channels. Because of the increased density of Na^+ channels at the nodes and the increased current along the axon to the nodes, the membrane at the nodes of Ranvier can reach depolarization threshold much faster than would be the case without the myelin sheath. The depolarization "jumps" from node to node, a process termed **saltatory conduction** from *saltare,* the Latin word for "to jump." The net result of myelination is that myelinated neurons are able to transmit action potentials faster. Conduction in nonmyelinated and myelinated axons is compared in **Fig. 6.7**.

The diameter of an axon contributes to how fast the neuron can transmit signals. Propagation of depolarization is related to the transmembrane resistance and capacitance and to the resistance down the axon. In a conductor, resistance falls as the diameter of the conductor increases. Therefore, there will be more current flow in larger-diameter axons. This means that the next segment of the membrane will reach threshold faster, but not because the actual ions are moving faster. One explanation offered for decreased resistance with increased diameter of the axon is the "skin effect," where varying (nondirect) current induces a back voltage that counters the flow of electrical charges at the center of the conductor, thus increasing resistance, and forcing current flow to occur at the surface (skin). Thus, larger-diameter axons have more "skin" area and, therefore, less resistance. Therefore, larger-diameter myelinated axons will transmit signals more quickly than smaller diameter and unmyelinated neurons.

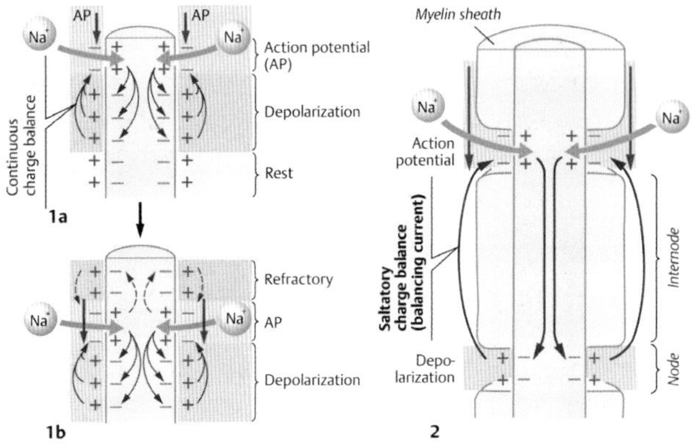

Fig 6.7 Continuous and saltatory propagation of action potentials. **(1a)** Na$^+$ enters the neuron at the starting location on the neuronal membrane, causing depolarization of the adjacent membrane. **(1b)** Na$^+$ then diffuses to the adjacent membrane, and the region of depolarization moves in the direction of the axon terminal. **(2)** Myelin insulation causes current to flow to the adjacent node of Ranvier, resulting in depolarization. Na$^+$ then enters at the next adjacent node of Ranvier, ~ 1 mm farther along the nerve fiber. From: Physiology: An Illustrated Review.

■ Neurotransmission

As mentioned previously, neurons communicate with neurons or target tissue such as muscles or glands through chemical synapses or electrical gap junctions. Chemical signaling employs neurotransmitters that must be synthesized, packaged, released, and then removed from the synapse. This process occurs within milliseconds. Neurotransmitters are the messengers, but not the message. Using a computational systems analogy, release of a neurotransmitter can be thought of as a binary or dichotomous event; release or no release. In this analogy, the neurotransmitter is similar to the value 1, and nonrelease of the neurotransmitter corresponds to 0, in a binary code where the sequences of 1s and 0s encode information. As information is encoded in a precise sequence of 1s and 0s in an

---

Box 6.4 Multiple Sclerosis

Multiple sclerosis (MS) has many variants and can affect neurons and glial cells in the brain. As described in **Chapter 5**, MS causes damage to myelin, the insulation around many axons in the brain. The functional result of MS is widespread neurologic damage to visual, sensory, and motor areas. MS is one of the main causes of **dysarthria**, a motor speech disorder characterized by deficits in speed, strength, range, timing, or accuracy of speech movements. Individuals with MS can have difficulty speaking and swallowing. The extent of the impairment will depend on where the site of damage occurs.

The myelin sheath, due to its high electrical resistance, prevents ions from going through the axonal membrane and ensures that more ions make it to the next node of Ranvier. This facilitates action potential propagation down the axon to its terminal. The loss of myelin in MS means that ions leak out of the axonal membrane before they reach the next node, leaving an insufficient ion concentration to depolarize the membrane and generate an action potential.

Interestingly, many patients with MS find that increased temperatures worsen their symptoms. Indeed, many years ago this response to high temperatures was used as a test for MS called the hot bathtub test. Individuals were placed in a hot bath to increase their body temperature, and worsening of symptoms and signs or development of new symptoms or signs was used as evidence of MS. Recall that generation of electrical potentials across the neuronal membrane depends on the diffusion rate of ions across the membrane, and the rate of diffusion is temperature-dependent. Higher temperatures increase the rate of diffusion and thus increase the amount of ions that can leak through areas of the neuronal membrane without myelin insulation.

electronic computer, patterns of electrical activity in the neuron determine patterns of neurotransmitter release. Additionally, as in a computer, networks of neurons integrate thousands of messages to orchestrate signaling for particular behaviors.

Neurotransmitter Packaging, Docking, and Release

Some neurotransmitters are synthesized in the cell body and transported down the axon to the axon terminal, whereas others are synthesized and/or packaged in the axon terminal. At the terminal, neurotransmitters are generally stored in packets called **vesicles**. These vesicles fuse to the cell membrane to release neurotransmitters into the synapse. When an action potential travels down the axon and reaches the axon terminal, voltage-gated calcium channels open and there is an influx of Ca^{2+} into the cell. Through a cascade of events, that influx of Ca^{2+} causes the vesicle to fuse to the cell membrane, and the neurotransmitter in that vesicle is released (**Fig. 6.8**). Several drugs work by blocking vesicular fusion or release.

Actions of Neurotransmitters

It is very important to remember that neurotransmitters themselves are not inherently excitatory or inhibitory. Rather, the effect of a neurotransmitter on a postsynaptic cell is determined by two fac-

tors: (1) other inputs received by the postsynaptic cell over space (spatial summation) or time (temporal summation), and (2) the actions of the postsynaptic receptor. When a neurotransmitter binds to a postsynaptic receptor, it may cause opening or closing of ion channels directly. This effect is said to be **ionotropic**. Ionotropic effects are rapid and of short duration. Neurotransmitters can also have an effect by binding to postsynaptic receptors that activate second messenger systems. These second-messenger effects are called **metabotropic**, have a longer time course, and tend to be more modulatory in nature. Metabotropic receptors use G-coupled proteins and enzymes to activate second messengers that can synthesize proteins and/or up- or downregulate the number of ion channels in the cell membrane. Some neurotransmitters actually bind to the presynaptic cell and alter the ability of the cell to release neurotransmitter. This process is mediated by a specific receptor, called an **autoreceptor**. Finally, **neuromodulators** are released by small groups of neurons and diffuse throughout the nervous system rather than having an effect only on the specific presynaptic or postsynaptic cell as in direct synaptic transmission. Neuromodulators can be the same neurotransmitters used in direct synaptic transmission, again showing how the effects of a neurotransmitter are determined by the receptor and not the neurotransmitter itself. Some behaviors that employ neuromodulation are learning, short-term memory, and reward.

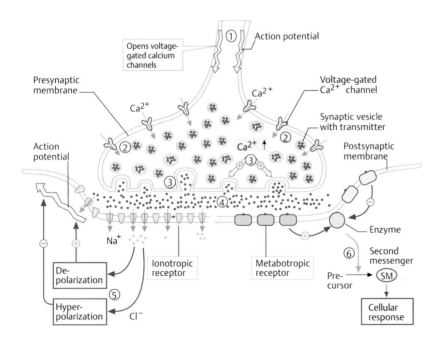

Fig. 6.8 Synaptic signal transmission. An action potential arriving at the presynaptic membrane **(1)** causes voltage-gated Ca^{2+} channels to open **(2)**. This increase in the intracellular Ca^{2+} concentration triggers the release of neurotransmitters from their storage vesicles into the synaptic cleft **(3)**. Neurotransmitter molecules then diffuse across the synaptic cleft **(4)** and bind with ionotropic or metabotropic receptors on the postsynaptic membrane. Ionotropic receptors are ligand-gated ion channels. Ligand (in this case, neurotransmitter) binding **(5)** causes the inflow of ions into the cell, resulting in either depolarization (inflow of cations) or hyperpolarization (inflow of anions). **(6)** Ligand binding to metabotropic receptors activates G proteins, which transduce a cellular response via second messenger molecules. From: Physiology: An Illustrated Review.

Box 6.5 Botulinum Toxin

Botulinum toxin is one of the world's most deadly poisons on a per weight basis, yet it is often injected to remove wrinkles by partially paralyzing muscles that pull the skin to cause wrinkles. Intramuscular injections of botulinum toxin are also a very important treatment for a number of disorders, including dystonia and spasticity. Typically, only tiny amounts of the toxin are injected into specific muscles, and botulinum toxin does not cross the blood-brain barrier, so generally there are no central nervous system or systemic effects.

For normal neuromuscular function, muscle contraction is activated by the release of acetylcholine from the alpha lower motor neuron onto the postsynaptic receptor on the muscle, as mentioned previously in Box 6.3. Specifically, action potentials generated in the alpha lower motor neuron are conducted to presynaptic terminals. Depolarization of the synaptic terminals causes a release of acetylcholine from vesicles. The released acetylcholine diffuses across the synaptic cleft to bind to ligand-gated Na^+ ionic conductance channels to generate a depolarization that ultimately results in muscle contraction.

Botulinum toxin binds to the neuronal presynaptic membrane and is taken into the neuron terminals. Inside the neuron, botulinum breaks apart the complex of proteins that enable synaptic vesicles containing acetylcholine to bind to the internal surface of the neuronal presynaptic terminal, a process necessary for the synaptic vesicles to open and release acetylcholine into the synaptic cleft. The result is muscle paralysis (Tighe and Schiavo 2013).

Controlled use of botulinum toxin, also known commercially as Botox (Allergan, Dublin, Ireland), can be highly therapeutic in the treatment of various conditions. In addition to cosmetic uses, Botox is used to treat a common communication disorder called spasmodic dysphonia. Spasmodic dysphonia, characterized by overactivation of muscles in the larynx, causes untimely closure (adductor spasmodic dysphonia) or opening (abductor spasmodic dysphonia) of the vocal folds during speech. This leads to either voice stoppages or periods of breathiness that interfere with speech intelligibility. This condition is extremely debilitating and stressful to the patient. Because the mechanisms that cause spasmodic dysphonia are not well-understood, pharmacologic therapy with Botox is currently the gold-standard treatment for temporary relief of the symptoms associated with the disorder. Botox is injected into the overactive laryngeal muscles to temporarily stop them from contracting. This treatment is widely used and successful, but the effect lasts only 3 to 6 months, requiring repeat injections into the larynx.

Major Types of Neurotransmitters

Hundreds of types of neurotransmitters have been identified, and this number will likely continue to increase with further scientific discovery. A noncomprehensive list of neurotransmitters is provided in **Table 6.2**. Neurotransmitters are synthesized in the cell and are often derived from our dietary intake. When neurotransmitters are released by the cell, transmission across the synaptic cleft usually takes fewer than 10 milliseconds. Neurons are often labeled by the type of neurotransmitter they release (e.g., the **dopaminergic** neurons in the substantia nigra and **noradrenergic** neurons in the locus coeruleus), but most individual neurons release at least two different kinds of neurotransmitters, and a neuron may respond to more types of neurotransmitters than it releases. After release and binding to the postsynaptic cell, neurotransmitters must be cleared from the synaptic space, which is achieved through a variety of mechanisms. The neurotransmitters can be inactivated by enzymes, be taken up by neighboring glial cells or the postsynaptic neuron, or diffuse into the extracellular space. They also can be taken back up by the presynaptic cell, using special membrane proteins. This **reuptake** recycles the neurotransmitter for subsequent use. Some neurotransmitters are subject to more than one mechanism. For example, the neurotransmitter acetylcholine is broken down by the enzyme **acetylcholinesterase (AChE)** into acetate and choline. Choline is taken back into the cell for reuse, while the acetate ion diffuses away.

■ Effects of Drugs and Disease on Neurotransmission

It is important to explore the physiology of neurotransmitters in order to understand how drugs can affect neurotransmission, downstream cell function, and, eventually, behavior.

Actions of Drugs at the Synapse

Drugs can act in many ways to alter synaptic transmission. Drugs affect the presynaptic cell by increasing the synthesis or release of a neurotransmitter or by blocking binding or release of a neu-

Table 6.2   Types of neurotransmitters

Name	Type of molecule	Site of synthesis
Neuroactive peptides		
Substance P	Neurokinin	Soma
Somatostatin	Large molecule	Soma
Enkephalins	Opioid	Soma
Endorphins	Opioid	Soma
Small molecules		
Gamma-aminobutyric acid (GABA)	Amino acid	Axon terminal
Glutamate	Amino acid	Axon terminal
Glycine	Amino acid	Axon terminal
Dopamine	Biogenic monoamine (catecholamine)	Axon terminal
Norepinephrine	Biogenic monoamine (catecholamine)	Axon terminal
Serotonin	Biogenic monoamine (indolamine)	Axon terminal
Acetylcholine	Biogenic monoamine	Axon terminal
Histamine	Biogenic monoamine	Axon terminal

Box 6.6   Special Case of Neurotransmission: The Endocochlear Potential

The action potential that takes place in the inner ear in response to sound is different from the action potential previously described and is termed the **endocochlear potential (Box Fig. 6.2)**. Vibration of the fluid in the cochlea causes localized shearing of the tectorial membrane relative to the basilar membrane, causing bending of the stereocilia at the tectorial end of the outer hair cells embedded in the basilar membrane **(1)**. This bending causes mechanosensitive cation channels in the stereocilia cell membrane to open, allowing K^+ to enter and depolarize outer hair cells. This depolarization causes outer hair cells to shorten, which changes the amplitude of the traveling sound wave, which then bends the stereocilia of the inner hair cells. Depolarization of inner hair cells occurs in the same manner as for outer hair cells and also causes opening of basolateral Ca^{2+} channels, increasing the cytosolic Ca^{2+} concentration. This process leads to the release of the neurotransmitter glutamate and subsequent conduction of impulses in afferent neurons to the central nervous system. Repolarization is achieved by the opening of K^+ channels on the perilymph side of the hair cell. Outflowing K^+ is taken up by K^+/Cl^- cotransporters in the supporting cells and recirculated via gap junctions to the stria vascularis **(2, 3)**. From: Physiology: An Illustrated Review.

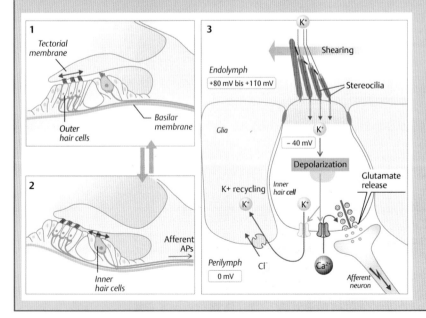

Box Fig. 6.2   Stimulation of hair cells by membrane deformation. Vibration of the fluid in the cochlea causes frequency-localized movement of the tectorial membrane relative to the basilar membrane, causing bending of the stereocilia of the outer hair cells **(1)**. This bending causes mechanosensitive cation channels in the stereocilia membrane to open, allowing K^+ to enter and depolarize the outer hair cells. This causes the outer hair cells to shorten. Repolarization is achieved by the opening of K^+ channels on the perilymph side of the hair cell.

rotransmitter. Drugs that act at the postsynaptic cell by directly stimulating a receptor are called **agonists**, and drugs that block the action of a neurotransmitter at the receptor are called **antagonists**. Other drugs block the breakdown of the neurotransmitter in the synapse, which most often increases the activity at that synapse. An example is selective serotonin reuptake inhibitors (SSRIs), which increase availability of serotonin in the synapse. Likewise, some drugs block the breakdown of a neurotransmitter, such as the anticholinesterase class of drugs that are often used in the treatment of Alzheimer's disease.

The ability of a drug to bind with the intended receptor is called **affinity**, and the ability of a drug to elicit a desired response is called **efficacy**. Drugs have combinations of affinity and efficacy. Because drugs can have multiple effects on neural transmission and behavior, they may be associated with undesirable side effects. Some of these side effects, however, have evolved into treatments for a variety of conditions. For example, the drug metoclopramide, which is a dopamine antagonist, is used as a gastrointestinal stimulant to treat nausea, vomiting, and reflux. Metoclopramide also, however, increases the breast milk hormone prolactin and thus breast milk supply. When an individual is taking metoclopramide for nausea and experiences unwanted lactation, this is considered a side effect. However, an individ-

---

Box 6.7 Neurotransmitters and Neuropharmacology

Neurotransmitter-based drug treatments have led to remarkable advances in the treatment of disease. However, many of these were developed without a complete understanding of the neurotransmitters or receptors impacted by these drugs. For example, medications derived from methylene blue, a dye, were accidentally discovered to improve mood disorders. These effects were discovered when methylene blue was administered to psychiatric patients to ensure compliance with prescription medications. If the patients took their medications that contained methylene blue, their urine turned blue. This application was long before it was known that methylene blue is a monoamine oxidase inhibitor (MAOI) capable of blocking the breakdown of amines such as serotonin. In another example, the neurologist Jean-Martin Charcot was using the extract of the belladonna plant for the treatment of Parkinson's disease in the late 1800s, long before anyone recognized that it was a precursor of drugs that block the acetylcholine receptor. Interestingly, levodopa (the precursor to dopamine) was initially used in humans because it reversed catatonia in rodents given reserpine, which blocks dopamine receptors. It was later discovered that patients with Parkinson's disease lost dopaminergic neurons in the substantia nigra.

The power of neuropharmacology was greatly enhanced by the recognition of chemical synaptic transmission. However, the physiology of nonchemical and gap junction contributions to neurotransmission is continuing to evolve. Research in the 1940s demonstrated that nervous system effects on various organs, such as the heart, could be mimicked by the application of neurotransmitters. For example, electrical stimulation of the vagus nerve causes the heartbeat to slow. Applying acetylcholine likewise slows the heart. This effect can be prevented by the administration of agents that block the acetylcholine receptor.

In some cases, research on chemical neurotransmission led to the incorrect inference that neurotransmitter function was synonymous with nervous system function, and neurological and psychiatric disorders were attributed to relative excesses or deficiencies of neurotransmitters. For example, the "dopamine hypothesis of schizophrenia" attributed schizophrenia to an excess of dopamine, whereas it was also believed that Parkinson's disease was simply a state of dopamine deficiency. These overly simple explanations were inaccurate (e.g., replacing dopamine does not fully reverse the signs of Parkinson's disease, any more than blocking dopamine reverses the signs of schizophrenia). These erroneous inferences have had lasting effects on treatment. The inference that signs of Parkinson's disease reflect a dopamine deficiency has led to a strange bit of reasoning that signs such as dysphagia, which do not respond to dopaminergic drugs, are caused by nondopaminergic mechanisms. However, this hypothesis assumes that pharmacologic dopamine replacement normalizes dopamine-dependent systems in the brain and, therefore, should completely correct any dopamine-related problems.

Neurotransmitters are critical to nervous system function and treatment of neurological diseases, but they are simply the messengers, not the message. It is now becoming increasingly recognized that the disabilities associated with many neurologic signs and psychiatric disorders are the result of misfiring or the loss of information in the nervous system, resulting from changes in the electrical potentials across neuronal membranes.

ual who would like to increase breast milk supply would consider this a benefit. Drugs can have major effects or side effects on speech, language, swallowing, hearing, and balance, and it is important for the speech-language pathologist and audiologist to be familiar with drug targets, desirable effects, and side effects.

Effects of Diseases on Neurophysiology

Many diseases, conditions, injuries, and medications have an impact on neuronal physiology. An overview of representative diseases and how these affect neuronal physiology is provided in **Table 6.3**. These effects can be at the level of the synapse, neuron, neural subsystem (e.g., autonomic nervous system),

Table 6.3   Examples of diseases, disorders, and injuries that affect neuronal function, communication, and swallowing

Condition	Neural substrate	Physiologic function impairment	Communication impairment
Epilepsy	Ion channels	Excitotoxicity, aberrant firing	Seizures, which can impair any aspect of cognitive, sensory, or motor function, depending on seizure focus, distribution of electrical disruption, age of onset, and duration of seizures
Sensorineural hearing loss	Inner hair cell	Impaired stimulation of cochlear nerve due to loss of inner hair cells	Hearing loss
Multiple sclerosis	Myelin; neuron	Reduced ability to propagate action potentials due to the breakdown of myelin and cell death in the brain and spinal cord	Impairment in any aspect of motor, sensory, or cognitive function, depending on site(s) and extent of demyelination and stage of the disease
Amyotrophic lateral sclerosis	Myelin; neuron	Loss of myelin in the brain and spinal cord, interfering with synaptic transmission, causing inability to move appropriately	Impaired motor function affecting respiration, swallowing, voice, and speech
Traumatic brain injury	Neurons, neuronal connections, neurotransmitter systems, glial cells	Damage to neurons and glial cells via mechanical injury and hypoxia (loss of oxygen), disrupting electrical signaling	Short- and long-term effects on hearing, speech, language, cognition, swallowing, balance, and voice, depending on site and extent of neurological damage
Alzheimer's disease	Neurons, neurotransmitter systems, beginning primarily in the hippocampus and progressing to widespread cortical regions	Neurofibrillary tangles and plaques, which interfere with basic cell metabolism and neurotransmission; cell death	Impairments in declarative learning and memory, manifesting primarily as word-finding and discourse-level impairments in the early to mid stages; impairments in all aspects of communication and swallowing dysfunction in the later stages
Stroke	Groups of neurons in cortical and subcortical structures	Hypoxia causing death of brain tissue in core of lesion, and potentially reversible suppression of firing in peripheral regions via loss of ATP to drive ion pumps	Deficits depend on site of lesion and extent of damage but often include impairments in movement, cognition, language, speech production, and swallowing dysfunction
Parkinson's disease	Neurons, systems of neurons, neuronal circuitry, dopamine and other neurotransmitters	Lewy bodies and oxidative stress, causing widespread cell death in the central and peripheral nervous systems; dopaminergic cells are particularly vulnerable; neuronal circuits have aberrant firing patterns	Motor speech impairment, cognitive and emotional dysfunction, dementia

or entire nervous system. For example, idiopathic Parkinson's disease historically was attributed to loss of dopamine in the basal ganglia, resulting in a cluster of classical motor signs. Currently, it is widely accepted that in addition to the loss of dopamine and other neurotransmitters, Parkinson's disease impairs neuronal function, leading to cell death and abnormal firing patterns not only in the central nervous system, but also in the peripheral nervous system. This widespread damage explains, at least in part, the deficits in movement, sensation, autonomic nervous system function, sleep, cognition, communication, and swallowing observed in Parkinson's disease. In other words, Parkinson's disease affects not only neurons but also how they function as circuits.

■ Putting It All Together

Neuroplasticity is the concept that the nervous system can change in an experience-dependent manner. Improved understanding of neuroplasticity has revolutionized rehabilitation. It was once assumed that after development, the nervous system was relatively static and did not extensively remodel after injury or disease. As you can imagine, interest in the development of strategies to rehabilitate the brain was, thus, lacking. If an individual suffered a stroke

or a neurodegenerative disease such as Parkinson's disease, it was generally assumed that the damaged tissue could not be changed and that compensation from other brain areas, if any, was insignificant. As such, rehabilitation of disorders of the brain was not common practice. However, with advances in technology and the observations and curiosity of clinicians and scientists, rehabilitation strategies have evolved to capitalize on the brain's ability not only to compensate for damage but also to change structure and function. These changes occur at the molecular level, within circuits, or within brain systems.

A famous concept in neuroscience was described by Hebb (1949):

Let us assume that the persistence or repetition of a reverberatory activity (or "trace") tends to induce lasting cellular changes that add to its stability. For example, when an axon of cell A is near enough to excite cell B and repeatedly or persistently takes part in firing it, some growth process or metabolic change takes place in one or both cells such that *A*'s efficiency, as one of the cells firing *B*, is increased.

This concept has been popularized as the phrase coined by Siegrid Löwel: "neurons wire together if they fire together" (Löwel and Singer 1992). Simply, activity-dependent changes in synaptic strength

---

Box 6.8   Deep Brain Stimulation

Deep brain stimulation (DBS) is a remarkable, indeed revolutionary treatment for neurologic and psychiatric disorders. DBS involves the permanent placement of electrodes in specific brain structures to provide electrical stimulation. There is considerable evidence that DBS exerts its benefit by generating action potentials in axons in the vicinity of the stimulating electrode, causing retrograde or backward-propagating action potentials, referred to as *antidromic conduction*. Normal conduction from the neuron cell body to the axon terminals is called *orthodromic conduction*.

Generation of action potentials in axons near the electrode is likely only the first step in the therapeutic effect of DBS, as action potentials initially generated in the axon propagate widely through the circuitry of the brain. The specific circuits affected and how those effects mediate the therapeutic mechanisms of action of DBS is unknown. We do know that the critical first step in the generation of action potentials by DBS likely involves voltage-gated ionic conductance channels,

particularly Na⁺ channels. Electrical stimulation at the surface of the electrode causes the production of ions that change the ratio of positive to negative charges across the neuronal membrane. The consequence is a depolarization of the neuronal membrane, which, if above the threshold level, will generate an action potential. Because of their geometry, axons are more susceptible to the depolarizing effects of DBS, which explains why DBS generates action potentials in axons passing by the electrode. This initial effect does not depend on neurotransmitters.

Interestingly, DBS protocols involved in the treatment of Parkinson's disease often involve high-frequency stimulation to an area in the basal ganglia called the subthalamic nucleus. Although it has been well documented that this approach benefits movement in the limbs by reducing tremor and **bradykinesia**, DBS does not improve speech or swallowing. In some cases, speech and swallowing actually worsen. This disparity between improvement for movement in the limbs but not in the head and neck is fascinating from a motor control standpoint.

are important in development, learning, memory, and recovery after disease or injury. Activity-dependent modulation of the synapse is one of the main principles of neuroplasticity.

For neuroplasticity to occur, a change in behavior and a change in the structure and function of the nervous system is required. A seminal review of the concepts of neuroplasticity, especially as they pertain to rehabilitation and can be applied to treating communication disorders, is discussed by Kleim and Jones (2008). How neuroplasticity occurs depends, of course, on the substrates involved. However, returning to the concepts described earlier in this chapter, exercise, drugs, or experience can affect all aspects of cellular function, including changing the excitability of the membrane, up- or downregulating receptors, changing the amount or release of neurotransmitter, changing the breakdown or uptake of neurotransmitter, speeding up or slowing down neural transmission, or even changing second messenger signaling. Thus, the development of treatments that address aberrant cell physiology upstream of behavior provides a significant opportunity in the treatment of nervous system diseases and disorders.

■ Suggested Readings

Bear MF, Connors BW, Paradiso MA. Neuroscience: Exploring the Brain, 3rd ed. Philadelphia, PA: Lippincott Williams and Wilkins; 2006

De Zeeuw CI, Hoogland TM. Reappraisal of Bergmann glial cells as modulators of cerebellar circuit function. *Frontiers in Cell Neuroscience, 9*, 246; 2015

Gundersen V, Storm-Mathisen J, Bergersen LH. Neuroglial transmission. *Physiological Reviews, 95*(3), 695–726; 2015

Hebb DO. The Organization of Behavior. New York, NY: Wiley & Sons; 1949

Kaune WT, Gillis MF. General properties of the interaction between animals and ELF electric fields. *Bioelectromagnetics, 2*, 1–11; 1981

Kleim JA, Jones TA. Principles of experience-dependent neural plasticity: implications for rehabilitation after brain damage. *Journal of Speech, Language, and Hearing Research, 51*, S225–S239; 2008

Lee CH, Ruben PC. Interaction between voltage-gated sodium channels and the neurotoxin, tetrodotoxin. *Channels, 2*(6), 407–412; 2008

Löwel S, Singer W. Selection of intrinsic horizontal connections in the visual cortex by correlated neuronal activity. *Science, 255*, 209–212; 1992

Montgomery EB Jr. Effects of GPi stimulation on human thalamic neuronal activity. *Clinical Neurophysiology, 117*, 2691–2702; 2006

Nicholls JG, Martin AR, Fuchs PA, Brown DA, Diamond ME, Weisblat DA. From Neuron to Brain, 5th ed. Cary, NC: Sinauer Associates; 2011

Rieke F, Warland D, de Ruyter van Steveninck R, Bialek W. Spikes: Exploring the Neural Code (Computational Neuroscience), reprint ed. Cambridge MA: MIT Press; 1999

Tighe AP, Schiavo G. Botulinum neurotoxins: mechanism of action. *Toxicon, 67*, 87–93; 2013

■ Study Questions

1. The fundamental operating element of the nervous system is the:

A. Neuron
B. Glial cell
C. Axon
D. Neurotransmitter
E. Brain

2. The part of the neuron in which information coming from other neurons and glial cells is received is the:

A. Dendrite
B. Axon
C. Axon terminal
D. Soma
E. Nucleolus

3. Where one neuron communicates electrically directly with another neuron is referred to as:

A. A synapse
B. A gap junction
C. An action potential
D. An enzymatic reaction
E. Transmission

4. Neuronal cell membranes are described as semipermeable because they:

A. Sometimes leak
B. Are formed by a lipid bilayer
C. Have embedded ion channels that can be opened and closed
D. Can be disrupted in disease
E. Are in a complex network

5. Which of the following is **not** a type of glial cell in the central nervous system?

A. Oligodendrocyte
B. Microglia
C. Ependymal cell
D. Astrocyte
E. Schwann cell

6. The resting cell membrane potential is determined primarily by:

A. Concentrations of chloride and sodium in the extracellular fluid
B. Movement of sodium and chloride along their concentration gradients
C. Movement of sodium and potassium along their electrical gradients
D. Concentrations of sodium and potassium in the intra- and extracellular fluid
E. Transport of sodium and chloride across the neuronal cell membrane

7. The main protein that actively moves cations across the cell membrane is:

A. Na^+, Ca^{2+}-ATPase
B. Na^+, Cl^--ATPase
C. Na^+, K^+-ATPase
D. K^+, Cl^--ATPase
E. ATP-independent Na^+, K^+ pump

8. Ion channels at which neurotransmitters bind are:

A. Voltage-gated
B. Autologous
C. Postsynaptic only
D. Ligand-gated
E. Presynaptic only

9. The depolarization phase of the action potential is primarily driven by:

A. Voltage-gated sodium channels
B. Ligand-gated sodium channels
C. Voltage-gated potassium channels
D. Ligand-gated potassium channels
E. Prolonged subthreshold depolarization of the cell membrane

10. The repolarization phase of the action potential is primarily driven by:

A. Ligand-gated sodium channels
B. Voltage-gated sodium channels
C. Voltage-gated potassium channels
D. Ligand-gated potassium channels
E. Prolonged subthreshold depolarization of the cell membrane

11. Temporal summation occurs when:

A. Inputs to the same section of the neuronal membrane occur very close in time
B. The axon hillock sums inputs to the axon that occur simultaneously
C. Inputs to adjacent sections of the neuronal membrane occur simultaneously
D. Postsynaptic muscle cells contract simultaneously
E. Neurons computationally sum inputs across the entire neuronal surface

12. Nodes of Ranvier:

A. Are one section of the axon in which there are no channels where sodium can leak out
B. Have the highest density of myelination of any section of the axon
C. Have a low concentration of voltage-gated sodium channels
D. Are the main action potential propagation segment of the axon
E. Are the product of myelination by oligodendrocytes

13. The main ion involved in docking of vesicles at the presynaptic membrane of the axon terminal is:

A. Calcium
B. Potassium
C. Sodium
D. Chloride
E. ATP

14. Neurotransmitters can be removed from the synapse by:

A. Diffusion away in the extracellular fluid
B. Uptake by local glial cells
C. Reuptake by presynaptic neurons
D. Enzymatic breakdown
E. All of the above

15. Drugs that stimulate a postsynaptic receptor are called

A. Antagonists
B. Neuromodulators
C. Binding agents
D. Agonists
E. Ionotropic

16. An input that causes a positive shift in the postsynaptic membrane potential is called:

A. A hyperpolarizing postsynaptic potential
B. An excitatory postsynaptic potential
C. A depolarizing postsynaptic potential
D. An inhibitory postsynaptic potential
E. A tetrodotoxin potential

17. When a neurotransmitter attaches to a receptor and initiates a sequence of metabolic reactions that are slower and longer lasting, this is called:

A. Metabotropic effect
B. Exocytosis effect
C. Ionotropic effect
D. Graded effect
E. None of the above

18. Glutamate is always an excitatory neurotransmitter.

A. True
B. False

19. These may open or close ion channels, alter production of activating proteins, or activate chromosomes:

A. Graded potentials
B. Excitatory postsynaptic potentials
C. Inhibitory postsynaptic potentials
D. Sodium-potassium pumps
E. Second messengers

20. An example of a monoamine neurotransmitter is:

A. Serotonin
B. Dopamine
C. Norepinephrine
D. All of the above
E. None of the above

■ Answers to Study Questions

1. The correct answer is (A) neuron. Recall that neurons encode, process, and transmit information.

2. The correct answer is (A), dendrite. The soma (D) is the cell body, and a nucleolus (E) is a cell body organelle. The axon (B) transmits signals away from the cell toward the axon terminal. The axon terminal (C) is where neurotransmitter is released.

3. The correct answer is (B), gap junction. Gap junctions are sometimes called electrical synapses, but in most cases, synapses in the human nervous system use neurotransmitters (chemical signaling).

4. The correct answer is (C) have embedded ion channels that can be opened and closed. The membrane is impermeable except when channels open, allowing ions to move across the membrane.

5. The correct answer is (E) Schwann cells. Schwann cells are the counterpart in the *peripheral* nervous system to oligodendrocytes.

6. The correct answer is (D) concentrations of sodium and potassium in the intra- and extracellular fluid. There is active transport of ions across the cell membrane (E), but for the resting membrane potential the ions involved are sodium and potassium, not sodium and chloride.

7. The correct answer is (C) Na^+, K^+-ATPase, which moves three Na^+ ions out, moves two K^+ ions in, and consumes one ATP molecule.

8. The correct answer is (D) ligand-gated. A ligand is a substance that binds to a receptor, such as a neurotransmitter.

9. The correct answer is (A) voltage-gated sodium channels. When these channels open, sodium enters the cell rapidly because of the concentration gradient, and the cell becomes rapidly depolarized (more positive). This is during the action potential, which primarily uses voltage-gated channels.

10. The correct answer is (C) voltage-gated potassium channels. When these channels open, potassium leaves the cell rapidly because of the concentration gradient, and the cell becomes rapidly repolarized (more negative). This is during the action potential, which primarily uses voltage-gated channels.

11. The correct answer is (A) inputs to the same section of the neuronal membrane occur very close in time. The word "temporal" refers to time.

12. The correct answer is (D) are the main action potential propagation segment of the axon. Nodes of Ranvier have no myelination and have the highest concentration of voltage-gated sodium channels on the axon to enable saltatory conduction.

13. The correct answer is (A) calcium.

14. The correct answer is (E) all of the above.

15. The correct answer is (D) agonists. Antagonists (A) inhibit activity at the postsynaptic cell.

16. The correct answer is (C) a depolarizing postsynaptic potential. Although these are often called excitatory postsynaptic potentials (B), "depolarizing" is a more accurate term. Depolarizing events are not always excitatory, and excitatory events are not always caused directly by depolarization.

17. The correct answer is (A) metabotropic effects.

18. The correct answer is (B) false, because the effect of a neurotransmitter is due to its *receptor*.

19. The correct answer is (E) second messengers.

20. The correct answer is (D); all of these are examples of monoamines.

7

Suprasegmental Motor Control

Erwin B. Montgomery Jr., Michelle R. Ciucci, and Lyn S. Turkstra

■ Chapter Summary

Speech and swallowing are motor phenomena. Consequently, an understanding of how disorders of the central nervous system (CNS) affect speech and swallowing ultimately must be explained at the level at which motor phenomena are generated; that is, the motor unit, which consists of alpha lower motor neurons (α-LMN) and the muscle fibers they innervate. Similarly, any treatment for speech and swallowing disorders of CNS origin ultimately must be understood by their effects on motor units. Other than perhaps the motor cortex, very little is known about how the CNS affects the physiology of the motor unit. Nonetheless, this does not relieve the speech-language pathologist and audiologist from at least understanding the challenges. Moving a muscle is complicated, especially for complex voluntary movements such as speaking, writing, singing, and swallowing. It is hard to imagine how the nervous system orchestrates force, timing, onset, and offset of muscle activity for multiple muscles during these voluntary activities. The alpha and gamma motor neurons that are part of the peripheral nerves that activate muscle fibers are the final link in a complex system of CNS structures that control voluntary movement. Thus, while a movement is *effected* through lower motor neurons, the force, timing, onset, and offset of voluntary muscle activity are controlled by structures in the central nervous system. These structures are referred to as *suprasegmental* structures (i.e., they interact in complex ways "above the segment" of the peripheral nerve, the spinal cord at the level at which peripheral nerves enter and exit, and the muscle), and include the motor cortex, basal ganglia, cerebellum, association cortex, brainstem nuclei reticular formation, and their interconnections. Damage to suprasegmental structures results in movement disorders such as Parkinson's disease and dystonia. Suprasegmental disorders also commonly affect speech, voice, and swallowing, often in ways that differ from effects on limb movements. In this chapter, we will discuss common suprasegmental disorders and how lesions to different parts of the suprasegmental motor control system result in patterns of signs and symptoms. Specifically, we will (1) present current theories about suprasegmental motor control and provide empirical data that show limitations of these theories and gaps in knowledge, (2) describe the function of the basal ganglia, (3) highlight limitations of current theories and introduce alternative theories that may advance our understanding of not only basic motor function but also movement disorders that affect speech, voice, and swallowing, and (4) relate these concepts to disorders managed by speech-language pathologists and audiologists.

■ Learning Objectives

- Understand the basic mechanisms by which force is generated to produce movement
- Describe the anatomy and physiology of the motor cortex and how movement-related information is represented and controlled by neurons of the motor cortex
- Explain how damage to the motor cortex produces the symptoms and signs resulting in the upper motor neuron syndrome

191

- Describe the anatomy and physiology of the cerebellar system and how cerebellar anatomy and physiology relate to clinical syndromes associated with cerebellar lesions

Putting It Into Practice

- Understand the relationships between the alpha lower motor neuron and other structures that provide information to the alpha lower motor neuron. These other structures include the gamma lower motor neuron, upper motor neuron, brainstem nuclei and reticular formation, basal ganglia, cerebellum, and association cortices.
- Describe the anatomy, neurochemistry, and physiology of the basal ganglia and explain why the basal ganglia must be understood as part of a network: the basal ganglia–thalamic–cortical system.
- Critically evaluate theories and hypotheses related to the physiology and pathophysiology of the basal ganglia–thalamic–cortical system, particularly concepts related to the pathophysiology of Parkinson's disease.
- Describe syndromes associated with lesions of the motor association cortices.

Introduction

Speech and swallowing disorders basically are disorders of motor control. The fundamental unit by which motor control is effected is the **motor unit (MU)**, which comprises the muscle fibers innervated by a single **alpha lower motor neuron** (α-LMN). The α-LMN is influenced by structures in the central nervous system that project to the α-LMN, such as the **motor cortex** and various nuclei in the **brainstem**. These structures in turn are affected by other regions of the cortex as well as subcortical structures such as the **basal ganglia** and **cerebellum**. Together, the cortex and subcortical structures represent the **suprasegmental** control system for the orchestration of α-LMN activities.

Unfortunately, very little is known about how the various suprasegmental structures orchestrate the activities of the motor unit, with the possible exception of the motor cortex. This lack of knowledge likely limits current therapies and impedes the development of future treatments. The temptation to discuss only what is simple or intuitive and what provides a patina of understanding often leads to "dumbing down" the material for the learner's sake. Although

we are unable to provide explicit answers as to how disorders of the CNS manifest in altered motor control in speech and swallowing, we hope that readers today will succeed in doing so in the future.

Theories, which form the basis of understanding, do not arise spontaneously. They require prior suppositions, perspectives, and modes of thinking, if only to make sense of the relevant observations. If the understanding of speech and swallowing problems associated with disorders of the CNS is to advance, it is necessary to also consider the suppositions, perspectives, and modes of thinking that have led to current notions of CNS **pathophysiology**. These discussions will take place predominantly in the context of disorders of the basal ganglia–thalamic–cortical system, for which theoretical developments are more advanced.

The Motor Unit and Segmental Motor Control

Before we discuss suprasegmental motor control, it may be helpful to review the function of the motor unit, which is discussed in much greater detail in **Chapter 8**. A motor unit is defined as one alpha lower motor neuron (α-LMN) and all the individual muscle fibers it innervates (**Fig. 7.1**). Any motor behavior is fundamentally implemented in the orchestration of motor units. The term *orchestration* is apt, given the complexities of motor unit control needed to execute complex speech, voice, and swallowing movements. To follow our analogy, if motor units are the orchestra, the conductors are structures in the central nervous system. The role of central nervous system structures in motor control is evidenced by the wide variety of central nervous system lesions that can impair motor function.

A useful conceptual approach is to consider the orchestration of motor units as **information**. In the most general sense, information can be defined as nonrandom state changes. For example, in English written text, each potential space in the sentence that could contain a character (letter of the alphabet, number, punctuation, or blank) is a state. The sequence of states then conveys information. The changes in the content of each state as the sequence of the text is read is not random. Otherwise the information would be meaningless.

When viewed in this context, normal motor control requires normal information, and misinformation is the cause of disorders. This stands in contrast to much current thinking of neurological disorders as relative excesses or deficiencies of function, ascribed to relative excesses or deficiencies of neurotransmitters or inhibition and excitation. It is likely that current and future treatments will be best understood as they relate to changes in information content. Consequently, the information content in the orchestration of motor unit activities are central. The subtlety and complexity of the information over multiple time scales will become apparent, and one might wonder in retrospect how simple, one-dimensional schemes of relative excess or deficiency were ever thought to be sufficient.

Consider the most articulate speaker or skilled singer, and you will appreciate the precision and complexity motor units must achieve. However, a motor unit can be only on or off, so how can it achieve complexity? It might be helpful to use an analogy from computer science. After all, the nervous system is essentially a very powerful supercomputer that can simultaneously assimilate, process, organize, and distribute information. In the nervous system, the term "information" refers to signals encoded in the changes in electrical potentials across the membrane within a neuron and among groups of neurons that are used to make decisions about executing movement.

Any motor behavior can be understood as a precise series of changes in the electrical potentials across the cell membranes of many neurons throughout the motor control systems that ultimately result in activations of individual motor units over time and in concert with other motor units. Just as one can analyze the written text by its syntax or set of rules that ensure nonrandom sequences of symbols, one can search for the syntax of the changes in the electrical potentials across the cell membrane of many linked neurons and muscles.

Just as the syntax in an English text operates over different levels, such as letter, word, sentence, paragraph, and narrative, the syntax of motor behavior operates at multiple levels. The most fundamental level that constitutes the syntax of motor behavior is the changes in electrical potential across the neuronal membrane. This is detailed in **Chapter 6**. In motor control, the change in electrical potential across the **action potential–initiating segment** controls **action potentials** in the α-LMNs. These action potentials are relayed to muscle fibers via the axons to the presynaptic terminals, which release the neurotransmitter **acetylcholine** onto the muscle fibers to initiate contraction of the muscle fiber. The precise pattern of acetylcholine release is determined by the pattern of changes in electrical potentials across the neuronal membrane of the presynaptic terminals as a consequence of action potentials generated in the α-LMNs. Muscle fibers in turn respond via contraction of an individ-

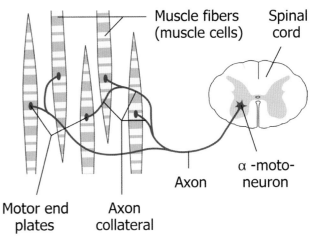

Fig. 7.1 Schematic representation of a motor unit. The cell body of the alpha lower motor neuron resides in the ventral gray matter of the spinal cord. The axon arising from the cell body exits the spinal cord through the ventral root to combine with the other axons to create the peripheral nerve. The motor unit comprises the muscle fibers that are innervated by a single alpha lower motor neuron.

ual muscle fiber, which is an **all-or-none response**. However, motor units vary in size, in the number of muscle fibers innervated by a single α-LMN, and in the force that is produced. As will be discussed later, which axons from the α-LMN have action potentials and how multiple action potentials are patterned in space over many axons and over time in individual axons is not random but is precisely controlled to achieve specific forces required for that movement. Using our computer analogy, the timing and locations of action potentials are nonrandom changes in state.

The α-LMN is a **lower motor neuron** because it is the last link in a series of complex circuits that can cause a muscle to contract. LMN activity can be affected by many types of inputs, which influence α-LMNs as well as **gamma lower motor neurons** (γ-LMNs) (see **Chapter 8**) by changing the electrical potential across their cell membranes. These other inputs are mostly in the form of synaptic contacts onto the **dendrites** and **cell body** (**soma**) of the LMN. Some inputs arise from sensory neurons and constitute a peripheral nervous system control over the LMN, and can cause an action potential or perhaps prevent it from happening. The γ-LMN can also activate muscle fibers in the **muscle spindle** sensory apparatus; these constitute the peripheral motor control system, as discussed in **Chapter 8**.

Other inputs to the α-LMN arise within the spinal cord (for spinal nerves) or in close proximity to the α-LMN cell body in the brainstem (for cranial nerves). For example, a **Renshaw cell** receives a depolarizing input from an α-LMN and in turn

Box 7.1   Muscles As Springs around a Joint

The γ-LMN innervates the muscle fiber within the muscle spindle (**intrafusal muscle fiber**) (**Box Fig. 7.1**). The muscle spindle is a sensory organ within the muscle that senses the stretch of the muscle or the rate of change in the stretch of the muscle and presumably informs the nervous system of the state of contraction of the muscles so as to achieve proper control of the muscles. The role of the spindle in motor control is problematic. Clearly, with active muscle contraction, the main muscle fibers shorten in length, and this would unload the muscle spindle, lessening the stretch and therefore reducing the output of the muscle spindle. Certain theories posit that the actual control of the muscles is done by setting the sensitivity of the muscle spindle. The final position of a limb or structure then depends on achieving a specific muscle spindle output, which is controlled by the γ-LMN. One could imagine the muscles as springs around a joint. The joint would rotate until the forces exerted by the opposing springs balanced. If one were to tighten one of the springs, for example by contracting the intrafusal muscle fiber by increasing the action potentials generated in the γ-LMN, the joint would rotate until a new equilibrium or balancing of the forces of the springs was obtained. However, when the dorsal roots of the spinal cord segment are cut, thereby removing information from the muscle spindles from the CNS, often there is no abnormality of the movements, which raises questions about the role of the muscle spindle information.

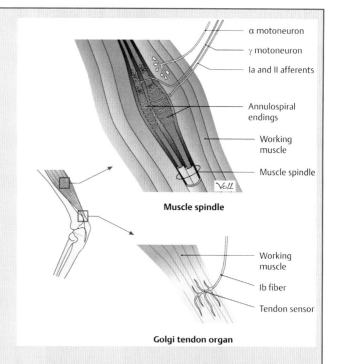

Box Fig. 7.1 Schematic representation of the muscle, muscle spindle, alpha and gamma lower motor neurons. As can be seen, the muscle spindles consist of specialized intrafusal muscle fibers. As the limb is rotated about a joint, the intrafusal muscle fibers are stretched or shortened. Sensory annulospiral nerve endings respond to the stretch intrafusal muscle fibers, thereby indicating the degree of joint rotation. The sensitivity of the muscle spindle is controlled by the degree of contraction of the intrafusal muscle fibers in response to action potentials in the γ-LMN.

sends a hyperpolarizing input back to the same α-LMN. It is hypothesized that this recurrent inhibition improves the temporal resolution in the pattern of action potentials generated by that α-LMN. **Interneurons**, neurons with processes wholly within the CNS, also provide input to α-LMNs. This level of local organization is called **segmental** motor control, and the circuitry of segmental motor control systems is the mechanism for many reflex behaviors observed in lesioned systems, such as the snouting reflex in adults with severe brain damage. Segmental motor control is relevant to our discussion here, as, according to some theories of motor control, discussed later in this chapter, the role of suprasegmental inputs is to modify these segmental reflex behaviors.

Box 7.2   Effects of Deep Brain Stimulation on Limb versus Speech Motor Function

Much of the discussion in this chapter is borrowed heavily from limb motor control. This borrowing is useful, because there is extensive research on limb motor control, and a great many useful insights and concepts have been achieved. However, it is not clear, nor should it be taken for granted, that limb motor control is an apt metaphor for motor control of speech, voice, and swallowing. Indeed, there are situations in which effects of a treatment or disease process may have different effects on limb than on speech motor function. An example is high-frequency **deep brain stimulation** (DBS) for treatment of Parkinson's disease, which can improve limb motor control but worsen speech and swallowing.

Suprasegmental Structures

Suprasegmental structures are defined as structures other than α-LMNs and γ-LMNs in the spinal cord and brainstem and local circuitry in which they are embedded. Suprasegmental structures include the **motor cortex**, **basal ganglia**, **cerebellum**, **associational cortex,** brainstem nuclei, brainstem, reticular formation, and interconnections among these structures. The importance of suprasegmental motor control is evident in the movement disorders that result from injury or disease affecting these structures. Many suprasegmental structures can be identified by their axonal connections to the α-LMNs and γ-LMNs. Some of these connections are listed in **Table 7.1**.

Orchestration of Motor Unit Activation

First-Order Motor Unit Control

Activations of individual motor units are not random but are executed according to the force required to apply torque around a joint, as in movements of the jaw, or pull on nonbony insertions, as in movements of the tongue, lips, or soft palate for speech and swallowing. Motor units are organized by size, which can range from just a few muscle fibers per α-LMN to several hundred. The amount of force generated by a single α-LMN is determined by the number of muscle fibers the α-LMN innervates.

Thus, small motor units generate only a small force, but the small force allows for fine resolution of the force required (see **Chapter 8**). When a force is required, small motor units activate first. As greater force is required, small motor units discharge more rapidly and larger motor units are recruited. This size-based order of motor unit recruitment is called the **Heinneman size principle**.

Initially, it was thought that the order of motor unit recruitment by size was solely a consequence of the size of the α-LMN. Small α-LMNs, associated with small motor units, were thought to be easier to excite than large α-LMNs associated with large motor units. The Heinneman size principle was thought to offload the task of ordering α-LMN recruitment onto α-LMNs, so suprasegmental systems had only to specify the force, and the biophysics of the α-LMNs controlled the recruitment order. We now know this is not the case. As an example, individuals with **Parkinson's disease** have an abnormal α-LMN recruitment order. Rather than small motor units being recruited first, large motor units may be recruited first. This abnormal recruitment can be made more normal by DBS in the vicinity of the **subthalamic nucleus** of the basal ganglia (**Box 7.3**). If recruitment order is entirely a segmental function, however, central nervous system stimulation should not affect it. Thus, it is likely that the basal ganglia–thalamic–cortical system participates in orderly recruitment and derecruitment of motor units. Indeed, the adverse effects of DBS in the vicinity of the subthalamic nucleus may reflect counterproductive changes in the orchestra-

Table 7.1 Axonal connections to the α-LMNs and γ-LMNs

Structure	Direct and indirect pathway to α-LMNs and γ-LMNs
Motor cortex, **supplementary motor area (SMA)**, and **primary somatosensory cortex** (the last projects primarily to the sensory relay nuclei of the nuclei gracilis and cuneatus)	Lateral and medial **corticospinal** and **corticobulbar tracts**; also called the **pyramidal tract**, as these fibers travel through the **pyramids** of the **medulla oblongata**
Reticular formation of the brainstem	Medial and lateral **reticulospinal tracts**
Fastigial nucleus of the cerebellum	**Fastigiospinal tract**
Vestibular nuclei	**Vestibulospinal tracts**
Red nucleus	**Rubrospinal tract**
Tectum of the brainstem	**Tectospinal tract**
Pyramidal system	Another term for the corticospinal and corticobulbar tracts
Extrapyramidal system	Suprasegmental pathways other than the corticospinal and corticobulbar tracts
Dentate, globose, and **emboliform nuclei** of the cerebellum	Project to the LMNs via the rubrospinal and reticulospinal tracts
Globus pallidus of the basal ganglia, internal segment	Projects to the LMNs via connections to the **pedunculopontine** nucleus

Box 7.3   Deep Brain Stimulation for Movement Disorders

DBS for movement disorders such as Parkinson's disease is probably the most remarkable therapeutic advance since the introduction of levodopa for Parkinson's disease. DBS is more effective for many disorders than medications, gene therapy, or even brain tissue transplants. The treatment involves the permanent placement of an array of electrical contacts in various brain targets and electrically stimulating the nervous system using a pacemaker-like device placed under the skin of the chest (**Box Fig. 7.2**).

Despite the remarkable benefits of DBS, its therapeutic mechanisms are unknown, largely because it is not known what neuronal abnormalities are to be corrected. Studies of the brain responses to DBS have demonstrated that most current concepts of motor control physiology and pathophysiology are incorrect. This necessitates great caution in attempting to use behavioral responses to DBS as a means of understanding the pathophysiology and physiology of nervous system structures.

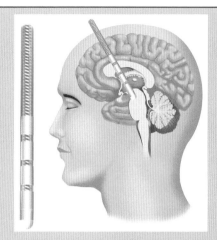

Box Fig. 7.2   The DBS lead contains a set of four metal contacts that serve as stimulating electrodes. The right side of the image shows a sagittal (side view) magnetic resonance imaging (MRI) scan of the brain, with eyes and nose at the left. As can be seen, the DBS lead is placed in the brain. In this case, the tip of the DBS lead is located in the vicinity of the subthalamic nucleus, a structure in the basal ganglia–thalamic–cortical system.

---

tion of motor units in the speech and swallowing articulators. These adverse effects often limit the therapeutic efficacy of DBS for many patients.

It is critical to appreciate the dynamics of motor unit control. Dynamics—the change in a system over time—can be considered a form of information or misinformation. In the case of first-order motor unit control, the dynamics must occur over a very short time scale. For example, a rapid ballistic movement requiring large forces may need to be accomplished in 30 milliseconds; thus, activation of multiple α-LMNs must occur repeatedly within that time. The dynamics of higher orders of motor unit activation occur over different and often longer time scales. The first-order level of motor control can be considered roughly analogous to the sequence of letters and spaces that define words.

Second-Order Motor Unit Control

Typically, multiple muscles operate around any one axis of movement, such as the center of rotation about a joint. Thus, actions of multiple muscles must be coordinated around that movement axis. Consider rapid flexion around the wrist joint from a starting position of wrist extension. Initially, the wrist extensor muscles are active to hold the wrist in extension against the elastic force of the stretched wrist flexor muscles. With the initiation of wrist

flexion, the wrist extensor muscles must derecruit so as not to oppose the subsequent wrist flexion. Subsequent to extensor muscle derecruitment, the flexor muscles must be recruited to begin wrist flexion. Initially, there is a burst of flexor muscle activation to overcome the inertia of the hand. However, if this burst continued, it would flex the wrist beyond its target. Consequently, after the initial burst of the flexor muscles, the motor units in the flexor muscle derecruit and the motor units in the extensor muscle are recruited again to prevent the wrist from overflexing. Once the extensor muscles have acted as a brake on the acceleration of wrist flexion, the extensor muscles derecruit. Finally, the flexor muscles are recruited to move the wrist to its final position. These changes in motor unit activations over different muscles—in this case, the wrist flexor and extensor muscles—is called the triphasic pattern (**Fig. 7.2**). The dynamics of second-order control of motor unit activation occur over a longer time scale than those of first-order control, as previously mentioned. Again by analogy to English text, the second order of motor unit control can be considered the organization of words into phrases and sentences.

Extensor muscles often are described as the antagonistic muscles opposing wrist flexion. However, it is important to note that, as can be seen from the foregoing description, this nomenclature is incorrect. In the case of ballistic movements, the wrist extensor muscles play an important role in achieving

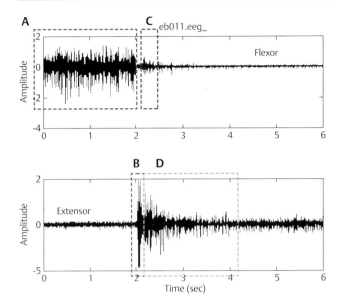

Fig. 7.2 Example of electrical activities generated by motor units in the wrist flexor and extensor muscles in an isometric task involving rapid wrist extension forces from a position in wrist flexion force.

precise wrist flexion. One can appreciate the effect of prior one-dimensional push-pull conceptualizations, in this case into agonist and antagonist muscles. As seen, however, this notion is incorrect.

Second-order control of joint rotations becomes even more complex in multijoint movements. An example is writing, which requires coordination of muscle actions across multiple joints and over space and time. Information regarding the recruitment and derecruitment of every muscle must capture all muscles acting across all joints. Suprasegmental disorders can affect this multijoint orchestration. For example, individuals with Parkinson's disease are impaired in making multijoint movements that evolve over time. When using American Sign Language, which requires movement to and between specific upper extremity positions to signify words, individuals with Parkinson's disease do not move fully to each position but rather move to intermediary positions (Tyrone et al 1999). Another clinical example is patients with cerebellar disorders, who show **decomposition of movement**, in which complex multijoint rotations that normally are executed simultaneously are broken down into simpler movements that are executed sequentially.

Third-Order Motor Unit Control

According to Newton's third law of motion, forces created by muscles in order to rotate a joint or move an object are associated with equal and opposite forces. Thus, rotational forces at one joint can lead to forces that act through the lever arms that form that joint. For example, in a limb with a distal and a proximal joint, rotation about the distal joint will produce a force that will act on the proximal joint (e.g., moving the finger in relation to the wrist will produce a force acting on the elbow). Proximal joints must have forces exerted on them to counteract the reactive forces from rotation about the distal joint. The central nervous system is able to estimate the degree of reactive forces that will be encountered and generate the necessary counterforce in anticipation of the primary joint rotation. The role of suprasegmental structures in this counterforce generation becomes evident when you lift a box that is lighter than you imagined: you prepare to generate force in muscles that will counter the upward lifting forces needed to move the box based on your expectation about the weight of the box. When much less upward lifting force is needed than expected, the lifting movement has more counterforce than needed, and the lifting movement is highly exaggerated.

Movements may change the body's center of gravity, stimulating movements to maintain the center of gravity over the base of support. Consider extending your arms in front of you. The weight of your arm moves from the side of your body to in front, which shifts your center of gravity forward. Forces are generated that move your body to bring the center of gravity back over your base of support. In this case, ankle plantar flexion rotates the upper body posteriorly to move the center of gravity posteriorly and over the base of support. Again, there is evidence that suprasegmental motor structures are involved in these third-order motor control functions. For example, individuals with Parkinson's disease have diminished ability to counteract shifts in their center of gravity. The time scales for motor unit activation sequences in third-order motor unit control are even longer than those of second- and first-order levels of control. Extending the analogy to English text, the third-order organization of motor control could be considered the organization of sentences into paragraphs.

Organizing Information across All Levels of Motor Unit Control

Information required for the orchestration of motor unit recruitment and derecruitment must account for all levels of motor control, from the simplest first-order motor unit activations to complex, third-order, multisegment movements over long durations. Furthermore, information for each level of motor control must be generated simultaneously. It is tempting to think that third-order control, particularly as it relates to movements that shift the center of gravity, can be orchestrated by reflexes alone. However, this does not appear to be the case. In the example given, changes in the activities of the muscles in the trunk and lower extremities are tailored to counteract the shift in the center of gravity even before the upper limbs are extended and, thus, even before there is any shift in the center of gravity.

Information for longer sequences of complex movements also is constructed simultaneously, as evidenced by anticipatory errors. For example, a person asked to repeat "beef noodles" several times rapidly is likely to say something like "neef boodles." Articulatory gestures for "n" that should be produced later in the utterance occur at the beginning, which would not be possible if motor unit activations for the phrase "beef noodles" were encoded sequentially.

The fact that all these different aspects of motor unit activations at different levels of control are active simultaneously means that the suprasegmental motor control system must be involved to achieve the different time scales of the different dynamics. Unfortunately, no currently accepted theory of suprasegmental motor control begins to account for these different dynamics beyond the scheme proposed later in this chapter.

■ General Anatomical Organization of the Suprasegmental Motor Control System

Fig. 7.3 illustrates the various components of the suprasegmental control system. Although these structures are described individually, this does not mean that each structure encodes or processes information in some unique way. Rather, as will be seen, all of these structures participate simultaneously in creating the information that ultimately will drive motor units to produce specific behaviors.

Organization Based on Projections to α-LMNs

Specific suprasegmental structures appear to play different motor control roles. For example, the medial reticular formation and midline cerebel-

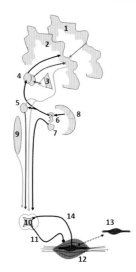

Fig. 7.3 Schematic representation of the suprasegmental control system. (1) associational cortex; (2) primary motor cortex; (3) basal ganglia; (4) thalamus (relay nuclei for the basal ganglia and cerebellum); (5) red nucleus; (6) dentate, globose, and emboliform nuclei of the cerebellum; (7) fastigial nucleus of the cerebellum; (8) cerebellar cortex; (9) brainstem nuclei, including the reticular formation; (10) spinal cord; (11) peripheral motor nerve; (12) muscle; (13) muscle spindle; and (14) peripheral sensory nerve from muscle spindle. Various descending pathways from the suprasegmental structures onto the spinal cord are described by their origin. The spinal cord and peripheral motor and sensory nerves are considered part of the segmental motor system.

lar structures appear to be involved in the control of posture and gait, whereas the motor cortex appears to play more of a role in the control of fine distal movements of the extremities, particularly the upper extremities. Interestingly, the control of motor units related to speech and swallowing appears to correlate better with those that control posture and gait rather than control of the distal upper extremities. This association can explain the patterns of disabilities associated with suprasegmental disorders such as Parkinson's disease. These different roles may relate to the pattern by which these structures project onto different groups of α-LMNs.

Projections from suprasegmental structures to α-LMNs vary according to the α-LMN target. For example, for α-LMNs to the distal musculature, most of the input is from the corticospinal tract. Similarly, the lateral reticulospinal tract tends to synapse more heavily onto α-LMNs projecting to the distal musculature (e.g., limb muscles). The anterior corticospinal tract and the rubrospinal, vestibulospinal, fastigiospinal, and medial reticulospinal tracts project more heavily to the α-LMNs that project to the proximal musculature (e.g., muscles of the trunk). This has important implications, as proximal muscles are more involved with counterforces to the reactions generated by distal joint rotations as well as postural control in response to displacement of the center of gravity. This arrangement has important implications for signs and symptoms associated with disorders of each of the descending pathways and lesions in structures that originate these pathways (discussed later in this chapter).

The Motor Cortex

As discussed in **Chapter 5**, the cerebral cortex is divided by infoldings known as **sulci** into ridges known as **gyri** and larger areas known as **lobes**. The primary motor cortex occupies the **precentral gyrus**. The primary motor cortex is designated as **Brodmann area 4** based on its cellular architecture. Like most areas of the cerebral cortex, it is organized in six layers or *laminae*, of which layer 5 contains cell bodies of neurons that project to the LMNs. These layer 5 neurons are therefore referred to as **upper motor neurons (UMNs)**. The other layers in Area 4 contain interneurons. For muscles innervated by spinal nerves, UMN axons with destinations in the spinal cord (corticospinal axons) project through the corona radiata, down the posterior limb of the **internal capsule**, through the crus cerebri (cerebral peduncle), the ventral pons, and the pyramids of the medulla. At that point, axons of the lateral corticospinal tract cross to the contralateral side via the decussation of the pyramids. Once crossed, the descending axons travel down the lateral funiculus of the spinal cord until they enter the ventral gray matter to synapse on LMNs (**Fig. 7.4**). The axons of the medial corticospinal tract maintain their laterality until they finally cross in the spinal cord, generally at the level of the α-LMN. For muscles innervated by cranial nerves, corticobulbar axons (which originate in the cortex and synapse with LMNs in the brainstem or "bulb") tend to cross near the level of the nuclei of the cranial nerves that they innervate. It is important to note that most of the brainstem nuclei serving the speech articulators receive bilateral input, with two exceptions: (1) the portion of the facial nerve nucleus that projects to the lower facial musculature receives only contralateral UMN input (**Fig. 7.5**); and (2) neurons that project to the hypoglossal nuclei have a heavier contralateral than ipsilateral UMN innervation. This organization has important clinical implications, as weakness of only the lower face (not the upper face) can be an indication of a UMN lesion. Also, axons from

the primary motor cortex project back to the ventral lateral thalamus, basal ganglia, red nucleus, and cerebellum.

The primary motor cortex receives inputs from the ipsilateral **ventral intermediate nucleus** of the thalamus and the contralateral cerebellum. The supplementary motor area, which is anterior to and projects to the primary motor cortex, receives afferents from the ventral thalamus pars oralis, which relays information from the basal ganglia and cerebellum. In addition, the primary motor

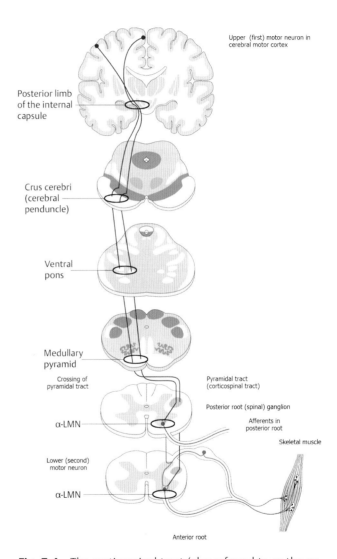

Fig. 7.4 The corticospinal tract (also referred to as the pyramidal tract, as the fibers pass through the pyramids of the medulla). The cell body of origin lies in the primary motor cortex (although a few axons originate in the supplementary motor area). These axons descend via the corona radiata to the posterior limb of the internal capsule, to the crus cerebri (or cerebral peduncle), through the ventral pons; cross the midline at the decussation of the medullary pyramids; and descend down the lateral funiculus of the spinal cord to terminate on the α-LMNs.

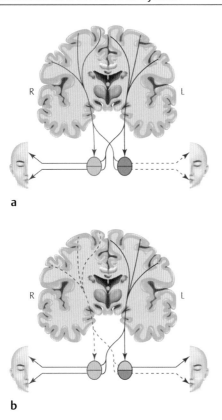

a

b

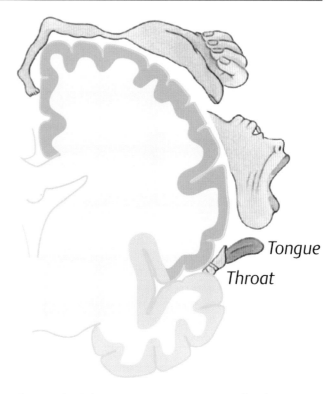

Fig. 7.6 Schematic representation of the motor homunculus.

Fig. 7.5 Schematic representation of the cortical innervation of the facial nerve nuclei and the nature of LMN and UMN facial weakness. One component of the facial nerve nuclei supplies the facial muscles for the upper half of the face, and the other component to the lower half. **(a)** A lesion of the facial nucleus or the facial nerve affects muscles of the upper and lower face as shown by the shaded areas. **(b)** Effects of a corticobulbar fiber lesion. Input to both the upper half and lower half of the contralateral facial nerve nucleus is lost. However, the component to the upper face still receives input from the ipsilateral corticobulbar fibers arising from the ipsilateral primary motor cortex. Consequently, the patient is able to move the upper face but not the lower face.

cortex receives input from other cortices, including ipsilateral primary sensory cortices, the premotor cortex, and contralateral motor cortex.

Although the layers of primary motor cortex are organized vertically, the cortex is also organized horizontally into columns. Each column is thought to be related to a specific function, such as the activation of a specific muscle. Various parts of the body are represented in vertical sequence along the precentral gyrus in an organizational scheme referred to as the motor **homunculus** (**Fig. 7.6**). The presumption is that the muscles are laid out on the motor cortex like keys on a piano, where each key is associated with a single note. Just as playing a piece of music involves information about which keys to strike at which time, so too are movements

orchestrated by activating sequences of columns in the homunculus.

The motor homunculus might suggest that the only role of UMNs is to control activations of motor units in specific muscles, but information encoded by UMNs specifies a variety of dimensions of movement. For example, a change in activity of some UMNs is associated with the direction of a movement rather than the muscles that would be activated. If a nonhuman primate is trained to make movements to different locations in extrapersonal space, extracellular action potentials will show activity changes correlated with onset of movement in a particular direction. Activity of other UMNs is related to the next movement in a sequence of movements.

The motor homunculus should not be construed as fixed. Rather, it is dynamic. For example, a motor cortex neuron preferentially related to the appearance of a go signal in one task may be preferentially related to the onset of muscle activity in another task (Montgomery et al 1992). Additionally, anesthesia of a limb, even for a few minutes, can drastically change the nature of the homunculus, a change that can be detected by electrical stimulation of UMNs or by neurometabolic imaging. This plasticity may be very important in understanding the natural history of speech and swallowing deficits associated with disorders of the upper motor

Box 7.4 Free Arm Movements to Visual Targets in Three-Dimensional Space

Encoding information on the direction of an intended movement was studied by recording action potentials generated by neurons in the motor cortex in a nonhuman primate **(Box Fig. 7.3)**. The primate would reach for a number of switches arranged in the space around it. Whenever the animal activated a switch, the moment of the event was recorded (A in the figure). In B, rasters of the time of onset of action potentials relative to the commencement of movements were generated. In the raster, there are rows of dots, where each dot represents the time of onset of an action potential generated in the motor cortex neuron. Each row represents a trial of the task. The increase in action potentials was greatest whenever the animal extended its reach to the space's lower left front corner and least—indeed, negative—whenever it extended its reach in the opposite direction. Increases were intermediate to other targets and varied with them. A tuning curve resolves with plotting of the direction of movement as a vector in such a way that its direction represents the direction of movement and its magnitude represents the change in neuronal discharge frequency (C). Using the tuning curve, the frequency of action potentials of a neuron in the motor cortex enables one to predict the direction of movement. For discharge frequencies that fall between the minimum and the maximum, however, different movement directions are possible. However, if one knows the tuning curve of each of the frequency of any neuronal action potentials one has recorded, the resultant vector·for addition of the vectors generated for each neuron (gray vectors in D) enables one to predict the movement shown in D. The yellow vector indicates the direction of the actual movement, and the red vector indicates the direction of the resultant vector.

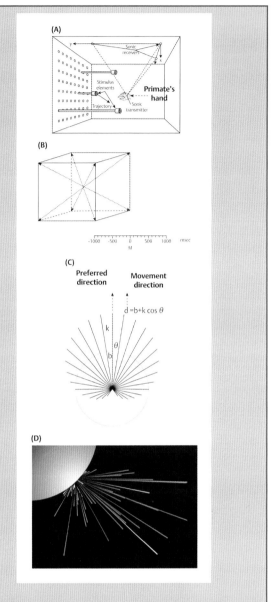

Box Fig. 7.3 Direction of arm movement encoded by changes in frequency of upper motor neuron action potentials. Details are described in the box text. (Modified from Schwartz et al 1988; Georgopoulos et al 1988).

neuron. A unique feature of the primary motor cortex is that the α-LMNs to the distal musculature are dependent on its output. Generally, α-LMNs do not generate action potentials to activate motor units on their own. Thus, loss of input from the primary motor cortex means that α-LMNs are likely to remain inactive, and consequently there is little activation of motor units related to distal musculature. This loss of driving results in paresis (weakness) or paralysis (total loss of voluntary movement) of the distal musculature.

The α-LMNs to the proximal musculature receive considerable descending input from sources other than UMNs, such as tectospinal and reticulospinal tract inputs, and thus can still be driven to produce movement in the event of UMN lesions. These inputs are referred to as *extrapyramidal*, as they include all fibers or tracts that do not pass through the pyramids of the medulla. A patient with a cortical stroke affecting UMNs in the motor cortex may have a lower facial weakness such that when the patient is asked to smile volitionally, one side of the mouth retracts less. However, in response to humor, both sides of the face may move equally. Likewise, a patient who cannot move her upper extremity in response to a command may reach up and cover her mouth when yawning. The degree of relative preservation of proximal motor function often depends on the rapidity over which the damage to the corticospinal and corticobulbar systems occurs. Patients with slowly progressive loss of UMNs typically retain much more of their proximal motor function compared to those with acute lesions.

Effects of Motor Cortex Lesions: the Upper Motor Neuron Syndrome

Lesions of the primary motor cortex and its efferent projections through the corticospinal and corticobulbar systems produce weakness, as just described, and also symptoms beyond impaired ability to generate a muscle force. Often there is increased **muscle tone**, defined as a resistance to passive movement. This increased muscle tone is velocity-dependent: resistance increases with increased velocity up to a certain point, at which muscle tone abruptly diminishes. This velocity dependence distinguishes the increased muscle tone associated with lesions of the motor cortex and its efferent projections from increased tone due to other causes, such as increased muscle tone with disorders of the basal ganglia as in Parkinson's disease. In addition, pathological reflexes such as the **Babinski sign** may appear, and superficial reflexes such as the **superficial abdominal** and **cremasteric reflexes** may disappear. In contrast, **deep tendon reflexes** may be increased. The combination of these symptoms and signs constitutes the **upper motor neuron syndrome**.

The mechanisms underlying the increased muscle tone and increased deep tendon reflexes in UMN syndrome are not precisely known. Evidence suggests that decreased inhibition of the α-LMNs renders them hyperexcitable in response to sensory input, such as muscle spindle activation when tapping (stretching) the muscle tendon at the patella (kneecap), as is often done in the neurological examination (**Fig. 7.7**). Decreased inhibition also could be due to the loss of motor cortex influence on other descending pathways such as the reticulospinal pathways (**Box 7.5**). The extent to which these effects are mediated by the α-LMN or γ-LMN systems is unknown.

As noted earlier in this chapter, because most cranial nerve nuclei in the brainstem receive bilateral UMN input, with the exception of the lower

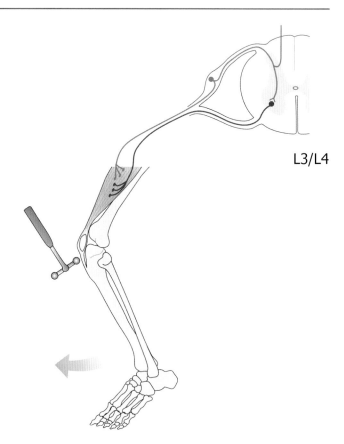

L3/L4

Fig. 7.7 Schematic representation of the deep tendon reflex. A tap to the patellar tendon just below the kneecap produces a rapid stretch of the quadriceps muscle as well as the intrafusal muscle fibers of its muscle spindles, which generates action potentials in the axons of the sensory nerves to the spinal cord, where the sensory axons synapse on α-LMNs whose axons synapse on fibers of the same muscle. Action potentials from the sensory axons generate action potentials in the α-LMNs, which result in contraction of the muscle and extension at the knee.

face (**Fig. 7.5**), unilateral UMN lesions rarely cause long-lasting and severe deficits in speech and swallowing. The intact UMN system on one side may not immediately compensate for a sudden or acute loss of the UMN system on the other side; thus, unilateral weakness may be evident acutely but resolve over time.

■ Basal Ganglia–Thalamic–Cortical System

Throughout the history of modern neurology, the pathophysiology reflected in the symptoms and signs of disorders and the physiology as inferred from the pathophysiology of the basal ganglia has been the archetype for understanding the role of suprasegmental structures in motor control. The great variety of syndromes and the relatively well-understood anatomy coupled with neurochemistry of disorders of the basal ganglia have fueled a great many theories of motor control.

We use the term *basal ganglia–thalamic–cortical system* instead of the more conventional term *basal ganglia* to avoid the **mereological fallacy:** attributing to a part the function of the whole, which is very common in neuroscience and neurology. Given the dynamics of the basal ganglia–thalamic–cortical system, it is highly unlikely that the basal ganglia act alone or have some unique property. Unfortunately most authors regard the basal ganglia as a physiologically or functionally independent entity, based primarily on anatomy rather than physiological considerations. For example, many authors describe the **caudate nucleus** and **putamen** as the *input stage* to the basal ganglia and the globus pallidus internal segment and **substantia nigra pars reticulata (SNr)** as the *output stage*. This categorization is anatomically reasonable but may be misleading with respect to physiology (**Fig. 7.8**).

Anatomically, the basal ganglia–thalamic–cortical system appears to comprise a number of anatomically distinct structures; however, this is a misconception predicated on the methods used to define the anatomy. For example, using a cell body stain to look at the macroscopic anatomy would suggest discrete anatomic structure that invites a discrete and localized anatomy (**Fig. 7.9**). However, when viewed from the perspective of anatomic interactions, the perception is anything but a discrete localized physiology.

From the perspective of a cell body stain, the anatomic structures include the caudate nucleus and putamen, together referred to as the (corpus) **striatum**. Neurons of the striatum are divided into two components: one component sends axons to the globus pallidus internal segment (GPi), and the other component sends axons to the globus pallidus external segment (GPe). Many current concepts of basal ganglia physiology and pathophysiology maintain these two striatal projections as distinct. The pathway from the striatum to the GPi and SNr

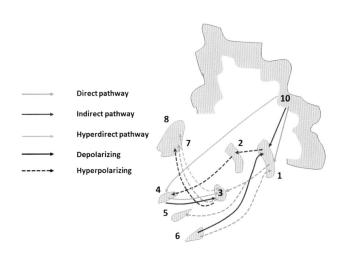

Fig. 7.8 Schematic representation of the basal ganglia–thalamic–cortical system. (1) putamen; (2) globus pallidus external segment (GPe); (3) globus pallidus internal segment (GPi); (4) subthalamic nucleus; (5) substantia nigra pars reticulata (SNr); (6) substantia nigra pars compacta (SNc); (7) ventral thalamus pars oralis; (8) parafascicular and centromedian nuclei of the thalamus; (9) supplementary motor area; (10) primary motor cortex. The interconnections represented in red are described as the indirect pathway, the green as the direct pathway, and the blue as the hyperdirect pathway.

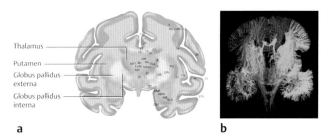

a   b

Fig. 7.9 Images demonstrating two approaches to under-standing the macroscopic anatomy of the brain, particularly the basal ganglia–thalamic–cortical system. **(a)** Image produced by a stain that shows neuronal cell bodies and gives the impression of a segregated, well-demarcated, and relatively simple organization (from a nonhuman primate, though very similar to humans). **(b)** Tractography created from MRI demonstrating the tracts that connect different structures; even so, it shows only a very limited number of tracts. The appearance is not as well segregated or demarcated and is anything but simple.

is called the **direct pathway**, and the pathway from the striatum to the GPe and then on to the subthalamic nucleus, GPi, and SNr is called the **indirect pathway**. This conventional nomenclature is inconsistent with actual anatomic facts, but it unfortunately continues to be included in current theories (**Fig. 7.10**). In addition, striatal axons project to the SNr and the **substantia nigra pars compacta (SNc)**.

The striatum receives input from most of the cerebral cortex and the **centromedian** and **parafascicular nuclei** of the thalamus. Axons from these brain regions release **glutamate** onto striatal neurons and cause postsynaptic depolarization. Striatal neurons also receive input from **dopaminergic** neurons in the SNc.

Within the striatum are interneurons (neurons that synapse within the nucleus in which they are embedded), predominantly **large aspiny neurons** that release acetylcholine. A smaller number of interneurons release **gamma-aminobutyric acid (GABA)**. The positive clinical response of Parkinson patients to anticholinergic drugs (drugs that block acetylcholine neurotransmission) suggests that large aspiny neurons play an important role in movement, although most theories regarding the physiology and pathophysiology of the basal ganglia–thalamic–cortical system fail to explain any role of the cholinergic interneurons.

Neurons in the striatum release GABA as a neurotransmitter and initially *hyperpolarize* target neurons in the substantia nigra and globus pallidus. As discussed in **Chapter 6**, hyperpolarization of the neuronal membrane reduces the probability of the postsynaptic neuron generating an action potential, so GABAergic striatal output neurons are

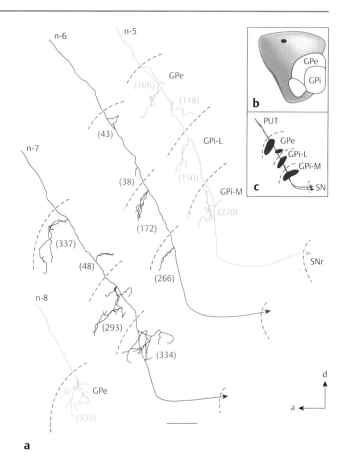

a

Fig. 7.10 Reconstructions along the sagittal plane of four singly labeled axons that project to GPe, GPi, and SNr and whose cell body is located in the matrix compartment of the putamen. **(a)** Three of them innervate GPe, GPi, and SNr (n-5, n-6, and n-7), whereas the other arborizes within GPe only (n-8). Neurons projecting to the three striatal targets yield several distinct arborizations within each pallidal segment: they have one or two collaterals that arborize within both anterior and posterior halves of GPe and GPi. The total number of terminal boutons in each target structure is indicated in parentheses. The exact location of the injection site in the putamen matrix compartment is indicated by the red spot in **(b)**, whereas the entire axonal trajectory of this neuron is illustrated in red in **(c)**, with thick red areas indicating the location of terminal fields in GPe and GPi. (Scale bar: 500 μm.) (Lévesque and Parent 2005.)

often referred to as "inhibitory." However, many postsynaptic neurons display rebound excitation and generate action potentials after the hyperpolarizing current (Plenz and Kital 1999; Nambu and Llinas 1994), so the term "inhibitory" is an inaccurate descriptor of the effects of striatal outputs on their targets. The functional significance of rebound excitation is not precisely known. However, considerable evidence from invertebrate neurophysiology suggests that postinhibitory rebound is critical to ongoing activities in neural circuits. In a sense, purely inhibitory circuits risk collapsing into no activity, while purely excitatory circuits risk chain reactions that would saturate and thus destroy information. Postinhibitory rebound excitation may limit activity and thus prevent saturation and circuit collapse, which would block the neuron from processing information.

The GPi receives input from the GPe and the subthalamic nucleus and projects to the ventral lateral thalamus and to the pedunculopontine nucleus of the brainstem tegmentum. GPi efferents release GABA, which hyperpolarizes postsynaptic membranes of the target neurons. GPe neurons receive input from a subgroup of striatal neurons and project to the GPi, subthalamic nucleus, and SNr and back to the striatum (Sato et al 2000). The subthalamic nucleus intervenes between the GPe and GPi. It receives input from the GPe and cerebral cortex and in turn projects to the GPi. The efferent neurons of the subthalamic nucleus release glutamate, which results in depolarization of the postsynaptic membranes of the target neurons.

The effects of dopamine on the main output neurons of the striatum, the **medium spiny neurons** (**MSNs**), are complex (Surmeier et al 2007). For MSNs that project to the GPe and those that project to the GPi, dopamine receptors are metabotropic receptors mediated by cAMP, but GPe neurons have D_2 **receptors** and GPi neurons have D_1 **receptors**. The general effect of dopamine on D_1-receptor-bearing striatal neurons appears to be increased responsiveness to corticospinal action potentials, resulting in increased probability of action potentials generated in the striatal neuron and projecting onto the neurons of the GPi. The general effect of dopamine on D_2 receptors is the opposite: to reduce the probability that the striatal neuron will generate action potentials in the event of action potentials in the presynaptic corticospinal neurons.

Inferring Function from Disease

Hypotheses about functions of brain structures often depend on the methods used to study function and structure. The earliest method of studying brain–behavior relations was to correlate a site of lesion with patient behavior: an anatomic–pathologic correlation. If patients had specific signs and symptoms after lesions to one part of the nervous system, the functions affected to produce those symptoms would be "localized" to that part of the nervous system. In other words, what the brain could not do without that brain structure was interpreted as evidence for the function of that structure. As has been the case since antiquity, nervous

---

Box 7.6   A Solution to the Inverse Problem

One approach to solving the inverse problem is to utilize John Stuart Mill's method of induction, referred to as the **method of difference**. According to this method, if in one case A, B, C and D (causal factors) are seen associated with w, x, y, and z (effects) and then in another case B, C, and D (but not A) are associated with x, y and z (but not w), than A is considered to be the cause of w. For example, consider an individual reading text while functional MRI (fMRI) is being recorded, showing activations in structures A, B, C, and D. Next, the individual is asked to read a text where the same letters of the previous text were randomized to something unintelligible. Now the fMRI scan shows activations only in structures B, C, and D. From Mill's method of difference, one might conclude that structure A is related to extracting meaning from the intelligible text. However, this method is fraught with difficulties. It presumes that A, B, C, D, w, x, y, and z are independent of each other, with the only dependence being between A and w.

Application to neurophysiology also presumes that the effects w, x, y, and z are independently discernible; that is, the observed variable is categorical. These effects would not be discernible if the effects shared any common mechanisms. This is extremely problematic when there are behaviors that typically involve complex synergies among a variety of α-LMNs. Even attempting to dissociate the components of the behaviors necessarily involves presuppositions and assumptions that often prove untenable.

Despite the problematic nature of reasoning from pathology in the manner of the method of difference, such reasoning is fundamental to scientific investigation. Indeed, the very concept of controls in scientific research is to provide an opportunity to utilize the method of difference (as well as other similar methods). For example, in the hypothetical example given above, removing meaning from the text but giving the same but randomized symbols to be read the second time serves as a control. The presumption is that every conceivable confounding fact, such as lighting, sounds from the MRI machine, among many others, is exactly the same in each condition. The only difference, the researcher hopes, is between meaningfulness in one text and absence of meaningfulness in the second text. However, such methods are only as robust as the cautions observed.

system physiology largely is inferred from reasoning the converse from pathological cases. For example, an individual with weakness of the right hand is found to have a tumor of the left precentral gyrus about halfway down on the lateral convexity. The symptoms and signs are not only a consequence of the functions that might be lost but also the result of the nervous system accommodating or compensating for that loss, which begins almost instantaneously after damage. The brain's incredible ability to compensate is shown by slow-growing lesions, which can have almost no clinical effects on the individual until they get very large.

The **inverse problem** is the difficulty of using observations to infer cause and effect when there are multiple causes that can produce the same effect. By analogy, a modern automobile could stop running for many reasons, and even experienced mechanics have difficulty diagnosing the cause just from the fact that the car has stopped running. There are many sources of information that the α-LMN converts to information to be encoded into muscular activity. It is impossible from observations of the organism to infer which source of information causes which particular muscular action.

For the sake of simplicity, we can assume that the observation variable is categorical. Note that it is not necessary that the observations be categorical; they can be continuous, allowing the use of correlations, as in Mill's **method of concomitant variations**. However, as will be seen, attempts to create categorical causes necessitates categorical effects. Indeed, modern neurology continues, in many situations, to follow Jackson's methods in conceptualizing neurological phenomena. Jackson maintained that symptoms of neurological disorders reflected either a loss of function (**negative symptoms**) or excessive function (**positive symptoms**). This is not surprising, as Jackson was heavily influenced by his studies of epilepsy, where convulsions are intuitively appreciated as excesses and the subsequent **postictal paralysis** (**Todd paralysis**) as deficit. Jackson's dichotomization (categorization into two exclusive categories) of observations produces a great economy of explanation. Note that the manifestations of a seizure and the absence of one in weakness or paralysis involved only a single explanation rather than multiple independent explanations.

The intuitive appeal of reducing the complexity of explanations goes back at least to Aristotle (385–322 BC). The Greek philosopher exposed the concept of **contraries**, where every force or element had its opposite, and it and its opposite defined the ends of a continuum. Consider a grayscale that goes from black to white. One is faced with an epistemic and ontological question. Are there as many objects (colors) as there are shades of gray, potentially infinite, or are there just two objects, black and white, with all the shades just admixtures of black and white? Aristotle's notion of contraries continued as Galen's (130–200 AD) notion of relative excesses and deficits of four bodily fluids or "humors"; it persists today in concepts such as Parkinson's disease being a relative deficit of dopamine and hyperkinetic disorders being a relative excess of dopamine. Although we caution about inferring function from lack of function, such as in the disease state, there are early voice, speech, and language deficits in Parkinson's disease (see Ciucci et al 2013).

In addition to lesion studies, another approach to determining anatomic-pathologic relationships is to stimulate an area of the nervous system and then infer the function of the area by the observed consequence of the stimulation. In 1870, Fritz and Hitzig applied electrical stimulation to the cortex of a canine and identified the motor cortex, as this area demonstrated the lowest threshold to produce a muscle contraction. What they did not recognize, however, was that stimulation of other brain regions also could produce muscle contractions. Thus, even in the 1870s there was controversy about whether the motor cortex was the unique generator of movement.

Today, we study anatomic-pathologic correlations using modern technology that can produce temporary and reversible "lesions." One such method is **transcranial magnetic stimulation (TMS)**, in which electrical stimulation applied to the skull temporarily blocks depolarization of neurons located under the stimulator. Another method is to have the individual perform tasks and record corresponding changes in the nervous system. These changes can range from altered generation of action potentials of individual neurons to evoked potentials and local field potentials, as seen in an electroencephalogram (EEG). Newer techniques image metabolic changes, such as oxygen utilization, as a surrogate for changes in neuronal activity. Each of these techniques has advantages and disadvantages. As a general principle, the further a method is from detecting changes in electrical potentials across the neuronal membrane, the more problematic it is as a means to draw conclusions about brain function. For example, fMRI relies on aggregate changes in blood oxygen levels, which are distant in time, space, and resolution from neuronal cell membrane changes.

Disorders of the Basal Ganglia–Thalamic–Cortical System

The approaches to inferring brain–behavior relations discussed in the preceding section underlie our current classification of movement disorders into **hypokinetic disorders**, those associated with a relative deficit or paucity of movement, and **hyperkinetic disorders**, associated with relative excess of movement. Parkinson's disease is the archetypical hypokinetic movement disorder, while **Huntington's disease** and **hemiballismus** are archetypical hyperkinetic disorders. Hyperkinetic syndromes can produce quick, jerky movements at proximal joints, described as **chorea**; slow, graceful movements, referred to as **athetosis**; wild flailing movements called **ballismus**; and slow, abnormal, sustained postures referred to as **dystonia**.

Signs of Parkinson's disease include **bradykinesia** (slowness of movement), **akinesia** (absence of movement), **resting tremor**, **rigidity**, and **postural instability**. Of these signs, bradykinesia is the most consistent and can result in severe disability and handicap. Bradykinesia can affect all types of movement, including speech. Speech in an individual with Parkinson's disease can be very slow and **hypophonic**. Akinesia can also affect any movement, and individuals with Parkinson's disease often display lack of facial expression (**masklike facies**), a limited range of intonation or inflections (**monotone speech**), and limited tongue, mandible, and pharyngeal movement during swallowing, along with limb signs such as reduced arm swing when walking.

Whether akinesia represents the extreme of bradykinesia is unknown. However, the effects of Parkinson's disease on postural stability may represent a qualitatively different phenomena from bradykinesia of the upper extremities. Although the postural reflexes are slowed, they may be qualitatively different. For example, research demonstrates that when one is pushed while standing, rotations about the hip or ankle are used to maintain the center of gravity over the base of support. The strategy used depends on how far the person is pushed; larger displacements result in rotation about the hip, whereas smaller displacements induce rotation about the ankles.

Parkinson's disease can affect both voluntary movements of the limbs and also postural stability and gait, and the distinction between these two types of movements is important for speech. Severity of deficits in voluntary limb movements is not strongly correlated with severity of gait and postural instability, and response to treatments differs as well. For example, DBS of the subthalamic nucleus can improve upper-extremity function remarkably yet worsen gait and postural stability. Interestingly, effects on speech more directly correlate with effects on gait than with effects on upper-extremity functions, consistent with evidence of fundamental differences between speech and limb motor control (Grimme et al 2011). The same may be true for swallowing.

Although the term "hypokinesia" is widely used to describe patients with Parkinson's disease, many behaviors in individuals with the disease suggest that "hypokinesia" may not be an accurate description. Individuals with Parkinson's disease demonstrate **hastening**, an irregular change in rhythm of movement that was first labeled *arrhythmokinesia* (Nakamura et al 1976). When asked to tap their finger along with a metronome that is gradually increasing in rate, patients with Parkinson's disease typically keep tapping at the initial rate and thus tap more slowly than the metronome as it increases in speed, until the metronome reaches a certain rate at which the patient begins to tap faster than the metronome until the metronome has increased its rate to that of the patients' finger tapping. Individuals with Parkinson's disease also may be slow in walking yet dance normally, or have slow and hypophonic speech but sing or swear normally. Patients with Parkinson's disease may move normally in some circumstances but be immobile in others, a phenomenon known as **kinesia paradoxica**. Deaf adults who used American Sign Language before they developed Parkinson's disease show altered, not just slowed signing movements. For example, rather than making sharp transitions between appropriate hand positions, individuals may hold intermediate positions between the appropriate signs. Patients treated with **levodopa** may have hyperkinesia with some movements and simultaneous bradykinesia with other movements. All of these phenomena are inconsistent with the notion of generalized slowing or hypokinesia in Parkinson's disease.

The next question is whether the term "hyperkinesia" is appropriate to describe patients with Huntington's or Parkinson's disease. Again, the answer is no. Individuals with Huntington's disease have bradykinesia, as measured by reaction times and movement velocities of intended movements. Patients with Parkinson's disease treated with levodopa may have simultaneous hypokinesia and bradykinesia. These observations strongly suggest that hyperkinesia and hypokinesia do not represent the extremes of a single, one-dimensional common continuum.

Models of the Basal Ganglia–Thalamic–Cortical Systems

Despite clear evidence such as that just discussed in the context of dyskinesias, discussions of basal ganglia physiology and pathophysiology often continue to invoke a one-dimensional, push-pull concept. It is well recognized that individuals will continue to believe a notion that is intuitive and will not be dissuaded even in the context of evidence to the contrary (Johnson-Laird 2009). As will be demonstrated, the intuitive appeal of the dichotomization of the clinical phenomenology of basal ganglia disorders is not due to the economy of clinical description but rather its consistency with notions related to the underlying pathophysiology.

The one-dimensional view of the basal ganglia as a push-pull system, exemplified by the foregoing discussion of hypokinesia and hyperkinesia, has persisted in science for decades, despite considerable evidence to the contrary. This dichotomization of the pathophysiological mechanisms underlying disorders of the basal ganglia began with the discovery that reserpine-induced **catatonia** in rodents, considered to be an extreme form of hypokinesia, could be reversed by levodopa, a discovery that led to the use of levodopa in individuals with Parkinson's disease. The subsequent demonstration that degeneration of the substantia nigra pars compacta, known to be associated with Parkinson's disease, led to loss of dopamine from the brain further solidified the use of levodopa in patients with Parkinson's disease, in addition to the discovery in the 1800s that agents that blocked the acetylcholine receptor improved symptoms and signs of Parkinson's disease.

These observations led to the cholinergic/dopaminergic imbalance theory of Parkinson's disease, popularized in the 1970s. This theory postulated that an excess of acetylcholine relative to dopamine resulted in hypokinetic disorders such as Parkinson's disease, and improvement could be accomplished by restoring the balance by either reducing the effects of acetylcholine with anticholinergic medications or increasing dopaminergic effects by administering levodopa to patients. Levodopa is converted to dopamine once it enters the brain and is used because dopamine is unable to cross the blood-brain barrier. It followed that in hyperkinetic disorders, an excess of dopamine relative to acetylcholine resulted in excess movements. Thus, drugs that blocked dopamine would restore the balance and reduce the hyperkinesia.

The cholinergic/dopaminergic imbalance theory achieved a remarkable and internally consistent notion of the pathophysiology of Parkinson's disease. In the 1980s, however, with increased knowledge of the anatomy and chemistry of the basal ganglia, the cholinergic/dopaminergic imbalance theory literally disappeared from conversation. It was replaced by theories extrapolated from anatomy and chemistry of basal ganglia structures and their connections, for example the **GPi rate theory**,

to be discussed next, where overactivity of the GPi neurons were thought to cause parkinsonism. These more recent theories were considered even though the replacement makes no mention of the role of acetylcholine in the pathophysiology of the basal ganglia. From that perspective, it is hard to see why these new theories are considered an improvement. It is a telling commentary on the human condition that a theory—even one that is incomplete and, as will be seen, inconsistent—is considered preferable to just saying "we don't know." So long as the theory explains the salient observations, many will appear to tolerate it despite its inability to explain other observations. The key, then, is what constitute the salient observations. The identification of the salient observations may have all to do with protecting current, intuitively appealing notions against refutation (Kuhn 1962).

As will be demonstrated, current theories regarding the pathophysiology (and subsequently, the physiology) of the basal ganglia are extrapolations from anatomy and chemistry and are inconsistent with physiologic function. Further, the anatomic considerations that form the basis for current theories are so highly selective and narrow as to misconceive the notions of physiology. One cannot say that these theories are justified by their heuristic value of providing a framework on which to organize therapeutic interventions. The problem is when such heuristic convenience leads to complacency.

The anatomic notions underlying current theories are shown in **Fig. 7.11**. The many millions of neurons comprised in the basal ganglia–thalamic–cortical system are reduced to seven or so structures, comprising the cortex and nuclei of the system. Further, each nucleus and the cortex are then linked by what are construed as anatomic connections between neurons of one structure to neurons of another. It is important to note that the connections illustrated in the figure are a small subset of the interconnections among neurons in these different structures.

Anatomically based theories, such as the GPi rate theory, generally reduce connections in the basal ganglia–thalamic–cortical system to three sets of connections via three pathways. As previously described, these are the indirect pathway, comprising the subset of striatal neurons that project to the GPe, which then projects to the subthalamic nucleus, which then projects to the GPi. The **direct pathway** constitutes the set of connections from striatal neurons to the GPi. Finally, there is the **hyperdirect pathway** from the cortex to the subthalamic nucleus and then to the GPi. Inconsistent with this simplified view of basal ganglia–

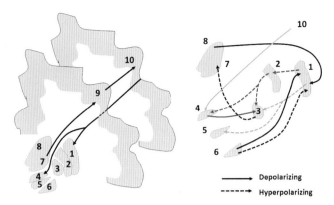

Fig. 7.11 Schematic representation of the basal ganglia–thalamic–cortical system. The various structures are represented as follows: (1) putamen (as representative of the striatum); (2) GPe; (3) GPi; (4) subthalamic nucleus; (5) SNr; (6) SNc (location of the cell bodies that use dopamine as their neurotransmitter); (7) ventral thalamus pars oralis; (8) parafascicular and centromedian nuclei of the thalamus; (9) supplementary motor area; and (10) primary motor cortex. Putative pathways within the basal ganglia–thalamic–cortical system include the direct pathway, which links a subset of putamen neurons to the GPi; the indirect pathway, which links another set of putamen neurons to the GPe, thence to the subthalamic nucleus and GPi; and the hyperdirect pathway from the cortex to the subthalamic nucleus and then on to the GPi.

thalamic–cortical system function is evidence that a significant number of striatal neurons project in both the direct and indirect pathways (Lévesque and Parent 2005). Other studies demonstrate that at least some and possibly nearly all striatal neurons express both D_1 and D_2 receptors (Aizman et al 2000). How is it that notions of direct, indirect, and hyperdirect pathways persist in face of overwhelming evidence to the contrary? The answer may have little to do with anatomic truths and more to do with economy of explanation of the current theories regarding the pathophysiology of basal ganglia disorders.

Anatomy of neurotransmitter systems has also been extrapolated to physiologic and pathophysiologic models of the basal ganglia–thalamic–cortical system. In this case, interactions among different structures are viewed as a product of inhibitory and excitatory neurotransmitters and their respective receptors (e.g., the GPi inhibits the thalamus via GABA). However, as discussed already, the notion of inhibitory and excitatory actions of neurotransmitters is a misconception. Although there may be a reduction in action potential generation in the postsynaptic neuron as a consequence of GABA-induced hyperpolarization, in many neurons, such as those in the subthalamic nucleus and the ventral lateral thalamus, rebound excitation produces

a net excitatory effect on the postsynaptic cell membrane. Thus, the nature of the neurotransmitter does not actually predict the electrophysiologic consequences of its release.

The GPi rate theory is another current theory of basal ganglia–thalamic–cortical physiology that is extrapolated from anatomy and chemistry. This theory posits that overactivity of the GPi suppresses thalamic neuronal activity, resulting in less activation of motor cortex and in subsequent hypokinesia, as seen in Parkinson's disease. This process begins when degeneration of substantia nigra neurons leads to loss of dopaminergic input to the striatum, causing loss of dopamine-mediated excitation of the striatal neurons that project to the GPi, and disinhibited GPi neurons then suppress activity of the ventral lateral thalamic relay neurons to the cortex (**Fig. 7.12**). Similarly, loss of dopamine-mediated inhibition of striatal neurons projecting to the GPe suppresses neuronal activities in the GPi. Reduced activity in the GPe reduces inhibition of the subthalamic nucleus and GPi, and disinhibition of the subthalamic nucleus further excites neurons of the GPi. Thus, the combined effects through the direct and indirect pathways is to increase the neuronal activity of the GPi.

The GPi rate theory is inconsistent with a number of observations. First, the neurotoxin **N-methyl-4-phenyl-1,2,3,6-tetrahydropyridine** (**MPTP**), which selectively destroys dopaminergic neurons, does not produce changes in neuronal activity as predicted by this theory (Montgomery 2007). Second, induction of experimental parkinsonism in nonhuman primates, using dopamine receptor-blocking agents or electrolytic lesions of the **nigrostriatal** axons, is not associated with the changes in neuronal activities predicted by this theory (Filion 1979). Third, DBS of the GPi increases the output of the GPi. Rather than worsening parkinsonism, as the theory predicts, symptoms actually improve.

The GPi rate theory also has been used to explain hyperkinetic disorders such as Huntington's disease, hemiballismus, and levodopa-induced hyperkinesia. The notion is that these disorders result in decreased neuronal activities in the GPi and subsequent disinhibition of the ventral lateral thalamus and overactivity of the motor cortex, leading to involuntary movements. However, **pallidotomy,** or the purposeful destruction of the GPi, *improves* hyperkinetic disorders, precisely the opposite of what is predicted by the GPi rate theory.

While there are likely a multitude of reasons for the failure of the GPi rate theory, one certainly may be the postinhibitory rebound excitation noted earlier, seen in subthalamic and ventral lateral thalamic neurons. The theory posits that movement should be associated with a reduction in neuronal activities in the GPi, but recordings of GPi neuronal activity show that 58 to 80% of GPi neurons increase their activity with movement. Further, the theory posits a reciprocal relationship between GPi and GPe activities; if most GPi neurons increase activity at movement onset, most GPe neurons should decrease activity at that time, but this is not the case (Zimnik et al 2015; Yoshida and Tanaka 2009; Gdowski et al 2007; Wannier et al 2002; Anderson and Horak 1985). Posthyperpolarization rebound excitation might explain this finding. Initial movement-related increases in globus pallidus activity might cause hyperpolarization of subthalamic nucleus neurons, but posthyperpolarization rebound excitation of subthalamic nucleus neurons results in a net increase in GPi neuronal activity, demonstrated in neuronal recordings in nonhuman primates.

The GPi rate theory also fails to acknowledge information processing within the basal ganglia–thalamic–cortical system. The theory suggests an open-loop mechanism in which the subcortical nuclei are arranged hierarchically; it is as though information is relayed from the cortex and intralaminar nuclei of the thalamus to the striatum. The striatum then processes information, which then is relayed to the GPi and GPe and is then relayed on to the next structure in the chain. However, recordings of extracellular action potentials and local field potentials in motor cortex and striatal neurons demonstrate that changes in neuronal activities occur nearly simultaneously in both structures during some tasks (Montgomery and Buchholz 1991; Brasted and Wise 2004; Fujii and Graybiel 2005).

Another theory of basal ganglia–thalamic–cortical function, referred to as the **beta oscillation theory**, is conceptually related to the GPi rate theory. The beta oscillation theory holds that excessive

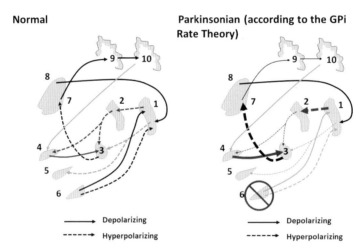

Fig. 7.12 Schematic representation of the basal ganglia–thalamic–cortical system in normal and in parkinsonism according to the GPi rate theory. The various structures are represented as follows: (1) putamen (as representative of the striatum); (2) GPe; (3) GPi; (4) subthalamic nucleus; (5) SNr; (6) SNc (location of the cell bodies that use dopamine as their neurotransmitter); (7) ventral thalamus pars oralis; (8) parafascicular and centromedian nuclei of the thalamus; (9) supplementary motor area; and (10) primary motor cortex. A primary assumption of the theory is that hyperpolarizing interactions, mediated by GABA, cause a net reduction in neuronal activities in the postsynaptic structures. However, this is not entirely true, as many neurons in the basal ganglia–thalamic–cortical system display posthyperpolarization rebound excitation, which can result in a net increase in neuronal activity in the postsynaptic structure. As applied to Parkinson's disease, degeneration of dopamine neurons (structure 6) results in the loss of hyperpolarizing inputs to a group of neurons in the putamen (structure 1). These groups of putamen neurons are thought to increase their activities and thereby increase hyperpolarization of neurons in the GPe (structure 2) via the indirect pathway (red arrows), represented by the connecting arrow of greater thickness. The putative decrease of neuronal activity in the GPe is posited to reduce the hyperpolarization of the subthalamic nucleus (structure 4) and the GPi (structure 3), represented by the thinner connecting arrows. The reduced hyperpolarization is thought to increase the activities in the subthalamic nucleus, which then further increases the neuronal activities of the globus pallidus internal segment, represented by the thicker connecting arrow. Similarly, loss of depolarizing inputs from the degenerated dopamine neurons of the substantia nigra pars compacta results in reduced activities in a portion of the putamen neurons that project to the globus pallidus internal segment via the direct pathway (green arrows). Thus, the reduction of activities in these putamen neurons decreases the hyperpolarization of the GPi neurons, leading to a posited increase in their activities. The net effect is to increase GPi activities that result in increased hyperpolarization of the ventral thalamus pars oralis neurons, represented by the thicker connecting arrow. The reduced activity in the thalamic relay neurons then reduces drive onto the neurons of the supplementary motor area, shown by the thinner connecting arrow, and then onto the primary motor area, presumably causing the bradykinesia and akinesia seen in parkinsonism.

neuronal activities produce oscillations in the beta frequencies in electrophysiological measures of neuronal activities, on the order of 20 Hz, and these oscillations interfere with movement, much as excessive neuronal activity in the GPi affects movement according to the GPi rate theory. However, a significant number of patients with Parkinson's disease do not have increased beta oscillatory activity, meaning that increased beta oscillations are not a necessary condition for parkinsonism. Further, if one assumes that DBS in the vicinity of the subthalamic nucleus drives neuronal activities in the GPi, then DBS in the beta frequencies should worsen parkinsonism. It does not and, in some cases, may improve motor function (Huang et al 2014). These findings suggest that increased beta oscillations are not a sufficient condition for parkinsonism.

The latencies in the transmission of information between neurons within the many circuits of the basal ganglia–thalamic–cortical system mean that in a closed circuit such as the direct pathway, information can traverse the entire circuit in 14 milliseconds. For information repeatedly traversing the circuit, the frequency is 71 Hz. In other words, the cortex influences the striatum 70 times during a 1-second movement. It also means that the striatum influences the cortex via the GPi and ventral lateral thalamus 70 times per second. Thus, the basal ganglia–thalamic–cortical system does not operate in a sequential and hierarchical manner. Rather, the operations are more akin to parallel and distributed processing.

It may be the case that the basal ganglia–thalamic–cortical system operates as a loosely coupled network of polysynaptic **nonlinear** oscillators operating over a range of frequencies, discussed later in this chapter. If true, it becomes less tenable to dichotomize basal ganglia functions into those attributed to the direct pathway and those attributed to the indirect pathway. For example, it has been argued that the direct pathway mediates movement initiation while the indirect pathway mediates movement termination. **Fig. 7.13** shows that striatal neurons demonstrate multiple signal changes associated with different aspects of a behavior. The initial change in striatal neuron activity is best related to the onset of the "go" signal, part of the direct pathway. However, later activity in the same neuron is best related to task completion, which, according to the hypothesis, should be a property of the indirect pathway.

Although information flow within the GPi and GPe may be segregated, it is only brief and not related to the **cycle** time of a typical behavior. For example, information exiting the GPi can reenter and go to the GPe 70 times during the course of a

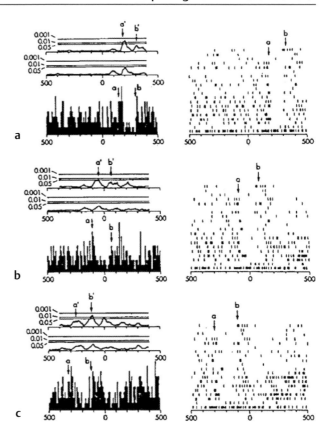

Fig. 7.13 Three sets of representations of the same dataset showing putamen neuron activity during the performance of a wrist flexion and extension task in a nonhuman primate. Data on the right represent perievent rasters in which each row corresponds to a sequence of neuronal action potentials for each trial of the task. These rows are summed vertically to form the histograms on the left. Over each summed histogram are two statistical measures relating the change in neuronal activity. In one method (top tracings), two adjacent sliding windows are compared by calculating the p-value of the differences in the content of the two windows. The lower tracing relates the activity of a sliding window to the baseline activity preceding the go signal. The associated graphs plot the p value of the statistical comparisons between windows. There are two peaks in histograms a' and b'. **(a)** The top set of rasters and histograms are centered on the go signal. **(b)** The middle set is centered on movement onset, **(c)** whereas the bottom set is centered on reaching the target. The peak a' is most consistently related to and follows the appearance of the go signal, whereas the peak b' is most consistently related to and precedes the movement of reaching the target, as demonstrated by a maximum p value (from Montgomery and Buchholz 1991).

1-second behavior, as previously stated. Even if the population of striatal neurons in the direct pathway were completely segregated from those of the indirect pathway, which they are not (Huerta-Ocampo et al 2014), afferents to the striatal neurons from the cortex and thalamus are not segregated. Further, fast-spiking interneurons in the striatum project to both pools of striatal output neurons, further blurring any distinction in the information processed within the different striatal output neurons. Thus, striatal neurons in both the direct and indirect pathways likely see the same information from the cortex and thalamus. At the very least, is it not clear that the information would differ between these two pathways?

There are other misconceptions engendered by the anatomic and chemical models that underlie theories such as the GPi rate theory. One misconception is that functions of suprasegmental structures are compartmentalized according to their anatomy. This is clear in descriptions of the striatum as being the "input" stage while the GPi and SNr are the "output" stages. Furthermore, the GPi is assigned the role of "allowing" intended movements and "inhibiting" unintended movements. Some theories, like those of John Hughlings Jackson, suggest that malfunction of the GPi would result in a loss of prevention in disallowing unintended movements, resulting in hyperkinetic disorders. An excess of GPi function would prevent intended movements, resulting in hypokinesia. Similarly, the direct pathway is considered to have the role of initiating movement, which it accomplishes by inhibition of the GPi, and the role of the indirect pathway is to stop movements once initiated by disinhibition of the GPe with subsequent disinhibition of the GPi and subthalamic nucleus.

The problem with these "anatomy as physiology" models is that the anatomical organization of the cortex and subcortical nuclei does not correspond with the physiology. With the exception of the striatal interneurons, the other neurons within each nucleus of the basal ganglia do not interact with each other, based on the lack of correlation in the neuronal discharges between pairs of simultaneously recorded neurons. Indeed, neurons in a particular structure interact more with neurons synapsing on them and with the neurons on which they synapse in the downstream structure than they do with each other. Thus, cooperation for processing information occurs between nuclei, not within nuclei. Does it then make sense to speak of the function of any particular structure, and refer to those structures and functions as "hierarchical"? Rather, functions are represented in circuits of neurons distributed across the basal ganglia–thalamic–cortical system.

The circuit-based model is supported by evidence that correlations between changes in neuronal activities and specific aspects or components of a behavior are similar throughout the basal ganglia–thalamic–cortical system (as shown in **Fig. 7.14**). For example, neurons active when flexing or extending the wrist can change their activities in

relation to the appearance of the go signal, movement onset, onset of electromyographic (EMG) activity in the appropriate muscles, or the wrist moving to the target. As shown in **Fig. 7.14**, neurons with each of these properties can be found in the motor cortex as well as in the striatum (Montgomery and Buchholz 1991).

Cumulatively, these data suggest that the basal ganglia–thalamic–cortical systems are best repre-

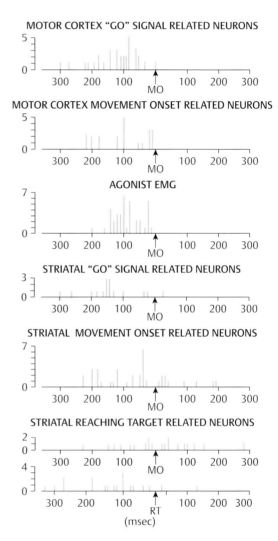

Fig. 7.14 Neurons recorded in the motor cortex and striatum in a nonhuman primate performing a wrist flexion and extension task. Neurons were categorized based on whether their change in action potential generation rate was best related to the appearance of a go signal, the onset of movement, the hand reaching the target, or the onset of agonist wrist flexor and extensor muscles. The time of onset relative to movement onset or reaching target is shown in the histogram. As can be seen, timing of the onset of neuronal activities for the same behavioral classification is the same for the motor cortex and striatum within the 10 ms time resolution available with these techniques (from Montgomery and Buchholz 1991).

sented by a number of circuits organized around a specific component of behavior, such as responding to a go signal or driving electromyographic (EMG) activities. Additionally, activations span all cortical regions and subcortical nuclei simultaneously rather than in a hierarchical sequence based on anatomical connections. Further, these data show that there is little value in parsing physiology among the direct, indirect, and hyperdirect pathways.

It is important to recognize that basal ganglia–thalamic–cortical circuits are not fixed but rather dynamic. A neuron may preferentially respond to the go signal in one task and then change to be preferentially related to movement onset in another task, at least in the motor cortex (Montgomery et al 1992). The dynamic nature of the behavioral properties of neurons argues for a dynamic physiology rather than a fixed anatomic circuit, at least at time scales shorter than the time required for anatomic changes. An analogy is the Internet, where hardwired connections between servers remain fixed, at least at time scales relevant to information transmission within the Internet, but information may be routed through different paths, electronically controlled, at any one time.

The dynamics of information encoding, represented by the correlation of changes in neuronal activities and behavioral events, argue that information is not intrinsic to the individual neuron but rather related to the network of physiologic interconnections. These physiologic interconnections are dynamic, as is the type of information processing. Such dynamics have been clearly demonstrated in the simplified nervous systems of invertebrates, where, for example, a neuron previously active in the operations of the pylorus can switch to activity related to cardiac function (Marder and Bucher 2007).

The Future of Basal Ganglia–Thalamic–Cortical Systems Theories

The ability of neurons to switch from one behavioral function to another suggests dynamism, yet with some degree of stability. **Complex systems** are capable of this combination of dynamism and stability. Complex systems involve large-scale, nonlinear interactions that allow rapid changes between states (e.g., **bifurcations**) that are relatively stable. This stability, however, is not permanent. These temporary states are referred to as *metastable states*. Schooling fish are an excellent example of a complex system: fish can scatter rapidly as a predator approaches but then rapidly coalesce to a relatively stable school formation. There is

evidence that neurons within the basal ganglia–thalamic–cortical system display bifurcations and metastable states consistent with complex systems. Complex systems can be implemented by networks of loosely coupled nonlinear oscillators. Networks of oscillators have additional, potentially important properties. The systems oscillators theory of the physiology and pathophysiology of the basal ganglia–thalamic–cortical system suggests that this system is a network of loosely coupled oscillators with neuronal activities across a range of different frequencies.

At the beginning of this chapter, motor unit recruitment was described as operating over different time scales. The first time scale was at the level of the individual muscle producing a single simple force, referred to as level 1. With the initial generation of force, small motor units are recruited and increase their discharge rate. As greater forces are required, progressively larger motor units are recruited. The second time scale is the level of the joint (level 2), with recruitment and derecruitment of motor units from multiple muscles for ballistic joint rotation and maintenance of joint rotation against countering elastic forces, and similar recruitment and derecruitment of the muscles initially antagonistic to the intended joint rotation. The third time scale (level 3) is at the level of complex, multijoint movements and reflects the time course of muscle recruitments and derecruitments across the time of these movements.

Each of these levels of motor unit orchestration can be considered as operating over different time scales, as evident by frequency analyses of motor unit activities over the time course of the behavior. The systems oscillators network theory, a complex systems theory, posits that motor control over each of these levels is affected by different sets of oscillators within the basal ganglia–thalamic–cortical system. There is evidence that the basal ganglia–thalamic–cortical system is involved in the first level of motor unit recruitment. In a study where patients produced a gradually increasing wrist flexion force, motor units were recorded and identified in the flexor carpi ulnaris muscle. In untreated patients with Parkinson's disease, the normal pattern of motor unit recruitment was not found. Indeed, in some cases, the largest motor unit was recruited first. This abnormal motor recruitment was corrected with high-frequency DBS of the subthalamic nucleus. This finding suggests that Parkinson's disease affects the first level of motor unit recruitment (as shown in **Fig. 7.15**). In the figure, the onset of different motor units as the subject exerts greater force is shown. In the case of DBS at 160 pulses per second, the normal pattern of recruitment is

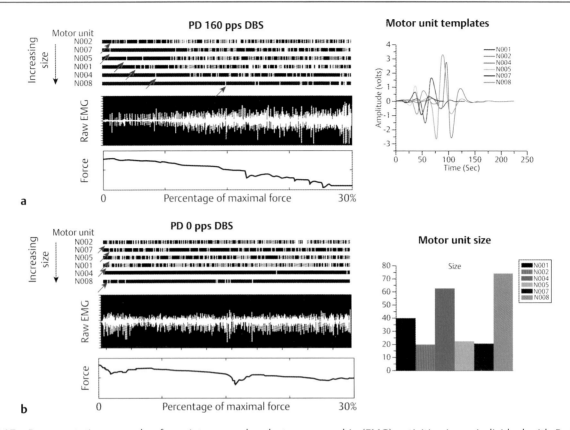

Fig. 7.15 Representative example of raw intramuscular electromyographic (EMG) activities in an individual with Parkinson's disease under conditions of 160 pps DBS (therapeutic) and 0 pps DBS. The same six motor units were identified under both conditions, and their waveforms and sizes are shown here. Waveform size was determined by measuring the area under the curve for each waveform. Motor unit discharge times are shown in the rasters, with one row for each motor unit and motor units ordered from smallest to largest along the Y-axis. Onset of motor unit activities is indicated by the red arrow. Graphs on the right show that waveforms associated with each motor unit are distinct in size and timing. **(a)** In the 160-pps DBS condition, there is an orderly recruitment of motor units (indicated by the red arrows), with smaller units recruited first, followed by progressively larger motor units, consistent with the Henneman size principle. **(b)** Under the 0-pps DBS condition, however, orderly recruitment of motor units is lost and the units are recruited nearly simultaneously, with large motor units recruited early in the task and at small forces.

seen by the successive onset of electromyographic (EMG) spikes of increasing amplitude. This pattern is not seen in the untreated patient off medications and with DBS at 0 pps.

The GPi rate theory and the beta oscillation theory do not explain how orchestration of motor unit recruitment is affected by Parkinson's disease or how DBS improves the different levels of orchestration of movement. By contrast, the systems oscillators network theory accounts for issues related to motor unit recruitment via excessive amounts of synchronization of neuronal activities within the basal ganglia. Increased synchronization would interfere with the ability of neurons to modulate their activities dynamically, thereby reducing the degrees of freedom or complexity of information processed by that system. Indeed, individuals with Parkinson's disease have reduced complexity of

neuronal activities in the subthalamic nucleus compared to patients with epilepsy (Vyas et al 2016).

Another theory of pathophysiology of hypokinetic disorders such as Parkinson's disease posits that excessive synchronization of neuronal activities is causal. However, this is not true, as DBS greatly synchronizes neuronal activities but improves, rather than worsens, motor control. Large numbers of neurons are activated with each pulse of the stimulation, so by definition, activities of neurons are synchronized. However, the nature of the synchronization is interesting. DBS is very inefficient at activating action potentials, at least as evidenced by recordings of action potentials during stimulation. Approximately 10% of DBS pulses actually result in **antidromic action potentials** (pulses that travel back toward the cell body rather than down the axon). Thus, the synchronization of neuronal activities is inefficient in that only a fraction of stimulation pulses activate axons, although when a pulse does activate axons, all are at a constant latency relative to the time of the stimulation pulse. This inefficient stimulation results in inefficient synchronization at the stimulation frequency as well as harmonics of the stimulation frequency. This suggests that **stochastic resonance** may be contributory. Stochastic resonance is a counterintuitive physical phenomenon whereby a signal embedded in noise can be improved by the addition of more noise. Stochastic resonance phenomena occur in many biological systems. For example, humans have lower hearing thresholds for pure tones in the presence of noise than pure tones alone (Zeng et al 2000). Stochastic resonance may be the mechanism by which transcranial direct current stimulation of the brain facilitates some types of learning (Fertonani et al 2011). However, the bandwidth of the added noise must be comparable to the noise obscuring the signal. Therefore, DBS may improve the signal-to-noise ratio of information that is ultimately transmitted to motor units for precise orchestration of motor unit activations.

In this context, stochastic resonance as just described is *positive resonance*. It is also possible that increased noise in a dysfunctional network of neural oscillators could cause abnormal stochastic resonance, causing an abnormally large signal-to-noise ratio in the information, which is disruptive. This type of positive stochastic resonance may be a mechanism underlying involuntary movements (Montgomery and Baker 2000). It also is possible to have negative resonance when signals are played back to reduce the noise rather than increase the signal, a method used by some noise-reduction headphones. In the case of hyperkinesia, DBS of the appropriate frequency could reduce the signal leading to involuntary movements via negative resonance. However, it is also possible that noisy synchronization at specific frequencies could reduce the normal or desired signal by negative resonance, thereby worsening the orchestration of motor unit recruitment and worsening symptoms.

This chapter has mostly focused on Parkinson's disease and hypokinesia because the neuronal mechanisms underlying the symptoms of these conditions are largely unknown. It is unlikely that these mechanisms are the converse of the mechanisms underlying hyperkinesia, as the two can coexist. Also, DBS in the vicinity of the GPi can improve both hyperkinetic as well as hypokinetic disorders. Hyperkinesias demonstrate specific orchestrations of motor unit recruitment and derecruitment, but this information is largely aberrant.

The Role of Dopamine in Basal Ganglia–Thalamic–Cortical Circuits

In our discussion of basal ganglia–thalamic–cortical circuits, it is important to address the role of the neurotransmitter dopamine, particularly given the number of diseases and disorders attributed to altered central nervous system dopamine levels. There is a tendency to attribute the pathophysiology of Parkinson's disease to dopamine deficiency. However, this would be a mistake. To be sure, most cases of Parkinson's disease are associated with loss of dopamine consequent to degeneration of neurons in the SNc, but this dopamine deficiency is not present in all cases. For example, parkinsonism can be produced by lesions of the GPe, the ventral thalamus pars oralis, or the supplementary motor area (SMA). Further, replacing dopamine in the striatum, by medication or cellular transplant, does not always improve the symptoms of Parkinson's disease.

Initial depletion of dopamine can result in an altered physiology that can also be induced by other pathological processes. Thus, the pathophysiology in Parkinson's disease is not from the initial abnormality in the substantia nigra but reflects subsequent self-organization of basal ganglia–thalamic–cortical dynamics in response to degeneration of SNc neurons. Describing the pathophysiology of Parkinson's disease as due to dopamine depletion is to confuse pathophysiology with **pathoetiology**. This is not just an issue of semantics, as evidenced by the fact that therapies directed at targets other than dopamine levels in the brain can be effective, including DBS.

■ Cerebellum

The cerebellum is an engineer's dream. The cytoarchitecture of the cerebellar cortex is one of the most regular and stereotyped in the nervous system. In other words, the "blueprint" of the cerebellum is easily appreciated. One would suspect that its physiology relative to motor control would be relatively straightforward. Yet, in reality less is known about the role of the cerebellum in motor control than about that of the basal ganglia–thalamic–cortical system. Few α-LMNs depend on direct innervation from axons projecting from the cerebellum, in contrast to the basal ganglia–thalamic–cortical system, and consequently, disorders of the cerebellum are not associated with deficient motor unit recruitment. Thus, disorders of the cerebellum are not associated with weakness *per se*. However, the cerebellum is involved with the precise orchestration of motor unit recruitment necessary for normal movement, as evident in movement disorders associated with lesions of the cerebellum and its efferent and afferent connections.

Anatomically, the cerebellum is composed of the cortex and the deep cerebellar nuclei and is located in the **posterior fossa** of the skull. The cerebellar cortex and deep cerebellar nuclei are connected to the rest of the brain by three bundles of fibers: the **superior**, **middle**, and **inferior cerebellar peduncles** (**Fig. 7.16**). The superior cerebellar peduncle is the major output pathway of the cerebellum. It projects to the contralateral cerebral cortex via the thalamus and red nucleus and to the vestibular nuclei in the brainstem. The middle cerebellar peduncle carries inputs to the cerebellum from widespread cortical regions via the pontine nuclei. The inferior cerebellar peduncle carries input to the cerebellum from the posterior columns of the spinal cord and the trigeminal nucleus in the brainstem but also has a small output or efferent projection in the juxtarestiform body.

The cerebellar cortex is divided in the superior-inferior plane by three clefts into the **paleocerebellum** or anterior lobe, the **neocerebellum** or posterior lobe, and the **archicerebellum**. The archicerebellum consists of the flocculonodular lobe and its connections with the vestibular system in the brainstem. The cerebellum also is divided transversely into the **vermal zone** in the midline, the **lateral** zone, and the **paravermal zone**, which is located between the vermal and lateral zones.

Although the gross anatomy suggests one description of the cerebellum whose organization is determined by various lobes, sulci, and gyri as just described, the physiology is quite different. The physiologic organization of the cerebellum is based on the afferent and efferent connections and the clinical syndromes associated with disorders of the cerebellum. The efferent connections from the cerebellar cortex are to the deep cerebellar and brainstem nuclei. These efferent connections are paralleled by the afferent connections. The organization based on the efferent and afferent connections combines the paleocerebellum with the neocerebellum and leaves the archicerebellum on its own. The archicerebellum receives information from and projects to the vestibular nuclei in the brainstem. It also receives input directly from the vestibular apparatus in the inner ear as well as visual inputs from the pretectal region and visual cortex. The vermal, paravermal, and lateral zones project to the **fastigial**, **interpositus** (consisting of the **globose** and **emboliform** nuclei in primates) and **dentate nuclei**, respectively. With the exception of the archicerebellum, outputs of the cerebellar cortex originate in these four deep cerebellar nuclei. The vermal zone, crossing the midline of the paleo- and neocerebellum, receives input primarily from the periphery and, in turn, has projections directly to the brainstem and spi-

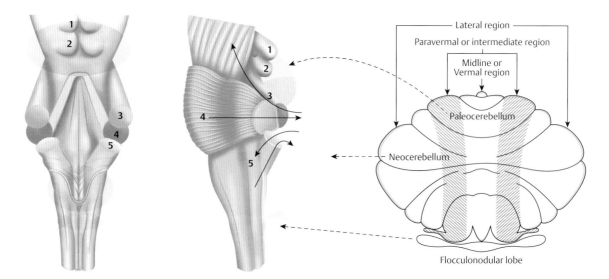

Fig. 7.16 Schematic representation of the anatomy of the cerebellum. The dorsal brainstem view shows the cerebellum as transparent to demonstrate the connections of the cerebellum to the brainstem. There are three main connections: the superior (3), middle (4), and inferior cerebellar peduncles (5). The superior peduncle is efferent (i.e., outflow from the deep cerebellar nuclei), while the middle cerebellar peduncle is afferent (i.e., input). The inferior peduncle is both input and output, with the output through the juxtarestiform body. Also represented are the superior (1) and inferior colliculi (2). The dorsal cortex view is from Montgomery et al (1985).

nal cord. For that reason the vermal zone is often referred to as the **spinocerebellum**. The lateral zone, primarily in the neocerebellum, has extensive inputs from the cerebral cortex and in turn projects to the motor cortex via the ventral intermediate nucleus of the thalamus. Based on these anatomical considerations, it is presumed that the lateral cerebellar zone is primarily involved with volitional movements. However, microstimulation of neurons in the lateral zone causes contraction of proximal muscles via direct projections from the cerebellum to the brainstem through the descending limb of the superior cerebellar peduncle, also called the **brachium conjunctivum,** suggesting control of postural muscles that anticipate changes in the center of gravity with volitional movements.

The neuronal architecture of the cerebellar cortex is remarkable for this stereotypy and regularity; the same basic circuity is found across the entire cerebellar cortex. The output of the cerebellar cortex is through the **Purkinje cell** (**Fig. 7.17**), which is regularly arrayed in the Purkinje cell layer of the cerebellar cortex. Purkinje cells then project to neurons in the deep cerebellar nuclei. Purkinje cells release the neurotransmitter GABA, which causes hyperpolarization of neurons in the deep cerebellar nuclei, thus reducing the probability of an action potential being generated by neurons of the deep cerebellar nuclei. However, there is evidence that there may be posthyperpolarization rebound excitation. Purkinje cells receive input from **climbing fibers** that originate in the **inferior olivary nucleus** in the brainstem. The axonal terminals of the climbing fibers arborize extensively among the Purkinje cell dendrites and exert a powerful depolarization that results in a sequence of action potentials referred to as a **complex spike**. These repetitive spikes are thought to play a role in learning.

Purkinje cells also receive information from axons of **granule cells**, and these axons form a parallel array, called **parallel fibers**, that traverse the gyri of the cerebellar cortex. Interdigitated among the parallel fibers are hyperpolarizing interneurons that also synapse on Purkinje cell dendrites. Granule cells receive inputs from the **pontine relay nuclei** of the brainstem via **mossy fibers**. The deep cerebellar nuclei receive **axon collaterals** from the climbing and mossy fibers.

It is remarkable, and certainly humbling, that despite the remarkably stereotypic and repetitive organization of the cerebellar cortex, we still know relatively little about cerebellar functions. Most of current theories about cerebellar physiology derive from observations of humans with cerebellar lesions, such as those studied by Gordon Holmes following World War I (Holmes 1939).

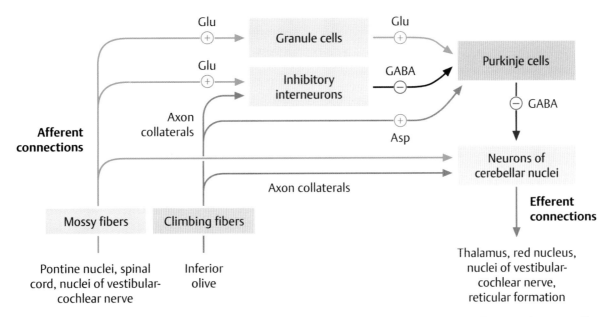

Fig. 7.17 Cellular anatomy and connections of the cerebellum. The primary inputs to the cerebellum are the mossy fibers and the climbing fibers. These afferents synapse on the granule cells and a series of inhibitory neurons. Afferents from the climbing fibers synapse on the inhibitory interneurons and also send collaterals to the Purkinje cells. The Purkinje cells are inhibitory onto the neurons of the deep cerebellar nuclei that are the source of the efferent connections from the cerebellum. It is important to note that the term "inhibitory" is used carefully. To be sure, the involved neurotransmitters produce hyperpolarization; however, many neurons display posthyperpolarization rebound excitation.

Cerebellar Disorders

Patients with lesions restricted to the cerebellum develop severe disruption of normal movement. They are slower to initiate movement (bradykinesia), and their movements are often imprecise (**dysmetric**) by undershooting (**hypometria**) or overshooting (**hypermetria**) targets. Hypometria is more common. These abnormal movement trajectories are evident on the finger-to-nose test, where the patient holds both arms outstretched and then is asked to touch the tip of the index finger to the tip of the nose. There is a tendency for the patient's fingertip to veer off course, requiring a corrective movement that itself may veer off course, in turn requiring a series of corrective movements. These patterns may also manifest as an abnormality in speech prosody, such as the sing-song quality of the speech of some patients with cerebellar disorders, or as dysarthria. The series of corrective movements may be the basis for the **action tremor** associated with cerebellar disorders. The awkward and ever-changing direction of movement is described as **ataxia**, which can be evident not only in limb and trunk movements but also in speech, voice, and swallowing. In addition to dysmetria, individuals with cerebellar lesions may show a breakdown of complex movements into a sequence of simpler movements (decomposition of movement). For example, reaching to grasp a cup requires joint rotations across multiple joints. Normally, these joint rotations are executed simultaneously to produce a smooth and continuous trajectory. However, with cerebellar disorders, multiple-joint rotations are not executed in an integrated and continuous manner but instead show decomposition of movement. Decomposition of movement may be related to the cerebellar sign of **scanning speech**, in which words are decomposed into separate syllables and spoken with equal or irregular stress.

Another symptom and sign related to cerebellar lesions is inability to perform a regular repetitive movement such as finger tapping, referred to as **dysdiadochokinesia**. Patients also demonstrate **hypotonia**, defined as decreased resistance to passive joint rotation. Lesion-related research on cerebellar function has generally been descriptive rather than providing a causal model. This is not to say that causal models have not been offered, but theories to date have been underdetermined by available facts (Manto 2009).

The regions of the body affected by cerebellar lesions relate to the cerebellar zone affected. For example, lesions of the neocerebellum typically result in motor disturbances of the distal extremities during intentional movements. Often gait and balance are not affected. In contrast, lesions of the anterior vermal zone produce symptoms and signs such as ataxia, primarily affecting posture and gait, while lesions in the posterior vermal zone affect oculomotor control. Lesions of the paravermal zone often affect a combination of these body regions. It is important to recognize, however, that the symptoms and signs typically associated with lesions of the cerebellum do not necessarily mean that the cerebellum is the primary site of the pathology. Lesions of cerebellar afferents and efferents can produce virtually identical symptoms and signs, including lesions of the contralateral motor cortex.

Considerable evidence suggests that the cerebellum is involved in cognitive and language functions, not unlike the basal ganglia–thalamic–cortical system. Schmahmann (1991) used the term "dysmetria of thought" to refer to a constellation of cognitive and language deficits occurring with cerebellar lesions, including executive function, visuospatial, and affective impairments, as well as agrammatism and anomia (Mariën et al 2014).

■ Association Cortex

Lesions of the association cortex—cortical regions outside the primary motor and sensory cortices—have been associated with a wide range of motor abnormalities termed **apraxias**. Apraxia is defined as an impairment in executing appropriate voluntary movements that is not due to weakness or loss of sensory function. Lesions must be outside of the motor cortex, as patients with motor cortex involvement are often paralyzed, so it is not possible to observe movement disorders. Movements in patients with apraxia typically appear normal, with no abnormalities in movement trajectory, as might be the case with lesions of the cerebellar system, and no slowing or involuntary movements, as may be observed with lesions of the basal ganglia–thalamic–cortical system.

Three general types of apraxia have been described: **kinetic** apraxia, typically affecting a limb and called **limb-kinetic apraxia**; **ideomotor** apraxia; and **ideational** apraxia. Limb-kinetic apraxia manifests as clumsiness of movement. Unlike other apraxias, limb-kinetic apraxia affects both voluntary and automatic movements. Ideomotor apraxia affects imitation of gestures and causes altered ability to demonstrate how tools are used. When asked to mime tool use, patients often use a body part as though it was the target object (e.g., when asked to show what a brush does, the patient will rake his fingers through his hair as though his hand were the brush). Automatic movements using the same objects such, as in activities of daily living, may be intact. Ideational apraxia affects the ability to execute a complex sequence of tasks voluntarily, and patients may make errors such as buttoning a shirt before putting it on, or breathing in rather than out when blowing out a candle.

Special cases of apraxia have also been described. For example, patients with constructional apraxia may have difficulty copying the drawing of an object. Dressing apraxia is demonstrated by a patient who puts clothing on inappropriately, such as putting arms in the wrong sleeves. Orofacial apraxia impairs the ability to carry out skilled orofacial movements such as imitating blowing out a candle. Apraxia of speech affects an individual's ability to speak, though other facial and lingual voluntary and involuntary movements may be normal.

■ Loss of Sensation

Disorders associated with the loss of sensation, such as a peripheral neuropathy, also affect movement. For example, the local anesthetic used in dental procedures will often impair speech. Other examples include an action tremor and ataxia that is nearly identical to that associated with lesions of the cerebellum and its efferents and afferents but improves under visual guidance. Patients with significant sensory loss can have what appear to be involuntary movements called pseudoathetosis when holding out their arms while the eyes are closed.

■ The Perils of Inferring Normal Brain Function from Patients with Brain Lesions

In the previous sections, we discussed suprasegmental functions as they have been identified in patients with lesions in those suprasegmental structures. We introduced the limitations of inferring the function of a brain region by what the brain does without it, and here we return to that topic with the goal of developing a conceptual framework for suprasegmental motor control.

Earlier in this chapter, we reviewed the lack of evidence to support one-to-one correspondence of a specific sign or symptom with damage to a specific brain region. For example, bradykinesia can be associated with lesions of (1) dopaminergic neurons of the SNc; (2) the GPe; (3) the ventral thalamus pars oralis; (4) the supplementary motor area; or (5) the

putamen. Similarly, the same motor abnormalities can be observed with lesions of (1) the cerebellar cortex; (2) the deep cerebellar nuclei; (3) the pontocerebellar nuclei; (4) the inferior olivary nucleus; (5) cortical input to the pontocerebellar nuclei; or (6) sensory pathways to the cerebellum.

We have a conceptual choice. Either there are as many different pathophysiological mechanisms as there are pathoetiologies, or there are few pathophysiological mechanisms that are engendered by different pathoetiologies. To be sure, the inverse problem generated by the common final pathway could result in the same phenomenon with different mechanisms just to the point of the final common pathway, such as the α-LMN. However, how the α-LMN produces the same behavior in the face of different mechanisms is problematic. Further, William of Occam's admonition that "it is vain to do with more that which can be done by fewer" suggests caution in positing a plethora of different mechanisms to explain behaviors.

Neurophysiologic studies can identify neurons with activities that are correlated with various aspects of motor behavior. For example, some neurons in the basal ganglia–thalamic–cortical system and cerebellum change activities with the onset of a signal to prepare to move, a go signal, muscular activity, and/or the movement reaching its goal. Further, timings of the onset of neuronal activities are not different among the different structures, as shown in **Fig. 7.14** and **Fig. 7.18** (Montgomery and Buchholz 1991; Thach 1975). Similarly, during a **saccadic** eye task, changes in activities of neurons of the GPi and GPe and the SNr are more alike than different (Shin and Sommer 2010).

Also striking is that patients with extensive lesions in suprasegmental structures other than motor cortex may have normal movements despite the lesion. For example, patients may have multiple infarctions in the basal ganglia without any obvious motor abnormalities. Similarly, young persons can recover from severe lesions of the cerebellum without obvious residual motor abnormalities. Indeed, persons born without a cerebellum are not unheard of. These phenomena are explained as the product of compensation by other brain structures. Structures compensating for the loss must have access to the same inputs and outputs as the lesioned structure, or at least be part of the same anatomic and physiologic network. Initially, it was thought that the basal ganglia–thalamic–cortical system reached the motor cortex through separate pathways than the cerebellum did, as the cerebellar relay nucleus in the thalamus is the ventral intermediate nucleus, while the relay for the basal ganglia system is the ventral thalamus pars oralis.

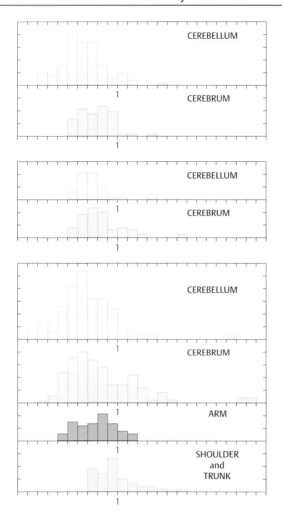

Fig. 7.18 Time-of-change histograms summarizing timing results. The three sets of histograms are from three monkeys and show the distribution of time of change (relative to change of force) of unit discharge in cerebellar nuclei and arm area motor cortex (monkeys 1 and 2), and muscles in the arm, shoulder, and trunk (monkey 3). The horizontal axis is time of change (in milliseconds) before or after change of force; scale is 20 m/division. The vertical axis is number of neural and EMG changes; scale is 5 neural changes/division. Units that changed for both flexion and extension are represented twice. For the first monkey, the histograms comprise 91 neural changes in cerebellar nuclei (48 neurons, 12 penetrations) and 52 changes in motor cortex (34 neurons, 10 penetrations). Within the cerebellar nuclei, 10 penetrations were in the dentate nucleus (37 neurons, 70 changes) and two penetrations were in the interpositus nuclei (11 neurons, 21 changes). For the second monkey, the histograms comprise 35 changes in the cerebellar nuclei (22 neurons, 6 penetrations) and 47 changes in motor cortex (32 neurons, 6 penetrations). Within the cerebellar nuclei, two penetrations were in interpositus nuclei (4 neurons, 6 changes); three penetrations were at the junction of interpositus and dentate nuclei (24 neurons, 35 changes), and only one penetration was well lateral in dentate nucleus (4 neurons, 6 changes). For the third monkey, the histograms comprise 130 changes (77 neurons, 19 penetrations), all in dentate nucleus; and 126 changes in motor cortex (78 neurons, 21 penetrations) (modified from Thach 1975).

However, there may be some overlap of cerebellar and pallidal efferents to the thalamus. In one study, multisynaptic anatomic tracers showed that the output of the dentate nucleus of the cerebellum projects to the striatum via the thalamus and that the subthalamic nucleus projects to the cerebellar cortex via the pontine relay nuclei (Bostan and Strick 2010). These findings suggest points of network integration.

Tracer studies in nonhuman primates have demonstrated that the supplementary motor area receives input primarily from the pallidal relay nuclei of the thalamus, but also from the cerebellar relay nuclei (Sakai et al 1999). Similarly, pallidal and cerebellar thalamic relay neurons project to the motor cortex, serving as another site of integration (Nambu et al 1988). In addition, both the striatum of the basal ganglia and the pontine nuclei of the cerebellar system receive inputs from wide areas of the cerebral cortex. Whether individual cortical projection neurons are segregated based on cerebellar or basal ganglia projections is unknown. In other words, it is not clear whether or to what extent the corticopontine fibers are collaterals of the corticostriatal fibers, although evidence in rodents suggests this may be the case (Mercier et al 1990).

It is problematic to infer differences in function from differences in anatomy between the basal ganglia–thalamic–cortical system and the cerebellar–cortical system when physiologic dynamics are considered, particularly cycle time. Cycle time is the time between repetitions of a process. For example, each pixel on a computer monitor is typically refreshed 60 times per second (i.e., the refresh rate is 60 Hz). However, the threshold frequency at which the human eye can detect a flicker is less than 60 Hz. Because the time it takes to refresh the screen is shorter than the time in which the eye can process the image, pixels appear to change smoothly. Similarly, if the propagation of one bit of information between two neurons in sequence takes approximately 3.5 ms, then for information to traverse the cortex–striatum–GPi–ventral thalamus pars oralis–cortex takes 14 ms. Information could repeatedly traverse this circuit 71 times in one second. Simply, this calculation suggests that during the course of a behavior lasting 1 second, information could reenter the motor cortex 71 times. Also, information initiated in one structure can go to more than one target. For example, information initiated in the basal ganglia 71 times also could go to the cerebellar system from the motor cortex 71 times. These dynamics argue against sharp categorization of these physiologic systems.

■ Is There a Motor Control Hierarchy?

Nearly every current theory of suprasegmental motor control is conceptually structured as a hierarchical and sequential process. At the bottom of this hierarchy are the α-LMNs, which passively relay information from higher structures. Above α-LMNs, interconnections within the spinal cord give rise to reflex mechanisms differing in both complexity and the level of the spinal cord at which they occur (indicated by the level of transection of the neural axis necessary to produce them by removal of conscious control). Above these structures are UMNs, above those are inputs from basal ganglia, and so on. This conceptual organization owes much to the work of Sir Charles Sherrington (1857–1952), although the ancient Greeks made reference to different types of "souls" (roughly equivalent to minds) that were implemented by different levels of the nervous system, a notion that might have been based on observations of decapitated animals and injured humans.

The most basic of Sherrington's spinal reflexes is the deep tendon reflex, in which the muscle tendon is suddenly stretched (by tapping on the tendon), which results in a rapid stretch of the muscle spindles. The stretched muscle spindle nerve endings generate axon potentials that are conducted to the spinal cord, where they synapse on α-LMNs, which in turn activate the muscles to produce a contraction of the muscle. These reflexes are greatly increased with transections of the spinal cord above the level of the spinal nerves. With other transections, other reflexes appear, such as the withdrawal reflex, which retracts the limb from a source of irritation. The crossed-extensor reflex is an elaboration of the withdrawal reflex in which the affected limb is withdrawn flexion, thereby removing a source of support if the limb is a leg, and the contralateral limb is simultaneously extended in order to maintain balance. Transections of different levels of the brainstem produce other types of postural reflexes. Lesions between the **inferior colliculi** and the **lateral vestibular nucleus** produce **decerebrate posturing**, with extension of the lower and upper extremities, whereas higher lesions produce **decorticate posturing**, with extension of the lower extremities and flexion of the upper extremities.

In Sherrington's view, each of the reflexes just described is organized in a hierarchy, with those above suppressing those just below. These reflexes were, then, the basic building blocks of motor control, and the orchestration of motor unit recruitment and derecruitment was implemented by variable control over the various reflexes. Indeed,

the dynamic descending control of the γ-LMN that innervates the intrafusal muscle fiber of the muscle spindle has been postulated to control movement by dynamically varying muscle spindle sensitivity, and thus feedback through the monosynaptic reflex mechanism just described.

There are a number of problems with the Sherringtonian notion of motor control through hierarchical control of basic reflex mechanisms. Most importantly, cutting the **posterior (dorsal) roots** to the spinal nerve, which mediate sensory input from the muscle spindles, often does not produce any observable movement deficits in nonhuman primates. This procedure, known as **dorsal rhizotomy**, is often done in children to reduce spasticity, without noticeable effects on motor function, although the effects may not be visible given the underlying pathology. There have also been reports of improved motor control following dorsal rhizotomy (Bakir et al 2013). Dorsal rhizotomy or removal of the **dorsal root ganglia** is also used for treatment of pain, and the rare reports of effects on motor function describe those effects as minor and transient (Taub et al 1995). A study in which local anesthetic was injected in the region of the posterior roots in order to anesthetize the sensory fibers selectively in normal subjects did not produce any significant motor abnormalities (Landau et al 1960).

These observations suggest that the reflexes described by Sherrington play little role in normal motor control. Sherrington made what the philosopher Gilbert Ryle (1900–1976) identified as a category error, commonly described as "comparing apples to oranges." In a sense, the reflexology of Sherrington was "apples," while normal motor control is "oranges." In research, the spinal cord preparations used by Sherrington are called "**reduced preparations**." These preparations are used to reduce the complexity of the subject one is attempting to study. Sherrington initially wanted to understand the role of the motor cortex and, finding it too difficult, went on to study spinal cord preparations.

The problem with using reduced preparations is that the dynamics are a function of the **degrees of freedom**, or the number of relevant variables in that preparation. Reduced preparations do not capture qualitative changes that occur when the complexity of any system reaches a certain threshold. The dynamics below that threshold, such as in reduced preparations, differ from the dynamics above that threshold. The dynamics in complex systems can be dramatically different from those in reduced preparations, a concept we will return to soon when we discuss the complex systems theory of motor control.

While the hierarchical organization in Sherrington's reflexology is questionable, so too is its claim that motor control is sequential. The concept of sequential processing is ubiquitous in motor control theories. For example, the description of the striatum as the "input" stage of the basal ganglia, with the GPi and SNr as the "output," is problematic. The foregoing discussion of duty cycle shows how such sequential hierarchical structure is not realistic, though it continues to be a mainstay of most discussions about the physiology of the basal ganglia–thalamic–cortical system.

Another inaccurate view of motor control that is still retained from Sherrington's reflexology is the notion of one-dimensional, push-pull dynamics that typifies most theories of motor control, at least as it relates to the basal ganglia–thalamic–cortical system. We introduced this on-or-off view earlier in the chapter in the context of hypo- vs. hyperkinetic disorders. Sherrington observed that reflexes are either increased or decreased. As mentioned, Jackson described symptoms and signs as either an *excess* or a *deficit* of function; for example, seizures are a manifestation of excessive function in the motor system, while paralysis reflects a deficit of motor function. The one-dimensional push-pull dynamic is an intuitively appealing device to reduce complexity. As already mentioned, this type of approach dates back to Aristotle's notion of contraries, which are not opposites but rather two extremes of the same single dimension. Any number of intervening properties can be obtained when the system is at different points along the single dimension. Galen followed this thinking when he described disease as relative excesses or deficiencies of different humors.

The one-dimensional conceptual approach still operates today. Hypokinetic disorders are attributed to a relative deficiency of dopamine and hyperkinetic disorders to a relative excess of dopamine, despite evidence noted earlier in the chapter that patients with hypokinesia due to Parkinson's disease remain bradykinetic even when the brain is flooded with dopamine, either from medication or from fetal dopamine cell transplants. Movements are either "allowed" or "blocked." In the GPi rate theory, the GPi has "excessive" neuronal discharge rates in hypokinetic disorders or "deficient" discharge rates in hyperkinetic disorders. Alternatively, there is a relative excess of beta oscillations in neuronal activities causing hypokinesia by interfering or blocking the normal dynamics. However, the changes in motor unit recruitment associated with Parkinson's disease, described previously, do not fit with a one-dimensional push-pull dynamic.

■ Complex Systems and Network of Oscillators Approach

We argue that to advance knowledge and understanding of motor control, we need new metaphors that are radically different from those offered by Aristotle some 2,300 years ago. One candidate is the metaphor of complex systems. Complex systems are determinant, in that the basic mechanisms are causal and not random or happenstance. Consider the formation of a snowflake. The variety of snowflakes is so astronomical that, statistically, there is a high probability that no two snowflakes are exactly the same, although all are six-pointed and symmetric. However, there are not separate physics for each snowflake. Rather, there is a relatively economical set of forces that generate all snowflakes. Because of the very large number of water molecules that make up each snowflake, the number of interactions among water molecules that create specific snowflake shapes is so large that they become a complex system. These interactions are nonlinear, further adding to their complexity and, thus, the variability in snowflake shapes. Clearly, these factors that generate complex systems are present in the nervous system, with the human brain containing approximately 86 billion neurons and each neuron making approximately 7,000 synapses on other neurons. The number of neurons in each nucleus of the motor system is considerably smaller but still substantial. Thus, the human nervous system clearly is large enough to be a complex system.

Critical to the dynamics of complex systems is nonlinearity in the interactions among the components. Linear systems generally have the property that when one parameter changes by a given factor (e.g., is doubled), the consequent parameter changes by the same factor (e.g., is also doubled). In the equation $y = x$, when the value of x is increased from 1 to 2, the value of y also is increased from 1 to 2; similarly, increasing x from 2 to 3 results in y increased from 2 to 3, or an increase of 50%. In the equation $y = x^2$, on the other hand, increasing x by one unit from 1 to 2 increases the value of y by 3 units, however, increasing x again by one unit from 2 to 3 increases y by 5 units. Thus, the relationship of y to x in $y = x^2$ is nonlinear. A major source of nonlinearities is systems describable by functions that incorporate time, particularly where rates of change with respect to time (for example, $y = dx/dt$, where dx/dt is the rate of change in x with respect to time) themselves change over time. As an example, consider the equation that describes a swinging pendulum, $\partial^2\theta/\partial t^2 + (g/l)\sin\theta = 0$, where

θ is the angle of the pendulum, g is the acceleration due to gravity, and l is the length of the pendulum. The rate at which the angle of the pendulum changes varies over time and depends on the present angle of the pendulum. This is a complicated enough equation; ordinary calculus cannot convert it to a simple algebraic equation for θ in terms of t. Now consider a system with a double pendulum, where the second pendulum is suspended from the swinging bottom of the first. Both pendulums exert reactive forces on each other in addition to the force on their own weights, producing a system that is chaotic, in that its behavior is unpredictable. The double-pendulum system acts like a complex system because of nonlinearites in the equations that describe its motions.

Neurons process information in highly nonlinear ways. For example, the thresholds for generation of an action potential impose nonlinearities because of discontinuity between subthreshold graded potentials and the rapid depolarization that occurs when the cell is depolarized to the threshold for generating an action potential. Similarly, refractory periods following generation of an action potential render the neuron unexcitable, when the same depolarization just before or just after might produce an action potential.

The dynamics of many complex systems have a number of important features that may provide metaphors for creating theories of suprasegmental motor control. For example, many complex systems achieve a remarkable degree of stability through self-organization into attractor states, much in the manner that water molecules self-organize to produce specific snowflakes. Further, the self-organizing states can display specific dynamics, such as an oscillator in what is called a limit cycle or multiple limit cycles. **Fig. 7.19** shows that a train of neuronal action potentials contains a number of frequencies simultaneously. It appears that there is a specific set of frequencies for time periods on the order of 1

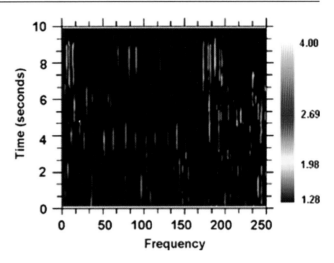

Fig. 7.19 Spectrogram showing the appearance and disappearance of significant frequencies in the discharge of a neuron recorded in the GPe in a nonhuman primate. The circular statistics method is applied repeatedly over 10 s (vertical axis) to 2-second windows, which are then moved through time at 0.2-second increments. The method is applied for periods (the inverse of the frequency) corresponding to frequencies from 1 to 250 Hz (horizontal axis). At every instant of time, multiple frequencies are represented in the neuronal spike train (verbatim from Montgomery and Gale 2008).

to 2 seconds, and then a relatively abrupt change to another set of frequencies. In complex systems theory, these abrupt changes are called bifurcations. Temporary states are called metastable states. Information can be encoded within each state; for example, in the set of frequencies and in the transitions between states, as shown in the figure.

The ability of a single neuron to entrain multiple frequencies simultaneously and to move between metastable states greatly increases the computational power of neurons and the networks in which they are embedded. This feature of neurons is critical because the potential number of movements is astronomical, perhaps even infinite.

Box 7.7   The Necker Cube

An example of a perceptual bifurcation is the Necker cube. **Box Fig. 7.4** shows a three-dimensional wire frame model of a cube. The shaded face can be seen either in the front of the cube or the back of the cube. The shaded surface appears to change suddenly or "pop" from one side to the other, but the viewer never sees a gradual transition from one position to the other.

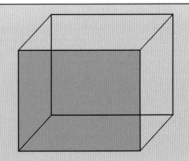

Box Fig. 7.4   Necker cube.

Another potentially important feature of complex systems is their dependence on initial conditions. This means that small changes in initial conditions can produce marked changes in final states achieved by the complex system. Conceptually, this phenomenon can increase the computational power of neurons and networks in which they are embedded. Thus, relatively small changes in neuronal activities within the motor system could result in very large changes in motor unit recruitment and derecruitment.

Complex systems can be implemented in networks of loosely coupled oscillators (Hoppensteadt and Izhikevich 1997). Such systems have a rich set of dynamics that include positive and negative resonance, **beat interactions**, and **oscillator phase changes**. Also, different oscillators can entrain each other. Another remarkable feature is that information encoded in the amplitudes of different loosely coupled oscillators can carry independent information much as in amplitude-modulated (AM) radio. For example, a set of oscillators can express information on multiple frequencies simultaneously so long as the frequencies are noncommensurate (i.e., the frequencies are not integer multiples of some other fundamental frequency; for example, 29 Hz and 67 Hz, which are prime numbers, but not 29 Hz and 58 Hz, where the latter is twice the former). This means that information entrained in the variations in amplitude of the 29-Hz oscillation is unaffected by information contained in the modulated amplitude of the 67-Hz signal.

In the case of neural oscillators, the same neuron's spike train contains multiple frequencies simultaneously, meaning that the same neuron can process different sets of information simultaneously. Again, this process greatly increases the computational power of the system. Further, the different frequencies entrained in the neuron's spike train may correlate with orchestration of motor unit recruitment and derecruitment at different time scales, allowing simultaneous processing of behaviors over different time scales. These features are well appreciated in **continuous harmonic oscillators** but become more robust in networks of **discrete oscillators**.

Applying these concepts to networks of neural oscillators suggests that the same neuron or set of neurons can process multiple streams of information independently and simultaneously, as long as the information operates over specific frequencies and time scales. If the basal ganglia–thalamic–cortical system is a set of nested oscillators, it can operate over different frequencies simultaneously, representing different time scale dynamics. Consequently, the basal ganglia–thalamic–cortical system could participate in the orchestration of α-LMN activations over different time scales, ranging from recruitment of individual motor units to the synergies of different muscles over multiple joints simultaneously. These time scales correspond to the first-, second-, and third-order levels of motor unit orchestration discussed at the beginning of this chapter.

Complex systems metaphors can account for many speech phenomena, such as anticipatory coarticulation errors in normal speech, such as saying "neef noodle" for "beef noodle"; within-person variability in articulatory errors in patients with motor speech disorders; and reductions in loudness and pitch complexity in individuals with Parkinson's disease, none of which can be explained by models that view motor control as a linear sequence of steps. To be sure, the orchestration of motor unit activities is precisely controlled over time.

Consider the situation of an operator of a tractor who must back up a trailer to a loading dock. Typically, a proficient human operator cannot explain how she does it, nor verbally direct a novice to do so. A computer system containing multiple neuron-like processing units that simply add the inputs to produce an output arranged in two layers can, after sufficient practice, succeed (**Fig. 7.20**). The training involves trial and error, with the error signal used to modify the synaptic weights of the inputs from neurons of one layer to neurons of the next layer. Once learning is complete, the synaptic weights are not further modified. It is problematic, however, to determine the precise role of any individual neuron at any stage of the process of backing the trailer up from the starting position to the final position at the dock. This illustration is not meant to argue that the nervous system is constructed in the manner shown in the figure, but rather to emphasize that a sequential and hierarchical level of organization is not necessary to explain what appears to be, at the surface, a sequential and hierarchical problem.

Most schematic representations of the basal ganglia–thalamic–cortical systems are shown as open circuits without specific closed-loop feedback. The systems oscillators theory closes these open circuits to produce reentrant circuits (**Fig. 7.21**). Different oscillators contain different nodes, so the time that it takes for a bit of information to traverse the different oscillators will vary. Thus, each oscillator will have a different inherent frequency. Each node contains multiple neurons that have a relatively low probability of discharge for any specific cycle of the oscillations. However, there are a sufficient number of neurons in each node to ensure that the oscillations will continue. Thus, the discharge rate of any particular neuron is some fraction of the intrinsic frequency of the oscillator in

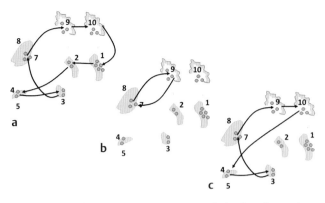

Fig. 7.21 Schematic representation of the basal ganglia–thalamic–cortical system. The various structures are represented as follows: (1) putamen (as representative of the striatum); (2) GPe; (3) GPi; (4) subthalamic nucleus; (5) SNr; (6) SNc (location of the cell bodies that use dopamine as their neurotransmitter); (7) ventral thalamus pars oralis; (8) parafascicular and centromedian nuclei of the thalamus; (9) supplementary motor area; (10) primary motor cortex. Oscillator A contains seven nodes, while oscillator B contains two nodes and oscillator C six nodes.

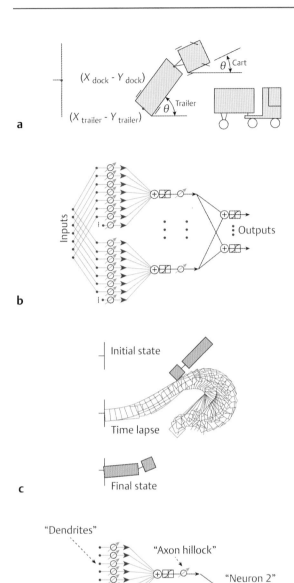

Fig. 7.20 **(a)** Schematic representation of a neural network solution to the computational problem of backing a tractor trailer, **(c)** up to a loading dock. **(b)** The neural network consists of 25 processing units arranged in two layers. The output layer drives a virtual tractor trailer, the position of which is sent to the input units. **(d)** Input to each unit is adjusted by a synaptic weight that experience can alter through the digital equivalent of dendrites. Weighted inputs are summed and submitted to a mathematical operation—a sigmoid function, to limit the magnitude of the outputs—which is analogous to an action potential–initiating segment. Actual output is compared to input. Any difference is an error signal, which propagates back through the neural network to change the synaptic weights. Unlike biologic neuronal action potentials, the digital equivalent of the output neuron generates output that ranges from a value of zero to one (some neurons produce a graded output), but the concept is the same (from Nguyen and Widrow 1990).

which the neuron is embedded. As different oscillators share the same nodes, the neurons within those shared nodes can participate in a number of different oscillators simultaneously. Thus, multiple frequencies are entrained in the spike train of any individual neuron, as shown in **Fig. 7.22**. With

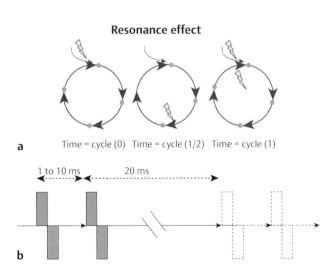

Fig. 7.22 **(a)** Schematic representation of the resonance effect. The first stimulation (conditioning pulse) causes an excitation to traverse the closed loop. If the second stimulation (test pulse) is delivered just as the excitation effect from the first or conditioning pulse returns to the original site, temporal summation on the neuronal cell membrane will amplify the response. **(b)** Schematic representation of the paired-pulse stimulus trains. The interstimulus interval represents a specific frequency (1/interval).

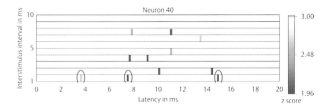

Fig. 7.23 Results from the paired-pulse experiments for a neuron recorded in the motor cortex of a nonhuman primate. Each row represents changes in the probability of neuronal discharge from baseline for each interstimulus interval of the paired-pulse stimulus. Colored bars represent any change with a z-score greater than 1.96 compared to baseline. The horizontal axis represents latency of the resonance effect after the second or test pulse of the pair.

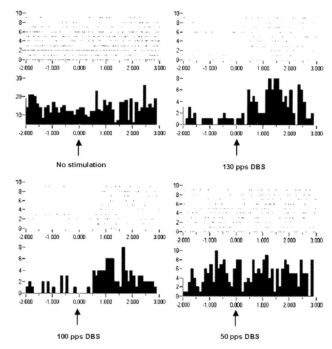

Fig. 7.24 Perievent rasters and histograms for a neuron recorded in the putamen of a nonhuman primate. In the no-stimulation condition, there is no meaningful modulation of neuronal activity with behavior (appearance of the "go" signal at time zero is indicated by the up-arrow). However, with 130 pps and to a lesser extent with 100 pps DBS, there is a consistent modulation of neuronal activities related to behavior, suggesting that DBS has "enlisted" the neuron into relating meaningfully to the behavior. This phenomenon is consistent with (but not proof of) a resonance effect (Montgomery and Gale 2008).

changes in the dynamics of the network of oscillators, the probability of a neuron discharging in any cycle of the associated oscillators can change, thereby producing changes in discharge frequencies associated with behaviors.

The systems oscillators theory is supported by evidence from transsynaptic anatomical tracer studies, in which tracers from cortical regions that project to the basal ganglia return to those same cortical regions, consistent with a closed loop. Electrophysiologic studies also support closed-loop circuitry and thus are consistent with the systems oscillators theory (**Fig. 7.23**).

The systems oscillators theory is consistent with effects of DBS at different frequencies. DBS can be viewed as another oscillator introduced into the set of oscillators that constitute the basal ganglia–thalamic–cortical system. Thus, the manner by which the stimulation interacts depends on the relative frequencies. In the early days of DBS therapy, it was thought that high-frequency stimulation improved movement disorders, while low-frequency stimulation either had no effect or could worsen symptoms. Later, the effects of stimulation frequencies were reconsidered as a product of the total electrical energy delivered, with progressively higher frequencies monotonically increasing the total electrical energy delivered. Neither of these accounts was correct.

A third account emerged from a study examining the effects of a wide range of DBS frequencies on the ability of patients with Parkinson's disease to open and close their hands rapidly (Huang et al 2014). The speed of hand opening and closing was measured at different stimulation frequencies. If the total electrical energy delivered was the controlling variable, then speed of hand opening and closing should have increased monotonically with increasing stimulation frequency. This was not

found; rather, there were a number of peaks in speed corresponding to specific frequencies within the range tested (2 to 180 pulses per second). This finding showed that DBS was interacting with frequency-dependent neuronal mechanisms. Thus, the effects of DBS could be the consequence of positive resonance with specific neural oscillators within the basal ganglia–thalamic–cortical system.

An example of possible resonance between DBS and neuronal activities is shown in **Fig. 7.24**. The neuron shown in the figure did not modulate its activities relative to a movement behavior in the no-stimulation condition, but did so with high-frequency stimulation in the range that is therapeutic for individuals with movement disorders, and also to a lesser extent with stimulation at lower frequencies. DBS at the right frequency increased the signal relative to the noise by stochastic resonance interactions.

This chapter primarily focused on motor functions of suprasegmental structures, but these structures also participate in many other nonmotor operations. For example, there are components

> ### Box 7.8 Deep Brain Stimulation
>
> DBS is a remarkable treatment for movement disorders associated with the basal ganglia and tremor secondary to cerebellar damage. DBS provides benefit when all attempts at alternative therapies fail, including medications and even fetal cell transplants. DBS involves the permanent implantation of an array of electrodes in the brain that provides electrical stimulation from an implanted pulse generator, much like a cardiac pacemaker. The therapeutic mechanisms of DBS action are unknown but probably involve activation of voltage-gated depolarizing ion channels that results in action potentials (see **Chapter 6**). The systems oscillators theory posits that DBS is another discrete oscillator that is introduced into the basal ganglia–thalamic–cortical system to interact with neural oscillators. Recordings of behavior-related neuronal activities in the putamen of nonhuman primates show that DBS-like stimulation of the sub-thalamic nucleus can improve the signal-to-noise ratio in the neuronal activities. If one mechanism of movement disorders such as Parkinson's disease is misinformation encoded in the sequences of action potentials, then increasing the signal-to-noise ratio may improve motor symptoms and signs. The systems oscillators theory suggests that DBS at different frequencies would interact with different neural oscillators within the basal ganglia–thalamic–cortical system to produce different effects. Contrary to the original hypotheses that high-frequency DBS improves, while low-frequency DBS worsens, the symptoms and signs of Parkinson's disease, recent studies show that DBS at many frequencies, including low frequencies, improves speed of hand opening and closing (Huang et al 2014). In addition, DBS is inefficient at producing action potentials in neurons. Approximately 10% of DBS pulses produce an antidromic action potential, but the driving of those antidromic action potentials is not random. Rather, it appears that the DBS pulse interacts with two intrinsic oscillators, one at 27 Hz and the other at 66 Hz.

within the basal ganglia that are related to limbic and cognitive functions. Also, the cerebellum has been implicated in language. Examples include cognitive functions associated with the cerebellum and conceptual impairments seen with lesions of the association cortex (Ikemoto et al 2015). Many of these nonmotor effects may be due to the fact that these structures receive input from throughout the cerebral cortex, which includes many regions that are not primarily motor in nature (Bostan et al 2013).

It probably is a misconception to think that motor, limbic, and cognitive operations are distinct and separate. For example, the limbic system involved in emotions may play a role in motor control, as evidenced by the phenomena of kinesia paradoxica. There is evidence that the motor cortex may play a role in memory (Smyrnis et al 1992). Neuronal recordings in the motor region of the subthalamic nucleus in patients with Parkinson's disease during a voicing task demonstrated changes in activities while voicing a meaningful sentence and not when producing related but nonmeaningful syllables. Changes in the neuronal activities suggested a relationship to the syntactical structure or, alternatively, to the prosody of the utterance (Watson and Montgomery 2006). However, this complexity should not be surprising given the role of the basal ganglia in programming sequential movements. It may very well be that in the evolutionary development of speech, the basal ganglia were coopted to control the sequential nature of speech such as in syntax and prosody.

■ Suggested Readings

Aizman O, Brismar H, Uhlén P, et al. Anatomical and physiological evidence for D1 and D2 dopamine receptor colocalization in neostriatal neurons. *Nature Neuroscience, 3*, 226–230; 2000

Anderson ME, Horak FB. Influence of the globus pallidus on arm movements in monkeys. III. Timing of movement-related information. *Journal of Neurophysiology, 54*, 433–448; 1985

Bakir MS, Gruschke F, Taylor WR, et al. Temporal but not spatial variability during gait is reduced after selective dorsal rhizotomy in children with cerebral palsy. *PLoS One, 8*, e69500; 2013

Bostan AC, Dum RP, Strick PL. Cerebellar networks with the cerebral cortex and basal ganglia. *Trends in Cognitive Sciences, 17*, 241–254; 2013

Bostan AC, Strick PL. The cerebellum and basal ganglia are interconnected. *Neuropsychology Review, 20*, 261–270; 2010

Brasted PJ, Wise SP. Comparison of learning-related neuronal activity in the dorsal premotor cortex and striatum. *European Journal of Neuroscience, 19*, 721–740; 2004

Ciucci MR, Grant LM, Rajamanickam EP, et al. Early identification and treatment of speech and swallowing disorders in Parkinson's disease. *Seminars in Speech-Language Pathology, 34*, 185–202; 2013

Fertonani A, Pirulli C, Miniussi C. Random noise stimulation improves neuroplasticity in perceptual learning. *Journal of Neuroscience, 31,* 15416–15423; 2011

Filion M. Effects of interruption of the nigrostriatal pathway and of dopaminergic agents on the spontaneous activity of globus pallidus neurons in the awake monkey. *Brain Research, 178,* 425–441; 1979

Fujii N, Graybiel AM. Time-varying covariance of neural activities recorded in striatum and frontal cortex as monkeys perform sequential-saccade tasks. *Proceedings of the National Academy of Sciences of the USA, 102,* 9032–9037; 2005

Gdowski MJ, Miller LE, Bastianen CA, Nenonene EK, Houk JC. Signaling patterns of globus pallidus internal segment neurons during forearm rotation. *Brain Research, 1155,* 56–69; 2007

Georgopoulos AP, Kettner RE, Schwartz AB. Primate motor cortex and free arm movements to visual targets in three-dimensional space. II. Coding of the direction of movement by a neuronal population. *Journal of Neuroscience, 8,* 2928–2937; 1988

Grimme B, Fuchs S, Perrier P, Schöner G. Limb versus speech motor control: a conceptual review. *Motor Control, 15,* 5–33; 2011

Holmes G. The cerebellum of man. *Brain, 62,* 1–30; 1939

Hoppensteadt FC, Izhikevich EM. Weakly Connected Neural Networks. Berlin, Germany: Springer, 1997

Huang H, Watts RL, Montgomery EB Jr. Effects of deep brain stimulation frequency on bradykinesia of Parkinson's disease. *Movement Disorders, 29,* 203–206; 2014

Huerta-Ocampo I, Mena-Segovia J, Bolam JP. Convergence of cortical and thalamic input to direct and indirect pathway medium spiny neurons in the striatum. *Brain Structure & Function, 219,* 1787–1800; 2014

Ikemoto S, Yang C, Tan A. Basal ganglia circuit loops, dopamine and motivation: A review and enquiry. *Behavioural Brain Research, 290,* 17–31; 2015

Johnson-Laird P. How We Reason. Oxford, UK: Oxford University Press; 2009

Kuhn T. The Structure of Scientific Revolutions. Chicago, IL: University of Chicago Press; 1962

Landau WM, Weaver RA, Hornbein TF. Fusimotor nerve function in man. Differential nerve block studies in normal subjects and in spasticity and rigidity. *Archives of Neurology, 3,* 10–23; 1960

Lévesque M, Parent A. The striatofugal fiber system in primates: a reevaluation of its organization based on single-axon tracing studies. *Proceedings of the National Academy of Sciences of the USA, 102,* 11888–11893; 2005

Manto M. Mechanisms of human cerebellar dysmetria: experimental evidence and current conceptual bases. *Journal of Neuroengineering and Rehabilitation, 6,* 10; 2009

Marder E, Bucher D. Understanding circuit dynamics using the stomatogastric nervous system of lobsters and crabs. *Annual Review of Physiology 69,* 291–316; 2007

Mariën P, Ackermann H, Adamaszek M, et al. Consensus paper: language and the cerebellum: an ongoing enigma. *Cerebellum, 13,* 386–410; 2014.

Mercier BE, Legg CR, Glickstein M. Basal ganglia and cerebellum receive different somatosensory information in rats. *Proceedings of the National Academy of Sciences of the USA, 87,* 4388–4392; 1990

Montgomery EB Jr. Basal ganglia physiology and pathophysiology: a reappraisal. *Parkinsonism and Related Disorders, 13,* 455–465; 2007

Montgomery EB Jr. Deep Brain Stimulation Programming: Mechanisms, Principles and Practice, 2nd ed. Oxford, UK: Oxford University Press; 2016

Montgomery EB Jr, Baker KB. Mechanisms of deep brain stimulation and future technical developments. *Neurological Research, 22,* 259–266. 2000

Montgomery EB Jr, Buchholz SR. The striatum and motor cortex in motor initiation and execution. *Brain Research, 549,* 222–229; 1991

Montgomery EB Jr, Gale JT. Mechanisms of action of deep brain stimulation (DBS). *Neuroscience and Biobehavioral Reviews, 32,* 388–407; 2008

Montgomery EB Jr, Clare MH, Sahrmann S, Buchholz SR, Hibbard LS, Landau WM. Neuronal multipotentiality: evidence for network representation of physiological function. *Brain Research, 580,* 49–61; 1992

Montgomery EB, Wall M, Henderson V. Principles of Neurologic Diagnosis. Boston, MA: Little, Brown and Co; 1985

Nakamura R, Nagasaki H, Narabayashi H. Arrhythmokinesia in parkinsonism. In: Birkmayer W, Hornykiewicz O, eds. Advances in Parkinsonism. Basel: Roche; 1976, 258–268

Nambu AR, Llinas R. Electrophysiology of globus pallidus neurons in vitro. *Journal of Neurophysiology 72,* 1127–1139; 1994

Nambu A, Yoshida S, Jinnai K. Projection on the motor cortex of thalamic neurons with pallidal input in the monkey. *Experimental Brain Research, 71,* 658–662; 1988

Nguyen DH, Widrow B. Neural networks for self-learning control systems. *IEEE Control Systems Magazine,* 18–23, April 1990

Plenz D, Kital ST. A basal ganglia pacemaker formed by the subthalamic nucleus and external globus pallidus. *Nature. 400*(6745), 677–682; 1999

Sakai ST, Inase M, Tanji J. Pallidal and cerebellar inputs to thalamocortical neurons projecting to the supplementary motor area in *Macaca fuscata*: a triple-labeling light microscopic study. *Anatomy and Embryology, 199,* 9–19; 1999

Sato F, Lavallée P, Lévesque M, Parent A. Single-axon tracing study of neurons of the external segment of the globus pallidus in primate. *Journal of Comparative Neurology, 417*(1), 17–31; 2000

Schmahmann J. An emerging concept. The cerebellar contribution to higher function. *Archives of Neurology,48,* 1178–1187; 1991

Schwartz AB, Kettner RE, Georgopoulos AP. Primate motor cortex and free arm movements to visual targets in three-dimensional space. I. Relations between single cell discharge and direction of movement. *Journal of Neuroscience, 8,* 2913–2927; 1988

Shin S, Sommer MA. Activity of neurons in monkey globus pallidus during oculomotor behavior compared with that in substantia nigra pars reticulata. *Journal of Neurophysiology, 103,* 1874–1887; 2010

Smyrnis N, Taira M, Ashe J, Georgopoulos AP. Motor cortical activity in a memorized delay task. *Experimental Brain Research, 92,* 139–151; 1992

Surmeier DJ, Ding J, Day M, Wang Z, Shen W. D1 and D2 dopamine-receptor modulation of striatal glutamatergic signaling in striatal medium spiny neurons. *Trends in Neurosciences, 30,* 228–235; 2007

Taub A, Robinson F, Taub E. Dorsal root ganglionectomy for intractable monoradicular sciatica. A series of 61 patients. *Stereotactic and Functional Neurosurgery, 65,* 106–110; 1995

Thach WT. Timing of activity in cerebellar dentate nucleus and cerebral motor cortex during prompt volitional movement. *Brain Research, 88,* 233–241; 1975

Tyrone ME, Kegl J, Poizner H. Interarticulator coordination in deaf signers with Parkinson's disease. *Neuropsychologia, 37,* 1271–1283; 1999

Vyas S, Huang H, Gale J, Sarma S, Montgomery E. Neuronal complexity in subthalamic nucleus is reduced in Parkinson's disease. *IEEE Transactions on Neural Systems and Rehabilitation Engineering, 24,* 36–45; 2016

Wannier T, Liu J, Morel A, Jouffrais C, Rouiller EM. Neuronal activity in primate striatum and pallidum related to bimanual motor actions. *Neuroreport, 13,* 143–147; 2002

Watson P, Montgomery EB Jr. The relationship dof neuronal activity within the sensori-motor region of the subthalamic nucleus to speech. *Brain and Language, 97,* 233–240; 2006

Yoshida A, Tanaka M. Enhanced modulation of neuronal activity during antisaccades in the primate globus pallidus. *Cerebral Cortex, 19,* 206–217; 2009

Zeng FG, Fu QJ, Morse R. Human hearing enhanced by noise. *Brain Research, 869,* 251–255; 2000

Zimnik AJ, Nora GJ, Desmurget M, Turner RS. Movement-related discharge in the macaque globus pallidus during high-frequency stimulation of the subthalamic nucleus. *Journal of Neuroscience, 35,* 3978–3989; 2015

■ Study Questions

1. A person presents with weakness and increased reflexes. Which of these would you expect to be damaged?

A. Basal ganglia
B. Cerebellum
C. Sensory neurons
D. Upper motor neurons
E. Lower motor neurons

2. The final common pathway is also known as the:

A. Neuromuscular junction
B. Upper motor neuron
C. Direct activation pathway
D. Lower motor neuron
E. Rubrospinal tract

3. This mediates skilled movements with an external target:

A. Primary motor area
B. Premotor area
C. Sensory area
D. Posterior parietal area
E. Supplementary motor area

4. Damage to the *left* cerebellum would cause:

A.   Rigidity and hypokinesia on the left side of the body
B.   Rigidity and hypokinesia on the right side of the body
C.   Incoordination on the left side of the body
D.   Incoordination on the right side of the body
E.   None of the above

5. If you have a lesion to the upper motor neurons on the right side of the brain, you will have:

A.   Drooping and weakness of the entire right side of the face
B.   Drooping and weakness of the lower right side of the face
C.   Drooping and weakness of the entire left side of the face
D.   Drooping and weakness of the lower left side of the face
E.   None of the above

6. This part of the sensorimotor system receives a copy of the motor plan and adjusts movements based on feedback from ongoing movement:

A.   Thalamus
B.   Premotor area
C.   Basal ganglia
D.   Cerebellum
E.   Primary motor area

7. Damage to the basal ganglia can cause:

A.   Ataxia
B.   Hypokinesia
C.   Hyperkinesia
D.   Hypokinesia or hyperkinesia
E.   Hypokinesia, hyperkinesia, or ataxia

8. The pyramidal system sets background muscle activity on which skilled movements are performed.

A.   True
B.   False

9. Which of these is part of the direct activation pathways or the pyramidal tract?

A.   Corticospinal tract
B.   Corticobulbar tract
C.   Corticospinal and corticobulbar tracts
D.   Rubrospinal tract
E.   Rubrospinal and corticobulbar tracts

10. Primary sensory areas (S1) do have some descending projections via the extrapyramidal system.

A.   True
B.   False

11. What part of the basal ganglia gets the major input from the cortex?

A.   Substantia nigra
B.   Striatum
C.   Nucleus accumbens
D.   Globus pallidus internal segment
E.   Subthalamic nucleus

12. The second-order neurons from the dorsal columns run in a tract called the:

A.   Spinothalamic tract
B.   Spinal trigeminal tract
C.   Medial longitudinal fasciculus
D.   Fasciculus cuneatus
E.   Medial lemniscus

13. When considering fine motor control, innervation ratio is important. An innervation ratio of 1:10 is better for fine motor control than a ratio of 1:100.

A.   True
B.   False

14. Which of these can exert an effect on a lower motor neuron?

A.   Upper motor neuron
B.   Interneuron
C.   Peripheral sensory neuron
D.   All of the above
E.   None of the above

15. The corticobulbar tract generally provides bilateral innervation to the muscles of the head and neck:

A.   True
B.   False

16. A lesion to the right basal ganglia causes deficits on the right side of the body.

A.   True
B.   False

17. Dysmetria, terminal tremor, incoordination, and ataxia are associated with lesions to the:

A. Basal ganglia
B. Thalamus
C. Motor cortex
D. Hypothalamus
E. Cerebellum

■ Answers to Study Questions

1. The correct answer is (D), upper motor neurons. Damage to upper or lower motor neurons can both cause weakness, but increased reflexes are a sign that upper motor neurons are involved.

2. The correct answer is (D), lower motor neuron. Activation of the lower motor neuron causes release of the neurotransmitter at the neuromuscular junction and thus muscle contraction. There are several ways the lower motor neuron can be activated, including by the direct activation pathway or reflexes.

3. The correct answer is (B), premotor area. The premotor area mediates skilled movments with an external target. The supplementary motor area is more involved with internally generated movements. Sensory areas, including the posterior parietal area all contribute to movement. Purposeful movement is then executed by the primary motor area.

4. The correct answer is (C), incoordination on the left side of the body. The left cerebellum has connections with the right side of the brain. The right side of the brain also controls sensorimotor function of the left side of the body. Because of these crossings, when you damage the cerebellum, you get damage to the ipsilateral (same) side of the body.

5. The correct answer is (C), drooping and weakness of the entire left side of the face. Remember, the face has a different pattern of innervation to the lower motor neurons from the upper motor neurons than most of the body (which is typically contralateral) or the head and neck (which is typically bilateral). The lower motor neurons associated with muscles of the upper face, such as the forehead, get bilateral innervation from upper motoneurons, which the lower motor neurons for the lower face get contralateral innervation from upper motor neurons. The only way to get damage to the entire face is by damaging the lower motor neuron (final common pathway) on that side of the face. With upper motor neuron damage, you get contralateral weakness of the lower face only. The upper face is preserved because of the contralateral innervation to the lower motor neurons.

6. The correct answer is (D), the cerebellum. The cerebellum is the major part of the brain that adjusts and coordinates ongoing movements using sensory feedback.

7. The correct answer is (D), hypokinesia or hyperkinesia, depending on the pattern.

8. The correct answer is (B), false. The extrapyramidal system sets up background activity and the pyramidal system mediates skilled movements. Both are necessary to achieve appropriate movement.

9. The correct answer is (C), the corticospinal and corticobulbar tracts are direct activation pathways.

10. The correct answer is (A), true. Sometimes we forget how much influence the sensory system has on motor control.

11. The correct answer is (B), striatum.

12. The correct answer is (C), medial longitudinal fasciculus.

13. The correct answer is (A), true. When you have fewer neurons to control, you can exert more finely tuned control.

14. The correct answer is (D), all of the above.

15. The correct answer is (A), true.

16. The correct answer is (B), false.

17. The correct answer is (E).

8

Peripheral Motor Control

Mary J. Sandage and David D. Pascoe

■ Chapter Summary

The study of peripheral motor control is essential to the understanding of muscle function for speech, swallowing, hearing, and balance. For both congenital and acquired disorders, speech-language pathologists and audiologists must have a working understanding of muscle physiology. The purpose of this chapter is to provide an overview of muscle anatomy and physiology through the lifespan to appreciate better the nature of impairment and the implications of rehabilitation programs on function. Specifically, we will (1) describe basic muscle anatomy and physiology as it relates to muscle function in general, (2) specify aspects of muscle development in infants and muscle decline with aging that are relevant to speech-language pathologists and audiologists, (3) address principles of muscle training and adaptations that occur with use and disuse, and (4) apply aspects of muscle physiology to clinical practice.

■ Learning Objectives

- Define anatomic and physiologic aspects of muscle cells
- Describe basic differences between muscle fiber types and their functions
- Describe muscle energy pathways (bioenergetics) and how muscle fuel is produced

- Understand muscle function in response to medications, toxins, and neuromuscular disease
- Describe how muscle tissue adapts to conditions of exercise, detraining/disuse, loss of tissue compensation, and aging

■ Putting It Into Practice

- Humans are not born with a fully intact neuromuscular system; this system continues to develop and become refined into early childhood, so that motor training interventions for infants and children should not mirror those for an adult.
- Muscle tissue has plasticity, which means that it is continually responding to the load that is imposed or the rest that is imposed with up- and downregulation of contractile metabolism and function. Principles of muscle training (specificity, overload, and reversibility) should be at the core of treatment programs that target improved muscle function in communication and swallowing disorders.
- Muscle tissue improvements are specific to the training the muscle receives. Therefore, if stronger velopharyngeal closure to reduce hypernasal speech is the desired clinical goal, the exercise protocol used by the speech-language pathologist should include activities that engage the velopharyngeal mechanism in speech tasks.

■ Introduction

Knowledge of anatomical structure and physiological function of muscle cells is critical to the speech-language pathologist and audiologist for understanding of motor control for speech, swallowing, hearing, and balance. Treatment programs for speech, voice, and swallowing increasingly focus on the role of muscle training for habilitation (improved skills and function) and rehabilitation (restoration of function after disease or injury). The speech-language pathologist and audiologist should have a comprehensive understanding of muscle morphology (anatomy) and function (physiology) that supports speech, swallowing, hearing, and balance function. This chapter focuses on (1) the structural components of the musculoskeletal system that provide the foundation for movement within the human body; and (2) the physiologic processes that integrate structure and function, produce fuel for muscular contractions, and provide the stimulus for training adaptations that improve functional movement. Muscle contraction is a highly orchestrated event, the knowledge of which is necessary to develop a greater understanding of neuromuscular disorders that can affect speech, swallowing, hearing, and balance. Additional aspects of muscle adaptations secondary to training, detraining, loss of tissue compensation, and aging are presented in the context of the skeletal muscle response to disease, injury, and recovery.

Broadly, muscle tissue can be divided into two groups: involuntary and voluntary. Smooth muscles and cardiac muscles fall into the involuntary muscle group, and their primary responsibility is to transport nutrients to cells, transport byproducts and waste from cellular activity, and support gas exchange of oxygen and carbon dioxide. Cardiac muscles work involuntarily to pump the appropriate blood flow to match work output. Smooth muscle works in a variety of systems, including the digestive system and the vascular system. Smooth muscle controls the diameter of blood vessels, thereby controlling blood flow and pressure. For example, blood can be directed to active tissues to match the need for oxygen and removal of carbon dioxide or directed toward the skin for thermoregulation. Under these conditions, less blood flow is available in the digestive tract. Smooth muscle also plays a critical role in the esophagus for swallowing.

Activation of skeletal muscles is voluntary. Skeletal muscle is recruited to develop the necessary and appropriate force outputs required to perform specific work or movement tasks. Skeletal muscle tissue, like cardiac muscle tissue, responds and adapts to specific physical demands placed upon tissues. This response is commonly referred to as the **specific adaptation to imposed demand (SAID)** principle. Plasticity of skeletal muscle tissue provides the theoretical basis for the development of muscle training programs used in communication science and disorders.

Much of what is currently known regarding muscle anatomy and physiology is derived from the study of skeletal muscle, cardiac muscle, and smooth muscle. Recently, there has been increased interest in the physiologic principles underlying muscle training interventions in treatment. As you can imagine, it is difficult to study muscles of the tongue, velum, or larynx in a living individual. Muscle biopsy, for example, is a well-established method used to study muscle physiology *in vivo* in the field of kinesiology. However, muscle biopsies are rarely performed *in vivo* in speech and hearing science. Disruption of muscle function may be too great in muscles used for airway protection or hearing. Basic knowledge regarding muscle tissue and its adaptability has the potential to provide important information on the prescription of specific exercises for patients with speech, swallowing, hearing, and balance disorders. This chapter provides an overview of muscle architecture and physiology, with particular attention given to skeletal muscle tissue, such as those tissues that constitute most muscles that support speech and swallowing.

■ Muscle Mechanics

Skeletal muscles are positioned to produce longitudinal movement through a shortening of their fiber structure that pulls on tendons or bones. When a muscle contracts, we do not recruit all the muscle fibers, but rather selected fibers within the muscle. The recruitment pattern may include hundreds to thousands of fibers appropriate for the movement task. The alignment of the muscle, more specifically the muscle fibers, develops force through a mechanical lever system. Muscles do not work in isolation; therefore, it is important to consider how muscles work in relation to the structures to which they are attached to produce movement. Skeletal muscles typically produce movement by acting on a joint that lies between the origin and insertion of the muscle. A muscle-joint complex makes up what could be considered a simple machine. Putting it another way, skeletal muscles apply a force to a lever system, resulting in movement. Bones act as lever arms, and the joint becomes the pivot point.

Three classes of levers are represented in the body. As shown in **Fig. 8.1a**, each of the three lever systems has a fulcrum (F), or pivot point, a load (L),

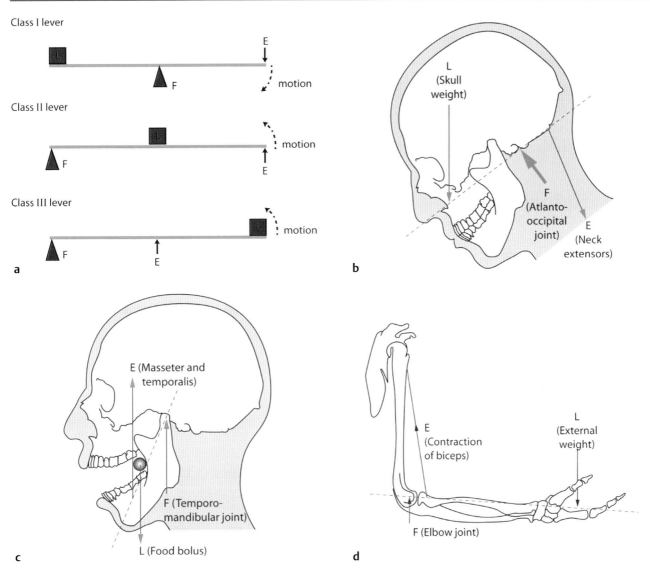

Fig. 8.1 Levers in the musculoskeletal system. **(a)** The three classes of levers. F is the fulcrum (pivot point), L is the load, and E is the effort applied. **(b)** Examples of Class I levers. **(c)** Examples of Class II levers. **(d)** Examples of Class III levers.

and applied effort (E). These levers are denoted as Class I, Class II, and Class III, all of which are represented in systems used for communication and hearing. As illustrated in **Fig. 8.1b**, movement of the head in a forward posture is an example of a Class I lever. In this example, the atlantooccipital joint is the pivot point (fulcrum), and the skull weight is the load, with the neck extensors providing the effort. Few examples of Class I levers exist in the body. In **Fig. 8.1c**, a Class II lever is shown, as the temporomandibular joint works as the pivot point for a food bolus, which serves as the load, with the effort applied via the masseter and temporalis muscles. Opening the jaw against resistance is another example of a Class II lever. The ossicular chain in the middle ear is also considered a Class II lever. A

Class III lever is illustrated in **Fig. 8.1d**, in a classic example of the elbow joint as the fulcrum and the lower arm and hand providing the external weight. This lever takes advantage of the length of the lever arm in which the effort is placed between the load and fulcrum. As such, the effort or muscular force travels a shorter distance than the load (greater range of motion, increased capacity for speed of movement). Class III levers are the most common in the human body and provide rapid movements with little muscle contraction distance.

Muscles vary greatly in size and shape. The tensor tympani, which is responsible for adjusting tension in the eardrum, has only a few hundred muscle fibers, whereas the principal calf muscle, gastrocnemius, has over a million muscle fibers (MacIntosh et

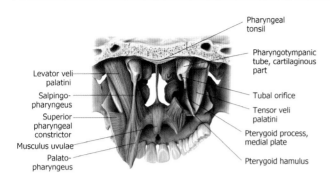

Fig. 8.2   The musculus uvulae provides central bulk to the velum during velar elevation, a feature of a fusiform muscle orientation.

al 2006). Muscle fiber number and size are consistent with function and the degree of force required. Muscles also differ in shape and orientation. Muscles in which the fibers are oriented in a longitudinal fashion to the belly of the muscle are described as having a **fusiform** shape. An example of a fusiform muscle is the musculus uvulae in the velum (**Fig. 8.2**). Contraction of individual muscle fibers in a fusiform-oriented muscle results in shortening of the muscle. Other muscle fibers are oriented in a fan-shaped or **pinnate** arrangement. Muscle fibers

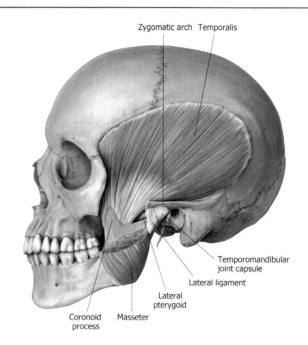

Fig. 8.3   The fanlike structure of the temporalis muscle contributes to greater force production.

arranged in a pinnate fashion are generally shorter than those in a fusiform muscle arrangement; however, the angle of pull on the associated tendon pro-

Box 8.1   Electromyography

When a muscle contracts, an electrical signal is produced that, when recorded, sounds like radio static. Electromyography (EMG) measures motor unit recruitment by determining the amount of electrical activity a muscle generates during contraction. EMG is used in research to study muscles of articulation, swallowing, and voicing; it is also used clinically to help diagnose and treat certain disorders of communication and swallowing. There are two EMG methods: surface electrodes (SEMG) and intramuscular needle or hooked-wire electrodes. SEMG is used when the electrical activity of the muscle can be detected through the skin. The masseter is an example of a muscle that can be studied using SEMG. Many of the muscles of interest for articulation, phonation, and swallowing are too small or located too deep to the skin surface to be detectable with SEMG; therefore, intramuscular EMG methods are preferred. Intramuscular EMG requires inserting a thin needle or hooked wire into the muscle of interest.

Clinically, EMG is frequently used to diagnose vocal fold paralysis. Once a vocal fold paralysis is suspected, needle or hooked-wire EMG can be used to determine whether a given laryngeal muscle is producing any electrical signal or not. Absence of electrical signal can confirm a suspected diagnosis of muscle paralysis. The timing of diagnostic EMG matters. If, for example, a unilateral vocal fold paralysis is suspected due to severing of the recurrent laryngeal nerve during surgical removal of the thyroid, EMG to confirm the paralysis should be deferred for about 1 month. Denervated muscles continue to have measurable electric activity for a short time after nerve damage, rendering EMG potentially misleading in the early days following nerve damage.

Another common clinical use of intramuscular EMG is EMG-guided botulinum toxin injections for the treatment of spasmodic dysphonia, a neurologic voice disorder. Injection of botulinum toxin into the upper airway requires precision to avoid breathing or swallowing impairment from the toxin. Given that the muscles most frequently injected with botulinum toxin (thyroarytenoid, lateral cricoarytenoid, and posterior cricoarytenoid muscles) are deeply placed within the upper airway, laryngologists and neurologists who conduct this procedure often prefer to determine proper muscle location via EMG prior to injecting the toxin.

vides a performance advantage. An example of the latter is the temporalis (**Fig. 8.3**), whose pinnated arrangement largely accounts for the significant strength of the jaw (McComas 1998).

■ The Motor Unit

The motor unit (discussed in **Chapter 7**) is the smallest functional unit, but not the smallest contractile unit, of a whole muscle that can be activated at any given time. The motor unit comprises the nerve that innervates the muscle (**alpha lower motor neuron**, α-LMN), the **neuromuscular junctions (NMJs)**, and the muscle fibers that are innervated by that motor neuron (**Fig. 8.4**). Each individual muscle fiber is innervated by a single motor neuron. However, a single motor neuron innervates a group of muscle fibers ranging in size from a few to thousands. The small muscles of the larynx, for example, are innervated by fewer motor neurons than the larger muscles in the legs. Motor units that innervate fewer fibers can provide discrete amounts of force that are important in fine motor skills, such as voicing. Given that a single motor neuron innervates a group of muscle fibers, it may be assumed that these fibers are grouped together, but this is not the case. Muscle fibers innervated by a single motor neuron are rarely located right next to each other and are instead distributed throughout the whole muscle. Electromyography is one means to study motor unit recruitment intramuscularly as described in **Box 8.1**.

Conscious activation of the motor unit can be initiated in the brain (cerebral cortex) or be the result of a reflex arc. The reflex arc, as illustrated in **Fig. 8.5**, has three components: afferent branch (sensory receptor and nerve); interneuron, which crosses the spinal cord and redirects the reflex response; and efferent branch (one or more nerves that link to muscular response). In communication and swallowing, the reflex arc is important for the pharyngeal reflex or gag response and swallowing reflex.

■ Motor Unit Development

Motor unit development is not complete at birth and continues for some time after birth. The fact that the neuromuscular system is still developing should be considered when developing an intervention for motor tasks, such as swallowing, in infants and small children. **Myospecificity**, or the manner in which a motor unit develops in the fetus through early childhood and during reinnervation, is a highly organized process. The generation of motor units is neither random nor solely due to mechanical factors such as limb mobility. In the embryonic stage, nerve–muscle specificity occurs before muscle fibers are fully developed. Evidence also suggests that neuronal specificity develops even if muscle location is surgically changed prior to the formation of the motor unit (Landmesser 1980). Growth of the nerve axon toward the specific muscle occurs while that muscle is still developing. Muscle formation is called **myogenesis**. When the axon has extended sufficiently to meet up with the muscle, the

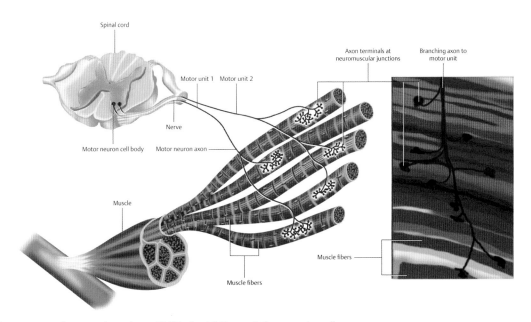

Fig. 8.4   The motor unit comprises the α-LMN, the NMJs, and the muscle cells.

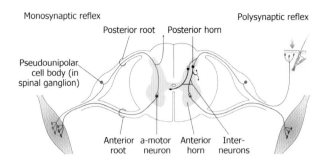

Fig. 8.5 Polysynaptic reflexes may be mediated by receptors inside of or remote from the muscle (e.g., skin); these receptors react via interneurons to stimulate muscle contraction. Muscular function at the unconscious (reflex) level is controlled by the gray matter of the spinal cord.

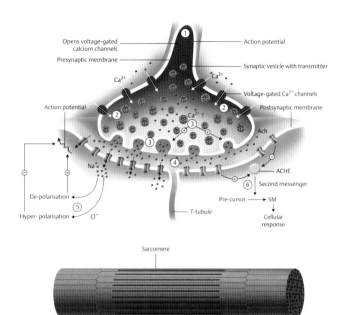

Fig. 8.6 Synaptic signal transmission. An action potential (AP) arriving at the presynaptic membrane (1) causes voltage-gated Ca^{2+} channels to open (2), admitting calcium ions to flow into the cell. This increase in intracellular $[Ca^{2+}]$ triggers the release of neurotransmitter molecules from their storage vesicles into the synaptic cleft (3). Neurotransmitter molecules then diffuse across the synaptic cleft (4) and bind with ionotropic or metabotropic receptors on the postsynaptic membrane. Ionotropic receptors are ligand-gated ion channels. Ligand (in this case, neurotransmitter) binding (5) causes the inflow of ions into the cell, resulting in either **depolarization** (inflow of **cations**) or **hyperpolarization** (inflow of **anions**). (6) Ligand binding to metabotropic receptors activates G proteins, which transduce a cellular response via second messenger molecules.

axon terminal converges in **synaptogenesis**, the formation of the synapse that bridges the nerve and the muscle cell. Synapse sites are likely selected through a combination of local signaling from neural cell adhesion molecules (NCAMs), which are found in abundance in embryonic and perinatal muscle (Covault et al 1986), and **acetylcholine (ACh) neurotransmitter** receptors that cover the muscle surface. Once the initial synapses are formed, a process of synapse elimination occurs, wherein only the synapses with the greatest accumulations of ACh receptors remain (Poo 1982; Fambrough 1979), leaving each axon terminal with a single synapse. This elimination process leaves behind the NMJ. The motor unit that is ultimately formed may be further delineated by muscle fiber type characteristics that are based on contractile and metabolic (energy) properties, as described subsequently in the discussion of muscle fiber types.

■ Excitation-Contraction Coupling

The nerve that innervates muscle fibers is a peripheral nerve that receives neural stimulation from the central nervous system (CNS). As the motor axon approaches a muscle fiber, it loses its **myelin sheath** and branches into small "twigs" that lie on the surface of the muscle fiber (MacIntosh et al 2006), terminating in **motor end plates**, as shown in **Fig. 8.4**. The juncture of the nerve "twig" and muscle cell, the NMJ, is a complex structure. As shown in **Fig. 8.6**, the motor end plate does not adhere directly to the surface of the muscle fiber. Instead, it approximates the surface of the muscle fiber, leaving a space between the motor end plate and muscle that is called the **synaptic cleft** or synapse. As described

in **Chapter 6**, the signal coming down the nerve axon to the NMJ is in the form of an electrical pulse known as an **action potential** (AP). To cross the physical gap between the nerve and the muscle tissue, this electrical pulse causes the release of neurotransmitter, transforming the nerve electrical signal into a chemical signal that diffuses across the gap. Muscle fiber activation involves the process of **excitation-contraction coupling**: excitation of the motor end plate precedes muscle fiber contraction. The neural impulse that triggers muscle fiber contraction is based on an all-or-none principle: either there is an AP or there is not. The threshold of excitation at the cell body of the α-LMN must exceed the minimum required for the AP to be generated and travel to the neuromuscular junction. If any impairment of the excitation-contraction coupling process occurs, atypical muscle contraction may occur (e.g., muscle paresis or weakness, fatigue, or paralysis).

The membrane that covers the motor end plate is called the **presynaptic membrane**. When an AP arrives at the axon terminal, the voltage-gated calcium (Ca²⁺) channels open up, allowing Ca²⁺ to enter into the axon terminal. Ca²⁺ and clathrin are required for the mobilization of ACh vesicles to the membrane, to which they fuse, releasing their contents into the synaptic cleft (**exocytosis**). Once in the synapse, ACh travels across the synaptic cleft; the space that separates the axon terminal from the muscle fiber surface is about 70 nanometers wide (MacIntosh et al 2006). This space contains **acetylcholinesterase (AChE)**, an enzyme that breaks ACh down into its two ingredients (choline and acetic acid), thus regulating how much ACh makes it across the synapse to the postsynaptic membrane. This is an important regulatory process that ensures that one action potential initiates only one contractile sequence.

Muscle anatomy has some distinctive nomenclature compared to that of other cells. The muscle cell outer membrane is called a **sarcolemma**, unlike other cells in which the cell membrane is called the plasmalemma. The sarcolemma that covers a muscle cell is populated with **postsynaptic acetylcholine receptors (AChRs)**. AChRs are not permanently fixed within the muscle fiber membrane but are grouped together around the NMJ. These postsynaptic receptors are responsible for perpetuating the impulse along the sarcolemma. The number and proximity of AChRs in the sarcolemma varies depending on muscle training, detraining, aging, and/or neuromuscular disease. AChRs are continually renewed and replaced with an average half-life of 8 to 11 days (Fambrough 1979). An adequate number of AChRs tightly arranged at the neuromuscular junction is necessary for optimal muscle contraction. In contrast to nerve tissue, electrical stimulation propagated to the muscle cell travels bilaterally away from the NMJ. The physiology, and therefore the effectiveness, of the NMJ can be altered by medications and toxins as described in **Box 8.2**.

Below the sarcolemma lies the sarcoplasm (corresponding to cytoplasm in other cells), in which the organelles, cellular proteins, and **myofibrils** are contained. Invaginations, or channels, within the sarcolemma called **transverse tubules (T-tubules)** travel deep into the muscle cell. T-tubules are responsible for carrying the neural signal transmitted across the NMJ to another network of channels, the **sarcoplasmic reticulum (SR)**. The SR, corresponding to the endoplasmic reticulum in other cells, serves vital regulatory functions within the muscle fiber, storing, releasing, and resequestering calcium (Ca²⁺) required for muscle contraction and relaxation. As shown in **Fig. 8.7**, the SR has a net-

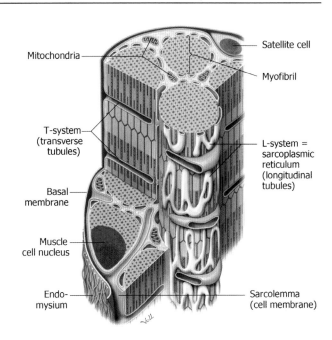

Fig. 8.7 Network of channels in muscle cell.

like appearance, enmeshing each myofibril deep to the SR structure. This arrangement is ideal for rapid availability of Ca²⁺ for muscle contraction and rapid reuptake of Ca²⁺ (via Ca²⁺-ATP pumps) when contraction ceases. Calcium is tightly regulated by the SR and is released only to initiate muscle contraction when the excitation component of excitation-contraction coupling has successfully taken place. Only with exposure to Ca²⁺ ions can the muscle contractile proteins attach to each other to produce force. As long as the contractile proteins are exposed to Ca²⁺, muscle contraction will occur.

■ Skeletal Muscle

Skeletal muscles are the primary muscles used for communication and swallowing. Skeletal muscles are highly organized structures consisting of bundles of muscle fibers, which are in turn, made of bundles of the smallest contractile units, **sarcomeres**. The end-to-end, or serial, arrangement of the sarcomeres enables the contraction distance of each sarcomere to be additive across the entire length of the fiber. Muscle fiber alignment, the number of fibers, metabolic fiber type, stimulation, and the manner in which fibers are recruited dictate the amount of force that can be produced by the muscle. As shown in **Fig. 8.8**, muscle cells are encased in an outer membrane called the sarcolemma. A unique aspect of muscle cell anatomy

Box 8.2 Neuromuscular Junction

The neuromuscular junction is complex in terms of both anatomy and physiology. Many opportunities exist for interruption or alteration of the transmission of a neural impulse to the muscle fiber, due to environmental agents, neurotransmitter inhibitors, and disease processes. Once a general understanding of NMJ physiology is established, the various mechanisms that interrupt excitation-contraction coupling become clearer. The degree to which neural transmission is negatively affected will have a lot to do with the point at which NMJ physiology is interrupted. The functional manifestations of NMJ interruption may vary from muscle weakness (paresis) or complete loss of muscle function (paralysis) to overstimulation of muscle fibers. There are several points at which transmission of the neural impulse may be interrupted or amplified: the presynaptic membrane, the synaptic cleft, and the postsynaptic membrane. As illustrated in (A) in **Box Fig. 8.1**, botulinum toxin interrupts packaging and release of the neurotransmitter acetylcholine (ACh) into the synaptic cleft. There are several forms of botulinum toxin in nature; two of these forms have come into medical use: type A (Botox, Allergan, Dublin, Ireland) and type B (Myobloc, US WorldMeds, Louisville, KY). Botulinum toxin is a reversible inhibitor, which means that its effect of preventing ACh vesicles from merging with the presynaptic membrane for exocytosis of ACh into the synaptic cleft slowly wears off. Botulinum toxin is used to treat spasmodic dys-phonia, a neurogenic voice disorder characterized by involuntary muscle spasms in intrinsic laryngeal muscles during connected speech.

An alternative location that NMJ function can be altered is the synaptic cleft between the pre- and post-synaptic membranes. As illustrated in image B in **Box Fig. 8.1**, organophosphate agents such as the nerve gas sarin prevent AChE, the "off switch" for the excitation signal, from clearing ACh from the synaptic cleft, preventing the muscle from ceasing to contract.

Postsynaptic ACh receptors can also be affected by toxins and neuromuscular disease. In image C in **Box Fig. 8.1**, snake venom neurotoxins such as bungarotoxin (produced by kraits) or cobratoxin (produced by cobras) bind to postsynaptic ACh receptors, competitively inhibiting binding of ACh to the postsynaptic membrane, preventing propagation of the neural impulse to the muscle fiber. NMJ alterations of the postsynaptic membrane also occur with the chronic autoimmune neuromuscular disease myasthenia gravis (MG), which is characterized by weakness of specific voluntary muscles that is not accompanied by general fatigue. As shown in image D in **Box Fig. 8.1**, in MG postsynaptic ACh receptors are fewer in number and partially blocked by antibodies, which result in weakened transmission of the neural impulse. Because MG can affect muscles of articulation, voice, and swallowing, therapy programs need to be designed to reduce muscle fatigue during exacerbation of the disease.

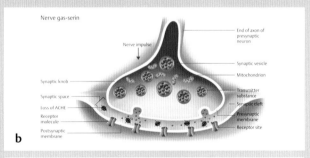

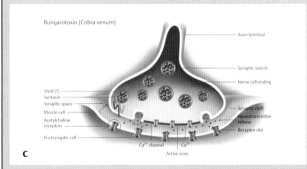

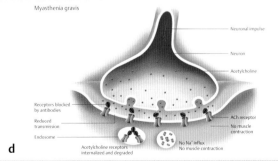

Box Fig. 8.1 Interference with excitation-contraction coupling in the NMJ. **(a)** Botulinum toxin prevents release of ACh into the synaptic cleft. **(b)** Sarin prevents AChE from resetting the excitation signal. **(c)** Snake venom neurotoxin prevents ACh from binding to AChRs on the postsynaptic membrane. **(d)** Antibodies bind to AChRs in MG.

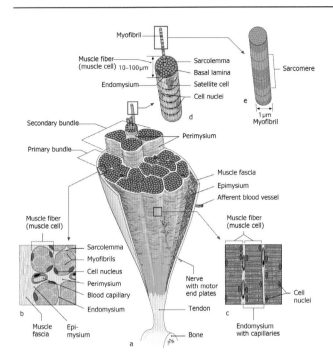

Fig. 8.8 Structure of a skeletal muscle. **(a)** Cross section of a skeletal muscle; **(b)** detail from (a) (cross section); **(c)** detail from (a) (longitudinal section); **(d)** structure of a muscle fiber (= muscle cell); **(e)** structure of a myofibril.

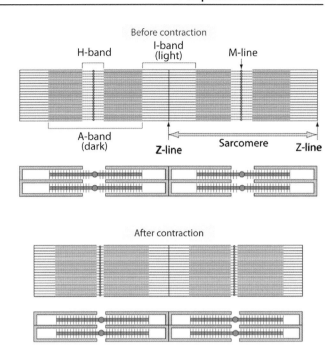

Fig. 8.9 Dark and light bands in striated muscle. Contraction reduces the widths of the I-band and H-band, but the width of the A-band remains unchanged.

is the presence of satellite cells, located above the sarcolemma, which play a key role in muscle repair and growth. New muscle fibers can be formed from activated satellite cells, and new nuclei can be contributed to existing muscle fibers during muscle growth (e.g., during strength training).

Deep to the SR lie the myofibrils, threadlike structures made up of serially arranged sarcomeres that contain the primary contractile proteins. Recruited myofibrils that make up the muscle fiber are responsible for producing contractile force. Skeletal muscles are striated; that is, under high magnification they are crossed by repeating differently colored stripes or bands. The coloration differences illuminate the architecture of the myofibrils that make up the muscle fiber and the sarcomeres that make up the myofibrils. As can be seen in **Fig. 8.9**, a diagram of two sarcomeres placed end to end, the juncture between two sarcomeres is called the **Z-line**, which is represented as a light band. The dark bands (**A-bands**) contain the primary contractile proteins: **actin** and **myosin**.

Muscle fibers are composed of bundled myofibrils, which are in turn composed of bundled sarcomeres arranged end to end. Muscle fiber length is variable and can change with the addition or elimination of sarcomeres at the end of the fiber. An example of sarcomere addition is during devel-

opment, when sarcomeres are added to lengthen muscle fibers as they adapt to skeletal growth. Conversely, sarcomeres can also be removed in response to chronic muscle shortening, as when a limb is immobilized in a cast and the muscle is not positioned at optimal resting length. Sarcomeres are uniformly organized with the primary contractile proteins, actin and myosin (**Fig. 8.10**). These two contractile proteins work together to engage the sarcomere in muscle contraction (shortening). Simply put, when contractile proteins are stimulated to contract, myosin adheres to the actin, and together these contractile proteins slide along each other in a corkscrew fashion to produce force within the muscle fiber. Actin, also referred to as the thin filament, when examined close-up, resembles two strings of pearls intertwined together. Actin is the location of the myosin head binding site. A long, regulatory protein called **tropomyosin** winds around the actin filament and covers the binding site for myosin, the thick filament (**Fig. 8.11**). Attached to this tropomyosin strand is a complex of three proteins called **troponin**. The three proteins each have regulatory functions. Troponin T holds the protein complex onto the tropomyosin strand. Troponin I maintains the position of the tropomyosin strand over the active sites. Troponin C has a strong affinity for Ca^{2+}; when calcium is released into the cell, troponin C pulls the tropo-

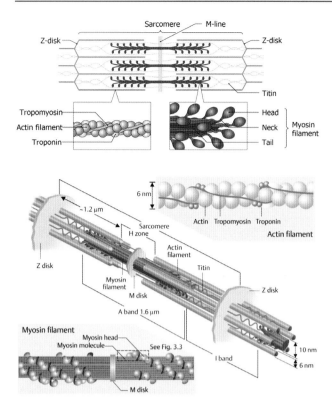

Fig. 8.10 Sarcomeres are bounded by Z-disks. The I-band contains only thin actin filaments. The A-band contains thick filaments and is where the actin and myosin filaments overlap. The H-zone contains only myosin filaments, which thicken toward the middle of the sarcomere to form the M-line. Actin is a globular protein molecule. Four hundred such molecules join to form F-actin, a beaded polymer chain. Two of the twisted protein chains combine to form an actin filament. Tropomyosin molecules joined end to end lie adjacent to the actin filaments, and a troponin molecule is attached every 40 nm or so. The sarcomere also has another system of filaments formed by the filamentous protein titin. Titin is anchored to the M-lines and Z-disks. Each myosin filament consists of bundles of myosin molecules.

myosin away from the myosin-binding sites. Actin filaments are positioned along the outside edges of the sarcomere. Myosin, the thick filaments, are positioned toward the center of the sarcomere. The overlap of actin and myosin creates the dark banding characteristic of striated muscle. Myosin filaments are called thick filaments because their individual architecture make this contractile protein appear darker than the thinner actin filament. A single myosin molecule is made up of a single tail with two globular heads attached at one end (**Fig. 8.12**). The myosin filament is made up of several hundred myosin molecule tails intertwined together, with the myosin heads sticking out to be available for attachment to the actin filament. Each myosin head contains a heavy chain of amino acids (proteins) and two light chains that are the point of attachment to the actin filament. Properties inherent to the myosin head are used for one method of muscle fiber typing.

The anatomy of the muscle fiber serves as the foundation for further description of excitation-contraction coupling. Once the neural impulse is transmitted to the muscle cell membrane, or sarcolemma, it is transported into the skeletal muscle cell by the T-tubules to the sarcoplasmic reticulum (SR), which then releases Ca^{2+} in the region of the myofilaments, actin and myosin—the second place Ca^{2+} plays an important role in excitation-contraction coupling, after its role in presynaptic release of ACh. Released Ca^{2+} binds to the troponin complex, lifting the tropomyosin away from the actin filament to expose the myosin binding site, allowing interaction between the myosin and actin filaments. When the neural impulse stops, Ca^{2+} is no longer released from the SR and is taken back up by Ca-ATP pumps in the SR and stored for later use. Ca^{2+} bound to the troponin complex is also released for uptake by the SR. Calcium availability is highly regulated in muscle cells. The return of Ca^{2+} to the

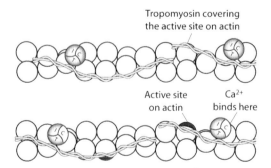

Fig. 8.11 Tropomyosin covering myosin binding site and troponin complex. Binding of calcium ions to troponin C shifts the tropomyosin molecule, uncovering the active sites on actin that bind to myosin heads.

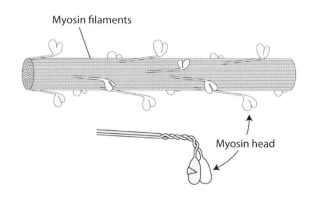

Fig. 8.12 Orientation of myosin filaments.

SR requires energy in the form of **adenosine triphosphate (ATP)**, one instance in which ATP is critical for muscle contraction/relaxation. With Ca^{2+} removed from the sarcoplasm, the myosin head can be separated from the actin filament if ATP is available. If ATP is unavailable, filaments will remain locked together in a state of rigor. The role of Ca^{2+} differs in smooth and cardiac muscles, which rely on external sources of Ca^{2+}.

Our current understanding of the interaction of myosin and actin was clarified by work conducted in the 1950s by two unrelated research groups. Andrew Huxley and Jean Hansen (1954), on the one hand, and Hugh Huxley (not related) and Rolf Niedergerke (1954), on the other, conducted experiments independently of each other, and both published their results in the same issue of *Nature*. Both groups proposed in their separate research papers that muscle contraction could be explained by a sliding movement of the actin and myosin filaments past each other, thus establishing the **sliding filament theory** of muscle contraction. When a muscle fiber shortens, the opposing actin filaments within each sarcomere slide along the myosin filaments positioned next to the actin (**Fig. 8.13**), where the actin filament can be seen to slide medially, engaging a larger percentage of the myosin filament during fiber shortening. For force production, the contractile proteins must do more than slide past one another. The manner in which myosin and actin fibers engage with each other, triggered by the release of Ca^{2+} as described in the previous paragraph, is explained by the **cross-bridge theory** of skeletal muscle. Observations of muscle contractions with electron micrographs indicated that the myosin heads attached momentarily to the actin filament, forming cross-bridges. Through a series of myosin head attachments to the actin filaments followed by a power stroke motion of the myosin head, the actin filament moved to a new position, as shown in **Fig. 8.14**. The effectiveness of this cross-bridge relationship between the two contractile proteins is largely influenced by the resting relative position of actin and myosin within each sarcomere.

■ Muscle Fiber Types

Skeletal muscle has several types of fibers often categorized by their biochemical properties, color (white and red), motor unit characteristics, and ability to produce force. Muscle energy requirements, force production capability, and fatigability are better understood with knowledge of muscle fiber typing. Knowledge of muscle fiber types that make up a particular muscle can provide improved understanding of how specific muscles may respond to training. This information can also be used to make predictions about muscle function. The human body comprises a continuum of

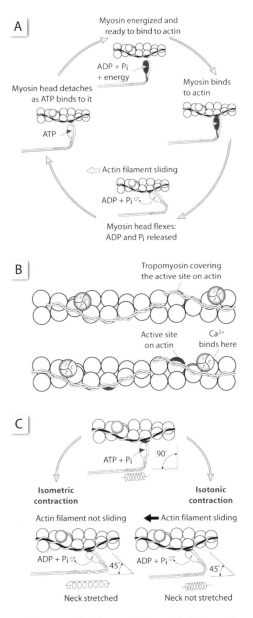

Fig. 8.14 The cross-bridge cycle in a skeletal muscle.

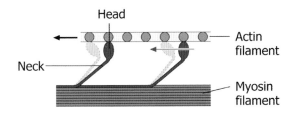

Fig. 8.13 Structure of a sarcomere: interaction between myosin heads and actin.

muscle fiber types and muscles providing an array of movement possibilities and discrete amounts of force. Despite this complexity, most descriptions of muscle fibers simplify the classification into three primary groups: fast-twitch, intermediate, and slow-twitch. Muscle fiber types are most often classified based on characteristics of force production and the ability to resist fatigue. Morphological aspects (features of form and structure) are delineated by differences in size, cell features, and vascular supply. The morphologic composition of muscle fibers is adaptable and can be altered by muscle training, detraining, disuse, electrical stimulation, and aging. The following section provides a description of the anatomical aspects of specific muscle fiber types, but it should be noted that muscle tissue is constantly adapting to changing demands.

Slow-twitch muscle fibers are generally considered to be the most resistant to fatigue, but have less ability to produce power. Slow-twitch fibers are typically called Type I fibers or slow-oxidative (SO) fibers. Refer to **Table 8.1** for a summary of labeling terminology and anatomic features of the muscle types. Slow-twitch fibers rely more on oxygen in producing energy, facilitated by an increased network of capillaries. Because of their greater reliance on oxygen, slow-twitch fibers have more **mitochondria**, the organelles in a cell that produce ATP and consume oxygen; they are often referred to as the "powerhouse" of the cell. With training, the number of capillaries and mitochondria increase, thereby increasing the exercise capacity of the muscle. These fibers are primarily used for endurance activities that require fatigue resistance and provide postural support.

Fast-twitch fibers are referred to as Type II fibers and are typically divided into two groups:

fast oxidative-glycolytic/fatigue-resistant (Type IIa) and fast-fatigable (Type IIx) as described in **Table 8.1**. An additional Type II muscle fiber type (IIL) has been identified in the intrinsic laryngeal skeletal muscles (Hoh 2005). Fast-twitch fibers are used primarily for muscle effort that requires power. Type II muscle fibers fatigue more quickly than slow-twitch fibers. Within the fast-twitch fiber group, Type IIa fibers are more fatigue-resistant than the fast-fatigable IIx fibers. Although fast-twitch fibers primarily rely on anaerobic sources of energy, IIa fibers have some reliance on the oxidative system to contribute to reduced fatigue. Structurally, these muscles have less capillary and mitochondrial density than Type I fibers. With strength training, fast-twitch fibers develop a larger cross-sectional area than Type I fibers. Fast-twitch fibers are generally used for muscle activities that require power over a short period of time, such as heavy lifting or propelling a bolus of food from the mouth into the pharynx for swallowing. Fast-twitch fibers may also play an important role in airway protection, as seen in rapid coughing in response to having food or liquid go down the wrong way. The muscle fiber complement of the intrinsic laryngeal muscles is described in **Box 8.3**.

■ Bioenergetics

All forms of human movement, including speech, breathing, and swallowing, in health and in recovery/rehabilitation, are energetic events, which means that these movements require energy. Muscles require energy in order to contract and relax. This energy comes in the form of ATP, the energy currency of the body. The ATP molecule consists

Table 8.1 Muscle fiber type characteristics

Characteristics	Muscle Fiber Types		
	Type I	Type IIa	Type IIx
Contractile properties	Slow-twitch	Fast-twitch	Fast-twitch
Fatigue resistance	High	Moderate	Low
Glycolytic capacity	Low	High	High
Oxidative capacity	High	Medium/high	Low
Metabolic properties	Slow, oxidative	Fast, oxidative, glycolytic	Fast, glycolytic
Exercise	Prolonged, moderate intensity	Shorter, high-intensity activity, stop-and-go activities	Shorter, high-intensity activity, stop-and-go activities
Sport	Distance running	Soccer, football, basketball	Basketball, soccer, football

Box 8.3 Muscle Fiber Types in the Human Larynx

The human larynx includes skeletal muscle fibers that in some respects are distinct from limb skeletal muscle. The muscle fiber complement of the intrinsic laryngeal skeletal muscles is well suited for the work required of these muscles for both the biologic role of airway protection and the nonbiologic role of communication. As can be seen in the graphs in **Box Fig. 8.2**, adapted from Rosenfield et al (1982), the lateral cricoarytenoid (LCA), interarytenoid (IA), and cricothyroid (CT) had a higher percentage of Type II muscle fibers in three cadavers investigated. This distribution makes functional sense given that these muscles are primarily responsible for rapid adduction of the vocal folds for airway protection and articulation. The thyroaryte-

noid (TA) had a more variable fiber type complement among the three cadavers. These differences may, in part, account for why there are individual differences in the ability to produce vocal power. However, production of vocal power is complex and encompasses far more than entrainment of the TA. The posterior cricoarytenoid (PCA) is distinct in that it clearly has a higher percentage of Type I fibers across the cadavers studied. Given that the PCA is primarily responsible for maintaining a patent (open) airway during most of our waking and sleeping time, it makes sense that this muscle would comprise more fatigue-resistant muscle fibers. Ultrafast muscle fibers, Type IIL (Tellis et al 2004), and slow tonic muscle fibers (Han et al 1999), which are precisely controlled and fatigue resistant, have also been identified in the IA and TA, respectively.

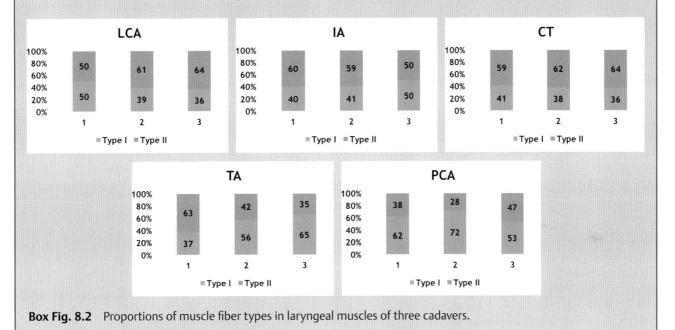

Box Fig. 8.2 Proportions of muscle fiber types in laryngeal muscles of three cadavers.

of adenosine (ribose sugar plus the RNA and DNA base adenine) bound to a chain of three phosphate groups, the last being attached by a particularly high-energy bond. When an enzyme breaks down (hydrolyzes) the ATP to adenosine diphosphate (ADP) and an inorganic phosphate ion, the energy of the bond is transferred to the enzyme, which can then do some mechanical work. Muscles often store a small amount of ATP for immediate use when muscles are called into action. Additional ATP required for continued muscle use, either through repeated power tasks or through endurance tasks, has to be made within the muscle cells themselves to keep the muscle working. The term **bioenergetics** refers to the process by which cells

(such as muscle cells) use oxygen from the air we breathe and molecules from the food and liquid we consume to obtain energy and store it in ATP. Two primary types of bioenergetics exist: anaerobic and aerobic. An overview of these pathways is provided in **Fig. 8.15**.

Anaerobic bioenergetic pathways do not require oxygen in the biochemical pathway to produce ATP. Two anaerobic pathways exist from which humans obtain fuel: the **immediate energy system** and **glycolysis**. These energy pathways are primarily used by Type II fibers for brief, high-intensity, or power tasks, such as lifting a heavy object or airway protection. The immediate energy system, so called because the energy sources it uses are

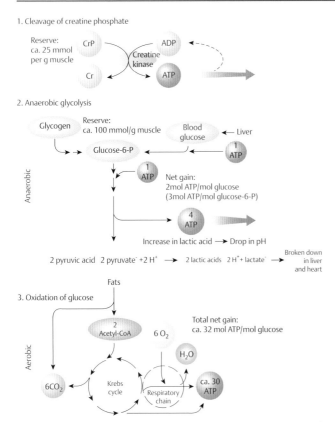

1. Cleavage of creatine phosphate

Reserve:
ca. 25 mmol
per g muscle

CrP   Creatine kinase   ADP

Cr   ATP

2. Anaerobic glycolysis

Glycogen   Reserve: ca. 100 mmol/g muscle   Blood glucose   ← Liver

Anaerobic

Glucose-6-P   1 ATP

1 ATP   Net gain:
2 mol ATP/mol glucose
(3 mol ATP/mol glucose-6-P)

4 ATP

Increase in lactic acid → Drop in pH

2 pyruvic acid   2 pyruvate$^-$ +2 H$^+$ ⟶ 2 lactic acids   2 H$^+$+ lactate$^-$ ⟶ Broken down in liver and heart

Fats

3. Oxidation of glucose

Aerobic

2 Acetyl-CoA   6 O$_2$ Total net gain: ca. 32 mol ATP/mol glucose

H$_2$O

6CO$_2$ Krebs cycle   Respiratory chain   ca. 30 ATP

Fig. 8.15 Anaerobic glycolysis (2) produces 4 ATP and feeds pyruvate into the aerobic oxidative phosphorylation process (3).

immediately available to support muscle contraction, is primarily used for power activities and is largely depleted within 30 seconds. The immediate energy system uses local muscle stores of ATP, creatine phosphate, or biochemical pathways that can provide immediate ATP for energy consumption. It is suited to quicker bouts of exercise as well as to such tasks as propelling a bolus of food from the back of the tongue, through the pharynx, and into the esophagus. Temporally, this is also the logical energy pathway for muscles of articulation during connected speech, which are entrained for only fractions of a second at a time as a speaker moves from voiced to voiceless phonemes, produces consonant blends, and marks punctuation in connected speech with pauses and breathing. This energy pathway, although rapidly depleted, can be restored during a short recovery period of ~ 2 minutes. As described in the Muscle Adaptations section of this chapter, muscle training can make the recovery of the immediate energy system more efficient by enhancing the storage potential of the muscle for energy substrates and increasing the concentrations of enzymes that increase the rate of biochemical reactions.

Muscle activity that lasts beyond the immediate energy system relies on both anaerobic glycolysis and aerobic metabolic pathways. Glycolysis is a non-oxidative (no oxygen required) pathway that is activated when muscle activity begins and can extend maximally for 30 to 45 seconds. Glycolysis relies on glucose, a simple sugar that is either imported into the cell from circulating blood or acquired by breaking down glycogen stored in muscle cells or the liver. Type II muscle fibers rely more heavily on glycolysis for production of ATP and, therefore, are more densely packed with the enzymes required to break down glucose or glycogen rapidly. For each glucose molecule, glycolysis will yield a net of two ATP and two electron transfer agents (nicotinamide adenine dinucleotide, reduced; NADH). Glycogen will provide three ATP and two electron transfer agents, as the ATP needed to bring glucose into the cell was already accounted for when the glucose molecule was brought into the muscle cell and incorporated into the glycogen. This nonoxidative yield from glycolysis is modest when compared to continued aerobic metabolism of glucose or fats. This glycolytic source of ATP is most useful for muscle activities sustained for up to about 2 minutes. One of the byproducts of glycolysis is lactate (La^{2+}), which, when released into the muscle, was formerly thought to cause muscle soreness. This is not the case, as lactate is a byproduct that is used as fuel (**Box 8.4**).

The aerobic energy pathway used by muscle tissue is called **oxidative phosphorylation**; this pathway is most efficient at delivering the largest quantity of ATP. Oxidative phosphorylation is initiated when muscle activity starts, but it does not take over as the primary source for ATP production until about 2 minutes or more into exercise. Energy sources used in oxidative phosphorylation include carbohydrates (sugars), fats, and amino acids. For the glucose molecules, glycolysis provides the entrance pathway to oxidative phosphorylation. Fats and proteins can enter the oxidative phosphorylation cycle without going through glycolysis. Oxidative phosphorylation is so efficient at producing energy that 36 to 38 ATP are produced from one glucose molecule, far more than the two produced by glycolysis. Production of ATP from fats provides even more energy, which varies according to the size of the fatty acid chains on the molecule.

To summarize, all three energy pathways are activated at the start of muscle activity. Depending on the intensity of exercise, the immediate energy system gradually gives way to glycolysis, which then gradually gives way to oxidative phosphorylation (**Fig. 8.16**). The initial energy requirements for muscular activity are handled by the immediate energy system and glycolysis, both

Box 8.4 The Fates of Lactate

Lactate, a byproduct of glycolysis (**Box Fig. 8.3**) has long been considered a waste product of high-intensity muscle activity. A persistent belief exists that large amounts of lactate accumulating in muscle tissue is a primary cause of muscle fatigue and soreness. These beliefs, however, are not supported by evidence. Research published since 2000 tells a different, more complex story of the four fates of lactate (Gladden 2004). Lactate is used in specific ways during exercise as a metabolic substrate for the manufacture of ATP and, after exercise, as stored glycogen in the liver. As shown in **Box Fig. 8.3**, during production of ATP in glycolysis, lactate is given off as a byproduct when pyruvate is formed. Pyruvate is a necessary metabolite for oxidative phosphorylation. At the point that lactate is given off, it can experience one of four fates: (1) it can be converted back to pyruvate for additional use in oxidative phosphorylation, (2) it can travel to neighboring muscle tissue for use as fuel, (3) it can travel to distant tissues such as the heart or other muscle cells for use as fuel, or (4) it can be converted back to stored glycogen in the liver via the Cori cycle. Therefore, circulating lactate plays a primary role as muscle fuel and stored glycogen. It is estimated that the majority of circulating lactate is oxidized in ATP metabolism and the rest is stored as glycogen or used to synthesize amino acids (Brooks et al 2005).

The clearance of lactate from muscle tissue and blood occurs quickly, as lactate moves down the

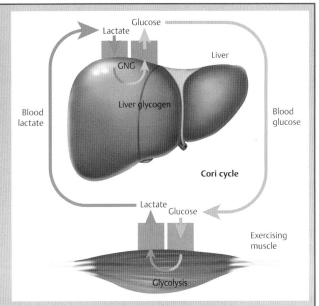

Box Fig. 8.3 Fates of lactate.

concentration gradient and according to the various pathways available for its removal. The accumulation of lactate occurs with exercise in which the production of lactate exceeds the rate of removal. For a highly trained individual, lactate clearance may occur in less time. Compelling evidence suggests that engaging in light exercise for a short period of time after the high intensity exercise increases lactate clearance (Menzies et al 2010). Therefore, if a patient describes muscle soreness after completing exercises prescribed for a communication disorder, lactate is not the cause.

---

anaerobic systems. Muscle tasks that last longer than 2 minutes are considered endurance tasks. One might assume that talking for several minutes would then translate to endurance activity. However, humans do not engage muscles of articulation, voicing, or swallowing for more than a few

seconds. Human communication and swallowing do not require continual muscle contraction, unlike muscles of the arms or legs, with the exception of the posterior cricoarytenoid (PCA), which is engaged for extended periods of time to maintain a patent airway.

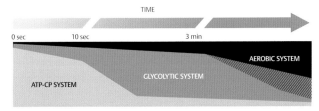

Fig. 8.16 At the onset of muscle activity, energy metabolism relies on the immediate energy system (ATP-CP system), which then gives over to glycolysis as exercise continues and finally to aerobic mechanisms for ATP production. All energy systems are at the ready to adjust to the workload required for the task.

■ Muscle Receptors

Activation of muscle fiber types and recruitment needs are based on the relationship of the work intensity and duration. Feedback mechanisms that carry information from the muscles back to the CNS are necessary for optimal muscle function. The two main types of sensory mechanisms are **muscle spindles** and the **Golgi tendon organ**.

Muscle spindles are sensory organs that detect changes in muscle length. This information is important for reflex responses and coordination of learned movements. They also provide proprioceptive feedback. Muscle proprioception provides sensory feedback important for performing muscle activities already learned, such as on-line adjustment of the articulatory muscles when a sound is not produced correctly. They also provide information for learning new and recovering lost motor behaviors. This feedback mechanism is faster than the auditory feedback loop and is important for rehabilitation in communication disorders and swallowing. As shown in **Fig. 8.17**, muscle spindles are found in the muscle belly, surrounded by and positioned in parallel with muscle fibers. Spindles are not as long as muscle fibers, which does not present a problem because the spindles are integrated with the connective tissue of the matrix. The number of muscle spindles per muscle varies, depending on the role that the muscle plays. Small muscles of the hand, typically engaged in fine motor tasks, have a dense supply of muscle spindles. Larger muscles of the body that generally engage in less precise movement have a less dense supply of muscle spindles. The muscle spindle is innervated by both afferent (sensory) and efferent (motor) nerve inputs. Based on muscle activ-

ity, the muscle spindle can regulate the action of the muscle by controlling the motor neurons that innervate the muscle fibers.

In addition to muscle movement, muscle spindles are also involved in muscle tone and tendon reflexes. For example, an individual with a neurological disorder that results in increased spindle activity may present with muscle spasticity when a limb is moved. Conversely, a reduction in muscle spindle activity can diminish reflex activity and decrease muscle tone.

The second primary sensory receptor in the skeletal muscle system is the Golgi tendon organ (GTO), first described by Camillo Golgi (who also discovered the Golgi stain for neurons and the Golgi apparatus for packaging proteins in cells). GTOs are fewer in number than muscle spindles and play a different role in muscle function. GTOs are responsible for communicating to the CNS how much force is being produced by the muscle on a tendon. GTOs are located at the junction of the muscle and the tendon, not in the belly of the muscle fiber, and each is connected to up to 25 muscle fibers. These muscle receptors are activated during activities of daily living, send-

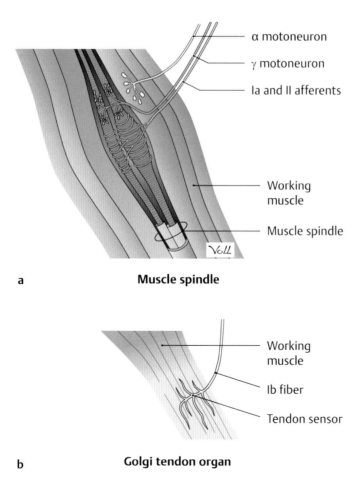

a   **Muscle spindle**

b   **Golgi tendon organ**

Fig. 8.17   **(a)** Muscle spindles are sensors that function to regulate muscle length. Group Ia afferent neurons coil around the nuclear chain and nuclear bag fibers (intrafusal fibers), whereas group II coil around nuclear chain fibers only. These coiled endings detect longitudinal stretching of intrafusal fibers and transmit information about their length (group II) and rate of change in length (group Ia) to the spinal cord. Efferent I3 motor neurons innervate both types of intrafusal fibers, allowing variation of their length and stretch sensitivity. **(b)** Golgi tendon organs are sensors found in tendons that function to regulate muscle tension. Group Ib afferent fibers that originate in Golgi tendon organs transmit information regarding muscle tension to inhibitory interneurons in the spinal cord. These interneurons inhibit motor neurons of the muscle from which the type Ib afferent impulse originated. They also activate antagonistic muscles via excitatory mechanisms. These factors combine to adjust muscle tension.

ing information back to the CNS during routine motor behaviors. Both GTOs and muscle spindles have been identified in the muscles of mastication, serving as a brake for the power generated during chewing, which would crush the teeth if unchecked.

Types of Muscle Contraction

When muscles are engaged in work, they do not always contract in the same manner. Muscle contraction can be divided into **isometric** and **isotonic** activity. Isometric muscle activity is characterized by tension generated in muscle tissue without any change in muscle length or joint angle. In other words, tension is built up in the muscle without any visible appearance of gross motor movement. This tension occurs when the resistance to movement is equal to the force applied. One use of isometric contraction is to stabilize a body segment and prevent it from being moved by external forces. Isotonic muscle action, on the other hand, is characterized by a change in muscle length, and it can be divided into two types: **concentric** and **eccentric**. Concentric muscle activity is characterized by muscle force that is exerted as the muscle shortens in length. In this context, the force is greater than the resistance, which causes the sliding filaments to contract to shorten the sarcomere. It is generally the kind of muscle movement used when moving against gravity or a resistance, such as lifting a weight. The angle of a joint changes in the direction of the muscle force applied. Eccentric muscle activity is characterized by muscle lengthening under tension and is used during muscle effort that requires a controlled descent against resistance (gravity). In this activity, the load or resistance is greater than the applied force, causing the sarcomere to be extended in length.

Motor Unit Recruitment

An additional aspect of motor unit function is the manner in which motor units are selected and put into service for muscle activity, known as motor unit recruitment. Motor units are progressively recruited to meet the demands placed upon muscles. Recall that each motor unit, innervated by a single motor neuron, comprises multiple muscle fibers, and each muscle contains multiple motor units. Activation of a single motor unit will result in a weak muscle contraction. Therefore, additional motor units must be recruited within a muscle or group of muscles to grade the force production response to the target muscle activity. This recruitment of motor units occurs in an orderly fashion and is described by the **size principle** (Mendell 2005). The size principle states that the smallest and slowest motor units are recruited first, followed by larger and faster motor units. The smallest and slowest motor units are those that have Type I or slow muscle fibers. Type II, or fast, muscle fibers are larger and faster than the slow fibers. Therefore, Type I muscle fibers are recruited first, followed by the larger, faster Type II muscle fibers.

Frequency of Motor Unit Stimulation

A lone motor unit can exert varying degrees of force depending on the frequency at which it is stimulated. The smallest contractile response that can be elicited in a single motor unit is called a **twitch** and occurs when a single AP is applied to the nerve innervating a motor unit. A simple twitch response has three phases, the first of which is a brief latent period called the electromechanical delay. This delay is the time during which the action potential is conducted into the T-tubules, Ca^{2+} is released into the sarcoplasm, Ca^{2+} binds to troponin, and cross-bridge cycling is initiated. The second phase of a simple twitch is the contraction phase, in which myosin binds to actin. The final phase is relaxation, but another AP delivered in rapid sequence prevents the relaxation phase of the twitch from occurring and causes another contraction instead, leading to an increase in force generation, called summation. If neural stimulation continues at high frequencies, the tension in the muscle fiber will reach its maximum possible level, called tetanus or tetanic contraction. (The disease tetanus, often due to wound infections, causes tetanic muscle contractions, sometimes powerful enough to break bones.) The transition from simple twitches, through summation, culminating in tetanic contraction is shown in **Fig. 8.18**. The degree to which a muscle fiber or motor unit is neurally stimulated is a component of the generation of muscle force.

Muscle Force Generation

Several factors contribute to force development in muscle tissue. The number of motor units (e.g., fibers recruited), fiber type (Type I or Type II), recruitment pattern, muscle twitch summation, and cross section of the fiber all influence the amount of force generated. Increased motor unit activation is associated with greater force.

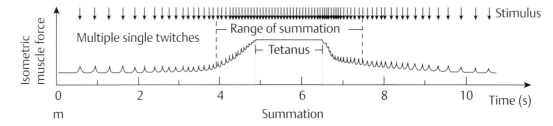

Fig. 8.18 When individual twitches are elicited by rapidly repeating stimuli, the muscle does not relax between stimuli and continuously contracts, referred to as a tetanic contraction or a tetanus. Muscle force is significantly greater in a tetanus than in a twitch because more cross-bridges are activated.

Type II motor units generate more force than Type I; therefore, engaging more Type II motor units results in increased force production. The greater the cross-sectional area of a muscle, the greater the force. During training, muscles can hypertrophy (increase in size) and become stronger. Additionally, force development in muscles must be matched or graded to the needs of the muscular activity. The force generation requirements for swallowing a bolus of food would exceed the requirements for producing the /p/ phoneme. To take this example further, the force generation requirements during swallowing are graded to match the texture of the bolus, with a puree requiring less force to propel the bolus of food toward the pharynx and a piece of steak requiring more.

Length-Tension Relationship

Another factor that contributes to generation of muscle force is the **length-tension relationship**. Tension development in muscle fibers is relative to the degree to which actin and myosin filaments overlap at the start of muscle contraction (**Fig. 8.19**). The percentage of tension in a sarcomere peaks at what can be considered the optimal resting length. Optimal length of a muscle fiber occurs when there is some overlap of the actin filaments with the thick myosin filaments, but not complete overlap. The amount of force produced is correlated to the number of myosin cross-bridges formed with actin; the more cross-bridges that can be formed result in more force generation. With too little overlap of actin to myosin, there is little opportunity for tension development, as the myosin heads have few closely approximated myosin-binding sites on the

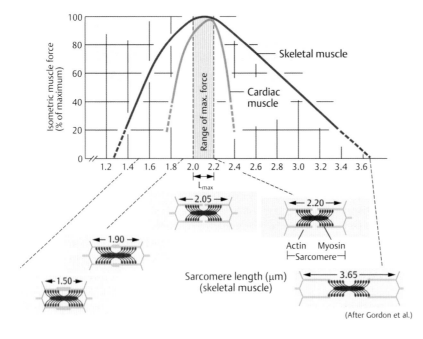

Fig. 8.19 Isometric muscle tension relative to sarcomere length. The length (L) and force (F), or tension, of a muscle are closely related. Because the active force is determined by the magnitude of all potential actin-myosin interactions, it varies with sarcomere length. Skeletal muscle can develop maximum (isometric) force (F_0) at its maximum resting length (L_{MAX}). When the sarcomeres shorten ($L < L_{MAX}$), part of the thin filaments overlap, allowing only forces smaller than F_0 to develop. When L is 70% of L_{MAX}, the thick filaments make contact with the Z disks, and F becomes even smaller. In addition, at nonphysiologic extensions ($L > L_{MAX}$) a muscle can develop only restricted force because the number of potentially available actin-myosin bridges is reduced.

actin filament to engage. Similarly, with too much overlap, there are few myosin-binding sites available because most of them are already occupied. Practically speaking, muscles that are markedly stretched or shortened beyond the optimal length (rest to 1.2 times resting length) generate less force.

Control of Shortening/Lengthening Velocity

The speed of muscle contraction also influences force development in motor units. The speed of force generation can be influenced by the type of muscle fibers engaged and the nature of muscle contraction. Twitch contraction speeds vary between muscle fiber types. Fast fibers, or Type II fibers, contract in a shorter period of time than Type I or slow fibers. Type II fibers release Ca^{2+} from the SR at a faster rate than Type I fibers do. Type II fibers also have higher adenosine triphosphatase (ATPase) enzyme activity than Type I fibers, which results in faster splitting of ATP for faster release of energy for contraction.

Load-Velocity Relationship

The relationship between the ability of muscles to produce force and the velocity of the movement follows a curvilinear path, as is illustrated in **Fig. 8.20**.

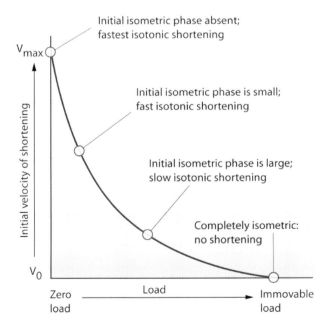

Fig. 8.20 As the load increases, muscle engagement shifts from reliance on fast isotonic shortening to complete reliance on isometric muscle contraction.

For example, the point at which the load and muscle force are equal results in an isometric contraction that has no fiber length changes or movement velocity. At the other extreme, a minimal load exists that does not hinder the development of maximal velocity. Not all muscle fiber types contribute to the force production, due to the fast velocity or speed of movement. The force-velocity curve describes the attainable force production as it is influenced by the resistive load and the fiber type recruitment.

A primary aspect of force-velocity relationships is the percentage of muscle fiber type engaged for the muscle activity. The velocity or speed of movement is faster in muscles that have a high percentage of fast or Type II fibers. As described previously, Type II fibers produce force at a faster rate than Type I or slow fibers because ATP is broken down faster and Ca^{2+} is released faster following neural stimulation. Therefore, if a motor unit has a higher percentage of fast fibers, the peak power that it can generate will be higher.

Control of Muscle Tension

Control of muscle tension is a complex process with contributions from the peripheral nervous system, afferent feedback mechanisms located within the motor units, differences between muscle fiber types, and adaptive responses of muscle tissue to training.

Fatigue

Exercise-related fatigue is defined as the reduced ability of muscle to produce force or power. Fatigue is an aspect of muscle function that has not been well described for communication and swallowing disorders. A general summary of muscle fatigue mechanisms are described here as a framework for understanding muscle training, which will be addressed in the next section. The mechanisms for muscle fatigue are often identified anatomically as central (brain, CNS) versus peripheral or by a substrate scheme that relates fatigue to the accumulation or depletion of various substances.

Central fatigue is related to elements of the central nervous system that may contribute to muscle fatigue: emotions, psychological factors contributing to perception of effort, brain waves, and descending motor pathways and interneurons in the brainstem and spinal cord. An example of central fatigue is the case of a prolonged task during which an individual's muscular performance could suffer due to attentiveness or volitional fatigue. Peripheral fatigue focuses on potential fatigue mechanisms identified for impulse conduction along the motor neuron, NMJ activity, neural impulse conduction into the muscle fiber, excitation-contraction coupling, and cross-bridge formation (MacIntosh et al 2006).

In general, muscle fatigue presents as a decline in speed and degree of force production as well as slowed relaxation time. Substrate fatigue classification factors include the reduction/depletion of ATP, blood glucose, glycogen, and creatine phosphate or the accumulation of lactate, hydrogen ions, and inorganic phosphate. Exercise-related fatigue is the result of the intensity and duration of muscular activity. In general, fatigue is the result of numerous factors combined to reduce the ability to maintain performance at maximal levels.

■ Skeletal Muscle Disease

With a working understanding of muscle anatomy, discussion of neuromuscular injuries and conditions that disrupt muscle development, alter cellular functions, and interfere with normal body functions is critical as a context for disease.

Muscular dystrophy (MD) is one such disease of muscle cells and is more common in males. MD is characterized by progressive weakening and wasting of muscles. This disease has many types, some of which are diagnosed in infancy, some around age 4 or 5, and others that have a later onset and a slower course of muscle wasting. MD is caused by mutations to the genes that support the production of proteins needed to form healthy muscle. Clinical considerations for MD are described in **Box 8.5**.

Many different metabolic diseases of muscle interfere with processing food for energy production needed for muscle function. McArdle's disease and Tarui's disease are metabolic diseases of muscle that both, in different ways, interfere with the breakdown and use of carbohydrates for production of ATP for muscle function.

Myasthenia gravis (MG), previously mentioned in **Box 8.2**, is an autoimmune disease whereby the immune system attacks the body's own tissues, primarily affecting the neuromuscular junction (NMJ). MG is characterized by a loss of postsynaptic acetylcholine receptors (AChRs). Fewer AChRs on the surface of the muscle cell makes it difficult for the muscle cell to receive and transmit the action potential sent from the central nervous system. Patients with MG present with muscle weakness that worsens with muscle activity such as swallowing and voicing. Typical symptoms for MG by subsystem are described in **Box 8.6**.

Box 8.5   Muscular Dystrophy

Muscular dystrophy (MD) is a group of genetic diseases characterized by progressive degeneration of skeletal muscles that result in progressive weakness. Some of the diagnoses included in this group are Duchenne MD, the most common form of pediatric-onset MD, and myotonic MD, the most common adult form. The onset of MD can range from infancy through adulthood, and the progression of the disease varies between individuals. Pediatric onset of MD is distinct from adult onset in that the child with MD is impeded from developing and refining motor skills for activities of daily living (ADLs), communication, and feeding/swallowing, whereas the adult is losing developed and refined skills. Treatment planning for the young child must balance the development of motor skill with the progressive loss of muscle function.

MD can affect muscles of articulation, breathing, voicing, resonance, feeding, and swallowing. Given this variability of onset and progression, evaluation and treatment of communication and swallowing disorders must be tailored to the specific needs of the individual. The efficacy of muscle exercise to improve functional ability in MD is controversial. There is some indication that lower-intensity limb skeletal muscle training may be of some benefit for improving limb strength and endurance; however, the research to date is limited. There is little evidence to support use of exercise for muscles of respiration, communication, feeding, or swallowing. Use of high-intensity exercise regimes for breathing and swallowing would likely be contraindicated in this population, given that high-intensity exercise may create muscle fatigue that could compromise airway protection.

Given this controversy, it is likely that continual reassessment and treatment adaptations related to communication and swallowing function are necessary. Use of adaptive technology to maintain functional communication may be the best treatment approach. For weakened respiratory muscles that may contribute to inadequate sound level, use of a personal amplifier may be beneficial. For weakened muscles of articulation, an augmentative and alternative communication (AAC) device may be indicated. If airway clearance becomes an issue because of weakened respiratory muscles, the pulmonologist may prescribe a cough assist machine to introduce a large volume of air into the airway during inhalation and then quickly reverse airflow to drive mucus out of the lungs.

Box 8.6 Myasthenia Gravis

There is a growing interest in the use of muscle training programs for improvement of respiratory, voice, and swallowing function. In many cases that involve decline of muscle function, as with the elderly, increased muscle activity can improve functional ability. However, this adaptation is not the case with individuals who have communication or swallowing impairment secondary to MG. MG is an autoimmune disorder that produces antibodies that block, alter, or destroy neuromuscular junction postsynaptic acetylcholine receptors (AChRs) in voluntary muscle. This disease is distinct in that the affected muscles rapidly fatigue with use, contraindicating the use of exercise as a therapy modality.

The clinical presentation and severity of MG are variable. When severe, MG can result in difficulty smiling, talking, chewing, swallowing, or breathing. Typical symptoms for MG by subsystem and the clinical implications are as follows:

Speech Breathing
Breathing symptoms include shortness of breath or difficulty taking a deep breath or coughing. Since taking a deep breath is difficult, inhalation may be insufficient for typical speech phrasing and adequate vocal loudness. Insufficient subglottic pressure generation may make these individuals particularly vulnerable to airway protection. Use of respiratory muscle resistance training devices is not indicated with this population. Shorter phrasing and frequent breaks from talking are appropriate intervention strategies.

Articulation
When muscles of articulation rapidly fatigue with use, an AAC system is helpful to assist with communication.

Voice and Resonance
Voice symptoms include hoarseness, breathy voice, vocal weakness, and sluggishness of vocal fold abduction. The primary voice symptom is breathiness. Insufficient loudness, particularly with ambient noise, may be a challenge. Use of an affordable, portable, lightweight personal amplifier may be the best recommendation.

Feeding and Swallowing
Involvement of oropharyngeal musculature is not uncommon. Timely consideration of myasthenia gravis in evaluating dysphagia is crucial to prevent complications and to improve the quality of life of these patients. The impact of MG on swallowing may occur gradually or suddenly. Swallowing muscles may become fatigued, particularly toward the end of a meal or when food requires a lot of chewing. Because airway protection may be compromised, these individuals are more likely to have silent aspiration. A clinical assessment of swallowing function may not be adequate to assess these individuals fully should they exhibit swallowing difficulty.

■ Physical Injury and Overuse

Muscle tissue can be damaged from external or internal causes. Internal causes can be secondary to overuse injuries that can include muscle tears or tendon ruptures. External causes can include crushed or lacerated muscle tissue and tissue damage secondary to extreme exposure to heat or cold.

A primary reason for internal muscle injury is repeated lengthening contractions. These types of muscle contractions are used in activities that require a muscle to contract in a brake-like fashion. An example of this activity would be the contractions in the biceps brachii while a heavy load is being lowered. Relative to communication, an example of this type of contraction might be the braking action of the infrahyoid muscles to slow engagement of the suprahyoid muscles during extreme voicing tasks. Physiologically, these lengthening contractions pull the actin filaments away from the center of the sarcomere. Extreme muscle behavior in this manner can result in muscle inflammation or, in severe cases, muscle cell necrosis (Jones et al 1986), which over time will be repaired by regeneration of muscle fiber components. Additionally, overstretch of the sarcomeres can disrupt the sarcolemma, swell and disrupt the T-tubule system, and distort the relationship of the contractile proteins (Friden and Lieber 2001).

Lengthening contractions in untrained individuals can cause muscle discomfort 24–48 hours after strenuous exercise, referred to as **delayed-onset muscle soreness (DOMS)**. As descibed in **Box 8.4**, lactate is not responsible for this soreness. The discomfort is more commonly attributed to microscopic tears in muscle tissue caused by excessive mechanical force placed on the muscle and connective tissue (Friden et al 1983).

Muscle injury due to external causes such as trauma or exposure to temperature extremes, although somewhat similar to the injury with use just described, generally results in increased necrosis. Following laceration or crushing of muscle tissue, a necrotic zone develops at the site of the injury, extending laterally from the injury site a few millimeters. In the necrotic zone, contractile proteins, muscle cell organelles, and tubular systems are initially destroyed before macrophages remove the debris. While this breakdown and clearance of damaged tissue is occurring, satellite cells activate to signal muscle cell repair. If muscle injury is sufficient enough to lose communication with the motor end plate, the muscle will become denervated, and downregulation of resting membrane potential and loss of AChRs will occur.

■ Muscle Adaptations

Like most other living tissues, muscles are in a constant state of synthesis and degradation, changing and adapting to meet the requirements imposed on the muscle. In other words, plasticity is an inherent characteristic of muscle. The number and types of muscle fibers activated within a whole muscle ideally match the desired muscle behavior. Selection of the right number of muscle fibers and in what order they are contracted is achieved through neuromuscular adaptations, motor learning, and training. For example, lifting a 2-pound weight requires fewer muscle fibers than lifting a 10-pound weight. Muscle physiology is more than activation and contraction of a muscle for a particular target behavior. It is also about the manner in which muscles can be trained to do certain work, how they respond to periods of no use, and what to expect during muscle recovery. Muscle training can upregulate muscle mechanisms, changing the muscle morphologically (size and organization), neurologically (how many fibers and what type of fibers in a motor unit), and bioenergetically (substrate storage, enzyme concentrations). Upregulated mechanisms of training can also be reversed in what can be termed detraining or disuse. This plasticity of muscle tissue is often overlooked during communication or swallowing habilitation or rehabilitation programming. In this section, the focus shifts from anatomic considerations to physiologic mechanisms of muscle function that underlie the ability to move muscles at the appropriate rate and force and how muscle tissue adapts to exercise, detraining, loss of tissue compensation, and aging.

Several concepts in exercise science guide the discussion of muscle adaptation: the **specificity principle** (SAID principle), the **overload principle**, and the **reversibility principle**. These concepts are important not only to the general understanding of muscle function but also to the role that speech-language pathologists and audiologists play in habilitation and rehabilitation of patients' muscle function.

Principles of Muscle Adaptation

As previously discussed, the SAID principle describes muscle-specific adaptations to imposed demand. It is a primary concept in muscle training. Muscle fibers are activated in sequence as described by the size principle; however, with practice, skilled movements (fine motor), force production (gross motor), and endurance can be trained for specific motor tasks. As the muscle learns the precise force and speed required for a task, motor unit recruitment progresses toward a more efficient recruitment pattern. Another way to describe this principle is through the concept of specificity of training; a target skill must be practiced for improvements in the target task to be realized. Generalization of training of a muscle should not be assumed to translate to another task, even one that uses the same muscle(s). An example of this specificity is the degree to which velar closure against the posterior pharyngeal wall varies by task. Velar closure for nonspeech activities such as blowing uses different pressures than does velar closure for speech-specific activities. Even within speech sounds, velar closure force is different between production of /s/ and production of /p/. It is for this reason that blowing activities are not useful for improving velopharyngeal function for speech; they lack specificity to the task.

The overload principle is a second principle that explains how muscles change in response to demands placed on them. Training should provide the optimal stress without exceeding the tolerance of the person in training. Thus, a muscle must be worked at a level beyond what it is accustomed to in order to upregulate those mechanisms of muscle efficiency and realize strength gains. The exercise regimen/training needs to include a plan that addresses intensity, duration, and frequency of muscle activity. Therefore, an overload approach can be implemented in a variety of ways. The amount of force produced for the target task can be increased as a means to increase exercise intensity. One way to provide increased muscle intensity for voice production could be to increase how loud the voice target is in therapy. Keeping intensity constant, overload can be achieved by increasing the duration of muscle activity and how often muscle activity occurs. Lower intensity with increased repetitions is one approach to overload. Fewer repetitions with maximal muscle effort is another approach to overload. The choice of muscle training approach should match the goals set for muscle behavior. Lee Silverman Voice Treatment is a voice therapy program that employs the principles of specificity and overload, as described in **Box 8.7**.

The opposite of the overload principle is the reversibility principle. The metabolic, morphologic, and neurologic mechanisms upregulated when muscle tissue is challenged can also be downregulated, lowering metabolic and morphological needs to match a reduced or absent work load. In exercise science, the general guideline is that as long as the muscle is working at 70% or greater of maximum ability, training is maintained. If the intensity of training falls below 70% for even two weeks, metabolic, morphologic, and neurologic mechanisms that have been maintained at a certain level will no longer be supported at that same level, and those metabolic, morphologic, and neurologic mechanisms will be downregulated. In general, muscle detraining results in decreased muscle strength and muscle mass. The specifics of this will be discussed subsequently in the Detraining Adaptations section.

Exercise Adaptations

The changes discussed are at the muscle tissue level following exercise, not cardiovascular changes that occur as a result of whole-body exercise such as running or rowing. No evidence exists that whole-body exercise such as running directly translates to improvements in communication or swallowing function, primarily because whole-body exercise lacks the specificity for the tasks.

Muscle adapts to exercise in specific ways depending on whether the activity is related to speed, force, or endurance, either individually or in combination. Exercise can facilitate morphologic (size and structure), neurologic, and bioenergetic changes to motor units. The morphological change that is most evident with strength training is muscle **hypertrophy**. Muscle hypertrophy is muscle enlargement that occurs secondary to strength training that occurs without the creation of new muscle fibers. Muscle size increases because of an increase in muscle fiber cross-sectional area, and this is most noticeable in Type II fibers, which realize greater change in cross-sectional area than Type I fibers. Increased muscle fiber size is due to growth and proliferation of the contractile proteins actin and myosin. Increase in muscle size is not due to increased number of muscle cells, which is called **hyperplasia**. Another morphological change that occurs secondary to exercise is a change in capillary density. With strength training, there may be a decrease in capillary density as a result of muscle fiber hypertrophy. With endurance training, capillary density may be increased to offload oxygen more quickly to muscle tissues that rely on oxygen as an energy substrate for oxidative phosphorylation. Mitochondrial density also increases in response to the increased requirement for ATP.

Muscle adaptations to exercise are also neurologic in nature, as can be seen in changes to motor unit recruitment patterns. In early strength training, neural recruitment is the primary means of strength gains during the first few weeks before muscle hypertrophy begins at 5 to 10 weeks. During the first 3 to 8 weeks of training, increased enzyme production to support muscle function is observed. With endurance training, motor units within a whole muscle may learn to cycle among themselves to offset fatigue. In other words, the muscle will "learn" that when a group of motor units is nearing fatigue, a new group of motor units

---

Box 8.7 Lee Silverman Voice Treatment and Muscle Training Principles

The Lee Silverman Voice Treatment (LSVT, LSVT Global, Tucson, AZ) program is an intensive therapy program designed for the treatment of speech and voice disorders associated with Parkinson's disease (PD; Mahler et al 2015). Individuals with PD may have difficulty being understood because of a soft voice and poor speech intelligibility. When evaluating this therapy program from the perspective of muscle training principles, this approach uses the principles of specificity and overload effectively to realize sig-

nificant improvement in vocal loudness and speech intelligibility. This program focuses on functional speech tasks, such as frequently used phrases, thus honoring the principle of specificity. With patients completing all of the therapy tasks at a louder level than typically employed, the communication mechanisms are employed at a level beyond which they are used to working, honoring the overload principle. By assigning regular posttherapy practice and scheduling follow-up appointments, the LSVT program also helps avoid reversibility of muscle adaptations realized during treatment.

should take over until it nears fatigue in turn, and so on. Muscle training can realize muscle efficiency to offset muscle fatigue. An additional muscle adaptation with exercise occurs at the NMJ, where the postsynaptic AChRs increase in number and proximity to the NMJ to facilitate more efficient and more fatigue-resistant transmission of the neural impulse to the muscle fiber.

In general, the tension that the muscle experiences and the total activity of the muscle determine the nature and extent of muscle adaption from exercise. Compelling evidence suggests that neural adaptations can occur without directly exercising a muscle. These adaptions have been demonstrated in studies of the crossover effect, in which strength increases were observed in the contralateral untrained limb (Carroll et al 2006). Imaginary exercise has also been found to result in significant increases in maximum voluntary contraction (Yue and Cole 1992).

Finally, bioenergetic adaptations occur in response to exercise. Bioenergetic efficiency is improved in part because of the morphologic changes just described. Increased mitochondrial and capillary density allow more rapid production and delivery of ATP to the engaged muscle tissues. Additional changes that occur in muscle fibers include an increase in local stores of bioenergetic enzymes used to produce ATP, glycogen, oxygen, and CP. Increased local availability of these bioenergetic enzymes and substrates translates to more efficient energy production for muscle tissue. The speed of ATP delivery is also increased as a result of muscle training. In general, muscles work efficiently with training, and these training adaptations, or upregulation of these mechanisms, will be maintained as long as muscle use continues at a constant or increased demand.

Detraining Adaptations

Detraining occurs when muscle use falls below 70% of maximum ability, triggering a downregulation of the morphologic, neurologic, and bioenergetic mechanisms that were upregulated during increased muscle activity. Detraining can range from no activity to reduced intensity or frequency of activity. After a short period of time, muscles become smaller with an overall decrease in muscle mass. The loss in muscle mass is due to downregulation of contractile protein fiber synthesis. Muscle tissue is in an ever-adaptable balance between synthesis and degradation, whereby a reduction in net synthesis will translate to loss of overall muscle volume. Over a longer period of time, fiber type

conversion may occur in the direction of slow to fast fiber characteristics. A muscle fiber is neurally innervated as a specific muscle fiber type, so, in that regard, the muscle fiber type will not change; however, characteristics of the muscle fiber may transition to become more like a different fiber type. Motor innervation is also reduced with detraining, resulting in decreased voluntary force production and the inability to recruit the motor unit population. The NMJ resting membrane potential also diminishes as the period of detraining extends.

Downregulation of metabolic, morphologic, and neurologic muscle mechanisms is not unlimited, and a new level of muscle homeostasis is generally achieved after about 30 days of sustained detraining. Once muscle tissue has reached the new state of equilibrium, barring denervation or neurological injury, the changes are reversible if muscle exercise is reinitiated.

Functionally, detraining results in performance changes in endurance, power, and flexibility. Although no empirical evidence describes changes to muscle morphology, neural function, or bioenergetics with a detraining model in the muscles of articulation, voice, or swallowing *in vivo*, there are clinical observations of reduced muscle ability following a period of prolonged disuse. For example, when an individual is not allowed to eat by mouth for an extended period of time, return to typical swallowing function may take time for the muscles to adapt to the increasing demand placed on them with advancement of dietary textures (e.g., moving from puree to a regular diet). Further, the stamina required to rely on oral intake for all caloric and nutritional needs may take time to recover.

A more extreme form of detraining is muscle disuse. Muscle disuse is characterized by complete or near complete unloading of the muscle. When a muscle is not engaged in any force production for a period of time, it undergoes the changes described for detraining, but to a greater degree. Disuse research has investigated muscle tissue changes that occur with limb immobilization, bed rest, paralysis, and space flight. A well-studied clinical example for disuse in a muscle of communication is the change to the diaphragm that occurs when an individual is placed on total ventilator assistance. Within 24 hours of being placed on total ventilator assistance, the diaphragm undergoes atrophy and decreased protein synthesis (Levine et al 2008). Further, the degree of muscle atrophy is correlated with the duration of mechanical ventilation (Powers et al 2013). This research has direct implications for the rehabilitation of patients weaned off of mechanical ventilation.

Loss of Tissue Compensation

Compensatory hypertrophy occurs when one muscle compensates for partial or total loss of its synergist. Exercise forces the compensating muscle to work harder than normal and in a manner to which it is not accustomed, resulting in adaptations to muscle morphology that may include muscle fiber type conversion to the muscle fiber type that is preferred for the target activity. For example, if the muscle tissue lost was used primarily for endurance activity, such as postural support, the compensating muscle tissue may slowly transition from fast-glycolytic fibers to fast oxidative-glycolytic and then finally to slow oxidative fiber types. Knowledge of compensatory hypertrophy can be applied in the head and neck cancer population, whereby rehabilitation of swallowing and communication may require residual structures following oncologic resection.

Muscle Adaptations in Aging

Skeletal muscle in older adults is characterized by morphologic and neurologic changes that may contribute, in part, to the decline in function that can be observed in both communication and swallowing. In general, skeletal muscles lose the ability to contract fast-twitch fibers efficiently and become slower and more oxidative with aging. Loss of muscle mass is common, characterized by smaller muscle fiber volume and increased percentage of connective tissue. Although women continue to rely primarily on neural mechanisms for strength gains, men in their older age also start to rely more on neural mechanisms than on testosterone-driven hypertrophy for strength gains. Neuromuscular junction changes also occur with aging and are characterized by overall loss of NMJs as nerve terminals withdraw from muscle fibers. Capillary density has also been observed to decline with aging, which may be secondary to a muscle fiber metabolic shift with aging. Evidence suggests that exercise, even into the ninth decade of life, can improve muscle function. Specifically, muscle adaptations that have been observed in the motor unit following exercise in old muscle include tightening up of the postsynaptic AChRs around motor end plates for more efficient propagation of the neural impulse into the muscle cell (Johnson et al 2013). In humans, significantly increased isometric and swallowing pressures have been found following an 8-week tongue resistance exercise program in older individuals who are at greater risk of developing swallowing disorder (Robbins et al 2005; Hind and Robbins 2013).

■ Suggested Readings

Brooks GA, Fahey TD, Baldwin KM. (2005). Exercise Physiology: Human Bioenergetics and Its Applications. New York, NY: McGraw-Hill; 2005.

Carroll TJ, Herbert RD, Munn J, Lee M, Gandevia SC. Contralateral effects of unilateral strength training: evidence and possible mechanisms. *Journal of Applied Physiology, 101*, 1514–1522; 2006

Covault J, Merlie JP, Goridis C, Sanes JR. Molecular forms of N-CAM and its RNA in developing and denervated skeletal muscle. *Journal of Cell Biology, 102*, 731–739; 1986

Fambrough DM. Control of acetylcholine receptors in skeletal muscle. *Physiological Reviews, 59*, 165–227; 1979

Friden J, Lieber R. Eccentric exercise-induced injuries to contractile and cytoskeletal muscle fibre components. *Acta Physiologica Scandinavica, 171*, 321–326; 2001

Friden J, Sjöström M, Ekblom B. Myofibrillar damage following intense eccentric exercise in man. *International Journal of Sports Medicine, 4*, 170–176; 1983

Gladden L. Lactate metabolism: a new paradigm for the third millennium. *Journal of Physiology, 558*, 5–30; 2004

Han Y, Wang J, Fischman DA, Biller HF, Sanders I. Slow tonic muscle fibers in the thyroarytenoid muscles of human vocal folds; a possible specialization for speech. *The Anatomical Record, 256*, 146–157; 1999

Hind JA, Robbins J. Oropharyngeal strengthening and rehabilitation of deglutitive disorders. In: Shaker R, Easterling C, Belafsky PC, Postma GN, eds. Manual of Diagnostic and Therapeutic Techniques for Disorders of Deglutition. Berlin, Germany: Springer; 2013, 237–255

Hoh JFY. Laryngeal muscle fibre types. *Acta Physiologica Scandinavica, 183*, 133–149; 2005

Huxley AF, Niedergerke R. Structural changes in muscle during contraction. *Nature, 173*, 971–973; 1954

Huxley H, Hanson J. Changes in the cross-striations of muscle during contraction and stretch and their structural interpretation. *Nature, 173*, 973–976; 1954

Johnson AM, Ciucci MR, Connor NP. Vocal training mitigates age-related changes within the vocal mechanism in old rats. *Journals of Gerontology Series A: Biological Sciences and Medical Sciences, 68*, 1458–1468; 2013

Jones D, Newham D, Round J, Tolfree S. Experimental human muscle damage: morphological changes in relation to other indices of damage. *The Journal of Physiology, 375,* 435–448; 1986

Landmesser LT. The generation of neuromuscular specificity. *Annual Review of Neuroscience, 3,* 279–302; 1980

Levine S, Nguyen T, Taylor N, et al. Rapid disuse atrophy of diaphragm fibers in mechanically ventilated humans. *New England Journal of Medicine, 358,* 1327–1335; 2008

Lieber RL. Skeletal Muscle Structure and Function: Implications for Rehabilitation and Sports Medicine. Philadelphia, PA: Williams & Wilkins; 1992

MacIntosh BR, Gardiner PF, McComas. Skeletal Muscle: Form and Function. Champaign, IL: Human Kinetics; 2006

Mahler LA, Ramig LO, Fox C. Evidence-based treatment of voice and speech disorders in Parkinson disease. *Current Opinion in Otolaryngology & Head and Neck Surgery, 23,* 209–215; 2015

McComas AJ. Oro-facial muscles: internal structure, function and ageing. *Gerodontology, 15,* 3–14; 1998

Mendell LM. The size principle: a rule describing the recruitment of motoneurons. *Journal of Neurophysiology, 93,* 3024–3026; 2005

Menzies P, Menzies C, McIntyre L, Paterson P, Wilson J, Kemi OJ. Blood lactate clearance during active recovery after an intense running bout depends on the intensity of the active recovery. *Journal of Sports Sciences, 28,* 975–982; 2010

Poo M-m. Rapid lateral diffusion of functional ACh receptors in embryonic muscle cell membrane. *Nature, 295,* 332–334; 1982

Powers SK, Howley ET. Exercise Physiology: Theory and Application to Fitness and Performance, 6th ed. Boston, MA: McGraw-Hill; 2007

Powers SK, Wiggs MP, Sollanek KJ, Smuder AJ. Ventilator-induced diaphragm dysfunction: cause and effect. *American Journal of Physiology—Regulatory, Integrative and Comparative Physiology, 305,* R464–R477; 2013

Robbins J, Gangnon RE, Theis SM, Kays SA, Hewitt AL, Hind JA. The effects of lingual exercise on swallowing in older adults. *Journal of the American Geriatrics Society, 53,* 1483–1489; 2005

Rosenfield DB, Miller RH, Sessions RB, Patten BM. Morphologic and histochemical characteristics of laryngeal muscle. *Archives of Otolaryngology, 108,* 662–666; 1982

Sale DG. Neural adaptation to resistance training. *Medicine and Science in Sports and Exercise, 20,* S135–S145; 1988

Schiaffino S, Reggiani C. Fiber types in mammalian skeletal muscles. *Physiological Reviews, 91,* 1447–1531; 2011

Tellis CM, Thekdi A, Rosen C, Sciote JJ. Anatomy and fiber type composition of human interarytenoid muscle. *Annals of Otology, Rhinology & Laryngology, 113,* 97–107; 2004

Yue G, Cole KJ. Strength increases from the motor program: comparison of training with maximal voluntary and imagined muscle contractions. *Journal of Neurophysiology, 67,* 1114–1123; 1992

■ Study Questions

1. Why are in vivo muscle biopsies not commonly used in speech and hearing science?

A. No equipment has been developed for the procedure at this time.
B. Muscle biopsies are relatively new techniques.
C. Removing a biopsy of a small muscle could greatly affect function of the muscle.
D. There is no need for in vivo biopsies in speech and hearing science.
E. Muscle biopsies are completed very commonly in speech and hearing science.

2. Which of the following refers to muscle formation:

A. Myogenesis
B. Myospecificity
C. Synaptogenesis
D. Synapse
E. Muscle genesis

3. The neurotransmitter that is required for muscle contraction is:

A. Acetylcholine
B. Acetylcholinesterase
C. Calcium
D. Sarcolemma
E. Sarcomeres

4. What causes acetylcholine vesicles to be released from the cell membrane?

A. Lactate entering the cell
B. Sodium leaving the cell
C. Acetylcholinesterase activity
D. Calcium entering the axon terminal
E. Calcium leaving the axon terminal

5. In a muscle cell, the postsynaptic membrane, or the _____, contains _____, which binds with acetylcholine to propagate the neural impulse.

A. Plasmalemma; acetylcholine
B. Sarcolemma; acetylcholine receptors
C. Acetylcholine receptors; plasmalemma
D. Acetylcholine receptors; sarcolemma
E. Sarcolemma; enzymes

6. List the muscle fiber types from most to least fatigue-resistant:

A. Type IIa, IIx, I
B. Type IIx, I, IIa
C. Type IIx, IIa, I
D. Type I, IIx, IIa
E. Type I, IIa, IIx

7. Which muscle fiber type(s) primarily relies on oxidative phosphorylation to produce ATP?

A. Type I
B. Type IIa
C. Type IIb
D. Type IIx
E. B and C

8. _____ muscle fibers are endurance fibers, while _____ are power fibers.

A. Type IIa, Type IIb
B. Type I, Type II
C. Type II, Type I
D. Type IIa, Type IIx
E. Type IIx, Type I

9. Which of the following is/are the energy system(s) that produces the most ATP per glucose molecule?

A. Oxidative phosphorylation
B. Immediate energy system
C. Glycolysis
D. A and B
E. B and C

10. Which of the following are changes that would occur in muscle tissue with training?

A. Hypertrophy
B. Amount of acetylcholine released into the synaptic cleft
C. Number and distribution of postsynaptic acetylcholine receptors in the sarcolemma
D. Increase in capillary density
E. All of the above

11. The first time calcium is important in muscle fiber contraction:

A. Bind to troponin complex, allowing the actin and myosin filaments to slide past each other, thus contracting the muscle fiber
B. Bind with sarcoplasmic reticulum to produce ATP
C. Enter into the axon terminal in order for acetylcholine to be released
D. Storing fuel for muscle contraction
E. Relaxing the muscle after contraction is complete

12. For motor unit recruitment, the size principle explains that _____ are recruited first, followed by _____:

A. Type II muscle fibers (smaller and slower); Type I muscle fibers (larger and faster)
B. Type II muscle fibers (larger and faster); Type I muscle fibers (smaller and slower)
C. Type I muscle fibers (larger and faster); Type II muscle fibers (smaller and slower)
D. Type I muscle fibers (smaller and slower); Type II muscle fibers (larger and faster)
E. Type I and II muscle fibers are recruited at the same time

13. Which of the following is an example of isometric muscle contraction?

A. Raising a 10-lb weight in a biceps curl
B. Lowering a 10-lb weight in a biceps curl
C. Holding a heavy box of textbooks
D. Touching your toes
E. Going down a flight of stairs

14. Which of the following is an example of concentric muscle contraction?

A. Raising a 10-lb weight in a biceps curl
B. Lowering a 10-lb weight in a biceps curl
C. Holding a heavy box of textbooks
D. Touching your toes
E. Going down a flight of stairs

15. Which of the following is an example of eccentric muscle contraction?

A. Raising a 10-lb weight in a biceps curl
B. Lowering a 10-lb weight in a biceps curl
C. Holding a heavy box of textbooks
D. Standing up after a leg squat
E. Going up flight of stairs

16. Which principle states that muscles need to be trained beyond the level at which they are used to without exceeding the tolerance of the individual?

A. Overload
B. Reversibility
C. Size
D. Specific adaptation to imposed demand
E. Delayed onset muscle soreness

17. Which principle describes the organization of motor unit recruitment?

A. Overload
B. Reversibility
C. Size
D. Specific adaptation to imposed demand
E. Delayed onset muscle soreness

18. Which of the following refers to muscle discomfort that occurs 24–48 hours after heavy exercise?

A. Overload
B. Reversibility
C. Size
D. Specific adaptation to imposed demand
E. Delayed onset muscle soreness

19. Which of the following interrupts the formation and release of acetylcholine into the synaptic cleft?

A. Black widow spider venom
B. Bungarotoxin
C. Botulinum toxin
D. Sarin gas
E. Myasthenia gravis

20. Which of the following are changes that occur to skeletal muscle with aging?

A. Reduced efficiency of fast-twitch fiber contraction
B. Loss of muscle mass
C. More reliance on neural mechanisms for strength in older males
D. Reduction in capillary density
E. All of the above

■ Answers to Study Questions

1. The correct answer is (C). Because the majority of the muscles in speech and hearing anatomy are very small, taking a biopsy even the size of a grain of rice could potentially have detrimental effects on the function of the remaining muscle. Equipment (A) and techniques (B) are currently in place to conduct muscle biopsies. In vivo biopsies would provide useful information (D), but the benefit is not worth the cost of muscle damage. Muscle biopsies are rarely conducted in speech and hearing science (E) on account of the risks mentioned previously.

2. The correct answer is (A). The definition of myogenesis is "muscle formation." Myospecificity (B) refers to motor unit development, synaptogenesis (C) refers to the formation of the synapse that bridges the nerve and muscle cell, or synapse (D), so answer choices B, C, and D are incorrect. Muscle genesis is not a real term (E).

3. The correct answer is (A). Acetylcholine is the neurotransmitter required for muscle contraction. Answer choices (B), (C), (D), and (E) are not neurotransmitters.

4. The correct answer is (D). Calcium entry into the axon terminal facilitates release of acetylcholine (ACh) vesicles from the presynaptic membrane. Lactate entering the cell (A) and sodium leaving the cell (B) do not cause release of ACh vesicles. Acetylcholinesterase breaks down acetylcholine in the synaptic cleft after it is released (C). Calcium leaving the axon terminal does not cause ACh to be released (E).

5. The correct answer is (B). Sarcolemma is the correct name for the cell membrane in muscle cells, not plasmalemma (A), and acetylcholine receptors bind with acetylcholine to propagate the neural impulse. The other answer choices are incorrect because they either contain incorrect terms or have the terms in the incorrect order.

6. The correct answer is (E). Type I muscle fibers are the most fatigue-resistant fibers because they depend on oxidative phosphorylation for energy. Type IIa are more fatigue-resistant than Type IIx because they contain a greater capacity for oxidative phosphorylation than Type IIx. The rest of the answer choices are incorrect because they list the fibers in the incorrect order.

7. The correct answer is (A). Type I muscle fibers rely more on oxidative phosphorylation than the other muscle fiber types do. Type IIa has some capacity to use oxidative phosphorylation, but not to the extent of Type I fibers (B, E). Type IIb fibers are transition fibers as is currently understood in the exercise science literature (C, E). Type IIx fibers rely primarily on anaerobic energy systems, not oxidative phosphorylation (D).

8. The correct answer is (B). Type I fibers are more endurance fibers and Type II are more power fibers. The remaining answer choices place the terms in the incorrect order or classify Type II fibers as endurance fibers, which is incorrect.

9. The correct answer is (A). Oxidative phosphorylation produces 36 to 38 ATP, while glycolysis produces 2 to 4 ATP (C, E). The immediate energy system also produces limited ATP and does not consume glucose (B, D).

10. The correct answer is (E). All of the answer choices are adaptations that occur to muscle fibers with training. Selecting only one of the answers does not completely answer the question.

11. The correct answer is (C). The first time calcium is important to muscle fiber contraction is when it enters the axon terminal in order for acetylcholine vesicles to be released into the synaptic cleft. Although (A) is a function of calcium in muscle contraction, this occurs after (C). Answer choices (B), (D), and (E) are not functions of calcium.

12. The correct answer is (D). Muscle fibers that are smaller and slower are recruited first, which are Type I muscle fibers. Muscle fibers that are larger and faster are recruited after the Type I fibers, which are Type II fibers. Answer choices (A), (B), and (C) either switch the properties of the muscle fibers or list them in the wrong order. Type I fibers are recruited before Type II fibers (E).

13. The correct answer is (C). Isometric muscle activity is characterized by tension that is built up in the muscle without any visible appearance of gross motor movement, as in holding a heavy box of textbooks in your arms. All other answers involve gross motor movement, making them incorrect answer choices.

14. The correct answer is (A). Concentric muscle movement is used when moving against gravity or a resistance, such as lifting a weight. Answer choices (B), (D), and (E) involve lowering movements, not raising. Answer choice (C) does not involve motor movement.

15. The correct answer is (B). Eccentric muscle activity is characterized by muscle lengthening under tension and is used during muscle efforts that require a controlled descent against resistance (gravity), such as lowering a weight. Answer choices (A), (D), and (E) involve raising movements, not lowering. Answer choice (C) does not involve motor movement.

16. The correct answer is (A). The overload principle states that a muscle must be worked at a level beyond what it is accustomed to in order to upregulate those mechanisms of muscle efficiency and realize strength gains. Answer choices (B) and (D) are principles involved in training, but they do not match the definition provided. Answer choice (C) is not a principle involved in training. Answer choice (E) is not a principle.

17. The correct answer is (C). The smallest and slowest motor units are recruited first, followed by larger and faster motor units, as explained by the size principle. Answer choices (A), (B), and (D) are principles, but they do not match the definition provided. Answer choice (E) is not a principle.

18. The correct answer is (E). Delayed onset muscle soreness describes how muscle tissue discomfort is experienced about 24–48 hours after eccentric muscle exercise. None of the other answer choices matches the definition provided.

19. The correct answer is (C). Botulinum toxin, as described in **Box 8.2**, prevents acetylcholine from forming into vesicles and being released into the synaptic cleft. All of the other answer choices inhibit correct NMJ function in other ways: black widow venom (not mentioned in the box) releases all of the acetylcholine into the synaptic cleft (A), bungarotoxin inhibits acetylcholine from binding with ACh receptors (B), sarin gas prevents ACh from being cleared from the synaptic cleft to enable another signal to be transmitted (D), and myasthenia gravis reduces the number of ACh receptors (E).

20. The correct answer is (E). All of the answer choices are adaptations to skeletal muscle that occur with the aging process. Selecting only one of the answer choices does not answer the question completely.

9

Sensory Systems

Richard D. Andreatta and Nicole M. Etter

■ Chapter Summary

The ability to detect and understand the world around us requires a means of receiving, transmitting, and interpreting a vast amount of information from the environment in which we exist. The study of anatomy and physiology of sensory systems is essential to the understanding of human action and perception. To appreciate the underlying normal or disordered nature of speech behaviors fully, a working knowledge of nervous system structures that enable individuals to detect and appreciate sensory events that arise from the therapeutic task is required. The purpose of this chapter is to provide a broad overview of the anatomic and functional features of the major sensory systems in the body. Specifically, we will characterize somatosensation, hearing, vestibular, visual, gustatory, and olfactory systems and discuss them in terms of their (1) basic anatomy, (2) transduction mechanisms, (3) central pathways, and (4) cortical areas mediating each type of sensation. Additionally, the chapter will provide a concise summary of universal aspects of sensory coding and perceptual factors applicable to all sensory systems, including (1) principles of psychophysics, (2) sensory coding in the nervous system, and (3) the basic mechanisms underlying the appreciation of modality, location, duration, and intensity of sensory inputs.

■ Learning Objectives

- Understand and describe the basic anatomic structures and pathways underlying each major sensory system
- Identify, compare, and contrast the mechanisms of sensory receptor transduction across all sensory systems
- Identify and describe universal attributes related to sensation and perception
- Describe the complexity and importance of sensation and perception to human behavior

■ Putting It Into Practice

- All perception begins with the transduction of real-world sensory events into the electrochemical language of the nervous system. Although the specific details may differ, all sensory systems generally encode and respond to four basic stimulus attributes: modality, location, intensity, and duration. Sensory systems form the basis for learning about the features and relationships that exist within our natural environment.
- Perception is relative and dynamically constructed by the brain. Our ability to create conceptual categories of knowledge is critically dependent upon sensations transduced by dedicated neural sensory systems.
- The early stages of learning any skilled motor behavior are dependent upon feedback derived

from sensory systems. As such, the integrity and health of sensory systems is paramount to normal development.

Introduction

How do you know something is real? How do you know you are holding this book and feeling it in your hands? How do you know the colors of the figures or that the words themselves exist? If you were blind, would colors exist in your mind? If you had no perception of touch, would any object exist from your point of view? Imagine being able to see something resting on your hand but not being able to feel it in any way; the moment you looked away from your hand, it would appear that the object ceased to exist. Does it exist or not? Does it exist visually, but not physically? Finally, one of the most perplexing questions ever asked in the history of mankind: If a tree falls in the woods and no one is around to hear it, does it make a sound?

You may be wondering what these hypothetical and philosophical questions have to do with the concrete biologic ideas of sensory systems. In fact, these questions and thought experiments fuel the spirit of inquiry for many who study sensation and perception. In reality, the questions posed in the preceding paragraph are not trivial at all. Questions such as these drive our scientific curiosity to seek out improved understanding of the role of sensation and perception in human behavior.

One of the most challenging concepts to grasp is the notion that the perception of our world (i.e., coming to know what is real and what exists and how to use these concepts functionally to behave) is totally dependent on the nervous system to transduce, transmit, integrate, and cognitively process a limited range of sensory inputs. We are born, effectively, a sensory "blank slate." Everything we learn about how we interact with our world, from the effects of gravity on our bodies to the spectrum of colors around us, to sounds and their meanings, to textures are based on our capacity to take information in and formulate it into a code that is understood by the electrochemical nature of the nervous system.

This chapter provides an overview of the major sensory systems and processing factors that enable us to encode, transmit, and appreciate sensory events. From the perspective of a practicing professional in communication sciences and disorders, it is important to appreciate that all forms of behavioral treatment rely on the premise that a client possesses the ability to detect and appreciate the

behavioral details of therapy activities. Sensory systems are, in fact, the only avenue through which carefully crafted treatments can be appreciated and understood by the patient. Without sensation and perception of what is being taught and demonstrated, the client will be unable to (1) internalize the specific details of the task, (2) make behavioral changes in response to what is taught, and (3) appreciate the nature of those changes with regard to the client's own performance.

The first section of this chapter reviews the organization of the general mechanisms of sensory coding that are universally applicable to all sensory systems. The second portion of the chapter provides an overview of the major sensory **modality** systems: the somatosensory, auditory/vestibular, visual, and chemical senses. For each sensory modality, the specialized peripheral structures, transduction mechanisms, and dedicated pathways through the nervous system are presented.

Sensation versus Perception

Sensation consists of the processes by which specialized neural structures known as **sensory receptors**, located throughout the body, come to be activated by environmental or internal stimuli and produce corresponding neural signals. Sensation is, at its simplest, a two-step process that transduces real-world energy of a stimulus event into signals carried by the nervous system and transmits them through the nervous system to the systems concerned with the stimulus. The first step, transduction, can be thought of as the receiving phase of the process, whereby specialized sensory receptors interact with real-world stimulus energies to convert them into the electrochemical "language" of the **central nervous system (CNS)**. After transduction, the converted raw inputs are subsequently transmitted through the nervous system in the form of electrical signals known as **action potentials** along dedicated axon pathways to specialized regions of the CNS.

If sensation consists of the reception and transmission of important stimulus features, **perception** is the interpretation of these raw inputs once they reach CNS locations. Perception is an integrative process actively constructed by the brain and dependent on past experiences with a given stimulus or set of stimuli. In short, it is a cognitive and conceptually based event. Concepts such as sounds, smells, colors, and tactile feelings are all cognitively constructed ideas and truly exist only within the network functioning of the brain itself. Pressure waves, chemicals, light waves, and mechanical features of an object, on the other hand, are the raw materials that we use to construct these conceptual categories. To complicate matters of perception further, the biologic systems and mechanisms that underlie our perceptual skills are far from perfect. The nervous system is not capable of creating a "carbon copy" of the environment. Considering the nearly infinite array of sensory stimuli available to us at every moment in time as we pass through our environment, we simply do not possess the biologic means of transducing every bit of information or every variation of a sensory signal that we may encounter at every second. Thus, perception requires us to develop conceptual categories that emerge throughout our lives as a consequence of repeated and variant experiences. The categories that we create help us predict and infer future events and interpret novel experiences based on our past experiences with similar events.

The nervous system samples the environment using a limited set of sensors and sensory systems. Our sensory systems detect only a small and narrow range of stimuli, with these stimuli becoming the raw materials upon which our cognitive world is built. What we perceive is highly constrained by the anatomic and physiologic characteristics of the peripheral sensory apparatus that interfaces with the environment. There are many information gaps in the sensory stream; thus, the brain must develop cognitive strategies to predict and infer from earlier experiences and fill in those sensory gaps.

"If a tree falls in the woods and there is no one around to hear it, is there a sound?" Technically, the answer is no. The falling tree results in changes in air pressure, but sound exists only if the right set of sensory receptors and a brain linked to those receptors with sufficient past experience with falling objects are in the vicinity to interpret those variations in air pressure.

■ Universal Aspects of Sensory Systems

A **sensory system** is defined as the collection of peripheral sensory receptors, neural pathways, and parts of the brain that are involved in the perception of a given modality, or type, of sensory stimulus. Behavioral and functional differences among sensory systems stem from different real-world energies that activate each pathway and the processing characteristics of the components constituting a given system. Because of these factors, each neuron along a sensory system is functionally related

to and participates exclusively toward the appreciation of a modality-specific **percept**. In other words, no matter how a neuron is activated within a given sensory system, the defined modality of the system will always be perceived. For example, if a photoreceptor is activated using a mechanical stimulus, we perceive flashes of light, not touch. If your head has ever been hit hard enough that you "saw stars," it was because the impact mechanically jostled the photoreceptors in your eye, triggering a spurious train of action potentials that activated visual regions of your **cerebral cortex**, giving you the perception of seeing flashes of light. Thus, perception is effectively localized and mapped by modality or class of sensation to specific cortical regions. Together, these ideas form what is referred to as the **labeled-line principle of sensory systems**, one of the foundational tenets of sensory neuroscience.

Quantifying Sensation and Perception

One of the experimental challenges of studying sensation and perception is the ability to quantify and correlate neuron activation along a sensory system to our internal and personal appreciation of a sensation resulting from that neuronal activity. In other words, how do we know that what I perceive as "red" is the same color you perceive as "red"? Why does a small cut on the skin cause someone mild discomfort, while in another person it results in great pain? Several key investigators throughout the past 150 years have defined quantifiable laws of perception that give us insight into our ability to detect, discriminate, and process sensory inputs.

Although the details of sensory reception and processing are different from one sensory modality to another, three basic conditions are applicable to almost all of the senses:

1. A physical stimulus of some type must be present to initiate sensation and perception.

2. Some form of peripheral apparatus and mechanism is required to transduce a physical event into a series of neuronal action potentials.

3. Some form of response to the signal, either conscious or unconscious, is needed to complete the cycle.

These basic steps are amenable to two distinct manners of investigation, leading to the evolution of two highly productive fields of study: psychophysics and sensory physiology. Psychophysics is the science that relates physical properties of a stimulus to our internal percepts. Sensory physiology, on the other hand, is more concerned with neural activity associated with a stimulus and how the stimulus is transduced and processed by specific regions of the nervous system.

Psychophysics has given us several ways to quantify subjective experiences, including measures of **sensory threshold**, detectability, and discrimination; **just-noticeable differences (JNDs)**; and **magnitude estimation**. These metrics are routinely incorporated into assessment methods to define the sensitivity and integrity of sensory systems. Sensory thresholds define the smallest magnitude of input required to detect a stimulus event. By plotting detection against intensity of a test stimulus, **psychometric functions** can be defined and utilized as normative measures for diagnostic purposes. Psychophysical experiments have shown us that threshold detection and discrimination are highly modulated based upon factors such as prior experience, practice, fatigue, and the context of stimulus presentation. We refer to such changes as a contextual shift in the psychometric function for a given form of sensory information. For example, pain from injuries sustained during contact sports such as football is commonly suppressed or attenuated. It is not uncommon for football players not to realize they have broken a bone during a game until they are changing out of their uniforms in the locker room.

Another critical discovery is the appreciation of stimulus intensity and its role for distinguishing between different magnitudes of common stimuli, such as distinguishing the brightness of two sources of light. Why is it easy to distinguish the brightness between a dim and a bright light source, whereas determining differences between two bright lights is difficult? Ernst Weber famously addressed this question in the early nineteenth century, suggesting a qualitative relation between discrimination and intensity. Weber's law states that the **just-noticeable difference (JND)** between two stimuli can be defined as $\Delta S = K \times S$, where K is a constant and ΔS is the minimal difference in strength between a reference stimulus and a second stimulus whereby a difference can be detected. This law essentially states that the magnitude of change needed to distinguish a difference between a reference and a second stimulus must increase as the magnitude of the reference intensity increases. In the mid-nineteenth century, Gustav Fechner refined Weber's law to characterize the relationship between stimulus magnitude and subjective stimulus intensity using a logarithmic scale according to Fechner's equation, defined as: $I = K \log[S/S_0]$, where I is the subjective intensity perceived by an individual, S_0 is the reference stimulus, and S is the comparison stimu-

lus. Stanley Smith Stevens, building upon work by Weber, Fechner, and other psychophysicists, determined that the subjective perception of stimuli is better characterized as a power function in the form of $I = K(S - S_0)^a$. In this equation, I is the intensity or magnitude perceived by the individual, K is a constant, S is the stimulus strength, and S_0 is the threshold amplitude of the stimulus. Over a limited range of intensities, Fechner's and Stevens's laws are in very close agreement. Stevens's equation, though, is a more accurate description of subjective intensity along the entire range of an experience. Intrinsic in both Stevens's and Fechner's equations is the notion that intensity measures depend on a comparison of a given stimulus input to a reference of the same modality. This basic comparison is the foundation for clinical assessment methods such as those found in clinical audiometry. A more detailed discussion on clinical audiometric methods and practices is provided in **Chapter 13**. Stevens continued to refine methods to quantify human perception by introducing tests of magnitude estimation, in which participants used a numeric scale to estimate the magnitude of a stimulus. If you are ever asked to rate your pain or discomfort on a scale from 1 to 10 at the doctor's office, you can thank Stevens (and Fechner) for this innovation. These types of assessment are quite robust and show that verbal reports of one's experience are reliable and repeatable within an individual or when assessing the same type of stimulus class.

The combination of psychophysics with sensory physiologic approaches has further advanced our understanding of human perception by bridging the gap between subjective experience and neuronal activation. Groundbreaking work by sensory physiologists such as Vernon Mountcastle in the 1960s and 1970s ushered in a new era of understanding of how perception is physiologically encoded by the nervous system. Using direct microelectrode recordings of sensory receptors and other neurons within a sensory system, Mountcastle was one of the first investigators to characterize statistically the neural signals generated by environmental stimuli corresponding to psychophysical data under perceptual task conditions. By recording neural activity at discrete locations and stages of information processing within a sensory system, it was discovered that all sensory systems neurally encode and respond to four basic stimulus attributes: modality, location, intensity, and duration. The details and mechanisms related to these four essential sensory attributes are presented in the following sections.

Stimulus Attributes Related to Perception

Modality

Modality is the general class and form of a sensory stimulus available to the nervous system. The major sensory modalities include touch and proprioception, pain and temperature, hearing and balance, vision, smell, and taste. Each modality is mediated by distinct groups or classes of sensory receptors throughout the body. Sensory receptors are dedicated anatomic components capable of transducing real-world stimulus energies into the electrochemical signals of the nervous system and are excellent at encoding specific stimulus features into trains of action potentials. The major classes of sensory receptors are defined by the form of energy or stimuli they transduce and include the following: **mechanoreceptors** (touch, hearing, balance, proprioception), **photoreceptors** (vision), **chemoreceptors** (smell, taste), **thermoreceptors** (temperature), and **nociceptors** (pain).

Within a modality, more than one type of sensory receptor is usually present in the body to record a particular portion of the total range of defining events. In other words, for each major modality, one can define a number of more discrete submodalities. A submodality represents a specific "quality" of a given class of sensation. For example, tactile sensations can feel like a flutter, or a stretch, or pressure; foods can taste salty or sweet; pictures can vary in their coloring or brightness. Underlying the ability to detect the variety of sensory qualities that exist is the notion that sensory receptors are "filters," highlighting a specific range of values within a complex stimulus and ignoring or attenuating the rest. For example, a given mechanoreceptor is not responsive to all forms of tactile energy, but rather is activated to a specific mechanical feature such as an edge, vibration, or stretching of skin.

Receptor function can also be physiologically characterized by constructing a **tuning curve**, which plots the activation level of a receptor (frequency of action potentials) against the intensity of the driving stimulus input. As with all tuning curves, the minimum intensity required to activate the receptors maximally can be quantified, as well as how the receptor varies its response to stimulus inputs that deviate from the optimal. Since sensory receptors are sensitive to a limited range of inputs, the direct implication is that many different types of receptors, with differing ranges of sensitivity, are needed to appreciate fully the nuances and complexities of naturally occurring sensory events.

Location

To determine the location and point of origin of a stimulus event, the brain must possess some means of mapping external space to central neural structures and representations. The simple position of a sensory receptor within a given sensory organ is a major factor conveying spatial properties (profile, contour, size) and location of a stimulus. At the core of this ability is a key anatomic and functional feature of a sensory neuron called the **receptive field**. A receptive field is defined as the skin area, region of space, or tonal space in which an adequate stimulus generates action potentials in a sensory neuron. Simply, the receptive field is the area or region of space being "monitored" by a sensory neuron. A stimulus that lands within the confines of a sensory receptor's receptive field will activate the receptor, whereas a stimulus falling outside of that region would result in no response from the receptor. As illustrated in **Fig. 9.1**, receptive fields are classified as small or large. Small receptive fields map onto a very small region of the sensory organ and are usually clustered together in tight groupings, producing a high density of sensors in a given body region. Together, these features enable individuals to detect and discriminate small variations in sensory input. Large receptive fields, on the other hand, span large areas of the sensory organ and do not allow precise localization of the stimulus or great discriminatory skill.

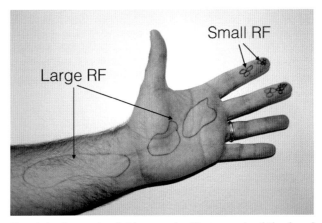

Fig. 9.1 Receptive field example. Photograph of the hand and arm illustrating small and large receptive fields at various locations on the skin.

The **two-point discrimination** test is a simple experiment to measure the size and density of receptive fields on your skin. In this test, an adjustable two-pronged probe is used to map the spatial resolution and, therefore, receptive field properties of the skin. You can make a simple test probe kit by uncurling 10 paper clips and bending them into the shape of a **V**. For each paper-clip probe, set the distance between the ends to different values from 1 to 10 mm in 1-mm increments. Begin by using the widest-spaced probe to touch the skin of your fingertip. Be sure that both points touch the skin simultaneously and that you are using a constant amount of contact pressure. Detecting the two points should be quite easy at this probe tip distance. Repeat this procedure using probes of decreasing distance until you find a probe that generates the perception of a single point when touched to the skin. When this happens, you have discovered a single receptive field. Attempt this experiment on other body parts such as the back of your hand, arm, and shoulder. You will soon discover that your sensitivity in detecting one or two points changes depending on location.

If you were to test all possible skin locations, the most sensitive areas of the body (i.e., those with the lowest detection/discrimination thresholds) are those involved in behaviors requiring great skill and a high need for detailed sensory information. The lips and the fingertips possess the lowest two-point thresholds, while the skin of the back and forearm have the highest. By default, sensory organs that possess dense numbers of small receptive fields are going to be represented by greater numbers of neurons and thus take up a disproportionately larger part of the central neural representation responsible for processing and integration. Put simply, the relationship between the size and density of receptive fields and the central neural representation of that body part are closely related. As such, the fingertips and the orofacial region possess high numbers of small receptive fields, which, in turn, provide the CNS with much more specific and detailed information regarding tactile events.

The physical dimensions of a receptive field help to define the spatial properties of a stimulus, such as its size and surface structure. Under natural conditions, a stimulus typically falls onto many receptive fields and many sensory receptors simultaneously. Under these conditions, some receptive fields are completely covered and others are only partially covered. The distribution of activated versus nonactivated receptive fields gives the nervous system an estimate of the relative size and profile of the stimulus. To accentuate the spatial features of a stimulus that lies on many receptive fields, the nervous system employs several mechanisms to enhance the contrast between activated and nonactivated receptive fields. The ability to enhance the differences among receptive fields is a common feature of sensory systems. One of the primary means to achieve contrast enhancement is to employ **lateral inhibition**. Under lateral inhibition, inhibitory interneurons at locations upstream from the sensory receptor, typically within central nuclei, suppress activity of nonactivated or weakly activated receptive fields surrounding those that are strongly activated.

Box 9.1 The Critical Value of Sensation

Sensation is at the heart of learning to produce and maintain the constituent behaviors underlying speech production and perception. The ability to appreciate our sensory environment is critically important for recognizing everything from the nuances of producing speech sounds to understanding an inspiring speaker or actors in a play. To produce just one independent phoneme, our entire system from respiration to voice to resonance and articulation must work in a rapid, precisely coordinated manner. This level of coordination requires that that the central nervous system possess reliable, accurate, and detailed information regarding the real-time state of the system during a behavior. If you could no longer feel where your tongue was or how it contacted your teeth to produce a specific sound, do you think you would be as accurate at making an /s/? High-fidelity sensory systems allow us to adaptively self-correct and maintain our speech production and perception skills to a high degree of competency.

A frequently used approach used in speech therapy is to shape accurate speech production skills by focusing on salient feedback to inform production attempts. Typically, patients are provided with sensory feedback through acoustic, visual, and tactile channels ("Did that sound right?" or "Put your tongue here" or "Watch my lips"). The central role of the clinician is to increase the sensory saliency of therapeutic activities by crafting intervention opportunities to increase patient access to quality sensory feedback. In turn, the quality of incoming sensory feedback and patient ability to process and use that information are paramount for adaptive and intelligible speech production.

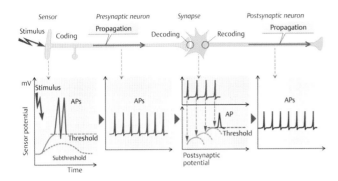

Fig. 9.2 Receptor potential and action potential generation. A stimulus event is transduced by a sensory receptor, leading to depolarization of the sensor. Receptor potential generation leads to action potential firing and the transmission of the stimulus down that axon. In turn, action potentials trigger neurotransmitter release at synapses with a second neuron downstream.

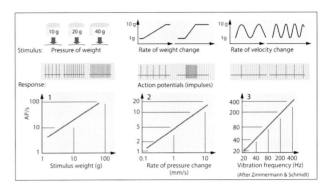

Fig. 9.3 Receptor coding of intensity. Three different stimulus examples (static weight, rate, or frequency) are used to illustrate the change in action potential firing rate with changes in stimulus intensity.

Intensity

Understanding stimulus intensity has much to do with how the nervous system translates or codes physical properties of real-world events. As previously discussed, sensory receptors are at the forefront of this process, but how exactly do these physical features get translated or mapped into differences in neuronal activity by the receptor? The receptor potential is the fundamental mechanism underlying this process.

The **receptor potential** is a graded change in membrane voltage of a sensory receptor produced by an adequate and appropriate form of real-world energy corresponding to the modality of the system. For example, a mechanoreceptor is activated through physical deformation or change in shape of its transducing element. Such change results in the opening of Na$^+$ and K$^+$ **ion channels**, initiating a depolarizing current into the sensory receptor. For the most part, receptor potentials are depolarizing events, with the exception of the visual system, where the graded response is hyperpolarizing. The receptor potential that is generated as a consequence of a stimulus reflects the "actual" moment when analog real-world stimuli are transformed into the electrochemical signal understood by the nervous system (**Fig. 9.2**).

All sensory receptors have a threshold of activation required to generate action potentials and subsequent transmission of the input toward the CNS. As illustrated in **Fig. 9.2**, if the stimulus-evoked receptor potential is of sufficient magnitude, the sensory receptor initiates a series of action potentials subsequently propagated down its **primary**

afferent axon toward the CNS. On the other hand, when a stimulus is very weak, it will not cause sufficient change in receptor potential to generate action potentials in the afferent axon. Under these conditions, the stimulus has a subthreshold effect on the sensory receptor. Subthreshold effects are quite interesting in that they clearly demonstrate how sensory receptors effectively filter low-level inputs, allowing the CNS to remain responsive to stronger inputs, which are likely to be more salient to ongoing behavior. Subthreshold effects are also interesting in that they confirm that the CNS is not a "copy machine" but rather extracts information out of the environment. For example, imagine watching a ladybug land on your hand. You can see the ladybug but have no tactile sense of the bug on your skin. Because of visual input, you are clearly aware that the ladybug exists and is on your skin. If your eyes were closed when the ladybug landed on you, would the ladybug still exist from your perspective? If you were relying on touch only, the answer is no. Awareness and perception require stimulus transmission to the CNS; transduction alone is insufficient to result in perception.

The strength and pattern of receptor potential in response to a stimulus sets the stage for transmission of a stimulus's features to the CNS. Intensity is a critical sensory feature that depends upon the graded nature of the receptor potential. As shown in **Fig. 9.3**, stronger stimuli result in greater changes in a sensory receptor potential, which in turn causes the receptor to generate greater numbers of action potentials at faster rates. Simply, a sensory receptor effectively "codes" changes in stimulus intensity through a change in the number and rate of action potential generation. Rate coding is a ubiquitous functional feature in the CNS and can be found operating in all sensory systems.

Duration

The temporal properties of a stimulus event are encoded by the patterns of action potential generation by a sensory receptor. A common functional aspect of sensory receptors is that they will adapt to a chronic and unchanging stimulus by decreasing firing rate. This phenomenon is referred to as receptor adaptation and is believed to be strongly related to our ability to adapt perceptually to sensory experiences. The manner in which a receptor adapts is characterized as either being slow or rapid (**Fig. 9.4**). **Slowly adapting (SA)** receptors begin firing at the onset of a stimulus event and remain active as long as the stimulus remains present within the receptive field. This form of adaptation is ideal for providing the nervous system with key information about the persistence of a stimulus. On the other hand, **rapidly adapting (RA)** receptors begin firing at the onset of a stimulus, but then immediately cease generating action potentials during a steady-state event. RA receptors are active only during dynamically changing stimulus events (onsets and offsets), and as such signal the rate at which a stimulus is presented. The firing patterns of RA receptor activity are the bases for motion perception in the visual system and vibration sense in somatosensory systems.

Organization of Sensory Systems

All sensory systems possess a common serial or hierarchical information-processing structure. For example, real-world sensations are transduced by a given class of specialized receptors, then transmitted centrally via dedicated and organized pathways, and lastly made available to unimodal primary sensory areas of the cerebral cortex. Each primary sensory cortical area shares a number of basic properties that summarize information-processing activity, giving us insight into how peripheral inputs will later be used to construct more complex unified perceptual abstractions. First, inputs to primary sensory areas come from the thalamic nuclei, making the thalamus an obligatory source of cortical input. Second, neurons in primary sensory areas are spatially or functionally organized to form a detailed topographic mapping or representation of the sensory surface of interest. For example, in the somatosensory system, the body surface is topographically represented in the cortex reflecting spatial and functional aspects of touch, whereas in the auditory system, sound frequency is mapped. Whether we are talking about the skin, the **cochlea**, or the retina, peripheral inputs are

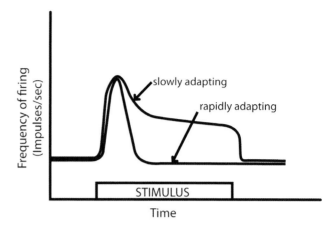

Fig. 9.4 Slow and rapid adaptation. Superimposed line drawings for both slow and rapid adaptation rates are shown.

ordered in primary sensory zones. Third, injury to a sensory map will cause a deficit or loss in function localized to the matching region of the peripheral sensory organ. For example, a lesion to the hand representation in the somatosensory cortex will result in paresthesias or sensory disturbances to the contralateral hand, not to the face or leg. Finally, although not exclusively, primary sensory areas process peripheral inputs that are contralateral to the physical location of the sensory receptor sheet.

From primary sensory areas, inputs are processed by a succession of "higher-order" sensory areas that possess different operational features, reflecting more complex abstraction and integration of initial sensory inputs. Higher-order areas receive input from lower-level cortical zones, have less precise topographical mappings of the periphery, and project back to primary sensory areas to actively modulate those areas' activity. Injuries to these zones do not cause deficits in signal detection but rather create complex perceptual and cognitive disturbances related to a sensory modality. The underlying reason for these complex disturbances lies in the fact that higher-order areas are organized in parallel to each other, processing common inputs found in primary areas in different ways simultaneously.

Several sensory systems (visual, somatosensory, and auditory systems) possess what are called dorsal and ventral processing streams. Simply, dorsal streams serve spatial functions, and ventral streams serve recognition operations. Thus, an injury to the dorsal stream of the visual system will cause anomalous perceptions in object motion but not in the color or shape of that same object. Imagine the perceptual disconnect if objects seemed to move erratically like scenes in a stop-motion film.

Active Regulation of Sensation and Perception by the CNS

We are capable of remarkable control and regulation of our own appreciation of an experience through changes in attentional state. When learning a new skill, such as driving a car for the first time, our attentional system actively suppresses vast quantities of sensory information from all sources to help keep our hands steady on the wheel, the car going straight, and our eyes on the road ahead. This type of attentional control occurs frequently during our daily lives. For example, if I tell you to start paying attention to how the sleeve of your shirt feels on your arm right now, suddenly what was once perceptually unnoticed, instantly becomes noticeable. Before I suggested this example to you, you were likely unaware of your shirt sleeve. Yet, tactile sensory receptors were still firing and centrally transmitting the details of the fabric as you moved your arm. The difference is that these inputs were not salient to you until you were made aware of them. By focusing your attention on your sleeve, you modulated your perceptual system to raise the already present tactile inputs coming from your arm to a higher level of conscious awareness. The ability to alter perception based upon the level of attention has major implications for exactly how and what we learn from our experiences in the world. Therapeutically, attention becomes a criti-

cal factor to manipulate directly during the course of treatment. If you consider that many treatment tasks are multimodal, attention to specific features or characteristics of a therapeutic task may allow modulation of perceptual systems to achieve the intended treatment goal better. During the course of treatment, the ebb and flow of patient attention must be considered to optimize learning.

■ The Somatosensory System

Holding the soft hand of a newborn baby, feeling the warmth of a summer's day on your face, having that itch you can't quite reach to scratch, sensing the pain from stubbing your toe, and even knowing how your body is moving as you walk across campus to get to your next class are all brought to you courtesy of the somatosensory system. Unlike other senses, which typically mediate one form of real-world stimuli and are localized to one discrete area of the body such as the eye or ear, the somatosensory system mediates a variety of stimulus energies (mechanical, thermal, chemical, and nociceptive) throughout the entire body surface, from within the viscera, sinuses, and cavities and throughout the musculoskeletal systems.

One of the founding fathers of neuroscience, Charles Sherrington, once characterized the somato-

---

Box 9.2   Anatomical Variants and Synesthesia

Can you see the words people speak? Do you associate sounds with specific colors? Synesthesia, or the union of the senses, refers to a neurologic state in which activation of one sensory pathway involuntarily triggers activation in a second sensory pathway. There are two major forms of synesthesia: associative and projecting. In projecting synesthesia, individuals report actually seeing colors, numbers, letters or shapes when a sensation pathway is stimulated, rather than just seeing it in their mind's eye. On the other hand, those with associative synesthesia report a strong, involuntary connection between a stimulus and a sensation; having a sense that two stimuli must belong together. One commonly reported associative synesthesia form is the experience of numbers and/or letters having an assigned color, referred to as graphemic synesthesia. People with graphemic synesthesia may describe remembering a telephone number or someone's name by its color representation.

Synesthesia was a popular research topic in the late nineteenth and early twentieth centuries and is experiencing a resurgence of interest these days. Although researchers have not yet reached a consensus, many scientists contend that synesthesia is not just the result of an overactive imagination but has a structural basis in neural connectivity. Individuals experiencing synesthesia may have increased neural activation or additional neural connectivity within and between sensory cortical areas compared to others. Further research in the area of synesthesia may provide scientists with key insight into brain connectivity and how sensory information is normally processed (Hupé and Dojat 2015).

Box Fig. 9.1   Example of graphemic synesthesia.

sensory system as having three principal responsibilities: (1) **exteroception**, (2) **interoception**, and (3) **proprioception**. In essence, Sherrington's conception enables you to frame the function of the system into sensations that arise from outside the body (exteroception), those that arise from within the body (interoception), and those that result in our awareness of how our body is moving through and is positioned in space (proprioception). This framework is critical to the study of the anatomic complexities of somatosensation and their perceptual consequences.

Using Sherrington's framework, the somatosensory system can be conceptualized as a collection of several subsenses or, more technically, submodalities. These submodalities of somatosensation include the sense of touch, proprioception, mechanical or chemically induced pain, and temperature. Each of these submodalities can be further subdivided into more specific forms, such as tactile stretch and pressure detection or hot and cold temperature sense. Together, transduction and simultaneous perceptual processing of these submodalities leads to exteroceptive, interoceptive, and proprioceptive cognitive awareness.

Exteroception enables direct sensation of interactions with the world as differing external environmental conditions are encountered. The main submodality in this category is touch, which includes specific sensory events such as pressure, contact, vibration, and directional motion on the skin. Included in exteroception is the sense of temperature and pain, often overlooked, yet critical for safe interactions with the environment. Receptor classes that mediate exteroceptive signals include mechanoreceptors, nociceptors, and thermoreceptors. Essentially, exteroception is any sense that would enable you to obtain information regarding the form, shape, heft, and safety of an object or environment.

Interoception, conversely, enables the detection and appreciation of the internal functioning of the body and the physical state of major visceral organ systems. Interoceptive signals typically do not rise to the level of consciousness, but they are critical for providing key information for autonomic control and monitoring of internal body systems. Occasionally, interoception does gain conscious awareness, as in the case of gastrointestinal discomfort after eating an ill-prepared meal. Interoception uses receptor classes such as chemoreceptors, nociceptors, and mechanoreceptors to transduce signals from cardiovascular, renal, digestive, and respiratory systems.

Finally, proprioception is the ability to detect and sense position and movement in the environment. Proprioceptive signals provide critical feedback to motor control systems that enable both learning and refining all forms of movements, both skilled and gross. Classically, proprioceptors have been considered to include only sensory end organs present within muscle tissue, tendons, joint capsules, and ligaments, as these endings are well situated to transduce changes in body position. Recent studies, however, question this exclusivity. Work by Edin during the early 1990s discovered that humans are capable of determining finger position and motion through the exclusive use of cutaneous exteroceptors. In the human orofacial system, the case for the use of other forms of proprioception is more compelling. Psychophysical studies in humans and various anatomic studies in primates confirmed that the lower face is devoid of all forms of "classical" proprioceptors. These data strongly suggest that cutaneous mechanoreceptors are well suited and fully capable of transducing the sensory consequences of movement and contraction of the facial musculature.

The remaining portion of this section will describe the anatomic features and pathways that lead from peripheral transduction of somatosensory stimulus energies to central processing and integrative locations where cognitive perception is formed. The anatomic pathways comprised in the somatosensory system include: (1) the **dorsal-column medial lemniscal (DCML) pathway**, (2) the **anterolateral system (ALS)**, and last (3) the **trigeminothalamic pathway** and **trigeminal lemniscus**. These three pathways can be functionally grouped into those that mediate touch and proprioception versus those that mediate pain and temperature. Furthermore, the specific region of the body that each path mediates can be used as a differentiating factor as well. The DCML pathway mediates touch and proprioception for all body zones inferior to the head, while the trigeminal lemniscus route mediates these same inputs arising from the head and vocal tract. Similarly, pain and temperature sense from body zones inferior to the head are mediated by the ALS, while these same sensibilities for areas of the head and vocal tract are mediated by the trigeminothalamic pathway. Together, these anatomic pathways form three parallel routes that enable the simultaneous transduction and processing of all aspects of an experience involving somatosensation.

As discussed previously, the parallel nature of these paths forms the anatomic basis for the somatosensory version of labeled-line theory, the ability to segregate different sensory aspects of an experience into dedicated processing routes. Keep in mind that transduction and transmission are

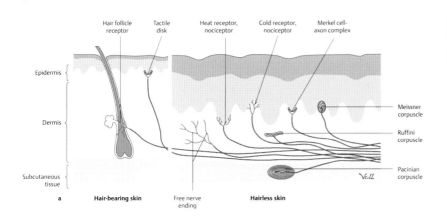

Fig. 9.5 Cutaneous mechanoreceptors. Nociceptors, thermoreceptors, free nerve endings, and mechanoreceptors are shown in the hairy and non-hairy skin.

only the beginning stages of perception. Only later do segregated inputs become holistically bound together with all other forms and modalities of sensation to help us develop conscious and cogent perception of a complex event or experience.

The Peripheral Somatosensory Apparatus: Sensory Receptors and the Primary Afferent

All three somatosensory pathways begin with a group of sensory receptors located either in the skin or the musculoskeletal system specifically tuned to transduce different forms and types of stimulus energies. These signals are then transmitted centrally toward the CNS along axons with differing diameters, degrees of myelination, and conduction velocities. Together, these first components of the somatosensory system (the sensory receptor plus the primary afferent) represent the first leg of a three-neuron system responsible for transmitting somatosensation from the outside world into the cerebral cortex.

Sensory Receptors of the Somatosensory System

Touch

Touch sensations arise from the outer skin and epidermal layers that line the oral mucosa, the vocal tract, and the laryngeal mucosa and lumen. In general, the skin can be subdivided into skin that possesses hair in some form (hairy skin, nonglabrous) and skin that does not have hair (glabrous). The vermilion border of the lip, palms of the hand, and soles of the feet are examples of glabrous skin, as is the epidermal lining of vocal tract structures. The skin provides a direct interface with external

events and is the most expansive sense organ of the body. Although touch sensations can be passive or imposed upon the skin surface, most forms of touch involve an active component whereby the skin is moved by the underlying musculature to synchronize motor control activity with the sensory consequences of volitional movement. Generally speaking, the ability to perform such synchronization is a crucial aspect underlying sensorimotor learning of skills and behaviors.

In the somatosensory system, mechanoreceptors form the principal sensory end organ that mediates tactile events such as pressure, directional stroking-type motion, vibration, flutter, and simple contact. Mechanoreceptors are sensory end organs that are sensitive to mechanical distortion, thus making the mechanoreceptor optimally suited for transducing tactile events from the environment. In the skin, five mechanoreceptor channels, mostly named for the European histologists who discovered them, are recognized: the (1) Meissner corpuscle, (2) Pacinian corpuscle, (3) Merkel disks, (4) Ruffini endings, and the (5) hair follicle receptor (**Fig. 9.5**).

Given the wide range of possible real-world stimulus energies available to us, mechanoreceptors vary in their (1) response to an ideal stimulating energy, (2) morphology, (3) receptive field size, and (4) embedded depth and proportion within the skin. Mechanoreceptors are distributed throughout the skin in different ratios and densities depending on the functional nature of the body zone. For example, the glabrous skin of the fingertips possesses a huge number of mechanoreceptive endings with small and closely packed receptive fields. This anatomy corresponds well to the exquisite sensitivity of the fingertips in the perception of textures and the ability to discriminate small changes in the surface features of objects. Similarly, the orofacial skin possesses receptor numbers that rival that of the hand, yet the proportion of specific receptor classes differs to support the behavioral need to transduce skin strain and stretch during speech and feeding behaviors. Finally, the skin of the forearm and the back possesses few or widely spaced tactile endings. Of the endings that are present, the majority possess large and wide receptive fields. In this case, we have the opposite condition: a body segment that is poorly able to transduce meaningful tactile information. Consider how often we use our backs or forearms to detect the shape or discriminate the texture of an object. This simple example highlights a critical feature of the somatosensory system; the number of sensory end organs in an area of skin, the size of their receptive fields, the adaptation properties of the receptor, and the form of energy each transduces are all critical factors that combine to contribute to our cognitive perception.

To transduce the wide range of stimulus energies that skin encounters under natural conditions, each type of cutaneous mechanoreceptor possesses a distinctive morphology and innervation pattern that enable it to transduce its particular range of tactile energy over its receptive field. By using controlled tactile inputs and determining the corresponding perception associated with these inputs, investigators in psychophysics and sensory physiology have defined the response characteristics of human cutaneous endings as described in the following paragraphs.

Merkel disks are found at the border of the epidermis and dermis and are clustered about papillary ridges in glabrous skin. Merkel disks possess small receptive fields, are innervated by slowly adapting type 1 (SA1) axon fibers, and are sensitive to edges and pointlike surfaces. In fact, these characteristics make the Merkel disk an ideal mechanoreceptor candidate to transduce the raised dot-pattern features used for reading Braille.

The Meissner corpuscle is characterized as globular in shape and is firmly attached to the papillary ridges via collagen fibers. This anatomic configuration provides an excellent substrate for detecting friction-type forces. Meissner corpuscles possess a small receptive field, are innervated by rapidly adapting type 1 (RA1) fibers, and are most sensitive to low-frequency vibration, object friction, and skin motion during movement. An example of the type of stimulus event that would engage primarily Meissner endings is the feel of your hand moving across the mesh of a window screen or the feel of a cup slipping out of your hand.

The Pacinian corpuscle (PC) is an onion-shaped receptor located deep within the dermis possessing a large receptive field and innervated by rapidly adapting type 2 (RA2) fibers. The encapsulation of the PC is believed to enable it to operate as a mechanical amplifier to high-frequency vibratory stimulation. The ideal stimuli to excite the PC are vibrational frequencies between 250 and 300 Hz. If you have ever felt on your skin the vibrations created by loud speakers during a rock concert, PCs were likely transmitting that sensation to your CNS.

Ruffini endings are stretch-sensitive spindle-shaped receptors that possess large receptive fields and are innervated by slowly adapting fibers. The Ruffini ending is ideally suited to detect stroking motion imposed on the skin as well as the direction of that motion. Imagine taking a pencil and lightly stroking the surface of your hand or feeling your lips produce a smile. The tactile information required to perceive such events are transduced by the Ruffini endings.

Finally, the hair follicle receptor is found only on nonglabrous skin and is typically innervated by free nerve endings (axon fibers with little to no myelination) that wrap around the lower shaft region of the hair-producing complex in the follicle. Hair follicle receptors activate in response to bending, pulling, or any other form of deflection of the hair shaft.

In summary, the five cutaneous mechanoreceptors transduce different salient features of a tactile experience. Receptors innervated by SA fibers are well suited to detect object pressure and tactile form, whereas receptors innervated by RA fibers are best suited to detect motion and vibratory-type activity. Thus, both SA- and RA-innervated cutaneous mechanoreceptors are needed to transduce the sensory consequences of functional and natural

Table 9.1 Cutaneous mechanoreceptors

Receptor	Sensation Detected	Adaptation
Pacinian corpuscles	Vibration	Very rapid
Hair follicles	Touch	Rapid
Meissner corpuscles	Touch	Rapid
Merkel disks	Pressure	Slow
Ruffini endings	Stretch	Slow

tactile behaviors. The different response features of the major classes of cutaneous mechanoreceptors are summarized in **Table 9.1**.

Proprioception

Proprioception consists of the ability to appreciate our body position, both statically and during movement. The two classically recognized proprioceptive endings in the somatosensory system are associated with the musculoskeletal system and are called the muscle spindle and the Golgi tendon organ (GTO). When critically considering the forms of sensory input required for the CNS to understand how we are moving or where our bodies are in space, appreciating how muscle tissue contracts, and how gravitational forces act on our bodies is critical. The muscle spindle and the GTO are well suited for transducing changes in muscle length and force, respectively.

As seen in **Fig. 9.6**, the muscle spindle consists of a football-shaped fibrous capsule containing several highly specialized fibers referred to as intrafusal fibers. The capsular structure of the muscle spindle is firmly embedded in and parallel to skeletal muscle fibers or extrafusal fibers, enabling the sensor to follow and detect muscle lengthening and contraction during action. Intrafusal fibers are innervated by a group of fast conducting axons referred to as group Ia afferents. These afferents are wrapped about the center of the intrafusal fibers and respond in a graded manner to tension changes within intrafusal fibers consequential to extrafusal activity.

One aspect of the muscle spindle that should be highlighted is the fact that muscle spindles regulate their own sensitivity dynamically during muscle contraction. Intrafusal fibers receive motor innervation via a class of motor neurons known as gamma lower motor neurons (γ-LMNs; **Fig. 9.6**). The γ-LMN system coactivates with the primary alpha lower motor neurons that innervate extrafusal fibers and ensures that the muscle spindle maintains a consistent level of tension to accommodate length changes caused by contraction or stretching. Essentially, the γ-LMN control system serves to take up the "slack" of the intrafusal fibers to maintain group Ia axon sensitivity and continuous activation.

Another critical factor to help the CNS appreciate its position in space is the effects of loading force on the skeleton. The second class of proprioceptors, GTOs, are ideally positioned within the dense fibrous tendon to transduce the loading or force exerted on the skeleton during muscle activity. As seen in **Fig. 9.6**, the GTO is positioned at the junction between the muscle and the tendon and is

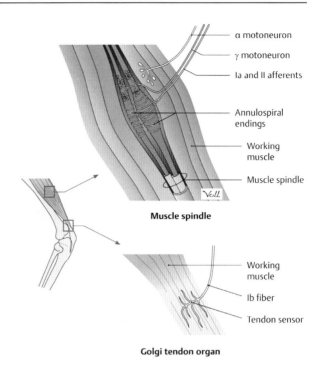

Fig. 9.6 Muscle spindles and Golgi tendon organs. Muscle spindles are sensors, innervated by group Ia afferents, that transduce static and dynamic muscle length changes. GTOs are found in tendons and operate to transduce muscle force. GTOs are innervated by group Ib afferents.

innervated by group Ib afferents. Within the GTO, fibers of the Ib afferent weave through and interdigitate with a meshwork of collagen fibers. When muscle contracts and loads the tendon, the collagen meshwork tightens and compresses the entwined Ib fibers, triggering depolarization in the afferent and signaling a graded loading input to the CNS.

In addition to the spindles and GTOs, proprioceptive inputs also arise from joint capsules and ligaments throughout the skeletal system. Afferents that innervate these zones are typically rapidly adapting mechanosensitive axons capable of transducing dynamic factors such as the angle, velocity, and direction of joint adjustment. Together with input from muscle spindles, GTOs, and cutaneous mechanoreceptors, the CNS integrates these movement-related inputs to form a map and appreciation of three-dimensional motion.

Temperature

Thermoreceptors, as the name implies, are sensitive to temperature changes in the environment and can transduce changes in ambient temperature as small as a hundredth of a degree Fahrenheit. Receptors responsible for the perception of normal ranges of temperature are located in the skin but are not distributed equally throughout the body. Thermo-receptor sensitivity and temperature direction (hot vs. cold) depends on neuronal expression of one of a family of similar ion channels, collectively known as the TRP (transient receptor potential) channels. To date, six TRP channel variants have been isolated and correlated to different temperature sensitivities from cold ($10°$ C) to hot ($> 50°$ C). Generally, only one TRP variant is expressed within a given thermoreceptor, accounting for the different degrees of temperature sensitivity and specificity throughout the body surface. As with most sensory systems, a swift change in the quality of an experience will generate the most vigorous perceptual response. Recall the temperature shock you have likely gone through when jumping into a pool after spending time sitting by the pool deck on a hot summer day. Temperature systems are particularly noticeable with regard to this functional aspect of sensation.

Pain

Why do we sense pain and what purpose does it serve? Life without the ability to perceive pain is in fact dangerous. From an evolutionary standpoint, pain perception and the ability to transduce noxious stimuli are what keep us alive. Imagine breaking a bone or burning your skin on a hot stove without any awareness of the event. These scenarios can occur in rare cases. Congenital insensitivity to pain is an extremely rare, genetically linked disorder in which an individual cannot sense any pain or even typical discomfort under any stimulus conditions. The genetic disorder targets nociceptors and appears to result in a curtailing of the depolarization mechanism necessary to trigger action potential generation in these neurons. Considering that low-level forms of **nociception** are critical to inform us of potential strain and injury to the body, routine daily events become potentially dangerous.

Now that you have a better appreciation for the importance of pain, we will discuss the peripheral mechanisms and structures responsible for transducing the critical submodality of nociception. Although pain and nociception are often confused, it is important at this point to clarify that they are not synonymous. Pain is a cognitive event. In other words, pain is the perceptual consequence of nociception, which is the processes and events that provide the raw stimuli to the CNS to appreciate pain. Pain is a perceptual quality that is highly regulated and modulated by the CNS. Nociceptors consist of free nerve endings of unmyelinated type C fibers or lightly myelinated type Aδ fibers and are responsible for the transduction of injurious events that lead to subjective perceptions of pain and discom-

fort. A variety of nociceptors transduce many forms of painful stimuli throughout the body including the skin, muscle, skeleton, internal organs, and the vascular system. Interestingly, the brain itself does not possess nociceptive endings. Nociceptors are triggered by inputs that have high likelihood of producing damage to tissues. Tissue injury can result from a host of different situations, including excessive temperature, exposure to chemical agents, and very strong tactile events. Mechanical nociceptors selectively transduce tactile inputs that mechanically damage tissue. Thermal nociceptors selectively transduce extreme levels of cold and heat. Finally, chemical nociceptors are triggered via chemical means and exposure. The majority of nociceptors, however, are multimodal and triggered by all forms of damaging inputs.

Generally, when tissue is damaged, many chemical agents are released by the damaged cells including neurotransmitters, cytokines, proteases, neurotrophins, histamines, and peptides. These agents initiate metabolic events that result in swelling, heat, redness, and increased vascular response to the injury site, as well as an increase or amplification of nociceptive reactivity. Importantly, peptides such as bradykinin can directly activate nociceptors, and substance P can induce vasodilation and further histamine release. These events are believed to contribute to hyperalgesia, a condition whereby injured tissues become exquisitely sensitive, triggering heightened pain responses to even non-noxious forms of stimulation.

Unique Anatomical Features of the Human Orofacial Region

With regard to speech production, the human lower face possess a unique set of anatomic and functional sensory characteristics that likely support orofacial behaviors such as speech and feeding. Histologic and electrophysiologic analyses have revealed that orofacial mechanoreceptors resemble those of the rapidly adapting type I (RA I) and the slowly adapting types I and II (SA I and II) receptor, typically found in the glabrous and nonglabrous skin of the hand. Conspicuously absent are Pacinian corpuscle (PC) type responses. The absence of PC end organs in the orofacial region has been confirmed through histologic, psychophysical, and electrophysiologic investigations in both humans and nonhuman primates.

Adding to the unique distribution of receptor types in the orofacial system, muscle spindles and GTOs are virtually nonexistent in the muscles of the lower face. Given the absence of these recep-

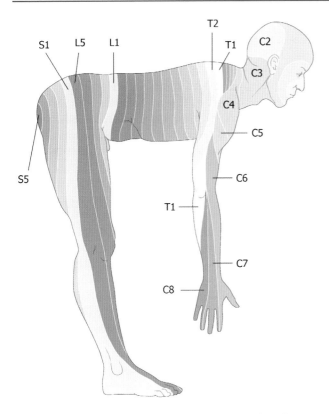

Fig. 9.7 Dermatomes are bandlike areas of skin that are innervated by primary afferents from a single pair of spinal nerves.

be broken down into two major systems: (1) axons that arise from cutaneous sources versus (2) those that arise from the musculoskeletal system. When discussing axons arising from the skin, fibers are ordered from largest to smallest in diameter in the following way: type Aα fibers, followed successively by the type Aβ, Aδ, and C fibers. Since conduction velocity is correlated to diameter, the same axon ordering also characterizes fibers from the fastest to the slowest conduction velocities. In discussing axons from the musculoskeletal system, axons are arranged into four groups: group I, II, III, and IV. Again, this order reflects the diameter and conduction velocity differences across groups. Generally speaking, proprioceptive endings are innervated by the fastest and largest-diameter axons (group I). These axons are capable of conduction speeds of well over 100 meters per second, equivalent to 250 miles per hour. Cutaneous mechanoreceptors are innervated by Aα and Aβ fibers with conduction velocities a bit slower, between 50 and 75 m/s (110–170 mph). Finally, pain and temperature receptors are typically innervated by the small-diameter and rather slowly conducting (0.5 to 2 m/s, 1.1–4.5 mph) type Aδ and C fibers.

Dermatomes

Primary afferents that arise from body areas below the head are housed within spinal nerves. Spinal nerves represent a mixture of afferents and efferents projecting to and from the spinal cord, respectively. Spinal nerves are arranged into right and left paired segments along the length of the spinal cord, with one pair of spinal nerves projecting from between a given set of adjacent vertebrae. We have 29 vertebrae in the ventral column and, therefore, 30 pairs of spinal nerves and segments. The peripheral distribution of receptors and spinal segments mirror each other in that one spinal segment provides the location for signal propagation from a discrete area of the body. These zones are referred to as **dermatomes**. Dermatomes are arranged in bands as shown in **Fig. 9.7**. Cutting the afferent fibers of a spinal nerve generally results in anesthesia of the associated dermatome on the skin.

tors and the fact that muscles of the lower face insert directly to the skin, several investigators have hypothesized an important role for cutaneous mechanoreceptor activity as an alternative means to convey proprioceptive sensibility to the face. The correlation between high numbers of stretch-sensitive SA units in facial skin, lack of spindles and GTOs in orofacial muscles, and the anatomic relationship between muscle and skin in the lower face, suggests that stretch-sensitive cutaneous receptors are fortuitously positioned to encode changes underlying muscle contraction and force generation in the face.

Innervation Zones of the Primary Afferent

As described previously, receptors are associated with an axon that projects centrally. This axon is known as the primary afferent and enters the CNS via the spinal cord or brainstem. Primary afferents vary in diameter and degree of myelination, which together strongly influences conduction velocity of action potential propagation. Nomenclature for axon type classification can be confusing, but can

Trigeminal Innervation Zones

For the head, somatosensory innervation follows the nerve distribution pattern of the trigeminal nerve (CN V). This nerve consists of three principal branches: the ophthalmic (V$_1$), maxillary (V$_2$), and mandibular (V$_3$) branches. Each branch serves different areas of the head and the face in the pattern shown in **Fig. 9.8**. In contrast to the DCML, cutaneous and proprioceptive inputs are segregated into different branches, with V$_1$ and V$_2$ mediating cutaneous inputs and V$_3$ mediating both cutaneous inputs from the lower facial skin and proprioceptive inputs from the mandibular musculature. Each branch enters into the brainstem to synapse onto three different sensory nuclei spanning the medulla, pons, and mesencephalon.

Central Somatosensory Pathways

Dorsal-Column Medial Lemniscal (DCML) System

The DCML is a somatotopically organized three-neuron pathway that exclusively mediates tactile sensation and proprioception from all regions of the body via the spinal cord. As shown in **Fig. 9.9**, the route of the primary afferent from the peripheral receptor (green line) is via the posterior (dorsal) root of each spinal nerve. The axons diverge toward posterior white matter of the spinal cord called the dorsal columns (more correctly, the dorsal or posterior funiculi). The dorsal columns are organized somatotopically into two major fasciculi: the **gracile** and **cuneate fasciculi**. Each fasciculus houses primary afferent axons from different regions of the body, with the gracile fasciculus carrying afferents from the lower limbs and lower trunk and the cuneate fasciculus carrying fibers from the upper trunk and upper extremities. The axons from the gracile and cuneate fasciculi project toward the medulla in the brainstem and terminate on neurons within the dorsal-column nuclei (also known as the posterior funicular nuclei), called the cuneate and gracile nuclei. The gracile and cuneate nuclei are the locations where the primary afferent

axons from the lower and upper body synapse onto the second neuron of the three-neuron DCML system. Dorsal-column nucleus neurons maintain the somatotopy of the pathway. Up until this point, all afferent inputs are ipsilaterally represented.

Neurons of the dorsal-column nuclei project axons across to the contralateral medulla at a location referred to as the internal arcuate. From this point onward, sensory input ascends contralaterally. It is at this point where the axons of the second-order neurons (the second leg of the three-neuron pathway) form the medial lemniscal pathway. This pathway extends from the medulla through the mesencephalon and into the diencephalon, where the axon fibers synapse onto the **ventral posterolateral (VPL) nucleus** of the thalamus. The VPL is one of many nuclei within the thalamus and is mapped to cutaneous and proprioceptive ascending inputs. The VPL maintains the somatotopic arrangement found throughout the DCML and is further organized into cutaneous and proprioceptive zones. Neurons within the VPL represent the final leg of the three-neuron system and are, therefore, called third-order neurons. These neurons project toward the cerebral cortex as **thalamocortical fibers**, innervating cells of the **postcentral gyrus**, functionally known as the **primary somatosensory cortex (S1)**. See **Table 9.2** for a summary of basic characteristics for the DCML.

Anterolateral System

The anterolateral system (ALS), also known as the **spinothalamic tract**, constitutes the principal pathway for the transmission of nociception and temperature sense as well as other submodalities including crude touch, tickle, and itch from the spinal cord. Like the DCML, the ALS is a three-neuron pathway that transmits inputs from peripheral

Table 9.2 DCML and ALS features

Somatosensory tract	Sensations projected	Types of afferent fibers	Course	Characteristics
DCML	Fine touch Pressure Two-point discrimination Vibration Proprioception	Aα and Aβ	Crosses in medulla	Preservation of modality specificity Precise mapping of body surface carried through all relays and onto the cortical surface High synaptic security
ALS	Temperature Pain Crude touch Tickle Itch	Aδ and C	Crosses in the spinal cord	Imprecise mapping of body surface Cross-modality (e.g., cutaneous and muscle) convergence Low synaptic security

(From *Physiology: An Illustrated Review*)

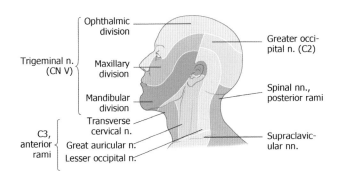

Fig. 9.8 Trigeminal innervation zones on the face. The three principal branches of the trigeminal nerve (CN V) innervate different spatial regions of the facial skin and scalp.

nociceptors and thermoreceptors. In contrast to the DCML, the ALS consists mostly of Aδ and C primary afferent fibers, which enter into the dorsal aspect of the spinal cord via the posterior roots and travel a short distance toward a region of dorsal gray matter of the spinal cord known as the substantia gelatinosa (**Fig. 9.9**; see purple line). At this location, the primary afferents synapse onto second-order neurons that then traverse the midline and enter the anterior and lateral spinothalamic tracts. From this point onward, the inputs for these submodalities are represented contralaterally. The anterolateral pathway continues through the spinal cord and brainstem to the thalamus, where second-order fibers synapse onto different regions of the VPL nucleus as well as on a secondary location known as the intralaminar nuclei of the thalamus. Finally, third-order thalamocortical projection fibers synapse on somatotopic regions of the postcentral gyrus, the anterior cingulate gyrus, and the insular lobe. A summary of basic characteristics of the ALS is shown in **Table 9.2**.

Trigeminal Lemniscus and the Trigeminothalamic Tract

The trigeminal lemniscus and the trigeminothalamic tract constitute the central pathways for touch/proprioception as well as pain and temperature, respectively, for the head. Primary afferents within the three main branches of the trigeminal nerve (CN V) project centrally toward the brainstem (**Fig. 9.8**). The cell bodies of these afferents are housed within the trigeminal ganglion, except for those from proprioceptive sources. In contrast to all other primary afferents, where the cell body is found within a peripheral ganglion, proprioceptive afferents from the mandibular muscles have cell bodies that exist within the central nervous system itself. The central targets of these primary afferents

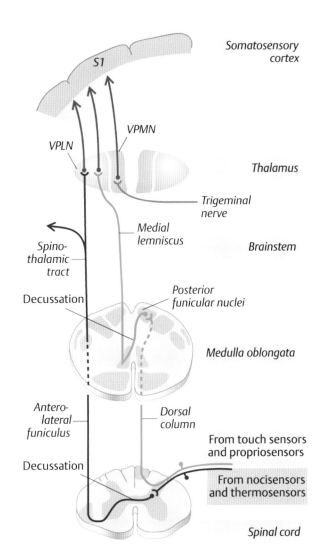

Fig. 9.9 DCML and ALS, central pathways. Touch and proprioceptive inputs are segregated from pain and temperature inputs in the somatosensory system. Both the DCML and the ALS ascend through the spinal cord in parallel toward the primary somatosensory cortex.

are the three nuclei constituting the trigeminal sensory complex (**Fig. 9.10**).

The trigeminal sensory complex consists of three separate nuclei spanning from the rostral end of the spinal cord to the mesencephalon. These nuclei are the spinal nucleus, the principal sensory nucleus, and the mesencephalic nucleus of the trigeminal nerve. Each nucleus mediates a different form of somatosensation: (1) The principal sensory nucleus is the target for cutaneous mechanoreceptive inputs arising from the skin, lips, and oral mucosa; (2) the mesencephalic nucleus is the target for proprioceptive inputs arising from the mandibular muscles; and (3) the spinal nucleus is the

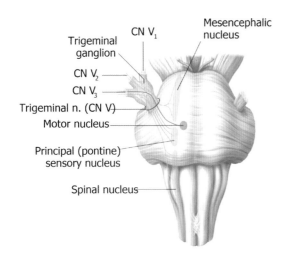

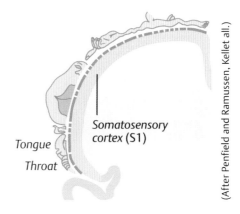

(After Penfield and Ramussen, Kellet all.)

Fig. 9.11 S1 somatotopic organization. Topographical distribution of the body surface is shown for the primary somatosensory cortex to illustrate differences in the size of neural populations subserving different regions of the skin. Note that regions with larger representations correspond to regions of the body used for highly skilled behaviors that require high levels of sensory feedback.

Fig. 9.10 Trigeminal sensory complex. Trigeminal sensory nuclei are divided into a spinal, a principal, and a mesencephalic nucleus, spanning the medulla and pons. Each nucleus mediates a different form of somatosensation.

input site for pain and temperature afferents from all regions of the head.

From the trigeminal sensory nuclei, second-order neurons project an axon across the midline to form the trigeminal lemniscus and trigeminothalamic tract. The trigeminal lemniscus transmits input from the principal and mesencephalic nuclei, while the parallel trigeminothalamic tract transmits inputs from the spinal nucleus. The eventual target for both pathways is the **ventral posteromedial (VPM) nucleus** of the thalamus. The VPM contains third-order neurons and, like the VPL in the DCML, is somatotopically mapped to afferents in the periphery. From the VPM, third-order neurons project to the most lateral zone of the postcentral gyrus, the cortical region for the face and vocal tract somatosensory representation. Thus, pathways from the peripheral facial mechanoreceptors to the principal and mesencephalic nuclei are analogous to the DCML, while nociceptive and thermoreceptive inputs to the spinal trigeminal nucleus are analogous to the ALS.

Somatosensory Cortex

Somatosensory representation of the contralateral side of the body occupies the region of the cerebral cortex referred to as the postcentral gyrus. Functionally, this area is the primary somatosensory cortex (abbreviated S1) and constitutes the primary receiving area for somatosensory information originating from slowly and rapidly adapting mechanoreceptive, proprioceptive, nociceptive, and

thermoreceptive afferent inputs. Generally, several architectonic and functional subareas within S1 have been described and include **Brodmann areas** 3a, 3b, 1, and 2. Each subarea within the somatosensory cortex (1) receives unique forms of somatosensory information from specific thalamic nuclei (VPL or VPM), (2) possesses some degree of reciprocal axon connectivity with other cortical and subcortical targets involved in sensorimotor control and processing, and (3) incorporates a complete somatotopic and functionally distinct representation of a specific part of the peripheral body. As shown in **Fig. 9.11**, the distribution of the body surface on S1 (the sensory **homunculus**) reflects differences in the size of neural populations serving different regions of the skin. As discussed previously, larger cortical representations correspond to areas of the body that require high levels of sensory feedback to support the performance of skilled sensorimotor behaviors.

In general, neurons in Brodmann area 3a respond to inputs from proprioceptive sources, whereas area 3b is activated by cutaneous mechanoreceptive endings. Area 1 receives direct projections from RA 1 (PC) receptors by way of the thalamus and extensive collateral inputs from the neighboring area 3b. Finally, area 2 contains a complex representation of both cutaneous and deep receptors, receiving inputs from adjacent somatosensory subareas and the thalamus. Generally, receptive fields for both areas 1 and 2 are larger and more complex, supporting the notion that these regions may hold higher-order integrative functions for perception, control, and learning.

With regard to the vocal tract, thalamocortical inputs originating from the face have been found to project into the most lateral extent of Brodmann area 3b. Neurons within the face representation of S1 alter their firing rate during a variety of oromotor control tasks. Experiments that have temporarily deactivated S1 in nonhuman primates have shown that fine control of orofacial movements is severely compromised by doing so. Damage to specific areas of S1 leads to deficits ranging from the inability to discriminate textures or the size of an object to poor regulation of precision force production and movement. These findings point to the important role of sensory feedback for the execution of precision and skilled activity.

■ The Visual System

As a testament to the critical importance of the visual system to human behavior, nearly 40% of all cortical area in the brain has some role in visual processing and integration. As such, the visual system is the most studied and best understood of the sensory systems, with a long history of discovery that has informed our appreciation of other sensory systems as well. The visual system transduces the electromagnetic energy of light (photons) into a representation of our optic world. Evolutionarily, vision is fundamental to our existence, as it assists in avoiding predators, identifying a mate, locating food, and building complex social structures in which to live. The purpose of this section is to provide an overview of some of the essential features of light transduction and transmission through the CNS and a brief discussion on major cortical structures involved in the processing of visual inputs.

The Retina

The eye is often compared to a digital camera, with the pupil being the aperture through which light enters, the cornea and lens providing the focusing assembly, and the retina operating as the digital sensor that records the image. The retina, however, not only operates as the site of light transduction but also functions as a low-level processor of visual stimuli, selecting out salient spatial and temporal features in the mediation of visually guided behavior.

As illustrated in **Fig. 9.12**, the retina is a layered or laminar structure consisting of three primary sheets of cells, with other layers present that consist of axon bundles and epithelium. The deepest cell layer (farthest from the pupil and lens) consists of the phototransducing cells known as **rods** and **cones**, followed immediately by the bipolar cells, and finally the retinal ganglion cells. This arrangement is rather odd, because this organization indicates that light must pass through the first two layers before it reaches the cells that transduce it. It has been posited that the reason for this inside-out organization resides in the fact that the retinal floor consists of a layer of pigmented epithelium. Since rods and cones are positioned directly on the pigmented surface, any light that is not transduced by the photoreceptors will be absorbed, reducing light scatter and blurring of the visual image.

The pattern of information flow in the retinal layers is as follows: the rods and cones synapse onto bipolar cells, which in turn synapse onto the retinal ganglion cells, which are ultimately responsible for initiating the transmission of the visual input via the optic nerve to central visual components. In addition, the retina possesses two other types of cells that are primarily positioned horizontally within the bipolar cell layer. These cells are known as the **horizontal** and **amacrine cells** and are chiefly responsible for enhancing detail contrast through processes of lateral inhibition.

The layout of the retina is fairly uniform except for two locations: the **fovea** and the optic disc. The fovea is a specialized region of the retina that corresponds to the center of the visual gaze. Within the region of the fovea, the three retinal layers are most densely populated; in addition, at the very center of the fovea is a small region known as the

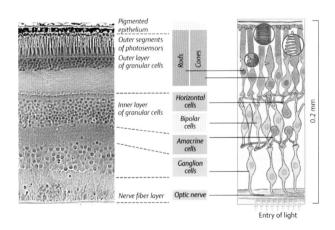

Fig. 9.12 Retinal layers. Three major cell types populate the retina, forming a laminar structure. Light entering into the eye must pass through the retinal ganglion cell and bipolar cell layers before even being transduced by the deepest layer of photoreceptors.

Box 9.3   Blind Spot

Draw and fill in a 1-cm diameter circle on the left side of a piece of paper and a small cross on the right-hand side of the page approximately 4 inches (10 cm) from the circle. Cover your right eye and fixate on the cross. Next, hold the paper approximately 12 inches (30 cm) from your face and gradually move it closer or farther away until you can no longer see the circle in your periphery. Notice that when you find your blind spot, you do not see "blackness," but rather you see nothing at all, similar to what an individual who is congenitally or totally blind would experience.

foveola, from which ganglion and bipolar cells are excluded to enable uninterrupted transmission of light to the deep phototransducing layer. The foveola is therefore the most sensitive region of the retinal surface, providing the sharpest and most unfiltered light transduction. The opposite is true for the optic disc, where all axons from the retinal ganglion cells converge to form the beginning of the optic nerve. The optic disc is devoid of any bipolar or phototransducing cells, forming what we colloquially refer to as our "blind spot." As described in **Box 9.3**, finding your blind spot is a simple experiment that enables you to experience blindness, if only for an instant.

The extent of external space that can be transduced by the retina is known as the **visual field**. The portion of the visual field mediated by one retina is known as a **hemifield**. The visual hemifield from each retina spans from 100° on the temporal aspect to approximately 60° on the nasal side, indicating that a significant portion of the visual field reflects visual input from both eyes simultaneously. This zone is the binocular region of vision and is the region of space where we possess the ability to detect visual depth. As shown in **Fig. 9.13**, if we were to divide the **binocular visual zone** in half, an image coming from the left side of the visual field would fall upon the temporal surface of the retina

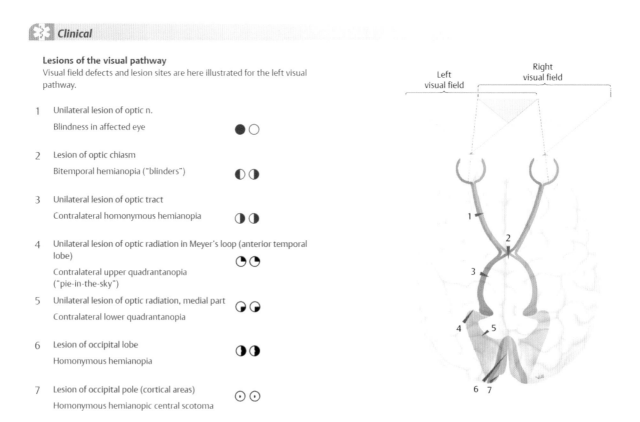

Clinical

Lesions of the visual pathway
Visual field defects and lesion sites are here illustrated for the left visual pathway.

1   Unilateral lesion of optic n.
    Blindness in affected eye

2   Lesion of optic chiasm
    Bitemporal hemianopia ("blinders")

3   Unilateral lesion of optic tract
    Contralateral homonymous hemianopia

4   Unilateral lesion of optic radiation in Meyer's loop (anterior temporal lobe)
    Contralateral upper quadrantanopia ("pie-in-the-sky")

5   Unilateral lesion of optic radiation, medial part
    Contralateral lower quadrantanopia

6   Lesion of occipital lobe
    Homonymous hemianopia

7   Lesion of occipital pole (cortical areas)
    Homonymous hemianopic central scotoma

Fig. 9.13   Visual fields and visual pathway lesion effects. Right and left visual hemifields are shown along with the overlapping binocular zone. Numbered arrowheads correspond to the table to the left of the illustration. This table describes the consequences of transection at different points along the visual system pathway.

of the right eye and the nasal surface of the retina on the left eye. In turn, an image coming from the right side of the binocular zone would fall upon the temporal surface of the retina of the left eye and the nasal surface of the right eye. Thus, each optic nerve contains axons transmitting visual inputs from both visual hemifields (see the purple and green shading of the optic nerves in **Fig. 9.13**). It is only at the **optic chiasm** that the axons from the nasal retinal surfaces cross to segregate visual input transmission from the left hemifield to the right optic tract and vice versa. In short, once optic nerve fibers cross in the optic chiasm, left hemifield input is processed by the right side of the brain and the right hemifield by the left side. Besides showing you the visual field distribution of the retinas under normal conditions, **Fig. 9.13** also illustrates and describes visual disturbances that occur if different points along the visual pathway are injured. By understanding the

organization of the visual pathway and how inputs are distributed across the retina, it is easy to localize, differentiate and describe the consequences of a variety of visual disturbances.

Light Transduction and Retinal Processing

Two important generalities inform our appreciation of visual input processing in the retina. First and foremost, retinal ganglion cells are the only class of cell in the retina that actually fire action potentials, forming the output pathway from the eye. The bipolar cells, rods, and cones function through graded changes in their membrane potentials. Neurotransmitter release from these cells is proportional to the change in each cell's membrane

---

Box 9.4 Glaucoma

Many of us have had the experience of going to an optometrist and enduring the annoying test where a puff of air is blown into the eye. This test actually has a purpose. The optometrist is testing for the level of pressure in your eyes and for the presence of glaucoma, a group of progressive diseases that damage the optic pathway and can result in visual distortions and in more severe cases, blindness (**Box Fig. 9.2**). One type of glaucoma, open-angle glaucoma, occurs when there is increased fluid pressure inside the eye that in turn presses on the optic nerve, causing losses in vision. Although not every person with increased intraocular pressure will develop glaucoma, it is important to control the pressure if noted. A subtype of open-angle glaucoma is low- or normal-tension glaucoma, which occurs even without increased intraocular pressure.

At first, individuals with glaucoma will most often not notice any symptoms of pain or vision loss. Glaucoma can present in one or both eyes by impacting peripheral vision at first and slowly moving more centrally, creating a tunnel-like visual field. If left untreated, individuals may eventually lose all vision in the affected eye. Glaucoma is most often associated with aging (individuals over 60 years), but can occur in younger individuals. African Americans over age 40 and individuals with a family history of glaucoma are at increased risk for open-angle glaucoma. The most effective approach to management of glaucoma is with early detection through routine screenings by your doctor, as there is no current cure for glaucoma.

Once vision has been lost, it cannot be restored. Currently, researchers are working to understand better how to mitigate the impact of this condition. (Hendry et al 2012)

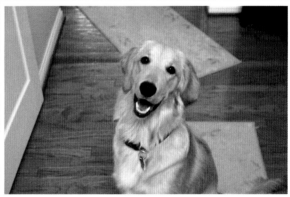

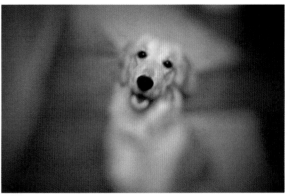

Box Fig. 9.2 Example of the effects of glaucoma on the visual field.

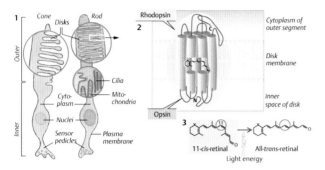

Fig. 9.14 Phototransduction mechanism. Structure of a photoreceptor is shown along with the molecular elements that form the transduction site for photons of light. Light energy produces a conformational change in the molecular structure of 11-*cis*-retinal, leading to a cascade of intracellular reactions that eventually hyperpolarize the rod or cone.

potential. Secondly, photoreceptors are the only cell types directly responsive to light energy.

The actual location where light is transduced into an electrochemical signal is the photoreceptive layer of the retina. There are two classes of photoreceptors: rods and cones. For the most part, rods are segregated to the peripheral regions of the retina, whereas cones populate the center and foveal regions. Rods are responsible for black-and-white vision when lighting conditions are dim, while cones are responsible for high-acuity color vision during daylight. Both photoreceptors share similar structural components consisting of an inner and outer segment, a cell body, and a synaptic terminal (**Fig. 9.14**). Rods and cones are distinguished from each other by length and shape, with rods being significantly longer and more flat-ended, while cones are shorter and more conically shaped.

Rods and cones have different sensitivities to light. The 100 million or so rods in the retina are highly responsive to light and in some cases can be activated through the reception of a single photon. Under dark or dim conditions, when light is scarce, the high light sensitivity of rods ensures that every available photon is used to support vision. As light levels increase, rods become saturated and no longer respond to variations in lighting levels. Cones, on the other hand, are far fewer in number (approximately 4 to 5 million) and mediate the appreciation of color. Cones are less sensitive to light, operate exclusively during daylight conditions, and are the bases for our keen visual acuity (the ability to distinguish two closely spaced objects from each other). In contrast to the single type of rod, humans have three variant types of cones, known as the L (long wavelength), M (medium), and S (short wavelength) cones. These designations characterize the

range of light energy each cone is most sensitive to. In general, long light wavelengths represent the red end of the spectrum, medium wavelengths the green range, and short wavelengths represent the blue end of the light spectrum.

The outer segments of the rod and cone possess specialized pigment molecules that enable each to capture photons of light. These pigment molecules are required to allow light inputs to trigger the necessary sequence of chemical events that leads to light transduction within the rod and cone. For rods, rhodopsin is the key molecular player in light transduction. This molecule consists of the protein opsin bound to a molecule of retinal. Rods transduce a range of wavelengths of light centered at about 500 nanometers (nm). Cones possess slightly different photopigments very similar to rhodopsin, known as photopsins. Each type of cone produces a photopsin with a different spectrum of light absorption sensitivity, accounting for the different color biases of the three types of cones. S cones have a photopsin variant that is biased to absorb the most light around 430 nm (blue), M cones absorb the most light in the 530 nm range (green), and finally, L cones absorb the longest wavelengths of light, 570 nm and longer (red). These wavelength values only represent the maximum sensitivity of each type of cone; like other sensory receptors, cones receive a range of wavelengths, creating overlap in responsiveness that provides the ability to represent all wavelengths of light in the visible spectrum with different proportions of the three cone signals (**Fig. 9.15**).

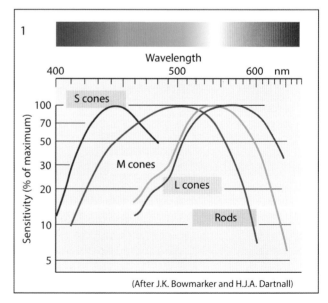

Fig. 9.15 Rod and cone light wavelength sensitivities. Light wavelength tuning curves are shown for each type of photoreceptor in the human retina.

As noted in previous sections, the process of transduction requires a stimulus to activate and depolarize a sensory receptor. In the visual system, however, the opposite condition exists. Light transduction, in fact, requires hyperpolarization of the photoreceptor. In dark conditions, rods and cones continually release the neurotransmitter **glutamate**, and operate differentially on two classes of bipolar cells. In turn, responsiveness of the retinal ganglion cell is dependent on the type of response profile of the connected bipolar cell. At rest, photoreceptors continuously generate a complex chemical known as **cyclic guanosine monophosphate (cGMP)**, which keeps cGMP-gated Na^+ and Ca^{2+} ion channels open, enabling the continuous diffusion of Na^+ and Ca^{2+} into the cell from the extracellular fluid. This is known as the dark current and keeps the photoreceptor effectively in a constant state of depolarization. When depolarized, photoreceptors release glutamate at their synapses. As shown in **Fig. 9.14**, when a photoreceptor pigment molecule absorbs a photon, the retinal component of the photopigment changes its shape. This shape change triggers a biochemical cascade within the cell via a **second messenger** system, a sequence of chemical reactions occurring within the neuron that leads to more complex and prolonged changes in the responsiveness and behavior of the neuron. The end product of the second messenger cascade in the photoreceptor is the activation of the enzyme phosphodiesterase, which converts cGMP into a nonfunctional form, GMP. The result of this step is to shut down the cGMP-gated Na^+ and Ca^{2+} channels, turning off the dark current, hyperpolarizing the photoreceptor and reducing the glutamate neurotransmitter release.

As mentioned earlier, bipolar cells are differentially affected by photoreceptor glutamate release. Bipolar cells that are hyperpolarized by photoreceptor hyperpolarization (decrease in glutamate) are known as OFF bipolar cells, while bipolar cells that are depolarized by the same event are referred to as ON bipolar cells. The difference in glutamate's effect on the ON or OFF bipolar cells lies with the type of glutamate receptor expressed by each bipolar-cell type. OFF bipolar cells possess classic ionotropic glutamatergic receptors, resulting in a standard depolarization of the cell. Conversely, the ON bipolar cell possesses metabotropic receptors that react to glutamate by hyperpolarizing the cell. In summary (**Fig. 9.16**), upon absorbing a photon of light, the photoreceptor hyperpolarizes and reduces glutamate release.

With less glutamate released, if the photoreceptor synapses onto an ON bipolar cell, the degree of hyperpolarization in the ON cell decreases. In other

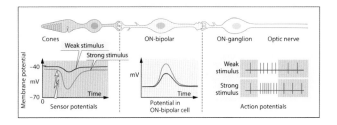

Fig. 9.16 ON bipolar cell. Connections between a photoreceptor, an ON bipolar cell, and a retinal ganglion cell are shown. Note that a strong hyperpolarization of the photoreceptor (blue trace) triggers a heightened depolarization of the ON bipolar cell, which in turn initiates a vigorous response from the ganglion cell.

words, the ON bipolar cell effectively is allowed to depolarize (becomes less hyperpolarized), thus increasing its own glutamate release. The greater release of glutamate by the ON bipolar cell subsequently drives activity of the retinal ganglion cell, and it generates action potentials down the optic nerve. **Fig. 9.16** illustrates the effects of photoreceptor hyperpolarization on the activity of an ON bipolar cell and its connected ganglion cell. A strong stimulus will generate powerful hyperpolarization of the cone, leading to a sharp curtailing of glutamate release (**Fig. 9.16**, left panel, blue trace). The ON bipolar cell reacts in an excitatory manner because the photoreceptor has reduced its expression of glutamate. Recall that ON bipolar cells are hyperpolarized by glutamate, and less glutamate released by the photoreceptor disinhibits the bipolar cell. Strong depolarization of the bipolar cell (**Fig. 9.16**, middle panel, blue trace) then increases the firing rate of the associated ganglion cell (**Fig. 9.16** right panel, bottom trace).

In the case of the OFF bipolar cell, reduced glutamate release by the photoreceptor effectively diminishes excitatory drive. Reduced OFF bipolar cell activity, in turn, produces a reduction in ganglion cell activity. Reduced ganglion cell activity decreases the rate of action potential generation down the optic nerve.

At this point, you may be wondering why ON and OFF bipolar cells even exist. Recall from the beginning of this chapter that the CNS possesses several mechanisms to enhance the contrast or differences between small variations of a stimulus event. In the visual system, ON and OFF bipolar cells are arranged in complex receptive field patterns in the retina to highlight features of the visual image. These highlighted features provide the CNS with details regarding motion, shape, orientation, and contrast. Our ability to detect the edges of an object or to distinguish objects in the visual foreground versus the background rely, in part, on the differential activity of the bipolar cells and the mapping of these outputs onto the retinal ganglion cells.

Central Visual Pathway

From the retina, visual inputs are directed centrally via the optic nerve in a retinotopic manner to the **primary visual cortex (V1)** in the occipital lobe. **Retinotopy** is the manner in which the patterns of inputs derived from the physical location of retinal ganglion cells are preserved at all subsequent visual processing locations. As discussed earlier, the optic nerve possesses axons transmitting visual inputs from both visual hemifields. It is only at the optic chiasm that optic nerve axons from each hemifield cross to segregate visual input from the left hemifield to the right **optic tract** and vice versa. The optic tract principally innervates the **lateral geniculate nucleus (LGN)** of the thalamus and the **superior colliculus (SC)** on the dorsal aspect of the mesencephalon. Retinal inputs routed through the LGN eventually terminate within the primary visual cortex, whereas those targeting the SC are involved in mediating reflexive head and eye-orienting behaviors. **Fig. 9.17** illustrates the major components of the central visual pathway.

The LGN is the obligatory thalamic relay en route to the visual cortex and receives retinotopically organized inputs from the optic tracts. Each LGN is a six-layered structure, with the first two layers known as the magnocellular layers (having large cells) and the remaining layers referred to as the parvocellular layers (having small cells). In a highly simplified description, the magnocellular layer cells receive retinal ganglion input related to image motion and low-contrast stimuli, while parvocellular layers receive inputs from retinal ganglion cells mediating color and high-contrast stimuli. LGN output neurons project a complete mapping of the contralateral hemifield posteriorly toward the occipital lobe via a massive bundle of axons known as the **optic radiations**. Besides input from the retina, the LGN also receives descending inputs from the primary visual cortex itself. This descending influence is believed to modify incoming visual inputs in a task-dependent manner and modulate the flow of visual information into the cortex. Top-down controlling influences of the cortex to lower-level processing regions of the CNS are common across all sensory systems. These descending effects clearly demonstrate that, regardless of modality, sensory transmission is far from passive but is actively regulated by the CNS.

The primary visual cortex (V1) is anatomically referred to as Brodmann area 17 (or sometimes, the striate cortex) and represents the first level of cortical visual processing. Inputs into V1 from the LGN are functionally organized into column-like collections of neurons known as right and left ocular dominance columns, reflecting the segregation of inputs from the visual hemifields and the LGN. Embedded within the ocular dominance columns is a second form of organization reflecting the preference of cortical neurons to respond to visual images in specific orientations. By using bars of light, investigators determined that clusters of cells within orientation columns were sensitive to specific orientations through 360° of space. Orientation columns are organized similar to a pinwheel of neurons that respond to slightly different visual orientations. Embedded within both ocular and orientation columns are also pockets of cells referred to as blobs, which are highly responsive to color inputs from parvocellular layers of the LGN. Together, the entire collection of ocular dominance columns, orientation columns, and blobs constitutes a processing unit called a hypercolumn.

The columnar organization of V1 holds many advantages for processing complex visual inputs. First, this organization minimizes the communication distance between neurons that possess similar function, allowing them to more easily share inputs that transmit related sensory attributes. Second, the columnar structure is highly efficient and max-

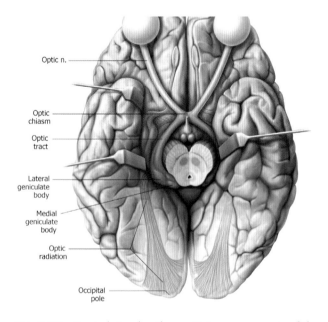

Optic n.

Optic chiasm

Optic tract

Lateral geniculate body

Medial geniculate body

Optic radiation

Occipital pole

Fig. 9.17   Central visual pathway. Major components of the visual pathway are shown in this ventral view of the cerebrum. The temporal lobes are retracted to reveal the optic tracts and innervation of the LGN.

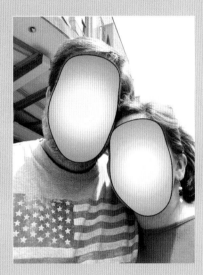
imizes brain volume and processing speed. Given the massive array of visual inputs available to the CNS at any moment in time, structural and functional efficiencies allow obtaining the greatest processing power by taking advantage of the fact that a given neuron will convey a combination of features of the visual image.

Dorsal and Ventral Visual Streams

Beyond the complexities of the initial processing of retinogeniculate input into V1, visual inputs are increasingly channeled into other cortical regions whose function is to extract information related to form, motion, color and depth. To date, nearly 30 cortical zones have been identified that contribute to visual processing. Collectively, these areas are known as extrastriate cortex, a catch-all term to denote any area outside of V1 that participates in visual processing. Discussing each of these areas is clearly beyond the scope of this chapter, but we can summarize them by describing two large-scale visual processing streams: one that projects dorsally from V1 toward parietal areas and a second that projects in parallel ventrally toward the temporal lobe. Neither of these streams is strictly hierarchical in its organization. Rather, the cortical zones that encompass each stream are organized functionally to construct increasingly complex visual representations from the raw visual inputs processed within V1. We will refer to these two streams as the dorsal and the ventral visual processing streams.

Dorsal Stream

The dorsal stream, colloquially referred to as the "where" pathway, appears to be involved in the processing of object motion and location (hence the "where" designation). Neurons within various subregions within the dorsal stream receive retinotopic inputs from V1. Cortical regions encompassed by the dorsal stream include the dorsal aspect of the occipital lobe and the inferior and superior parietal lobules. These areas respond preferentially to the direction of object motion. Among the types of motion that are processed in the dorsal stream are linear, rotational, and circular movement. It is hypothesized that the dorsal stream serves three important behavioral roles: (1) motion perception, (2) direction of eye position in the visual field, and (3) environmental navigation.

Evidence for dorsal stream activity in humans stems from cases of selective brain injury to parietal lobe areas, resulting in a selective loss of motion detection. In cases of stroke to the parietal cortex, individuals present with normal visual acuity but may have a severe deficit in visually detecting movement. Imagine the perceptual disconnect of not being able to detect the motion of an object. Living in such a state would be synonymous to living in a world of photographic still-shots or within a stop-motion or clay animation film. Think about seeing a person walking toward you on the street. At one moment you would see the person at some distance from you, and the next moment the person would appear right next to you.

Ventral Stream

The ventral stream, colloquially referred to as the "what" pathway, appears to be involved in the processing of object features and structure (hence the "what" designation). Neurons within various subregions of the ventral stream receive retinotopic inputs from V1. The ventral stream consists of cortical areas along the ventral occipital lobe and extending into the middle and inferior gyri of the temporal lobe. Not only does the ventral stream encode object structure; advanced forms of color perception also appear to be a component of this pathway's output. Achromatopsia is a rare condition, caused by cortical damage at the juncture of the posterior temporal lobe and the occipital lobe, whereby the perception of color vision is lost even though retinal input into the visual system remains intact. Individuals with this syndrome often describe living in a world where everything takes on a shade of gray. In addition, individuals with this syndrome have deficits identifying object form. Another fascinating syndrome that further highlights the complexity and detail of form abstraction by the ventral stream is a condition known as prosopagnosia. Prosopagnosia emerges from a selective lesion to an area of the inferior temporal gyrus known as the fusiform area. Under normal conditions, the fusiform area is highly selective for complex objects that resemble faces. For example, in nonhuman primates, the specificity of this zone is so discrete that certain profile views of faces are differentially encoded. Individuals with this syndrome possess normal vision in every other manner, except for the ability to identify and recognize a face.

Box 9.6   Hearing and Aging: Presbycusis

Damage to the sound-transducing cochlear hair cells can be caused by exposure to intense sounds, such as loud music during a concert, jet engines, gunfire, or even listening to music through headphones at excessively loud volumes. However, hair cells can also be damaged through repeated exposure to less intense sounds over long periods of time—say, a lifetime'a worth. Age-related hearing loss, or presbycusis, consists of a loss of hair cell sensitivity beginning near the oval window. The hair cells nearest the oval window are responsible for encoding high-frequency sounds, the critical acoustic feature of many consonants. Presbycusis is the most common type of sensorineural hearing loss, occurs bilaterally, and begins around 40 years of age. Because of the loss of high-frequency information, individuals with presbycusis often complain of difficulty understanding speech over the phone, when the speaker is using a microphone in a large lecture hall, or when there is extensive background noise.

However, individuals may have no difficulty in one-on-one conversations in quiet environments. The best way to prevent presbycusis is to protect your ears by using noise-canceling headphones or earplugs when exposed to loud sounds. Although not terribly fashionable in some cases, wearing ear protection during your lifetime is vital for preserving the integrity of your auditory system. Protect those hair cells!

(Hendry et al 2012)

CAUTION
Hair Cell
Protection Zone

Box Fig. 9.4   Hair cell protection zone.

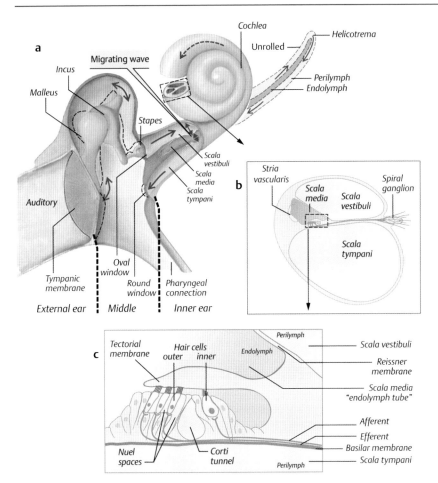

Fig. 9.18 Anatomy of the middle and inner ear. **(a)** Middle ear and inner ear are shown. The cochlea is shown both in its natural spiral form and unwound. **(b)** Cross section of the cochlea. **(c)** Organ of Corti. Note position of the inner and outer hair cells.

■ The Auditory-Vestibular Systems

The Auditory System

Many of the joys in life are dependent upon the auditory sensory system, with its amazing capacity to transduce, transmit, and process minute variations in air pressure into the infinite array of sounds that color our world. More critically, the auditory system takes center stage for the development and lifelong maintenance of the most complex behavior that humans can perform: speech. Human hearing begins with the mechanical funneling of sound pressure variations (acoustic inputs) from the outer ear, through the middle ear, and into the inner ear. We will focus on the auditory events that begin with the inner ear, specifically within a critical structure for sound transduction: the **organ of Corti (OoC)**. The function and anatomy of the outer and middle ear are presented in greater detail in **Chapter 13**.

Basic Structure of the Cochlea

As illustrated in **Fig. 9.18**, the inner ear, or cochlea, consists of three parallel fluid-filled tubes or chambers that are coiled to resemble the shape of a snail shell. This structure is embedded within the bony matrix of the petrous segment of the temporal bone and is approximately the size of an eraser on the top of a pencil. A cross-sectional view of the cochlea shows the arrangement of the three chambers: the **scala vestibuli**, **scala media**, and **scala tympani**. The scala vestibuli possesses a small membrane-covered opening known as the oval window, which communicates directly with the end of the ossicular bony chain of the middle ear. The oval window functions as the point of transduction of mechanical ossicular motion into hydraulic disturbances within the cochlea. The scala tympani communicates with the scalae vestibuli at the apical end of the coiled chambers and has a second membrane-covered opening known as the round window. Given that the scala vestibuli and tympani are joined, changes in hydraulic pressure that are created at the oval window are subsequently relieved by membrane

Box 9.7   Basilar Membrane Dynamics

Imagine a beach where a group of surfers are hanging out catching some waves. Surfers know that as a wave approaches the shoreline, the size and amplitude of that wave will hit a maximal point and then quickly fade as the water rolls up onto the sand. The size of the ocean swell depends on the physical surface features of the shoreline. Surfers count on this fact to harness the point of maximal ocean swell to catch a great ride. This scenario plays out in a metaphorically similar way when sound input is introduced into the cochlea. The sound pressure disturbance introduced at the oval window moves from the base of the BM toward its apex in a wavelike manner. As shown in **Fig. 9.19**, this traveling wave increases in amplitude until it reaches a maximal point of motion that is best suited to the physical features (stiffness) of the BM. After this point, the wave quickly dies out because the structure of the BM can no longer support vibration of that frequency. Who knew that surfing and hearing had so much in common?

bowing or displacement at the round window in a complementary manner. Finally, situated between the previous two chambers is the scala media, or cochlear duct, home to two of the key sound-transducing structures in the system: the OoC and the **basilar membrane (BM)**.

Basilar Membrane

The ability to understand the physiology behind the transduction of acoustic stimuli depends centrally on an appreciation of the anatomical features and response characteristics of a membrane that forms part of the floor of the scala media: the BM. The BM possesses three critical mechanical features that, when combined together, provide it with the ability to vibrate in specific locations to acoustic signals of different frequencies. The BM, from its base to its apex, varies in a graded and continuous manner in three properties: its thickness, stiffness, and width. The end of the BM closest to the oval and round windows (the base) is far thicker, stiffer, and narrower than its opposite end (apex), even though the cochlea itself is wider. Why are these simple anatomical features so important? Simply put, mechanical systems that are floppy, long, and thin tend to resonate at lower frequencies when excited by some disturbance. Think of how the end of a flag on a flagpole moves in the wind. It flops and flutters in large-amplitude waves to the air moving past it. On the other hand, mechanical systems that are stiff, thick, and short will tend to resonate at higher frequencies when excited by a disturbance. In this case, think of clamping one end of a ruler (preferably a metal ruler) to a table with a small portion of the other end hanging over the table edge. If you try to "strum" the unclamped end of the ruler with your hand, it will vibrate very quickly, weakly, and then stop. Because the mechanical properties of the BM vary gradually from base to apex, different frequencies of vibration will produce specific patterns of maximal motion on the membrane. This mapping of frequency of vibration onto location on the BM is the reason that the brain is able to detect different frequencies of sound and relate them to each other. In short, the BM "maps" acoustic frequencies from high to low proceeding from the base to the apex (**Fig. 9.19**). The human BM maps frequencies from 20 Hz at the apex up to 20

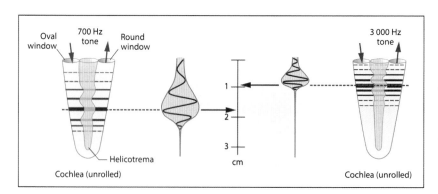

Fig. 9.19 Basilar membrane dynamics. An uncoiled basilar membrane is schematically shown with respect to two excitation frequencies. Note that the input frequencies cause BM motion at different locations from its basal to apical end. Lower frequencies resonate toward the apical end, while higher frequencies resonate toward the basal end.

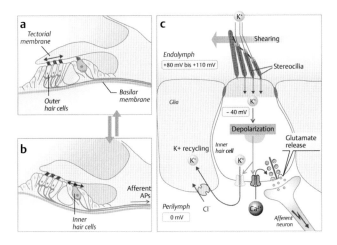

Fig. 9.20 Hair cell shearing action and depolarization. Panels **(a)** and **(b)** depict the back-and-forth motion of the organ of Corti relative to the tectorial membrane. This action generates a bending force upon the embedded stereocilia. In panel **(c)**, the hair cell structure is depicted. The hair cell is shown undergoing depolarization when the stereocilia are bent toward the kinocilium.

kHz at its base. We can say that the BM is a type of frequency analyzer—a system capable of resolving a complex acoustic stimulus into its constituent frequency components. This important functional aspect of the BM sets the stage for the emergence of **tonotopy**, the systematic organization of acoustic processing according to frequency in the auditory system.

Organ of Corti and the Hair Cells: Structure and Function

The OoC is a band of specialized epithelium running along the length of the BM that functions as the transduction site for acoustic stimuli. The OoC possesses two types of mechanoreceptive cells known as the outer and inner hair cells. Technically, **hair cells** are not neurons but a highly specialized form of epithelium. Hair cells do not possess an axon and do not generate action potentials. Instead, hair cells generate graded receptor potential changes when stimulated. The **inner hair cells (IHCs)** number approximately 3,000 to 4,000 and form a single row down the length of the OoC, positioned closest to the central axis of the cochlear spiral. The **outer hair cells (OHCs)**, numbering approximately 12,500, are organized into three distinct rows and are located distally to the IHC.

Hair cells derive their name from the fact that shafts of interlinked hairlike structures called **stereocilia** extend from their top surfaces. As illustrated in **Fig. 9.20** (panel 3), stereocilia are arranged in bundles with one longer shaft, the **kinocilium**, positioned at one edge of the bundle. The stereocilia are the location where hydromechanical energy is converted into electrochemical neural impulses.

Box 9.8   Outer Hair Cells

What is the purpose of the OHCs? The OHCs play a special role in the process of sound transduction that we typically would not expect in a sensory system. OHCs appear to amplify the resolution of low-amplitude acoustic input through *efferent* (motor) input from the CNS, giving the OHCs their functional designation as cochlear amplifiers. An efferent action potential into the OHC produces a conformational change in the structural proteins making up its cytoskeleton, changing the overall shape, stiffness, and length of the cell. If you recall, OHCs are physically linked to the tectorial membrane as well as anchored to the BM. This places the OHC in an ideal position to alter or "tune" the responsiveness of basilar and tectorial membrane motion and in turn change the sensitivity of the IHC to acoustic inputs. OHC adjustments are exceptionally fast, allowing for tuning changes to follow the timing of incoming acoustic inputs.

The discovery of this tuning system was based on clinical research that demonstrated reduced IHC sensitivity when individuals were administered a powerful antibiotic known as kanamycin, an ototoxic agent that damages OHCs but not IHCs. IHC sensitivity changes could therefore be altered only if the OHC had a role in adjusting the sensitivity of the BM. A second line of evidence for the tuning role of OHCs came from investigations on the source of a phenomenon known as spontaneous otoacoustic emissions. If an extremely sensitive microphone is placed within the ear canal, in roughly 50 to 70% of individuals, it is possible to record the spontaneous production of faint tones. The mechanism behind the OHCs' tuning function appears to be related to excitability changes to the internal potential of the cell through efferent inputs. It does not appear that processes using cellular metabolic products such as ATP are involved in this activity.

At the tips of the stereocilia are protein filaments known as **tip links**, which attach to adjacent stereocilia and are associated with ion channels that open (depolarizing the cell) when the stereocilia shafts are bent toward the kinocilium and close (hyperpolarizing the cell) when the shaft is bent in the opposite direction. When the hair cell is depolarized, calcium enters the cell at its base and initiates glutamate release onto peripheral terminals of afferent fibers of the vestibulocochlear nerve (CN VIII) (**Fig. 9.20**, panel 3).

The hair cells are innervated by synaptic terminals of the vestibulocochlear nerve (CN VIII), which respond to the graded changes of the hair cell's receptor potential with graded production of action potentials. The vestibulocochlear nerve cell possesses a peripheral and a central axon, with a cell body situated in between (bipolar cell type) located within the spiral ganglion, which runs along the outside of the cochlea. Inputs from the peripheral axon branch propagate through the cell body and into the central axon branch. The central axon branches form the cochlear (auditory) branch of the vestibulocochlear nerve (CN VIII), which enters the brainstem to synapse upon the **cochlear nuclei** in the medulla. Approximately 95% of the afferent innervation in the cochlear branch is from the IHCs, with the remaining 5% coming from the OHCs. This distribution strongly indicates that the inner hair cell is mostly responsible for transducing sound.

Central Auditory Pathways

The central auditory pathway (CAP) consists of several nuclei and axon pathways that ascend within the brainstem. The CAP begins with auditory nerve fibers that project from the cochlea into the brainstem, where they synapse onto neurons of the cochlear nuclei. Neurons from the cochlear nuclei project bilaterally into nuclei in the pons called the **superior olivary complex (SOC)**. This is the first place where information from both ears converges upon common neurons in the CAP. Binaural information is critically important for determining the location of a sound in space. From the SOC, auditory input transmission continues to the **inferior colliculus** in the auditory midbrain. The outputs of the inferior colliculus are then sent to the **medial geniculate body** and finally to the auditory cortex in the temporal lobe. The following section will describe some key operating and structural features of the CAP structures (**Fig. 9.21**).

The Auditory Nerve and the Cochlear Nuclei

The tonotopic organization of the BM is represented equally by the hair cells of the OoC as well as the primary afferent fibers of the auditory nerve (the cochlear branch of the vestibulocochlear nerve, CN VIII). Because specific cochlear branch fibers (peripheral axons of spiral ganglion cells) synapse onto specific hair cells, these fibers are frequency-specific, mirroring the tonotopic organization of the BM. Thus, frequency in the auditory system is coded as a function of place and position of the afferent terminal on the BM. As shown in **Fig. 9.22**, stimulus intensity is coded through variations in the rate of action potential generation within an afferent fiber and through the recruitment of greater numbers of afferent terminals.

The auditory nerve projects in a tonotopic manner to the cochlear nuclei in the medulla (**Fig. 9.23**). The cochlear nuclei (CN) consist of two major divisions: the ventral and dorsal CN. The ventral CN is further subdivided into the posteroventral and anteroventral CN. Each division of the CN possesses a complete tonotopic mapping of afferent fibers from the cochlea, with high-frequency inputs mapped onto dorsal aspects and low-frequency inputs mapped onto ventral aspects of each nucleus.

The ventral CN is populated by three different cell types that each encode spectral and temporal features of acoustic inputs: bushy, stellate, and octopus cells. Bushy cells come in two forms (small and large), each processing and extracting different acoustic features and projecting to different locations in the brainstem. The small bushy cells receive high-frequency inputs and project bilaterally to the lateral aspect of the superior olivary complex (LSOC). The LSOC is active during the detection of interaural intensity differences and is a participant in the sound localization of high-frequency inputs. Large bushy cells receive low-frequency inputs and project bilaterally to the medial aspect of the superior olivary complex (MSOC). The MSOC is active during the detection of interaural timing differences and is a participant in the sound localization of low-frequency inputs. Stellate cells feed back onto other regions of the CN and encode spectral information of acoustic inputs. Lastly, the octopus cells drive neurons at several contralateral locations upstream from the CN and are believed to encode sound onsets and the periodic nature of sounds, two factors critical for sound pattern detection. In fact, data indicate that synchronous firing of populations of octopus cells can be produced by sounds with inherent periodicities, such as vowels and music.

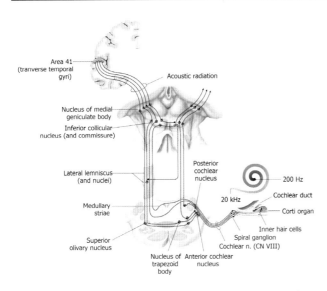

Fig. 9.21 Central auditory pathway structures. Central auditory components are shown from the cochlea through the auditory cortex. Lines depict axon pathways interconnecting each CAP structure.

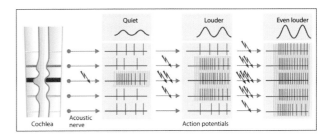

Fig. 9.22 Intensity coding in the cochlea. Intensity of sound is encoded in two ways: first, through an increase in the firing rate of an individual auditory nerve fiber; second, through recruitment of additional adjacent fibers.

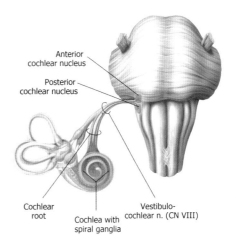

Fig. 9.23 Cochlear nuclei. Auditory nerve fibers project to the cochlear nuclei at the junction of the medulla and the pons.

The dorsal CN appears to integrate sound input along with somatosensory and vestibular information regarding the position and motion of the head. Several investigators suggest that the dorsal CN likely assists in the interpretation of sound spectral cues for purposes of localization. Animals use spectral cues to help them differentiate self-generated sounds as they move through their environment from those sounds that have greater saliency to their behavior. While moving through a forest, it is more important to pay attention to the sound of a potential predator than to the sound of your own feet.

The Superior Olivary Complex and Sound Localization

The best studied and understood function of the SOC is that of sound localization. As has been mentioned, the CN projects distinctly and tonotopically to various locations within the superior olivary complex, suggesting that the mechanisms for low- versus high-frequency sound localization may be different. Indeed, this is exactly the case. Sound is localized in a duplex manner depending on the range of frequencies requiring localization. Low-frequency sounds (20 to 2,000 Hz) use differences in time between the reception of sound at each ear, whereas high-frequency sounds (> 2,000 Hz) use interaural intensity differences between the ears to localize a source.

The differences between the use of these two processes has much to do with the physical nature of sound wavelengths for low versus high frequen-

cies. Imagine you are listening to a woman who is standing to your right singing a pitch. The typical fundamental frequency for a woman is approximately 225 Hz, which would be equivalent to an effective sound wavelength of approximately 152 cm. If the diameter of your head is 20 cm, there is a time delay of approximately 0.5 milliseconds for sound to reach your left ear. Of course, if she moves directly in front of you, you would detect no delay in the pitch reaching your two ears. The key takeaway is that as long as a sound wavelength is longer than the diameter of your head, you can take advantage of interaural time delays to localize sound. As discussed earlier, the medial SOC receives low-frequency inputs from the CN, suggesting that the circuitry required to recognize time difference between the right and left ear exists within this nucleus (**Fig. 9.24**, left panel).

Now imagine that you are listening to a speaker playing a 10,000-Hz pure tone to your right. The wavelength of this sound is approximately 3.5 cm, considerably shorter than the diameter of your head. This suggests that time delay difference would not be effective to localize this sound. It is simply happening too quickly. For high-frequency sounds, the auditory system uses interaural intensity differences instead of time delay differences. This method counts on your head acting as an acoustic shadow, causing a slight decrease in the intensity of a sound as it travels from one side of your head to the other. As noted earlier, the lateral SOC receives high-frequency inputs from the CN, suggesting that the circuitry required to recognize intensity difference between the right and left ear exists within this nucleus (**Fig. 9.24**, right panel).

The Inferior Colliculus

Consider this dilemma for a moment: Three-dimensional space is not encoded in any way by the tonotopic arrangement of the BM, nor the auditory afferent fibers that synapse onto the hair cells. Yet we are quite adept at localizing sound in our three-dimensional environment. How is this possible? How does a two-dimensional representation of frequency on the BM become transformed into a signal that conveys the nature of our multidimensional auditory space? The inferior colliculus (IC), located in the dorsal aspect of the mesencephalon, appears to be the location in the CAP that integrates auditory inputs from lower levels of the brainstem to synthesize our perception of auditory space (**Fig. 9.21**). The IC receives inputs directly from the contralateral CN and bilaterally from the SOC. These regions heavily process and extract critical information from sound inputs including spectral features, timing, and location. What emerges from

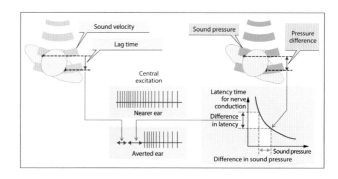

Fig. 9.24 Interaural time and intensity differences. Mechanisms of sound localization are frequency dependent. Low-frequency sound localization uses differences in interaural timing (left panel) to determine location source. High-frequency sound localization uses interaural intensity differences (right panel) to determine location source.

the binaural integration of lower-level inputs in the IC is a calculated representation of the physical features of auditory space. Experiments in owls, whose echolocation skills to find prey in complex environments are legendary, demonstrate that IC neurons are active to sounds emanating from a preferred vertical (elevation) as well as horizontal (azimuth) location.

Experiments in a variety of mammalian species have demonstrated that IC neurons are also tuned to respond to frequency-modulated sounds or to sounds of certain durations. These acoustic factors are typical of environmental sounds that hold biological importance to animals (e.g., helping them find a mate, escape from predators, or communicate among their group). These two IC cell response

---

Box 9.9 Cochlear Implants

Cochlear implants (CIs) have been a successful neuroprosthetic means of restoring partial hearing to children and adults with profound or complete sensorineural hearing loss. Cochlear implants have two main components: one that sits externally on the ear and a second internal component that is surgically placed under the skin and threaded into the cochlea of the implanted ear. CIs consist of a microphone that records sound; a signal processor that filters and boosts the strength of the signal, and a transmitter and receiver system for conveying the processed sound to a thin electrode array. At the electrode array, electrical impulses operate to stimulate auditory nerve afferent terminals, thus initiating sound transmission centrally. The electrode arrays are constructed so that they span the entire length of the basilar membrane, providing electrical stimulation across a wide range of frequencies.

It is important to remember that CIs do not restore normal hearing. The process of normal sound transduction involves the coordinated activity of literally thousands of hair cells. The best a CI can do is replace a tiny fraction of those hair cell inputs. Individuals with CIs may be able to achieve good speech recognition and comprehension in person or on the telephone, as well as improve their ability to hear environmental sounds. After the surgical procedure, individuals with CIs must go through a period of training to learn how to discriminate these new inputs into meaningful sounds.

(National Institutes of Health)

features should catch your attention, for one critical reason: both factors also underlie the acoustic properties of speech sounds. Thus, it appears that early stages of speech perception may occur within the IC even before acoustic inputs reach the auditory cortex.

The Medial Geniculate Body

The medial geniculate body (MGB) receives input almost exclusively from the IC, with some lesser projections from lower CAP levels (**Fig. 9.21**). The MGB is the first location in the CAP where neurons are activated by specific combinations of frequencies. Experiments in the echolocating bat suggest that the tonotopy of lower levels of the CAP is harnessed by MGB neurons to respond to sound patterns with unique spectral signatures. In addition, MGB neurons are responsive to time intervals between the presentations of two frequencies. Once more, echolocating bat experiments have demonstrated that these mammals assess distance to a target by calculating the time delay between the presentations of calls as the animal homes in on prey. Recordings from MGB neurons demonstrate a response preference to specific delays. When the entire population of time-sensitive neurons is taken into account, one can readily see that a whole array of distances are encoded through differential neuron MGB activity. From the perspective of speech, changes in combinations of **formant** frequencies are what distinguish phonemes from each other. Furthermore, the ability to detect temporally related coarticulatory factors is critical for the segmentation and perception of running speech. Together, MGB spectral and temporal response characteristics suggest that these neurons may play an important role in facilitating speech perception.

The Auditory Cortex

From the MGB, projection neurons precisely innervate the superior temporal gyrus, home of the **primary auditory cortex (A1)**, corresponding to Brodmann areas 41 and 42. The auditory cortex possesses a tonotopic representation of the BM and the cochlea. Auditory cortical neurons responsive to low-frequency sounds are located rostrally in the cortex, while those mapped to higher frequencies are found more caudal. Besides frequency, many other acoustic features are mapped onto A1, including loudness changes, frequency modulations, and binaural interactions. Finally, posterior to A1 in the human is Wernicke's area, a major component of the perisylvian language zone responsible for the comprehension and perception of speech.

Recent experiments suggest that A1 activity is far richer than simply that related to processing frequency information. For example, recent data suggests that cortical areas surrounding A1 may be active in pitch perception, both for musical purposes and, more critically, for vocalization and speech. Pitch perception may play an important role in discriminating multiple speech sounds when they possess similar spectral qualities and are produced from the same location in space.

Another example of the complexity of auditory processing is the recognition that auditory cortical areas are arranged into dedicated processing systems. Like the visual system, the cortical auditory system appears to possess "what" and "where" information-processing streams. Although the details of these processing streams are still under investigation and debate, it appears as if a ventral (what) stream that passes through the temporal lobe to prefrontal cortical areas may be involved in identifying auditory objects through spectral analysis. A dorsal (where) stream obtains input from A1 and routes processing through the posterior parietal cortex, eventually reaching prefrontal cortical areas as well. The dorsal stream is likely specialized to locate sound sources, detect sound motion, and segregate sources of sound from each other.

■ The Vestibular System

When functioning well, we have little conscious awareness of the vestibular system, but when things go awry, our entire world can be literally turned upside down. In simple terms, the vestibular system's activity is to keep us upright and moving smoothly through the gravity field on earth. Underlying this seemingly simple activity is a host of complex mechanisms that detect and transduce factors such as momentum and acceleration of the head in both angular and linear dimensions. These signals are then passed to various regions of the brainstem, cerebellum, and somatosensory cortex to coordinate the musculoskeletal and motor control systems to maintain our posture and balance in the face of changing environmental conditions.

Like the auditory system, the vestibular system uses hair cells as its principal transducing elements. The vestibular hair cells transduce the mechanical energy created by head motion and transmit these inputs centrally via excitatory synapses with axon terminals of the vestibular division of the vestibulocochlear nerve (CN VIII). The mechanism of hair cell transduction and excitability changes in the vestibular system is almost identical to that in the cochlea. The vestibular hair cells are located within the vestibular labyrinth, which is divided into two chief sensory elements: the **semicircular canals** and **otolith organs** (**Fig. 9.25**). The semicircular canals are designed to detect and transduce head rotation and angular acceleration, while the otolith organs detect linear acceleration.

Transduction of Linear Motion by Otolith Organs

The otolith organs consist of the **utricle** and the **saccule** (**Fig. 9.25**, **Fig. 9.26**). These chambers, situated at the base of the vestibular labyrinth, are well suited to detect linear acceleration as well as the static position of the head relative to gravity. Acceleration generates an inertial counterforce proportional to the acceleration and to the mass of an object, and it is these forces that are detected by the hair cells within the otolith organs. The hair cells are situated within a layer of epithelium called the **macula** and positioned in different orientations. The utricle macula is positioned horizontally with the hair cells pointing up toward the the top of the head and oriented on an anterior-posterior axis. With the head in an upright starting position, the hair cells of the utricle respond to backward and forward accelerations, such as one would experience in stop-and-go traffic on a busy street. In the saccule, the macula is oriented 90° degrees to the utricle. Again, with the head in an upright position, saccule hair cells respond to upward and downward accelerations, such as one would experience riding in an elevator. The stereocilia of the otolith hair cells are embedded within a gelatinous structure known

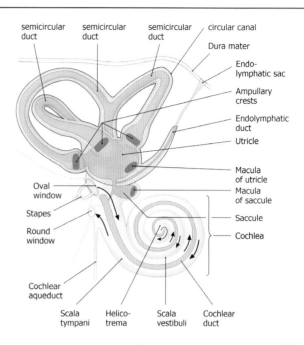

Fig. 9.25 Major structural components of the vestibular system are shown. Note the locations of the ampullae, utricle, and saccule at the base of the semicircular canals.

as the **otolithic membrane**, reminiscent of the tectorial membrane in the cochlea. The otolithic membrane is covered with inert particles and rocklike crystals of calcium carbonate called **otoconia** (**Fig. 9.26** panel 4), that add mass and inertia to the top of the otolithic membrane. So the next time someone asks whether you have rocks in your head, you can answer "Yes."

The translation of the otoconia-encrusted membrane relative to the membranous labyrinth is responsible for generating the shearing forces

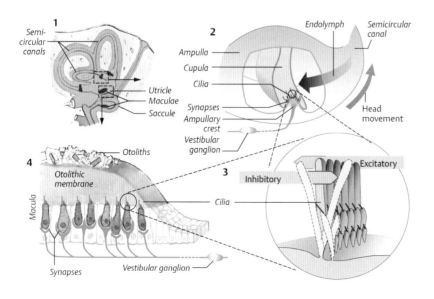

Fig. 9.26 Semicircular canal and otolith organ physiology. Overview of the transduction structure and events leading to rotational and linear acceleration detection in the semicircular canals and otolith organs. (1) Semicircular canals and otolith organs. (2) Transduction within the ampulla and cupula of the semicircular canals. (3) Stereocilia deflection is a common event for both rotational and linear acceleration transduction. (4) Otolith organ otoconia shown as a layer on top of the gelatinous tissue of the otolithic membrane.

needed to modify the excitability of the hair cells. Suppose you tilt your head forward; say, to look at your feet. As you start tilting forward, gravity pulls on the otoconia. The gelatinous membrane allows the otoconia to move relative to the stereocilia beneath (imagine a bowl of Jell-O with large slices of fruit on the top; if you tilt the sheet, the heavy fruit layer will move in the direction of the tilt relative to the bottom of the bowl). The end result of this action is to create shearing-type forces within the membrane that bend the embedded stereocilia of the hair cell. As in all hair cells, stereocilia deflection will mechanically gate ion channels. As shown in **Fig. 9.26** (panel 3), depending on the deflection direction of the stereocilia, the hair cell will be either depolarized (deflection toward kinocilium) or hyperpolarized (deflection away from kinocilium).

Measurement of Angular Acceleration by Semicircular Canals

Considering that the head sits on a pivot point created by the atlas and axis of the cervical vertebrae, any motion of the head about this rotational axis will generate angular accelerations. Behaviors such as shaking your head "no" or nodding in approval are examples of rotational axis motion. The semicircular canals are positioned roughly in three mutually perpendicular planes similar to X, Y, Z coordinates, meaning that they are able to transduce the magnitude and direction of rotational motion around all three basic anatomic axes and convey these measures toward the brain. Each semicircular canal will be maximally sensitive to rotational forces in its plane.

At one end, the semicircular canal opens into the utricle, and at the other end the canals terminate in structures known as an **ampulla** (**Fig. 9.26**, panels 1 and 2). Within the ampulla, there is a sheet of thickened epithelium known as the ampullary crista, in which the hair cells are embedded. Rising up from the crista and crossing the entire length of the ampulla lumen is a sail-like gelatinous stalk, called the **cupula**, that contains the stereocilia of the ampullary hair cells. The configuration of the cupula within the ampulla is similar to that of a hydraulic diaphragm. Imagine a clear, fluid-filled plastic tube with a small flexible rubber diaphragm situated in the center of the tube. As you tilt the tube from side to side, you will notice that the displacement of the fluid in the tube presses on the flexible diaphragm, causing it to bulge out in the direction of the tilt. Likewise, with sudden rotation of the head, the endolymph fluid is displaced rela-

tive to the labyrinth, thus placing hydraulic pressure on the cupula. Because the ampullary hair cell stereocilia are encased in the cupula, displacing the cupula bends the hair cells, resulting in excitability changes that transduce parameters of rotation (**Fig. 9.26**, panel 2).

Although the functions of the two main vestibular systems were described separately, it is important to realize that under natural conditions, these systems are simultaneously activated. This results in a complex neural pattern of excitatory and inhibitory activity among the vestibular neural structures. For example, imagine that you are turning to stand up from the dinner table. As you begin to shift your body around the chair, the horizontally oriented semicircular canals are strongly engaged, producing inputs to tell the CNS that you are indeed turning. Next, as you shift your weight forward, the utricle is excited and transduces your slight forward motion. Finally, as you start standing up, the hair cells of the saccule indicate to the CNS a change in your vertical position. As you can see, such a simple act requires the integrated activity of both vestibular sensory systems.

Central Vestibular Pathway

At rest, the vestibular nerves are tonically active equally on each side of the body. The equal degree of activity within these nerves indicates to the CNS that the head is still. Motion of the head disturbs this relative equilibrium and generates a short-term change in excitability that correlates with position, orientation, and motion of the head. The vestibular nerves project to a collection of four **vestibular nuclei** (lateral, medial, superior, and inferior) located in the dorsal medulla and partially in the pons (**Fig. 9.27**). Vestibular nuclei receive inputs from a variety of sources besides the vestibular nerves, including the cerebellum and the somatosensory and the visual systems. As shown in **Fig. 9.27**, the output from the vestibular nuclei targets the **ventral posterior (VP) nuclei** of the thalamus (part of the ventral line nuclei discussed in the somatosensory system) (not shown in **Fig. 9.27**), the **flocculonodular lobe** of the cerebellum (via vestibulocerebellar fibers), and cranial nerve nuclei III, IV, and VI (all active in mediating eye motion).

Each of the subdivisions of the vestibular nuclear complex has a unique function and contribution to vestibular activity. The superior and medial nuclei primarily mediate our gaze reflex response through inputs derived from the semicircular canals and outputs directed to brainstem nuclei responsible for oculomotor control (cranial nerves III, IV, and

VI). The lateral nucleus receives inputs from both the otolith organs and the semicircular canals and outputs to the **vestibulospinal tracts**. The **lateral vestibulospinal tract** receives output from the otolith organs and innervates lower motor neurons in the spinal cord, controlling muscles of the trunk and lower limb extensor muscles to maintain postural control of the body. The **medial vestibulospinal tract** receives output from the semicircular canals via the medial vestibular nucleus and innervates muscles of the neck to adjust head position while the body moves. Finally, the inferior vestibular nucleus obtains the majority of its inputs from the otolith organs and outputs to the cerebellum via vestibulocerebellar fibers and to the brainstem **reticular formation**. Vestibular outputs to the cerebellum enable this structure to coordinate and smoothly adjust evolving body movement to changes in head and eye position.

Although the chief function of the vestibular nuclei is autonomic in nature, these nuclei also possess projections, by way of the thalamus, that terminate in Brodmann areas 3a and 2 of the primary somatosensory cortex. These same cortical zones also receive inputs from visual areas of the parietal lobe and from proprioceptive endings. Together, this combination of inputs into area 3a and area 2 may facilitate the blending of critical data related to motion and position in space. It is hypothesized that such an integration of sensory information may aid the cortex in creating an appreciation for self-generated movement in relation to the outside environment.

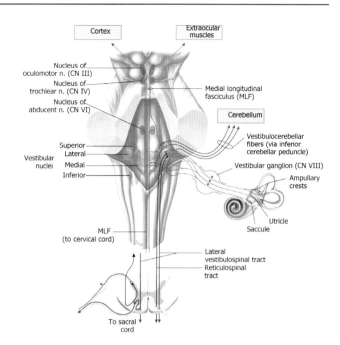

Fig. 9.27 Vestibular central targets; central projections from the vestibular nerve.

The Chemical Senses

Our chemical senses of taste and smell detect a variety of ambient molecules and encode these inputs to provide important information regarding our environment. Although humans tend to rely more on visual and hearing cues during behavior, our chemical senses are used to indicate the presence of pleasurable experiences (freshly baked

---

Box 9.10   Benign Paroxysmal Positional Vertigo (BPPV)

While not life threatening, disorders in our vestibular system make it difficult to maintain our balance and can have a dramatic impact on our quality of life. Benign paroxysmal positional vertigo (BPPV) is a vestibular disorder that can cause vertigo and sudden dizziness when there is a change in the position of your head. For example, if you hear a noise and turn your head to see what is happening, you may suddenly become dizzy and disoriented. When we turn our heads, the fluid within the vestibular system mechanically activates sensory receptors that provide the brain with information regarding the position, rotation, and acceleration of our heads. For individu-

als with BPPV, the otoconia of the otolith organs can collect and clump together in one area of the system. When the head turns, the clump of otoconia moves erratically and stimulates receptors to send false signals to the brain regarding our position.

Aside from vertigo, individuals with BPPV may experience nystagmus (involuntary eye movements), imbalance, lightheadedness, and nausea with even the slightest movement of their heads. BPPV can occur after certain types of surgery or trauma, but most cases are idiopathic. BPPV can be treated by specialists who are trained in using specific head positions to move the otoconia out of the impacted areas of the vestibular system.

(Fife et al 2008)

chocolate chip cookies), invoke powerful memories (your mother's favorite perfume or the smell of the ocean), or even indicate possible danger (the smell of a gas leak or the taste of spoiled food). There are an incredibly vast number of smells and flavors that we are able not only to identify, but also to discriminate to give us clues about our current environment. Alterations in olfaction or gustatory sensation can have an impact on our safety, nutritional status, and overall quality of life.

Smell is the psychological interpretation of odors perceived primarily by the nose and is processed through our olfactory system. Our sense of taste is the perception of salty, sweet, sour, bitter, and umami by the tongue and other pharyngeal components and processed through the gustatory system. We perceive smell or taste from **odorant** or **tastant** molecules through specialized sensory cells in the nose, mouth, and oropharynx that can encode chemical stimuli. Our sense of smell is almost always necessary for the perception of taste; this is why food may taste bland when you have a stuffy nose. Physiologically, there is overlap between the two systems, given that our perception of flavor is influenced by the integration of both taste and smell. Although the two systems share some similarities, such as their ability to regenerate sensory neurons throughout our lifespan, their peripheral and central neural pathways for encoding, detecting, and discriminating chemical stimuli are distinct.

Olfactory System

Information about the air we breathe and food we eat is cognitively interpreted as smell by our olfactory system. Although olfactory capabilities of humans are somewhat limited compared to other species (such as dogs), we can still perceive thousands of different odorant molecules, even at concentrations as low as 1 part per 10 million. The pinnacle of olfaction sensitivity in the human is best exemplified by wine connoisseurs or perfumers, who specialize in detecting tiny differences in odors between multiple scents. Such a nose can be very valuable indeed!

Olfactory Receptors and Transduction Mechanism

The set of chemoreceptors used for olfaction are located in a small area of epithelial tissue at the roof of the nasal cavity in approximately a 5-cm^2 area on each side of the nose (**Fig. 9.28**). Olfactory epithelium consists of three main cell types: olfactory sensory neurons, supporting cells, and basal stem cells. The supporting cells aid in secretion of mucus to coat the olfactory epithelium. Mucus is important for transducing specific odorants by providing the necessary molecular and ionic environment for detection to occur. Olfactory neurons are unique among other sensory nerve endings in that they have an average life span of only 30 to 60 days and undergo constant renewal and replacement. Olfactory basal stem cells are responsible for regeneration of these sensory neurons.

Olfactory receptors are bipolar neurons located within the olfactory epithelium that act as both a receptor and a first-order afferent. Olfactory receptors possess a peripheral branch that proceeds to the epithelial surface and a central axon that projects to the **olfactory bulb**. It is estimated that there are between 10 and 20 million olfactory receptor neurons in the nasal cavity. At the proximal end of the olfactory receptor neuron is a thin unmyelinated axon that joins with other axons, passes through the cribriform plate of the ethmoid bone, and forms the first-order synapse in the olfactory bulb. This relationship offers a close association between our environment and the CNS, making the olfactory system highly susceptible to infections, toxins, and trauma.

Olfactory receptors are exquisitely sensitive and can detect the faintest smell; however, they can adapt quite rapidly and lose their responsiveness. Consider a particularly strong smell you have encountered, such as a too infrequently emptied garbage bin behind a restaurant. At first, the smell is overwhelmingly strong, but then begins to fade slowly. You might ask people who live nearby about the smell and they might reply, "You get used to it." More likely, individuals in these cases have gone

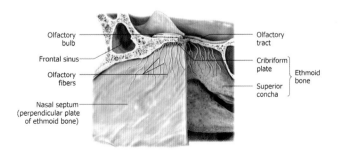

Fig. 9.28 Olfactory bulb fibers are shown protruding through the ethmoid cribriform plate into the nasal cavity.

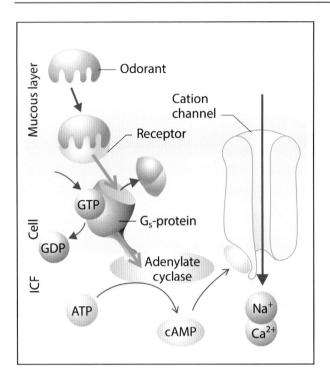

Fig. 9.29 Odorant reception and transduction. Schematic of the chemical cascade required to trigger ion channel opening and current flow in the presence of an odorant. Intracellular fluid (ICF) shows second-messenger system activation needed to open the ion channel.

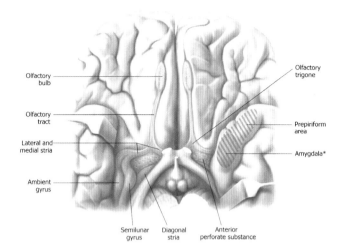

Fig. 9.30 Olfactory system. A ventral view of the major components of the olfactory system.

through a process of olfactory adaptation. In the presence of a specific odorant, the olfactory cells begin to fatigue and no longer fire action potentials. In fact, olfactory cells lose their sensitivity to a specific chemical odor by up to 50% in the first second of an exposure. Breathing through the mouth in the presence of a strong odor is an often used strategy to avoid intense smells. Unfortunately, this strategy does not prevent you from detecting the noxious odor. You will still perceive the odor due in part to retronasal olfaction, where odorants are detected from the oral and pharyngeal cavities alone. Retronasal olfaction plays an important role in fully appreciating the flavors of food, which may explain why some confuse the loss of smell with a loss in gustatory or taste sensation.

The first step in olfactory sensation is the movement of odorants through the nasal passages via breathing or sniffing. These actions bring the odorant molecules into contact with the olfactory epithelium. The perceptual strength of an odor can, in part, be explained by the velocity at which the odor molecules move and the volume of the odorant in the air. Sniffing may increase air flow turbulence at the epithelium, but it may also prime the

olfactory system for the incoming olfactory information. Hydrophilic odorants dissolve into the watery mucus, while hydrophobic molecules must first interact with binding proteins to be transported across the mucosal lining. As shown in **Fig. 9.29**, odorant molecules eventually will bind to an olfactory receptor, activating an olfactory-specific G-protein second messenger pathway. The resulting intracellular chemical cascade initiates an influx of Na^+ and Ca^{2+} and the efflux of K^+, depolarizing the cell and triggering action potential firing.

From this point, second-order neurons leave the olfactory bulb and project along the **olfactory tract (CN I)**, eventually synapsing onto the primary olfactory cortex. Some portions of the trigeminal nerve (CN V), specifically the ophthalmic and maxillary branches, contribute to olfaction by detecting specific noxious irritants such as ammonia. These fibers are involved in nasal reflexes such as sneezing or reflexively holding your breath when a noxious odor is detected. Connections between trigeminal chemoreceptors and the olfactory system occur in the thalamus.

Central Olfactory Pathway

The primary olfactory cortex consists of a collection of structures including the anterior olfactory nucleus, the piriform cortex, anterior cortical nucleus of the amygdala, the periamygdaloid complex, and the rostral entorhinal cortex (**Fig. 9.30**). It does not appear that there is topographic distribution from the olfactory bulb to the cortex. In fact, each region of the olfactory cortex can receive information from all areas of the olfactory bulb. Interestingly, the olfactory system sends information directly to cortical structures without first passing through the thalamus, a unique feature in sensory transduction. However, many connections between primary and secondary olfactory cortices do occur through the nuclei in the dorsal medial thalamus.

The primary and secondary olfactory structures share a reciprocal relationship with one another as well as with higher brain structures. For example, the piriform cortex can encode higher-order representations of smells, including qualities related to identification and familiarity of a smell, and the coordination of smell information with vision and taste. Additionally, fibers from the olfactory complex project directly to the lateral hypothalamus and hippocampus, providing a critical link between olfaction, learning, and behavior. These interrelationships might help to explain why certain smells tend to elicit strong memories.

Gustatory System

Gustation is the sensory perception of taste. We use taste primarily during feeding to assess the quality of food we take in and to avoid toxic or potentially harmful foods. In order for taste perception to occur, soluble chemicals must come into contact with sensory receptors. The primary sensory receptors for taste are several thousand **taste buds** located primarily on the surface of the anterior two-thirds

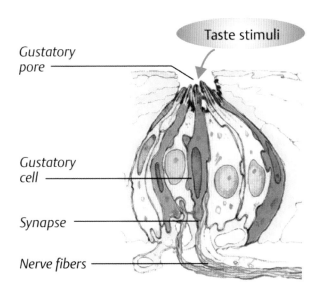

Fig. 9.31 Taste bud structure. Major components of a taste bud are shown.

of the tongue. Limited numbers of buds can also be found on the posterior tongue as well as on the surfaces of the pharynx, larynx, soft palate, epiglottis, and upper portions of the esophagus.

Gustatory Receptors and Transduction

A taste bud is a collection of 50 to 100 taste cells that congregate together in a barrel-shaped grouping (**Fig. 9.31**). Taste cells are arranged in a concentric fashion around a central taste pore. Microvilli containing membrane receptors project into the taste pore, where they interact with the chemical tastants. Each taste bud or receptor cell may be innervated by multiple afferent fibers. In turn, a single gustatory nerve fiber may innervate cells in more than one taste bud.

In vertebrates, taste receptor cells are considered modified epithelial cells. Four morphologically distinct cell types are found in each taste bud: basal cells, dark cells, light cells, and intermediate cells. Taste cells have a very short lifespan; in rats, the lifespan of a taste cell is approximately 10 days. Basal cells are responsible for continually repopulating taste receptor cells. The other three nonbasal cell types are all referred to as simply taste cells and may reflect the various stages of development of a new taste cell, with the light cell classification representing the most mature form of the cell.

The vast majority of taste buds are located within structures on the surface of the tongue called papillae, which are defined based on their shape and have particular locations on the lingual epithelium. There are three types of papillae on the tongue surface that carry taste buds: fungiform, foliate, and circumvallate. Fungiform papillae are located on the anterior two-thirds of the tongue and resemble a club or mushroom. The chorda tympani branch of the facial nerve (CN VII) innervates these papillae. The foliate papillae can be found on the lateral surface of the tongue and are also innervated by the facial nerve (CN VII). Posteriorly positioned foliate papillae are innervated by the glossopharyngeal nerve (CN IX). Lastly, circumvallate papillae are located in the midline of the posterior tongue and are innervated by the glossopharyngeal nerve (CN IX). (There are also filiform papillae, with a hairlike appearance, which do not carry taste buds.) Taste buds located on the epiglottis and esophagus are innervated by the vagus nerve (CN X).

There are five primary taste qualities that we can perceive: sweet, sour, salty, bitter and umami (a savorylike taste quality perceived by mammals and elicited by glutamate). In mammals, gustatory nerve fibers respond to a broad class of taste stimuli, not just one taste quality, contradicting the often cited fallacy of the tongue being divided into taste quadrants where only one taste quality can be perceived. In fact, all taste bud populations are able to perceive each of the five taste qualities, with each taste quality perceived or mediated through different mechanisms. However, groups of nerve fibers seem to show a "preference" for certain taste qualities, demonstrating a greater response in their presence. For example, fibers of the facial nerve (CN VII) are most responsive to sweet and salty stimuli, while fibers of the glossopharyngeal nerve (CN IX) are more responsive to sour and bitter stimuli.

Taste perception begins when tastants are dissolved in saliva. Saliva is vitally important in taste transduction by acting to move the solubilized taste molecules to the taste receptor cells, initiating the process of transduction. Additionally, saliva helps to remove the previous chemical tastants once stimulation has already occurred. When the saliva carrying the chemical tastants washes over a receptor, the molecule binds with a receptor on the microvilli of the cell and causes either a hyperpolarization or a depolarization of the receptor. During depolarization, an influx of Ca^{2+} into the receptor cell causes release of neurotransmitter into the synaptic cleft. From here, the process of taste transduction varies based on the taste quality. Although the mechanism is not completely clear in humans, salty taste qualities are perceived through direct interaction between the tastants and Na^+ ion channel activity. Acidic (sour) taste qualities involve multiple pathways involving voltage-dependent potassium (K^+) channels. Finally, sweet, bitter, and umami qualities involve specific membrane receptors activating G-protein second-messenger systems and depolarization of the cell membrane through voltage-dependent calcium (Ca^{2+}) channels.

The different mechanisms used for processing varying taste qualities enable separate, yet simultaneous perception of tastes that, in combination with olfaction, can enable complex appreciation of flavors. As with olfaction, there is a process of adaptation to the continued presence of tastant stimuli. However, gustatory adaptation is class-specific. For example, prolonged exposure to a sour taste quality will decrease the stimulation response to other sour tastants but not necessarily to sweet, salty, bitter, or umami stimuli.

Central Gustatory Pathway

Using **Fig. 9.32** as a guide, all afferent fibers for taste terminate in the rostral segment of the **nucleus of the solitary tract (NST)** located in the medulla. The NST region is often referred to as the gustatory nucleus. Second-order taste neurons project from this region to the **parabrachial nuclei (PBN)** of the pons and terminate in the thalamus. Fibers then project to the insular cortex and frontal operculum. A second projection from the pons connects multiple areas in the ventral forebrain including the lateral hypothalamus, amygdala, and nucleus of the stria terminalis. All gustatory pathways follow an ipsilateral course, a distinct organizational feature of gustation that is different from the other senses.

Dysfunction in the Chemical Senses

Olfactory and gustatory dysfunction can occur as a function of aging, disease, or infection. Changes in olfaction can be perceived as a total loss of smell (anosmia) or incomplete loss of perceived smell (partial anosmia or hyposmia). Other dysfunctions

---

Box 9.11 Xerostomia

Xerostomia is the perceived sensation of dry mouth and may range from a mild decrease in saliva, which an individual finds annoying, to the complete loss of salivary production, harming health and quality of life. Xerostomia is a common side effect of radiation therapy but may also be associated with aging, Parkinson's disease, trauma to the oral cavity, Sjögren's syndrome, exposure to tobacco, or methamphetamine use or as a side effect to certain over-the-counter and prescription medications. Patients experiencing xerostomia find it difficult to produce the amount of saliva necessary to chew, swallow, and properly digest food.

Lack of saliva may even have an impact on the clarity of speech. More importantly, dry mouth can lead to an increased risk of poor oral health and hygiene, mouth sores, bad breath (halitosis), and difficulty wearing dentures.

Some individuals may find relief by increasing water intake, chewing sugarless gum, avoiding tobacco and alcohol, and using over-the-counter dry mouth moisturizing fluids. Consistent and high-quality oral care is also imperative to maintain good oral hygiene and prevent oral disease.

(Plemons et al 2014)

may occur that distort our sense of smell. For example, a person may perceive the scent of something rotten when smelling a rose, as in **dysosmias**, or they may perceive the smell of roses when none are actually present, as in **phantosmias**. Although less common, alterations in the sense of perceived smell may occur after head trauma, particularly in injuries that occur due to a sudden acceleration or deceleration causing a stretch or strain to the ventral cortex. Any loss in smell associated with head trauma is usually recovered within the first year after trauma.

Loss of perceived taste may be caused by upper respiratory infections, head trauma, drug use, or idiopathic causes. Our sense of taste may also be impacted by problems with chewing associated with tooth loss, the outfit of dentures, and reduction or impairments in saliva production. Changes in taste and smell can impact the desire and enjoyment during meals and can lead to a decline in nutritional status and quality of life.

Age-Related Changes to the Chemical Senses

It is estimated that over half of the population over 65 years experiences some significant loss in olfaction capacity. Changes in olfactory sensation with age can lead to difficulty in smell detection and discrimination. In typical aging, there is a decrease in the number of fibers in the olfactory bulb and the number of olfactory receptors. As discussed previously, mammals can replace olfactory receptor neurons using basal stem cells after the neurons undergo apoptosis or cell death. However, this process degenerates with aging, leading to a decrease in the total number of receptors available. Olfactory decline with aging can also be the result of ossification and closure of the foramina of the ethmoid cribriform plate, repeated viral infections, or the early development of neurodegenerative diseases. Changes in olfactory sensation tend to be greater and more severe in men than in women, but this can greatly depend on a variety of life choices, such as smoking behavior, and other health-related causes.

Taste disorders associated with aging are less prevalent than olfactory disorders, likely because gustatory dysfunctions can masquerade as deficits in olfaction. Many of our favorite flavors (coffee, chocolate, and pizza, to name a few) actually require stimulation to the olfactory nerve during deglutition (see the mention of retronasal olfaction). Damage to portions of the nasal cavity may decrease our ability to perceive these complex flavors while leaving only somatosensory sensations

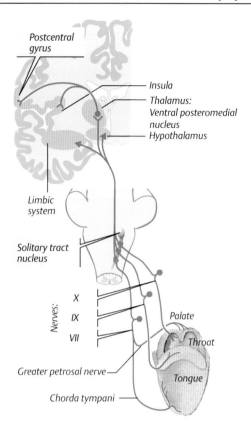

Fig 9.32 Gustatory pathways. Gustatory afferent projections to central targets including the solitary tract nucleus, thalamus and postcentral gyrus.

and primary taste qualities (e.g., sweet, sour, bitter) intact. Because of the redundant innervation of taste buds from the facial (CN VII), glossopharyngeal (CN IX), and vagus (CN X) nerves, primary taste qualities are more resilient to pathology and trauma-related events.

■ Suggested Readings

Barlow SM. Real-time modulation of speech-orofacial motor performance by means of motion sense. *Journal of Communication Disorders, 31*, 511–534; 1998

Edin BB. Strain-sensitive mechanoreceptors in the human skin provide kinaesthetic information. In: Franzén O, Johansson RS, Terenius L, eds. Somesthesis and the Neurobiology of the Sensorimotor Cortex: Advances in Life Sciences. Basel, Switzerland: Birkhäuser Verlag; 1996: 283–294

Fife TD, Iverson DJ, Lempert T, et al. Practice parameter: therapies for benign paroxysmal positional vertigo (an evidence-based review): Report of the Quality Standards Subcommittee of the American Academy of Neurology. *Neurology*, *70*, 2067–2074; 2008

Gescheider GA. Psychophysics: The Fundamentals, 3rd ed. Mahwah, NJ: L. Erlbaum Associates; 1997

Hendry C, Farley A, McLafferty E. Anatomy and physiology of the senses. *Nursing Standard*, *27*(5), 35–42; 2012

Hupé JM, Dojat M. A critical review of the neuroimaging literature on synesthesia. *Frontiers in Human Neuroscience*, *9*, 103; 2015

Kandel ER, Schwartz JH, Jessell TM, Siegelbaum SA, Hudspeth AJ. Principles of Neural Science, 5th ed. New York, NY: McGraw Hill; 2013

Mountcastle VB. The Sensory Hand: Neural Mechanisms in Somatosensation. Cambridge, MA: Harvard University Press; 2005

National Institutes of Health. National Institutes of Deafness and Other Communications Disorders. www.nidcd.nih.gov/health/hearing/pages/coch.aspx

Pickles JO. An Introduction to the Physiology of Hearing, 3rd ed. New York, NY: Academic Press; 2008

Plemons JM, Al-Hashimi I, Marek CL. Managing xerostomia and salivary gland hypofunction: executive summary of a report from the American Dental Association Council on Scientific Affairs. *Journal of the American Dental Association*, *145*, 867–873; 2014

Squire LR, Berg D, Bloom FE, du Lac S, Ghosh A, Spitzer NC, eds. Fundamental Neuroscience, 4th ed. Boston, MA: Elsevier/Academic Press; 2013

■ Study Questions

1. Sensation can be thought of as:

A. A cognitive event
B. The quantifiable signals that arise from sensory stimuli
C. Mechanical features of an object or event
D. A series of action potentials
E. The regions of the cortex that processes external inputs

2. Sensory systems are defined as the:

A. Collections of cortical areas that process stimuli
B. Sensory receptors located in the periphery
C. Psychophysical features for a modality
D. Collections of all neurons that contribute to processing sensory inputs of modality
E. Manner in which real-world inputs are organized in the CNS

3. The difference between the study areas of psychophysics and sensory physiology lies with:

A. The manner in which perception is studied
B. The manner in which sensory processing is defined
C. The idea that sensations can be quantified using instrumentation
D. The areas of the brain that are investigated
E. The form of tools used to quantify perception

4. Modality of a sensory system refers to:

A. A general class of stimulus energy transduced by the CNS
B. The sensory inputs that help you localize inputs
C. The submodalities that define the quality of sensations
D. The major classes of receptors underlying a sensory event
E. The form and shape of a sensory receptor

5. Receptive fields define an area of the sensory sheet monitored by:

A. Sensory systems
B. Small or large sensory neurons
C. A single sensory receptor
D. Multiple groups of sensory receptors
E. The primary cortical areas of the brain.

6. A sensory receptor's response to intensity changes is best understood by appreciating the characteristics of its:

A. Ion channels
B. Action potential generation
C. Distribution of Na^+ and K^+
D. Threshold of receptor activation
E. Receptor potential

7. Proprioception and pain appreciation are two sensations mediated by the:

A. Auditory system
B. Somatosensory system
C. Thermoregulatory system
D. Hydrodynamic receptor system
E. Nociceptive system

8. The DCML and the ALS mediate which of the following forms of somatosensory inputs?

A. Pain and temperature
B. Touch and proprioception
C. Exteroception and interoception
D. Tactile and nociception
E. Nociception and exteroception

9. Unlike other sensory receptors, photoreceptors require which unique neural event to develop for transduction to occur?

A. Light must shine on the photoreceptor.
B. The photoreceptor must be hyperpolarized.
C. The photoreceptor must be depolarized.
D. Bipolar and retinal ganglion cells must be present and active.
E. Cones and rods must be segregated from each other in the retina.

10. The primary visual cortex is structurally and functionally organized into hypercolumns. Which of the following major features of visual stimuli is directly encoded in this structure?

A. Brightness
B. Gray scale
C. Shadows
D. Orientation
E. Faces

11. In the visual system, the dorsal stream functions to provide what main form of complex visual perception?

A. Color of an object
B. Form of an object
C. Motion of an object
D. Name of an object
E. Use of an object

12. The foveola is a critical structure of the retina for which of the following reasons?

A. It contains a concentration of rods that support vision in dark conditions.
B. It possesses four distinct layers of cells to maximize light transmission.
C. It contains a concentration of cones enabling precise transduction of light in daylight.
D. It represents the location where the optic nerve begins.
E. It contains high numbers of both rods and cones to transduce light optimally in the human.

13. The graded nature of the basilar membrane's structural features indicates that:

A. Frequency is place dependent.
B. The cochlea responds to frequencies of only certain intensity.
C. The organ of Corti is not the true site of auditory stimulus transduction.
D. The BM can only resonate one frequency at a time.
E. Hair cell activity is key to the processes of transducing multiple frequencies.

14. OHCs play which following crucial role during sound transduction?

A. They transduce all sound inputs entering the cochlea.
B. They function to tune the sensitivity of the BM to sound inputs.
C. They allow the transduction of sound intensity.
D. They are the origin of the auditory nerve.
E. They are the source of fluid production within the cochlea.

15. The inferior colliculus performs what function in the context of the central auditory pathway?

A. Transforms sound input into a map of frequency
B. Helps in the localization of sound
C. Creates a three-dimensional map of auditory space
D. Transduces intensity of sound
E. Localizes specific frequency patterns

16. The SOC functions to localize sound in a frequency-dependent manner using which of the following mechanisms?

A. Interaural timing differences to detect high-frequency inputs
B. Interaural intensity differences to localize both high- and low-frequency sounds
C. Basilar membrane amplitude differences
D. Interaural intensity differences to localize high-frequency sounds
E. Spectral differences to localize complex sounds

17. The otolith organs are able to transduce what form of acceleration of the head?

A. Rotational acceleration
B. Only vertical linear acceleration
C. Only horizontal linear acceleration
D. Rotational and linear acceleration
E. Both horizontal and vertical linear acceleration

18. The vestibular nuclei project to the following structures:

A. Ventral posterolateral thalamic nucleus
B. Medulla
C. Optic (CN II) and oculomotor (CN III) nerves
D. Flocculonodular lobe of the cerebellum
E. Trigeminal system

19. The following set of cranial nerves transduce gustatory sense:

A. Trigeminal (CN V), facial (CN VII), and hypoglossal (CN XII)
B. Abducens (CN VI), facial (CN VII), and vagus (CN X)
C. Glossopharyngeal (CN IX) and vagus (CN X)
D. Facial (CN VII) and glossopharyngeal (CN IX)
E. Only glossopharyngeal (CN IX)

20. Changes in olfactory sensation with age can lead to difficulty in smell detection. What is a main cause of this difficulty?

A. Reduced area in the cortex for processing smell
B. Changes to the size of the nasal cavity
C. Lack of attentional skills
D. Loss of interest in smelling things due to dietary changes
E. Reduced numbers of olfactory sensory receptors

■ Answers to Study Questions

1. The correct answer is (B). Sensations are defined as real-world stimulus events that can be quantified objectively through instrumentation and the recording of a subject's response. The other responses are incomplete or incorrect.

2. The correct answer is (D). A given sensory system requires that all components, from receptor to cortical area, be accounted for to explain the processing of an input. The other choices are components of the concept, but by themselves are not complete.

3. The correct answer is (A). While all the other choices are partially valid, they do not capture the core difference between these areas. Only (A) is a broad enough response to answer the question.

4. The correct answer is (A). This is the actual definition of the term. The other choices are components of the concept but by themselves are not complete.

5. The correct answer is (C). Receptive fields are by definition innervated by a single afferent and sensory receptor. No other choice is consistent with the definition of a receptive field.

6. The correct answer is (E). While all other choices are a part of the answer, only (E) completely satisfies the question. The receptor potential is the key to understanding how receptors translate stimulus magnitude into different rates of action potential firing.

7. The correct answer is (B). The somatosensory system mediates touch, proprioception, pain, and temperature sensations. No other choice mediates both of the examples in the question.

8. The correct answer is (D). The DCML mediates tactile inputs while the ALS mediates nociception. No other choice contains the correct combination of sensations.

9. The correct answer is (B). Of all the choices available, only (B) is unique to photoreceptors compared to other sensory receptors as stated in the question.

10. The correct answer is (D). Orientation is directly coded in the primary visual cortex as part of the hypercolumn complex. All the choices are visual features that are abstracted either prior to or after V1.

11. The correct answer is (C). The dorsal stream cortical areas code for spatially related features such as object motion. Answer choices (A) and (B) are more likely to be coded within the ventral stream. Answer choices (D) and (E) pertain to processing that goes well beyond the sensory areas.

12. The correct answer is (C). The foveola possess the highest concentration of cones, and they are unobstructed by the bipolar and retinal ganglion layers. All other choices are incorrect or incomplete.

13. The correct answer is (A). The graded changes in stiffness and thickness of the BM indicates that specific frequency resonances depend on the physical nature of the BM at every location. All other responses are either incorrect or are offering an incomplete idea.

14. The correct answer is (B). OHCs receive efferent input that allows these cells to dynamically change the physical relationship between the BM and the tectorial membrane, thus changing the response sensitivity of the BM to vibratory inputs. All other choices are incorrect or vague.

15. The correct answer is (C). The IC is believed to create a 3-D map of auditory space through the integration of inputs coming from the SOC and the CN. The other choices in the question either are incorrect or are not functions specific only to the IC.

16. The correct answer is (D). Interaural intensity differences are used to localize high-frequency sound inputs. All other choices are incorrect.

17. The correct answer is (E). Only (E) possesses the correct combination of responses. Otolith organs transduce linear acceleration of the head and neck.

18. The correct answer is (D). Of the choices provided, only (D) is correct. The vestibular nuclei project heavily to the cerebellum and help this structure to smooth and coordinate movement patterns in real time.

19. The correct answer is (D). Only (D) possesses the correct combination of cranial nerves in the choice.

20. The correct answer is (E). Reduced numbers of sensory receptors as well as ossification of the cribriform plate are two main factors reducing one's sensitivity to odorants. All other responses are incorrect.

Part III

The Anatomy and Physiology of Speech and Language, Swallowing, Hearing, and Balance

10

Respiration

Erin P. Silverman and Bari Hoffman Ruddy

■ Chapter Summary

Respiration sustains life, and the pace of our breathing reflects the body's continual adaptation to an ever-changing environment. When we are excited or fearful, our breath quickens. When we relax or rest, it slows, ushering in feelings of calm and peace. The study of the anatomy and physiology of respiration is essential to our understanding of the human body, as well as of what it means to be human. Respiration is the power source for voice and speech and responds in specific ways to the actions of coughing and swallowing. The purpose of this chapter is to provide a framework for understanding of the speech and nonspeech functions of the human respiratory system. Specifically, we will (1) provide an overview of respiratory anatomy and physiology; (2) discuss conditions that adversely affect the respiratory system; and (3) describe the physiologic principles underlying therapeutic management of speech- and nonspeech-related respiratory dysfunction by the speech-language pathologist.

■ Learning Objectives

- Describe the anatomy and physiology of the human respiratory system
- Understand the functional contributions of respiratory system structures to gas exchange
- Explain the contributions of respiratory system structures to the physiological processes underlying airway protection

- Describe the contributions of the respiratory system to voice and speech production
- Explain the effects of respiratory dysfunction on voice, speech, swallowing, and cognitive processes

■ Putting It Into Practice

- The respiratory system assists in the regulation of blood pH, filters potentially harmful microorganisms from the outside environment, assists with immune system functions, regulates core body temperature, enables the sense of smell, and is the driving force behind the uniquely human functions of voice and speech.
- The therapeutic management of disorders of voice, speech, and swallowing requires a comprehensive understanding of respiratory system mechanics, pressure-volume relationships, respiratory muscle function, and the impact of respiratory dysfunction on voice, speech, and swallowing across the lifespan.
- Speech-language pathologists often work on multidisciplinary teams involving pulmonologists, respiratory physiologists, and respiratory therapists in the management of patients with respiratory dysfunction. The speech-language pathologist provides a critical role in providing counseling and therapeutic management of the speech- and nonspeech-related functions of the respiratory system, including those related to speech, voice, and swallow function.

■ Introduction

At the most fundamental level, the human respiratory system supports life through the exchange of oxygen (O_2) and carbon dioxide (CO_2) between the external (atmospheric) and internal (corporeal) environments while maintaining the life-sustaining balance of acidity and alkalinity within body fluids. The metabolic processes that support life require a continual supply of O_2 in order to produce **adenosine triphosphate (ATP)**, a coenzyme that functions as the energy currency for cells and their activities. In addition to consuming O_2, production of ATP releases CO_2 into the intracellular fluid, or cytosol, where, if not removed, it lowers the **pH** to acidic levels incompatible with cell viability. The continual processes of the supply of O_2 and removal of CO_2 are accomplished through the cooperative actions of the cardiovascular (heart) and respiratory (**lungs**) systems. The repeated processes of inhalation and exhalation replenish O_2 (inhalation) and remove CO_2 (exhalation). Following inhalation, oxygen-rich blood is pumped by the heart through the arterial system to tissues. Following transfer of O_2 to the cells, depleted blood returns to the lungs carrying high levels of CO_2, which are then removed by the lungs, from the body, via exhalation.

Beyond the cellular and life-sustaining functions of gas exchange and maintaining pH balance, the respiratory system serves many other functions. The upper respiratory tract filters and humidifies inhaled air, protecting the lungs from contact with foreign organisms. Sensory receptors embedded in the epithelial tissues that line the nasal cavity transmit neural impulses, generated through contact with chemical stimuli contained within the inhaled air, to the brain, producing the sense of smell. Exhalation removes excess heat and moisture from the body, thereby assisting in regulation of body temperature. Respiration is also the driving force behind coughing, an important mechanism of airway defense that removes excess secretions or foreign matter from the lungs. Finally, voice and speech are the result of dynamic shaping of acoustic waves that consist of exhaled air transformed into acoustic waveforms by the **vocal folds**.

Changes to the respiratory system that occur as a result of normal aging, injury, disease, or medical interventions can have mild to profound effects on any or all of these processes. With regard to the diagnosis and treatment of swallowing disorders, an evolving understanding of the shared neurologic substrates of coughing and swallowing has influenced the professional scope of practice, shifting focus from swallow-specific approaches to diagnosis and treatment to methods that address

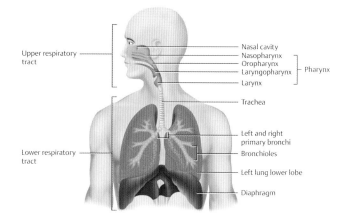

Fig. 10.1   Upper and lower respiratory systems.

a continuum of airway protective behaviors, from preventative (swallow) to corrective (cough) (Troche et al 2014).

Structurally, the respiratory system can be subdivided into the **upper respiratory system**, consisting of the nose and **pharynx** (particularly the oropharynx and nasopharynx); the **larynx**; and the **lower respiratory system**, consisting of the **trachea**, bronchi, and lungs (West 2012). See **Fig. 10.1**.

Upper Respiratory System

Air enters the respiratory tract through the mouth and nose, which warms and filters inhaled air. The oral and nasal cavities merge to form the throat, or pharynx, through which air passes as it is inhaled into the lower respiratory tract (West 2012). Positioned inferior to the skull base and anterior to the oral cavity, the nose consists of paired nasal cavities, separated medially by a cartilaginous wall known as the **nasal septum**. Posteriorly, where the septum meets the skull base, this partition is bony, consisting of portions of the ethmoid bone, the vomer, the nasal crest of the maxilla, and the palatine bone. The **paranasal sinuses** are air-filled chambers that lie within the bones of the skull and face surrounding the nasal cavities. Closest to the nasal cavities are the **maxillary sinuses**, situated laterally to the nasal cavity on either side. Other paired sinuses include the **ethmoidal air cells** (located superiorly and posteriorly to the nasal cavities, between the eye sockets), **sphenoidal sinuses** (within the sphenoid bone in the center of the skull), and **frontal sinuses** (housed superior to the eyes and nose within the frontal bone, which defines the forehead). The paranasal sinuses serve to lighten the skull, warm and humidify inhaled air, and amplify speech by resonating the acoustic waves generated by the larynx.

The nasal cavities are further equipped with **nasal conchae** (also called turbinates), three projections from the nasal septum that run from front to back, subdividing each nasal cavity into inferior, middle, and superior regions. The mucosa-lined nasal conchae effectively increase the surface area of the inside of the nose, similarly to the way the sulci and gyri increase the surface area of the cerebral cortex, which allows greater contact between air that is inhaled through the nose and the mucosal lining of the nasal cavity. The lower nasal concha is the largest of the three conchae and serves an important function in the warming and humidification of inhaled air. The next largest is the curved middle nasal concha, followed by the relatively narrow superior nasal concha.

The most inferior portion of the upper airway is the larynx, positioned on top of the trachea. The larynx serves as a valve. It is capable of opening to allow air into the lower respiratory tract, and closing to protect the lower airways from damage that may result from the inhalation of foreign objects. Tight, sustained closure of the larynx is necessary to build up air pressure within the **thoracic cavity**. Laryngeal closure and the accumulation of pressure below the glottis make up the **Valsalva maneuver,** which is crucial for stabilization of the trunk and to protect the spine during high-effort tasks that involve lifting or bearing down.

In humans, voicing is a secondary or nonbiological function of the larynx, developed over the course of evolution. The vocal folds are anchored to cartilages inside the larynx. The vocal folds can be opened (abducted) and closed (adducted), enabling the larynx to act as a valve, separating the upper airway from the lower airway and lungs. A detailed overview of the structure and function of the larynx is presented in **Chapter 11**.

Lower Respiratory System and Associated Structures

The human airway is often referred to as "treelike" in appearance; it progressively divides into multiple narrower and shorter branches that penetrate progressively deeper into the lungs (**Fig. 10.2**). The larynx sits at the superior end of this (upside down) tree. Just inferior to the larynx is the trachea (**Fig. 10.3**). Going back to the tree analogy, the larynx and the 16 cartilaginous rings of the trachea serve as the trunk, from which the first pulmonary branches, the right and left principal **bronchi**, arise. Unlike a tree, the bronchi (and subsequent branches) are

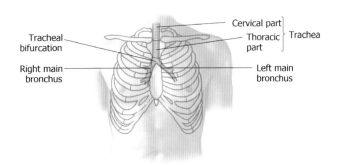

Fig. 10.2 Relationship of trachea to bronchial tree.

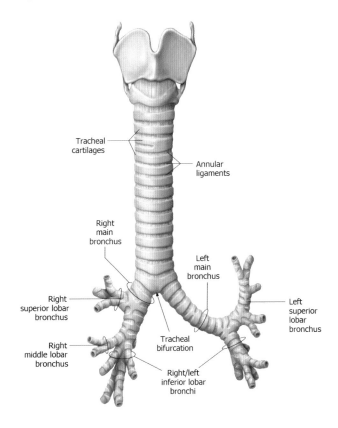

Fig. 10.3 Trachea, relationship to bronchi, and projection into the thoracic cavity.

not solid. They are hollow tubes, reinforced with a series of grossly circular rings made of cartilage and muscle and covered by epithelial and glandular tissues. These branches serve to transport gases into and out of the lungs.

The lungs are paired, roughly cone-shaped organs located inside the chest wall or thoracic cavity. Though paired, the lungs are not identical. The right lung is larger than the left lung in order to accommodate the heart (**Fig. 10.4**). The lungs begin at approximately the level of the clavicle and extend

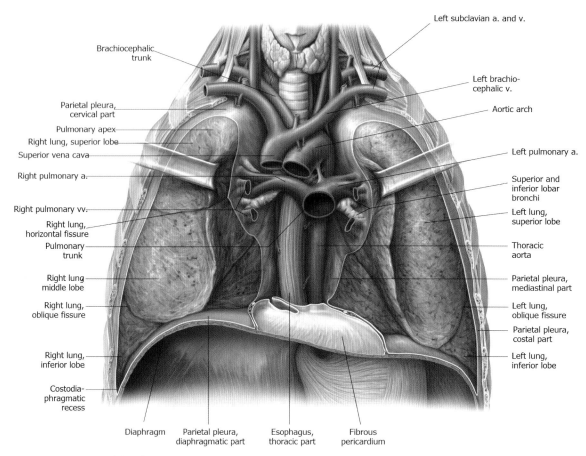

Fig. 10.4 Anterior view of the thoracic cavity showing the lungs retracted from the midline. The left and right lungs normally occupy the full volume available to them in the thoracic cavity. Note that the left lung is smaller than the right because of the asymmetrical position of the heart.

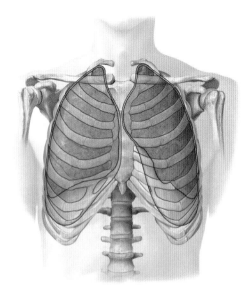

Fig. 10.5 The relationship of the lungs (dark purple shading) to the pleural cavity (lighter blue shading). The pleural cavity is the narrow, fluid-filled space between the visceral and parietal pleurae of each lung.

downward to the **diaphragm**. Anteriorly, laterally, and posteriorly, the **costal surface** of the lungs faces the concave inner surface of the rib cage. The lungs are separated from each other by the **mediastinum**, a membranous compartment containing the heart, blood vessels, esophagus, trachea, phrenic and cardiac nerves, thoracic duct, thymus, and numerous lymph nodes. The mediastinum protects the lungs. Separation of the lungs means that, should one lung collapse or otherwise fail, the likelihood that the other lung would do the same is reduced, minimizing the risk of complete respiratory failure or death. The lung root or **hilum** is a triangle-shaped depression located in the medial (mediastinal) surface of each lung and is where the bronchi enter the lung. Nerves, pulmonary blood vessels, and lymphatic vessels also enter the lungs through the hilum (West 2012).

During respiration, the human lungs continually inflate and then deflate. The lungs contain no muscle tissue and do not modify their shape independently. Lung expansion occurs as a result of a close coupling between the lungs and the surrounding rib cage. This coupling is achieved through a process known as **pleural linkage.** Surrounding nearly three-quarters of the total surface area of each lung is a two-layer **pleural membrane** that attaches each lung to the inside of the thoracic cavity. The outer layer of the pleural membrane is called the **parietal pleura**, which lines the inner wall of the thoracic cavity. The inner layer is called the **visceral pleura** and covers the lungs themselves. In between the parietal and visceral pleurae is the **pleural cavity**, which contains a thin layer of **pleural fluid**. Under normal conditions, this fluid maintains a surface tension between the parietal and visceral pleura. This tension holds the two membranous surfaces together, enabling the lungs to adhere to the inside of the thoracic cavity. The pleural fluid also acts as a lubricant, and under normal conditions the parietal and visceral pleura freely slide alongside each other as the lungs inflate as a result of thoracic expansion and deflate when the thoracic cavity returns to its resting, nonexpanded state. The lungs and thoracic

cavity move as a unit during the cyclical process of breathing but never actually touch (**Fig. 10.5**).

Pleural linkage also counteracts the natural recoil pressures within the lungs and thoracic cavity. The term **hydrostasis** refers to the manner in which equal and opposing pressures generated by proximal liquids create equilibrium. The natural tendency of the thoracic cavity is to expand; however, the **hydrostatic** force generated by the pleural fluid mitigates this tendency, keeping the thorax somewhat retracted. Similarly, the natural tendency of the lungs, which contain no muscle tissue, is to collapse. Pleural linkage of the lungs to the thoracic cavity and the resultant hydrostatic forces counteract this tendency, keeping the lungs partially expanded. The end product of this linkage is a durable balance between the expanding elastic force of the thorax and the collapsing elastic force of the lung. Disruption of pleural linkage can cause partial or total lung collapse, known clinically as **pneumothorax** as air is admitted into the pleural cavity. Pneumothorax can result from any force

Box 10.1   Disorders of the Pleural Membranes and Pleural Cavity

Pleurisy is inflammation of the pleural membrane. Often, this condition results in the accumulation of excess pleural fluid, referred to as pleural effusion, but it can also occur in isolation (Kass et al 2007). Patients with pleurisy often experience sharp chest pain, typically localized to one side. This pain typically increases during movement of the rib cage during breathing, coughing, or changing positions. Pleurisy can result from a variety of conditions including lung infection or pneumonia, lung cancer, pulmonary embolism (blood clot within the lungs), or connective tissue disorders such as lupus (Kass et al 2007). Occasionally, patients undergoing radiation therapy for cancer develop pleurisy. Although symptoms typically improve with improvement of the underlying condition, in some cases, severe pleural effusion must be removed via a **thoracentesis** (Kass et al 2007).

The pleural space can also be infiltrated by blood (hemothorax), pus, or air (pneumothorax). Pneumothorax is commonly caused by a penetrating injury (e.g., surgical incision, gunshot wound) to the pleural membrane (Papagiannis et al 2015). If air breaks the fluid surface tension bonds between the parietal and visceral pleural, partial or total collapse of the affected lung, known as **atelectasis**, is likely. Treatment typically involves evacuation of the pneumothorax and reinflation of the lung (Papagiannis et al 2015).

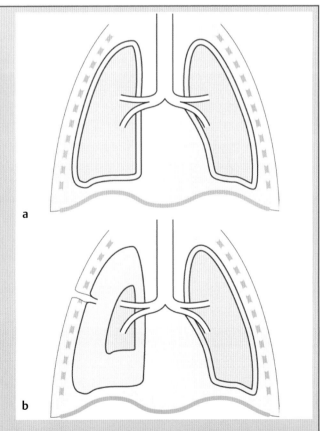

Box Fig. 10.1 Pneumothorax. **(a)** Normal lung and pleural space. **(b)** Collapsed right lung and enlarged pleural space, a condition referred to as atelectasis.

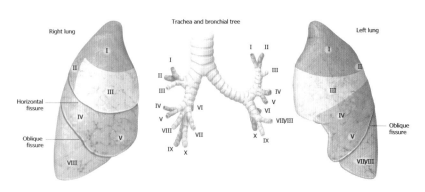

Fig. 10.6 Tracheobronchial tree and relationship to bronchopulmonary segments. The ten tertiary bronchi are labeled according to the bronchopulmonary segments that they supply.

that penetrates the thoracic wall (e.g., blast injury, fractured rib, knife or gunshot wound) and occasionally occurs as a symptom of pulmonary disease such as cystic fibrosis (CF) or chronic obstructive pulmonary disease (COPD).

The pulmonary branches of the right and left lungs are not identical. In the right lung, the right principal bronchus gives rise to three **lobar bronchi**, one for each of the three lobes of the right lung. The left principal bronchus subdivides into two lobar branches that penetrate the two lobes of the left lung. Lobar bronchi are referred to as sec-

ondary bronchi. Each lobar bronchus further subdivides into tertiary, **segmental bronchi**, which penetrate each of the ten bronchopulmonary segments (**Fig. 10.6**). These segments are separated by connective tissue. Similar to how the mediastinum protects the lungs from collapse of both lungs should one lung become damaged, the connective tissues that separate the bronchopulmonary segments allows single segments to sustain damage, or even removal, without affecting the other segments (West, 2012).

The segmental bronchi divide into progressively smaller bronchi, then **bronchioles** (which no longer have cartilage in their walls), then **terminal bronchioles**, **respiratory bronchioles**, **alveolar ducts**, and finally **alveolar sacs** and **alveoli**. Alveoli are considered the terminal airway (top of the "tree") and site of gas exchange between the respiratory and circulatory systems (**Fig. 10.7**). Each alveolus is a cup-shaped pouch made from extremely thin simple squamous epithelial tissue anchored to a similarly thin basement membrane. The epithe-

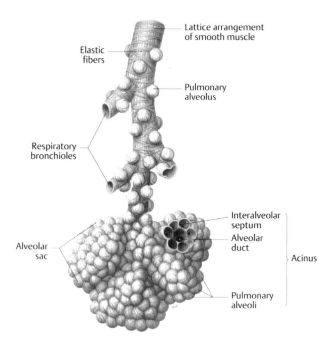

Fig. 10.7 Division of the bronchi into respiratory bronchioles, alveolar sacs, and pulmonary alveoli. Alveoli first appear within the respiratory bronchioles as isolated structures but become more numerous, appearing in clusters or sacs, toward the more distal end of the bronchial tree. The alveolar walls, composed of squamous epithelium, are the site of gas exchange within the lungs.

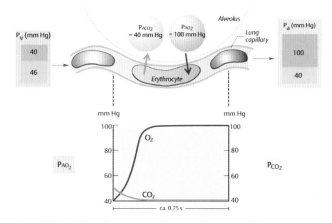

Fig. 10.8 Alveolar gas exchange. P_v = partial pressure of venous blood. P_a = partial pressure of arterial blood. PAO_2 = alveolar partial pressure of oxygen. $PACO_2$ = alveolar partial pressure of carbon dioxide.

lial tissues are composed of **type 1 alveolar cells**, where actual gas exchange occurs; **type 2 alveolar cells**, containing microvilli that produce alveolar fluid (**pulmonary surfactant**) to decrease the surface tension of the alveolus, thereby preventing collapse; and **alveolar macrophages**, which continually remove waste products and foreign cells and particles from the alveolar wall. Two or more alveoli that share a common opening into the duct are referred to as an alveolar sac. Capillary beds surround each alveolus, supplying blood to lung tissue. Capillary beds contain a lower concentration of oxygen (O_2) and a higher concentration of carbon dioxide (CO_2) than alveoli do. When blood flows through the capillary bed, it takes in oxygen from the alveolus, increasing the partial pressure of blood O_2, and gives up CO_2, decreasing the partial pressure of blood CO_2 (**Fig. 10.8**). This exchange is the process of **diffusion** and is discussed in greater detail later in this chapter.

Bones of Respiration

At the most superior aspect of the thoracic cavity are the sternum and clavicle. The sternum has three bony processes where muscles attach that aid in respiration: the manubrium, body, and xiphoid process. The clavicle, commonly referred to as the "collar bone," is actually two bones that extend from the manubrium and serve as attachment sites for muscles including the deltoid, trapezius, subclavius, pectoralis major, sternocleidomastoid, sternohyoid, and trapezius muscles (West 2012).

Muscles of Respiration

The diaphragm is a thick sheet of skeletal muscle and connective tissue that is positioned at the floor of the thoracic cavity, separating the thoracic cavity from the abdominal cavity. The diaphragm is the principal muscle of **inspiration**. The diaphragm separates the thoracic and abdominal cavities (**Fig. 10.9**). The diaphragm is attached posteriorly to the lumbar vertebrae of the spinal column and the lower ribs. Anteriorly it is attached to the xiphoid process of the sternum. The diaphragm is innervated by the **phrenic nerves** derived from spinal nerves C3 through C5.

Second only to the diaphragm in importance, the **external intercostal muscles** play a key role in active inspiration. Located between the ribs, the external intercostal muscles are active during inhalation, expanding the rib cage. Each of the external intercostals originates along the inferior border of

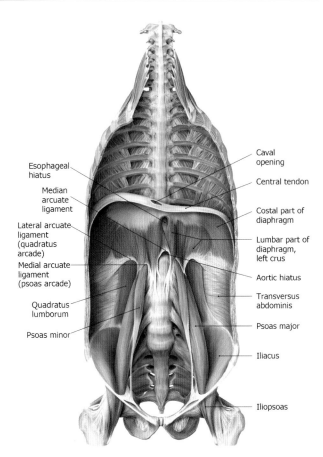

Fig. 10.9 Anterior view of the thoracic and abdominal cavities showing a coronal section of the diaphragm, positioned at the floor of the thoracic cavity and separating the thoracic and abdominal cavities

a rib and inserts into the superior border of the rib that lies just below (**Fig. 10.10**). The internal intercostal muscles are located beneath the external intercostal muscles and are active during forced exhalation, compressing the thoracic cavity. The external and internal intercostals cross in opposite directions, thereby exerting opposing forces on the thoracic cavity. Lastly, the individual muscles that form the abdominal wall are also important for respiration. This multilayered muscular structure connects to the ribs and the pelvic girdle and is active during high-effort (including cough) or sustained expiratory tasks.

Blood Vessels and Airways

Pulmonary blood vessels, much like the airways themselves, are a series of tubes, composed primarily of smooth muscle tissue, that form progressively smaller branches as they penetrate deeper into the lung (**Fig. 10.11**).

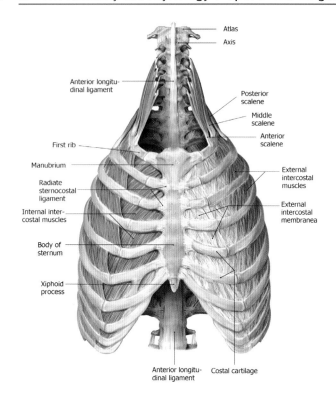

Fig. 10.10   The intercostal muscles line the rib cage. The external intercostals, when contracted, pull the rib cage up and out, expanding the thoracic cavity horizontally.

The **pulmonary artery** receives oxygen-depleted blood directly from the right side of the heart. This blood is transported down to the most **distal** regions of the lung, where the capillary beds meet the alveoli and gas exchange occurs across the exceptionally thin blood-gas barrier that these two structures form.

Functional Organization of the Respiratory System: Respiratory Physiology

The respiratory system can be subdivided into separate functional components. These components serve various respiratory and nonrespiratory functions. In this section, we will discuss tissue oxygenation as well as mechanisms for protecting the lungs including conduction/filtration and airway protection. Nonrespiratory functions, including those that give rise to voice and speech, as well as regulation of intrathoracic pressure and a variety of other functions not related to tissue oxygenation, will be presented.

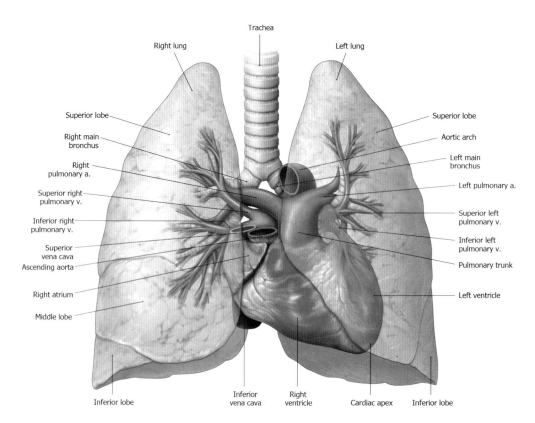

Fig. 10.11   Distribution of main pulmonary arteries and veins (anterior view).

Respiration and Tissue Oxygenation

The respiratory assembly is composed of the lungs and associated tissues (e.g., terminal bronchioles, alveolar ducts, alveolar sacs, and alveoli) that serve as the site of gas exchange between the lungs and blood to oxygenate tissues. The process of respiration involves the movement of air in response to a driving force. This force exists as a pressure gradient or differential between the pressure of the air within the lung alveoli, or alveolar pressure, and the pressure of the air in the outside environment, referred to as **atmospheric pressure**. Two distinct forces change alveolar pressure. First, displacement of respiratory structures generates passive recoil forces that, if not countered, return the affected structures to pre-displacement equilibrium. Passive forces are always present within the lungs, which tends toward collapse, and chest wall, which tends toward expansion. These forces are passive and therefore not under neural control. At rest, these opposing recoil forces are balanced through the pleural linkage of the lungs to the inner surface of the thoracic cavity (West 2012). Secondly, alveolar pressures are altered through active, contractile forces generated by respiratory muscles. Active forces are intermittently present and occur under both conscious voluntary and unconscious involuntary and automatic control (West 2012).

The ability of a structure to be displaced is referred to as **compliance**. Displacement of the lungs and chest wall changes lung volumes and pressures. These changes are illustrated by the **relaxation pressure curve** (**Fig. 10.12**). The X-axis represents pressure, typically expressed in cm H_2O or mm Hg, generated by the human airways (e.g., lungs coupled to thoracic cavity). The Y-axis represents the volume of air contained within the lungs as a percentage of vital capacity (VC), the volume of air maximally inhaled and exhaled from the lungs. The volume of air contained within the lungs at the end of tidal **expiration** with the respiratory muscles relaxed is referred to as **functional residual capacity** (FRC) (Lalley 2013). At FRC, the respiratory structures are at rest, meaning that the passive recoil forces present within the lung are balanced by those within the chest wall. Under normal conditions, the compliance of the chest wall is high, meaning that it is readily displaced and inhalation is unencumbered. At this moment of rest, the human lungs are filled to approximately 40% of total lung capacity (TLC) (Sapienza and Hoffman-Ruddy 2013). Departure from FRC progressively increases passive recoil forces in the lungs and chest wall, requiring the introduction of active muscular forces on the paired lung–chest wall unit. Specifically, as

Speech pressure curve

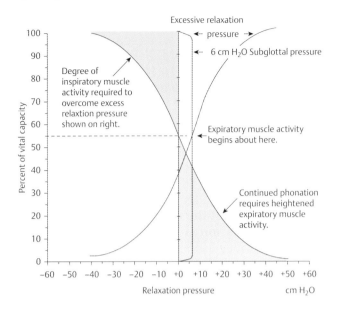

Fig. 10.12   Relaxation pressure curve.

lung volume increases above FRC, passive recoil forces in the lungs and chest wall increase, pushing the lungs and chest cavity toward collapse, and compliance decreases. Below FRC, lung volumes decrease, as do passive recoil forces that pull the lungs and chest wall toward expansion.

Active Inspiration

Lung inflation or inspiration can only occur in the presence of negative alveolar air pressure. Conversely, air flow out of the lungs or expiration requires an alveolar pressure greater than atmospheric pressure (West 2012; Hixon 1987). Volume and pressure share an inverse relationship; that is, as one increases, the other decreases when temperature is constant. This relationship is known as **Boyle's law.** Simply, when lung volume increases, alveolar pressure decreases (West 2012; Hixon 1987). Chest wall expansion increases volume of the thoracic cavity, thereby increasing the volume of the lungs coupled to the thoracic cavity via pleural linkage and lowering alveolar pressure. Principles of pressure equalization describe how air flows from regions of high partial pressure into areas of low partial pressure until pressure is equalized. The flow of air from the outside environment into the lungs is an example of this phenomenon (**Fig. 10.13**) (West 2012).

The primary muscle of inspiration is the diaphragm. At rest and prior to inspiration, the diaphragm is a domelike structure. During active inspiration, the diaphragm contracts and flattens, enlarging the thoracic cavity vertically. At the same time, the external intercostals contract and lift the ribs upward and outward, enlarging the thoracic cavity horizontally (**Fig. 10.14**; Hixon 1987).

Inspiration increases both the volume of the thoracic cavity and the recoil forces within the lungs to accommodate the inspired air. As air flows into the lungs, alveolar pressure increases, eventually exceeding atmospheric pressure. **Total lung capacity (TLC)** is the maximum volume of gas contained in the lungs and is reached following maximal inspiration (Lalley 2013). TLC is determined by the strength of the inspiratory muscles as well as elastic recoil forces within the thoracic cavity and lungs (Lalley 2013). At TLC, chest wall compliance is extremely low because the lungs are filled to maximum capacity. At TLC, elastic recoil forces within the lungs and chest wall are very high and, if unopposed by active muscular forces, the tendency of the lungs and chest wall will be to return to equi-

librium or FRC. As the body ages, the recoil forces of the thoracic cavity decrease as respiratory muscle strength decreases. However, TLC remains fairly stable with aging, as these changes in respiratory muscle strength are offset by reduced inward recoil forces of the lung secondary to elastic airway connective tissue loss (Lalley 2013).

In contrast to active inspiration, expiration can be either passive or active. At the end of inspiration, lung volume, alveolar pressure, and passive recoil forces are elevated. When the muscles of inspiration relax at the conclusion of the inspiratory cycle, these recoil forces, which are now unopposed by inspiratory muscle activity, exert influence over the lungs and chest wall to return to FRC as air is passively exhaled from the lungs (West 2012).

In contrast to passive expiration, active expiration involves expiratory muscle activity (West 2012). Active exhalation occurs when high-velocity airflows are produced (e.g., to clear the airways), when exhalation must be sustained over longer periods of time (e.g., during conversational speech or singing), or at low lung volumes, when passive recoil forces within the lungs and chest wall are high (West 2012). The principal muscles of active expiration are the abdominals and internal intercostal muscles. Contraction of the expiratory musculature reduces the volume of the thoracic cavity and maintains elevated alveolar pressures, causing air to continue to flow from the lungs into the outside environment (West 2012). When exhalation

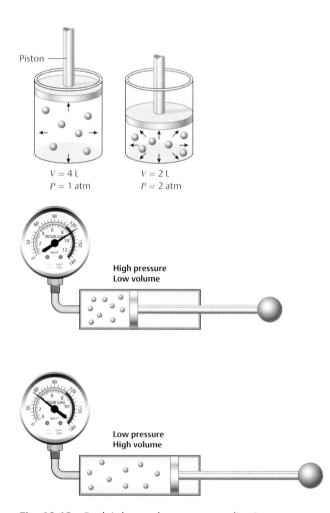

Piston

$V = 4$ L
$P = 1$ atm

$V = 2$ L
$P = 2$ atm

High pressure
Low volume

Low pressure
High volume

Fig. 10.13 Boyle's law and pressure equalization.

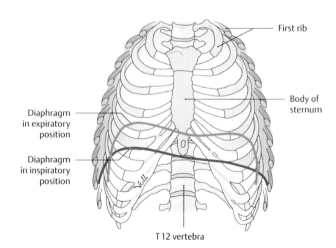

First rib

Body of sternum

Diaphragm in expiratory position

Diaphragm in inspiratory position

T 12 vertebra

Fig. 10.14 The mechanics of respiration. When the diaphragm contracts on inspiration (red line), the ribs are elevated by contraction of the external intercostal muscles. This contraction expands the thoracic cavity transversely and anteriorly. Lowering of the diaphragm causes the thoracic cavity to expand inferiorly. When the diaphragm is relaxed during expiration (blue line), the thoracic cavity contracts in all dimensions.

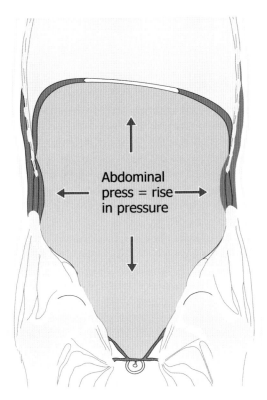

Fig. 10.15 Active expiration. The abdominal muscles are able to increase intra-abdominal pressure (increasing subglottal air pressure for speech) by reducing the volume of the abdominal cavity, compressing the viscera, which then displace superiorly, displacing the diaphragm further into the thoracic cavity and further lowering the volume of the thoracic cavity.

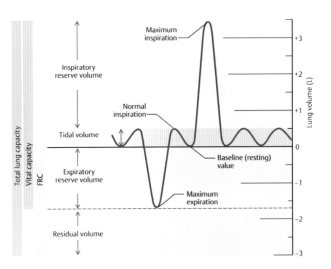

Fig. 10.16 A normal spirogram. VC = vital capacity; IC = inspiratory capacity; ERV = expiratory reserve volume; TV = tidal volume; IRV = inspiratory reserve volume.

is sustained over time, lung volumes continue to decrease as passive recoil forces increase and are increasingly opposed by the active forces of the expiratory musculature (**Fig. 10.15**; West 2012). This interplay is discussed in greater detail within the section of this chapter dealing with cough and respiration for voice and speech.

Between FRC and TLC, a number of specific lung capacities exist, with corresponding lung volumes expressed as a percentage of TLC. During quiet, or tidal, breathing, the volume of air repeatedly inhaled and exhaled is referred to as **tidal volume** (V_T). The volume of air that can be actively inhaled beyond tidal inspiration is the **inspiratory reserve volume** (IRV). The volume of air forcefully exhaled beyond tidal expiration is the **expiratory reserve volume** (ERV) (West 2012).

Following a maximal, forced expiration the lungs may feel "empty." However, a **residual volume** (RV) of air remains in the lungs that cannot be exhaled (West 2012). Two factors determine RV: the strength of expiratory muscles that oppose pas-

sive recoil forces within the chest wall at low lung volumes, and the extent to which the small airways collapse, trapping gas in alveoli during forced expiration (Lalley 2013). With advancing age and decreased expiratory muscle strength, opposition to outward chest recoil decreases, thereby increasing RV (Lalley 2013). **Vital capacity** (VC) is the maximum volume of air that can be passed in and out of the lungs. Mathematically, VC can be thought of as TLC – RV, and because RV increases with age, VC decreases with age (Lalley 2013). In addition to age-related changes, these volumes or capacities vary considerably among individuals as a result of differences in size and stature, in addition to other factors. A diagram of lung volumes and capacities is provided as **Fig. 10.16**.

At rest, the average adult will complete approximately 15 breaths per minute. An average cycle of inhalation and exhalation will move approximately 500 mL (V_T) of air in and out of the lungs. Approximately 70% of V_T reaches the terminal regions of the alveoli and is directly involved in gas exchange. This percentage of V_T can be used to determine the **alveolar ventilation rate** or the volume of air (per minute) involved in gas exchange within the respiratory zone. The remaining 30% of V_T never enters the respiratory zone and is not involved in gas exchange, remaining within the conducting structures of the upper and lower airways (West 2012).

Multiplying V_T by the number of breaths per minute yields the **minute ventilation** (MV), or volume of gas exchanged per minute of breathing. During tidal breathing in adults, MV is approximately 6 liters per minute (500 mL × 15 breaths per

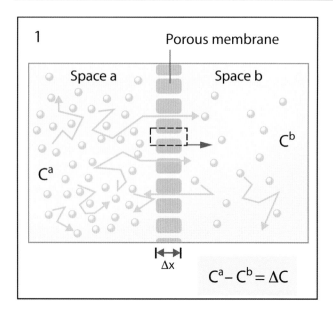

Fig. 10.17 Diffusion through a porous membrane such as the capillary bed lining the walls of the alveoli. Gases diffuse from areas of high concentration (area a; partial pressure or concentration of substance within area a denoted as C^a) to areas of low concentration (area b; partial pressure or concentration of substance within area b denoted as C^b). The rate of diffusion increases relative to the difference between C^a and C^b (expressed as delta C or ΔC).

minute=7,500 mL/min) (West 2012). Conditions that adversely impact the respiratory system typically result in lower-than-expected MV values.

Gas Exchange in Tissue

Gas exchange inside tissues is referred to as **internal respiration** because it takes place within body tissues, not the lungs or **peripheral gas exchange**. The process of O_2 moving from the lungs into the blood takes place according to principles of diffusion. Specifically, gases such as O_2 and CO_2 move from areas of high to low concentration (**Fig. 10.17**).

Blood traveling to tissues from the lungs contains relatively high concentrations of O_2 (approximately 20%) and low concentrations of CO_2. Metabolic activities within tissues consume O_2, leaving low residual concentration of O_2, and produce CO_2, so levels of CO_2 in tissues tend to be high. O_2 diffuses from the blood and into tissues, and CO_2 diffuses from tissues into blood. The volumes of O_2 and CO_2 exchanged at the junction of the capillary bed and alveoli is potentially affected by a number of factors. The magnitude of O_2 concentration in the blood or CO_2 concentration in the tissues affects diffusion; lower concentrations result in lower volumes of diffused gases. Conversely, higher concentrations pro-duce larger volumes of diffused gas. In areas of the body where blood flow is low, less diffusion occurs. When tissues are at work and maintaining high levels of metabolism (the chemical processes which convert substances obtained from the environment into energy for use in driving bodily processes), diffusion rates of O_2 and CO_2 are higher than in tissues at rest (Stickland et al 2013).

Passive diffusion of O_2 and CO_2 occurs across the union of the capillary beds and alveoli, referred to as the respiratory membrane. The exceptionally thin structure of this membrane (~ 0.5 µm) allows rapid and unimpeded gas exchange. The respiratory membrane consists of four distinct layers. O_2 transferring from the alveolus into blood first passes through the alveolar wall, the **epithelial basement membrane**, the **capillary basement membrane**, and finally the **capillary epithelium**, a single layer of cells anchored to the capillary basement membrane. Inside the capillary bed, every red blood cell makes brief physical contact with two to three alveoli and sheds CO_2 while taking in O_2 from the alveolar gas via passive diffusion (West 2012). Red blood cells contain high levels of the protein hemoglobin. Hemoglobin is important for transport of O_2 from the lungs to tissues; however, the concentration of hemoglobin within the blood and therefore the ability of the blood to transport O_2 can be affected by a number of factors such as blood pH and temperature. During normal gas exchange, hemoglobin is loaded to near-capacity (97.5%) with O_2, much more O_2 than is required by the tissues (West 2012). **Respiratory acidosis**, or reduced blood pH, is an example of one condition that can reduce the concentration of blood hemoglobin (Epstein and Singh 2001). Increased body temperature, such as during exercise, can also decrease the concentration of blood hemoglobin due to increased demand by the tissues.

Transportation of CO_2 from the Tissues to the Lungs

Once CO_2 moves from tissues into the bloodstream via diffusion, a small percentage (~ 10%) of the total CO_2 dissolves into blood plasma cells. An additional 60% of total CO_2 binds with H_2O to produce bicarbonate (HCO_3^-) ions as well as free hydrogen (H^+) ions. As these ions are transported to the lungs, their relative concentration within blood helps maintain **homeostasis** through stabilization of blood pH within an optimal, narrow range (**Fig. 10.18**; West 2012).

The remaining ~ 30% of CO_2 binds to hemoglobin, now free from O_2 following diffusion into the tissue.

CO₂ is then transported back to the lungs where it diffuses across into the alveoli and is exhaled (West 2012).

Air Conduction and Filtration

During respiration, extremely large volumes of air (typically around 10,000 liters per day) are exchanged between the body and outside environment. Air that enters the body from the outside environment can contain any number of potentially harmful substances (dust, pollen, bacteria, etc.) which, if allowed to enter the lungs, could result in injury or death. The conduction and filtra-

tion assembly consists of the nose, pharynx, larynx, trachea, bronchi, and sub-bronchial structures (e.g., bronchioles and terminal bronchioles) (West 2012). This assembly filters, moistens, and warms air from the atmosphere and directs it to the lungs. On exhalation, this assembly directs exhaled air from the lungs back into the atmosphere (West 2012).

The upper and lower airways are lined with mucosal tissue that produces mucus secretions, commonly referred to as **phlegm**. These secretions form a protective barrier between the delicate tissues of the inner airway lining and the air passing through the airway during inhalation and exhalation (Button and Button 2013). Mucus also moisturizes the inner surfaces of the upper and lower respiratory tracts. Specialized epithelial (goblet) cells and submucosal glands located within the mucosa produce mucus, which consists primarily of water, proteins, antiseptic enzymes, and non-organic salts (Button Button 2013). As air passes through the upper and lower airways, small particles of foreign matter such as pollen, dust, and bacteria become embedded within the sticky mucus and are thereby prevented from entering the distal airway (**Fig. 10.19**). The mucus, with its trapped particles, that lines the inner surfaces of the lower airways is gradually propelled upward toward the pharynx and mouth, where it is expectorated or, more commonly, swallowed. This move-

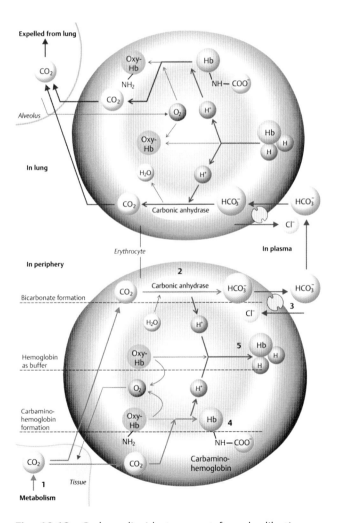

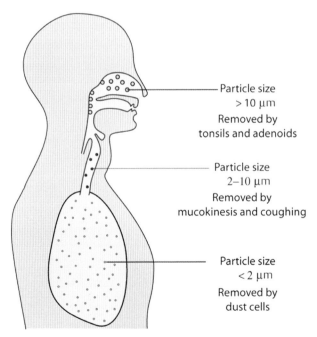

Fig. 10.18 Carbon dioxide transport from bodily tissues. CO₂ accumulates within cells as a byproduct of metabolism. (1) Upon diffusion into red blood cells CO₂ combines with water (H₂O) to form H⁺ and HCO₃[−]. (2) HCO₃[−] is removed from the red blood cell. (3) CO₂ also forms carbaminohemoglobin. (4) H⁺ ions are buffered by hemoglobin. (5) This diffusion occurs in the opposite direction in the lung, with CO₂ diffusing from the blood and into the alveoli.

Fig. 10.19 Filtration of exogenous substances by the respiratory system. Moving from the upper to lower divisions of the respiratory system, protective mechanisms exist to detect and remove progressively smaller particles.

ment is referred to as the **mucociliary escalator** and consists of the paired actions of mucus produced by goblet cells and ciliated epithelium and is yet another line of defense against foreign bodies entering the lungs (Button and Button 2013).

Production of excessive mucus is a common symptom of many diseases and is one component of a larger activation of the immune system in the presence of a pathogen. Mucus that clogs the airway or impedes breathing can be unpleasant or, in severe cases, life threatening. Normally clear in color and somewhat watery in consistency, mucus produced in response to invasion by viral or bacterial agents can be thick with altered viscosity and may vary in color from shades of yellow to dark green.

Airway Protection

The airway protection assembly protects the lungs from damage through close coordination among muscles and other structures active during swallowing and coughing (Troche et al 2014). Cough protects the lungs by removing secretions or foreign material from the airway. Cough is classically defined as a temporal sequence of inspiration, compression, and expulsion that can be thought of as either voluntary or reflexive (Bolser and Davenport 2002). A brainstem neural network generates the stereotypical cough pattern. Immediately prior to cough onset, this neural network is reconfigured to generate a cough-specific respiratory motor pattern. Evidence supporting integrated neural control of cough and breathing includes the convergence of central cough and respiratory neural networks (Bolser and Davenport 2002). This convergence further suggests that

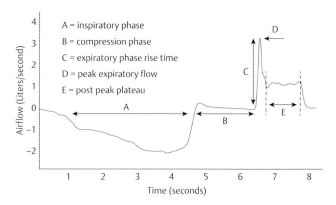

Fig. 10.20 Cough aerodynamic waveform (Kim et al 2009).

cough dysfunction can affect other airway defense mechanisms such as swallow. Cough motor pattern is a coordinated series of respiratory, laryngeal, and pharyngeal muscle activities that can be identified and characterized by electromyography of inspiratory and expiratory muscles as well as by direct sampling of airway pressures and flows (**Fig. 10.20**). In the case of reflexive cough, the cough neural network is activated by stimulation of airway afferents (Bolser and Davenport 2002). Following activation, however, various aspects of cough are mediated by the cortex (Janssens et al 2014).

The **urge-to-cough (UTC)** is a conscious perception of respiratory stimulation/sensation through neural gating of subcortical afferents into the cerebral cortex (Bolser 2010; Davenport 2008, 2009). Gating refers to the idea that the brain takes an active role in determining which stimuli are elevated to the level of conscious awareness and which are not. Although cough is typically thought of as reflexive and under brainstem control, a con-

---

Box 10.2 Cystic Fibrosis

CF is an incurable genetic disorder involving many bodily systems, including marked effects on respiratory function (Dodge 2015). Although many people carry any one of thousands of genetic mutations responsible for CF, relatively few are born with active disease. CF is an **autosomal recessive** disorder, meaning that both parents must be carriers of the same mutation. A child born as a result of such a pairing will have a one in four (25%) chance of having the disease. CF is life limiting, with most individuals succumbing to respiratory infection or failure by the third to fifth decade of life (Dodge 2015).

Individuals with CF demonstrate a wide range of symptoms from the disease. Within the lungs, the ge-

netic mutation present in CF causes the lungs to produce abnormally thick or viscous mucus (Dodge 2015). Normally, mucus production and movement protects the lungs through removal of foreign substances or pathogens. In CF, mucus accumulates in the lungs to the point where mucociliary clearance is drastically reduced, resulting in infection and inflammation. Individuals with CF suffer from frequent, severe respiratory infections, worsening over time. No cure for CF has been developed, so medical management is primarily directed to managing symptoms of the disease. Future efforts toward genetic manipulation may allow for the replacement of the damaged portion of the gene responsible for CF, preventing the development of the disease from the earliest of stages (Dodge 2015).

sciously perceived UTC precedes the cough motor response, enabling behavioral adaptation of cough, including conscious suppression, according to specific circumstances (Hegland et al 2011). Anecdotally, one can imagine many situations where cough cannot be suppressed, so it is instead modified. Movie theaters or auditoriums are settings where a loud, explosive cough would be socially inappropriate. Other times, the situation and not the setting determine cough modification. Most people have experienced the unpleasant sensation of having to cough during a ceremony, movie, or performance. In settings and situations such as these, people decrease the intensity or loudness of cough, if cough cannot be suppressed. These types of modifications are examples of cortical regulation and modification of "reflexive" or "stimulus-evoked" cough. Areas reported to be active during UTC include discriminative and affective brain areas including the somatosensory cortices, anterior cingulate gyrus, amygdala, orbitofrontal cortex, supplementary motor area, cerebellum, and insular cortex (Dicpinigaitis et al 2012). The significant role of the cerebral cortex in the control of voluntary and stimulus-evoked cough has been demonstrated empirically in healthy human participants via functional magnetic resonance imaging (fMRI) studies as well as via study of cough in patients with neurologic disease, including stroke and Parkinson disease. UTC varies in a dose-dependent manner in accordance with the intensity of cough trigger, with stronger stimuli evoking a stronger UTC. The UTC threshold is critical for airway clearance. Increased UTC threshold results in seeding of the airways with micro-aspirates including foreign matter. Frequently, this seeding leads directly to the development of a lung infection (**Fig. 10.21**).

UTC is also a **homeostatic emotion** (Bolser 2010; Davenport 2008, 2009). This term refers to subjective, affective ("emotional") experiences related to temperature, itch, visceral distension (e.g., of bladder, stomach, rectum, or esophagus), muscle ache, hunger, thirst, breathlessness or dyspnea, and sensual touch. Homeostatic emotion is important because it functions under two key principles: (1) whenever homeostasis of the body is threatened, the brain is informed that local regulation mechanisms may not be sufficient, and (2) producing an affective-motivational drive to carry out homeostatic behavior (Bolser 2010; Davenport 2008, 2009). The latter aspect warrants the use of the term "emotion" because sensations signaling a need are typically experienced as unpleasant and aversive, providing the drive for action. When this action satisfies the perceived need, a pleasing sensation of relief or satisfaction is experienced.

Clinical and experimental findings indicate an intrinsic and reciprocal relationship between anxiety and respiration (Van den Bergh et al 2012). Dyspnea is accompanied by fear and anxiety (De Peuter et al 2004). It is a defining symptom of panic attacks and occurs in healthy persons with high levels of negative emotions. Fear augments respiratory drive and can trigger hyperventilation, a process in which fear and dyspnea maintain one another. Emotional states of fear and anxiety are defense system activations capable of modulating the perception of dyspnea (De Peuter et al 2004). Although the terms "fear" and "anxiety" are often used interchangeably, they represent functionally distinct states. Fear is an immediate alarm reaction to a specific, imminent threat, characterized by escape impulses that mobilize for action and result in a surge of sympathetic activation and attentional narrowing

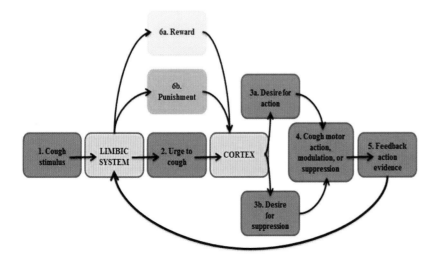

Fig. 10.21 The urge-to-cough: inputs from cortical and subcortical structures (Bolser 2010; Davenport 2008, 2009).

Box 10.3   Aging and Cough

Aging and age-related diseases (e.g., stroke, neurodegenerative conditions), are associated with skeletal muscle atrophy or sarcopenia (Wang and Bai 2012). Sarcopenic changes in muscle composition after the age of 50 include, on average, decreases of between 25% and 30% in total muscle mass, with functional decreases in strength and capacity as early as age 30. These changes comprise more than simple atrophy of fibers; they reflect a loss of fibers (Wang and Bai 2012). Additionally, age-related shifts in the relative percentage of different fiber types is observed. Initially, decreases in fibers responsible for the generation of large-magnitude force (type II) are observed, followed by decreases in fatigue-resistant (type I) fibers (Wang and Bai 2012). Changes to the lungs themselves include loss of elastin fibers within the bronchioles and widening of the alveoli (Lalley 2013; Rabello et al 1996). Reduced total capillary surface area within the lungs is associated with reduced efficiency of gas exchange (Lalley 2013). In addition to neuromuscular changes, the ability of the chest wall to expand decreases with age as a consequence of calcification of the vertebrae and rib cage, narrowing of intervertebral disk spaces, and onset of osteoporosis (Janssens et al 1999).

Age-related reductions in force-generating capacities within respiratory musculature, coupled with reduced chest wall compliance, frequently translates into reduced maximal inspiratory and expiratory pressures in the elderly (Wijesinghe and Dow 2006). These changes lead to increased susceptibility to fatigue and decreased cough strength and effectiveness (Ebihara et al 2012). Disruption of the cough motor pattern is known as dystussia. Reduced expiratory muscle strength associated with age typically results in reduced expiratory pressures and subglottal pressure (Ebihara et al 2012). Reduced glottal closure is commonly observed in the elderly. Incomplete glottal closure prior to the expulsive phase of cough will result in positive compression-phase airflow leak (**Box Fig. 10.2**), a common symptom of dystussia in elderly individuals. Decreased peak expiratory airflow and mean expiratory plateau-phase airflow are also characteristic of dystussia in the elderly (Ebihara et al 2012). Incomplete glottal closure and the resultant positive compression-phase airflow leak further reduces subglottal pressure, effectively slowing cough airflow acceleration and reducing peak flow rates during the expulsive phase of cough. These alternations to the cough motor pattern reduce the "shearing" effect of cough, weakening cough, and inhibiting forces of airway clearance (Ebihara et al 2012).

Lung infections are the sixth leading cause of death among Americans and Europeans. Although lung infections can occur at any age, there are a number of age-related risk factors. Consequently, lung infections are most frequently observed in adults aged 65 and older, with exponential increases in the very elderly. Lung infection-related deaths are among the top 15 causes of mortality in the United States. As recently as 2010, chronic lower respiratory diseases were third, influenza and pneumonia were ninth, and pneumonitis due to aspiration of solids and liquids was fifteenth. Death rates secondary to pneumonia or chronic lower respiratory disease also increase exponentially with age, in direct relationship to increases in lung infections. Continued efforts to understand the etiologies, and strategies for prevention, of lung infections in the elderly will decrease disease-related morbidity and mortality. Symptoms of dystussia, coupled with age-related declines in immune function, place elderly individuals, and particularly the frail elderly, at exceptionally high risk for lung infections and resultant death.

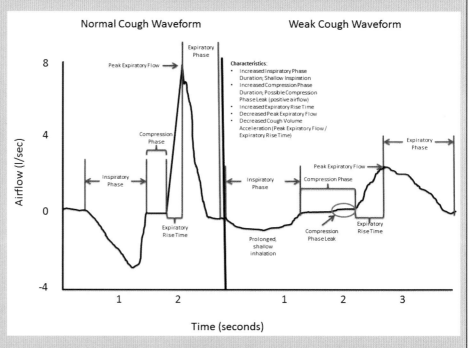

Box Fig. 10.2 Normal versus weakened cough. Note the changes in slope of inhalation and expulsion. Loss of air during the compression phase is also characteristic of weak cough.

Box 10.4 Pulmonary Nontuberculous Mycobacteria Infections in the Elderly, or Lady Windermere Syndrome

Pulmonary infection with nontuberculous mycobacteria (pNTM) is a well-recognized and well-characterized cause of chronic pulmonary infection. Rates of pulmonary infection with NTM are increasing throughout all regions within the United States as well as in specific international regions including Toronto, Ontario, and Queensland, Australia (Kahn et al 2007; Marras et al 2003). A recent examination of 2.3 million Medicare beneficiaries enrolled between 1997 and 2007 revealed that the prevalence of pNTM is increasing significantly across all regions of the United States with point prevalence estimates of cases per 100,000 individuals (Cassidy et al 2009). Although pNTM is increasing among both men and women, the incidence of pNTM disease has shifted from middle-aged men with COPD and cavitary lung disease to thin, elderly white women with bronchiectasis and nodular lung disease. Consequently, the disease has been dubbed "Lady Windermere's syndrome" after the fictitious Lady Windermere, a character in the Oscar Wilde play *Lady Windermere's Fan*, published in 1893 (Iseman 1996; Kasthoori et al 2008). In the play, Lady Windermere represents the proper Victorian-era woman, and the term is meant to evoke the idea that elderly women with pNTM infections have these infections because they purposefully suppress expectoration and coughing out of fear of attracting unwanted attention. It is unknown whether Lady Windermere's syndrome exists as a manifestation of this social behavior or as a consequence of weakness and deficient airway protection (Kim et al 2008; Billinger et al 2009).

Risk of hospitalization from pNTM is greater among women and increases exponentially with age. The biological mechanisms underlying the epidemiology of pNTM disease are unknown. Within the United States, those infected with pNTM are overwhelmingly white females who typically demonstrate no immune deficiencies and have low body mass index (BMI). Characteristic symptoms are fatigue, cough, and production of mucopurulent sputum. Elderly women with pNTM disease have generally been thin most of their lives and often report additional weight loss associated with the pulmonary infection. Low BMI is also a risk factor for tuberculosis (TB), a more severe pulmonary infection caused by the more virulent *Mycobacterium tuberculosis*. Malnutrition is a risk factor common to both TB and NTM and is associated with poor immune responses to these mycobacteria. Of note, protein and calorie malnutrition is also associated with sarcopenia.

Treatment of pNTM often requires at least three antibiotic medications for at least 12 to 18 months, and toxicity from these medications is common. For many, pNTM is incurable and relapse of disease due to reinfection with new isolates is common, suggesting a limited role for acquired immune responses. However, these reinfections might be preventable if modifiable risk factors can be identified and addressed. Elderly women with pNTM are often functionally limited due to their recurrent pulmonary disease. Other patient groups at risk for NTM infection include those with COPD, primary ciliary dyskinesia, or CF. Each of these conditions is associated with poor airway clearance, suggesting that inability to clear secretions from the lungs is, at the very least, one mechanism in the pathophysiology of NTM infections. The increasing prevalence of pNTM bears a direct, positive correlation to measures of clinical burden in this population. A recent investigation sought to assess costs associated with NTM disease treatment and to identify risk factors associated with increased costs. Patients with pNTM infections demonstrated increased use of antibiotic medications, with a median of five (range 1–10) antibiotics. Adverse treatment effects were observed in up to 50% of those prescribed common antibiotics and up to 100% with uncommonly used antibiotics. Treatment costs for pNTM infections are comparable to those found with other chronic infectious diseases such as HIV/AIDS.

---

towards the threat. Anxiety is a future-oriented, apprehensive state to a range of potential, uncertain threats, characterized by free-floating attentional vigilance (De Peuter et al 2014). Although no research has directly compared the influence of fear to that of anxiety on UTC, a review of the literature suggests UTC may be an important factor governing cough behavior (Bolser 2010; Davenport 2008, 2009). Disordered cough, or **dystussia**, and its associated physical and psychologic symptoms are crucial predictors of increased vulnerability to lung infection. The relationship between breathing, dystussia, and the emergence of lung infections are not fully understood. Furthermore, the extent to which these deficits represent a manifestation of disordered sensory afferents, impaired sensory-motor integration, or disrupted motor capacity is also unknown.

If foreign particles in inhaled air produce a cough stimulus that surpasses the cough sensory threshold, a cough response consisting of a gated sequence of stereotypical motor behaviors is elicited. Initial inspiration serves to increase lung volume. Next, the vocal folds adduct, closing the glottis and so halting transglottal airflow, referred to as the compression phase. During the compression phase, subglottic pressure, which is essential for high-velocity cough expiratory airflow, increases. The glottis then opens rapidly at the onset of the cough expiratory phase. This opening is characterized by transient, high-velocity peak airflow which creates shearing and turbulence within the airways. Following peak expiratory airflow, sustained expiratory airflow then perpetuates forces of airway clearance (Hegland et al 2013).

Functional Organization of the Respiratory System: Nonrespiratory Physiology

Voicing and Speech

The voice and speech mechanism includes the lungs, larynx, pharynx, nose, and oral structures including the lips, teeth, and tongue as well as hard and soft palate. This assembly interacts with air exhaled from the lungs, transforming it to produce a dynamic acoustic waveform used for human vocalization and communication. As with nonspeech respiration, breathing for speech requires that alveolar pressure be lower than atmospheric pressure for inhalation. Speech and nonspeech respiration differ both in regard to the goal of each process and the manner in which respiratory structures operate in order to accomplish the respective goals.

The previously described active and passive forces that control nonspeech respiration also control the specialized demands of voice and speech tasks and require additional, active (muscular) control over both inhalation and exhalation. Speech production variations, such as changes in pitch or loudness, production of voiced versus voiceless phonemes, or sustaining phonation over time, require active modification of respiratory forces. In particular, voicing at high or low lung capacities requires specialized recruitment of muscle groups in order to oppose the high recoil forces present at either extreme of the relaxation-pressure curve.

Inhalation in anticipation of voicing may differ markedly from inhalation for tidal breathing because of the need to create, and sustain, appropriate **subglottal air pressure** for voicing (Sapienza and Roddy 2013). Subglottal air pressure is the partial pressure of exhaled air beneath a closed glottis. The minimum amount of subglottal air pressure required to initiate vocal fold vibration is referred to as the **phonation threshold pressure** (PTP) (Hixon 1987). Average PTP for healthy adults without vocal pathology is approximately 2 cm H_2O (Jiang

et al 1999). Once sufficient pressure is generated to meet PTP and vocal fold vibration is initiated, control over subglottal pressure is necessary to control pitch and loudness.

Once sufficient subglottal pressure is generated to meet or exceed PTP and vocal fold vibration begins, the frequency of vibration (cycles per second or Hz) determines the perceptual quality of pitch, referred to as **fundamental frequency** (F_0) and can vary relative to a multitude of intrinsic (e.g. sex, age, hormonal factors, etc.) and extrinsic/environmental factors. Beyond F_0, pitch can be altered across a relatively wide range via two main mechanisms. The first involves lengthening of the vocal folds. In addition, pitch can also be altered via changes to subglottal pressure. Increasing subglottal pressure increases the vibratory frequency of the vocal folds, perceptually increasing pitch.

The **amplitude** of vocal fold vibration, measured in decibels (dB), quantifies the level of acoustic power produced during vocal fold vibration and corresponds to the perceptual quality of loudness. As with frequency, the amplitude of vocal fold vibration can be altered through changes in subglottal pressure. Subglottal pressure during conversation at "typical" loudness levels is around 7 to 10 cm H_2O (Sapienza and Ruddy 2013). The production of progressively louder voice requires correspondingly progressive increases in subglottal pressure.

Increasing subglottal pressure requires inhaling to a higher lung volume (Hixon 1987) requiring activation of the muscles of inhalation to overcome passive recoil forces present in the lungs and chest wall, expanding these structures to accommodate higher lung volume (Sapienza and Ruddy 2013). Following inhalation, the vocal folds adduct, closing off the upper and lower airways in order to generate sufficient levels of subglottal pressure prior to initiation of vocal fold vibration. At high lung volumes, this vibration is initiated under correspondingly high passive recoil forces present within the lungs and chest wall (Hixon 1987). If left unopposed, these high recoil forces will cause rapid loss of lung air volume via passive exhalation as recoil forces influence the thoracic cavity to rapidly return to its resting state. During sustained voicing, this loss of thoracic volume and resultant loss of lung volume are prevented through continued activation of the muscles of inhalation during the initial, high-lung-volume phase of exhalation (Hixon 1987). This activation of the inspiratory muscles is an example of the application of active (muscular) forces to overcome passive recoil forces within the respiratory system.

As exhalation continues and lung volumes decline and approach FRC, passive recoil forces attenuate as the lungs and chest wall move progressively closer to a state of equilibrium (Hixon 1987). However, just as active, muscular forces were required at high lung volumes to counter the tendency of the thoracic cavity to lose volume and return to its resting state, maintaining or exceeding PTP at low lung volumes necessitates recruitment of expiratory musculature to compress the thoracic cavity and increase subglottal pressure (Hixon 1987). When exhalation continues at lung volumes below FRC, these passive recoil forces increase as the lungs and chest wall are displaced from FRC, their point of equilibrium, in the direction of expansion (Hixon 1987). Increasing passive recoil forces at low lung volumes require similar increases in active, muscular forces from the expiratory muscles if exhalation is to continue to overcome the passive recoil forces.

Respiratory muscle strength can decrease as a result of age, disuse, or deconditioning or as a consequence of neuromuscular disease. However, because these muscles are composed of skeletal muscle tissue, they are also capable of increasing force-generating capacity in response to principles of muscular strength training. Respiratory muscle strength training (RMST) consists of the process of increasing the contractile forces within inspiratory (**inspiratory muscle strength training**, or **IMST**) or expiratory (**expiratory muscle strength training** or **EMST**) muscles (Sapienza 2008).

Intrathoracic Pressure Regulation

The assembly that regulates intrathoracic pressure includes the larynx and vocal folds and lungs. During exhalation, the vocal folds close tightly, temporarily closing off air flow between the upper and lower respiratory tracts. With continued exhalation against a closed glottis, intra-abdominal pressure (IAP) increases (West 2012). High IAP stabilizes the thoracic cavity and spine during high-effort tasks such as lifting, coughing, defecation, or childbirth (Hackett and Chow 2013). These pressures are maintained over the duration of the high-effort task, providing a stable base against which the upper and lower extremities can move, assisting in the support of heavy loads and helping protect the lower back from damage (Hackett and Chow 2013).

Other Nonrespiratory Functions

Immunoprotection

The lungs are the first point of contact for inhaled pathogens and particles and are therefore a crucial site for the staging of immunologic defense responses. In addition to the nonspecific defense mechanisms present within the respiratory system such as the mucociliary escalator, antimicrobial substances, structural barriers, and alveolar macrophages, specific **immunologic defense mechanisms** exist (Joseph et al 2013; Nicod 1999). Whereas nonspecific mechanisms react in a uniform manner to a wide range of respiratory system penetrants, immunologic defense mechanisms are more specific and develop in response to exposure to specific pathogenic stimuli. Exposures that result in the development of immunologic defense mechanisms occur over the course of development, either naturally (e.g., contracting a viral disease, placental transfer of immunity to certain pathogens from mother to child) or artificially (e.g., vaccination). Immunologic defense mechanisms are a form of acquired immunity, characterized by the body's ability to recognize and respond to antigens produced by a pathogen (Nicod 1999). Antigens activate an immune response, causing the release of antibodies (Nicod 1999).

At birth, very few antibodies are produced and released. Consequently, newborn babies are highly dependent on antibodies transferred from their mothers for the first few weeks of life outside the womb. Beginning shortly after birth, the body is exposed to a wide range of pathogens, dramatically increasing the rate at which antibodies are created. This rapid synthesis of antibodies continues at a high rate until early adulthood, where it slows to a rate that is perpetuated over the remainder of the lifetime (Nicod 1999).

Specific immunologic defenses within the lungs are activated to resolve threats posed by invading pathogens and minimizing damage and inflammation to lung tissue (Nicod 1999). Invading pathogens are detected by receptors on the respiratory epithelium, subsequently stimulating the release of antimicrobial substances or the production of **cytokines**, small proteins that affect cellular activity and are used for signaling (Nicod 1999). In the case of immunologic defense mechanisms within the lungs, these cytokines signal for the release of **T cells**, white blood cells that destroy pathogens through a complex series of coordinated actions (Nicod 1999).

Circulatory System Filtration

The extremely small diameter of pulmonary capillaries (~ 7 µm) filters blood-borne substances from systemic circulation. Pulmonary capillaries protect pulmonary circulation by destroying blood clots. Inside the capillary, a component of blood plasma is

Box 10.5   Respiratory Muscle Strength Training

Respiratory muscle strength training (RMST) is a family of therapies that focus on increasing the force-generating capacity of muscles that are active during inspiration or expiration through targeted exercise protocols that exploit the ability of these muscles to undergo specific transformations in response to exercise stimulation (Sapienza 2008).

When a skeletal muscle is "loaded," or forced to generate contractile forces above and beyond those generated during "typical use," a number of adaptations occur over time. Early adaptations, or those that occur immediately following the initiation and repetition of an exercise, are behavioral in nature (MacDougall et al 1980). With practice, the muscles involved in executing a particular task display increased coordination and efficiency. Within several weeks, if the exercise is repeated regularly, changes to the structure of the muscle occur. These changes include muscle fiber growth, or **hypertrophy**, as well as shifts in the relative concentration of type I versus type II fibers in the muscle itself (MacDougall et al 1980). Generally speaking, as a muscle increases its force-generating properties, there is a shift toward greater numbers of fatigue-resistant type I fibers. If the exercise is continued over time, changes may also be observed at the neuronal level, including **synaptogenesis**, or the formation of new synapses between neurons, as well as increased dendritic branching (Sale 1988). Whereas rapid increases in force-generating capacity (or "strength") of the muscle are typically evidenced during the early stages of beginning an exercise protocol, these gains tend over time to plateau or continue to increase at a slower rate. Unfortunately, once the exercise is discontinued, following a brief period of maintenance that can last anywhere from 5 to 31 weeks, each of the processes described previously reverses. This reversal is referred to as a **detraining effect** and culminates with the muscle returning to its previous level of force-generating capacity, loss of synapses and dendrites, atrophy, and shifts in muscle fiber composition back toward more fatigable type II fibers (MacDougall et al 1980).

RMST protocols target the muscles of inspiration (primarily the diaphragm and external intercostals), muscles of expiration (primarily the abdominals and internal intercostals), or both, and may be referred to as IMST, EMST, or **inspiratory-expiratory muscle strength training (IMST-EMST)** (Sapienza 2008). These protocols are generally carried out through use of a handheld exercise device or "trainer." Available RMST devices operate under principles of resistive or pressure threshold training and are widely available commercially without a prescription (Sapienza 2008; Sapienza and Wheeler 2006).

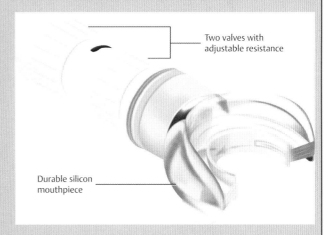

Two valves with adjustable resistance

Durable silicon mouthpiece

Box Fig. 10.3   RMST, resistive trainer example.

Resistive trainers train inspiration, and all operate under a similar principle of airflow resistance. Individuals are instructed to inhale through the device multiple times per day; typical IMST protocols involve five sets of five inhalations per day, repeated three to five days per week. Airway resistance is the opposition to flow caused by friction (West 2012). Strength increases are attained through progressively increasing resistance to airflow through the device, causing muscles of inspiration to generate increased contractile forces in order to overcome this resistance (**Box Fig. 10.3**). Resistive trainers all feature a range of orifices or openings, from wide diameter to small diameter, through which air must pass as it is inhaled (Sapienza 2008). As training progresses, resistance to inhalation is increased through use of progressively smaller and smaller orifices. To understand this progression better, imagine the difficulty of breathing (with your nose plugged) through a wide-diameter straw. Now contrast that with inhaling through a cocktail straw. The cocktail straw provides much more resistance to airflow due to its narrow diameter. One consideration when using resistive trainers is that the diameter of the orifice is not the only factor involved in establishing target resistance to inhalation. Two additional factors—the viscosity of the gas that is flowing and the nature of the flow (smooth or laminar or fast and turbulent)—are critical to determine resistance to flow according to **Poiseuille's law,**

$$R = 8l\eta/\pi r^4$$

where l = length of the tube (in this case, the trainer), η = the viscosity of the gas (in this case air) being passed, and r = the radius of the tube (West 2012). Given that the viscosity of the gas (air) is invariable, we can effectively ignore that variable when determining resistance. However, the third factor, reflective of the nature of the airflow, cannot be ignored. Faster rates of airflow through a closed structure will produce higher turbulence with correspondingly increased resistance (West 2012). Conversely, slowing the rate of airflow through a closed structure decreases turbulence and decreases resistance (West 2012). From a clinical standpoint, to apply a consistent resistance to airflow through a resistive trainer, the rate at which the individual must inhale must be kept constant across repetitions (Sapienza 2008). Consciously or subconsciously altering inhalation rate to lessen resistance will effectively reduce the load placed on the muscles of inspiration, potentially reducing the strengthening effect of the exercise (Sapienza 2008).

In contrast to resistive trainers, pressure threshold trainers (**Box Fig. 10.4**) train either inspiration or expiration. As with resistive training, during pressure threshold training the individual being trained is instructed to inhale or exhale through the pressure threshold device multiple times daily (Sapienza 2008). Also as with resistive training, most pressure threshold training protocols require inhalations or exhalations to be repeated over five sets of five inhalations per day, repeated three to five days per week. Unlike resistive trainers, however, the load imposed on target muscles by the pressure threshold trainer is independent of flow rate through the device (Sapienza 2008). Pressure threshold trainers feature a calibrated internal spring attached to a one-way valve. Shortening or elongating the spring increases or decreases the pressure that is applied to the one-way valve, holding it closed (Sapienza 2008). To open the valve and pass air through the device, individuals must inhale or exhale with sufficient pressure to exceed the pressure setting of the internal spring. Inspiratory rate is irrelevant; the magnitude of air pressure generated is the critical variable. This feature may improve training outcomes during RMST, as it provides a consistent, externally imposed load on the muscles being trained (Sapienza 2008).

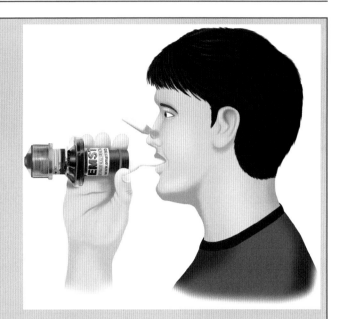

Box Fig. 10.4 RMST, pressure threshold trainer example.

IMST increases the force-generating properties of the diaphragm and external intercostals and, therefore, is frequently applied when the clinical concern revolves around adequate ventilation or overcoming upper airway resistance typically brought about through narrowing or obstruction of upper airway structures (Sapienza 2008). EMST increases the force-generating properties of the abdominal muscles and internal intercostals and may, therefore, be indicated when the clinical concern is increasing airway clearance, cough strength, or vocal loudness (Sapienza 2008). Additional evidence suggests that EMST may exert a positive effect on the pharyngeal phase of swallowing by increasing the force-generating capacity of the submental muscle group, an assembly of muscles that anchor the hyolaryngeal complex to the lower jaw and tongue and are important for displacing the laryngeal complex and airway closure during the pharyngeal phase of swallowing (Laciuga et al 2014). Additional, anecdotal evidence suggests that EMST may reduce or eliminate snoring, although the exact mechanism underlying this outcome is not yet understood.

converted into **fibrinolysin**, an enzyme that breaks down **fibrin**, an insoluble protein found in blood clots. **Heparin**, an anticoagulant frequently used in medical settings to prevent the formation of blood clots, occurs naturally in the lung, where it breaks down small emboli as they occur. Conversely, in the case of unwanted blood loss, the lungs produce **thromboplastin**, which promotes blood coagulation (Joseph et al 2013).

Pharmacokinetics

Various drugs are removed from the body through the lungs; that is, the lungs serve a critical nonrespiratory pharmacokinetic (from Greek *pharmakon*, drug, and *kinesis*, movement or motion) function. **Pulmonary extraction** is the process of removing drugs from the systemic circulation through the lungs. By removing chemicals from the body, the lungs act as a buffer, preventing sudden systemic increases in drugs administered intravenously. In some cases, the lungs metabolize or chemically transform drugs that are administered via inhalation (Joseph et al 2013). The lungs also serve as a binding site, holding onto the drug before releasing it back into circulation. Pulmonary extraction takes place primarily within the endothelial cells lining the delicate capillary bed that surrounds the alveoli. The endothelium demonstrates high levels of metabolic activity and is capable of breaking down chemical material. Pulmonary extraction can metabolize only small amounts of drugs at a time (Joseph et al 2013).

This capacity for pulmonary extraction can be both beneficial and harmful. One example of the benefits of pulmonary extraction or uptake is the binding of intravenous drugs to pulmonary endothelium, buffering the release of these drugs into the general circulation. Pulmonary extraction can have adverse effects when excessive amounts of certain drugs accumulate within the epithelium, increasing the likelihood of dangerous toxicity (Joseph et al 2013).

Respiratory administration via inhalation, rather than intravenous administration, of drugs has the advantage of enabling the drug to enter the systemic circulation quickly. To avoid toxic accumulations, the drug may be administered as a **prodrug**, an inactive compound chemically transformed into an active drug inside the body. Steroids are occasionally administered this way to minimize potential adverse side effects. Other drugs take advantage of the transformative properties of the lungs through direct delivery, via inhalation, to the therapeutic target within the lung (Joseph et al 2013).

Uptake and Transformation of Endogenous and Exogenous Substances

Along with the heart, the lungs are the place through which all blood contained within the human body must circulate, and they metabolize a wide range of substances contained within the blood. **Vasoactive** substances regulate blood pressure by altering vascular tone along a continuum from vasodilation (widening of blood vessels, which lowers blood pressure) to vasoconstriction (narrowing of blood vessels, which causes blood pressure to rise). Many of these substances are either partially inactivated or completely removed from systemic circulation by the lungs. The lungs also regulate blood pressure by converting angiotension I to angiotension II, described in the next section (Joseph et al 2013).

Homeostasis and Blood Pressure

Systemic blood pressure that is neither too high (hypertension) nor too low (hypotension) is maintained through a complex hormonal network referred to as the **renin–angiotensin–aldosterone system (RAAS)** (Kuba et al 2006). The human body increases systemic blood pressure through any combination of the following events: (1) vasoconstriction, (2) increasing the volume of blood that is circulating within the body, or (3) a combination of vasoconstriction and increased blood volume. When low blood pressure threatens homeostasis, **baroreceptors** (*baro-* = pressure) inside the blood vessels and kidneys are activated. This activation stimulates the release of **renin**, an enzyme that acts as a catalyst for the transformation of the inert precursor protein angiotensinogen, manufactured by the liver, to angiotensin I (Kuba et al 2006). When angiotensin I reaches the lungs, it interacts with an enzyme called angiotensin-converting enzyme (ACE) and becomes the powerful hormone angiotensin II (Kuba et al 2006). Angiotensin II enters the systemic circulation, where it exerts widespread effects over numerous systems including the cardiovascular (by inducing vasoconstriction), nervous (by increasing thirst and desire for salt, which will cause water retention and increase blood volume), adrenal (by stimulating production of aldosterone), and renal (where aldosterone causes the kidneys to retain sodium and release potassium); all these effects contribute to raising blood pressure (Kuba et al 2006).

Homeostasis and Blood Reserves

The highly vascularized tissue of the lung is extremely compliant and therefore is able to accommodate large volumes of blood returning via the venous system (Fishman 1966). Changes in activity, posture, or overall blood volume can increase the volume of blood returning to the lungs. At resting heart rate, the pulmonary vasculature is not fully perfused with blood. However, when heart rate increases, as during exercise, perfusion increases and additional regions of pulmonary vasculature receive incoming blood (Fishman 1966). This process is referred to as **pulmonary recruitment** and by taking on greater volumes of blood, the lungs help prevent a "back loading" of blood that could produce dangerous increases in pulmonary arterial pressures. The pulmonary vasculature is composed of extremely thin tissues that are able to stretch and deform. This process is called **pulmonary distention**, and, in combination with pulmonary recruitment, enables the lung to handle blood volumes between 500 and 1,000 milliliters.

The lungs also serve as a reservoir for blood (Fishman 1966). Activation of the autonomic nervous system ("fight or flight" or "rest and digest") influences how much blood is stored within the pulmonary vasculature. During sympathetic ("fight or flight") activation, both heart and respiratory rate increase, increasing the volume of pulmonary blood. Forceful inhalation also causes blood to leave the systemic circulation and enter the lungs (Fishman 1966). Parasympathetic ("rest and digest") activation has the opposite effect, causing blood to leave the lungs and enter the systemic circulation. Changes in posture or body position, as well as increases in IAP, can cause several hundred milliliters of blood to flow out of the lungs, back into systemic circulation (Fishman1966).

Homeostasis and O_2 Reserves

Homeostasis is maintained through a balanced exchange of O_2 and CO_2 between the blood and tissues. Low concentrations of O_2 in the blood produce a condition known as **hypoxia** (or hypoxemia) (Piper and Yee 2014). Hypoxia can be extremely dangerous because, in most cases, it only takes a matter of minutes to cause serious or permanent injury. Hypoxia is a common symptom of restrictive or obstructive lung disease, poisoning, use of medicines that suppress respiration, strangulation or choking, suffocation, heart dysfunction (insufficient pumping of blood), and anemia (insufficient number of red blood cells) (Piper and Yee 2014). Individuals who experience hypoxia frequently display changes in complexion, sometimes becoming very pale, blue in the face, or even flushed; dyspnea; heavy or rapid breathing; confusion; wheezing or stridor; and excessive coughing (Piper and Yee 2014). Prolonged coughing can actually exacerbate hypoxia by increasing systemic consumption of O_2. Any individual displaying signs or symptoms of hypoxia should receive prompt medical attention, and in instances where likelihood of hypoxia is increased (e.g., prior to administration of anesthesia for surgery), pure oxygen is provided to the patient (Bateman and Leach 1998). This treatment allows higher than normal (100% versus 20%) concentrations of O_2 to enter the systemic circulation, eventually reaching tissues where it is needed, provided the heart continued to beat, circulating blood (Bateman and Leach 1998).

A number of mechanisms assist the body in preventing hypoxia and maintaining stable levels of O_2 within tissues. Low levels of O_2 within the systemic circulation are detected by sensory receptors in the kidneys, which then excrete the hormone **erythropoietin**, which increases production of hemoglobin-containing red blood cells within bone marrow, yielding increased total blood volume and, therefore, more capacity to deliver O_2 to tissues (Souma et al 2015).

Hemoglobin is one of two proteins that bind and transport O_2 molecules; the other is myoglobin, discussed in the next paragraph (West 2012). The hemoglobin protein is contained within all red blood cells. As previously discussed, O_2 from inhaled air diffuses across alveolar and capillary walls in the lungs, binds hemoglobin, and is returned through the pulmonary venous system to the heart, which pumps it out to the rest of the body, where it diffuses from the blood into tissue (West 2012). Hemoglobin is capable of carrying extremely high concentrations of O_2 from the lungs. The immediate need for more O_2, such as when beginning a vigorous physical activity, is detected by specialized sensors located in the carotid artery and aorta. These sensors then activate respiratory centers within the central nervous system, increasing respiratory rate, thereby increasing the rate of delivery of O_2 to the blood, and more hemoglobin molecules loaded with O_2 are delivered to tissues where it is needed (West 2012).

Myoglobin (*myo-*, muscle) is a protein present in aerobic (oxygen-consuming) muscle tissue and serves as an additional binding site for O_2 and additional O_2 reserve within muscle tissue (West 2012). When a muscle contracts, O_2 is consumed to produce of cellular energy (in the form of ATP). Myoglobin proteins release small amounts of O_2 in order to increase the concentration of intracellular O_2 and assist with the maintenance of homeostasis at the cellular level (Kamga et al 2012).

If these mechanisms fail and reduced levels of blood O_2 persist for extended periods of time, capillary beds can expand to cover a greater surface area, producing more potential sites for diffusion of O_2 from the blood into the tissue (West 2012). In addition to individuals with chronically low concentrations of blood O_2 secondary to conditions such as cardiovascular or respiratory disease, this increased surface area can also occur in individuals who live (or athletes who train for extended periods of time) at high altitudes, where atmospheric pressure is reduced.

As discussed previously, FRC is the volume of air that remains within the lungs after the expiratory phase of tidal breathing. FRC serves as an additional physiologic reserve for O_2. Within this reservoir, O_2 and CO_2 are constantly exchanged through all phases of the respiratory cycle (Villars et al 2002). If respiration ceases, O_2 within the FRC reservoir continues to diffuse into the bloodstream; this reservoir of O_2 accounts for why animals survive for a number of minutes following respiratory cessation. Considering that the human body requires approximately 250 mL of O_2 per minute to survive, and the human FRC contains approximately 2500 mL of air at all times, at the point breathing stops the FRC would contain approximately 500 mL of O_2 (because atmospheric air is approximately 20% O_2), which would provide approximately 1 to 2 minutes of O_2 supply for the body. This reservoir, in addition to average concentrations of O_2 within arterial blood (approximately 100%) and even venous blood (approximately 75%), could potentially support cellular metabolism for an additional period of time that, in most people, would amount to four to five minutes (Bateman and Leach 1998).

Homeostasis and Blood pH

CO_2 that diffuses from body tissues and into the blood binds with water (H_2O). The ensuing chemical reaction produces a bicarbonate ion (HCO_3^-) as well as a free hydrogen ion (H^+). HCO_3^- acts as a **pH buffer**, maintaining the blood at a level of trace alkalinity (between 7.35 and 7.45) (West 2012). This chemical reaction is represented by the following formula:

$$H_2O + CO_2 \leftrightarrow HCO_3^- + H^+$$

The two-way nature of this equation is crucial for the maintenance of blood pH. If blood pH falls below this narrow range, a dangerous clinical condition known as acidosis occurs (West 2012). Respiratory acidosis is caused by accumulation of CO_2 within tissue. Common causes of respiratory acidosis are lung disease, chest injury, respiratory restriction (as a result of obesity, for example), respiratory muscle weakness, or drug and/or alcohol use. Symptoms of respiratory acidosis include fatigue, somnolence, dyspnea, and confusion (West 2012). The body can correct for acidosis by increasing respiratory rate, leading to increased CO_2 exhalation, reduced H^+ concentration, and increased blood alkalinity. On the other hand, blood can also become too

---

Box 10.6   Compression-Only Cardiopulmonary Resuscitation

Beginning in the mid-2000s, questions arose regarding traditional cardiopulmonary resuscitation (CPR). Historically, CPR consisted of a series of chest compressions in order to cause blood to circulate within the body, interrupted by two rescue breaths to allow oxygen to enter the lungs. Exhaled air contains anywhere from 14 to 16% O_2. In contrast, air that we inhale from the atmosphere consists of approximately 20% O_2. When administered by a skilled practitioner of CPR, the process can be very effective at preventing brain death and organ damage in individuals who have no heartbeat and who have stopped breathing. Unfortunately, the vast majority of people are not experts at CPR. CPR can be rendered less effective through improper administration. Taking too long to administer rescue breaths can reduce or stop blood from circulating. If the victim is not positioned so that the airway is opened and esophageal opening occluded, rescue breaths may inflate the stomach rather than the lungs.

These risks, among others, have shifted the manner in which nonmedical personnel are being trained to administer CPR.

As described previously, a number of O_2 reserves exist within the body even after breathing stops. The combined concentrations of O_2 contained within the arterial bloodstream, venous bloodstream, and FRC are sufficient to sustain metabolic activities at the cellular level for approximately 4 to 5 minutes. However, in order for this vital exchange of O_2 for CO_2 to occur, blood containing O_2 must reach the tissues. Compression-only CPR maximizes blood circulation so that these residual O_2 reserves may reach target tissues (Panchal et al 2013). Of primary importance is the brain, which will suffer permanent damage if deprived of O_2 for one minute or more. By administering only compressions to circulate systemic blood, a novice practitioner of CPR may be able to sustain metabolic activity within the brain and other crucial organs for as many as four to five minutes, perhaps enough time for emergency medical personnel to arrive (Panchal et al 2013).

alkaline, referred to as **alkalemia** (West 2012). The body compensates for alkalemia by slowing respiratory rate, resulting in less CO_2 exhaled, thus increasing the concentration of H^+, which shifts blood pH downward. Aside from its role in maintaining blood pH, H^+ produced during this reaction binds to hemoglobin, allowing O_2 to be released and diffuse from the blood and into tissues (West 2012).

Thermoregulation

Thermoregulation is the maintenance of core body temperature within a narrow range that, in mammals, is compatible with life. Thermoregulation is challenged by temperature variations in the outside environment as well as changes in activity. When body temperature increases to abnormally high levels, hyperthermia, literally "overheating," can occur (Robertshaw 1985). Conversely, the inability to maintain normal core temperature within a cold environment is referred to as hypothermia.

Humans and other mammals are **endothermic**, meaning they are able to thermoregulate via internal metabolic means. Many body structures and processes are involved in thermoregulation (Robertshaw 1985). The respiratory system cools the body by exhaling excess heat. Humans also perspire, which allows excess heat to evaporate from the skin surface. Animals that do not possess sweat glands and are therefore unable to perspire for thermoregulation rely much more heavily on evaporating heat via exhalation and will pant, or breathe rapidly, maximizing gas exchange and heat transfer (Robertshaw 1985).

Connection between Venous and Arterial Systems

The lungs act as a "bridge" between the venous and arterial systems. Deoxygenated blood returns to the heart through the superior and inferior venae cavae into the right atrium, from which atrial contraction pumps it through the right atrioventricular (tricuspid) valve and into the right ventricle of the heart. On ventricular contraction, the right ventricle pumps the deoxygenated blood through the pulmonary semilunar valve into the right and left pulmonary arteries, which direct it to the corresponding lungs. Inside the lungs, blood is oxygenated through processes of diffusion and exchange as discussed previously. It then returns to the heart through the pulmonary veins, normally the only veins in the body that carry oxygenated blood.

There are four pulmonary veins, two arising from each lung. Pulmonary veins carry oxygenated blood back into the left atrium of the heart, where atrial contraction pulls it through the left atrioventricular (mitral) valve into the left ventricle. Ventricular contraction ejects the oxygenated blood into the aorta and the arterial division of the systemic circulatory system (West 2012).

Lung cells are themselves supplied with oxygenated blood and nutrients through an entirely separate bronchial circulatory system that also removes waste products (West 2012). Bronchial circulation is a separate system from the pulmonary circulatory system, yet interrelated. Oxygenated blood is delivered to the lungs through the bronchial arteries. Exchange of O_2 for CO_2 and other waste products occurs within pulmonary capillaries. Deoxygenated blood then returns to the heart through either the pulmonary vein (which carries approximately 87% of returning circulation) or bronchial vein (which carries the other 13%) (West 2012). Because both the bronchial and pulmonary circulatory systems supply blood to the lungs, circulatory redundancy protects the respiratory system from damage.

Sensorineural Control of Respiration

Breathing functions under both involuntary and voluntary control, enabling continued respiration during all stages of consciousness, as well as reconfiguration of respiration in response to specialized needs (e.g., taking a deep breath before diving into a swimming pool). The repetitive cycle of inhalation and exhalation is controlled by a **central pattern generator (CPG)**, consisting of associated neurons located within two divisions of the brainstem: the pons and medulla. The **medullary respiratory center** resides in the **reticular formation** and consists of three main components. The **pre-Bötzinger complex (preBötC)** in the ventrolateral medulla generates the regular rhythm of respiration, generating regular and repetitive "bursts" of neuronal impulses that stimulate the muscles of inspiration to contract. The preBötC operates in concert with the **dorsal** and **ventral respiratory groups**, active during inspiration and expiration, respectively. The ventral respiratory group is particularly crucial for forceful or sustained expiration, such as is required for speech or airway clearance. The **apneustic center**, located in the lower pons, assists in inspiration by exciting the dorsal respiratory group within the medulla. The **pneumotaxic center** of the upper pons has the opposite role, functioning to inhibit inspiration, thereby reducing respiratory volume and rate (Guyenet and Bayliss 2015).

The cerebral cortex can override the actions of these brainstem centers, temporarily changing respiratory function. In addition, the respiratory system receives inputs from the limbic system (control center for emotional expression) and hypothalamus (which regulates the autonomic nervous system). Because of these connections, changes in emotional state (e.g., fear or excitement) and arousal are almost always accompanied by corresponding changes in respiratory function (Dempsey and Smith 2014). See **Fig. 10.22**.

Peripheral chemoreceptors are located within blood vessels and serve to detect changes in concentration of various chemicals vital to homeostasis, including O_2, CO_2, and blood glucose. In contrast to sensory organs that detect substances existing outside the body (**exteroceptors**), peripheral chemoreceptors sense changes to the internal environ-

ment and are therefore considered **interoceptors** (Guyenet 2014). These chemoreceptors take the form of cell clusters located within the aortic arch (known as the **aortic body**) and common carotid artery (known as the **carotid body**), areas of high blood flow. Blood flow contacts the aortic and carotid bodies through capillary beds. Low O_2 levels within arterial blood flow trigger cell bodies to transmit signals through the afferent division of the glossopharyngeal nerve (CN IX) into the respiratory control center located within the ventral medullary region of the brainstem to increase the respiratory rate, thereby raising blood O_2 (Guyenet 2014).

Central chemoreceptors are medullary neurons that reside proximal to the respiratory control center. Using a negative feedback loop, the central chemoreceptors are activated when the pH of nearby cerebrospinal fluid (CSF) varies from the narrow range of normal values. These changes in pH are the direct result of changes in blood O_2 or CO_2 levels. In

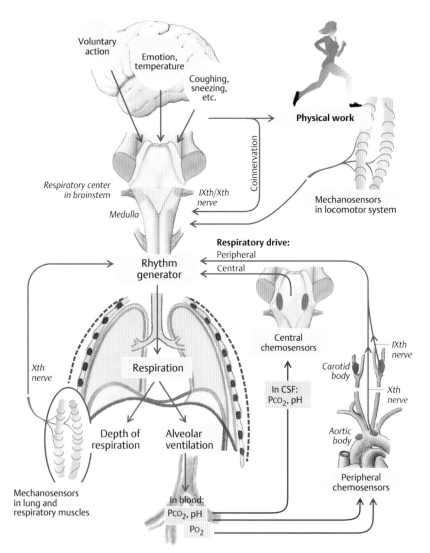

Fig. 10.22 Respiratory control and stimulation. Central pattern generators (CPGs) within the medulla repeatedly excite spinal motor neurons that control ventilation. The activity of these motor neurons is also affected by feedback from central chemoreceptors (which respond to changes in CO_2 concentrations within the cerebrospinal fluid [CSF]) and peripheral chemoreceptors (which respond to changes in CO_2 concentrations within the blood). In addition to this, mechanoreceptors within the intercostal muscles that line the rib cage respond to stretching of the thoracic cavity and therefore can modify the depth of breathing. Inputs from the cortex are able to modify respiratory patterns in response to emotion, during reflexive gestures such as coughing or sneezing, and during respiration for speech or singing.

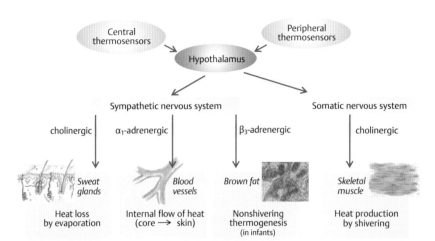

Fig. 10.23 Sensory receptors within the skin, spinal cord, and hypothalamus serve to regulate body temperature by activation, or deactivation, of a number of physiological processes including perspiration, vasodilation or constriction, and thermogenesis.

the case of **hypercapnic hypoxia**, increased blood CO_2 lowers blood pH (**Fig. 10.23**; Guyenet 2014).

The respiratory system responds rapidly to changes in O_2–CO_2 balance within the blood, blood pH, and increases in physical activity. These responses are crucial in that they serve to reestablish homeostasis. Under normal conditions, the partial pressure of CO_2 (PCO_2) within arterial blood exists within a very narrow range of 35 to 45 mm Hg. When PCO_2 levels increase beyond this narrow range, the increase is detected by central and peripheral chemoreceptors, which signal brainstem CPGs to increase respiratory rate to elevate partial pressure of O_2 (PO_2) within the blood, reestablishing homeostasis. Below-normal arterial blood levels of PCO_2 are suggestive of hyperventilation. Central and peripheral chemoreceptors detect the change and signal the brainstem CPGs to reduce the respiratory rate, allowing PCO_2 to rise to normal levels. Interestingly, trained athletes, divers, and individuals who spend extended periods of time at high altitudes can develop reduced sensitivity to PCO_2 and override normal respiratory responses to hypoventilation.

The range of normal PO_2 within arterial blood is a bit wider than with PCO_2, ranging from 75 to 100 mm Hg. Because this range is so wide, respiratory responses to altered PO_2 are uncommon in most conditions. One exception is the respiratory response to low PO_2 at extremely high altitudes. Low PO_2 is suggestive of hypoventilation. Once low PO_2 is detected by peripheral chemoreceptors within the carotid artery and aorta (there are no central receptors for PO_2, unlike PCO_2), brainstem CPGs increase respiratory rate. High-altitude climbers who ascend without supplemental O_2 frequently have an extremely high respiratory rate. There are, however, limits to this adaptation, and high-altitude climbers are at

increased risk of hypoxia, loss of consciousness, persistent brain damage, and death.

Patients with severe lung disease often lose sensitivity to hypoxic states and frequently demonstrate reduced hypoxic drive to increase the respiratory rate, in spite of chronically low PO_2 and high PCO_2 within arterial blood. Because of this reduced hypoxic drive, if these patients are provided a high concentration of O_2, respiratory rate decreases to extremely reduced levels (West 2012). It can be difficult to differentiate between respiratory responses to reduced PCO_2 and pH. pH of arterial blood has an extremely narrow range of 7.38 to 7.42, and if the pH falls below this critical range, the body enters a state of acidosis, and respiratory rate is signaled to increase. In all but extreme alterations in arterial blood pH, the change is detected by peripheral chemoreceptors, which in turn signal to increase ventilation (West 2012).

Dramatic increases in physical activity, such as those that occur during vigorous exercise, result in prompt and sustained increases in ventilation, which produce dramatic increases in O_2 consumption. Arterial PCO_2 does not increase during exercise and may actually decrease slightly during extremely vigorous exercise. Arterial blood pH remains stable during mild to moderate-intensity exercise but can decrease because of the release of lactic acid when exercise is extremely vigorous (West 2012).

There are three main types of sensory receptors located in the lungs: **pulmonary stretch receptors**, **irritant receptors**, and **J-receptors** (**juxtacapillary receptors**) (Lee and Yu 2014). Though each receptor type is specialized for detection of specific stimuli, all work in concert to control and alter breathing in response to internal and external environmental triggers. Pulmonary stretch receptors are located within the smooth muscle–lined walls of the bronchi and are slow-adapting receptors, meaning that they respond to sustained, repeated stimulation over time. They prevent overinflation of the lungs by triggering the **Hering-Breuer inflation reflex**, which signals the inspiratory control center within the medulla and pneumotaxic center within the pons, inhibiting inspiration and reducing respiratory rate (Lee and Yu 2014). Additionally, stimulation of pulmonary stretch receptors stimulates the production of **pulmonary surfactant**, which enhances the ability of the lungs to stretch and expand while simultaneously preventing lung collapse (Rugonyi et al 2008).

Pulmonary irritant receptors are present within epithelial tissue throughout the respiratory system where they sense, and respond to, inhaled chemical or mechanical irritants such as dust, pollen, smoke, irritating gases, or cold air (Lee and Yu 2014). The sensitivity of these receptors to particular stimuli varies relative to their location within the respiratory tract. Within the central airway, irritant receptors respond more selectively to mechanical irritants, whereas in the distal airways, they respond to chemical irritants. These receptors are rapidly adapting, meaning that their sensitivity will decrease in the presence of continual stimulation. When stimulated, irritant receptor cells communicate via the afferent (sensory) division of the vagus nerve (CN X) to brainstem respiratory control centers, resulting in any number of respiratory responses, including hyperpnea (deep and rapid breathing), cough, or bronchoconstriction (Lee and Yu 2014).

J-receptors (juxtacapillary receptors, also called pulmonary C-fiber receptors, are located within the walls of the alveoli, adjacent to the capillary bed where diffusion of blood gases occurs, and they are also found in other locations throughout the airway including the nasopharynx, larynx, and bronchi. These receptors respond to accumulation of fluid within the lung (**pulmonary edema**) as well as accumulation of blood within the capillary bed. When stimulated, J-receptors signal respiratory control centers in the brainstem, increasing respiratory rate and stimulating the perception of dyspnea, or difficulty breathing (Lee and Yu, 2014).

A multitude of other receptors are present throughout the respiratory system, and each serves some specialized function for respiratory control. Sensory receptors in the nose are sensitive to both mechanical and chemical stimuli and can produce a variety of reflex responses including sneezing, apnea, laryngeal closure or narrowing, bronchodilation, bronchoconstriction, increases in blood pressure (hypertension), increases in heart rate (**tachycardia**), and mucus secretion (West 2012; Loehrl 2005).

Laryngeal sensory receptors are highly diverse, responding to a variety of chemical and mechanical stimuli. Type I (rapidly adapting) receptors respond to both mechanical and chemical stimuli. Type II (slowly adapting) receptors respond selectively to mechanical inputs. Additional specialized receptors for pain and movement (for example, during voicing tasks) are also present in the larynx. Laryngeal reflex responses include cough, the expiratory reflex (forceful expiration of air from the lungs that is not preceded by inspiration), apnea (pause in breathing), bronchoconstriction, and secretion of mucus within the lower airways (Shaker 1995).

Respiratory Dysfunction: Disease and Age

A range of diseases and conditions affect the human respiratory system, producing abnormal breathing syndromes that vary relative to the body structures that are affected. Respiration can change secondary to changes in the airways, alveoli and interstitial tissue, pulmonary blood vessels, the pleural linings of the lungs and thoracic cavity, or the chest wall. Abnormal breathing syndromes manifest as either a consequence of altered central control of respiration or structural deviations that impede normal respiratory function.

Respiratory dysfunction, regardless of etiology, frequently results in severely reduced or impaired gas exchange, collectively referred to as hypoventilation. Hypoventilation is characterized by slow or shallow breathing and is a common symptom of reduced central nervous system function, cerebrovascular accident (CVA), obesity (due to increased external pressure placed on the thoracic cavity by increased weight), obstructive or central sleep apnea, deformities of the chest wall that prevent normal range of movement of the rib cage during breathing, COPD, or congenital hypoventilation syndrome (a rare disorder affecting children) (Piper and Yee 2014). Like hyperventilation, hypoventilation disrupts the O_2–CO_2 balance within the blood, resulting in abnormally high levels of CO_2, which may cause dizziness, weakness, or, in severe cases, loss of consciousness (Piper and Yee 2014).

Sleep apnea can be either obstructive or central in nature (Paiva and Attarian 2014). Obstructive sleep apnea (OSA) is characterized by partial collapse of the upper airway that disrupts sleep. Over time, OSA can exert wide ranging adverse effects on the body, particularly the cardiovascular system. Central sleep apnea (CSA) results when the brain does not properly regulate respiration during sleep, resulting in irregular patterns of inhalation and exhalation that disrupt sleep and, in extreme cases, can be fatal (Paiva and Attarian 2014).

Extreme obesity can interfere with thoracic expansion during breathing, causing dyspnea, low levels of O_2 and increased levels of CO_2 in the blood (Jones et al 2015; Böing and Randarath 2015). Aside from obesity, a range of neurogenic diseases are associated with hypoventilation, including amyotrophic lateral sclerosis (ALS, or Lou Gehrig's disease), muscular dystrophy (MD), Parkinson's disease (PD), and myasthenia gravis (MG), among others. Treatment of chronic hypoventilation is typically directed at treating the underlying disease process (Böing and Randarath 2015). The cardinal clinical sign of all hypoventilation syndromes is dyspnea.

Dyspnea

"Dyspnea" is a general term for shortness of breath, breathlessness, or air hunger; it is the perception of discomfort and fear (for example, of suffocation) that typically manifests as a symptom of an underlying condition such as hypoxia or hypercapnia resulting from asthma, pneumonia, congestive heart failure (CHF), COPD, or other lung diseases (Mahler and O'Donnell 2015). Dyspnea is a frequent symptom of panic attacks and may accompany increased levels of anxiety. The magnitude of the dyspnea sensation is variable, typically increasing during periods of increased stress or physical activity (Mahler and O'Donnell 2015). Because of the relationship between dyspnea severity and physical activity, individuals with dyspnea may exhibit a learned avoidance of exercise or other physically demanding tasks. Reduced levels of physical activity frequently result in further reductions in respiratory capacity and health, which in turn further exacerbate the perception of dyspnea and its effects on activities of daily living and quality of life (Mahler and O'Donnell, 2015).

Chronic Obstructive Pulmonary Disease

COPD comprises a family of respiratory diseases, including emphysema, asthma, and chronic bronchitis, that interfere with the ability to exhale completely, causing air to remain in the lungs. Additionally, in COPD, narrowing occurs in the upper airway as a compensatory mechanism in an attempt to regulate airflow and maintain lung volume during voice production. Self-reported symptoms in patients with COPD suggest both respiratory and laryngeal involvement and include dyspnea, reduced vocal loudness, and vocal hoarseness (Sapienza and Ruddy 2013).

COPD is typically associated with smoking or exposure to secondhand smoke, but it can also result from allergic or genetic conditions. In addition to respiratory symptoms of COPD itself, indi-

viduals with COPD typically have one or more of the following comorbidities: cardiovascular diseases (CVDs), metabolic disorders, osteoporosis, skeletal muscle dysfunction, anxiety/depression, cognitive impairment, gastrointestinal (GI) diseases, and respiratory conditions such as asthma, bronchiectasis, pulmonary fibrosis and lung cancer (Divo et al 2012; Negewo et al 2015; Patel and Hurst 2011). Individuals with severe COPD may also display excessive levels of fear and anxiety associated with suffocation and frequently avoid physically demanding activities that might potentially increase respiratory burden (Rose et al 2002). One form of COPD, chronic bronchitis, features persistent productive cough (Braman 2002).

Asthma

Airway inflammation is a key feature of asthma. Occasionally, this inflammation is accompanied by spasms (referred to as bronchial hyperresponsiveness), wheezing/stridor, or dyspnea. Asthma attacks can result from any number of factors including allergies, dust, pollen, systemic infection, or environmental pollution. Although asthma symptoms are reversible and symptoms typically abate with time and in response to medications to dilate and reduce airway obstruction, repeated bouts of asthma can cause damage to lung tissue over time (Fireman 2003).

Acute Bronchitis

Acute bronchitis consists of a temporary infection of the airways. In over 90% of instances, the infection is caused by a virus, rendering the symptoms nonresponsive to antibiotic therapy. Symptoms mimic chronic bronchitis but improve as the infection abates, typically within a period of around 3 weeks (Albert 2010).

Cystic Fibrosis

CF (**Box 10.2**) is a genetic condition involving drying of airway surface tissues and impairment of mucociliary clearance (Cohen-Cymberknoh et al 2013). The summation of these two processes results in the accumulation of thick mucus in the airway that is difficult or impossible to clear via normal mechanisms such as cough. Consequently, individuals with CF endure repeated lung infections. CF is typically a life-limiting condition, with a predicted median survival of 50 years for individuals born with the condition after the year 2000 (Hulzebos et al 2014).

Box 10.7   Improving Dyspnea in COPD

Patients with COPD frequently report high levels of breathlessness or dyspnea during rest and, especially, following physical activity such as day-to-day functional tasks or exercise. This dyspnea is related to their inability to exhale completely, which in turn contributes to overinflation of the lungs, also known as intrinsic positive end expiratory pressure (PEEP). A simple behavioral task commonly used to help patients with COPD exhale more completely is called **pursed-lip breathing**. Pursed-lip breathing is exhaling while the lips are pursed, as if about to take liquid through a straw. The patient breathes in through the nose while counting slowly to two, then exhales through pursed lips while counting slowly to four. By narrowing the space through which the patient must exhale (by pursing the lips), preserved positive air pressures are preserved into the airways, holding the airways open and allowing for more air to be exhaled prior to the next breath. This process is known as applied PEEP and helps to lessen the effects of intrinsic PEEP. As an alternative to pursed-lip breathing, a low-pressure-threshold PEEP device has been investigated to reduce perceived dyspnea in individuals with COPD following physical activity or exercise.

(Martin AD, Davenport PW. Extrinsic threshold PEEP reduces post-exercise dyspnea in COPD patients: a placebo-controlled, double-blind cross-over study. *Cardiopulmonary Physical Therapy Journal*, 22, 5–10; 2011)

Pneumonia

Pneumonia consists of an infection of the aveoli, the site of gas exchange within the lungs. Typically, pneumonia results from a bacterial infection, although viral etiologies are also common. Specific forms of pneumonia exist, including community-acquired pneumonia (infection spread among nonhospitalized individuals), hospital-acquired or nosocomial pneumonia (infection that develops following hospitalization), ventilator-assisted pneumonia (infection in patients on ventilator support), and aspiration pneumonia, which is an infection brought about by passage of food or liquid into the lower airways (Alcón et al 2005). Specific infectious agents may also result in pneumonia. One such example is tuberculosis, caused by the bacterium *Mycobacterium tuberculosis* (Venketaraman et al 2015).

Pulmonary Edema

Pulmonary edema results when fluid accumulates in the alveoli and surrounding tissue. This condition can occur as a symptom of heart failure as the heart is unable to transport fluid effectively away from the lungs (cardiogenic pulmonary edema) or as a result of physical injury to lung tissue (noncardiogenic pulmonary edema). Treatments and prognosis vary relative to the type of pulmonary edema (Murray 2011).

Lung Cancer

Lung cancer can develop in any part of the lungs and is linked to smoking or genetic factors. Globally, it is responsible for more deaths than any other type of cancer (Islami et al 2015). Mesothelioma is a rare form of lung cancer that affects the pleural linings of the lungs and thoracic cavity and has been associated with exposure to asbestos (Markowitz 2015). Lung cancer consists of rapid and uncontrolled growth of cancer cells, which in turn crowd out healthy lung cells and thereby disrupt normal lung functions including gas exchange.

Acute Respiratory Distress Syndrome

Acute respiratory distress syndrome (ARDS) or milder variants, occasionally referred to as acute lung injury, consists of sudden-onset hypoxemia associated with disease or injury. In many cases, patients with ARDS require assistance to ventilate and may be placed on a mechanical ventilator temporarily (Hager 2015).

Pneumoconiosis

Pneumoconiosis is caused by inhalation of foreign particles, such as coal dust or asbestos, into the lungs. In some cases, symptoms of pneumoconiosis are brought about as a result of irritation to the lungs caused by these inhaled particles. Conversely, the particles may cause changes within lung tissue (e.g., pulmonary fibrosis) that yield respiratory symptoms. Onset is typically gradual after months or years of exposure to irritant inhalants (Cullinan and Reid 2013).

Interstitial Lung Disease

Interstitial lung disease (ILD) is a class of lung disease involving the interstitium, the delicate lining of the alveoli. Examples of ILD include sarcoidosis and idiopathic pulmonary fibrosis. Because the alveoli are the site of gas exchange, ILD has the potential to exert widespread systemic effects and frequently results in death (Meyer 2014).

Pulmonary Embolism

A pulmonary embolism (PE) is a blood clot in the lungs. The clinical presentation of patients with PE can range from mild to extremely severe, in which cases thrombolytic therapy or surgery is necessary (Limbrey and Howard 2015). Thrombolytic therapy involves the administration of **lytic** medications to dissolve blood clots through release of enzymes that cut through the fibrin proteins that cause blood to coagulate. Conditions that impair circulation or increase the risk of a deep vein thrombosis may potentially give rise to PE, and common symptoms include dyspnea and low levels of oxygen within the blood.

Pulmonary Hypertension

Pulmonary hypertension consists of high blood pressures within pulmonary arteries. Common symptoms include dyspnea and chest pain. Pulmonary hypertension can be further categorized according to the assumed cause of the condition, as in pulmonary arterial hypertension (PAH), pulmonary hypertension due to left heart disease, pulmonary hypertension due to chronic lung disease, chronic thromboembolic pulmonary hypertension, and pulmonary hypertension due to multiple factors (Low et al 2015; Simonneau et al 2013)

Pleural Effusion

Pleural effusion (PE) involves accumulation of fluid within the pleural space between the lungs and thoracic wall (Na 2014; Light 1992). Severe PE can interfere with thoracic expansion, preventing adequate ventilation and causing dyspnea. If it does not resolve on its own or in response to medica-

tion, the effusion may need to be drained (Suárez and Gilart 2013).

Pneumothorax

Pneumothorax, or "collapsed lung" (**Box 10.1**), means the presence of air within the pleural space between the lung and thoracic wall, breaking the pleural linkage that binds the lung to the inner wall of the thoracic cavity and causing the lung to collapse. Treatment of pneumothorax can range from relatively noninvasive draining of the pleural space to more invasive techniques to seal the air leak (Slade 2014).

Hyperventilation

Hyperventilation is the process of abnormally rapid breathing and can be caused by panic or anxiety, traumatic brain injury (TBI), cerebrovascular accident (CVA, particularly within the regions of the brainstem that function to regulate respiratory rate), excessive caffeine intake, or overuse of stimulant drugs (Folgering 1999). Hyperventilation disrupts the O_2–CO_2 balance within the blood and may result in abnormally low levels of CO_2 along with accompanying symptoms such as dizziness, weakness, and paresthesia (e.g., abnormal sensation of tingling or prickling in the extremities). These symptoms typically resolve once respiratory rate is normalized (Folgering 1999).

Cheyne-Stokes Respiration

Cheyne-Stokes respiration is characterized by 10- to 20-second episodes of apnea followed by periods of hyperventilation approximately equal in length (Naughton 2012). Cheyne-Stokes respiration can manifest as a symptom of brain damage, severe heart disease, or high altitudes (and particularly during sleep at high altitudes). Some controversy exists as to the causes of Cheyne-Stokes respiration. However, in animal models, it can be induced by increasing the distance that blood must travel from the lung to the brain (Naughton 2012). This increased distance produces a delay in central chemoreceptors detecting the drop in O_2 and increase in CO_2 that occurs as a consequence of the long apneic pause. The extended period of hyperventilation that follows is believed to be a compensatory response, where the brain signals a dramatic increase in respiratory rate to correct the O_2–CO_2 balance (Naughton 2012).

The Aging Respiratory System

Marked variations in respiratory function exist among the elderly (Zeleznik 2003), and it is unclear which variations exist as a direct consequence of age and which occur secondary to the comorbidities associated with advancing age (Lalley 2013). Beginning around age 50, loss of muscle mass starts to affect most of the major muscles of respiration, affecting the expiratory more than inspiratory muscles (Lalley 2013). Loss of muscle thickness within both the internal and external intercostal muscles is common, and, although the diaphragm typically maintains its cross-sectional area (Lalley 2013), changes to chest wall morphology reduce diaphragm curvature (Zaugg and Luccinetti 2000). In addition to changes in curvature of the diaphragm, demyelination of large myelinated phrenic nerve fibers and changes in muscle fiber composition weaken the diaphragm (Miller 2010; Lalley 2013). Pulmonary vasculature begins to stiffen beginning around the third decade of life, resulting in gradual increases in pulmonary arterial pressure (Taylor and Johnson 2010).

Respiratory Effects on Disordered Speech, Language, or Swallowing

The production of voice requires generation and maintenance of adequate levels of subglottal air pressure, estimated to be 4 to 5 cm H_2O (Kunze 1964) or 7 to 10 cm H_2O (Sapienza and Ruddy 2013). Any condition that interferes with respiration has the potential to impact voice and speech adversely (Hixon and Hoit 2005). Individuals who experience dyspnea may not be able to generate or sustain adequate subglottal pressure for voice and speech. Consequently, the speech signal is typically soft and limited in duration to single words or short phrases. A range of voice and speech tasks, including conversation, raising the voice, speaking to a group, talking in a noisy place, and singing, can exacerbate dyspnea (Binazzi et al 2011). Conditions such as spinal cord injury, neuromuscular, or degenerative diseases such as multiple sclerosis (MS) frequently result in progressively reduced muscle strength. Respiratory muscle weakness reduces the ability of inspiratory and expiratory muscles to generate the active forces required to counter the passive recoil forces present in the lungs and chest wall. Reduced ability to counter these forces reduces the patient's ability to alter patterns of inhalation and/or exhalation for voicing or airway clearance. Reduced inspiratory muscle strength may prevent inhalation to high lung volumes, necessary for the generation of high subglottal air pressures for varying vocal pitch or loudness or for clearing the airway of foreign matter during cough. Those affected by inspiratory muscle weakness may demonstrate an inability to increase voicing pitch or loudness, potentially resulting in speech communication that is inappropriately soft or monotone. Severe inspiratory muscle weakness that interferes with effective gas exchange may carry higher-order cognitive linguistic consequences as a result of reduced supplies of O_2 to neural tissues.

Reduced expiratory muscle strength carries potentially life-threatening effects as a result of an inability to clear the airway of foreign matter through cough. Cough is a forced expiratory maneuver involving rapid release of subglottal pressure to produce shearing forces necessary to remove unwanted material. With regard to voice and speech, reduced expiratory muscle strength potentially impacts the ability to sustain phonation and low (below FRC) lung volumes. Continued phonation requires that exhalation be sustained in order to meet or exceed PTP. Additionally, expiratory muscles must activate at low lung volumes in order to oppose the passive recoil forces present in the lung and chest wall that pull the lung and chest wall unit back to a state of equilibrium.

The physiologic processes of breathing and swallow are intimately related (Martin-Harris et al 2005), with most swallows occurring mid-expiration. During pharyngeal swallow there is a brief apneic (respiratory) pause where the vocal folds close completely in order to prevent food or liquid from entering the lower airway. This pause is then normally followed by additional expiration prior to inspiring (Martin-Harris et al 2005). Individuals with respiratory impairment who demonstrate chronically low blood oxygen levels may find this pause uncomfortable, as it interrupts respiration for a brief period of time. Consequently, these individuals may demonstrate excessive fatigue while eating as well as disruption of normal respiratory-swallow temporal relationships. The relationships that exist between respiratory and swallow patterning suggest a need for treatment approaches that address these two physiological processes in functional, rather than isolated, contexts (Martin-Harris 2008).

Cognitive dysfunction is associated with many forms of lung disease and is a central extrapulmonary symptom of COPD (Cleutjens et al 2014). The reasons behind this association are unclear but may include common etiologic factors such as smoking or hypertension or as a result of ineffective oxygenation of brain tissue (Dodd 2015). Consequently, individuals with respiratory disease or dysfunction may exhibit cognitive linguistic deficits including impairments in comprehension, memory, attention, or higher cognitive abilities.

Elevated resistive forces in the larynx and upper and lower airways, such as those found in patients with adductor spasmodic dysphonia (ADSD), muscle tension dysphonia, laryngeal webbing, subglottal stenosis, laryngeal papilloma, or bilateral vocal fold paralysis, can restrict airflow and increase laryngeal airway resistance. If the larynx is likened to a valve, then these conditions display an "overtight" valve, which will exert considerable influences on voice and speech (Sapienza and Ruddy 2013).

Conversely, low laryngeal airway resistance (a "leaky" valve) can also exert negative effects on voice and speech. Conditions that potentially produce low airway resistance include hypofunctional voice disorders, abductor spasmodic dysphonia (ABSD), unilateral vocal fold paralysis, paresis, and other condition that interfere with normal patterns of vocal fold closure (Saarinen et al 2001). Low laryngeal airway resistance interferes with the ability to control the expiratory airflow for voicing, airway protection, or regulation of intrathoracic pressures, because of inadequate (or hypofunctional) vocal fold movement.

Although abnormalities in laryngeal airway resistance are essentially disorders of the larynx, they are included within this chapter because of the ways in which the respiratory system will frequently adapt, changing respiratory function in response to the dysfunction at the level of the larynx. Abnormally high or low laryngeal airway resistance can be initially detected via visual examination of the larynx, then verified through endoscopic examination of the vocal folds during voicing tasks as well as the sampling of airflows produced during voice and speech tasks (Sapienza and Ruddy, 2013). Characterization of high or low laryngeal airway resistance through these types of measures has been completed in a range of patient groups, including patients with vocal nodules (Sapienza and Stathopoulos 1994) and adductor spasmodic dysphonia (Finnegan et al 1996; Plant and Hillel 1998; Witsell et al 1994).

During respiration for voice and speech, the larynx, lungs, and thoracic cavity are anatomically, and functionally linked. The respiratory system will adapt to low laryngeal airway resistance by increasing lung airflows during voicing tasks, increasing recruitment of active expiratory muscle forces to maximize phonation over a single exhalation, many times resulting in abnormal phrasing of connected speech productions (Sapienza and Ruddy 2013).

■ Suggested Readings

Albert RH. Diagnosis and treatment of acute bronchitis. *American Family Physician, 82,* 1345–1350; 2010

Alcón A, Fàbregas N, Torres A. Pathophysiology of pneumonia. *Clinics in Chest Medicine, 26,* 39–46; 2005

Bateman NT, Leach RM. Acute oxygen therapy. *BMJ : British Medical Journal, 317,* 798–801, 1998.

Billinger ME, Olivier KN, Viboud C, et al. Nontuberculous mycobacteria-associated lung disease in hospitalized persons, United States, 1998–2005. *Emerging Infectious Diseases,15,* 1562–1569; 2009

Binazzi B, Lanini B, Romagnoli I, et al. Dyspnea during speech in chronic obstructive pulmonary disease patients: effects of pulmonary rehabilitation. *Respiration, 81,* 379–385; 2011

Böing S, Randerath WJ. Chronic hypoventilation syndromes and sleep-related hypoventilation. *Journal of Thoracic Disease, 7,* 1273–1285; 2015

Bolser DC. A streetcar named urge-to-cough. *Journal of Applied Physiology, 108,* 1030–1031; 2010

Bolser DC, Davenport PW. Functional organization of the central cough generation mechanism. *Pulmonary Pharmacology and Therapeutics, 15,* 221–225; 2002

Braman SS. Chronic cough due to chronic bronchitis: ACCP evidence-based clinical practice guidelines. *Chest, 129,* 104S–115S; 2002

Brunner E, Friedrich G, Kiesler K, Chibidziura-Priesching J, Gugatschka M. Subjective breathing impairment in unilateral vocal fold paralysis. *Folia Phoniatrica et Logopaedica, 63,* 142–146; 2011

Button BM, Button B. Structure and function of the mucus clearance system of the lung. *Cold Spring Harbor Perspectives in Medicine, 3*; 2013

Cassidy PM, Hedberg K, Saulson A, McNelly E, Winthrop KL. Nontuberculous mycobacterial disease prevalence and risk factors: a changing epidemiology. *Clinical Infectious Diseases, 49,* e124–e129; 2009

Cleutjens FA, Janssen DJ, Ponds RW, Dijkstra JB, and Wouters EF. Cognitive-pulmonary disease. *Biomedical Research International, 2014,* 697825; 2014

Cohen-Cymberknoh M, Kerem E, Ferkol T, Elizur A. Airway inflammation in cystic fibrosis: molecular mechanisms and clinical implications. *Thorax, 68,* 1157–1162; 2013

Cullinan P, Reid P. Pneumoconiosis. *Primary Care Respiratory Journal, 22,* 249–252; 2013

Davenport PW. Urge-to-cough: what can it teach us about cough? *Lung, 186 Suppl 1,* S107–S111; 2008

Davenport PW. Clinical cough I: the urge-to-cough: a respiratory sensation. *Handbook of Experimental Pharmacology, 187,* 263–276; 2009

Dempsey JA, Smith CA. Pathophysiology of human ventilatory control. *European Respiratory Journal, 44,* 495–512; 2014

De Peuter S, Van Diest I, Lemaigre V, Verleden G, Demedts M, Van den Bergh O. Dyspnea: the role of psychological processes. *Clinical Psychology Review, 24,* 557–581; 2004

Dicpinigaitis PV, Rhoton WA, Bhat R, Negassa A. Investigation of the urge-to-cough sensation in healthy volunteers. *Respirology. 17,* 337–341; 2012

Divo M, Cote C, de Torres JP, et al. Comorbidities and risk of mortality in patients with chronic obstructive pulmonary disease. *American Journal of Respiratory and Critical Care Medicine, 186,* 155–161; 2012

Dodd JW. Lung disease as a determinate of cognitive decline and dementia. *Alzheimer's Research and Therapy, 7,* 32; 2015

Dodge JA. A millennial view of cystic fibrosis. *Developmental Period Medicine, 19,* 9–13; 2015

Ebihara S, Ebihara T, Kohzuki M. Effect of aging on cough and swallowing reflexes: implications for preventing aspiration pneumonia. *Lung, 190,* 29–33; 2012

Epstein SK, Singh N. Respiratory acidosis. *Respiratory Care, 46,* 366–383; 2001

Finnegan EM, Luschei ES, Barkmeier JM, Hoffman HT. Sources of error in estimation of laryngeal airway resistance in persons with spasmodic dysphonia. *Journal of Speech and Hearing Research, 39,* 105–113; 1996

Fireman P. Understanding asthma pathophysiology. *Allergy and Asthma Proceedings, 24,* 79–83; 2003

Fishman AP. The volume of blood in the lungs. *Circulation, 33,* 835–838; 1966

Flesch JD, Dine CJ. Lung volumes: measurement, clinical use, and coding. *Chest, 142,* 506–510; 2012

Folgering H. The pathophysiology of hyperventilation syndrome. *Monaldi Archives for Chest Disease, 54,* 365–372; 1999.

Goldman JM, Rose LS, Morgan, MD, Denison DM. Measurement of abdominal wall compliance in normal subjects and tetraplegic patients. *Thorax, 41,* 513–518; 1986

Guyenet PG. Regulation of breathing and autonomic outflows by chemoreceptors. *Comprehensive Physiology 4,* 1511–1562; 2014

Guyenet PG, and Bayliss DA. Neural control of breathing and CO_2 homeostasis. *Neuron, 87,* 946–961; 2015

Hackett DA, Chow CM. The Valsalva maneuver: its effect on intra-abdominal pressure and safety issues during resistance exercise. *Journal of Strength and Conditioning Research, 27,* 2338–2345; 2013

Hager DN. Recent advances in the management of the acute respiratory distress syndrome. *Clinics in Chest Medicine, 36,* 481–496; 2015

Hegland KW, Pitts T, Bolser DC, Davenport PW. Urge to cough with voluntary suppression following mechanical pharyngeal stimulation. *Bratislavské Lekárske Listy, 112,* 109–114; 2011

Hegland KW, Troche MS, Davenport PW. Cough expired volume and airflow rates during sequential induced cough. *Frontiers in Physiology 4,* 167; 2013

Hillman RE, Holmberg EB, Perkell JS, Walsh M, Vaughan C. Objective assessment of vocal hyperfunction: An experimental framework and initial results. *Journal of Speech and Hearing Research, 32,* 373–392; 1998

Hixon TJ. Respiratory Function in Speech and Song. Boston, MA: College-Hill Press/Little, Brown; 1987

Hixon TJ, Goldman MD, Mead J. Kinematics of the chest wall during speech production: Volume displacement for the rib cage, abdomen and lung. *Journal of Speech and Hearing Research, 19,* 297–356; 1973

Hixon TJ, Hoit JD. *Evaluation and Management of Speech Breathing Disorders Principles and Methods.* San Diego, CA: Plural Publishing; 2005

Hoit JD. Influence of body position on breathing and its implications for the evaluation and treatment of speech and voice disorders. *Journal of Voice, 9,* 341–347; 1995

Hulzebos EH, Bomhof-Roordink H, van de Weert-van Leeuwen PB, et al. Prediction of mortality in adolescents with cystic fibrosis. *Medicine & Science in Sports & Exercise, 46,* 2047–2052; 2014

Iseman MD. That's no lady. *Chest, 109,* 1411; 1996

Islami F, Torre LA, Jemal A. Global trends of lung cancer mortality and smoking prevalence. *Translational Lung Cancer Research, 4,* 327–338; 2015

Janssens JP, Pache JC, Nicod LP. Physiological changes in respiratory function associated with ageing. *European Respiratory Journal, 13,* 197–205; 1999.

Janssens T, Silva M, Davenport PW, Van Diest I, Dupont LJ, Van den Bergh O. Attentional modulation of reflex cough. *Chest, 146,* 135–141; 2014.

Jiang J, O'Mara T, Conley D, Hanson D. Phonation threshold pressure measurements during phonation by airflow interruption. *Laryngoscope, 109,* 425–432; 1999.

Johns DP, Walters JA, Walters EH. Diagnosis and early detection of COPD using spirometry. *Journal of Thoracic Disease, 6,* 1557–1569; 2014

Jones SF, Brito V, and Ghamande S. Obesity hypoventilation syndrome in the critically ill. *Critical Care Clinics, 31,* 419–434; 2015

Joseph D, Puttaswamy RK, Krovvidi H. Non-respiratory functions of the lung. *Continuing Education in Anaesthesia, Critical Care & Pain, 13,* 98–102; 2013

Kahn , Wang , Marras. ; 2007

Kamga C, Krishnamurthy S, Shiva S. Myoglobin and mitochondria: a relationship bound by oxygen and nitric oxide. *Nitric Oxide, 26,* 251–258; 2012

Kass SM, Williams PM, Reamy BV. Pleurisy. *American Family Physician, 75,* 1357–1364; 2007

Kasthoori JJ, Liam CK, Wastie ML. Lady Windermere syndrome: an inappropriate eponym for an increasingly important condition. *Singapore Medical Journal, 49,* e47–e49; 2008

Kim J, Davenport PW, Sapienza CM. Effect of expiratory muscle strength training on elderly cough function. *Archives of Gerontology and Geriatrics, 48,* 361–366; 2009

Kim RD, Greenberg DE, Ehrmantraut ME, et al. Pulmonary nontuberculous mycobacterial disease: prospective study of a distinct preexisting syndrome. *American Journal of Respiratory and Critical Care Medicine, 178,* 1066–1074; 2008

Kuba K, Imai Y, Penninger JM. Angiotensin-converting enzyme 2 in lung diseases. *Current Opinion in Pharmacology, 6,* 271–276; 2006.

Kunze LH. Evaluation of methods of estimating subglottal air pressure. *Journal of Speech and Hearing Research, 7,* 151–164; 1964

Laciuga H, Rosenbek JC, Davenport PW, Sapienza CM. Functional outcomes associated with expiratory muscle strength training: narrative review. *Journal of Rehabilitation Research and Development, 51,* 535–546; 2014

Lalley PM. The aging respiratory system—pulmonary structure, function, and neural control. *Respiratory Physiology & Neurobiology, 187,* 199–210; 2013

Lee L, Friesen M, Lambert IR, Loudon RG. Evaluation of dyspnea during physical and speech activities in patients with pulmonary diseases. *Chest, 113,* 625–632; 1998

Lee LY, Yu J. Sensory nerves in lung and airways. *Comprehensive Physiology, 4,* 287–324; 2014

Light RW. Pleural diseases. *Disease-a-Month, 38,* 266–331; 1992

Limbrey R, Howard L. Developments in the management and treatment of pulmonary embolism. *European Respiratory Review 24,* 484–497; 2015

Loehrl TA. Autonomic function and dysfunction of the nose and sinuses. *Otolaryngologic Clinics of North America, 38,* 1155–1161; 2005

Low AT, Medford AR, Millar AB, Tulloh RM. Lung function in pulmonary hypertension. *Respiratory Medicine, 109,* 1244–1249; 2015

MacDougall JD, Elder GC, Sale DG, Moroz JR, Sutton JR. Effects of strength training and immobilization on human muscle fibres. *European Journal of Applied Physiology and Occupational Physiology, 43,* 25–34; 1980

Mahler DA, O'Donnell DE. Recent advances in dyspnea. *Chest, 147,* 232–241; 2015

Markowitz S. Asbestos-related lung cancer and malignant mesothelioma of the pleura: selected current issues. *Seminars in Respiratory and Critical Care Medicine, 36,* 334–346; 2015

Marras TK, Chedore P, Ying AM, Jamieson F. Isolation prevalence of pulmonary non-tuberculous mycobacteria in Ontario, 1997–2003. *Thorax, 62,* 661–666; 2003

Martin-Harris B. Clinical implications of respiratory–swallowing interactions. *Current Opinion in Otolaryngology & Head and Neck Surgery, 16,* 194–199; 2008

Martin-Harris B, Brodsky MB, Michel Y, et al. Breathing and swallowing dynamics across the adult lifespan. *Archives of Otolaryngology—Head and Neck Surgery, 131,* 762–770; 2005

Meyer KC. Diagnosis and management of interstitial lung disease. *Translational Respiratory Medicine, 2,* 4; 2014

Miller MR. Structural and physiological age-associated changes in aging lungs. *Seminars in Respiratory and Critical Care Medicine, 31,* 521–527; 2010

Murdoch BE, Pitt G, Theodoros DG, Ward EC. Real-time continuous visual biofeedback in the treatment of speech breathing disorders following childhood traumatic brain injury: Report of one case. *Pediatric Rehabilitation, 3,* 5–20; 1999

Murray JF. Pulmonary edema: pathophysiology and diagnosis. *International Journal of Tuberculosis and Lung Disease, 15,* 155–160; 2011

Na MJ. Diagnostic tools of pleural effusion. *Tuberculosis and Respiratory Diseases, 76,* 199–210; 2014

Naughton MT. Cheyne-Stokes respiration: friend or foe? *Thorax, 67,* 357–360; 2012

Negewo NA, Gibson PG, and McDonald VM. COPD and its comorbidities: impact, measurement and mechanisms. *Respirology, 20,* 1160–1171; 2015

Nicod LP. Pulmonary defense mechanisms. *Respiration, 66,* 2–11; 1999

Panchal AR, Bobrow BJ, Spaite DW, et al. Chest compression-only cardiopulmonary resuscitation performed by lay rescuers for adult out-of-hospital cardiac arrest due to non-cardiac aetiologies. *Resuscitation, 84,* 435–439; 2013.

Papagiannis A, Lazaridis G, Zarogoulidis K, et al. Pneumothorax: an up to date "introduction." *Annals of Translational Medicine, 3,* 53; 2015.

Parker MJ. Interpreting spirometry: the basics. *Otolaryngologic Clinics of North America, 47,* 39–53; 2014

Patel ARC, Hurst JR. Extrapulmonary comorbidities in chronic obstructive pulmonary disease: state of the art. *Expert Review of Respiratory Medicine, 5,* 647–662; 2011

Paiva T, Attarian H. Obstructive sleep apnea and other sleep-related syndromes. *Handbook of Clinical Neurology, 119,* 251–271; 2014

Piper AJ, Yee BJ. Hypoventilation syndromes. *Comprehensive Physiology, 4,* 1639–1676; 2014

Plant RL, Hillel AD. Direct measurement of subglottic pressure and laryngeal resistance in normal subjects and in spasmodic dysphonia. *Journal of Voice, 12,* 300–314; 1998

Rabello CM, Jobe AH, Eisele JW, Ikegami M. Alveolar and tissue surfactant pool sizes in humans. *American Journal of Respiratory and Critical Care Medicine, 154,* 625–628; 1996

Robertshaw D. Mechanisms for the control of respiratory evaporative heat loss in panting animals. *Journal of Applied Physiology, 101,* 664–668; 1985.

Rose C, Wallace L, Dickson R, et al. The most effective psychologically-based treatments to reduce anxiety and panic inpatients with chronic obstructive pulmonary disease (COPD): a systematic review. *Patient Education and Counseling, 47,* 311–318; 2002

Rugonyi S, Biswas SC, and Hall SB. The biophysical function of pulmonary surfactant. *Respiratory Physiology & Neurobiology, 163,* 244–255; 2008

Saarinen A, Rihkanen H, Malmberg LP, Pekkanen L, Sovijarvi AR. Disturbances in airflow dynamics and tracheal sounds during forced and quiet breathing in subjects with unilateral vocal fold paralysis. *Clinical Physiology, 21,* 712–717; 2001

Sale DG. Neural adaptation to resistance training. *Medicine & Science in Sports & Exercise 20,* S135–S145; 1988

Sapienza CM. (2008). Respiratory muscle strength training applications. *Current Opinion in Otolaryngology & Head and Neck Surgery, 16,* 216–220; 2008

Sapienza CM, Hoffman-Ruddy. *Voice Disorders.* San Diego, CA: Plural Publishing; 2013.

Sapienza, CM, Stathopoulos ET. Respiratory and laryngeal measures of children during vocal intensity variation. *Journal of the Acoustical Society of America, 94,* 2531–2543; 1994.

Sapienza CM, Wheeler K. Respiratory muscle strength training: functional outcomes versus plasticity. *Seminars in Speech and Language, 27,* 236–244; 2006

Sapienza CM, Stathopoulos ET, Brown WS. Speech breathing during reading in women with vocal nodules. *Journal of Voice, 11,* 195–201; 1997

Shaker R. Airway protective mechanisms: current concepts. *Dysphagia, 10,* 216–227; 1995

Sheel AW, Romer LM. Ventilation and respiratory mechanics. *Comprehensive Physiology, 2,* 1093–1142; 2012

Simonneau G, Gatzoulis MA, Adatia I, et al. Updated clinical classification of pulmonary hypertension. *Journal of the American College of Cardiologists, 62,* D34–D41; 2013

Slade M. Management of pneumothorax and prolonged air leak. *Seminars in Respiratory and Critical Care Medicine, 35,* 706–714; 2014

Solomon NP, DiMattia MS. Effects of a vocally fatiguing task and systemic hydration on phonation threshold pressure. *Journal of Voice, 14,* 341–362; 2000

Souma T, Suzuki N, Yamamoto M. Renal erythropoietin-producing cells in health and disease. *Frontiers in Physiology, 6,* 167; 2015

Stickland MK, Lindinger MI, Olfert IM, Heigenhauser GJ, Hopkins SR. Pulmonary gas exchange and acid-base balance during exercise. *Comprehensive Physiology, 3,* 693–739; 2013

Suárez PM, Gilart JL. Pleurodesis in the treatment of pneumothorax and pleural effusion. *Monaldi Archives for Chest Disease, 79,* 81–86; 2013

Taylor BJ, Johnson BD. The pulmonary circulation and exercise responses in the elderly. *Seminars in Respiratory and Critical Care Medicine, 31,* 528–538; 2010

Troche MS, Brandimore AE, Godoy J, Hegland KW. A framework for understanding shared substrates of airway protection. *Journal of Applied Oral Science, 22,* 251–260; 2014

Van den Bergh O, Van Diest I, Dupont L, Davenport PW. On the psychology of cough. *Lung, 190,* 55–61; 2012.

van der Velden VH, Hulsmann AR. Autonomic innervation of human airways: structure, function, and pathophysiology in asthma. *Neuroimmunomodulation, 6,* 145–159; 1999

Venketaraman V, Kaushal D, and Saviola B. *Mycobacterium tuberculosis. Journal of Immunology Research, 2015,* 857598; 2015

Villars PS, Kanusky JT, Levitzky MG. Functional residual capacity: the human windbag. *AANA Journal, 70,* 399–407; 2002

Wang C, Bai L. Sarcopenia in the elderly: basic and clinical issues. *Geriatrics and Gerontology International, 12,* 388–396; 2012.

West JW. Pulmonary *Pathophysiology: The Essentials,* 8th ed. Philadelphia, PA: Lippincott Williams and Wilkins; 2012

West N, Popkess-Vawter S. The subjective and psychosocial nature of breathlessness. *Journal of Advanced Nursing, 20,* 622–626; 1994

Wijesinghe M, Dow L. The effect of aging on the respiratory skeletal muscles. In: Pathy MSJ, Sinclair AJ, and Morley JE (eds.), Principles and Practice of Geriatric Medicine. Hoboken, NJ: John Wiley & Sons, Ltd; 2006, Chapter 59

Witsell DL, Weissler MC, Donovan MK, Howard JF, Martinkosky SJ. Measurement of laryngeal resistance in the evaluation of botulinum toxin injection for treatment of focal laryngeal dystonia. *Laryngoscope, 104,* 8–11; 1994

Zaugg M, Luccinetti E. Respiratory function in the elderly. *Anesthesiology Clinics of North America, 18,* 47–58; 2000.

Zeleznik J. Normative aging of the respiratory system. *Clinics in Geriatric Medicine, 19,* 1–18; 2003

Zemlin WR. Speech and Hearing Science: Anatomy and Physiology (4th ed.). Boston, MA: Allyn and Bacon; 1996

■ Study Questions

1. At rest the diaphragm sits in a(n) _____ position.

A. Domed
B. Flattened
C. Abducted
D. Adducted

2. The site of gas exchange in the lungs is at the:

A. Alveolar sac
B. Bronchioles
C. Alveoli
D. Alveolar ducts

3. Inspiration is _____.
Expiration is _____.

A. Always active, active or passive depending on lung volumes
B. Always active, always passive
C. Always passive, active or passive depending on lung volumes
D. Always passive, always active

4. True or False: Pulmonary function testing requires that the patient inhale to maximum capacity ("total lung capacity"), then exhale until the lungs are emptied of all air.

5. The mucosal tissue of the lung produces phlegm, which serves to:

A. Moisturize the inner surface of the respiratory tract
B. Protect the lining of the airway from particles that exist within inhaled air
C. Deliver oxygen to airway epithelial cells
D. Both A and B

6. Functional residual capacity is defined as:

A. The additional air that can be inhaled with maximum effort after a normal (tidal) inspiration
B. The volume of air present in the lungs after a normal (tidal) exhalation
C. The volume of air remaining in the lungs after maximal expiration
D. The total volume of air that can be exhaled after a maximal inhalation

7. The membrane that covers the surface of the lungs, connecting them to the inner surface of the thoracic cavity, is called the:

A. Respiratory pleura
B. Pleural linking tissue
C. Visceral pleura
D. Parietal pleura

8. The diaphragm is innervated by:

A. Cranial nerves III, IV, and V
B. Spinal nerves C3, C4, and C5
C. The first cranial nerve
D. The first spinal nerve

9. Shortness of breath or "air hunger" is referred to clinically as:

A. Dyspepsia
B. Dysrespia
C. Diphenia
D. Dyspnea

10. True or False: Individuals with chronic obstructive pulmonary disease (COPD) often exhibit psychoemotional symptoms that are related to their condition.

11. Respiratory muscle strength training increases the strength of respiratory muscles by forcing them to generate contractile forces that are greater than those generated during "typical use." This process of forcing increased contractile force generation is called _____ and is a necessary component of any program to increase strength.

A. Loading
B. Specificity
C. Transference
D. Contraction

12. Expiratory muscle strength training (EMST) primarily targets:

A. The diaphragm
B. The diaphragm and external intercostals
C. The abdominal complex and internal intercostals
D. The abdominal complex

13. Changing the diameter of the orifice on a resistive trainer changes the resistance to airflow through that orifice. These changes can be explained according to:

A. The Bernoulli effect
B. Poiseuille's law
C. Resistive modulation principles
D. Principles of flow viscosity

14. True or False: The muscle loading that is imposed during pressure threshold training is dependent on the rate at which air is inhaled or exhaled through the device, with slower inhalation decreasing loading and faster inhalation increasing load.

15. Age-related weakening of respiratory muscles is referred to as:

A. Atrophy
B. Hypertrophy
C. Sarcopenia
D. Sarcoidosis

16. Weakened cough is sometimes referred to as:

A. Dyspnea
B. Dystussia
C. Dysphagia
D. Dysarthria

17. What is the oxygen content of exhaled air?

A. 0%
B. 14 to 16%
C. 25 to 27%
D. 5 to 7%

18. If both the mother and father carry a recessive gene for cystic fibrosis (CF), there is a _____ percent chance that their child will have the disease.

A. 5
B. 10
C. 25
D. 50

19. Normal subglottal pressure necessary to initiate vocal fold vibration is approximately:

A. 4 to 10 cm H_2O
B. 15 to 20 cm H_2O
C. 25 to 30 cm H_2O
D. Over 30 cm H_2O

20. True or False: Respiratory muscle weakness can adversely impact voice and speech.

■ Answers to Study Questions

1. The correct answer is (A). The diaphragm is a dome-shaped sheet of muscle at rest. Upon contraction, the diaphragm flattens (B), effectively increasing the volume of the thoracic cavity and facilitating airflow from outside the body, into the lungs. The terms "abducted (abduction)" (C) and "adducted (adduction)" (D) are most often used to described the positioning of the true vocal folds as either open (abducted) or closed (adducted) within the laryngeal vestibule.

2. The correct answer is (C). The trachea ("windpipe") divides into the right and left bronchial trees. In the right lung this bronchial tree has three bronchi (one for each lobe), whereas in the left lung there are only two. Each of the five lobar bronchi (three in the right lung and two in the left) further subdivides into segmental bronchi, the respiratory bronchioles (B), then alveolar ducts (D), then alveolar sacs (A). Two or more alveoli opening on the same alveolar duct constitute an alveolar sac. The alveolus is a cup-shaped structure surrounded by capillary beds, enabling diffusional gas exchange to and from the lungs.

3. The correct answer is (A). Inspiration is always active, meaning that in order for inspiration to occur, muscles that enlarge the thoracic cavity must contract. The primary muscles of inspiration are the diaphragm and external intercostals. During tidal breathing, expiration is passive, meaning that no muscular action is needed. This is because following inspiration, the alveolar (lung) air pressure is greater than atmospheric (outside the body) air pressure. This causes air from inside the lungs to flow out of the lungs. In order to produce connected speech, the expiratory airflow must be carefully controlled and expiration must be allowed to continue even when alveolar pressure is lower than atmospheric pressure. In these instances, expiration is active. The abdominal muscles and internal intercostals contract, compressing the thoracic cavity and allowing for continuation of the expiratory airflow.

4. The correct answer is False. Intact lungs will always contain a set volume of air that cannot be exhaled. This is known as the residual volume. Exhaling the expiratory reserve volume of air will result in the feeling of there being no more air in the lungs; however, the residual volume remains.

5. The correct answer is (D). Mucus, or phlegm, forms a protective barrier between the lining of the inner airways and inhaled air (B). Because phlegm is composed primarily of water, it also moisturizes the lining of the inner airways (A) while trapping potentially harmful inhaled substances.

6. The correct answer is (B). Vital capacity is the total volume of air that can be exhaled after a maximal inhalation (D). Inspiratory reserve volume refers to the additional air that can be inhaled with maximum effort after a normal (tidal) inspiration (A). Residual volume is the volume of air remaining in the lungs after maximal expiration (C).

7. The correct answer is (C). The lungs are coupled with the inner surface of the chest wall via pleural linkage. Here, the visceral pleura, which surrounds the lungs, adheres to the parietal pleura, which lines the inner surface of the chest wall (D). The visceral and parietal pleura are not in direct contact but rather are joined as a result of surface tension that exists within the pleural fluid that exists between the two layers. This bond allows the lungs and chest wall to move as a connected unit.

8. The correct answer is (B). The phrenic nerve, which is the nerve that conveys motor information to the diaphragm while also carrying sensory information from the diaphragm to the central nervous system, arises from spinal nerves C3, C4, and C5 as part of the cervical plexus. There are both right and left phrenic nerves, innervating the right and left sides of the diaphragm, respectively.

9. The correct answer is (D). Dyspnea is a general term for shortness of breath or "air hunger" and typically manifests as a symptom of an underlying condition such as chronic obstructive pulmonary disease (COPD), asthma, or congestive heart failure (CHF). Dyspnea typically increases with physical activity and lessens during periods of rest or inactivity.

10. The correct answer is True. Anxiety and fear of suffocation or death are common psychoemotional symptoms of COPD. When present, these emotions may increase the perceived burden of breathing above and beyond the burden imposed by the disease itself.

11. The correct answer is (A). When a skeletal muscle is loaded, it is forced to produce contractile forces above and beyond those generated during "typical use" functions. Over time, the muscle will adapt to this loading by changes in muscle fiber composition as well as size. These adaptations serve to increase the contractile forces generated by the muscle, referred to as increases in strength. Without loading, these adaptations do not occur and significant increases in strength will not be realized.

12. The correct answer is (C). Expiratory muscle strength training (EMST) primarily targets the abdominal complex and internal intercostals. These muscles serve to decrease the volume of the thoracic cavity during forced exhalation manuvers. In contrast, inspiratory muscle strength training (IMST) primarily targets the diaphragm and external intercostals, muscles which on contraction serve to increase the volume of the thoracic cavity.

13. The correct answer is (B). Poiseuille's law determines the resistance to flow through a tube through consideration of three factors: the diameter of the orifice, viscosity of the gas flowing through the orifice, and the relative turbulence of the gas as it flows. The Bernoulli effect (A) is most commonly referenced when discussing physical properties governing vocal fold vibration.

14. The correct answer is False. The load imposed on respiratory muscles during pressure threshold training functions independently of the pattern of breathing itself. Pressure threshold trainers feature an internal, one-way valve that is held shut by a calibrated spring. In order to open (and air to pass through the trainer), the air pressure generated during inhalation or exhalation must exceed the setting of this spring. Inhaling more slowly, or more quickly, will not affect the muscular loading, in contrast to the case with resistive trainers.

15. The correct answer is (C). Aging and age-related diseases are associated with skeletal muscle atrophy or sarcopenia. Measurable decreases in muscle strength can begin as early as age 30 and typically increase over time. The effects of sarcopenia can be lessened through targeted application of muscle-strengthening protocols, although they can never be completely eliminated.

16. The correct answer is (B). Disordered cough, or dystussia, can be brought about through disruption of any of the key components of effective cough. These include adequate sensory perception of the need or urge to cough, ability to inhale an adequate volume of air prior to cough, the ability to form a tight glottal closure during the compression phase of cough, or the ability to generate high velocity peak cough airflows during cough. Dystussia impairs airway defense, potentially placing the individual at increased risk of uncompensated aspiration or other lung infection.

17. The correct answer is (B). Air that is exhaled from the lungs typically contains anywhere from 14 to 16% oxygen. By comparison, the air we inhale contains approximately 20% oxygen. The oxygen content of exhaled air administered during cardiopulmonary resuscitation (CPR) helps prevent brain death and irreversible organ damage.

18. The correct answer is (C). CF is an autosomal recessive disorder, meaning that both parents must be carriers of the same recessive mutation in order for their child to actively display the condition. A child born as a result of this pairing will have a 1 in 4 (25%) chance of having CF. Individuals with CF produce exceptionally thick mucus that is difficult to clear. This contributes to frequent lung infections with likely decreases in life expectancy.

19. The correct answer is (A). Prior to the onset of phonation, the vocal folds close, or adduct. This causes air pressure to build in the area below the vocal folds, known as the subglottal region. Once air pressure reaches a critical level, anywhere from 4 to 10 cm H_2O, the vocal folds will be forced apart and voicing can begin. This is known clinically as the phonation pressure threshold (PTP).

20. The correct answer is True. Respiration is the driving force behind voice and speech. Without the ability to generate adequate subglottal respiratory pressures, phonation cannot occur. Prolonged activation of muscles of inhalation and exhalation enables the speaker to control the rate with which air is exhaled from the lungs. During voicing, this air is used to drive vocal fold vibration. Consequently, disorders of the respiratory system will exert potentially devastating effects on voice and speech.

11

Phonation

Christopher R. Watts

■ Chapter Summary

The larynx provides an important biological function that includes breathing and airway protection and serves as the major organ of voice production. Phonation involves the modulation of airflow at the glottis and the transformation of aerodynamic to acoustic energy. Phonation is a tool that enables us to interact and influence the world around us. In addition to linguistic messages, our voice carries information that enables listeners to infer mood, sex, age, and other nonlinguistic characteristics. The study of anatomy and physiology of phonation is critical to the understanding of the role of the larynx during voice production. Additionally, knowledge of the physiologic mechanisms underlying the various life-sustaining biological functions of the larynx is an essential competency of the speech-language pathologist. This chapter provides an overview of laryngeal anatomy and physiology and a comprehensive overview of the biological and nonbiological functions of the larynx. Specifically, the chapter describes the cartilaginous framework, connective tissues and muscles, and nervous system pathways that support the biologic and nonbiologic functions of the larynx, and it discusses the role of the speech-language pathologist in the management of individuals with voice disorders.

■ Learning Objectives

- Describe the biological and nonbiological functions of the larynx

- Understand the peripheral and central nervous system control of laryngeal function
- Identify the intrinsic and extrinsic laryngeal muscles and describe their respective contributions to laryngeal physiology
- Describe the layered structure of the vocal folds and the role of aerodynamic forces in voice production
- Explain the influences of age and sex on characteristics of phonation

■ Putting It Into Practice

- The larynx consists of cartilage, muscle, and other connective tissues. The larynx provides important life-sustaining biological functions such as respiration and airway protection. Its most important nonbiological function is voice production.
- Phonation is the result of muscular and aerodynamic forces. Changes in phonatory physiology and voice quality occur during early development and as a result of aging.
- Dysphonia is a perceptual sign or symptom of an underlying physiological impairment. The etiology of dysphonia can be functional, organic, or neurologic in nature. Speech-language pathologists play an important role in the management of individuals with voice disorders.

■ Introduction

Voice production or **phonation** comprises the physiologic process of modulation of airflow by the **vocal folds** to produce acoustic sound energy (Titze 1994). Phonation occurs within the **larynx** or "voice box." The larynx consists of cartilage, muscle, ligaments, and other tissue that divide the respiratory tract into upper (pharynx, oral and nasal cavities) and lower (trachea, bronchi, and lungs) segments. As illustrated in **Fig. 11.1**, the larynx is located centrally in the anterior portion of the neck below the mandible. When the larynx is healthy and structurally intact, phonation results in age- and sex-appropriate sound. If asked to describe this voice, a listener may say that the voice sounds "normal." However, if there is structural damage to the vocal folds or if the physiology of voice production is abnormal, the resulting sound will be perceptually "abnormal." This is referred to as **dysphonia**. This chapter will focus on the anatomy and physiology of the larynx. The information presented in this chapter will provide a foundation for the speech-language pathologist to apply knowledge regarding the various conditions underlying abnormal structure and function of the structures involved in phonation.

■ Anatomy of Phonation

Biologic Functions of the Larynx

The larynx is essentially a tube with an opening on each end and an inner valve. The valve is created by the vocal folds. The openings are located at the top (superior) and bottom (inferior) of the larynx. The adult larynx (**Fig. 11.2**) is located centrally in the anterior neck anterior to the cervical vertebrae (C3–C6) and separated from the vertebrae by the posterior **pharyngeal cavity** and pharyngeal walls. The superior opening of the larynx is referred to as the **laryngeal vestibule** (**Fig. 11.3**) and is continuous with the pharyngeal cavity. The laryngeal vestibule forms the superior border of the laryngeal tube. The inferior opening is continuous with the trachea which is part of the lower airway.

The functions of the larynx are important for health, physical activity, and communication. Functions associated with the domains of health and physical activity are referred to as "biologic" functions of the larynx. These biologic functions include acting as a valve that opens and closes as well as a pressure generator. When positioned as an open valve, the larynx allows the passage of air between the upper and lower respiratory tracts during respiration. When closed, the larynx can prevent air from reaching the upper or lower respiratory tract (e.g., holding your breath to swim underwater) and can also prevent food or liquid from reach-

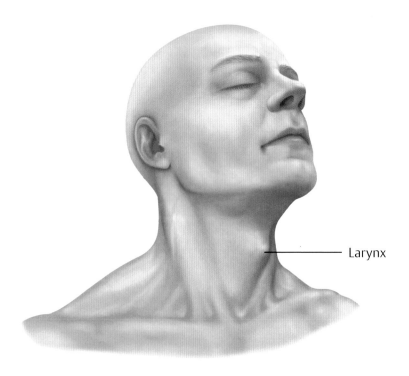

Larynx

Fig. 11.1   The location of the larynx in the anterior neck. The bulbous projection, called "Adam's apple," is part of the thyroid cartilage and is more noticeable in males than in females because of its size and angle.

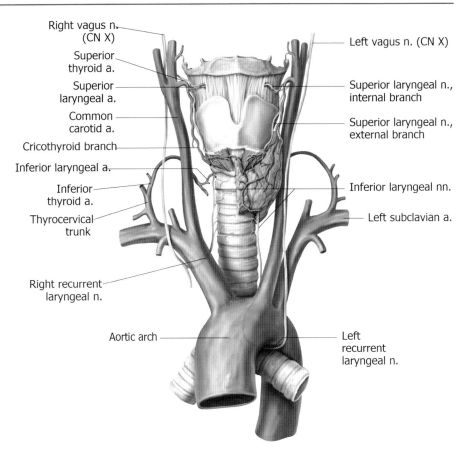

Fig. 11.2 Anterior view of the larynx in the midline of the neck. The larynx is continuous with the trachea inferiorly and with the pharyngeal cavity superiorly.

Labels for Fig. 11.2:
- Right vagus n. (CN X)
- Superior thyroid a.
- Superior laryngeal a.
- Common carotid a.
- Cricothyroid branch
- Inferior laryngeal a.
- Inferior thyroid a.
- Thyrocervical trunk
- Right recurrent laryngeal n.
- Aortic arch
- Left vagus n. (CN X)
- Superior laryngeal n., internal branch
- Superior laryngeal n., external branch
- Inferior laryngeal nn.
- Left subclavian a.
- Left recurrent laryngeal n.

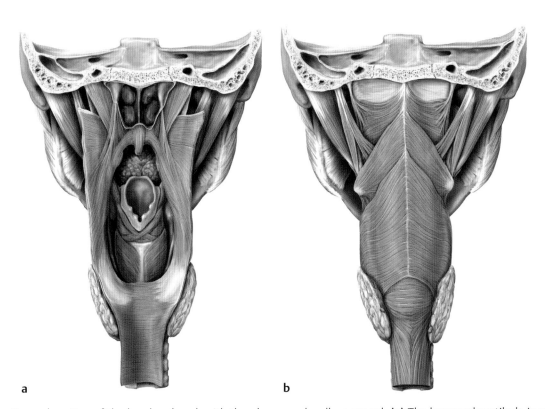

a   b

Fig. 11.3 Coronal section of the head and neck with the pharyngeal walls removed. **(a)** The laryngeal vestibule is continuous with the pharyngeal cavity above. **(b)** The esophagus is located immediately posterior and inferior to the larynx and runs parallel to the trachea (which it obscures in this image).

ing the lower respiratory tract during swallowing. When closed, the larynx can also act as a pressure generator, enabling expulsion of mucus or foreign substances from the lower airway (e.g., coughing or throat clearing). Additionally, if you take a deep breath and then close your larynx to trap the air below, the thorax (chest) is firmly fixed so that muscular effort can be maximally transferred to the limbs. This helps us to lift heavy objects.

Nonbiologic Functions of the Larynx

Not all functions of the larynx are associated with health or physical activity. The larynx also plays a very important nonbiological role in communication. Phonation allows us to produce various types of sounds during **speech** production. In speech, some sounds are said to be *voiced*, meaning that they are produced with phonation. Conversely, some speech sounds are *unvoiced*, meaning that they are produced without phonation. An example of an unvoiced sound is the /s/ sound in the word "sip," compared to the /z/ sound in "zip," which is voiced. Beyond voiced or voiceless sounds, fine control of the vocal folds enables us to change both the pitch and loudness of voice.

Phonation also conveys paralinguistic information about a speaker's disposition, sex, age, personality, and health. The larynx is directly connected to the emotional centers of our brain, and our emotional disposition is often con-veyed through the acoustic properties of voice. For example, when we are speaking to someone regarding an idea that we are excited about, typically, we produce sound more loudly than if we were not excited. This increased loudness serves as a signal to the listener. Another example is an individual giving an emotional speech who finds it difficult to talk without voice breaks (e.g., the speaker "chokes up"). It is often very easy to gauge how a speaker is feeling simply by listening to their voice. In this way, a voice can also tell us a great deal about a person's health status. Additionally, the vibratory characteristics of the vocal folds change with maturation and signal a speaker's age. This provides you with clues to understand whether you are speaking to an elderly adult or a young child simply by listening to the characteristics of the person's voice.

Laryngeal Development

During embryonic development, the laryngeal structures are formed from the branchial complex which includes the **branchial**, or **pharyngeal**, **arches**. Specifically, the fourth and sixth pharyngeal arches develop into the cartilages, muscles, ligaments, nerves, and vascular supply of the larynx (**Table 11.1**). The process of differentiation of laryngeal structures begins during the third gestational week, when the fourth pharyngeal arch begins to develop. **Fig. 11.4** shows the fourth pha-

Table 11.1   Structures forming out of the pharyngeal arches

Pharyngeal arch	Nerve	Muscles	Skeletal and ligamentous elements
First (mandibular arch)	CN V_3 (mandibular nerve from the trigeminal)	Masticatory muscles: Temporalis Masseter Lateral pterygoid Medial pterygoid Mylohyoid Digastric (anterior belly) Tensor tympani Tensor veli palatini	Malleus and incus Portions of the mandible Meckel cartilage Sphenomandibular ligament Anterior ligament of malleus
Second (hyoid arch)	CN VII (facial nerve)	Muscles of facial expression Stylohyoid Digastric (posterior belly) Stapedius	Stapes Styloid process of the temporal bone Lesser cornu of hyoid bone
Third	CN IX (glossopharyngeal nerve)	Stylopharyngeus	Greater cornu of hyoid bone Lower part of hyoid body
Fourth and sixth	CN X (superior and recurrent laryngeal nerve)	Pharyngeal and laryngeal muscles	Laryngeal skeleton (thyroid, cricoid, arytenoid, corniculate, and cuneiform cartilages)

Source: Schuenke et al 2015, Table 1.11E

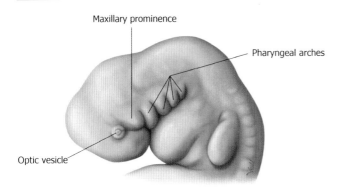

Fig. 11.4 Formation of the pharyngeal arches in a 5-week-old embryo.

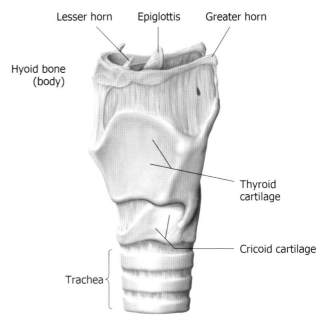

Fig. 11.5 A lateral view of the larynx showing the thyroid cartilage in relation to the hyoid bone, from which the thyroid is suspended.

ryngeal arch at the fifth gestational week in relation to the first, second, and third pharyngeal arches, which together form many of the structures within the head and neck. Laryngeal development continues through the tenth week of gestation, when the major elements of the laryngeal framework and associated structures are formed. From this point through adulthood, the macroscopic elements of the larynx remain consistent. The size and microscopic structure of the larynx continue to change, however, throughout prenatal development, childhood, puberty, adulthood, and advancing age.

The Laryngeal Framework

Stripped of all connective tissue and muscles, the core of the laryngeal framework is composed of six cartilages. These cartilages are suspended from a bone superiorly and connected to the trachea inferiorly. See **Table 11.2** for a list of the laryngeal cartilages along with their salient characteristics. The cartilaginous framework includes the thyroid cartilage, cricoid cartilage, arytenoid cartilages (paired), epiglottis, corniculate cartilages (paired), and cuneiform cartilages (paired). This entire structure is suspended from the **hyoid bone**, as shown in **Fig. 11.5** and **Fig. 11.6**.

The **thyroid cartilage** has been likened to the shape of a plow or a shield (**Fig. 11.7**). Like most of

Table 11.2 Names and characteristics of the laryngeal cartilages

Cartilage	Paired or Unpaired	Shape	Functions
Thyroid	Unpaired	Plow / shield	Anterior attachment for the vocal folds Pivots anteriorly and inferiorly to lengthen the vocal folds Attachment for the laryngeal muscles
Cricoid	Unpaired	Ring	Connects the larynx to the trachea Attachment for the laryngeal muscles Foundation for the laryngeal joints
Arytenoid	Paired	Pyramid	Posterior attachment for the vocal folds Pivots medially (adducts) and laterally (abducts) to move the vocal folds Attachment for the laryngeal muscles
Epiglottis	Unpaired	Leaf	Protects the laryngeal vestibule during swallowing Attachment for the laryngeal muscles and ligaments
Corniculate	Paired	Cone	Structural support for laryngeal tissue
Cuneiform	Paired	Wedge	Structural support for laryngeal tissue

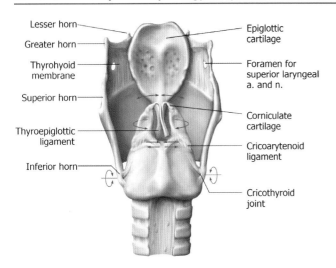

Fig. 11.6 A posterior view of the laryngeal cartilages.

the laryngeal cartilages, the thyroid cartilage is composed of an extracellular matrix filled with collagen proteins and chondrocytes. During development, two broad plates (thyroid laminae) come together and fuse at midline. Some studies suggest that the width of the thyroid lamina is greater in males as early as the second trimester (Gawlikowska-Sroka et al, 2010). This sexual dimorphism in laryngeal size continues through pre- and postnatal development but is most pronounced during and after puberty. Fusion of the thyroid laminae is incomplete superiorly, leaving a midline notch referred to as the **thyroid notch**. The thyroid notch is especially larger in males. The central line along which the two thyroid plates fuse just below the thyroid notch is called the **laryngeal prominence**. This prominence is often referred to as "Adam's apple," and it is more prominent in males due to the angle at which the left and right thyroid plates fuse; the angle is more acute in males. Just below the thyroid notch, on the inner surface of the thyroid, is a landmark called the **anterior commissure**, which is the anterior point of attachment for the vocal folds. At the posterior margins of the thyroid cartilage, there are superior and inferior projections called **thyroid horns** (or thyroid *cornua*, Latin for "horns"). The thyroid horns serve as points of attachment or articulation for ligaments, muscles, and other cartilages. The superior thyroid horns attach via a ligament to the hyoid bone. Along with other membranes, this ligament helps to suspend the thyroid cartilage and the entire larynx from the hyoid bone. The inferior thyroid horns communicate with the cricoid cartilage, enabling the thyroid cartilage to pivot anteriorly (forward) and inferiorly (downward).

The **cricoid cartilage** is located inferiorly to the thyroid cartilage and sits on top of the trachea. It is attached to the trachea by the **cricotracheal membrane**, also referred to as the cricotracheal ligament.

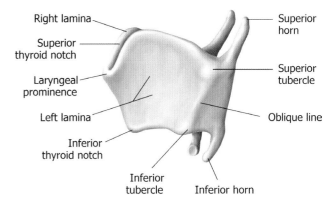

Fig. 11.7 The thyroid cartilage.

Its shape has been compared to a signet ring, with a thin anterior lamina and a lateral rim that arches upward on the sides to form an enclosed circle that joins at a broad posterior lamina. The posterior lamina is located inside the posterior inferior margins of the thyroid cartilage. On both lateral arches are articular facets (a **facet** is a small, smooth area on the surface of cartilage or bone). These articular facets form the **cricothyroid joints** (**Fig. 11.8**), the point where the left and right inferior horns of the thyroid cartilage articulate with the left and right lateral arches of the cricoid. On the superior surface of the posterior cricoid lamina are two additional facets where the cricoid and arytenoid cartilages articulate with each other and form the **cricoarytenoid joints.**

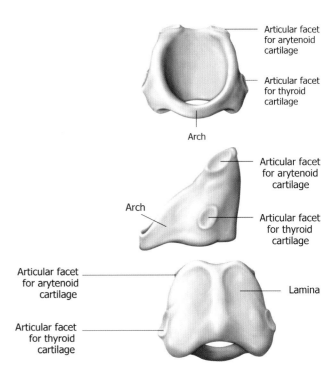

Fig. 11.8 The cricoid cartilage is shaped like a ring, with two articular facets on the lateral arches forming the cricothyroid joints.

The **arytenoid cartilages** are paired, pyramidal (triangular) cartilages, each with a superior apex and two processes (projections) at the base (**Fig. 11.9**). The **vocal process** of the arytenoid cartilages projects anteriorly, while the **muscular process** projects posterolaterally. The vocal process serves as the posterior attachment of the vocal folds; the vocal folds also attach anteriorly to the thyroid cartilage. The muscular process serves as an attachment site for laryngeal muscles. The arytenoids are located on top of the cricoid cartilage at the cricoarytenoid joint.

At the apex of each arytenoid are facets that form the articulation point for the **corniculate cartilages**. The corniculate cartilages are triangular or cone-shaped but have a curved apex. The corniculate cartilages have no obvious function other than possibly serving as structural scaffolding for laryngeal tissue. The smallest cartilages of the larynx are the **cuneiform cartilages**. The cuneiforms are embedded in tissue that surrounds the laryngeal vestibule, and, perhaps like the corniculate cartilages, they serve as scaffolding to support laryngeal tissues. Anatomic structures that have no obvious function or purpose are said to be vestigial; both the corniculate and cuneiform cartilages are commonly referred to as vestigial cartilages.

The thyroid, cricoid, and arytenoid cartilages are types of **hyaline cartilage.** Hyaline cartilage becomes harder with age as it begins to ossify or turn into bone. The corniculate and cuneiform cartilages are **elastic cartilages**. This type of cartilage consists primarily of elastin fibers, which allow a degree of flexibility. Because it contains more elastin than collagen, elastic cartilage does not ossify to the same degree as hyaline cartilage with advancing age.

The **epiglottis** is also an elastic cartilage of the larynx (**Fig. 11.10**). The epiglottis is leaf-shaped and serves to cover the laryngeal vestibule and direct food posteriorly towards the esophagus during swallowing. The superior surface of the epiglottis is broad and thick and narrows inferiorly. At its most inferior point, it becomes very narrow, forming a petiolus (stalk), and is attached

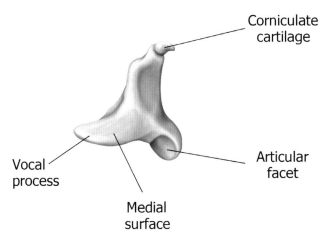

Fig. 11.9 The arytenoid cartilage showing apex, muscular process, and vocal process.

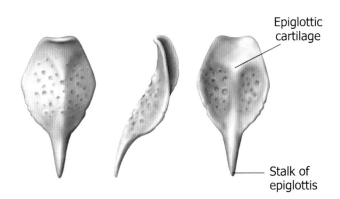

Fig. 11.10 The epiglottis.

to the thyroid cartilage by the thyroepiglottic ligament. At this point, the surface of the epiglottis forms a rounded projection known as the epiglottic tubercle. The epiglottis is not actively involved in phonation. However, it may contribute to resonance, as the elastic tissue of the epiglottis takes up space, can absorb acoustic energy, and influence vocal tract resonance. During swallowing, the larynx elevates superiorly and anteriorly due to the contraction of muscles located above the larynx, which attach to the hyoid bone. This upward and forward laryngeal excursion causes the superior portion of the epiglottis to invert and cover the laryngeal vestibule. The mechanics of swallowing are presented in greater detail in **Chapter 14**.

The hyoid bone (see **Fig. 11.5**), the only bone in the human body that does not articulate with another bone, is suspended in the neck through connections to muscles originating from the mandible and skull, muscles originating from the sternum and scapula, and to the thyroid cartilage. In addition to serving as a superior connection for the larynx, the hyoid bone acts as a point of attachment for the base of the tongue and epiglottis. The depression formed where these three structures come together is called the **vallecula**. The vallecula serves to catch food or liquid that spills over the tongue. The hyoid bone consists of a broad body in the middle, which narrows to form the **greater cornu** (greater horn) on each side. At the point where the hyoid body meets the greater cornu is another small superior projection called the **lesser cornu**. The greater and lesser cornua are sites of attachment for muscles that connect the hyoid to the rest of the body.

Membranes and Ligaments of the Larynx

In addition to the cartilaginous framework, the larynx contains a number of connective tissues including ligaments, membranes, and epithelium that cover and connect the laryngeal cartilages. At the most inferior aspect of the larynx, where the cricoid cartilage meets the trachea, a band of connective tissue called the cricotracheal ligament or cricotracheal membrane (**Fig. 11.11**) connects the cricoid cartilage to the first tracheal ring. The cricoid cartilage is also connected superiorly to the thyroid and arytenoid cartilages via the **cricothyroid ligament** (**Fig. 11.11**). This thick sheet of connective tissue, also known as the **conus elasticus**, cricothyroid membrane, and cricovocal membrane (**Fig. 11.12**), is composed of both collagen and elastin fibers and can be divided into two different parts: (1) the **median cricothyroid ligament** (**Fig. 11.11**), which is the thickened portion connecting the anterior arch of the cricoid to the posterior inferior undersurface of the thyroid, and (2) the **lateral cricothyroid ligament**, which is a thinner sheet of membrane originating from the cricoid arch and connecting to the thyroid and vocal processes of the arytenoids. The cricothyroid ligament covers the framework of the larynx below the level of the vocal folds. **Table 11.3** lists the membranes and ligaments of the larynx along with their points of attachment and key functions.

The vocal folds themselves are considered connective tissue, as the middle two layers of the vocal folds are collectively referred to as the **vocal ligament** (**Fig. 11.12**). The vocal ligament is paired and attaches to the vocal process of the arytenoid posteriorly and the anterior commissure of the thyroid cartilage anteriorly. The vocal ligament consists of varying concentrations of collagen and elastic fibers that connect the various functional layers of the vocal folds together (discussed subsequently under Vocal Fold Structure). The vocal folds form a border between the cricothyroid ligament, which covers the subglottal laryngeal regions, and a broad sheet of membrane covering the supraglottal regions of the larynx called the **quadrangular membrane**.

The connection between the cricoid cartilage and arytenoid cartilages is strengthened by a band of collagen-rich tissue called the **cricoarytenoid ligament**. This ligament originates on the superior surface of the posterior cricoid lamina on each side and courses at an angle to attach at the posterior and medial aspects of the arytenoid cartilage base. The cricoarytenoid ligament serves to strengthen the cricoarytenoid joint and is thought to play an important role in the control of vocal fold abduction and adduction by limiting rotation of the arytenoid cartilages at the cricoarytenoid joint. It has also been suggested that voice impairments can result from abnormalities in the structure or function of the cricoarytenoid ligament (Reidenbach 1995).

The thyroid cartilage is connected to the hyoid bone via the **thyrohyoid membrane**. This membrane attaches at the superior internal border of the thyroid cartilage and spans across the superior thyroid cornua bilaterally. It courses superiorly to the upper margin of the hyoid bone body and greater cornu. The middle portion of the thyrohyoid membrane is thickened and called the **median thyrohyoid ligament**, while the lateral portion of the membrane, at the greater thyroid horn, is also

Table 11.3 Membranes and ligaments of the larynx

Name	Attachments / Functions
Cricotracheal ligament	Inferior rim of cricoid to first tracheal ring; connects the inferior larynx to trachea
Cricothyroid ligament	Also known as conus elasticus; connects laryngeal structures below the vocal folds
Median cricothyroid ligament	Thickened medial division of the cricothyroid ligament, connecting the cricoid arch to middle thyroid lamina at inferior border
Lateral cricothyroid ligament	Thinner lateral division of the cricothyroid ligament, connecting the cricoid to lateral thyroid lamina at inferior border
Vocal ligament	Ligament extending from the anterior commissure of the thyroid to the vocal process of arytenoid; connects the vocal fold cover to the vocal fold body
Cricoarytenoid ligament	Midline of posterior cricoid lamina to base of arytenoid; stabilizes the cricoarytenoid joint
Quadrangular membrane	Broad sheet of membrane coursing upward from the arytenoids to epiglottis; covers and connects the laryngeal structures above the level of the vocal folds
Ventricular ligament	Also known as the vestibular ligament; runs from the thyroid cartilage above the anterior commissure to the anterior surface of the arytenoid cartilage above the vocal process; adducts via muscle contraction to prevent food/liquid from entering lower airway during swallowing
Aryepiglottic folds	Thickened superior borders of the quadrangular membrane; forms the laryngeal vestibule and houses the cuneiform cartilages
Thyrohyoid membrane	Extends from the superior borders of thyroid to the inferior border of the hyoid bone Connects larynx to the hyoid bone; the larynx is considered to be suspended from the hyoid via this membrane
Median thyrohyoid ligament	Thickened medial division of the thyrohyoid membrane, connecting the thyroid lamina to the body and cornu of the hyoid bone
Lateral thyrohyoid ligament	Thickened lateral division of the thyrohyoid membrane, connecting the superior thyroid cornu to the greater cornu of the hyoid bone
Thyroepiglottic ligament	Extends from the thyroid cartilage just below the notch to the petiolus of the epiglottis; connects the epiglottis to the thyroid cartilage
Hyoepiglottic ligament	Extends from the hyoid bone body to the middle portion of the epiglottis; connects the epiglottis to the hyoid bone; when the hyoid bone elevates during swallowing, the connection via this ligament results in epiglottic inversion, which covers the laryngeal vestibule

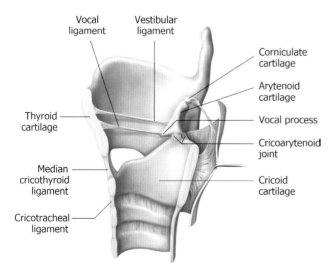

Fig. 11.11 Lateral view of the cartilaginous framework of the larynx, showing the various ligaments that connect the laryngeal structures together.

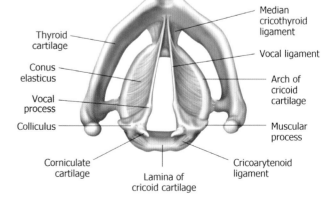

Fig. 11.12 Superior view of the median cricothyroid ligament and lateral cricothyroid ligament (conus elasticus).

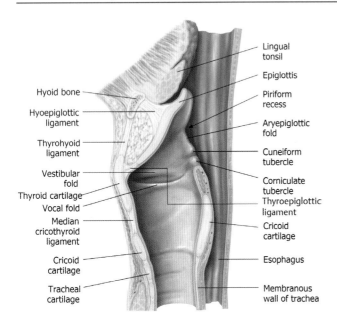

Fig. 11.13   Sagittal section through the larynx showing the vestibular (or ventricular) folds, which are formed by the inferior thickened tissue of the quadrangular membrane.

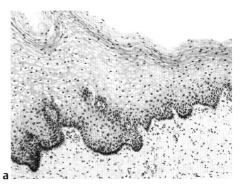

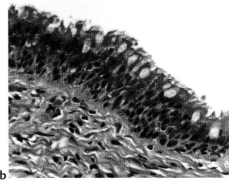

Fig. 11.14   (a) Pseudostratified, ciliated, columnar epithelium, also called respiratory epithelium, covering most of the larynx; **(b)** stratified squamous epithelium, covering the vocal folds and immediate surrounding regions.

thickened and referred to as the **lateral thyrohyoid ligament**.

The inferior petiolus of the epiglottis is connected to the thyroid cartilage just below the thyroid notch by the **thyroepiglottic ligament** (**Fig. 11.13**). The middle of the epiglottis is also connected to the hyoid bone by the **hyoepiglottic ligament** (**Fig. 11.13**), which divides the vallecula into left and right halves. The valleculae channel liquid and food around the lateral margins of the larynx into the pharynx, and can also act as a protective "holding area" for liquid or food that is prematurely spilled over the tongue prior to swallowing.

All of the cartilages, ligaments, muscles, and other tissue of the larynx are covered with a layer of epithelium. Most of the larynx is covered with respiratory epithelium, which is a type of pseudostratified, ciliated, columnar epithelium (**Fig. 11.14**) whose cilia move in a coordinated manner to drive mucus secretions (which hydrate and lubricate tissue in addition to trapping foreign particles) superiorly and out of the larynx. The vocal folds are covered with stratified squamous epithelium (**Fig. 11.14**). The epithelial cells of the vocal fold epithelium are frequently shed during phonation or coughing. The microstructure of the vocal fold epithelium is also characterized by microridges, which resemble tire treads and are thought to retain lubricating mucus.

Vocal Fold Structure

The vocal folds are paired structures located within the larynx that are capable of being moved toward the midline (**adducted**) and away from the midline (**abducted**) as well as lengthening and shortening. At rest (i.e., when one is quietly breathing and not producing sound), the vocal folds are abducted. The space between the two vocal folds is referred to as the **glottis**. The space below is referred to as the subglottis and the space above is referred to as the supraglottis. **Fig. 11.15** is a coronal section through the larynx showing the vocal folds in relation to the supraglottis and subglottis, the epithelial lining of the vocal fold and larynx, and the **vocalis muscle**. In adults, the vocal fold comprises five layers, as shown in **Fig. 11.16**, that can be differentiated from one another based on the concentrations of cells and extracellular proteins. The five layers of the vocal fold, from the surface to the deepest layer, are:

1. Epithelium
2. Superficial layer of the lamina propria
3. Intermediate layer of the lamina propria
4. Deep layer of the lamina propria
5. Vocalis muscle

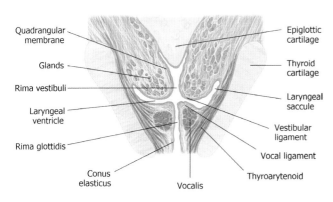

Fig. 11.15 Coronal section of the larynx.

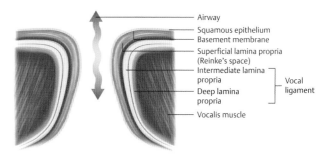

Fig. 11.16 The five layers of the vocal fold: the squamous epithelium, superficial lamina propria, intermediate lamina propria, deep lamina propria, and muscle. Together the intermediate and deep layers of the lamina propria form the vocal ligament.

The outermost layer of the vocal fold consists of stratified squamous epithelium. The surface of the vocal fold epithelium is covered with mucus, which acts as a protective barrier for the tissue underneath. This "blanket" of mucus is thought to protect the epithelium from exposure to inhaled particles and promote optimal vocal fold vibratory properties. Hydrating fluids on the surface of the vocal folds decrease the amount of air pressure required for vibration, also known as **phonation threshold pressure (PTP)**. Surface fluid moves across the vocal fold epithelium. These surface secretions come not only from the lower airway, but also from the vocal folds themselves via ion and water fluxes that cause the movement of fluid from the epithelium to the lumen (Leydon et al 2009).

Between the squamous vocal fold epithelium and the **superficial lamina propria (SLP)** is an important region called the **basement membrane zone (BMZ)**. This region contains fibrous proteins, primarily collagens that anchor the epithelium to the SLP (Gray 2000). Disruption of the BMZ secondary to trauma to the vocal fold tissues (e.g., phonotrauma) is thought to be associated with the development of benign vocal fold lesions such as vocal fold nodules.

The SLP is often described as "gelatinous" and is also referred to as the **Reinke space** after the German professor Freidrich Reinke, who first described this layer. Compared to the deeper layers of the vocal fold, the SLP is pliable and contains relatively few fibrous proteins. Collagen and elastin are two of the most abundant types of fibrous proteins in the larynx and vocal folds. Collagen is stiff and elastin is more elastic. Both collagen and elastin are sparse in the SLP. The SLP also contains **ground substance**, the substance found outside the cells other than the fibrous proteins. Unlike collagen and elastin, proteins that make up ground substance do not provide much resistance to movement and are thought to be similar to the consistency of gelatin.

The **intermediate lamina propria (ILP)** is histologically distinct from the layers lateral and deep due to higher concentrations of elastin fibers. The ILP is stiffer than the SLP, but more pliable than the layer below it. The fourth structural layer, the **deep lamina propria (DLP)**, is stiffer than the ILP due to higher concentrations of collagen fibers. Elastin and collagen fibers in the ILP and DLP course horizontally from the vocal process to the anterior commissure. Together, the ILP and DLP form the **vocal ligament**, which provides structural integrity as well as elastic properties to the vocal folds, so that the vocal folds can lengthen without tearing away from the arytenoid cartilage. When the vocal folds are lengthened to increase pitch, the vocal ligament bears the stress applied to the vocal fold tissue. The vocal ligament serves as a transition between the first two vocal fold layers (epithelium and SLP) and the deepest layer (vocalis muscle). This stiffness gradient influences how the vocal folds vibrate, which influences the resulting sound produced during phonation (Gray 2000; Titze 1994).

The deepest structural layer of the vocal folds is the **vocalis muscle (VM)**. The vocalis muscle is actually a division of a larger muscle, the thyroarytenoid muscle, which is described in the section "The Muscles of the Larynx." The VM courses parallel to the vocal ligament and is connected to the vocal process of the arytenoid posteriorly and to the anterior commissure anteriorly. The VM is attached to the vocal ligament by strands of collagen in the DLP. When this muscle contracts, it affects the tension of the vocal ligament and thickness of the vocal fold cover across its entire length, influencing the frequency of vocal fold vibration. Imagine stretching out a rubber band. The thickness of the band decreases when stretched.

Box 11.2   Congenital Laryngeal Webs

Laryngeal webs are bridges of tissue that connect the left and right vocal folds, most commonly at the anterior commissure. Multiple causes of laryngeal webs have been described, including congenital and acquired (e.g., due to irritation from an endotracheal tube or vocal fold surgery) etiologies. Congenital webs are present at birth and are thought to result from incomplete prenatal vocal fold development. Congenital webs can result from idiopathic (unknown) causes or due to genetic abnormalities that interfere with normal development.

The effect of a laryngeal web on voice production depends on the extent of the web. Small webs connecting the left and right vocal folds at the anterior com-

missure only ("microwebs") may have minimal if any noticeable effects on voice or breathing. However, larger webs that extend into the midmembranous region of the vocal folds can interfere with breathing and voice production. Treatment for laryngeal webs depends on the degree of impairment of breathing or voice. Surgical procedures are an option for dissecting the web to release the left and right vocal folds. Once the web has been resected, surgeons typically place some material on the free edges of the vocal folds to prevent the web from reforming. The proximity of the vocal folds to each other anteriorly and their complete adduction during phonation and nonspeech vocalizations places the tissue at risk for reformation of the web.

Although the majority of the layers of the lamina propria have low cellular content, the vocal fold regions at the anterior and posterior margins contain high concentrations of cells, primarily fibroblasts. These regions of high cellular content are called the anterior and posterior **macula flava**. The fibroblasts within the macula flava are responsible for producing much of the extracellular matrix including elastin, collagen, and hyaluronic acid.

Although structurally the vocal folds comprise five layers, during phonation these layers can be grouped into three functional components: the vocal fold cover (epithelium + SLP), the vocal ligament (ILP + DLP), and the VM or vocal fold body. The vocal fold cover is viscous and moves relatively freely when a force is applied to it. The vocal fold body is stiff and serves as a foundation over which the cover can oscillate. The vocal ligament connects the cover to the body. With regard to vocal physiology, it is important to consider the vocal folds as three-dimensional structures with an inferior border of tissue that courses upward to a superior border of tissue. The lower and upper edges can be seen in **Fig. 11.15** as the medial edges of vocal fold tissue inferior to the thyroarytenoid muscle and the tissue superior to the thyroarytenoid muscle, respectively.

The Muscles of the Larynx

To produce phonation, the left and right vocal folds approximate toward midline. Vocal fold adduction requires activation of laryngeal muscles to move the vocal folds from a resting position to an adducted position so that aerodynamic forces can act upon them. Laryngeal muscles also alter the length, tension, and density of the vocal folds. During connected speech, the vocal folds are rapidly abducted during voiceless sounds and then rapidly adducted for voiced sounds.

These movements are the result of highly coordinated neuromuscular activity. Groups of laryngeal muscles work in tandem. Specifically, the **extrinsic laryngeal muscles** largely act to position and stabilize the larynx in the vertical plane (e.g., elevating or depressing the larynx in the neck), while the **intrinsic laryngeal muscles** reposition and move the vocal folds.

Extrinsic Laryngeal Muscles

All muscles have a point of origin and termination. As a muscle contracts, the point of origin is typically fixed and the point of termination is typically movable. Thus, the point of termination moves toward the point of origin because of muscle fiber shortening. Many muscles of the body are named after their anatomical points of origin and termination, and this is true for many of the laryngeal muscles. The point of origin for one group of laryngeal muscles is outside the larynx, and their point of termination is on either the hyoid bone or the thyroid cartilage. These are known as the extrinsic laryngeal muscles.

The extrinsic muscles of the larynx are divided into the **laryngeal elevators** and **laryngeal depressors**. The laryngeal elevators originate above the larynx and are referred to as **suprahyoid muscles**. The laryngeal depressors have their point of origin below the larynx and are referred to as **infrahyoid muscles**. The laryngeal elevators and depressors can work either independently or synergistically. One coordinated function of the infrahyoid and suprahyoid extrinsic laryngeal muscles is to position the larynx in the vertical plane at the midline of the neck. Together, these muscles act like the chin strap on a football helmet, to hold the larynx in place. For this reason, the extrinsic laryngeal muscles are sometimes referred to as strap muscles. Contraction of elevators and depressors tends to elevate or depress the larynx, respec-

Table 11.4 Laryngeal elevators (suprahyoids)

Muscle		Origin	Insertion		Innervation	Action
Digastric	Anterior belly	Mandible (digastric fossa)	Via an intermediate tendon with a fibrous loop	Hyoid bone (body)	Mylohyoid n. (from CN V₃)	Elevates hyoid bone (during swallowing), assists in opening mandible
	Posterior belly	Temporal bone (mastoid notch, medial to mastoid process)			Facial n. (CN VII)	
Stylohyoid		Temporal bone (styloid process)	Via a split tendon			
Mylohyoid		Mandible (mylohyoid line)	Via median tendon of insertion (mylohyoid raphe)		Mylohyoid n. (from CN V₃)	Tightens and elevates oral floor, draws hyoid bone forward (during swallowing), assists in opening mandible and moving it side to side (mastication)
Geniohyoid		Mandible (inferior mental spine)	Body of hyoid bone		Anterior ramus of C1 via hypoglossal n. (CN XII)	Draws hyoid bone forward (during swallowing), assists in opening mandible
Hyoglossus		Hyoid bone (superior border of greater cornu)	Sides of tongue		Hypoglossal n. (CN XII)	Depresses the tongue

Source: Gilroy, *Atlas of Anatomy*, 2nd ed., Table 38.1. © 2017 Thieme Medical Publishers.

tively. The laryngeal elevators consist of four primary muscles (**Table 11.4**). A fifth muscle, the **hyoglossus**, is considered a suprahyoid muscle as it attaches to the hyoid bone from above, but it is not a laryngeal elevator, as contraction of this muscle does not influence laryngeal movement during voice or swallowing.

The prefix "genio" relates to the chin or mandible. Several of the laryngeal elevators originate on the medial surface of the mandible at specific landmarks. These include the midline **inferior mental spines** (small protuberances on the internal surface of the mandible), **digastric fossa** (*fossa* is Latin for "ditch" or "depression"; the digastric fossae are depressions located inferior and lateral to the inferior mental spines), and the **mylohyoid line** (a thin line running horizontally across the inside of the mandible (**Fig. 11.17**).

The **geniohyoid muscle** (**Fig. 11.18**) is a paired muscle that originates on the inferior midline of the internal mandibular surface at the inferior mental spine. The muscle fibers of the geniohyoid course downward to insert onto the body of the hyoid bone.

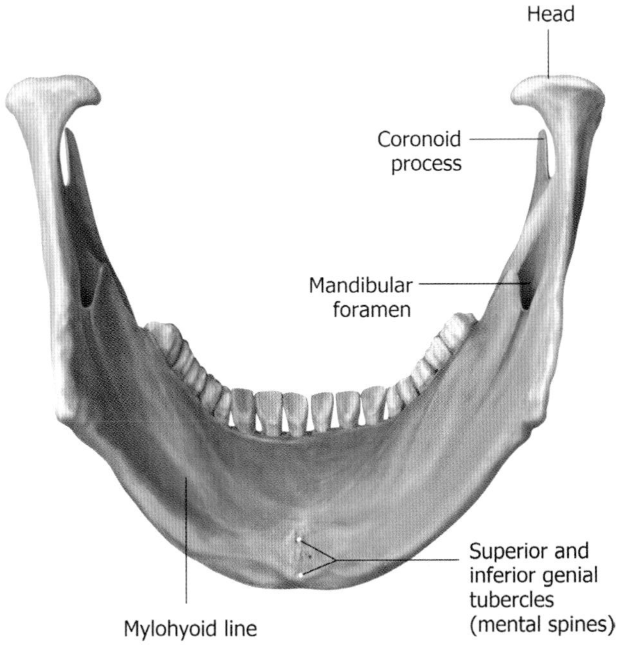

Fig. 11.17 The mandible showing the mylohyoid line and superior mental spines.

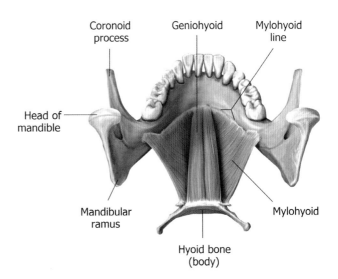

Fig. 11.18 The geniohyoid and mylohyoid muscles.

When the geniohyoid contracts, it moves the hyoid bone in a superior (upward) and anterior (forward) direction. Because the larynx is suspended from the hyoid bone by ligament and membrane, the larynx will also elevate. This superior and anterior movement of the larynx is called **hyolaryngeal excursion**. If the larynx is fixed in place due to activation of other muscles, contraction of the geniohyoid can also depress the mandible (e.g., open the jaw).

The **mylohyoid muscle** (**Fig. 11.18**, **Fig. 11.19**) also originates on the inner surface of the mandible. However, its origin is spread out across this inner surface along the mylohyoid line. It is a broad, thick sheet of muscle that forms the floor of the oral cavity. Like the geniohyoid, the mylohyoid muscle can act as a mandibular depressor, depending on the activation of other muscles. When the mandible is closed, contraction of the mylohyoid muscle results in hyolaryngeal excursion superiorly and anteriorly.

The **stylohyoid muscle** (**Fig. 11.19**) originates from the **styloid process** of the temporal bone of the skull. It courses inferiorly to insert on the body and greater cornu of the hyoid bone. Contraction of the stylohyoid muscle results in superior and posterior movement of the hyoid bone and laryngeal complex.

The **digastric muscle** (**Fig. 11.19**) is somewhat of a sling, as it consists of anterior and posterior divisions or bellies. "Digastric" comes from the Greek for "two bellies." The anterior belly of the digastric originates at the digastric fossa of the mandible. The posterior belly of the digastric originates at the **mastoid process** of the temporal bone. Both bellies course inferiorly toward the hyoid bone, where they are joined together by the intermediate tendon. A broad layer of connective tissue called the **suprahyoid aponeurosis** then connects the intermediate tendon to the body and greater cornua of the hyoid bone. Although the two bellies are controlled by different nerves, they are thought to work in concert as laryngeal elevators. However, because of their different points of origin, if contracting individually, the anterior digastric would pull the larynx superiorly and anteriorly, while the posterior digastric would pull the larynx superiorly and posteriorly. Like the geniohyoid and mylohyoid muscles, the anterior digastric can also act as a mandibular depressor.

The laryngeal depressors consist of four primary muscles (**Table 11.5**). All of these muscles have their origin below the hyoid bone and are referred to as infrahyoid muscles. The **sternohyoid muscle** (**Fig. 11.19**) originates on the posterior superior portion of the manubrium of the sternum, or breast bone, in the center of the chest. The manubrium is the thick broad sheet of bone that forms the most superior aspect of the sternum. Muscle fibers of the sternohyoid are also connected to the clavicle, or collarbone, by a ligament called the **sternoclavicular ligament**. Because of its orientation, contraction of the sternohyoid depresses the hyoid bone and larynx.

The **sternothyroid muscle** (**Fig. 11.19**) originates on the posterior surface of the manubrium just below the sternothyroid. It courses superiorly to terminate on the lateral thyroid lamina and exerts a downward pull on the thyroid cartilage.

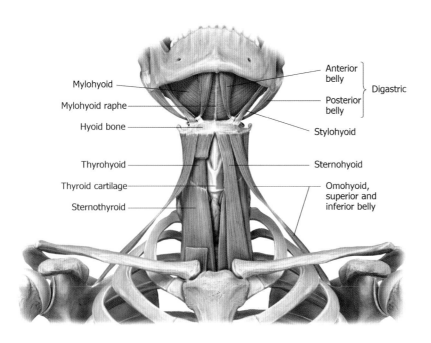

Fig. 11.19 Laryngeal elevators (suprahyoid muscles) and depressors (infrahyoid muscles) in relation to the hyoid bone.

Table 11.5 Laryngeal depressors (infrahyoids)

Muscle	Origin	Insertion	Innervation	Action
Omohyoid	Scapula (superior border)	Hyoid bone (body)	Ansa cervicalis of cervical plexus (C1–C3)	Depresses (fixes) hyoid, draws larynx and hyoid down for phonation and terminal phases of swallowing*
Sternohyoid	Manubrium and sternoclavicular joint (posterior surface)			
Sternothyroid	Manubrium (posterior surface)	Thyroid cartilage (oblique line)	Ansa cervicalis (C2–C3)	
Thyrohyoid	Thyroid cartilage (oblique line)	Hyoid bone (body)	C1 via hypoglossal n. (CN XII)	Depresses and fixes hyoid, raises the larynx during swallowing

*The omohyoid also tenses the cervical fascia (with an intermediate tendon)

Source: Gilroy, *Atlas of Anatomy*, 2nd ed., Table 39.4. © 2017 Thieme Medical Publishers.

The **omohyoid muscle** (**Fig. 11.19**) is like the digastric muscle in that it also has two bellies. The inferior belly of the omohyoid originates on the superior border of the clavicle. After coursing superiorly a short distance, it becomes a fibrous tendon that connects to the superior belly, which continues to course upward to terminate on the body of the hyoid bone, lateral to the sternohyoid attachment.

The **thyrohyoid** (**Fig. 11.19**) muscle acts as a depressor or elevator of the larynx. It originates on the thyroid lamina and terminates on the greater cornu of the hyoid bone. When this muscle contracts, its fibers shorten to decrease the distance between thyroid and hyoid. Depending on what the other extrinsic muscles are doing, this action can either depress the hyoid bone and larynx or elevate the thyroid cartilage. It is an important muscle for swallowing, where it acts as an elevator of the larynx during the pharyngeal phase of swallowing. However, when the other laryngeal elevators are not contracting, it can depress the larynx. The thyrohyoid is likely activated when you phonate at the lowest pitch possible.

Intrinsic Laryngeal Muscles

The intrinsic laryngeal muscles have both their origins and their insertions within the larynx itself, and these muscles influence the shape of the laryngeal tube. For example, they can adduct or abduct the vocal folds, lengthen the vocal folds, adduct the false vocal folds, or narrow the laryngeal vestibule. The intrinsic laryngeal muscles require precise coordination for speech. Both Type I (slow-twitch) and Type II (fast-twitch) muscle fibers are present in laryngeal muscles. Different concentrations of these types of muscle fibers exist in the various laryngeal muscles. The origin, insertion, and function of each intrinsic laryngeal muscle are shown in **Table 11.6**. The posterior cricoarytenoid muscle, the abductor of the vocal folds, contains more Type I fibers than Type II. The muscles that actively adduct, tense, and relax the vocal folds, such as the thyroarytenoid and cricothyroid muscles, contain more fast-twitch Type II muscle fibers. These varying concentrations of muscle fiber types help to explain the physiologic role of the intrinsic laryn-

Table 11.6 Intrinsic laryngeal muscles

Intrinsic muscles of the larynx			
Muscle	Origin	Insertion	Function
Vocalis (thyrovocalis)	Anterior commissure of thyroid	Vocal process of arytenoid	Tensor or relaxer
Muscularis (thyromuscularis)	Anterior commissure of thyroid	Muscular process of arytenoid	Adductor
Lateral cricoarytenoid	Anterolateral arch of cricoid	Thyroid lamina	Adductor
Interarytenoid	Arytenoid	Contralateral arytenoid	Adductor
Cricothyroid	Lateral arch of cricoid	Muscular process of arytenoid	Tensor
Posterior cricoarytenoid	Posterior lamina of cricoid	Muscular process of arytenoid	Abductor
Thyroepiglottic	Anterior commissure of thyroid	Aryepiglottic folds	Widens laryngeal vestibule
Aryepiglottic	Apex of arytenoid	Aryepiglottic folds	Pulls epiglottis posteriorly
Ventricular	Thyroid	Arytenoid	Adducts ventricular folds

Box 11.3   Spasmodic Dysphonia

Spasmodic dysphonia (SD) is a neurological voice disorder thought to be caused by dysfunction in the subcortical regions of the brain. SD is classified as a focal dystonia, and its clinical manifestation is characterized by intermittent hyperadduction ("adductor SD") or hyperabduction ("abductor SD") of the vocal folds. In adductor SD, the voice sounds strained and strangled with intermittent voice breaks and is typically accompanied by hyperfunctional muscular effort. In abductor SD, the voice sounds intermittently breathy with voice breaks and accompanying vocal hyperfunction.

Primary treatment for SD involves injections of botulinum toxin (BT) into the laryngeal muscles. Typically, an otolaryngologist uses electromyography and/or endoscopy to ensure accurate placement of BT. In the first week after BT injections, the voice may become breathy. This breathiness improves and the severity of the laryngeal dystonia is reduced, enabling less effortful voice production with fewer voice breaks. Unfortunately, BT injections do not cure SD. The effects of BT are temporary, and patients typically return for repeat injections every 3 to 6 months.

geal muscles during speech as well as the other biologic functions of the larynx.

There are five intrinsic laryngeal muscles, all of which, except for a portion of one, are paired. The **thyroarytenoid muscle** (TA; **Fig. 11.20**) is an important intrinsic laryngeal muscle with at least two distinct divisions: the vocalis or thyrovocalis muscle and the thyromuscularis or muscularis muscle. Both divisions attach anteriorly to the anterior commissure of the thyroid cartilage. The vocalis muscle is medial to the muscularis with its origin at the anterior commissure of the thyroid cartilage and posterior termination at the vocal process of the arytenoid cartilage. The vocalis is also the body of the vocal folds. When this muscle contracts, if it does not compete against other muscles that tense the vocal folds, it shortens the vocal folds, causing

the vocal ligament to become less tense and the vocal fold cover to become thicker. When other muscles lengthen and tense the vocal folds, contraction of the vocalis will increase tension in the vocal ligament and vocal fold cover and is said to act as a tensor of the vocal folds. As such, depending on the activity of other intrinsic laryngeal muscles, the vocalis can act as a tensor or a relaxer of the vocal folds.

The **muscularis muscle** (or thyromuscularis) also originates at the anterior commissure of the thyroid cartilage, but it terminates on the muscular process of the arytenoids posteriorly. When this muscle contracts, it pulls the muscular process, moving it anterolaterally. Because the muscular process and vocal process of the arytenoids are oriented at a 60° angle to each other, when the muscular process is pulled anterolaterally, the vocal process rotates medially and the vocal folds adduct. Therefore, the muscularis is classified as a vocal fold *adductor*. The TA muscle thus consists of a medial division, the vocalis, which tenses or relaxes the vocal fold tissue, and a lateral division, the muscularis, which adducts the vocal folds. As such, the TA can be labeled as a tensor (vocalis), a relaxer (vocalis), and an adductor (muscularis) of the vocal folds.

The **cricothyroid muscle** (CT; **Fig. 11.21**) is a paired muscle that originates on the lateral arch of the cricoid and terminates on the inner surface of the thyroid lamina. Like the TA, the CT has two divisions. The **pars obliqua** courses at an angle from the cricoid to the thyroid, while the **pars recta** courses vertically. Unlike the divisions of the TA, the pars obliqua and pars recta always contract together. These contractions adjust the thyroid cartilage to lengthen and increase tension of the vocal folds. When the CT contracts, the orientation of the muscle causes a pull on the thyroid cartilage antero-

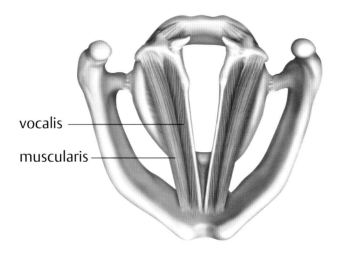

vocalis

muscularis

Fig. 11.20 The thyroarytenoid muscle showing its two divisions: the thyrovocalis (vocalis) and thyromuscularis (muscularis).

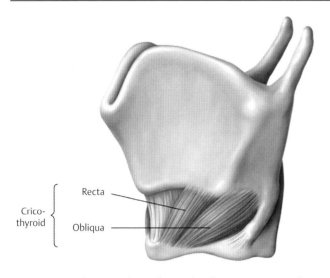

Fig. 11.21 The cricothyroid muscle showing its two divisions: the pars recta and pars obliqua.

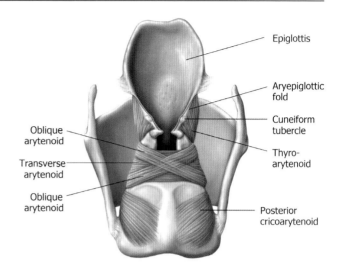

Fig. 11.22 Posterior view of the larynx showing the interarytenoids (oblique and transverse) and posterior cricoarytenoid.

inferiorly. The thyroid cartilage can move forward and downward because the thyroid articulates with the cricoid at the cricothyroid joint. Recall that the anterior ends of the vocal folds are attached to the thyroid cartilage. When the thyroid moves forward and down, the vocal folds lengthen. This lengthening stretches the vocal ligament and vocal fold tissue, resulting in increased tension and lower density. Because of this action, the CT is referred to as a tensor of the vocal folds.

The **interarytenoid muscle** (IA; **Fig. 11.22**), or arytenoid muscle, also has subdivisions similar to the TA and CT. A paired subdivision, the oblique IA, originates at the base of one arytenoid cartilage and courses at a vertical angle to the apex of the opposite arytenoid. The left and right oblique IA fibers cross each other forming an **X**. Some oblique IA muscle fibers continue past the apex of the opposite arytenoid cartilage to form the aryepiglottic muscle. The transverse IA is unpaired and consists of a sheet of muscle originating along the vertical length of one arytenoid cartilage and coursing horizontally to terminate along the vertical length of the opposite arytenoid. The two divisions of the IA contract together to move the two arytenoid cartilages closer to each other and adduct the vocal folds. As such, the IA is considered a vocal fold adductor.

The **lateral cricoarytenoid** (LCA; **Fig. 11.23**) muscle is a paired muscle originating on the lateral arches of the cricoid cartilage. It terminates on the muscular process of the arytenoid cartilage and pulls the muscular processes anterolaterally, which adducts the vocal folds. As such, the LCA is classified as a vocal fold *adductor*.

The **posterior cricoarytenoid** (PCA; **Fig. 11.22**, **Fig. 11.23**) muscle is a paired muscle originating on the posterior lamina of the cricoid cartilage. The muscle fibers course obliquely in a superior direction, terminating on the muscular process of each arytenoid. Because of their orientation, contraction causes the vocal process and arytenoid cartilage to move laterally to abduct the vocal folds. The PCA is the only vocal fold *abductor*.

The **thyroepiglottic muscle**, also known as the superior thyroarytenoid muscle, can be regarded as either another division of the TA or as its own separate muscle. It originates on the thyroid cartilage somewhat superiorly to the vocalis and muscularis, but courses obliquely to terminate on the sides of the epiglottis and aryepiglottic folds. This muscle does not influence vocal fold position, length, or

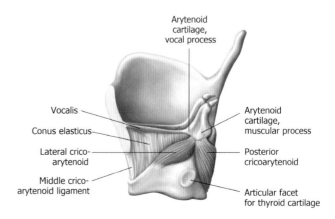

Fig. 11.23 Lateral view of larynx showing lateral and posterior cricoarytenoid muscles.

tension. Because of its orientation, when this muscle contracts, it widens the laryngeal vestibule.

The **aryepiglottic muscle** consists of muscle fibers that are extensions of the oblique IA. As such, this muscle can be thought of as originating at the apex of the arytenoid cartilages and terminating near the aryepiglottic folds lateral to the epiglottis. Although this muscle is not well understood, one possible function is to pull the epiglottis posteriorly and downward during swallowing. However, this movement also occurs during phonation. Whether or how the aryepiglottic contracts independently of the oblique IA has yet to be established.

Another intrinsic laryngeal muscle that receives little attention, because it has not been well defined anatomically, is the **ventricular muscle**. The fibers of this muscle are located along the length of the ventricular folds and are thought to be innervated by the internal division of the vagus nerve (CN X). The muscle fibers that make up the ventricular muscle may be another superior division of the TA muscle. Some suggest that the ventricular muscle is responsible for medial compression of the false vocal folds, as seen in patients with muscle tension dysphonia. The ventricular muscle may also be active during swallowing, when the laryngeal valve seals to prevent food or liquid from entering the lower airway.

Peripheral Neural Supply to the Larynx

Phonation is influenced by contraction of skeletal muscles, including the intrinsic laryngeal muscles, which change the shape of the glottis, and extrinsic laryngeal muscles, which stabilize the larynx in the vertical dimension. Skeletal muscle function is influenced by peripheral nerves, which contain motor and sensory fibers that are in communication with the central nervous system. The laryngeal muscles are all innervated by cranial nerves, which originate in the brainstem and travel to the muscles in the head and neck. Of the 12 pairs of cranial nerves, by far the most important for laryngeal function is the tenth, called the **vagus nerve (CN X)**. CN X serves both somatic and autonomic functions. This nerve has over ten distinct branches, but three are critical for phonation: the pharyngeal branch, the superior laryngeal nerve, and the recurrent laryngeal nerve.

The cell bodies for the somatic motor neurons in each of these branches reside in the **nucleus ambiguus** located in the medulla oblongata. Axons leave the nucleus ambiguus, exit through the skull, and travel toward structures of the oropharynx and larynx. The **pharyngeal branch** of CN X is a motor branch whose fibers form part of the pharyngeal plexus. As part of this plexus, the pharyngeal branch provides motor innervation to muscles of the pharynx (superior, middle, and inferior pharyngeal constrictors) and the soft palate, including the **levator veli palatini,** the main elevator of the soft palate. This branch is critical for velar elevation, which closes the nasal cavity off from the oral and pharyngeal cavities during both speech and swallowing.

Just above the thyroid cartilage, the **superior laryngeal nerve (SLN)** further subdivides into two divisions: the external and internal branches. The **external branch** of the SLN (ESLN) is a motor branch innervating the cricothyroid muscle, a tensor of the vocal folds. This branch also innervates the inferior pharyngeal constrictor and cricopharyngeus muscles, which together form the upper esophageal sphincter (UES). The **internal branch** of the SLN (ISLN) is a sensory branch that is the main sensory nerve for the mucous membranes of the epiglottis, base of the tongue, and larynx above the level of the vocal folds.

The **recurrent laryngeal nerve (RLN)** is the main motor nerve innervating the intrinsic laryngeal muscles including the thyroarytenoid, lateral and posterior cricoarytenoids, and interarytenoids, with the exception of the cricothyroid. The RLN also provides sensory information for the larynx below the level of the vocal folds. This branch of CN X is longer on the left side of the body than on the right, because it courses inferiorly around the aorta. The length of the left RLN and the distance it travels makes this branch of CN X more prone to injury, particularly following cardiac or thoracic surgery.

The extrinsic laryngeal muscles are also innervated by peripheral cranial nerves, including the **trigeminal (CN V)**, **facial (CN VII)**, and **hypoglossal (CN XII)** nerves. Motor innervation to most of the suprahyoid muscles is supplied by the trigeminal (anterior digastric and mylohyoid) and facial nerves (posterior digastric and stylohyoid). The geniohyoid is supplied by motor fibers traveling with the hypoglossal nerve as part of the **ansa cervicalis**. Motor innervation to most of the infrahyoid muscles is supplied by the hypoglossal nerve via the ansa cervicalis, including the thyrohyoid, sternothyroid, sternohyoid, and omohyoid muscles. In theory, these extrinsic laryngeal muscles can influence voice quality and vocal function, as their activation influences intrinsic laryngeal muscle activity (i.e., if the larynx is held in a high position, the intrinsic laryngeal muscles may have to activate with greater force, range, tension, or rate to achieve a target voice behavior).

Central Neural Supply to the Larynx

Cranial nerves are peripheral nerves that communicate with the central nervous system. The motor components of peripheral nerves (cranial and spinal) are referred to as lower motor neurons (LMN). Lower motor neurons are controlled by motor pathways in the central nervous system, consisting of upper motor neurons (UMN). The communication between LMN and UMN occurs in the brainstem, where peripheral and central nerves meet. Simply, to speak, UMN pathways communicate with the cell bodies of cranial motor nerves in the brainstem and spinal nerves in the thoracic region for respiration. When the cranial nerve is stimulated by a UMN, an action potential travels through the axon. The axons of cranial nerves exit the brainstem and travel toward their target muscles to elicit muscle activity. Voice production and speech are complex sensorimotor processes requiring sensory feedback and integrated motor pathways. During speech production, the central nervous system must coordinate respiratory, laryngeal, pharyngeal, and oral muscles in ways that differ from nonspeech tasks. The CNS modulates laryngeal muscle activity during nonspeech tasks including inspiration, expiration, cough, sniff, laughter, primal noises (grunts, groans, sighs, wails, etc.), and swallowing. The peripheral nerves involved in these tasks contribute both sensory and motor branches to the muscles, which become active during these processes.

Voluntary vocalizations require integration of neural networks at cortical, subcortical, and brainstem levels. Because respiratory, laryngeal, and oral muscular transitions during speech production are so rapid (i.e., voice onset after a voiceless phoneme can occur in less than 20 ms, and adjustments in F0 can occur even faster), some theories suggest that stored memories for spatial and temporal speech targets exist in cortical regions, which are accessed (motor planning) and modified (programmed) via feedforward (open-loop) mechanisms (Van der Merwe, 1997).

Vocalization during speech production involves activation of the **premotor cortex** (including the **supplementary motor** area and the **Broca area**), the **primary motor cortex**, and **auditory cortical regions** (in the temporal lobe, including the **Wernicke area**), with bilateral cortical activity but dominant activation in the left hemisphere. Additional evidence suggests that the auditory side channel (feedback) also influences ongoing voice production. Research illustrating the pitch-shift reflex, where a speaker automatically adjusts vocal fold vibratory frequency when the pitch that the speaker hears is altered, has also supported this theory (Liu et al 2010).

In nonhuman primates, research has shown that a region in the midbrain known as the **periaqueductal gray** (PAG) matter, which has connections to the limbic system (the regions of cortex and subcortical structures that control emotional responses), is a gateway for vocalization. The PAG communicates with the nuclei of spinal nerves in the spinal cord and cranial nerves in the brainstem, such as the nucleus ambiguus of the vagus nerve (CN X), which influences respiratory and laryngeal behaviors (Jürgens and Zwirner 1996). This network (limbic regions–PAG–brainstem nuclei) is likely involved in newborn infant vocalizations. This network may also be responsible for adult vocalization responses to emotional stimuli, such as pain, fear, and passion.

Humans must learn to reproduce the spoken speech and language patterns that they are exposed to. Babies often practice speech patterns through **babbling**, which evolves into speech as their motor system matures alongside their language networks. As already mentioned, the cortical regions involved in spoken language include the premotor cortex, primary motor cortex, and temporal lobe. Recall that these regions are not just responsible for laryngeal behavior. Vocalization also requires precise coordination of respiratory and laryngeal muscles. Additionally, these two subsystems must be further coordinated with pharyngeal and oral muscles to articulate and resonate speech sounds.

This human motor speech and vocal network is unlike any other in the animal world. One reason that we are able to produce speech sounds for oral language is that only humans have direct neural connections between the primary motor cortex in the frontal lobe and the nuclei of the vagus nerve (CN X) as a component of the **pyramidal pathway** or **direct activation pathway**. In the human nervous system, neurons in the primary motor cortex communicate directly with cranial nerve nuclei controlling the laryngeal muscles. Thus, humans are "wired" in a way that is different from all other animals on earth.

Learning and skilled use of the laryngeal muscles for speech and sound production also requires activity of subcortical structures. Among these, the **basal ganglia** (BGs) are critically important. The BGs are connected via networks to the motor regions of the cerebral cortex, the cerebellum, and the brainstem nuclei including the nuclei of the cranial nerves. When one is learning skilled movements such as speech, the BGs are important for integrating and modulating aspects of movement, such as rate and tone, as well as facilitating voluntary movement initiation. These same functions are controlled by the BGs once speech is learned, and when the BGs are impaired, as in Parkinson's disease, abnormalities occur in speech, including rate, tone, and articulatory precision. In fact, Parkinson's disease results in a unique voice disorder resulting from rigidity in the vocal fold and respiratory muscles.

The **cerebellum** is also important during the process of speech motor learning and skilled speech production. It, too, connects with the brainstem and cortex through neural networks. The cerebellum is thought to facilitate coordination and synergy between muscles and systems involved in speech and voice production, helping to make movement smooth. When the cerebellar pathways are damaged, motor irregularities are observed in the range of movement, velocity of movement, and smoothness of movement (e.g., motor tremor occurs, especially as a structure approaches its target position). The speech consequences of this impairment are manifested in articulatory imprecision and prosodic abnormalities.

At the lowest CNS level (brainstem), peripheral cranial nerves that influence laryngeal muscles are responsive to sensory stimulation from the PNS, which connects to the CNS in reflex loops. Involuntary laryngeal movement during spontaneous cough, for example, can be triggered by **pattern generators** in the brainstem that are responsive to sensory stimulation. Pattern generators in the brainstem are nuclei that cause a cascade of muscular activity in the same temporal order and frequency each time. Sensory neurons from the pharyngeal plexus—pharyngeal branches of glossopharyngeal (CN IX) and pharyngeal branch of vagus (CN X)—and the internal branch of the SLN of the vagus (CN X) are important components of these reflex loops. If while eating or swallowing you have ever felt something "go down the wrong way," you may have experienced a temporary cessation of breathing, called a **laryngospasm**. This reflexive action occurs when the vocal folds or the area in the trachea just below the vocal folds detects penetration of food, liquid, or another substance.

Nonspeech laryngeal behaviors, such as coughing, can also be produced voluntarily. **Perisylvian regions** (areas of cortex surrounding the sylvian fissure) are active during voluntary cough (Simonyan et al 2007). The same cortical regions become active during voluntary sniffing, where the vocal folds abduct maximally. This voluntary motor control of nonspeech laryngeal behavior enable us to modulate reflexive laryngeal responses (i.e., for reflexive cough or laryngospasm), which may help to explain why voice therapy can be very effective for conditions such as **chronic cough** and **paradoxical vocal fold motion** (or vocal cord dysfunction).

■ Physiology of Phonation

Vibratory Cycle

Vocal fold vibration can be thought of as a **self-oscillating system**, where the power source (e.g., airflow from the lungs) is steady, but the dynamic motion of the vocal folds is sufficient to maintain cyclic back-and-forth movement as long as the power source is available. You will recall that the vocal folds consist of functional layers, including a cover and a body. The physiological properties of the vocal fold cover, including its pliability, elasticity, and geometry, allow variable intraglottal pressures, which, along with influences from the supraglottic and subglottic spaces, create the dynamic forces that drive oscillation during voice production.

At the onset of phonation, the vocal folds are adducted at midline. In this posture, the vocal folds can be considered at a position of minimum displacement. A cycle of vocal fold vibration, or one **vibratory cycle**, begins when subglottic air pressure opens the adducted vocal folds. As air flows through the glottis,

---

Box 11.4   Paradoxical Vocal Fold Motion (Vocal Cord Dysfunction)

Paradoxical vocal fold motion (PVFM), also known as vocal cord dysfunction (VCD), is an idiopathic disorder characterized by involuntary vocal fold adduction during inspiration. Multiple triggers for PVFM have been described and may include physical exertion, noxious odors, and acid reflux, among others. Many individuals with PVFM suffer for years before they are accurately diagnosed. The most common misdiagnosis is asthma. The major difference, however, is that asthma narrows the lower airways, while PVFM is a narrowing at the level of the glottis. This difference explains why inhaled steroids have no effect on PVFM.

One major reason why PVFM is often misdiagnosed relates to the difficulty in observing an actual episode during an evaluation. The visual signs of PVFM are clear; the glottis is narrowed, often with just a small posterior gap during inhalation, but many patients are unable to elicit an episode of PVFM voluntarily. Once a diagnosis is made, however, respiratory retraining therapy is quite effective. Individuals are instructed to identify relevant triggers, identify their physical reactions to these triggers, and learn breath control strategies to prevent and/or reduce the severity of PVFM episodes.

the vocal fold tissue will reach a point of maximum lateral displacement and return to the midline position. Thus, the cycle of vocal fold vibration begins with a **closed phase**, where the vocal folds are at a point of minimum displacement, followed by an **opening phase**, where the vocal folds move laterally, followed by a brief period with the vocal folds at a point of maximum displacement from midline, followed by a **closing phase**, where they return to midline. **Fig. 11.24** shows an endoscopic view of the vocal folds during the vibratory cycle.

Laryngeal Physiology and Biomechanics

One way to conceptualize vocal fold physiology during phonation is to imagine the vocal folds consisting of an upper and lower edge, which form the vocal fold cover with the vocalis muscle deep to the cover, forming the body of the vocal folds. This concept has been described as the "**three-mass model**" of phonation (Story and Titze 1995) and helps us understand how different forces and phenomena influence vocal fold vibration during phonation (**Fig. 11.25**). In this model, the lower edge ($m1$) and upper edge ($m2$) of the vocal folds move independently but are connected to the body (m) via the vocal ligament and surrounding tissue. The properties of the vocal ligament and tissues between the cover and body (and tissue between $m1$ and $m2$) are characterized by varying degrees of stiffness and resistance. These properties are represented by the coiled springs.

Fig. 11.26 further illustrates a coronal cross section of the vocal folds along with a tracing of airflow through the glottis (**transglottal airflow**) at the different phases of vibration. Forces must be applied to the

vocal fold tissues that set them into motion and maintain oscillation, including both muscular and aerodynamic forces. As the vocal folds move from a closed phase to an opening phase, air begins to flow through the glottis. Airflow through the glottis increases (see the Y-axis in **Fig. 11.26**) as the upper and lower edges of the vocal folds open. As the vocal fold edges close, airflow begins to decrease until the lower vocal fold edges completely shut off the flow of air (see "closed phase" in **Fig. 11.26**). Throughout the process of vocal fold oscillation, this vertical phase difference between the upper and lower edges is maintained.

Before vocal fold vibration can occur, an aerodynamic pressure needs to be generated to act as the power source for oscillation. To generate this pressure, exhalation of air from the lungs using muscles of respiration is required. At the same time, the vocal folds must be adducted towards the midline via the LCA, IA, and muscularis muscles. The CT and vocalis muscles must also contract to set the required tension of the vocal folds. The degree to which the adductor muscles contract creates a "**medial compression**" force between the left and right vocal folds, and the amount of medial compression is in part dependent upon the intended vocal loudness and quality (e.g., normal, breathy, rough, strained). As the vocal folds approach midline, the glottis narrows and restricts the airflow.

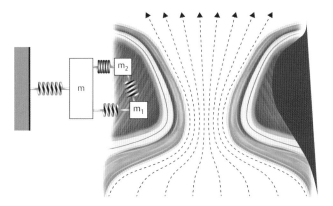

Fig. 11.25 Vocal fold three-mass model showing lower edge ($m1$), upper edge ($m2$), and vocal fold body (m).

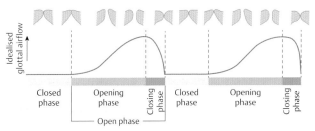

Fig. 11.26 The upper and lower edges of the vocal folds during vibration (top) and the airflow characteristics at various points during the vibratory cycle (bottom).

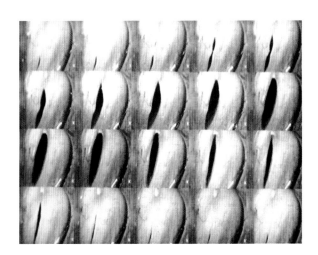

Fig. 11.24 View of vocal folds from above as they move through a cycle of vibration.

Box 11.5   Vocal Fold Nodules

Vocal nodules are bilateral masses that occur in the middle of the membranous portion of the vocal folds. True vocal fold nodules are bilateral and typically quasi-symmetrical, which distinguish them from other midmembranous lesions, such as polyps and cysts. Because they tend to occur in the same region, which happens to be the region of greatest impact stress during phonation, they are generally considered to be caused by phonotrauma, or excessive trauma to the vocal folds due to repeated and prolonged voice use. Vocal nodules start out as small swellings in the vocal fold cover, but over time they can become larger and stiffer. Nodules that have existed for a long time may be large, stiff, and resistant to voice therapy. Vo-

cal nodules often occur in individuals with profound vocal demands. These include speakers who use their voices as part of their job, including teachers, clergy, cheerleaders, singers, and other speakers (referred to as "professional voice users").

Vocal nodules usually respond well to voice therapy. Voice therapy for vocal nodules typically includes both a focus on vocal hygiene (taking care of the voice through healthy behaviors) and physiologic voice therapy (learning more efficient ways to phonate to reduce the impact stress on the vocal fold tissues). Physiologic voice therapy often includes training in the rebalancing of physical effort among the respiratory system, larynx, and upper respiratory tract in order to produce a more efficient voice.

The pressure of air flowing through a narrowing passage begins to increase immediately within and below the obstruction—in this case, the vocal folds. As the vocal folds adduct to midline, the flow of air becomes completely blocked, and the pressure below the glottis, increases rapidly. As the respiratory muscles continue to drive exhalation, the subglottal pressure becomes high enough to overcome the medial compression of the adductors and the tension forces of the CT and vocalis. When this occurs, the vocal folds begin to open, starting at the lower edge. Pressurized air then flows through the vocal folds at a high velocity, separating the tissue along its vertical dimension from the lower edge to the upper edge.

As the vocal folds begin to separate, the properties of airflow within the glottis will not be consistent throughout the subsequent phases of vibration. During the opening phase, the lower edge of the vocal folds will initially be displaced farther from midline than the upper edge. This causes the airflow at the superior glottis to converge, and this glottal shape is referred to as a **convergent glottis**. In a convergent glottis, air pressure is greater at the upper edges than at the lower edges due to the constricted intraglottal space superiorly. Conversely, during the closing phase, the upper edge of the vocal folds is displaced farther from midline than the lower edge, causing airflow at the superior glottis to diverge. This glottal shape is referred to as a **divergent glottis**. Intraglottal pressure is greater at the lower edges in a divergent glottis. The properties of transglottal airflow in a convergent and a divergent glottis are shown in **Fig. 11.27**. The different positions of the upper edge and lower edge during the different phases of the vibratory cycle result in continuously varying **intraglottal pressure differentials** between those two regions, which creates

forces necessary to sustain oscillation (Titze 1994). During the closing phase of vibration, intraglottal **flow separation vortices**, or small "whirlwinds," are created along the vocal fold walls near the upper edges in a divergent glottis. These vortices are characterized by extreme low pressure, so they further help to "suck" the two vocal folds back together near the end of the vibratory cycle (Khosla et al 2009).

Other forces also influence vocal fold vibration during phonation. At the beginning of a vibratory cycle, vocal fold tissue is displaced laterally from midline. Because vocal fold tissue is elastic (able to displace and then return to its original position), the vocal folds return to midline due to **elastic recoil**. At the same time, the vocal folds are influenced by the **Bernoulli effect** during the closing phase of the vibratory cycle. According to the Bernoulli principle, fluid pressure in a flow decreases immediately behind and perpendicular to a region of increased flow velocity. Compared to the subglottal and supraglottal spaces, the velocity of airflow within the narrowed glottis is increased during phonation. A negative pressure is created immediately behind the high-velocity flow of air within the glottis. This negative pressure has the effect of "sucking" the vocal folds back together. However, it is important to note

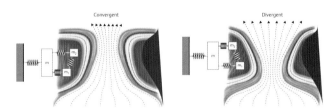

Fig. 11.27 Characteristics of airflow in convergent and divergent glottal shapes.

that, although negative pressures created via the Bernoulli effect exist during phonation, their importance for maintaining vocal fold oscillation has come into question. This influence of aerodynamic phenomena (pressure, flow, the Bernoulli effect) and tissue elasticity on vocal fold vibratory behavior has traditionally been termed the **myoelastic-aerodynamic theory** of phonation (van den Berg 1958).

In addition to the aerodynamic and muscular forces generated in the subglottic and intraglottic regions, forces above the vocal folds (supraglottis) also influence vocal fold physiology. The vocal folds are often referred to as the sound source of voice production. The regions above the vocal folds are referred to as the sound filter. The traditional **source-filter theory** explains how vocal tract shape (the filter) influences voiced sound (from the source) by resonating certain frequencies and attenuating others (Fant 1960). In a traditional source-filter model, the physiology of the source is independent of what is happening in the filter above it. That is, the filter influences the product of the source (acoustic energy traveling up through the vocal tract) but not how the source produces that product (e.g., phonation). However, current theories and models provide evidence that the supraglottal filter does indeed influence vocal fold vibration. For example, certain vocal tract shapes combined with certain phonation frequencies can destabilize vocal fold oscillation and create irregular vibration, producing sudden frequency jumps (Titze 2008b). At many fundamental frequencies, the supraglottal pressures generated by manipulations in the vocal tract act as a force, called **inertive reactance**, that influences the flow of air through the glottis during vibration. This effect subsequently influences the spectrum of sound produced during phonation, increasing the amplitude of selected harmonic frequencies (Titze 2008b). Supraglottal aerodynamic forces also vary during the cycles of vibration, and this variation has the effect of influencing intraglottal pressures. For example, at the beginning of the opening phase of vibration, when the upper vocal fold edge is closed, the column of air immediately above the glottis (i.e., in the vestibule) has no inertia. This column of motionless air acts to increase intraglottal pressures, which facilitates the separation of one vocal fold from the other (Titze 2008a).

In summary, both muscular and aerodynamic forces influence the physiology of phonation, including the characteristics of vocal fold movement during the various phases of vibration. Subglottal forces, intraglottal forces, and supraglottal forces all interact with each other to influence phonation. By manipulating muscular effort, timing, and coordination, a speaker or singer can take advantage of these interactions to produce a more efficient voice. However, inappropriate effort or an imbalance in the coordi-

nation between sub-, intra-, and supraglottal forces can disrupt phonation, resulting in a less efficient or less effective voice and, in some cases, dysphonia.

■ Characteristics of Acoustic Energy in Phonation

The acoustic energy produced during phonation is a sound wave created by the repeated opening and closing of the vocal folds. If you took a microphone and placed it immediately above the vocal folds, before the vocal tract filtered the acoustic energy, the acoustic properties of the sound waves would have distinctive characteristics. These characteristics can change depending on how a speaker controls muscular and aerodynamic forces. An important concept is that phonation results in the creation of **complex acoustic sound waves**. A complex wave (or complex tone) is one that comprises more than one frequency: a base frequency (called the **fundamental frequency** and denoted F0) and integer multiples of the base (e.g., 2 × F0, 3 × F0, . . .) called **harmonic frequencies** or harmonics. An example of an idealized acoustic spectrum produced by voice production is shown in **Fig. 11.28.**

In an idealized, normal voice (e.g., one without dysphonia), one cycle of vocal fold vibration produces one pulse of acoustic energy, which is characterized by an F0 and many harmonic frequencies, with very few nonharmonic frequencies. The fundamental frequency will typically contain the most energy, while subsequent harmonics drop in energy at a rate of 12 dB per octave (Fant 1960). When nonharmonic frequen-

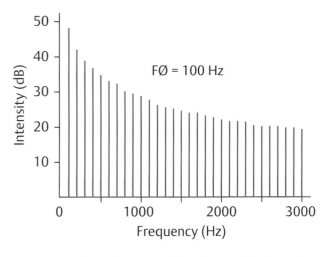

Fig. 11.28 Idealized spectrum of sound created by phonation. This spectrum represents characteristics of the *sound source*.

cies are produced, it creates acoustic "noise." Nonharmonic frequencies can arise from segments of a vocal fold, an entire vocal fold, or even both vocal folds if they are stiff and/or do not vibrate in a typical manner. Additionally, nonharmonic frequencies can be present whenever there is a glottal gap that creates an air leak during phonation. This type of phonation and the noise that results is often referred to as aperiodicity and **aperiodic energy**, respectively. Every speaker produces some acoustic noise during phonation, but typically voices that are perceived as "normal" produce less noise than voices perceived as "adysphonic."

As vocal fold oscillation continues, subsequent acoustic pulses are created, resulting in a continuous sound wave. This wave of acoustic energy travels through the larynx and upper vocal tract, where it is modified via articulation and resonance. Resonance filters the sound produced at the glottis and modifies the energy of the various harmonic and nonharmonic frequencies. If you measured the sound spectrum (the energy levels of the different frequencies) at the mouth, it would look very different from the spectrum measured directly above the glottis because of resonance.

Fig. 11.29 illustrates two acoustic waveforms from a speaker producing a sustained vowel sound. The X-axis shows time, and the Y-axis shows sound amplitude. In healthy normal voice production (top window), the vocal folds oscillate in a periodic manner where each cycle of vibration takes close to the same amount of time (period of vibration) as the cycle before it and after it. In addition, the amplitude of the sound energy created during each cycle of vibration is relatively similar during normal voice production. In dysphonic voices (bottom window), the periodicity of vibration is reduced such that the

vibration and amplitude during cycles of vibration are irregular. Listeners often perceive this irregular type of phonation as sounding "rough." If there is a glottal gap during phonation (e.g., the vocal folds do not close completely during vibration), or if vibratory irregularity is increased, it can introduce numerous nonharmonic frequencies into the sound wave, resulting in a perceptually "breathy" voice quality. Roughness and breathiness in the voice often results in the perceptual impression termed "hoarseness."

Control of Fundamental Frequency

Vocal fundamental frequency (F0) is a measurement of the number of vibratory cycles that occur during phonation over a certain period of time, and it also represents the base (fundamental) frequency of the complex acoustic sound wave that is produced during phonation. F0 is measured in **hertz** (Hz), or cycles per second. F0 is a physical phenomenon representing mass moving back and forth over time, and this movement can be quantified. However, our perception of F0 is psychological, and we refer to this perception as "**pitch**." Pitch is the result of subjective psychological processing of frequency. Our perception of pitch does not directly correlate with the physical properties of vibration, and the way one person perceives pitch can be different from how another perceives it, even when both listeners are exposed to the same F0. Frequency and pitch are related in a curvilinear manner as illustrated in **Fig. 11.30**. At low F0, small changes in frequency result in a change in the perception of pitch. However, at higher F0, it takes a much larger change in frequency before a listener will perceive a change in pitch.

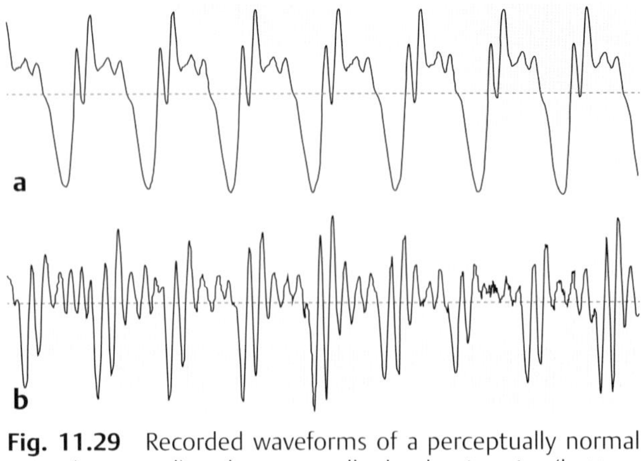

Fig. 11.29 Recorded waveforms of a perceptually normal voice (top panel) and perceptually dysphonic voice (bottom panel). Vocal fold vibratory cycle boundaries are located at the deepest valleys in the waveform. Note the periodicity (regularity) of vibratory cycles in the normal voice and the reduction in periodicity in the dysphonic voice.

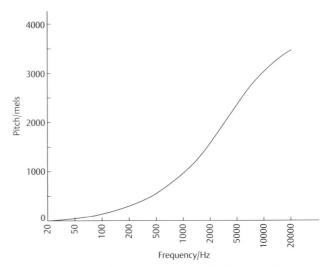

Fig. 11.30 The relationship between fundamental frequency (F0) and perceived pitch.

FO during phonation is controlled by the actions of the intrinsic laryngeal muscles, specifically coordination of the vocalis and CT muscles. At very low FO, both the vocalis and CT are engaged, but at the lower ends of their contraction range. When the muscles are engaged in this manner, the vocal fold cover is thick but very loose and pliable, and the vocal ligament vibrates along with the cover. The result is the production of a low FO, due to low tension in the vocal fold tissue and greater vibrating mass. If the CT is only minimally engaged, additional contraction of the vocalis results in a lower FO as tension in the vocal fold cover is further reduced.

With increasing FO, the CT contracts, but the majority of work is accomplished by the vocalis. With the CT engaged, additional contraction of the vocalis results in higher FO as tension in the vocal fold cover increases. Continued contraction of the vocalis with subtle increases in CT activity lengthens the vocal folds, and increases tension of the cover further. Increased tension along with lower density results in higher frequency of vocal fold vibration. Although both the vocalis and CT are active when going from lower to higher FO, the ratio of contraction activity is greatest for the vocalis throughout most of the frequency range (Titze 1994).

When FO is near the maximum of a speaker's physiologic abilities, the perceived pitch is often described as the "**falsetto**" register. As phonation begins to near falsetto, the CT rather than the vocalis becomes increasingly active. Further contraction of the CT continues to increase vocal fold tension and thin the vocal fold cover. At very high fundamental frequencies, the vocal fold cover is mostly involved in vocal fold oscillation.

In addition to intrinsic laryngeal muscle activity, the degree of airflow from the lungs by activity in the respiratory muscles can influence fundamental frequency. As the amount of airflow from the lungs increases, FO increases. Increased respiratory flow tends to translate to increased subglottal pressure, and a near-linear relationship between subglottal pressure and FO has been described (Titze and Sundberg 1992). To control FO, coordinated activity of the vocalis, CT, and respiratory muscles is required, with the vocalis and CT influencing vocal fold tension, length, and vocal fold density and the respiratory muscles influencing the amount of air flow from the lungs.

Control of Vocal Intensity

Vocal intensity is the amount of acoustic power generated by the vibrating vocal folds, typically measured in decibels (dB). The acoustic energy produced during phonation consists of many different frequencies, both harmonic and nonharmonic. Each frequency in the spectrum of sound has a level of intensity, all of which sum together to form an average intensity for the sound wave. Vocal intensity produced at the glottal sound source during phonation is influenced by subglottal pressure, the degree of medial compression, and longitudinal tension of the vocal folds. Once acoustic energy is generated at the glottis and the acoustic sound wave begins to travel through the vocal tract, the intensity of different frequencies in the spectrum is influenced by resonance that occurs in the supraglottal space.

Subglottal pressure influences vocal intensity as well as FO. Increased subglottal pressure typically results in increased intensity (Titze and Sundberg 1992; Plant and Younger 2000). Speakers manipulate respiratory and laryngeal muscles to influence subglottal airflow and medial compression forces. For a typical speaker, greater intensity requires increased respiratory drive and/or increased contraction of the adductor muscles. Likewise, any gap along the length of the glottis can cause air leakage, which may result in loss of vocal intensity and increased breathiness.

Medial compression forces along with vocal fold tension influence the vibratory dynamics of the vocal folds. These dynamics also influence vocal intensity. When the opening phase is temporally balanced with the closing and closed phases, speakers generate greater vocal intensity compared to an imbalanced relationship, such as prolonged closed or opening phases (Sundberg et al 1993). When impairment causes glottal gaps, such as vocal fold paralysis or changes related to advancing age (e.g., presbylaryngis), the vocal folds do not close completely and there is often decreased vocal intensity.

Voice Quality

When listening to someone speaking, we process a number of features in the acoustic sound spectrum. Among these features is the linguistic message embedded in the speech sounds, the suprasegmental features embedded in the prosody of speech, and the quality of the speaker's voice. The term "**voice quality**" is somewhat ambiguous in that it can be defined in many different ways. In most contexts, voice quality refers to the auditory-perceptual awareness of acoustic features related to frequency (pitch), intensity (loudness), and **timbre** of a speaker's voice. The perception of voice quality is a psychologic process unique to each listener. However, current research suggests that most listeners use multidimensional information embedded in the acoustic spectrum when making perceptual judgments about a speaker's overall voice quality (Awan and Roy 2006; Awan et al 2009; Kreiman et al 1994).

One salient acoustic feature that most listeners can directly detect is pitch, which is the psychologic correlate of fundamental frequency. That is, as a speaker alters F0, a listener's perception of vocal pitch will also change. Experienced (e.g., adult) listeners are somewhat biased in their perception of pitch because they have a long history of experience with pitch perception. Because of this bias, listeners generally have perceptual expectations for a pitch appropriate to an individual speaker's sex and age. For example, a listener generally expects a female to exhibit a perceived pitch higher than that of a typical male speaker. When a speaker's pitch matches a listener's expectation for sex and age, the conscious perception of pitch remains in the background, and the listener typically does not actively contemplate it. If perceptual expectations are not met, however, as if a man speaks with a perceived pitch that is much higher than the typical range for adult males or if a young child speaks with an extremely low pitch, the listener's attention is drawn to that perceptual attribute.

Another salient feature related to the perception of voice quality is vocal **loudness**, which is the psychologic correlate of intensity. In typical conversation, speakers produce a vocal intensity between 65 and 75 dB. In certain contexts, such as speaking in a library or speaking over loud background noise, a listener will accept deviations from this typical range of perceived conversational loudness. However, if a speaker produces voice with an intensity that is perceived as too loud or too soft for a given context, the perception of loudness will be raised to a conscious level. It is also important to remember that sometimes a listener perceives reduced loudness not because of something wrong with the speaker, but because the listener has decreased hearing acuity.

Many features related to the perception of voice quality fall into the category of timbre. The terms "timbre" and "voice quality" are often used interchangeably. Timbre specifically concerns the attributes of sound that contribute to its unique perceptual identity distinct from pitch or loudness. As an example, if your mother or father calls you on the phone, you automatically recognize the voice based on the timbre, among other things. Timbre is influenced by a number of factors including laryngeal anatomy, physiology of phonation, anatomy of the supraglottal vocal tract, and control of resonance. The properties that influence perceptions of timbre originate at the sound source (vocal folds) but are highly influenced by the sound filter (the supraglottal vocal tract).

The perception of timbre is influenced by acoustic properties in the sound spectrum. Although F0 and average intensity are part of the spectrum and will directly influence perception of pitch and loudness, it is the intensity relationships and temporal patterns among **the harmonic frequencies** in addition to the presence of nonharmonic frequencies that influence the perception of timbre. Our understanding of how the spectrum influences perception of timbre is broadly understood, but evolving. One spectral property that has a profound effect on timbre is the presence of high-frequency nonharmonic energy. Nonharmonic energy is referred to as noise, and a little bit of noise is present in every voice. However, if high-frequency nonharmonic energy is strong (e.g., it has sufficient intensity), it competes with harmonic energy in the spectrum and is perceived as a "breathy" timbre. An extreme example of breathy voice is whispered sound production.

Temporal patterns of the spectrum also influence timbre and the overall perception of voice quality. **Phonation periodicity** refers to the regularity of vibration and the resulting acoustic spectrum over time. Voices perceived as "normal" are typically characterized by a large degree of periodicity of vibration and the acoustic spectrum. Vocal fold lesions or inappropriate use of the voice can cause disturbances to phonation periodicity. In such cases, the vibration frequency (e.g., the amount of time it takes to complete a cycle of vibration) and sound intensity generated at each cycle of vibration can vary widely from one cycle to the next. These cycle-to-cycle deviations in vibratory frequency and sound intensity are referred to as "perturbations" in phonation periodicity. When perturbation is excessive, listeners often perceive the voice as "rough." Many voice disorders cause both increased nonharmonic energy and phonation perturbations, resulting in perceived elements of breathiness and roughness in the voice. When both roughness and breathiness are present in a voice, the overall perceived quality is often referred to as "hoarse" (Watts et al 2007). Hoarseness is sometimes used, however, as a general descriptor for any voice quality that deviates from expected perceptions.

In addition to pitch, loudness, and timbre other acoustic features of voice impact a listener's perception of overall voice quality. One example is **voice breaks**, which can occur when the vocal folds temporarily fail to vibrate during the production of voiced sounds (e.g., think of the word "begin," but instead of producing /g/ the speaker produces /k/ because their vocal folds did not vibrate during that sound). Another example is **vocal tremor**, which is caused by rhythmic hyperkinetic muscular activity. This rhythmic muscular activation influences vocal fold vibration, and its effects on frequency and intensity will be embedded into the acoustic spectrum. Listeners will often perceive vocal tremor as a "shaky" aspect to the voice.

Vocal Registers

Vocal registers are perceptually distinct categories of voice quality and are typically considered in the context of the singing voice, but can relate to any form of voice production, including the speaking voice. Definitions and labels for vocal registers have varied widely over the years. A broad definition for vocal registers is a range of sequential vocal fundamental frequencies produced with the same perceived voice quality and where there is little or no overlap in F0 between contiguous registers (Colton and Hollien 1972). Although vocal registers are an overtly perceptual phenomenon, a great deal of research has focused on the physiology underlying vocal registers and the resulting acoustic spectrum, which influences vocal register perception.

The specific number and labels for registers have been debated for decades (Roubeau et al 2009). For the sake of simplicity, five different registers will be presented, organized from lowest F0 range to highest. **Pulse register** represents the lowest range of F0 that speakers can produce. Pulse register is produced by complete relaxation of the CT muscle while maximally contracting the vocalis, which has the effect of thickening the vocal fold cover (Titze 1994). With a thick cover and very little tension in the vocal ligament, the vocal folds vibrate at their lowest frequencies. When they vibrate at an F0 around 70 Hz or lower, the perception of pulse register is often referred to as **vocal fry** and, colloquially, as a "creaky" voice. It is given the name of "pulse" register because the listener is almost able to perceive the individual glottal pulses that result from phonation.

Chest register or chest voice is produced over a broad range of lower F0 and represents the typical frequency range used during speech. In the singing voice, the perception of timbre during the production of chest register is sometimes referred to as "heavy" or "rich." Chest register receives its name from the location of the sensations that singers or speakers feel when they produce this register (i.e. in the chest). Chest register is produced by coordination of CT and vocalis muscle activity, but the predominant contraction that controls F0 throughout the range of chest register frequencies is the vocalis (Titze 1994).

Head register or head voice is produced with a range of higher F0. Similar to chest voice, the name is derived from where sensations are felt during production. Listeners describe their perception of head register as "lighter" or "higher" than chest voice. To produce this register, speakers or singers coordinate contraction of the CT and vocalis, but the predominant contraction controlling vocal fold tension and frequency of vibration is the CT. Contraction of the CT has the effect of lengthening, thinning, and tensing the vocal folds, resulting in decreased vibrating mass, which oscillates at higher frequencies.

Falsetto register is the highest frequency range that an individual can produce while singing or speaking. "Falsetto" literally means "false register," and, although this label can refer to male or female voices, it is most often applied to the highest frequencies produced by males. The equivalent in females is sometimes referred to as whistle or flute register. Falsetto is produced primarily through maximal contraction of the CT without opposition from the vocalis (Titze 1994). The vocal folds approximate each other during the production of falsetto, but their medial edges are in minimal contact due to extreme lengthening and tension applied to the tissue. The amount of vocal fold mass in contact during falsetto is less than in other vocal registers, which also translates to higher degrees of transglottal airflow (Murry et al 1998).

In singing, the repertoire or style of singer may require frequencies that straddle register boundaries. Typically, when head and chest register are produced interchangeably, the perception is referred to as **mixed register**. In this register, the singer can produce higher F0 but maintain the perception of vibration or energy in the chest region. The borders of this register can be easily detected in unskilled vocalists by having them glide up from their lowest to highest frequencies. A voice break will often occur at the boundary between chest and head registers. In skilled vocalists, however, this break may be imperceptible; they can control the vocal mechanism to produce a seamless transition between chest and head register and move back and forth across different F0 values during the production of mixed register. Mixed register is produced through the dynamic interplay and coordination of the vocalis and CT muscles.

Age and Sex Differences in the Anatomy and Physiology of the Larynx

As individuals mature from childhood to adolescence to adulthood, their bodies add mass, length, and definition. The brain, organs, and glands develop into mature form through childhood to early adult-hood. This process is also true of the larynx and vocal folds. Two broad stages of laryngeal and vocal fold development can be identified to characterize age and sex differences across the lifespan: development and aging. Laryngeal and vocal fold development persists from the embryonic stage through early adulthood, when morphological characteristics of structures and tissues become stable. During mid- to late adulthood, laryngeal tissues begin to change in a complex process known colloquially as aging. Development and aging have distinct effects on vocal physiology and phonation quality.

Laryngeal growth during the prepubertal and pubertal periods is driven by hormonal influences and is linearly related to increase in body height (Kahane 1982). As laryngeal cartilages mature, they increase in height, width, and length, although their shape remains relatively stable from birth through adulthood. In a newborn, the larynx is positioned higher in the neck than in an adult and will reach final position only after puberty. Full maturity is reached around the third decade of life. At birth, the inferior portion of the larynx (i.e., the cricoid cartilage) is situated at the level of the third cervical vertebra. Prior to and during puberty, the larynx continues to descend lower into the pharynx. Once physical maturity is reached in the third decade of life, the inferior larynx is located at the level of the sixth cervical vertebra.

Other head and neck structures mature as well, including the oral and pharyngeal cavities, which influence articulation and resonance. Within the larynx, the vocal folds continue to change before, during, and after puberty through the teenage years and into early adulthood (Kahane 1982). In cadaveric studies, the vocal folds in newborns are 2.5 to 3 mm long, with no difference between males and females. In adults, vocal fold length ranges from 17 to 21 mm in males and from 11 to 15 mm in females (Hirano et al 1983). The length of newborn vocal folds as measured *in vivo* averages approximately 7.9 mm and 7.2 mm in males and females, respectively. In young adults (17 years of age), total vocal fold length is approximately 22.8 mm in males and 19.8 mm in females on average (Rogers et al 2014). The portion of the vocal fold attached to the vocal process of the arytenoid, referred to as the **cartilaginous vocal fold** (or cartilaginous glottis), is much shorter than the remainder of the vocal fold (the **membranous vocal fold**), although the length ratio of these two components remains stable throughout development (Rogers et al 2014). From pre- to postpubescence, male vocal folds increase in length by nearly double the increase in length of female vocal folds, a 63% increase in

length compared to a 34% increase, respectively (Kahane 1982).

Laryngeal cartilages also change with age. Once humans reach physical maturity, the laryngeal cartilages begin a progressive process of hardening called **endochondral ossification**; the cartilages slowly become more bonelike. The thyroid, cricoid, and arytenoid cartilages consist of hyaline cartilage, an extracellular matrix containing primarily collagen and glycosaminoglycans, in addition to chondrocytes, which are the cells that produce these extracellular matrices. In children and young adults, the hyaline cartilages of the larynx are firm, but not like bone. With age, minerals are deposited in the matrix of the cartilage as a result of cell death and repair, and these minerals eventually form bone. This process begins at the borders of laryngeal cartilages and progresses toward the centers. Interestingly, laryngeal cartilage ossification is more advanced in males (Claassen et al 2014).

Newborn infant vocal fold structure is very different from that in the adult. Overall, the vocal folds of infants are shorter, contain less mass, and are characterized by a uniform layer of lamina propria compared to the differentiated layers of adult vocal folds. The newborn lamina propria consists of a single layer, which begins to differentiate within a few months into a bilaminar structure. In the second through seventh years of life, the vocal fold lamina propria further subdivides into three layers with different cellular concentrations. At age 5, the cellular concentrations of the vocal fold emerge that distinguish the superficial, intermediate, and deep layers of lamina propria (Rogers et al 2014). Throughout childhood and into adolescence, the mature trilaminar structure of the adult vocal fold will evolve, characterized by greater concentrations of collagen in the deep lamina propria, greater concentrations of elastin in the intermediate lamina propria, and greater concentrations of ground substance with less collagen and elastin in the superficial lamina propria (Hartnick et al 2005). Elastin and collagen within the lamina propria form the vocal ligament between the ages of 1 and 4 years, with full development in the teenage years after puberty (Stemple et al 2000). The vocal fold epithelium is also thinner in infants than in adults (Boone et al 2014)

Age and Sex Differences in the Production of Voice and Voice Quality

The physical changes that occur during human development influence the physiology of phonation. As cartilages enlarge, the larynx descends, vocal fold tissue matures, nervous system motor control is refined, and the properties of vocal function change. As humans mature from adolescence into adulthood, both age and sex influence characteristics of voice production. Fundamental frequency, frequency range, and voice quality are similar for both sexes and diverge only slightly throughout the childhood years. At puberty, significant growth in respiratory, laryngeal, and upper respiratory tract structures occur, which causes a divergence in voice characteristics as a function of sex. After puberty, vocal physiology and voice quality differs between sexes. Additionally, as humans mature from adulthood to advanced age, respiratory, laryngeal, and vocal tract structures undergo another period of change, which further influences vocal physiology and voice quality.

A number of characteristics related to the physiology of phonation are affected by the sex of a speaker, although these characteristics seem to be most prominent in early and middle adulthood. The frequency of vocal fold vibration is impacted by mass, length, and tension of the vocal folds. Prior to puberty, children have shorter vocal folds with less mass, characterized by thinner vocal fold tissue that has yet to organize into a distinct five-layered structure. In both sexes, F0 decreases slowly with increasing age (Titze 1994). Through puberty and into adolescence, F0 in both males and females drops dramatically as the vocal folds mature and lengthen. Growth at puberty is more extensive in males, and as such, the F0 drops significantly more than in females. The typical adult male F0 is approximately 125 Hz, while the adult female F0 is approximately 225 Hz, although significant variability exists (Baken and Orlikoff 1999).

One way to measure phonatory physiology is to examine how the vocal folds contact each other during vibration. Phonation contact patterns can be influenced by muscular physiology and vocal fold structure among other variables, which in turn can be influenced by the sex of a speaker. Speaker sex can influence vocal fold contact patterns and the resulting acoustic spectral characteristics. The vocal folds of females tend to stay in contact with each other for shorter periods of time within a vibratory cycle (Ma and Love 2010; Awan and Awan 2013). Additionally, females' vocal folds remain open for a longer duration of time during phonation than do those of males (Hanson and Chuang 1999). As the vocal folds enter the closing phase of vocal fold vibration, female vocal folds approximate each other in a more linear fashion from bottom to top than male vocal folds do (Titze 1989). Structurally, a more persistent posterior glottal gap during the closed phase of vibration has been described in females, and traditionally it has been considered a normal variation (Linville 1992). However, these differences should always be interpreted with caution, as the imaging methods that have been used to describe these differences often employ imaging modalities that include the insertion of an endoscope in the mouth with the tongue held and protruded anteriorly, which in itself can change phonatory dynamics. There may also exist functional differences in closure patterns related to cultural standards, gender-related expectations for voice quality, and even personality differences across speakers.

These physiological and structural differences between male and female vocal folds influence phonation quality. In prepubescent children, parameters such as frequency, intensity, and other spectral characteristics of voice do not reliably predict perceptions of speaker sex. In adults, differences in voice quality evolve that signal the sex of a speaker. In addition to differences in F0, females tend to produce voice with increased spectral noise (nonharmonic frequencies) that is perceived as more "breathy" than that of males (Klatt and Klatt 1990). Female speakers also produce vocalizations during connected speech that are softer (lower intensity) than those of male speakers.

◼ Measurement of Laryngeal Function

The anatomy and physiology underlying laryngeal function during phonation has been measured for various purposes utilizing many different modalities. Reasons for the measurement of laryngeal function include the need to obtain diagnostic information related to laryngeal impairment, to further knowledge regarding laryngeal function for scientific discovery, and to measure outcomes following treatment.

Auditory-Perceptual Analysis

Auditory perceptual analysis relies on the human auditory system to make judgments about perceptual dimensions of voice quality. This type of analysis requires a listener to hear a live or recorded speaker produce different utterances and rate various characteristics of voice based on perceptions of how those characteristics compare with an internal representation of a "normal" voice. The most common characteristics measured using auditory-perceptual analysis include pitch, loudness, breathiness, roughness, and overall severity of dysphonia.

Auditory-perceptual judgments of phonation are often used to characterize a deviation in voice quality. For example, speakers will often seek treatment for a voice problem after noticing an auditory-perceptual change in their voice quality. Additionally, a voice that is severely dysphonic will often be identified as perceptually different from normal by most listeners. However, the degree of dysphonia perceived by different listeners can vary widely, which is an inherent limitation of these measurements.

Perceptual ratings of voice quality exhibit large degrees of variability, both between and within listeners. This variability challenges the reliability of auditory-perceptual measurements. Tools have been developed to create a more structured and guided method for auditory-perceptual ratings. One such tool is the Consensus Auditory Perceptual Evaluation of Voice (CAPE-V), developed by a committee of clinical and scientific experts in vocal function and validated in subsequent research (Zraick et al 2011). This tool, illustrated in **Fig. 11.31**, rates five primary perceptual dimensions (roughness, breathiness, strain, pitch, and loudness) and the overall perceptual dysphonic severity along a 100-mm visual analog scale. These dimensions represent the most salient deviant characteristics in the majority of individuals with dysphonia. To use the tool, a listener places a tick mark along the scale representing the perceived degree of deviation from an idealized "normal" voice, which would be located on the far left of the scale. Any deviation from normal would result in a tick along the scale toward the right. The perceived difference from normal is then measured in millimeters by measuring the distance between the tick mark and the left side of the line.

Aerodynamic Analysis

Phonation is the result of aerodynamic forces that produce audible acoustic energy via modulation of airflow by the vocal folds. Changes in the aerodynamic properties of flow and pressure are often present after laryngeal pathology or when physiologic imbalances in the respiratory or laryngeal systems have occurred. From a clinical perspective, quantification of the aerodynamic forces underlying phonation provides important information that can be used to improve diagnostic precision, inform treatment planning, provide a means of biofeedback during treatment, and enable the measurement of treatment outcomes (Baken and Orlikoff 1999).

Concensus Auditory-Perceptual Evaluation of Voice (CAPE-V)

Vocal Tasks

- Sustained vowels
  - /a/
  - /i/
- Six sentences
  - The blue spot is on the key again.
  - How Hard did he hit him?
  - We were away a year ago.
  - We eat eggs every Easter.
  - My mama makes lemon muffins.
  - Peter will keep at the peak.
- Spontaneous speech

Perceptual Domains - 100 mm scale

- Overall severity
- Roughness
- Breathiness
- Strain
- Pitch
- Loudness

Fig. 11.31 Examples of rigid and flexible endoscopes used for laryngoscopy.

Aerodynamic measurements of laryngeal function include the parameters of volume, flow, pressure, and vocal efficiency. Two measurements often used to assess air volume for voice and speech include **vital capacity** (VC) and **phonation volume**. Vital capacity is a measure of the maximum amount of air that can be expelled from the lungs after a maximum inhalation and represents the amount of air available for phonation. Vital capacity is influenced by a number of factors including sex, age, and height as well as health conditions that restrict lung capacity. Normal values for healthy adults range between 3 and 5 L. Vital capacity is lower in children because of decreased lung size.

Phonation volume is related to vital capacity but represents the available amount of air used during phonation (typically measured during the production of a sustained vowel). It is measured using a spirometer in a similar manner as vital capacity. In addition to sex, age, height, and conditions that alter lung function, phonation volume can be impacted by laryngeal disorders, whereas vital capacity is typically not affected. Phonation volume is usually lower than vital capacity for the simple reason that during voice production, not all of the available air is used for vocal fold vibration. Between 45 and 90% of vital capacity is employed during sustained phonation, and much less is used during conversational speech (Yanagihara and Koike 1967; Rau and Beckett 1984; Baken and Orlikoff, 1999).

Measurements of airflow are used to quantify how efficiently the vocal folds valve air from the lungs during phonation. In the context of phonation, airflow represents the volume of air that flows through the glottis across a specific period of time. Airflow is measured in liters per second (L/s) or milliliters per second (mL/s). Airflows are typically higher in individuals with incomplete glottal closure and lower in individuals with hyperfunctional closure of the glottis during phonation.

Phonation quotient (PQ) has been used to assess airflow in normal and dysphonic speakers. Phonation quotient is derived by dividing vital capacity by maximum phonation time (VC/MPT), which is acquired by using a timer to measure the maximum amount of time a speaker can prolong a vowel sound. Similar to airflow, phonation quotient is expressed in L/s or mL/s. Phonation quotient is higher in males than in females, approximately 135 mL/s and 125 mL/s, respectively. Phonation quotient is sensitive to laryngeal disease, as increased values are often measured in individuals with voice disorders (Iwata and von Leden 1970). Using phonation quotient, clinicians can calculate another measurement called **estimated mean flow rate** (EMFR), which predicts airflow rate measurements. The formula for calculating EMFR is 77 + (0.236 × PQ), which results in measurements that are lower than the original PQ but correlate well with direct measures of airflow during phonation (Rau and Beckett, 1984).

At the onset of phonation, the narrowing glottis increases subglottal pressure. Subglottal pressure is important, as it represents the aerodynamic energy required to initiate vocal fold oscillation. **Pressure** is the force applied per unit area that acts perpendicular to that area (Baken and Orlikoff 1999). Most applications for clinical voice evaluation measure air pressure in centimeters of water (cm H_2O). Adducted vocal folds block the flow of subglottal air by sealing the larynx in a horizontal plane. The subglottal pressure presents a force distributed across the vocal fold tissue, which eventually separates the vocal folds in the vertical plane (inferior to superior) to initiate the opening phase of vocal fold vibration.

Phonation threshold pressure (PTP) represents the absolute minimum amount of pressure needed to set the vocal folds into oscillation, and it is known to be increased in many voice disorders. To measure PTP, speakers are instructed to produce voice at their minimum intensity level, just above a whisper. Measurement of pressure during voicing and speech is influenced by many factors including fundamental frequency and vocal intensity. In general, speakers who exhibit hyperfunctional closure during voice production exhibit increased subglottal pressure, as increased pressure is required

to overcome the resistance at the level of the vocal folds. Conversely, speakers with incomplete glottal closure also present with increased subglottal pressure, but for a different reason. In these cases, greater pressures are needed to set flaccid or incompletely adducted vocal folds into motion.

Voicing efficiency is another aerodynamic measurement that provides important clinical information. Voicing efficiency (also called "vocal efficiency") represents the amount of work required to convert aerodynamic energy into acoustic energy. These measures can also be thought of as indices of how efficiently the vocal folds control aerodynamic energy. Voicing efficiency can be measured in many different ways; one measure of voicing efficiency compares the measured subglottal pressure and transglottal airflow as a function of sound intensity (Zraick et al 2012). PQ has also been used as a measure of voicing efficiency, as it represents the ratio of available air to the duration over which the air is utilized for phonation.

Additional measures that have been used as representations of voicing efficiency include maximum phonation time (MPT) and **s/z ratio**. The s/z ratio compares the maximum sustained duration of an unvoiced sound /s/ to a voiced sound /z/. In theory, individuals with altered vocal fold anatomy or physiology have more difficulty sustaining /z/, as it requires vocal fold vibration to control the aerodynamic energy, whereas the /s/ does not. Some studies have found the s/z ratio to be a valid predictor of vocal fold lesions (Eckel and Boone 1981). Advantages and limitations exist for all aerodynamic measures (Baken and Orlikoff 1999). To date, no individual measure or set of aerodynamic measures has been demonstrated to be clinically more important or more cost-effective than others.

Acoustic Analysis

The end product of phonation is acoustic energy. Acoustic energy created during phonation consists of a series of pressure waves that travel out of the mouth and/or nose and radiate through air within the immediate surrounding environment. Because phonation results in a complex sound wave, the acoustic energy patterns resulting from phonation are characterized by many different frequencies, each possessing a certain amplitude or sound pressure. The relationships between the frequencies in the sound wave and their respective amplitudes influence not only the identity of the sound (e.g., whether it was an /u/ or an /a/ sound) but also sound quality.

The acoustic wave produced during phonation is influenced by many factors, including the health of the vocal folds and how the speaker controls the respiratory and laryngeal muscles during voice production. Acoustic measures have been used as indirect measures of phonatory physiology. By studying the frequency and amplitude characteristics of the radiated sound wave, a number of inferences can be made regarding how phonation is controlled and whether vocal fold lesions may be altering phonatory physiology.

Sound waves are captured using a recording device, typically a microphone that transduces the acoustic energy into electrical energy, which is then converted into a digital signal. Digital sound files are representations of the original analog signal that code the instantaneous amplitude values of the sound wave over time, measured at very short intervals, in digital form (e.g., as a series of binary numbers). **Fig. 11.29** shows a computer display of the sound waveform with time on the X-axis and sound amplitude (in dB) on the Y-axis.

From the digital waveform, F0 can be calculated by measuring the period of vibration. The period (P) is the amount of time for the vocal folds to complete one cycle of vibration. Because F0 is measured in Hz (cycles per second), knowing the vibration period allows calculation of F0 using the formula: F0 = 1/P. In **Fig. 11.29**, the period of vibration, particularly in the top panel, is clearly discernable for each cycle and can be measured in time along the X-axis. F0 is measured as the average rate of vocal fold vibration across a specific time duration. Measurement of F0 is an important clinical measure because it is affected by laryngeal impairment. Additionally, speech-language pathologists are often interested in the range of F0 that a speaker can produce. This measurement is referred to as the **physiologic voice range** and is also significantly affected by altered vocal fold anatomy and physiology. Specifically, most voice disorders are associated with a reduced physiologic voice range. A speaker with a healthy vocal mechanism should produce a frequency range of at least two octaves or 24 semitones.

Recall that **Fig. 11.29** shows sound amplitude along the Y-axis. The overall average amplitude can be derived from the average amplitude of each vibratory cycle. This measure is referred to as "**vocal intensity**" or "**sound intensity**," and its perceptual correlate is loudness. Sound amplitude is also a clinically relevant measure, as it is affected by many voice disorders. For example, presbylaryngis, or changes in voice due to aging, can result in glottal insufficiency. Glottal insufficiency typically results in the perception of reduced loudness, which can be quantified by measuring vocal intensity.

Acoustic analysis also allows the acquisition of measurements that are used to infer vibratory dynamics and the degree of glottal closure. Vibratory dynamics include the regularity or **periodicity** of vocal fold vibration. If vocal fold vibration is periodic or quasiperiodic, the period of vibration and amplitude of vibration from one cycle to the next should be similar. In fact, in voices that are perceived as "normal," cycle-to-cycle frequency and amplitude characteristics are very similar; notice in the top panel of **Fig. 11.29** how each vibratory cycle closely resembles the one before it and after it, both in period of vibration and in amplitude. However, if the period of vibration or amplitude of vibration varies widely from one cycle to the next, vibration is aperiodic and perceived as roughness, breathiness, or hoarseness. Decreased periodicity can be appreciated in the bottom panel of **Fig. 11.29**, particularly in the last few vibratory cycles.

When vibration periodicity is altered, it is said to be "perturbed." Perturbation is some change in the behavior of a physical system. Subtle changes in phonation frequency and amplitude from cycle to cycle are referred to as measures of **frequency perturbation** (also known as "**jitter**") and **amplitude perturbation** (also known as "**shimmer**"), respectively. Frequency and amplitude perturbations are normal; every voice is characterized by small fluctuations in frequency and amplitude from cycle to cycle. These small perturbations are largely imperceptible. Voice disorders can increase frequency and amplitude perturbations. For example, in a perceptually rough voice, increased measures of jitter and shimmer are common.

Frequency and amplitude perturbations can be measured from the acoustic waveform and plotted as a function of time, referred to as the "time domain." Additionally, **spectral acoustic analyses** can be performed using the sound spectrum. The acoustic sound spectrum for any sound is acquired by processing frequency components and amplitudes of those frequencies at a specific point in time. The visual graph is often referred to as an "amplitude spectrum," with amplitude on the Y-axis and frequency on the X-axis. **Fig. 11.28** is an example of an acoustic spectrum for a vowel sound; this type of display is said to be in the "frequency domain."

Nonharmonic frequencies are also referred to as "noise," and measures of spectral tilt, which compute a ratio of the average low-frequency energy to the average high-frequency energy, are known as measures of **harmonics-to-noise ratio**. In healthy normal voices, this ratio is large, but in many dysphonic voices, this ratio is smaller.

Endoscopic Analysis

Endoscopy consists of procedures that enable visualization inside the body (*endo* = inside, and *-scopy* = observation). The instruments used to perform these procedures are called **endoscopes**, and they can be rigid or can be made flexible to enter curved passages within the body, as shown in **Fig. 11.31**. Otolaryngologists and speech-language pathologists perform a type of endoscopy called **laryngoscopy** or **indirect laryngoscopy** using a rigid endoscope, a flexible endoscope, or simply a mirror that reflects an indirect, reversed image of the larynx. Otolaryngologists perform **direct laryngoscopy** in an operating room with the patient positioned supine, using a special type of rigid **laryngoscope** placed into the patient's mouth. The physician can obtain a direct line-of-sight view of the larynx and vocal folds. A microscope is attached to enable close inspection of the vocal folds during a procedure called **microlaryngoscopy**.

Indirect laryngoscopy can be performed in an office setting. Rigid endoscopes are placed into the mouth, as shown in **Fig. 11.32**, in the area of the oropharynx where the endoscope tip has an unobstructed view of the larynx below. If a flexible endoscope is used, it is passed through the nasal cavity into the region of the nasopharynx for laryngeal visualization. Observations of the larynx using either rigid or flexible endoscopes can be performed using two different light sources: constant and stroboscopic light. Constant light allows the assessment of laryngeal appearance including color, structure, and gross movement. In a normal healthy larynx, the color of laryngeal tissues should be light pink (as opposed to red, when they are inflamed) and the vocal fold tissue pearly white. The laryngeal structures should be shaped appropriately and free of any lesions. The arytenoid cartilages should adduct and abduct, and the vocal folds should lengthen with increased pitch.

Stroboscopic light is used to view vibratory dynamics during phonation. This procedure is sometimes referred to as **laryngeal videostroboscopy**. Because the vocal folds vibrate at rates faster than the visual system can process, a strobe light is used to create a visual illusion of continuous vibration. In actuality, the strobe light is timed to flash slightly slower or slightly faster than the patient's F0 such that the endoscope lens reflects images that occur in successive vibratory cycles rather than a single cycle. The visual system processes these images as occurring continuously rather than discretely, and the examiner can observe characteristics of the various phases of vibration. Under stroboscopic light, five main vibratory characteristics are often evaluated:

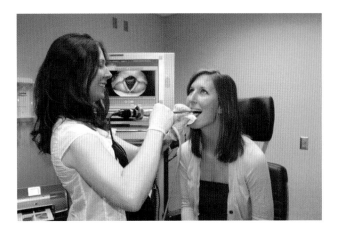

Fig. 11.32 Indirect laryngoscopy performed using a rigid endoscope.

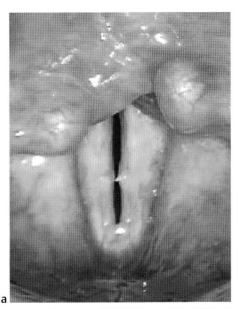

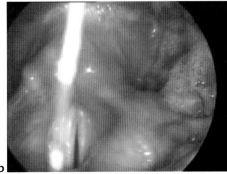

Fig. 11.33 (a, b) Images obtained using laryngeal videostroboscopy showing an hourglass closure pattern in a patient with vocal fold nodules.

- Symmetry: the degree to which the left and right vocal folds mirror one another as they move away and return to midline
- Amplitude: the degree to which the left and right vocal folds are displaced from midline during the opening phase of vibration
- Periodicity: the regularity of vibration across successive vibratory cycles
- Mucosal wave: the vibratory characteristics of the vocal fold cover, which is displaced from inferior to superior and then across the horizontal surface of each vocal fold, from medial to lateral, during a cycle of vibration
- Closure: the degree to which the vocal folds approximate each other

Vocal fold lesions result in unique patterns of vibratory dynamics, and laryngeal videostroboscopy is a powerful diagnostic tool. For example, vocal fold nodules often cause an hourglass closure pattern during phonation, as shown in **Fig. 11.33**.

■ References

Awan SN, Awan JA. The effect of gender on measures of electroglottographic contact quotient. *Journal of Voice, 27,* 433–440; 2013

Awan SN, Roy N. Toward the development of an objective index of dysphonia severity: a four-factor acoustic model. *Clinical Linguistics & Phonetics, 20,* 35–49; 2006

Awan SN, Roy N, Dromey C. Estimating dysphonia severity in continuous speech: application of a multi-parameter spectral/cepstral model. *Clinical Linguistics & Phonetics, 23,* 825–841; 2009

Baken RJ, Orlikoff RL. Clinical Measurement of Speech and Voice, 2nd ed. San Diego, CA: Cengage Learning; 1999

Boone DR, McFarlane SC, Von Berg SL, Zraick RI. The Voice and Voice Therapy, 9th ed. Washington, DC: Pearson Higher Education; 2014

Claassen H, Schicht M, Sel S, Paulsen F. Special pattern of endochondral ossification in human laryngeal cartilages: X-ray and light-microscopic studies on thyroid cartilage. *Clinical Anatomy, 27,* 423–430; 2014

Colton RH, Hollien H. Phonational range in the modal and falsetto registers. *Journal of Speech and Hearing Research, 15,* 708–713; 1972

Eckel FC, Boone DR. The s/z ratio as an indicator of laryngeal pathology. *Journal of Speech and Hearing Disorders, 46,* 147–149; 1981.

Fant G. Acoustic Theory of Speech Production. The Hague, Netherlands: Mouton; 1960

Gawlikowska-Sroka A, Miklaszewska D, Dzieciolowska-Baran E, Kamienska E, Sroczynski T, Poziomkowska-Gesicka I. Changes of laryngeal parameters during intrauterine life. *European Journal of Medical Research, 15 Suppl 2,* 41–45; 2010

Gray SD. Cellular physiology of the vocal folds. *Otolaryngologic Clinics of North America, 33,* 679–698; 2000

Hanson HM, Chuang ES. Glottal characteristics of male speakers: acoustic correlates and comparison with female data. *Journal of the Acoustical Society of America, 106,* 1064–1077; 1999.

Happak W, Zrunek M, Pechmann U, Streinzer W.. Comparative histochemistry of human and sheep laryngeal muscles. *Acta Oto-Laryngologica 107,* 283–288; 1989

Hartnick CJ, Rehbar R, Prasad V. Development and maturation of the pediatric human vocal fold lamina propria. *Laryngoscope, 115,* 4–15; 2005

Hirano M. Clinical Examination of Voice. New York, NY: Springer-Verlag; 1981

Hirano M, Kurita S, Nakashima T. Growth, development, and aging of human vocal folds. In: Abbs J, ed. Vocal Fold Physiology. San Diego, CA: College Hill Press; 1983, 23–43

Iwata S, von Leden H. Phonation quotient in patients with laryngeal diseases. *Folia Phoniatrica, 22,* 117–128; 1970

Jürgens U, Zwirner P. The role of the periaqueductal grey in limbic and neocortical vocal fold control. *Neuroreport, 7,* 2921–2923; 1996

Kahane JC. Growth of the human prepubertal and pubertal larynx. *Journal of Speech and Hearing Research, 25,* 446–455; 1982

Khosla S, Murugappan S, Paniello R, Ying J, Gutmark E. Role of vortices in voice production: normal versus asymmetric tension. *Laryngoscope, 119,* 216–221; 2009

Klatt DH, Klatt LC. Analysis, synthesis, and perception of voice quality variations among female and male talkers. *Journal of the Acoustical Society of America, 87,* 820–857; 1990.

Kreiman J, Gerratt BR, Berke GS. The multidimensional nature of pathologic vocal quality. *Journal of the Acoustical Society of America, 96,* 1291–1302; 1994

Leydon C, Sivasankar M, Falciglia DL, Atkins C, and Fisher KV. Vocal fold surface hydration: a review. *Journal of Voice, 23,* 658–665; 2009

Linville SE. Glottal gap configurations in two age groups of women. *Journal of Speech and Hearing Research, 35,* 1209–1215; 1992

Liu H, Auger J, Larson CR. Voice fundamental frequency modulates vocal response to pitch perturbations during English speech. *Journal of the Acoustical Society of America, 127,* EL1–EL5; 2010

Ma EP, Love AL. Electroglottographic evaluation of age and gender effects during sustained phonation and connected speech. *Journal of Voice, 24,* 146–152; 2010

Murry T, Xu JJ, Woodson GE. Glottal configuration associated with fundamental frequency and vocal register. *Journal of Voice, 12,* 44–49; 1998

Plant RL, Younger RM. The interrelationship of subglottic air pressure, fundamental frequency, and vocal intensity during speech. *Journal of Voice, 14,* 170–177; 2000

Rau D, Beckett RL. Aerodynamic assessment of vocal function using hand-held spirometers. *Journal of Speech and Hearing Disorders, 49,* 183–188; 1984

Reidenbach MM. The cricoarytenoid ligament: its morphology and possible implications for vocal cord movements. *Surgical and Radiologic Anatomy, 17,* 307–310; 1995

Rogers DJ, Setlur J, Raol N, Maurer R, Hartnick CJ. Evaluation of true vocal fold growth as a function of age. *Otolaryngology—Head and Neck Surgery, 151,* 681–686; 2014

Roubeau B, Henrich N, Castellengo M. Laryngeal vibratory mechanisms: the notion of vocal register revisited. *Journal of Voice, 23,* 425–438; 2009

Schuenke M, Schulte E, Schumacher U, eds. Thieme Atlas of Anatomy, Volume 1. General Anatomy and Musculoskeletal System, 2nd ed. New York: Thieme; 2015

Simonyan K, Saad ZS, Loucks TM, Poletto CJ, Ludlow CL. Functional neuroanatomy of human voluntary cough and sniff production. *Neuroimage, 37,* 401–409; 2007

Smitheran JR, Hixon TJ. A clinical method for estimating laryngeal airway resistance during vowel production. *Journal of Speech and Hearing Research, 36,* 138–146; 1981

Stemple J, Glaze LE, Gerdeman BK. Clinical Voice Pathology: Theory and Management, 3rd ed. San Diego, CA: Cengage Learning; 2000.

Story BH, Titze IR. Voice simulation with a body-cover model of the vocal folds. *Journal of the Acoustical Society of America, 97,* 1249–1260; 1995

Sundberg J, Titze I, Scherer R. Phonatory control in male singing: a study of the effects of subglottal pressure, fundamental frequency, and mode of phonation on the voice source. *Journal of Voice, 7,* 15–29; 1993

Titze IR. Physiologic and acoustic differences between male and female voices. *Journal of the Acoustical Society of America, 85,* 1699–1707; 1989.

Titze IR. Principles of Voice Production. Upper Saddle River, NJ: Prentice-Hall; 1994

Titze IR. The human instrument. *Scientific American, 298,* 94–101; 2008a

Titze IR. Nonlinear source-filter coupling in phonation: theory. *Journal of the Acoustical Society of America 123,* 2733–2749; 2008b

Titze IR, Sundberg J. Vocal intensity in speakers and singers. *Journal of the Acoustical Society of America, 91,* 2936–2945; 1992.

van den Berg J. Myoelastic-aerodynamic theory of voice production. *Journal of Speech and Hearing Research, 1,* 227–244; 1958

Van der Merwe A. A theoretical framework for the characterization of pathological speech sensorimotor control. In: McNeil MR (ed.), Clinical Management of Sensorimotor Speech Disorders. New York, NY: Thieme; 1997

Watts CR, Awan SN, Marler JA. An investigation of voice quality in individuals with inherited elastin gene abnormalities. *Clinical Linguistics & Phonetics, 22,* 199–213; 2008

Wu YZ, Crumley RL, Armstrong WB, Caiozzo VJ. New perspectives about human laryngeal muscle: single-fiber analyses and interspecies comparisons. *Archives of Otolaryngology—Head & Neck Surgery, 126,* 857–864; 2000

Yanagihara N, Koike Y. The regulation of sustained phonation. *Folia Phoniatrica, 19,* 1–18; 1967

Zraick RI, Kempster GB, Connor NP, et al. Establishing validity of the Consensus Auditory-Perceptual Evaluation of Voice (CAPE-V). *American Journal of Speech-Language Pathology, 20,* 14–22; 2011

Zraick RI, Smith-Olinde L, Schotts LL. Adult normative data for the KayPentax phonatory aerodynamic system model 6600. *Journal of Voice, 26,* 164–176; 2012

■ Suggested Readings

Aronson AE, Bless D. Clinical Voice Disorders. New York, NY: Thieme; 2009

Baken RJ, Orlikoff RL. Clinical Measurement of Speech and Voice, 2nd ed. San Diego, CA: Cengage Learning; 1999

Kendall KA, Leonard RJ. Laryngeal Evaluation. New York, NY: Thieme; 2010

Koyama T, Kawasaki M, Ogura JH. Mechanics of voice production. I. Regulation of vocal intensity. *Laryngoscope, 79,* 337–354; 1969

Koyama T, Harvey JE, Ogura JH. Mechanics of voice production. II. Regulation of pitch. *Laryngoscope, 81,* 45–65; 1971

Kreiman J, Gerratt BR. Sources of listener disagreement in voice quality assessment. *Journal of the Acoustical Society of America, 108,* 1867–1876; 2000

Ludlow CL. Central nervous system control of the laryngeal muscles in humans. *Respiratory Physiology & Neurobiology, 147,* 205–222; 2005

Titze IR. Principles of Voice Production. Upper Saddle River, NJ: Prentice-Hall; 1994

■ Study Questions

1. Which of the following is a nonbiologic function of the larynx?

A. Impounding air to fixate the thorax
B. Acting as a valve for respiration
C. Serving as a vibratory source for voice production
D. Creating subglottal pressure to generate a cough
E. All of the above

2. Which cartilage serves as the anterior attachment for the vocal folds?

A. Thyroid
B. Arytenoid
C. Cricoid
D. Epiglottis
E. None of the above

3. Which cartilage serves as the posterior attachment for the vocal folds?

A. Thyroid
B. Arytenoid
C. Cricoid
D. Epiglottis
E. Only C and E

4. The vocal folds consist of a layered structure, functionally divided into the cover, vocal ligament, and body. Which layers make up the vocal ligament?

A. Epithelium and superficial lamina propria
B. Intermediate and deep lamina propria
C. Deep lamina propria and vocalis muscle
D. Vocalis muscle and epithelium
E. None of the above

5. Which of the following muscles adduct (close) the vocal folds?

A. Posterior cricoarytenoid and interarytenoid
B. Lateral cricoarytenoid, interarytenoid, and thyroarytenoid (vocalis)
C. Lateral cricoarytenoid, interarytenoid, and thyroarytenoid (muscularis)
D. Posterior cricoarytenoid, lateral cricoarytenoid, and interarytenoid
E. Interarytenoid and thyrohyoid

6. Which of the following muscles is a tensor of the vocal folds?

A. Cricothyroid
B. Posterior cricoarytenoid
C. Lateral cricoarytenoid
D. Interarytenoid
E. None of the above

7. Which of the following helps to sustain vocal fold vibration during phonation?

A. Nasal resonance
B. Intraglottal vortices
C. Voice quality
D. The epiglottis
E. Lung capacity

8. What is fundamental frequency?

A. The highest frequency an individual is able to produce
B. The range of frequencies fundamental to the larynx
C. The basic frequency someone is able to perceive
D. The lowest frequency produced by a vibrating object
E. All of the above

9. What unit of measurement is used to quantify frequency?

A. Decibels
B. Milliliters
C. Hertz
D. Amperes
E. Centimeters

10. Aperiodicity, or irregularity, of vocal fold vibration will often be perceived as:

A. Roughness
B. Breathiness
C. Loud voice
D. Soft voice
E. Old voice

11. Which of the following is the primary sensory nerve for the larynx?

A. The pharyngeal branch of the vagus nerve (CN X)
B. The recurrent laryngeal branch of the vagus nerve (CN X)
C. The internal branch of the superior laryngeal nerve (of the vagus)
D. The external branch of the superior laryngeal nerve (of the vagus)
E. The glossopharyngeal nerve

12. True or False: The layered structure of the vocal folds is fully developed at birth.

13. Which of the following areas in the central nervous system drives emotional vocal responses?

A. Broca area
B. Periaqueductal gray matter
C. Nucleus ambiguus
D. Occipital lobe
E. The basal ganglia

14. Which of the following are suprahyoid muscles that elevate the larynx?

A. Omohyoid and thyrohyoid
B. Thyrohyoid and sternothyroid
C. Geniohyoid and mylohyoid
D. Digastric and sternothyroid
E. Diaphragm and external intercostals

15. The opening into the larynx, which is the space encircled by the aryepiglottic folds, is known as the:

A. Laryngeal valve
B. Laryngeal vestibule
C. Laryngeal hole
D. Trachea
E. Diaphragm

16. The space in-between the left and right true vocal folds is known as the:

A. Glottis
B. Trachea
C. Larynx
D. Vestibule
E. Ventricle

17. Supraglottal pressures are generated by manipulations in the vocal tract and act as a force on the vocal folds that influences vibration. This force is called:

A. Resonance
B. Frequency
C. Pitch
D. Inertive reactance
E. None of the above

18. Which of the following is the psychologic correlate of frequency?

A. Loudness
B. Quality
C. Pitch
D. Intensity
E. Timbre

19. Which of the following individuals would have the lowest natural fundamental frequency?

A. Male children
B. Male adults
C. Female children
D. Female adults
E. All would be the same

20. The larynx is suspended from ligaments and membranes attached to a bone, called the:

A. Hyoid bone
B. Temporal bone
C. Laryngeal bone
D. Frontal bone
E. Posterior bone

■ Answers to Study Questions

1. The correct answer is (C). The nonbiologic function of the larynx relates to voice production for communication purposes. It is considered an "overlaid" or secondary function of the larynx and is not necessary for survival. Although communication without a voice can be difficult, many other means of communication exist and are used on a daily basis.

   The other answers are incorrect because impounding air (A), respiration (B), and cough (D) are all biologic functions needed for survival. They are needed to function during daily life activities.

2. The correct answer is (A). The vocal folds attach anteriorly to the thyroid cartilage and posteriorly to the arytenoid cartilages. Anterior movement of the thyroid cartilage will cause the vocal folds to elongate with increased tension.

   (B) is incorrect because the vocal folds attach to the arytenoids posteriorly. (C) is incorrect because, while the cricoid cartilage can change the length of the vocal folds, they are not directly attached to it. (D) is incorrect because the epiglottis lies above the vocal folds.

3. The correct answer is (B). The vocal folds attach to the arytenoids posteriorly at the vocal process. Lateral and medial movements of the vocal process will cause the vocal folds to abduct and adduct, respectively.

   (A) is incorrect because the vocal folds attach to the thyroid anteriorly. (C) is incorrect because, while the cricoid cartilage can change the length of the vocal folds, they are not directly attached to it. (D) is incorrect because the epiglottis lies above the vocal folds.

4. The correct answer is (B). The intermediate and deep layers of the lamina propria collectively form the vocal ligament. The vocal ligament serves to connect the vocal fold cover to the body, in addition to absorbing physical stress caused by manipulations to vocal fold length and tension.

   The other answer choices are incorrect because the epithelium and superficial lamina propria make up the vocal fold cover (A, D). The vocalis muscle (C, D) is considered the body of the vocal fold and is connected to the cover by the vocal ligament.

5. The correct answer is (C). Contraction of the LCA, IA, and TA (muscularis) will move the vocal process medially, causing the vocal folds to adduct. The number of motor units recruited in each muscle during contraction will determine the degree of medial compression during vocal fold closure. Medial compression is one factor that can influence subglottal pressure during phonation.

   The other answer choices are incorrect. The posterior cricoarytenoid muscle is an abductor of the vocal folds (A, D). The thyrohyoid is an extrinsic laryngeal muscle that affects vertical position, not the position of the glottis (E). The TA (vocalis) adjusts the tension on the vocal folds; it does not adduct them. The only three muscles that actively adduct the vocal folds are the lateral cricoarytenoid, interarytenoid, and thyroarytenoid.

6. The correct answer is (A). The cricothyroid and thyroarytenoid (vocalis) serve as vocal fold tensors. A dynamic interplay between these muscles allows a speaker or singer to adjust fundamental frequency to produce speech prosody and the various transitions between musical notes.

   The other answer choices are incorrect. The posterior cricoarytenoid is an abductor of the vocal folds (B). The lateral cricoarytenoid is an adductor of the vocal folds (C). The interarytenoid is an adductor of the vocal folds (D). Both the cricothyroid and thyroarytenoid can be considered vocal fold adductors.

7. The correct answer is (B). Intraglottal vortices occur as the superior edges of the vocal folds separate during the opening phase of vocal fold vibration (e.g., during a divergent glottis). These "whirlwinds" create focal points of extreme negative pressure, which will assist in closing the superior edges during the subsequent closing phase of vibration.

   The other answer choices are incorrect. Nasal resonance affects speech quality and may influence inertive reactance, but its relationship to sustained vibration is less clear (B). Voice quality is a product of vocal fold vibration, not an influence on vocal fold vibration (C). The epiglottis does not actively influence vocal fold vibration, although it can absorb sound and act as a resonator of sound energy (D). Lung capacity determines the amount of air available to power the vocal folds, but does not directly cause sustained vocal fold vibration (E).

8. The correct answer is (D). Phonation results in acoustic energy characterized by a spectrum of sound. This sound spectrum consists of the amplitude at a fundamental frequency, amplitudes at integer multiples of the fundamental, called harmonics, and amplitudes at nonharmonic frequencies (noise). The lowest frequency and, in most cases, the frequency with the strongest amplitude is the fundamental.

The other answer choices are incorrect. The highest and lowest frequencies an individual is able to produce are often referred to as the "physiological frequency range" (A). The "range" of frequencies encompasses all of the different notes an individual is able to produce (B). The perception of frequency is known as "pitch" and is a psychological phenomenon, whereas frequency is a physical phenomenon that can be objectively measured (C).

9. The correct answer is (C). Hertz (Hz) is a measurement of cycles per second. For example, adult male vocal folds vibrate at a lower frequency than adult female vocal folds, which translates to male vocal folds completing fewer cycles per second (fewer hertz) than adult female vocal folds.

The other answer choices are incorrect. The decibel is a unit of measurement for sound intensity (A). Milliliters are a measurement of volume (B). Amperes are a measurement of electric current (D). Centimeters are a measurement of length (E).

10. The correct answer is (A). The perception of roughness is associated with an acoustic spectrum characterized by irregularity. The physiologic correlate of this spectral irregularity is aperiodic cycles of vibration, where the frequency and intensity of successive vibratory cycles are very different.

The other answer choices are incorrect. Perceptions of breathiness are typically related to glottal insufficiency, which allows too much air to escape during phonation (B). A loud voice is perceived as exactly that: too loud, resulting from excessive sound intensity (C). A soft voice is perceived as exactly that: too soft, resulting from insufficient sound intensity (D). An "old" voice is often perceived when a combination of factors are present, including glottal insufficiency resulting in breathiness and low volume, in addition to increased vibratory perturbation (E).

11. The correct answer is (C). The vagus nerve (CN X) has numerous branches, including the pharyngeal branch, the recurrent laryngeal nerve, and the superior laryngeal nerve. The superior laryngeal nerve itself branches into the external division and internal division. The internal branch of the superior laryngeal nerve provides the sensory receptors to the mucosa throughout the laryngeal region.

The other answer choices are incorrect. The pharyngeal branch of the vagus nerve (CN X) supplies motor innervation to the region of the velum (A). The recurrent laryngeal branch supplies motor innervation to all intrinsic laryngeal muscles except the cricothyroid (B). The external branch of the superior laryngeal nerve supplies motor innervation to the cricothyroid muscle (D). The glossopharyngeal nerve forms part of the pharyngeal plexus, which provides motor and sensory innervation to the oropharyngeal region (E).

12. The correct answer is False. Newborns possess a homogenous vocal fold structure that begins to differentiate during infancy and continues through the teenage years. A mature, multilayered vocal fold structure is not present until early adulthood.

13. The correct answer is (B). The periaqueductal gray matter is intimately linked to the limbic system in the central nervous system. The networks of the limbic system regulate emotional responses to environmental stimuli.

The other answer choices are incorrect. The Broca area is responsible for volitional expression of language (A). The nucleus ambiguus contains the cell bodies of the peripheral vagus nerve and would be influenced by activity in the periaqueductal gray matter (C). The occipital lobe is primarily involved in visual functions (D). The basal ganglia are part of the extrapyramidal control circuits but do not directly drive emotional vocal responses (E).

14. The correct answer is (C). The geniohyoid and mylohyoid originate at the inner surface of the mandible, attaching to the hyoid bone inferiorly. When they contract, their muscle fibers shorten, raising the hyoid bone. As the hyoid bone elevates, it also raises the larynx, which is suspended from the hyoid bone by membranes and ligaments.

The other answer choices are incorrect. The omohyoid is an extrinsic laryngeal depressor (A). The thyrohyoid muscle has its point of origin below the hyoid, but it can act as a depressor or elevator depending on the action of other muscles (A, B). The digastric muscle is a laryngeal elevator, but the sternothyroid is a laryngeal depressor (D). The diaphragm and external intercostal muscles are active during inspiration and do not manipulate laryngeal position (E).

15. The correct answer is (B). A vestibule is an opening to a space. The most superior region of the larynx is surrounded by the epiglottis and aryepiglottic folds. These encircle an open space, called the laryngeal vestibule, which effectively serves as the superior opening to the larynx.

The other answer choices are incorrect. The term "laryngeal valve" refers to the valving function of the larynx for respiration (A). The term "laryngeal hole" is rarely, if ever, applied to the larynx (C). The trachea is located inferior to the larynx (D). The diaphragm is inferior to the larynx and is a muscle of respiration (E).

16. The correct answer is (A). The glottis is the space between the vocal folds. Muscular action can serve to open the glottis or close the glottis. A patient with vocal fold paralysis that impairs the ability to close the vocal folds is said to have "glottal insufficiency."

The other answer choices are incorrect. The trachea is located inferior to the larynx (B). The larynx houses the two vocal folds (C). The (laryngeal) vestibule is the opening to the larynx (D). The (laryngeal) ventricles are located superior to the vocal folds, and are positioned in between the true and false vocal folds (E).

17. The correct answer is (D). When the anterior vocal tract is narrowed and the regions above the vocal folds are widened, it creates a backward directed pressure and impedance matching of intraglottal and supraglottal resistance, via a physical phenomenon known as inertive reactance. Inertive reactance serves to help separate the vocal folds during vibration and also amplify the resulting acoustic energy.

The other answer choices are incorrect. Resonance is the selective amplification and filtering of specific frequencies within the acoustic sound spectrum (A). Frequency is the rate of vibration of an object, and is not a pressure or force (B). Pitch is the psychologic correlate of frequency, not a force (C).

18. The correct answer is (C). Pitch and loudness are the psychologic correlates of frequency and intensity, respectively. The perception of pitch is not perfectly linear: higher frequencies will require a larger separation before a listener will perceive two different pitches. Pitch is experienced by a listener, while frequency is a physical phenomenon that can be objectively measured.

The other answer choices are incorrect. Loudness is the psychologic correlate of sound intensity (A). Voice quality is a perceptual phenomenon that is influenced by many factors, not only frequency (B). Intensity refers to sound power, not frequency (D). Timbre is another term for quality and is a perceptual phenomenon (E).

19. The correct answer is (B). Adult male vocal folds manifest greater mass than female vocal folds. Objects with greater mass will vibrate at lower frequencies than those with less mass.

The other answer choices are incorrect. Male children and female children often manifest similar fundamental frequencies until they reach puberty (A, C). Female adults typically manifest the highest fundamental frequency, due in part to smaller and thinner tissue, which vibrates at faster rates (D).

20. The correct answer is (A). The larynx is suspended from the hyoid bone. As the hyoid elevates and depresses, the larynx will move with it. Laryngeal position is thought to be important for efficient voice production because it can affect the flexibility and efficiency of the intrinsic laryngeal muscles during phonation.

The other answer choices are incorrect. The temporal bone is located superior to the larynx but is part of the skull (B). There is no such bone called the "laryngeal bone" (C). The frontal bone is part of the skull and is not connected to the larynx (D). The "posterior bone" does not exist (E).

12

Articulation and Resonance

Kate Bunton and Jessica E. Huber

■ Chapter Summary

The study of the anatomy and physiology of articulation and resonance is essential to the understanding of speech production and swallowing function. The purpose of this chapter is to present the skeletal and muscular anatomy of the articulatory and resonance systems along with the physiology of these structures for articulation and resonance. Specifically, we will (1) describe the structure and location of bones, muscles, and nerves in the articulatory and resonance systems, (2) present the dynamic physiologic processes involved in articulation and resonance, (3) introduce the source-filter theory of speech production, the concepts of coordinated articulation, and mechanisms of feedback in the articulatory system, and (4) highlight techniques used to study articulation and resonance.

■ Learning Objectives

- Understand the anatomy and physiology of the articulatory and resonance systems
- Describe the anatomic structures supporting articulation and resonance and their specific contributions to the physiology of speech production

■ Putting It Into Practice

- Speech production is an amazingly complex process in which rapid, precise movements of the larynx, tongue, jaw, lips, and velum are orchestrated to modify the shape of the airspace called the vocal tract. These movements produce a continuous flow of distinct sounds recognized as speech.
- Speech-language pathologists should have a working knowledge of the role of specific skeletal and muscular structures that make up the articulation and resonance systems to understand speech production difficulties and recognize the underlying structural contributions to these deficits.
- The study of anatomy and physiology of the articulatory and resonance systems provides the speech-language pathologist with the knowledge necessary to identify disorders related to articulation and resonance and to make evidence-based treatment decisions regarding habilitation.

■ Introduction

The act of producing speech is an extremely complex task. We produce speech at a rate of approximately 175 words per minute. We produce ~ 20 speech sounds per second. To produce speech at such a rapid rate, the structures of the vocal tract move in synchrony, which involves coordination of hundreds of neural impulses and muscle contractions. Speech production, for most, is automatic and effortless, yet the complexity of speech production can be fully appreciated only through careful examination of the underlying mechanisms involved in producing speech.

Articulation is defined as the act of moving various parts of the vocal tract to produce different sounds. As you learned in the preceding chapters, the respiratory and phonatory systems work together to produce sound. These sounds vary in intensity and frequency but cannot be recognized as speech without a vocal tract. It is the adjustments to the shape and subsequent modifications of the acoustic properties of the vocal tract that shape these sounds into recognizable speech. The anatomic structures within the vocal tract that transform these sounds into speech are collectively referred to as the articulatory and **resonance** systems.

This chapter begins with an introduction to the gross anatomy of the vocal tract, followed by a discussion of the skeletal structures in the head and neck important for speech production, the anatomic location and action of key muscles, and discussion of the importance of each articulator in speech production. Anatomic and physiologic changes in the vocal tract from infancy to adulthood are also highlighted. Finally, a brief overview of the various measurement approaches used to study speech production and a discussion of coordinated articulation are provided.

posteriorly. The **oral cavity** is also oriented horizontally. The oral cavity extends from the lips anteriorly to the palatoglossal arches posteriorly, and from the hard and soft palate superiorly to the tongue inferiorly. The **pharyngeal cavity** is vertically oriented and extends from the base of skull to the superior border of the cricoid cartilage of the larynx. The pharyngeal cavity can be divided into three sections: the **nasopharynx**, **oropharynx**, and **laryngopharynx**. The **velopharyngeal port** divides the nasopharynx from the oropharynx. The division between the oropharynx and the laryngopharynx is at the level of the base of the tongue and epiglottis.

The nasal cavity includes the nose and two chambers separated at the midline by the nasal septum. Each chamber contains a number of important landmarks that will be discussed later in the chapter, including the superior, middle and inferior **conchae** and corresponding **meatuses** (also called nasal passages). The oral cavity has several anatomical structures and landmarks (**Fig. 12.2**) including the lips, teeth, **alveolar ridge**, hard palate, soft palate (or velum), uvula, tongue, and **mandible** (lower jaw). Each of these structures is described in detail in subsequent sections. The pharyngeal cavity is unremarkable in terms of anatomical structures and landmarks but is an intricate and complex network of muscles. With the oral and nasal cavities oriented horizontally and the pharyngeal cavity oriented vertically, the human vocal tract resembles a capital

■ Anatomy of the Articulatory/Resonance System

Three primary cavities form the vocal tract: the nasal, oral, and pharyngeal cavities (**Fig. 12.1**). The **nasal cavity** runs horizontally from the nostrils anteriorly to the uppermost portion of the pharynx

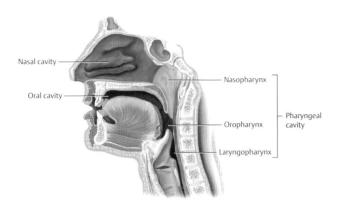

Fig. 12.1 Organization of the vocal tract, midsagittal section, left lateral view.

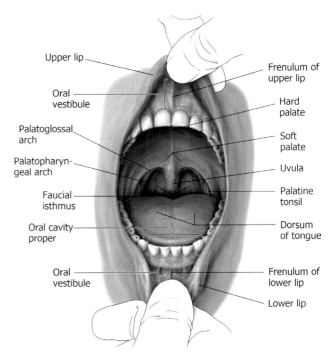

Fig. 12.2 Oral cavity.

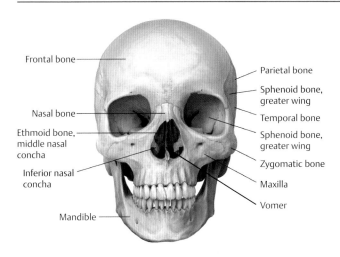

Fig. 12.3   Cranial bones, anterior view.

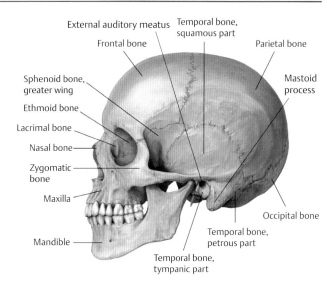

Fig. 12.4   Lateral view of the cranial bones.

F. In an adult male, the distance between the vocal folds and the lips is approximately 17 cm (Story et al 1996), and the length of the oral cavity and pharyngeal cavity are roughly equal for an adult male (Vorperian et al 2009). The adult female vocal tract is shorter, at 12 cm (Story et al 1998; Story 2005), with about 60% of the length in the oral cavity and 40% in the pharyngeal cavity (Vorperian et al 2009).

Eight primary articulators produce changes in the shape of the vocal tract. Some of the articulators are *mobile,* meaning that they can be moved by muscle contraction; they include the lips, velum, tongue, mandible, and pharynx. The remaining articulators are *immobile* and include the teeth, alveolar ridge, and hard palate. The *immobile* articulators are important because they represent a point of contact for other articulators. In producing speech, we move a mobile articulator to make contact with or approximate another articulator, which can be mobile or immobile.

Bones of the Neurocranium and Viscerocranium

As you learned in **Chapter 1**, the neurocranium (or simply cranium) includes eight bones (**Fig. 12.3**, **Fig. 12.4**): the unpaired ethmoid, sphenoid, **frontal**, and occipital bones and paired parietal and temporal bones. The viscerocranium or facial skeleton consists of fourteen bones (**Fig. 12.3**, **Fig. 12.4**): the unpaired mandible and **vomer** and paired **maxilla**; nasal, **palatine**, lacrimal, and **zygomatic bones**; and inferior nasal conchae. Finally, six miscellaneous bones are housed in the temporal bone, three tiny bones on each side, critical for hearing: the incus, malleus, and stapes. These bones are discussed in detail in **Chapter 13**. Some anatomists include the hyoid bone under the miscellaneous category,

as it is more closely related to the tongue than to the larynx. However, because the hyoid bone does not articulate directly with any other bones of the skull, it is not included here. Additional information about the hyoid bone can be found in **Chapter 11**.

The gross anatomy of the skull reveals several landmarks. The orbits of the eyes, or eye sockets, are prominent cavities where the eyeballs reside. The orbits are not a single bone but instead are composed of parts of the ethmoid, frontal, lacrimal, maxillary, palatine, sphenoid, and zygomatic bones (**Fig. 12.5**). The nasal cavity is divided by a vertical partition of bone. This partition is called the bony nasal septum and is made up of two bones: the ethmoid bone (specifically, the perpendicular plate) and the vomer. Along the edge of the nasal cavity are three scrolls of bone known as the nasal conchae (or turbinates). The upper two conchae (superior and medial) are part of the ethmoid bone, while the inferior nasal concha is an independent bone.

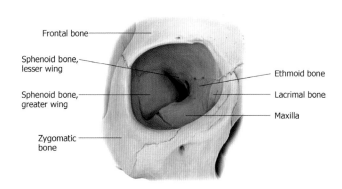

Fig. 12.5   Bones of the right orbit.

On the exterior of the skull you will notice several landmarks: the **frons** (forehead), **occiput** (posteriormost portion of the skull) and **vertex** (superior tip of the skull). Along the sides of the skull, where the viscerocranium ends and the neurocranium begins, are depressions called **temporal fossae**; in this area, commonly referred to as the temples, the external form of the head is defined by soft tissue structures that overlie the skull. Just lateral to and below each orbit is a prominent bone structure called the **zygomatic arch**, often referred to as the cheekbone (**Fig. 12.4**). The zygomatic arch is not a singular bone but rather is formed by parts of two bones: temporal and zygomatic.

On each side of the skull, immediately posterior to where the mandible articulates with the skull, is a small opening. This opening is the bony **external auditory meatus** (**Fig. 12.4**), the opening of the ear. Immediately posterior and inferior to the external auditory meatus is a rounded protuberance called the **mastoid process** (**Fig. 12.4**). Medial to the external auditory meatus on the inferior surface of the skull is a sharp bone projection known as the **styloid process**. On the midline at the base of skull is a large hole, the **foramen magnum**, through which the spinal cord passes (**Fig. 12.6**).

Facial Bones

Mandible

The mandible is a singular bone that makes up the lower jaw (**Fig. 12.7**). It begins as a paired bone but fuses at the midline during embryonic development. Several landmarks are of interest on both the inner and outer surfaces of the mandible. Starting with the outer surface, the point of fusion of the right and left halves is the **mental symphysis**, marking the midline of the mandible. Inferior to the mental symphysis is the **mental protuberance**, and inferior and lateral to the protuberance are the **mental tubercles**, the prominences in the bone of the mandible that form the chin ("mental" in all these names comes from the Latin word *mentum*, "chin," not *mens* "mind"). Lateral to the tubercle on either side is the **mental foramen**, the opening through which the mental nerve, arising from the mandibular branch of the trigeminal nerve (CN V_3), passes. On the internal surface (**Fig. 12.8**), the mylohyoid line, the attachment point for the mylohyoid muscle, is visible. The **mandibular foramen** is also visible; it is the opening to the canal through which the mental nerve, arising from the mandibular branch of the trigeminal nerve, travels on its way to the mental foramen. The lateral portion of the mandible is referred to as the **corpus** (**Fig. 12.7**) or body. In a healthy mandible, the teeth are located on the upper surface of the corpus on the alveolar arch. The mandibular **ramus** on either side rises at an angle of approximately 90° from the corpus. The area where the corpus and ramus are joined is the **angle** of the mandible, forming the angle of the lower jaw. The **coronoid process** on the anterior side of the top of the ramus is an important muscle attachment point. On the posterior side of the top of the ramus, the prominent head of the **condylar process** articulates with the temporal bone of the skull, permitting rotation of the mandible. This joint is referred to as the **temporomandibular joint (TMJ)**. The anterior surface of the condylar process also marks the point of attachment of the **lateral pterygoid** muscle. The condylar and coronoid processes are separated by the mandibular notch.

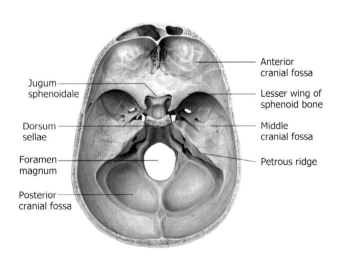

Fig. 12.6   Interior of the base of skull.

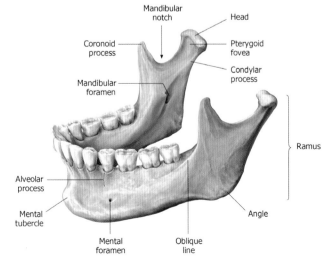

Fig. 12.7   Mandible.

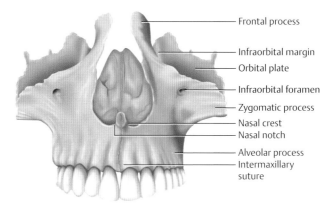

Fig. 12.9   Maxilla, anterior view.

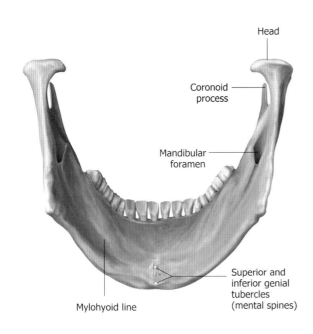

Fig. 12.8   Mandible, posterior view.

Maxillae

The paired **maxillae** (singular, maxilla), or maxillary bones, make up the upper jaw. These bones make up most of the roof of the mouth (hard palate), nose, and upper dental ridge. The maxilla articulates with nine other bones (**Fig. 12.3**) including the ethmoid bone, frontal bone, inferior nasal concha, lacrimal bone, nasal bone, palatine bone, vomer, zygomatic bone, and opposite maxilla. There are a number of significant landmarks on the maxilla, which are logically named. For example, the frontal process of the maxilla articulates with the frontal bone.

The anterior view of the maxilla can be seen in **Fig. 12.9**. The first significant landmark is the frontal process. The frontal process is the most superior point of the maxilla. This process can be felt by placing your finger at the nasal side of your eye and feeling for the infraorbital margin from there to the lower midpoint of the eye. The orbital surface of the maxilla projects into your eye socket and provides support for your eyeball (**Fig. 12.5**). Just inferior to the orbit is the **infraorbital foramen**, the opening for the infraorbital nerve, arising from the maxillary branch of the trigeminal nerve (CN V_2). This nerve provides sensory innervation for the lower eyelid, upper lip, and nasal alae (lateral sides of the nostril). The lateral margin of the orbit consists of the zygomatic process of the maxillary bone, which articulates with the zygomatic bone to form the zygomatic arch. The anterior nasal spine

(nasal crest) is at the midline of the maxilla. Lateral to the nasal spine on the right and left is the nasal notch. The alveolar ridge is the part of the maxilla that holds the teeth in a healthy adult.

If the left and right maxillae are disarticulated to view the medial portion (**Fig. 12.10**), the maxillary sinus, palatine process, and inner margin of the alveolar process can be seen. **Fig. 12.11** shows the inferior view of the maxillae. The left and right palatine processes of the maxillae articulate at the **intermaxillary suture,** also known as the median palatine suture. This suture marks the point of a **cleft** of the hard palate. The palatine process makes up three-fourths of the hard palate, with the other one-fourth being the horizontal plate of the palatine bone. The **transverse palatine suture** marks the location where the palatine processes of the maxillae join with the horizontal plates of the palatine bones.

The incisive foramen in the anterior aspect of the hard palate serves as an opening for the nasopalatine nerve innervating the nasal mucosa. The **premaxilla** is defined by the area anterior to the premaxillary suture to the incisive foramen and alveolar process (**Fig. 12.11**). The premaxilla is difficult to see in an adult skull, but it is an important landmark because a cleft of the lip occurs at this location and may include the lip, alveolar bone, and the region of the premaxillary suture. A cleft can be unilateral or bilateral, but in virtually all cases it will occur at this suture.

Nasal Bones

The nasal bones (**Fig. 12.3**) are small and make up the superior nasal surface. The nasal bones articulate with the frontal bones superiorly, the maxillae laterally, the perpendicular plate of the ethmoid bone medially, and the nasal septal cartilage.

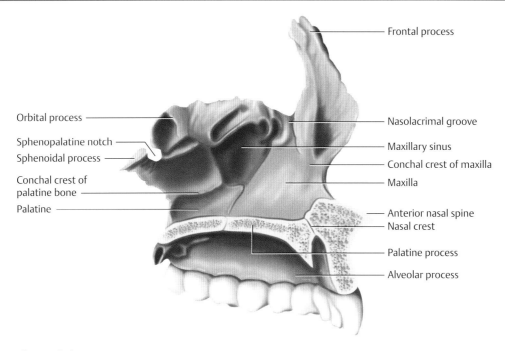

Fig. 12.10   Maxilla, medial view.

Palatine Bones and Inferior Nasal Conchae

As discussed previously, the posterior one-fourth of the hard palate is made up of the horizontal plate of the palatine bone (**Fig. 12.11**). In the ventral view, the articulated palatine bones parallel the nasal cavity, defined by the maxillae. The posterior nasal spine and nasal crest provide midline correlates to the anterior nasal spine and nasal crest of the maxilla, and the horizontal plate parallels the palatine processes of the maxillae. In the lateral view, the perpendicular plate makes up the posterior wall of the nasal cavity. The orbital process makes up a small portion of the orbital wall. The

Box 12.1   Cleft Lip and Palate

Cleft lip and cleft palate are congenital anomalies of the mouth and lip that occur in the first 3 months of pregnancy. They are the second most common birth defect in the United States, affecting one in 700 infants. Cleft lip and palate are caused by an interaction between genetic and environmental factors. In cleft lip, the two sides of the lip do not fuse together as they should during fetal development about 5 or 6 weeks into pregnancy. With cleft palate, the roof of the mouth fails to form completely around 8 to 12 weeks into pregnancy. A child may be born with a cleft lip, a cleft palate, or both a cleft lip and cleft palate. Cleft lip alone does not cause speech problems. The hard and soft palate separate the mouth from the nose. Typical development of the hard and soft palate coupled with the muscular closure of the velopharyngeal port enable us to achieve appropriate oral/nasal resonance during speech production. A child born with a cleft palate, however, is unable to close off the nasal cavity for speech production. Prior to surgical palatal repair, children will vocalize using primarily nasalized vowels and consonants that sound like /m/ or /n/. Following repair, children may still have difficulty building oral pressure for plosive and fricative sounds. Many children require secondary surgery to assist in closure of the velopharyngeal port for speech. For some of these children, even the secondary surgery is not successful in providing adequate velopharyngeal port closure. In those cases, a prosthesis called a palatal obturator can be used. The palatal obturator is attached to the upper teeth, much like an orthodontic retainer. It runs along the hard palate and has a bulb on the end in the area of the velopharyngeal port. The bulb is raised into the velopharyngeal port, and the children use the existing muscles and tissue to close the velopharyngeal port around the bulb. Because cleft palate can cause changes to the development of the bony structure of the face, some children with cleft palate require surgery to move the maxilla anteriorly to provide a more typical face shape. The speech-language pathologist will work together with the parents of these children to encourage vocalizations and provide cues about place and manner of production to help the child develop a full repertoire of speech sounds.

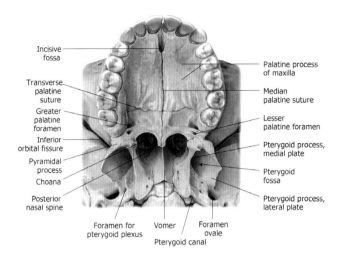

Fig. 12.11 Hard palate, inferior view.

inferior nasal conchae (singular, concha) are small, scroll-like bones that articulate with the maxilla, palatine, and ethmoid bones (**Fig. 12.3**). The middle and upper nasal conchae, processes of the ethmoid bone, are superior correlates of the inferior concha, all of which have important function in mammals. The mucosal lining covering the nasal conchae is the thickest anywhere in the nose and has a rich vascular supply. Air passing over the nasal conchae is warmed and humidified before reaching the delicate tissues of the respiratory system.

Vomer

The vomer (**Fig. 12.3**) is a singular bone located at the midline that makes up the inferior and posterior part of the nasal septum. The nasal septum divides the two nasal cavities. The vomer has the appearance of a knife blade with its point aimed toward the front. It joins the sphenoid rostrum and the perpendicular plate of the ethmoid bone at its posterosuperior margin and with the maxillae and palate bones at its inferior margin. The posterior **ala** of the vomer marks the midline boundary of the nasal cavities. The complete nasal septum consists of the perpendicular plate of the ethmoid, the vomer, and the septal cartilage.

Zygomatic Bone

The zygomatic bone is the prominent structure we identify as the cheekbone (**Fig. 12.4**). The zygomatic bone articulates with the maxilla, frontal bone, and sphenoid bone (although the latter articulation is not visible on the external surface of the facial

skeleton), which make up the lateral orbit, and with the temporal bone.

At the base of the orbital margin is the maxillary process, the point where the maxilla and zygomatic bones meet. The temporal process is seen laterally as the zygomatic bones project posteriorly, forming half of the zygomatic arch, a bridge over the temporal fossa. The zygomatic arch consists of two parts: the temporal process of the zygomatic bone and the zygomatic process of the temporal bone. The frontal process of the zygomatic bone articulates with the frontal and sphenoid bones.

Lacrimal Bones

The small lacrimal bones are almost completely hidden inside the skull. They articulate with the maxillae, frontal bone, nasal bone, and inferior conchae and make up a small portion of the lateral nasal wall and the medial orbit (**Fig. 12.5**).

Hyoid Bone

The hyoid bone is discussed in detail in **Chapter 11** because of its biomechanical linkage with the larynx, but it rightfully belongs in this chapter as well, as it serves as the point of attachment for muscles of the tongue and jaw. The role of the hyoid bone as an anchor point for articulatory and phonatory muscles demonstrates the interconnectedness of the phonatory and articulatory systems.

Cranial Bones

Frontal Bone

The frontal bone is a single bone that makes up the bony forehead, anterior cranial case, and supraorbital region (**Fig. 12.3**, **Fig. 12.4**). Near the middle of the skull, the coronal suture marks the point of articulation of the frontal and parietal bones. The frontal bone also articulates with the zygomatic bones, nasal bones, lacrimal bones, ethmoid bone, and sphenoid bone. The portion of the frontal bone in the orbital region creates the superior surface of the orbit.

Parietal Bones

The paired parietal bones overlie the parietal lobes of the cerebrum and form the middle portion of the braincase. These bones join at the midline by the sagittal suture, which runs from the frontal bone to the occipital bone (**Fig. 12.4**). The parietal bones

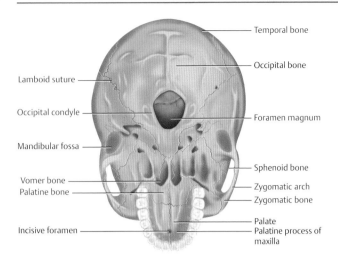

Fig. 12.12   Occipital bone.

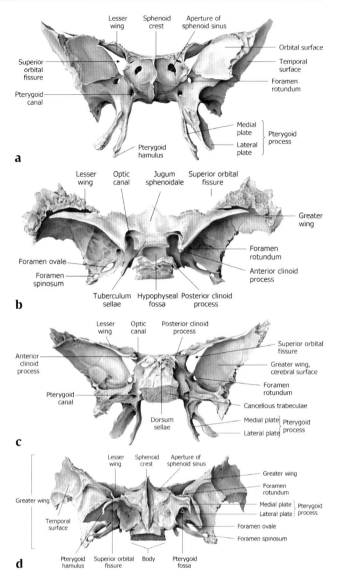

Fig. 12.13   Sphenoid bone. (a) Anterior view, (b) superior view, (c) posterior view, (d) inferior view.

are separated from the occipital bone by the lambdoid suture. The squamosal suture forms the union between parietal and temporal bones and marks the lateral margin of the parietal bone.

Occipital Bone

The unpaired occipital bone overlies the occipital lobe of the brain and makes up the posterior braincase (**Fig. 12.4**). It articulates with the temporal, parietal, and sphenoid bones. The basilar aspect of the occipital bone articulates with the corpus of the sphenoid. The external occipital protuberance is a posterior midline prominence. The most significant landmarks of the occipital bone are visible inferiorly (**Fig.12.12**). The occipital bone forms the base of the skull, with the foramen magnum providing the opening for the spinal cord and the beginning of the medulla oblongata. The condyles mark the resting point for the first cervical vertebra.

Temporal Bone

The temporal bone can be found on the lateral skull, separated from the parietal bone by the squamosal suture and from the occipital bone by the occipitomastoid suture (**Fig. 12.4**). The temporal bone is extremely dense and can be divided into four segments: the squamous, tympanic, mastoid, and petrous portions. The squamous portion, which borders the squamosal suture, is fan-shaped and thin. The inferior margin includes the roof of the external auditory meatus and the middle ear. Anteriorly, the zygomatic process arises from the squamous portion, articulating with the temporal process of the zygomatic bone to form the zygomatic arch. Inferior to the base of the zygomatic process is the

mandibular fossa of the temporal bone, with which the condyloid process of the mandible articulates to form the temporomandibular joint. The tympanic portion includes the anterior and inferior walls of the external auditory meatus. The prominent styloid process protrudes inferior to the external auditory meatus and medial to the mastoid process. A small opening between the mastoid and styloid processes, called the stylomastoid foramen, is the opening where the motor portion of the facial nerve (CN VII) passes on its way to the facial muscles. The petrous portion of the temporal bone includes the cochlea and semicircular canals. The medial surface of the petrous portion contains the internal auditory meatus, through which the vestibulocochlear nerve (CN VIII) passes on its way to the brainstem.

The mastoid portion makes up the posterior part of the temporal bone. Air cells in the mastoid portion communicate with the tympanic **antrum**.

The temporal fossa is a region that includes a portion of the temporal, parietal, sphenoid, and frontal bones. This entire region marks the point of origin of the fan-shaped **temporalis** muscle.

Sphenoid Bone

The sphenoid bone is a complex single bone, consisting of a corpus and three pairs of processes: the greater wings, lesser wings, and pterygoid processes. The sphenoid also contains numerous **foramina** (openings) through which nerves and blood vessels pass. The sphenoid bone can be seen from four different views in **Fig. 12.13**.

The lesser and greater wings of the sphenoid are striking landmarks, as they look like the wings of a bat. The lesser wings arise from the corpus and partially cover the **optic canal**. The greater wings arise from the posterior corpus, making up a portion of the orbit. The greater wings form a portion of the anterolateral skull and articulate with the frontal and temporal bones.

Projecting inferiorly from the greater wing and corpus are the lateral and medial pterygoid plates. The scaphoid fossa between the medial and lateral plates is the attachment point for one of the muscles of mastication (**medial pterygoid** muscle) and the **tensor veli palatini** muscle. A hamulus (hook) projects from the medial lamina, and the tendon of the tensor veli palatini passes around the hamulus on its course to the soft palate. The openings of the superior sphenoid are particularly important. For example, the optic canal carries the optic nerve (CN II), and the **foramen ovale** provides the opening for the mandibular branch of the trigeminal nerve (CN V_3). The maxillary branch of the trigeminal nerve (CN V_2) passes through the **foramen rotundum**, and the **superior orbital fissure** carries the oculomotor nerve (CN III), the trochlear nerve (CN IV), several branches of the ophthalmic branch of the trigeminal nerve (CN V_1), and the abducens nerve (CN VI). The body of the sphenoid includes the anteriorly placed **jugum** and the **chiasmic groove** that accommodates the optic chiasm, the optic nerve after it has left the optic canal on its way from the eye.

Ethmoid Bone

The ethmoid bone is a complex, delicate bone housed entirely within the space of the cranial, nasal, and orbital areas (**Fig. 12.14**). When viewed anteriorly,

the superior surface is dominated by the **crista galli** protruding into the cranial space. The perpendicular plate projects inferiorly and makes up the superior part of the nasal septum. The middle and superior nasal conchae are also part of the ethmoid bone, located lateral to this plate within each nasal cavity. On both sides of the perpendicular plate and perpendicular to it are the cribriform plates. The cribriform plates separate the nasal and cranial cavities and provide openings for the olfactory nerve fibers as they enter the cranial space. The very thin lateral orbital plates articulate with the frontal bone, lacrimal bone, and maxilla to form the medial orbit.

Nose and Nasal Cavities

The nose is defined as the prominent organ in the center of the face. The upper part constitutes the organ of smell, and the lower part the beginning of the respiratory tract, in which the air is warmed, moistened, and cleaned. Terms used to describe the gross anatomy of the nose include the tip (apex); the base,

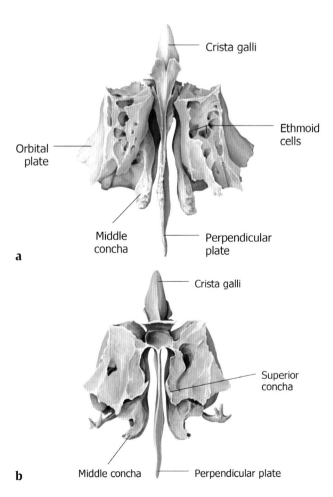

Fig. 12.14 Ethmoid bone, **(a)** anterior and **(b)** posterior.

which includes the nostrils (nares); the root, where the nasal bones join the frontal bone; the dorsum (located between the root and the tip); and the bridge (the upper part of the dorsum). Only the bridge of the nose has a bony framework. The inferior two-thirds have a strong cartilaginous framework (**Fig. 12.15**).

The cartilages of the nose include the septal, lateral, and major and minor alar cartilages (**Fig. 12.15**). The major alar cartilage forms much of the tip of the nose, with the smaller minor alar cartilages, located lateral to the major alae, contributing to the shape of the nose. The division of the base into two separate nostrils is completed by part of the septal cartilage. The lateral nasal cartilages are located in the middle third of the nose, between the nasal bones superiorly and the major alar cartilages inferiorly.

Two narrow, approximately symmetrical chambers in the nose are separated by the nasal septum. The nasal vestibule is a slight dilation just inside the opening of the nostril. The nasal cavities communicate with the outside by way of the nostrils (nares) and with the nasopharynx by way of the **choanae**. The lateral walls of the nasal cavities are composed of the superior, middle, and inferior nasal conchae, and their corresponding nasal passages or **meatuses**, which are named for their overlying conchae (**Fig. 12.16**). This labyrinthine structure greatly increases the surface area of the

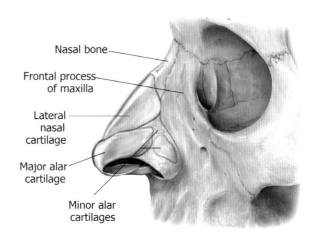

Fig. 12.15   Skeleton of the nose.

nasal cavities, which is critical for managing temperature and humidity and filtering particles out of incoming air.

The lateral walls of the nasal cavities also contain a number of **orifices** (openings) through which the nasal cavities communicate with the **paranasal sinuses**:

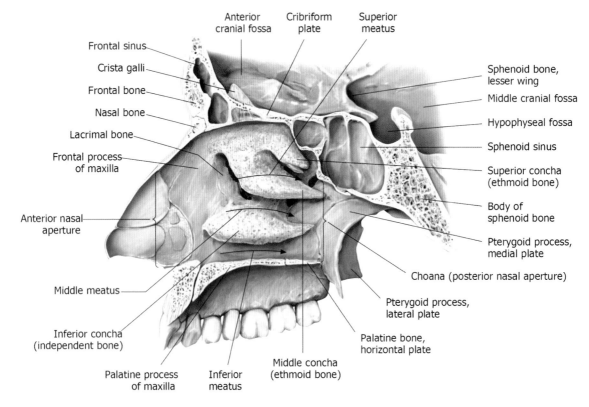

Fig. 12.16   Lateral wall of the right nasal cavity.

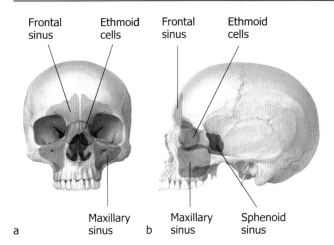

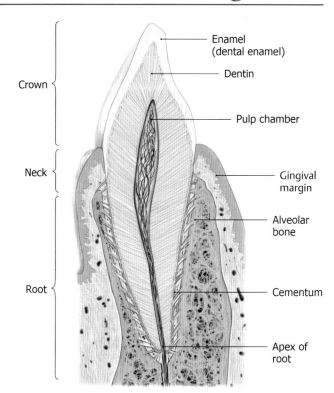

Fig. 12.17 Projection of the paranasal sinuses onto the skull; **(a)** frontal view; **(b)** lateral view.

Fig. 12.18 Histology of a tooth.

five paired sets of cavities, lined with a mucosal tissue that secretes fluid to keep them moist, which normally drain into the nasal cavity. The sinuses include the sphenoid sinus, frontal sinus, anterior ethmoidal air cells, middle ethmoidal air cells, and maxillary sinus (**Fig. 12.17**). One other structure empties into the nasal cavity: the **nasolacrimal duct**, close to the anterior portion of the nasal cavity. This duct is the reason crying makes the nose run; the nasolacrimal duct carries away tears from the eyes.

Teeth

The teeth, housed within the alveoli of the mandible and maxilla, serve both biologic and nonbiologic functions. Biologically, the teeth are essential for chewing, and thus a precursor of the digestive process (see **Chapter 14**). Nonbiologic functions include a contribution to the structure of the face as well as normal speech production. The teeth are particularly important for the production of some consonants, for example /f, v, θ, ð/, but also play an important role in the production of almost all sounds, including vowels.

Humans develop two sets of teeth during their life. The first set, called primary (also referred to as deciduous, temporary, milk, or baby teeth), consists of 20 teeth and develops early in childhood. Eruption of the second set, called permanent teeth, occurs during late childhood, resulting in a full complement of 32 teeth. These teeth are maintained throughout the lifespan, except for disease, infection, or damage.

The tooth is divided into three parts: a crown, a root, and a neck (**Fig. 12.18**). The crown is the part of the tooth that protrudes from the gums (gingivae) into the oral cavity and is covered by **enamel**,

which is the surface you brush every day. The root comprises about two-thirds of the tooth and resides below the surface of the gums, or **gingival margin**. The root is much softer than the crown and is covered by **cementum**. The neck is an ill-defined region at the transition between the enamel-covered crown and the cementum-covered root.

There are four general types of teeth: **incisors, canines, premolars,** and **molars** (**Fig. 12.19**). The incisors are the eight teeth in the front and center of the oral cavity; four upper and four lower. These incisors are typically the first primary teeth to erupt in children, at around 6 months of age. They are replaced by permanent teeth between 6 and 8 years of age. The four canines are the sharpest teeth and appear between 16 and 20 months of age, with the upper canines preceding the lower canines. For permanent teeth, the order is reversed—the lower canines erupt around age 9, and the upper canines erupt between 11 and 12 years of age. In the permanent teeth, four premolars, or bicuspids, are located on each side of the mouth: two on the upper and two on the lower jaw. There are no premolars in the primary set. The first premolars appear around age 10 and the second premolars a year later. The molars are the largest teeth and are located most posteriorly. There are eight molars in the primary teeth (four upper, four lower) and twelve in the

Primary vs. Permanent teeth eruption

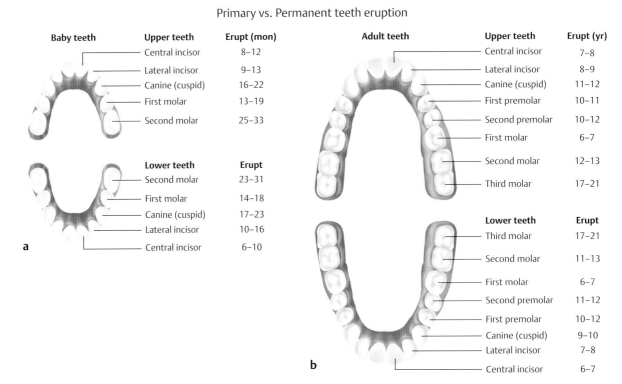

Baby teeth	Upper teeth	Erupt (mon)
	Central incisor	8–12
	Lateral incisor	9–13
	Canine (cuspid)	16–22
	First molar	13–19
	Second molar	25–33

	Lower teeth	Erupt
	Second molar	23–31
	First molar	14–18
	Canine (cuspid)	17–23
	Lateral incisor	10–16
a	Central incisor	6–10

Adult teeth	Upper teeth	Erupt (yr)
	Central incisor	7–8
	Lateral incisor	8–9
	Canine (cuspid)	11–12
	First premolar	10–11
	Second premolar	10–12
	First molar	6–7
	Second molar	12–13
	Third molar	17–21

	Lower teeth	Erupt
	Third molar	17–21
	Second molar	11–13
	First molar	6–7
	Second premolar	11–12
	First premolar	10–12
	Canine (cuspid)	9–10
	Lateral incisor	7–8
b	Central incisor	6–7

Fig. 12.19 **(a)** Primary versus **(b)** permanent teeth.

permanent set (six upper, six lower). The first two primary molars appear between 12 and 15 months of age. These primary molars are replaced around age 6 by the first permanent molars, with the second permanent molars coming in between 11 and 13 years of age. The third molars, more commonly referred to as the wisdom teeth, are the last teeth to develop and typically do not erupt until age 18 to 20. Some people never develop third molars at all. Wisdom teeth often cause crowding and require extraction.

Because of the curved nature of the dental arches, application of conventional anatomic descriptive terms (anterior, posterior, medial, lateral) is cumbersome. Therefore, dental anatomists have named the five surfaces of each tooth (**Fig. 12.20**). The biting surface, where the tooth comes in contact with the opposing tooth, is called the **occlusal** surface. The surface of the tooth that faces the center of the oral cavity is referred to as the **lingual** surface because it faces the tongue. The opposite surface, which faces the cheek wall (buccal wall), is referred to as the **labial** surface for the incisors and canine teeth and the **buccal** surface for the premolars and molars. Except for the last molar, the other two surfaces of a tooth are in contact, or nearly so, with adjacent teeth. The tooth surfaces in contact are collectively referred to as the approximal surfaces.

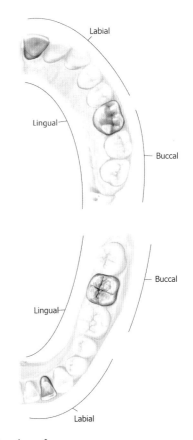

Fig. 12.20 Tooth surfaces.

In the typical skull, the upper, maxillary arch has a slightly larger diameter and is longer than the lower, mandibular arch. The larger size of the maxillary arch creates a normal relationship between the upper and lower teeth involving a small maxillary **overbite**. In other words, the upper arch overlaps and confines the lower arch such that the upper incisors and canines, and to a lesser extent the premolars, bite to the outside of the lower teeth. The amount of overlap by which the upper incisors lie labial (anterior) to the lower incisors is the **overjet**, typically 2 to 3 mm.

Occlusion is the complete joining or contact in a position of rest of the occlusal (biting) surfaces of the upper and lower teeth. In 1899, Edward H. Angle proposed a system of three main types of occlusion (**Fig. 12.21**). Class I occlusion is considered normal (**a**); the cusps of the first mandibular molars are ahead and inside of the corresponding cusps of the opposing maxillary teeth. This occlusion provides a normal facial profile. Class II malocclusion occurs when the cusps of the first mandibular molars are behind and inside the opposing molars of the maxillary arch (**b**). Class II is the most common type of occlusal discrepancy and is found in about 45% of the population. A Class II malocclusion results in an increased overjet and may give the appearance of a receding chin (**c**). Class III malocclusion occurs when the cusps of the first mandibular molar are a tooth (or more) ahead of the opposing maxillary incisors, giving the appearance of a protruding jaw.

Individual teeth can be misaligned as well. If a tooth is rotated or twisted on its long axis, it has undergone toriversion. If it tilts toward the lips, it is referred to as labioverted, whereas tilting toward the tongue is called linguaverted. When a tooth tilts away from the midline of the dental arch, it is considered to be distoverted, but if it tilts toward the midline, it is considered mesioverted. When a tooth does not erupt sufficiently to contact its match on the opposite arch, it is said to be infraverted. If a tooth erupts too far, it is said to be supraverted. In some cases, the teeth on the posterior arch prevent anterior contact of the front teeth, resulting in a condition called open bite. If supraversion prevents

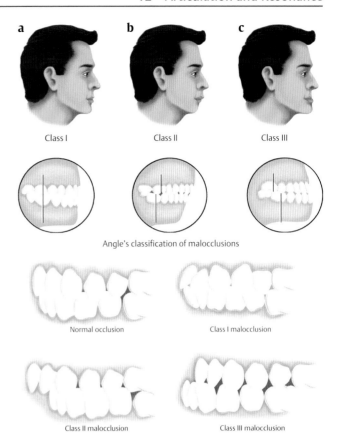

Fig. 12.21 Angle classification of dental occlusion. **(a)** Class I occlusion. **(b)** Class II malocclusion. **(c)** Class III malocclusion.

the posterior teeth from occlusion, this is referred to as a closed bite.

Innervation of Articulatory Structures

All of the structures of the vocal tract are located in the head and neck. Therefore, innervation for the velum, tongue, mandible, face, nose, and pharynx arises from the cranial nerves. Innervation for individual muscles is included in the muscle tables shown in the following section. At least seven of the twelve cranial nerves are important for speech production: the trigeminal (CN V), facial (CN VII), vestibulocochlear (CN VIII), glossopharyngeal (CN IX),

---

Box 12.2 Dental Anomalies

A number of developmental dental anomalies can occur in children. Children may be born with supernumerary teeth (teeth in addition to the normal number) or teeth that are smaller than appropriate for the size of their dental arch (microdontia). Teeth may fuse together at the root or crown. Some children may have extremely thin or missing enamel on the surface of the tooth (amelogenesis imperfecta). Many of these anomalies present as part of a syndrome. Therefore, it is important that the speech-language pathologist pay attention to the teeth during the oral mechanism exam.

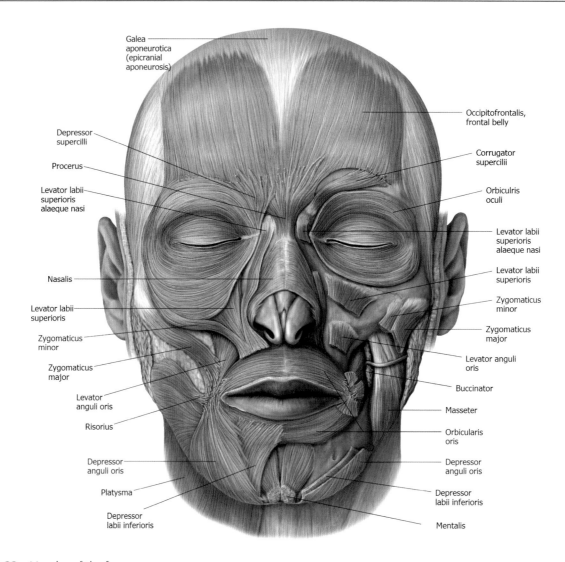

Galea aponeurotica (epicranial aponeurosis)

Depressor supercilli

Procerus

Levator labii superioris alaeque nasi

Nasalis

Levator labii superioris

Zygomaticus minor

Zygomaticus major

Levator anguli oris

Risorius

Depressor anguli oris

Platysma

Depressor labii inferioris

Occipitofrontalis, frontal belly

Corrugator supercilii

Orbiculris oculi

Levator labii superioris alaeque nasi

Levator labii superioris

Zygomaticus minor

Zygomaticus major

Levator anguli oris

Buccinator

Masseter

Orbicularis oris

Depressor anguli oris

Depressor labii inferioris

Mentalis

Fig. 12.22 Muscles of the face.

vagus (CN X), cranial root of accessory (CN XI), and hypoglossal (CN XII).

Muscles of the Face

The muscles of the face are responsible for moving the face and facial expressions (**Fig. 12.22**, **Fig. 12.23**; **Table 12.1**). The muscles near the lips are important for producing speech sounds, particularly bilabials, labiodentals, and vowels with lip rounding. In addition to speech production, these muscles are integral in the breakdown of food and formation of a bolus during the oral preparatory phase of a swallow as well as oral transport of the bolus. All of the muscles of the face are innervated by the facial nerve (CN VII).

The **orbicularis oris** (**Fig. 12.22**) is a prominent facial muscle with fibers originating from the maxilla, mandible, and deep layers of the skin. The fibers run around the upper and lower lips, forming an oral sphincter. They insert into the mucosa of the upper and lower lips. Many of the other muscles of the face that act on the lips interdigitate with the fibers of the orbicularis oris. This muscle is responsible for lip puckering and tight lip closure. This muscle is particularly important for creating a lip seal to allow for intraoral pressure buildup to oral plosives such as /p/ and /b/. It is also very important for creating a tight lip seal during the oral phases of swallowing.

Several of the muscles of the face are involved in pulling the lips superiorly and/or laterally. Lateral movement of the lips results in lip spreading, as for the vowel /i/, while superior and lateral movement of the lips results in smiling. The **risorius**

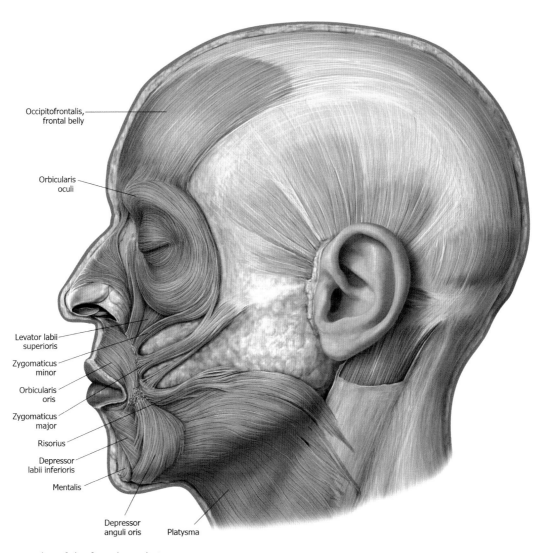

Fig. 12.23 Muscles of the face, lateral view.

Occipitofrontalis, frontal belly

Orbicularis oculi

Levator labii superioris

Zygomaticus minor

Orbicularis oris

Zygomaticus major

Risorius

Depressor labii inferioris

Mentalis

Depressor anguli oris

Platysma

(**Fig. 12.23**) starts in the fascia in the area of the cheek, over the **masseter** muscle, and the **platysma** muscle. It runs medially to insert into the corner of the mouth and the fascia inferior and anterior to the ear. This muscle draws the angle of the mouth laterally. The **buccinator** (**Fig. 12.24**) arises from the mandible, the pterygomandibular raphe (a portion of the buccopharyngeal fascia), and the alveolar processes of the mandible and maxilla. It travels medially to insert into the angle of the mouth. This muscle pulls the lips laterally, but it has a second important function. The buccinator tenses the cheek and presses the cheek against the teeth during chewing, keeps the cheek from being bitten during chewing, and assists with bolus formation by keeping food from falling into the lateral sulci (pockets between the cheek and teeth). The **levator labii superioris** (**Fig. 12.25**) has its origin in the frontal process of the maxilla, infraorbital region, and zygomatic bone. It runs inferiorly and medially to insert into the skin of the upper lip and the alar cartilage of the nose. The levator labii superioris raises the upper lip and the angle of the mouth. It can also dilate the nostril through its attachment to the alar cartilage. Lying deep to the levator labii superioris is the **incisivus labii superioris** muscle. This muscle starts on the maxilla near the canine and runs laterally, along the orbicularis oris to insert into the corner of the mouth, interdigitating with the other muscle fibers in that area. The incisivus labii superioris elevates the corner of the mouth. The **levator labii superioris aleque nasi** (**Fig. 12.22**) has two bellies. Both bellies start on the anterior surface of the maxilla and run inferiorly. The nasal belly inserts into the alar cartilage, and contraction of this belly opens the nostril. The

Table 12.1   Muscles of the face

Muscle	Origin	Insertion	Action	Innervation
Buccinator	Mandible and maxilla	Angle of mouth	Pulls corner of mouth laterally, tenses cheek	Facial nerve (CN VII)
Depressor anguli oris	Mandible	Angle of mouth	Depresses corner of mouth, assists in lip closure	Facial nerve (CN VII)
Depressor labii inferioris	Mandible	Lower lip	Pulls the lip inferiorly and laterally	Facial nerve (CN VII)
Frontalis	Front scalp	Eyebrows	Raises eyebrows	Facial nerve (CN VII)
Incisivus labii inferioris	Mandible	Corner of mouth	Depresses corner of mouth	Facial nerve (CN VII)
Incisivus labii superioris	Maxilla	Corner of mouth	Raises corner of mouth	Facial nerve (CN VII)
Levator anguli oris	Maxilla	Corner of mouth	Raises corner of mouth, assists in lip closure	Facial nerve (CN VII)
Levator labii superioris	Maxilla, infraorbital region, zygomatic bone	Upper lip, alar cartilage	Elevates upper lip, opens nostril	Facial nerve (CN VII)
Levator labii superioris alaeque nasi	Maxilla	Upper lip, alar cartilage	Elevates upper lip, opens nostril	Facial nerve (CN VII)
Mentalis	Mandible	Orbicularis oris, skin of chin	Depresses and protrudes lower lip	Facial nerve (CN VII)
Orbicularis oculi	Medial angle of eye, lacrimal bone	Skin on orbit of eye	Closes the eye	Facial nerve (CN VII)
Orbicularis oris	Mandible, maxilla	Mucosa of upper and lower lips	Closes and puckers the lips	Facial nerve (CN VII)
Platysma	Neck	Mandible, cheek, angle of mouth, orbicularis oris	Tenses lower face and neck, depresses corner of the mouth	Facial nerve (CN VII)
Risorius	Cheek, masseter platysma	Corner of mouth, near ear	Pulls corner of mouth laterally	Facial nerve (CN VII)
Zygomaticus major	Zygomatic bone	Corner of mouth	Raises corner of mouth	Facial nerve (CN VII)
Zygomaticus minor	Zygomatic bone	Orbicularis oris	Elevates upper lip	Facial nerve (CN VII)

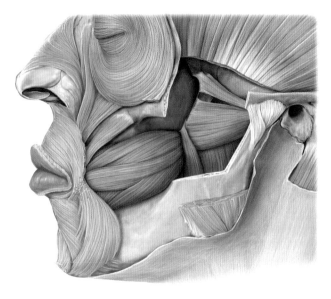

Fig. 12.24   Buccinator muscle.

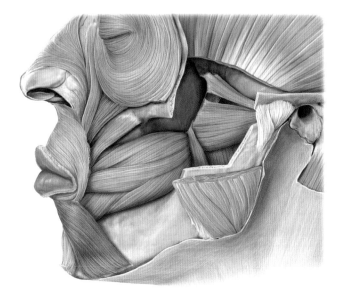

Fig. 12.25   Levator labii superioris and depressor labii inferioris.

labial belly inserts into the upper lip, interdigitating with the orbicularis oris; its contraction elevates the upper lip. The zygomaticus muscle (**Fig. 12.26**) has two parts, a major and a minor**. Zygomaticus major** runs inferiorly and medially from the zygomatic bone to the angle of the mouth, where it interdigitates with the orbicularis oris. It serves to draw the angle of the mouth superiorly and laterally. **Zygomaticus minor** is a much smaller muscle, located superior to zygomaticus major, that runs inferiorly and medially from the zygomatic bone to the orbicularis oris and raises the upper lip. **Levator anguli oris** (**Fig. 12.27**) starts at the infraorbital margin of the maxilla and runs inferiorly and medially to insert at the angle of the mouth, interdigitating with the orbicularis oris. This muscle moves the corner of the mouth superiorly and laterally. It also compresses the lips together to assist in lip closure for speech and swallowing.

Several muscles of the face pull the lips inferiorly and/or laterally. The **mentalis** (**Fig. 12.28**) runs from the anterior surface of the mandible, near the midline, superiorly to the skin of the chin and the fibers of the orbicularis oris. The mentalis depresses and protrudes the lower lip to produce a pouting facial expression, and it also raises the skin over the chin. **Depressor labii inferioris** (**Fig. 12.25**) is lateral to the mentalis. It starts on the anterior surface of the mandible and runs superiorly and medially to insert into the lower lip, merging with the orbicularis oris and the levator labii superioris. This muscle pulls the lip inferiorly and laterally, resulting in frowning. Deep to the depressor labii inferioris is the **incisivus labii inferioris** muscle. This muscle starts on the mandible

near the lateral incisor and runs laterally near the fibers of the orbicularis oris to insert on the corner of the mouth. The incisivus labii inferioris pulls the corner of the mouth inferiorly. **Depressor anguli oris** (**Fig. 12.27**) starts on the outer surface of the mandible, runs superiorly and medially to insert into the angle of the mouth, and interdigitates with the orbicularis oris. This muscle can move the corner of the mouth inferiorly and laterally. It also can compress the lips together, assisting with lip closure. The **platysma** (**Fig. 12.23**) is a broad muscle sheet that originates in the neck region on the superficial fascia of the deltoid (shoulder) and pectoral (chest) regions. It runs superiorly and medially to insert into the mandible, skin of the cheek, angle of the mouth, and the orbicularis oris. This muscle tenses the skin of the lower face and neck, pulls the corners of the mouth inferiorly, and assists with depression of the mandible.

Two other muscles of the face are important for facial expression but are not involved in lip movement. Like the orbicularis oris, the **orbicularis oculi** (**Fig. 12.29**) forms a sphincter, but instead of contracting around the lips, the orbicularis oculi contracts around the eye. It starts at the medial orbital edge, the medial palpebral ligament between the nose and the medial angle of the eye, and the lacrimal bone. It runs around the eye and inserts into the skin around the orbit of the eye and the tarsal plate (a structure that forms the "skeleton" of the eyelid). This muscle is responsible for both gently and tightly closing the eyelids. The **frontalis** muscle (**Fig. 12.30**) is the frontal belly of the occipitofrontalis, a scalp muscle. The frontalis has no bony attachments. It runs from the anterior epicranial aponeurosis inferiorly to the skin

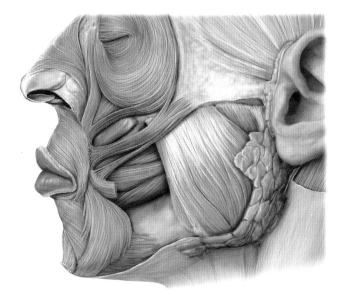

Fig. 12.26 Zygomaticus muscle.

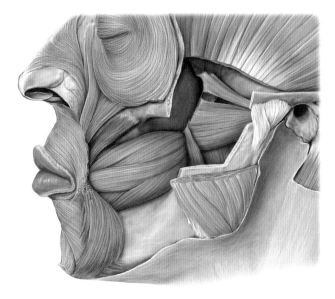

Fig. 12.27 Levator anguli oris and depressor anguli oris.

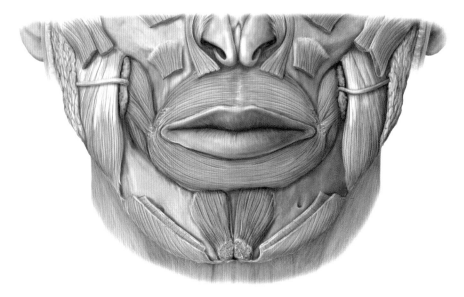

Fig. 12.28   Mentalis muscle.

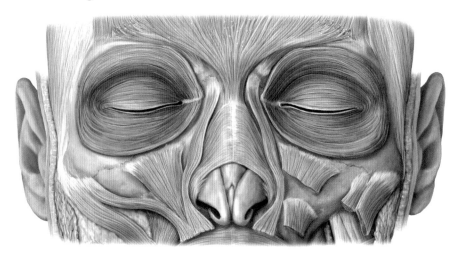

Fig. 12.29   Orbicularis oculi.

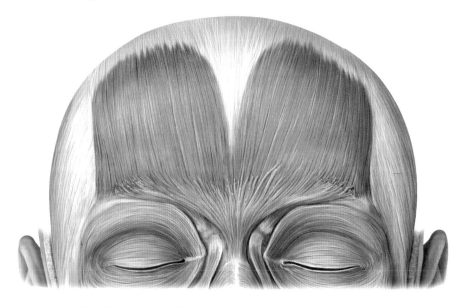

Fig. 12.30   Frontalis muscle.

of the eyebrows. This muscle raises the eyebrows, resulting in a surprised facial expression, and creates wrinkles in the forehead.

The Lips As an Articulator

The lips are a movable articulator, consisting primarily of the orbicularis oris muscles. It is not clear whether the upper and lower lips are controlled individually or whether they are activated as a unit (Smith 1992). The orbicularis oris muscle serves as the insertion for several facial muscles, including the buccinator, depressor anguli oris, depressor labii inferioris, incisivus labii inferioris, incisivus labii superioris, levator anguli oris, levator labii superioris, levator labii superioris alaeque nasi, mentalis, risorius, zygomaticus major, and zygomaticus minor. All of these muscles work on the lips in various combinations to produce a wide range of lip movements. One particular movement, important for speech production, is lip rounding. Lip rounding is accomplished primarily by contraction of the orbicularis oris muscles, which act as a sphincter. Lip rounding is important for production of vowel sounds, such as /u/ and /oʊ/, as well as consonant sounds such as /w/. Lip rounding is almost always accompanied by lip protrusion. Lip protrusion changes the resonant properties of the vocal tract and is accomplished by contraction of the depressor labii inferioris, levator labii superioris, mentalis, and zygomaticus minor muscles.

The lips are also important for production of bilabial consonants, including /p/, /b/, and /m/. The word "bilabial" implies that the two lips come in contact with each other during production of the sound. For /p/ and /b/, the lips must remain closed while pressure builds up in the oral cavity. Labiodental consonants /f/ and /v/ involve placement of the lower lip against the upper teeth to create turbulence, which the listener perceives as noise.

Muscles of the Jaw

The muscles of the jaw function in both speech and swallowing. In speech, small movements of the jaw assist in differentiation among a variety of consonants and vowels, along with tongue and lip movement. In swallowing, jaw muscles are critical for food breakdown and bolus formation. In general, the muscles of the jaw can be divided into two broad categories: those that close the jaw and those that open the jaw (**Table 12.2**). Almost all of the jaw muscles are innervated by the trigeminal nerve (CN V), with one exception: the **geniohyoid**, which is innervated by a branch of the first cervical spinal nerve.

Three muscles are responsible for jaw closing: the masseter, temporalis, and medial pterygoid. The masseter (**Fig. 12.31**) is a large muscle on the lateral aspect of the face, superficial to the mandible. When you clench your jaw, the bulk of the muscle can be felt under the skin. The masseter begins on the medial surface and inferior border of the zygomatic arch and runs inferiorly and laterally to insert on the angle, lateral side, and the coronoid process of the mandible. In addition to closing the jaw, this muscle also protrudes the jaw. The temporalis (**Fig. 12.31**) is a broad, fan-shaped muscle on the surface of the temporal bone. The temporalis originates on the temporal fossa and temporal fascia over the temporal bone and runs inferiorly to attach to the coronoid process and the anterior portion of the ramus of the mandible. In addition to closing the jaw, this muscle also retracts the jaw. The medial pterygoid (**Fig. 12.32**) starts at the lateral pterygoid

Table 12.2 Muscles of the jaw

Muscle	Origin	Insertion	Action	Innervation
Anterior belly of digastric	Mandible	Intermediate tendon on hyoid	Opens jaw, raises hyoid	Trigeminal nerve (CN V)
Geniohyoid	Mandible	Body of hyoid	Opens jaw, raises hyoid	First cervical nerve
Lateral pterygoid	Sphenoid bone	Condyle of mandible, TMJ	Closes jaw	Trigeminal nerve (CN V)
Masseter	Zygomatic arch	Coronoid process, angle and body of mandible	Closes jaw	Trigeminal nerve (CN V)
Medial pterygoid	Maxilla, sphenoid bone, palatine bone	Medial aspect of ramus and angle of mandible	Closes jaw	Trigeminal nerve (CN V)
Mylohyoid	Mandible	Body of hyoid	Opens jaw, raises hyoid	Trigeminal nerve (CN V)
Temporalis	Temporal bone	Coronoid process and ramus of mandible	Closes jaw	Trigeminal nerve (CN V)

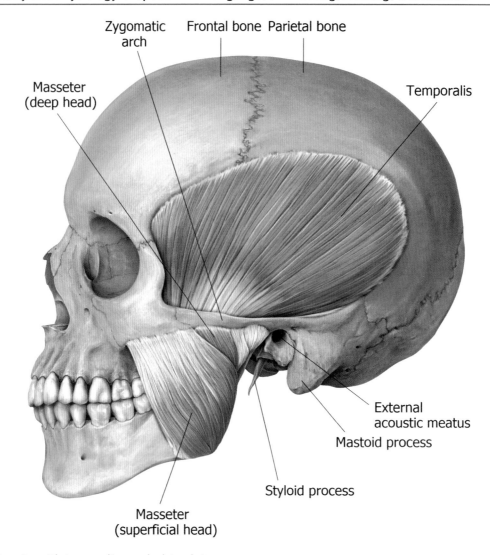

Fig. 12.31   Masseter with temporalis muscle, lateral view.

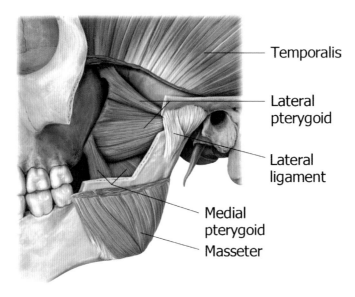

Fig. 12.32   Medial and lateral pterygoid muscles.

plate of the sphenoid bone, the pyramidal process of the palatine bone near the lateral pterygoid plate, and the inferior and posterior aspect of the maxilla. It runs laterally and inferiorly to insert on the medial aspect of the ramus and angle of the mandible. Essentially, the masseter and medial pterygoid attach to the mandible in similar locations. The difference is that the masseter attaches on the lateral aspect of the mandible and the medial pterygoid attaches on the medial aspect of the mandible (**Fig. 12.33**). In addition to closing the jaw, this muscle also protrudes the jaw.

Four muscles are responsible for opening the jaw. The lateral pterygoid (**Fig. 12.32**; **Fig. 12.33**) originates at the greater wing of the sphenoid and the lateral side of the lateral pterygoid plate of the sphenoid bone. It runs laterally and superiorly to insert on the neck of the condyle of the mandible and the articular disk and capsule of the TMJ. In addition to opening the jaw, this muscle also protrudes the jaw. The anterior belly of the digastric, the **mylohyoid**, and the geniohyoid also open the jaw (**Fig. 12.34**). These muscles pull down on the mandible when the hyoid bone is stabilized.

Temporomandibular Joint

The TMJ is a synovial joint. The distinguishing feature of a synovial joint is that it includes some form of joint cavity containing synovial fluid. The TMJ is formed by the articulation of the condyle of the mandible with the temporal bone in the mandibular fossa (**Fig. 12.35**). The surfaces of the joint are lined with fibrocartilage, which is unusual for a synovial joint, as most are lined with hyaline cartilage. Fibrocartilage can withstand more stretching or distortion than other types of cartilage can; thus, it is found in joints that withstand great forces of

movement, such as the jaw, the vertebral column, and the knee joint. The joint has an articular disk in the middle of the joint cavity. The fibrous layer of the joint capsule has a thickened portion called the lateral ligament that strengthens the joint laterally. The stylomandibular ligament runs from the styloid process of the temporal bone to the angle of the mandible (**Fig. 12.36**). The sphenomandibular ligament runs from the sphenoid bone to the lingula of the mandible. The mandibular fossa is a concave depression in the squamous portion of the temporal bone. Specifically, the TMJ is classified as a ginglymoarthrodial joint. This type of joint allows for a hingelike movement with some limited gliding. The joint is set in such a way that the mandible moves vertically (i.e., opening and closing), anteroposteriorly (i.e., protruding and retracting), and transversely (i.e., from side to side). All of these movements are utilized during speech production and chewing.

The Mandible as an Articulator

Movement of the mandible results in changes in the size of the oral cavity but also assists in positioning of the lips and tongue. The mandible is an important articulator in its supportive role of carrying the lips, tongue, and teeth to their targets on the maxilla (lips, teeth, alveolar ridge, and hard palate). During normal speech production, adjustments of the mandible are relatively small. However, paralysis of the muscles can have a devastating impact on intelligible speech.

During speech production, the muscles of mandibular elevation (temporalis, masseter, and medial pterygoid) and mandibular depression (anterior belly of digastric, mylohyoid, geniohyoid, and lateral pterygoid) stay in a dynamic balance so that a

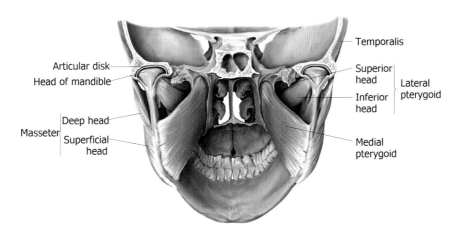

Fig. 12.33 Masticatory muscle sling.

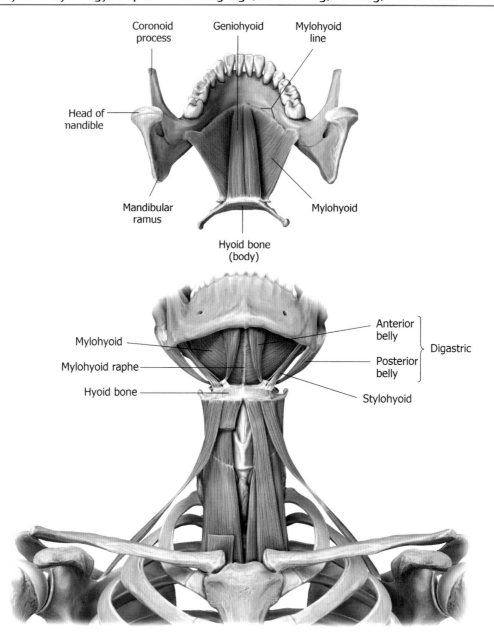

Fig. 12.34   Suprahyoid and infrahyoid muscles.

slight modification of muscle activation and inhibition by antagonists permits a quick adjustment of the mandible. In fact, electromyographic studies demonstrate that the mandibular elevators and depressors co-contract during speech production to provide fine control of the small movements of the jaw associated with speech (Smith 1992). The masseter and temporalis are less active during speech production than the medial pterygoid is (Smith 1992). Additionally, the anterior belly of the digastric is very active during speech (Smith 1992). Depression of the mandible seems to be a function of not only the classically defined mandibular depressors but, to a significant extent, the infrahyoid musculature as well. The hyoid moves quite a bit with depression of the mandible.

Velopharyngeal Muscles

The velopharyngeal muscles are involved in both speech and swallowing. In speech, these muscles close the velopharyngeal opening, or velopharyngeal port, for all oral sounds. In swallowing, these muscles close off the velopharyngeal port so that food and liquid do not enter the nasal cavity. Most velopharyngeal muscles are innervated

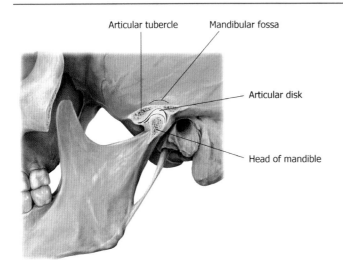

Fig. 12.35 Temporomandibular joint.

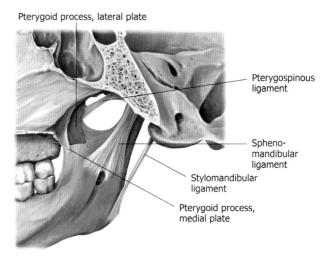

Fig. 12.36 Ligaments of the TMJ.

by the cranial part of the accessory nerve (CN XI) and the pharyngeal branch of the vagus nerve (CN X). Together, these two nerves are often called the pharyngeal plexus. There are two exceptions. The tensor veli palatini is innervated by the mandibular nerve of the trigeminal nerve (CN V₃), and the **palatoglossus** muscle is innervated by the hypoglossal nerve (CN XII).

Many muscles are involved in closing the velopharyngeal port (**Table 12.3**). The tensor veli palatini (**Fig. 12.37**, **Fig. 12.38**) starts at the scaphoid fossa of the medial pterygoid plate, the spine of the sphenoid bones, and the eustachian tube (auditory tube, pharyngotympanic tube). It runs inferiorly, hooks around the hamulus of the medial pterygoid plate, and spreads out to form a sheet of connective tissue known as the palatine aponeurosis, making up much of the soft palate. The tensor veli palatini dilates (opens) the eustachian tube and may

also tense the soft palate. The levator veli palatini (**Fig. 12.37**, **Fig. 12.38**) originates from the petrous portion of the temporal bone and the cartilage of the eustachian tube. It travels inferiorly and anteriorly to insert into the superior aspect of the palatine aponeurosis. The levator veli palatini elevates the soft palate. The **musculus uvulae** (**Fig. 12.37**, **Fig. 12.38**) is a small muscle that originates from the posterior nasal spine and inserts into the palatine aponeurosis and the mucosa of the uvula. This muscle shortens the uvula, pulling it superiorly. Contraction of the musculus uvulae can be thought of as adding bulk to the nasal surface of the velum, and when viewed from above, looks like a "knuckling up" of tissue in the soft palate. This bulging or bunching of tissue is sometimes helpful in making contact between the soft palate and the posterior pharyngeal wall for complete velopharyngeal closure.

Table 12.3 Muscles of the soft palate

Muscle	Origin	Insertion	Action	Innervation
Levator veli palatini	Temporal bone, eustachian tube	Palatine aponeurosis	Elevates soft palate	Accessory (CN XI) and vagus (CN X) nerves
Musculus uvulae	Posterior nasal spine	Palatine aponeurosis	Adds bulk and stiffness to velum	Accessory (CN XI) and vagus (CN X) nerves
Tensor veli palatini	Sphenoid bone, eustachian tube	Palatine aponeurosis	Dilates the eustachian tubes; tenses soft palate	Trigeminal nerve (CN V₃)
Palatoglossus	Palatine aponeurosis	Sides of tongue	Pulls soft palate toward tongue, elevates back of tongue	Hypoglossal nerve (CN XII)
Palatopharyngeus	Palatal aponeurosis and posterior margin of hard palate	Upper border of thyroid cartilage	Narrows the pharynx and lowering the soft palate	Accessory (CN XI) and vagus (CN X) nerves

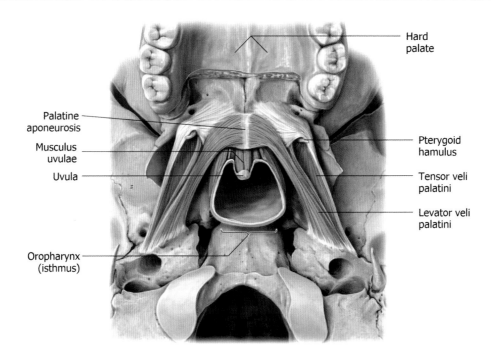

Fig. 12.37   Muscles of the soft palate, inferior view.

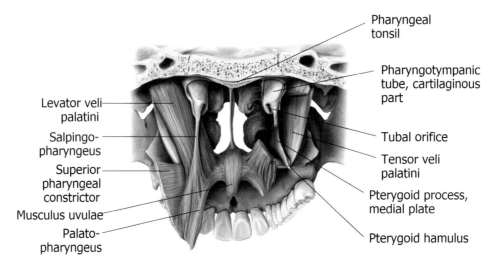

Fig. 12.38   Velopharyngeal muscles, posterior view.

Several pharyngeal muscles are also involved in velopharyngeal port function. The **palatopharyngeus** tenses the soft palate. The **superior** and **middle pharyngeal constrictors** enclose the nasopharynx and oropharynx, respectively (**Fig. 12.39**). Contraction of these muscles results in a narrowing of the port via movement of the lateral pharyngeal walls.

The palatoglossus runs from the palatine aponeurosis to the lateral edge of the tongue. This muscle forms the anterior faucial (palatoglossal) arch

(**Fig. 12.2**). This muscle is involved in pulling the soft palate toward the tongue. However, gravity is a prime mover in the opening of the velopharyngeal port, not muscle contraction.

The Velum (Soft Palate) as an Articulator

The velum is composed of muscular tissue and plays an active role in speech production. The velum is important for production of velar consonant

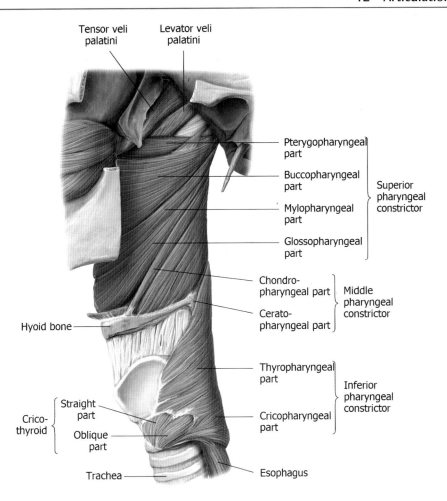

Fig. 12.39 Pharyngeal musculature.

sounds: /k/, /g/, and /ŋ/. For these sounds, the back of the tongue elevates to approximate the velum. The primary role of the velum, however, is to assist in regulation of oral/nasal resonance. In conjunction with the posterior pharyngeal wall and primarily the superior pharyngeal constrictor, the velum elevates as part of the velopharyngeal mechanism. When the velopharyngeal port is open, some of the acoustic energy is diverted into the nasal cavity and the remainder travels though the oral cavity. When the velopharyngeal port is closed, the nasal cavity is sealed off from the oral cavity so that all sound travels through the oral cavity. As the sound travels through the nasal and/or oral cavity, it changes as a result of the resonant properties of the cavities. In English, almost all consonant sounds are produced with a closed velopharyngeal port, meaning that the oral cavity shapes the sound. Only three consonant sounds in English, /m/, /n/, and /ŋ/, are produced with the velopharyngeal port open. For these sounds, the resonant properties of both the oral and nasal cavities shape the sound. These three sounds have a characteristic nasal quality or nasal murmur.

In summary, closing of the velopharyngeal port is caused by contraction of the levator veli palatini, palatopharyngeus, musculus uvulae, and superior and middle pharyngeal constrictors. The soft palate is positioned within the nasopharynx and oropharynx through contraction of the levator veli palatini, palatoglossus, and palatopharyngeus. Opening of the velopharyngeal port is primarily driven by gravity when speakers are in an upright position.

Normal patterns of velopharyngeal port closure include coronal closure, caused primarily by anterior-posterior movement of the soft palate toward the posterior pharyngeal wall. Sagittal closure is caused by lateral wall movement, narrowing the port laterally, resulting from contraction of the superior and middle constrictors. Circumferential closure is the result of both anterior-posterior movement of the soft palate and lateral wall movement, so that the lateral walls close around the elevated soft palate. Circular closure can also be achieved with the **Passavant ridge**. In this case, as the soft palate moves posteriorly to contact the posterior pharyngeal wall, a small portion of the posterior pharyngeal wall bulges anteriorly to contact the soft palate. That bulge in the posterior wall is called the Passavant ridge. In very young children, the soft palate will contact the pharyngeal tonsil (commonly called the **adenoids**) (**Fig. 12.40**). As the pharyngeal tonsil tissue atrophies, patterns of velopharyngeal closure change. Removal of the pharyngeal tonsil alters the anatomy, and it can take 6 to 12 months for children to adjust velopharyngeal closure appropriately. In the interim, children may sound mildly **hypernasal**.

The degree of velopharyngeal port closure during speech varies according to phonetic context. The velopharyngeal port is open for the nasal consonants. However, velopharyngeal port closure is not necessarily complete for the production of nonnasal sounds. A degree of opening is maintained for production of low vowels /ɛ/, /æ/, /ɔ/, /ɑ/, although not as much as for nasal consonants. Similarly, a smaller degree of velopharyngeal port opening is maintained for high vowels /i/, /ɪ/, /u/, /ʊ/. Differences in the degree of closure are related to the mechanical linkage of the soft palate and tongue.

Closure is greatest for the plosive consonants /p/, /b/, /t/, /d/, /k/, /g/ relative to other oral consonants. Complete closure is needed, as these sounds require the highest intraoral air pressure. Complete velopharyngeal port closure is not required for proper balance between oral and nasal resonance. If the balance shifts toward more nasal than oral resonance (e.g., the velopharyngeal port is too open or the opening occurs at an unexpected location during speech production), listeners perceive hypernasal speech. Conversely, speech produced with no velopharyngeal port opening may result in **hyponasal** speech. Moll (1962) estimated that normal speakers exhibit 14% opening of the velopharyngeal port during production of the vowel /i/, compared to 37% for the vowels /ɑ/ and /æ/. When you consider how rapidly speech is produced and the distribution of nasal consonants throughout speech, you realize how important the timing of velopharyngeal port opening and closure is to achieve the proper balance of oral and nasal resonance.

Tongue

The tongue is an intricate structure, and its importance for speech production cannot be emphasized enough. It is a massive structure that occupies the floor of the mouth. The tongue can be divided into three primary regions (**Fig. 12.41**). The most anterior portion is referred to as the **apex** or tip. The largest part of the tongue, in the middle, is called the body of the tongue. The base of the tongue is the portion that resides in the oropharynx. The superior surface is referred to as the **dorsum**. The tongue root is the posterior and inferior part of the tongue, forming the anterior wall of the pharynx. The portion of the tongue that resides in the oral cavity accounts for approximately two-thirds of the surface of the tongue, with the remaining one-third residing in the oropharynx.

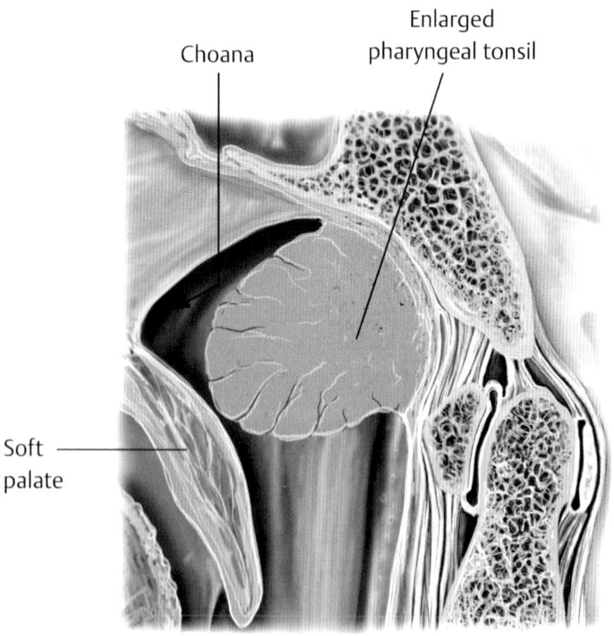

Fig. 12.40 Abnormal pharyngeal tonsil enlargement in children.

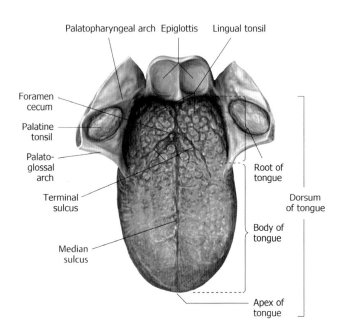

Fig. 12.41 Structures of the tongue.

Box 12.3   Children with Cerebral Palsy

Children with cerebral palsy often have difficulty moving the tongue for articulation as well as limited closure of the velopharyngeal port. As a result, their speech can be difficult to understand. Although it may be tempting to attempt to strengthen the speech muscles using non-speech tasks, research suggests that nonspeech tasks do not improve speech production or speech intelligibility. Speech is highly coordinated and is unlike any other task we perform with our articulatory muscles. Therefore, it is important that speech-language pathologists target coordinated speech movements when working with children to improve speech production skills.

The mucous membrane covering the tongue dorsum has several prominent landmarks. The **median sulcus**, which runs longitudinally, divides the tongue into right and left sides. Underlying this sulcus is the **median fibrous septum**, which divides the tongue into two halves but, more importantly, serves as the point of origin for a number of muscles of the tongue. The fibrous septum originates at the body of the hyoid, via the hyoglossal membrane, and courses the length of the tongue. The posterior portion of the tongue is covered with lingual papillae, small prominences of various shapes on the surface of the tongue, some of which carry taste buds. The terminal sulcus marks the posterior palatine surface, and the center of this groove is referred to as the **foramen cecum**, a deep recess in the tongue.

Inferior to the membranous lining of the pharyngeal surface of the tongue is the lingual tonsil, a region of lymphoid tissue, which is part of the immune system and is important for fighting infection. The **Waldeyer ring** is a ring of lymphoid tissue located in the nasopharynx and oropharynx surrounding the entrance to the aerodigestive tract (**Fig. 12.42**). This ring includes two palatine tonsils, the pharyngeal tonsil (adenoids), the lateral bands

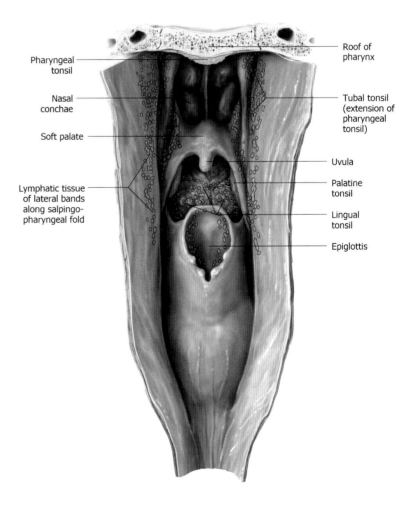

Pharyngeal tonsil

Nasal conchae

Soft palate

Lymphatic tissue of lateral bands along salpingo-pharyngeal fold

Roof of pharynx

Tubal tonsil (extension of pharyngeal tonsil)

Uvula

Palatine tonsil

Lingual tonsil

Epiglottis

Fig. 12.42 Posterior view of the opened pharynx showing the Waldeyer ring.

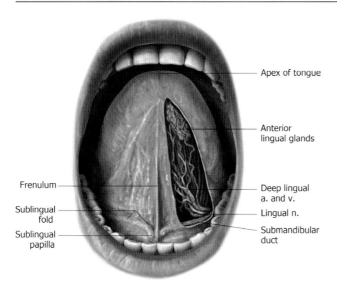

Fig. 12.43   Inferior surface of the tongue.

on the lateral walls of the oropharynx, and the lingual tonsil at the base of tongue. The Waldeyer ring grows until approximately age 11 and then decreases spontaneously.

The tongue is covered with taste buds to convey gustatory information including the sensation of sweet, sour, salty, bitter, and umami tastes (the five primary taste qualities). The taste buds are located in the various papillae found on the tongue and around the oral cavity. All types of taste can be detected by all taste bud populations, although some anatomists have suggested that there are regions of concentration for specific types of tastes. For example, the anterior tongue is sensitive to both sweet and sour while the sides of the tongue are most sensitive to sour taste. Bitter tastes are generally sensed near the terminal sulcus. As discussed in **Chapter 9**, this division does not appear to be due to the taste bud populations but to the nerves carrying the taste sensations.

Three important landmarks reside on the inferior surface of the tongue (**Fig. 12.43**). The lingual frenulum joins the inferior tongue and the mandible, perhaps stabilizing the tongue during movement. The transverse band of tissue on either side of the tongue (the sublingual folds) contains the ducts for the sublingual salivary glands. Just lateral to the lingual frenulum are the ducts for the submandibular salivary glands, which are hidden under the mucosa on the inner surface of the mandible. There is a rich vascular supply on the undersurface of the tongue as well.

The Tongue as a Muscular Hydrostat

The bulk of the tongue is composed of muscle tissue. Some of the muscles are housed entirely within the tongue itself and are referred to as intrinsic muscles. Other muscles originate on structures outside the tongue but attach to some part of the tongue and are called extrinsic muscles. The tongue has minimal skeletal support except from the hyoid bone and the mandible; the tongue connects to the mandible through the corium, the deep inner layer of skin on the medial surface of the mandible that contains connective tissue, blood vessels, and fat. The tongue can change shape and position without changing its overall volume. When either the intrinsic or extrinsic muscles of the tongue contract, the tongue acts as a fluid-filled structure that is incompressible. If you hold a water balloon and compress one end, the balloon changes shape and the liquid moves to the other end of the balloon, but no liquid escapes. The tongue is not filled with liquid, but is composed of muscle tissue that behaves in a similar way. This architecture is referred to as a **muscular hydrostat** and is similar to the structure of elephant trunks and octopus tentacles (Kier and Smith 1985; Smith and Kier 1989).

Box 12.4   Ankyloglossia (Tongue-Tie)

The lingual frenulum is a band of tissue that connects the tongue to the floor of the mouth and assists in stabilizing the tongue. Occasionally, the frenulum may be unusually short, thick, or tight and limit movement of the tongue tip; this condition is referred to as ankyloglossia or tongue-tie. During speech, difficulty elevating the tongue for phonemes that require palatal or alveolar contact may be most apparent. Additionally, the tongue may appear heart-shaped on protrusion.

This shape is created by the excessive tension at the midline of the tongue by the short frenulum. When newborn feeding problems or childhood articulation difficulties exist, a surgical procedure called a frenectomy (also known as a frenotomy) can be performed if medically necessary. The evidence for improvement in outcomes is low to insufficient. Speech-language pathologists may also be asked to work with these children before or after surgery.

The corium provides leverage for nine muscles (four intrinsic and five extrinsic) to move the tongue. As the tongue changes shape and position, inward displacement in one area of the tongue results in outward displacements in another area, thereby preserving the volume of the tongue. The hydrostatic property of the tongue allows it to perform a range of movements including protruding, retracting, elevating, depressing, bulging, centralizing, curling, flattening, grooving, lateralizing, and moving from side to side.

Intrinsic Muscles

The intrinsic muscles of the tongue include two pairs of muscles that run longitudinally, a muscle that courses transversely, and one that courses vertically. The intrinsic muscles interact in a complex fashion to produce the rapid articulations needed for speech production. The intrinsic muscles of the tongue are pictured in **Fig. 12.44** (lateral view) as well as **Fig. 12.45** (coronal section). These muscles are also highlighted in **Table 12.4**. All of the intrinsic muscles of the tongue are innervated by the hypoglossal nerve (CN XII).

Fig. 12.44 Muscles of the tongue, left lateral view.

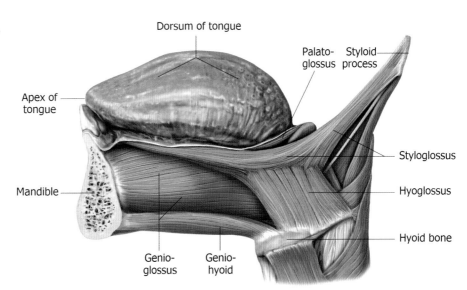

Fig. 12.45 Muscles of the tongue, coronal section, anterior view.

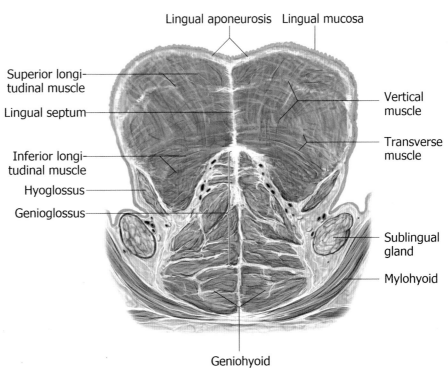

Table 12.4   Intrinsic muscles of the tongue

Muscle	Origin	Insertion	Action	Innervation
Inferior longitudinal	Root of tongue, body of hyoid	Apex of tongue	Depresses tongue tip, assists in tongue retraction	Hypoglossal nerve (CN XII)
Superior longitudinal	Submucous layer of epiglottis, hyoid, median fibrous septum	Lateral edges and apex of tongue	Elevates tongue tip, assists in tongue retraction	Hypoglossal nerve (CN XII)
Transverse	Median fibrous septum	Sides of tongue	Narrows tongue	Hypoglossal nerve (CN XII)
Vertical	Base of tongue	Membranous cover of tongue	Flattens tongue	Hypoglossal nerve (CN XII)

The **superior longitudinal muscle** courses the length of the tongue, constituting the upper layer of the tongue. This muscle originates from the fibrous submucous layer near the epiglottis, from the hyoid, and from the median fibrous septum. Its fibers fan anteriorly and laterally to insert into the lateral margins of the tongue and the region of the apex. The fibers of the superior longitudinal muscle serve to elevate the tip of the tongue when contracted and assist in retraction of the tongue if co-contracted with the inferior longitudinal muscle. If only one superior longitudinal muscle contracts, the tongue pulls toward the side of the contraction.

The **inferior longitudinal muscle** originates at the root of the tongue and the corpus of the hyoid, with fibers coursing to the apex of the tongue. This muscle occupies the lower sides of the tongue but is not seen in the medial tongue base. The inferior longitudinal muscle pulls the tip of the tongue inferiorly and assists in retraction of the tongue if co-contracted with the superior longitudinal muscle.

The **transverse muscles of the tongue** provide a mechanism for narrowing the tongue. The fibers originate at the median fibrous septum and course laterally to insert into the sides of the tongue in the submucous tissue. Some transverse fibers continue as the palatopharyngeus muscle. When the transverse muscles of the tongue contract, the edges of the tongue pull toward the midline, narrowing the tongue.

The **vertical muscles of the tongue** course at right angles to the transverse muscles and flatten the tongue. Fibers of the vertical muscle course from the base of tongue and insert into the membranous cover. The fibers of the transverse and vertical muscles interweave, and contraction of the vertical muscles pulls the tongue inferiorly into the floor of the mouth.

Extrinsic Muscles

The extrinsic muscles of the tongue move the tongue as a unit and complement the precise articulatory movements controlled by the intrinsic muscles. More generally, the extrinsic muscles posture the tongue for articulation. The extrinsic tongue muscles can be seen in the lateral view (**Fig. 12.44**) as well as the coronal section shown in **Fig. 12.45**. These muscles are also highlighted in **Table 12.5**. All extrinsic muscles are also innervated by the hypoglossal nerve (CN XII).

Box 12.5   Neuromuscular Disease and Tongue Function

Deficits associated with weakened articulatory muscles can have a significant effect on speech intelligibility. In a number of motor neuron diseases, such as amyotrophic lateral sclerosis (also known as Lou Gehrig's disease), muscles of the tongue can be especially impacted. Individuals may be unable to move their tongue far enough to produce speech sounds correctly, particularly palatal and alveolar consonants and vowels farther from the middle of the vowel space. Instead, they will produce speech sounds that are less distinct, because they cannot move their tongue to the appropriate place in the oral cavity. For example, vowels can all sound more like /ʌ/ than the intended target. Individuals often compensate for tongue weakness by moving their jaw more. The genioglossus muscle makes up the bulk of the tongue and is attached to the jaw. Therefore, the jaw can be moved to help place the tongue in the superior-inferior aspect of the oral cavity. These diseases are often progressive, and therapy typically involves work with patients and their families to develop augmentative and alternative methods of communication.

Table 12.5 Extrinsic muscles of the tongue

Muscle	Origin	Insertion	Action	Innervation
Chondroglossus	Lesser cornu of hyoid bone	Intrinsic tongue muscles	Depresses tongue	Hypoglossal nerve (CN XII)
Genioglossus	Inner surface of mandible near midline	Tongue tip and dorsum, corpus of hyoid	Retracts and protrudes tongue	Hypoglossal nerve (CN XII)
Hyoglossus	Cornu and lateral body of hyoid	Sides of tongue	Depresses sides of tongue	Hypoglossal nerve (CN XII)
Styloglossus	Styloid process	Sides of tongue	Retracts and elevates tongue	Hypoglossal nerve (CN XII)
Palatoglossus	Palatine aponeurosis	Sides of tongue	Pulls soft palate toward tongue, elevates back of tongue	Hypoglossal nerve (CN XII)

The **genioglossus** is the primary mover of the tongue and makes up the deep bulk of the tongue. The genioglossus originates on the inner mandibular surface at the symphysis and fans to insert into the tip and dorsum of the tongue as well as the corpus of the hyoid bone. The genioglossus occupies the medial position of the tongue. The inferior longitudinal muscles, the **hyoglossus**, and the **styloglossus** lie lateral to the genioglossus. Fibers of the genioglossus insert along the entire surface of the tongue but are sparse near the tip. Because the origin of the muscle is on the inner surface of the mandible, contraction brings the fibers closer to the inner surface of the mandible. Thus, contraction of the anterior genioglossus fibers results in retraction of the tongue, whereas contraction of the posterior fibers draws the tongue anteriorly to assist in protrusion. If both the anterior and posterior fibers contract simultaneously, the middle portion of the tongue pulls toward the floor of the mouth and produces cupping along the length of the tongue.

The **palatoglossus** may be functionally defined as a muscle of the tongue or of the velum. Based on its origin, it is more closely associated with the velum, but it is important to recognize its dual purpose. Contraction of the palatoglossus can depress the soft palate or elevate the posterior aspect of the tongue. The hyoglossus, as the name implies, arises from the length of the cornu and lateral body of the hyoid. It courses upward to insert into the sides of the tongue between the styloglossus and the inferior longitudinal muscles. Contraction of the hyoglossus muscle pulls the sides of the tongue inferiorly, acting as an antagonist to the palatoglossus muscle. The **chondroglossus** muscle is often considered part of the hyoglossus muscle. It originates on the lesser cornu of the hyoid bone and courses up to interdigitate with the intrinsic muscles of the tongue, medial to the point of insertion of the hyoglossus, and depresses the tongue. The styloglossus originates from the anterolateral

margin of the styloid process of the temporal bone, coursing anteriorly and inferiorly to insert into the inferior sides of the tongue. It divides in two portions: one interdigitating with the inferior longitudinal muscle and the other with the fibers of the hyoglossus. Contraction of the styloglossus pulls the tongue posteriorly and superiorly.

The Tongue as an Articulator

The tongue is involved in the production of most sounds in American English and is therefore, arguably the most important of the articulators. The two groups of muscles in the tongue, the intrinsic and extrinsic muscles, work together to achieve target articulator movements. Essentially, the extrinsic muscles set the basic posture of the tongue, and the intrinsic muscles are responsible for fine articulatory movements. For speech, at least 10 basic actions are required:

1. Tongue tip elevation: Elevation of the tongue is the primary responsibility of the superior longitudinal muscles of the tongue. When the fibers contract, the tip and lateral margins of the tongue are elevated.

2. Tongue tip depression: Depression of the tongue tip is primarily accomplished by constriction of the inferior longitudinal muscles. Their course along the lateral margins of the lower tongue enables them to depress the tip and sides of the tongue.

3. Tongue protrusion: Tongue protrusion requires contraction of the posterior genioglossus and at least two intrinsic muscles. Contraction of the posterior genioglossus moves the tongue anteriorly but does not point the tongue. To make the tongue point, assistance from the vertical and transverse intrinsic muscles is required. To deviate the tongue (superiorly, inferiorly, or to the sides) also requires

constriction of the superior and inferior longitudinal intrinsic muscles. Contraction of only the posterior genioglossus leaves the tongue hanging down from the open mouth.

4. Tongue retraction: Retraction of the body of the tongue involves both the intrinsic and extrinsic muscles. The anterior genioglossus pulls the protruded tongue into the oral cavity, and co-contraction of the superior and inferior longitudinal muscles shortens the tongue. To retract the tongue into the pharyngeal space, as in swallowing, the styloglossus must contract.

5. Tongue tip deviation, left or right: Movement of the tongue tip to the left or right requires contraction of the superior and inferior longitudinal muscles on the side you wish to move your tongue toward (e.g., left constriction to move left).

6. Lateral margin relaxation: The lateral margins of the tongue must be relaxed to produce the sound /l/ even as the tongue is protruded to the anterior alveolar ridge and elevated slightly. A slight contraction of the posterior genioglossus moves the tongue anteriorly, and the superior longitudinal muscle elevates the tip. Contraction of the transverse intrinsic muscles of the tongue pulls the sides medially away from the lateral gum ridge, allowing the lateral margins of the tongue to relax.

7. Central tongue grooving: The amount of tongue grooving is controlled by the magnitude of muscle contraction. Depression of the medial tongue is accomplished by the contraction of the entire genioglossus in conjunction with the vertical intrinsic fibers. A more moderate groove involves the genioglossus to a lesser degree but still employs the vertical muscles. A broad groove can be accomplished by contraction of the superior longitudinal muscle, elevating the sides of the tongue as well.

8. Posterior tongue elevation: The palatoglossus muscles insert into the sides of the tongue, and upon contraction, the sides of the tongue are elevated. Contraction of the transverse muscles in the posterior tongue assists in bunching the tongue in that region.

9. Tongue body depression: Contraction of the genioglossus depresses the medial tongue. Additional contraction of the hyoglossus and chondroglossus depresses the tongue, assuming the hyoid is fixed by the infrahyoid muscles.

10. Tongue narrowing: The transverse fibers coursing from the median fibrous septum to the lateral margins of the tongue are important for narrowing the tongue.

Although the tongue is capable of generating a great deal of force through contraction, we typically use only about 20% of its potential force during speech production (Muller et al 1985).

Muscles of the Pharynx

The muscles of the pharynx are important for modifying the cross-sectional area of the pharynx during speech production (**Fig. 12.38**, **Fig. 12.39**; **Table 12.6**). The muscles of the pharynx are innervated by the accessory nerve (CN XI) and the pharyngeal branch of the vagus nerve (CN X) via the pharyngeal plexus. The **inferior pharyngeal constrictor** is located most inferiorly. Fibers of the muscle arise from the sides of the thyroid and cricoid cartilages and diverge in a fanlike configuration as they course posteriorly and medially and interdigitate with fibers of the paired muscle from the opposite side at the median **pharyngeal raphe** (connective tissue running down the posterior aspect of the pharynx). The middle and upper fibers rise obliquely, whereas the lower fibers run horizontally and inferiorly and are continuous with those of the esophagus. When the inferior constrictor contracts, it pulls the inferior part of the posterior wall of the pharynx anteriorly and the sides of the lower pharynx anteriorly and medially, resulting in decreased cross-sectional area of the lower pharynx.

The middle pharyngeal constrictor is located midway along the length of the pharynx, between the inferior and superior pharyngeal constrictors, at about the level of the oropharynx. Fibers of the muscle arise from the greater and lesser horns of the hyoid bone and the stylohyoid ligament. Fibers course posteriorly and medially and insert into the median pharyngeal raphe. The uppermost fibers of the middle constrictor course obliquely superiorly and overlap with the lower fibers of the superior pharyngeal constrictor, while the inferior fibers run obliquely inferior to the fibers of the inferior constrictor muscle. When the middle constrictor muscle contracts, the cross-sectional area of the oropharynx is decreased by pulling anteriorly on the posterior pharyngeal wall and anteriorly and medially on the lateral pharyngeal wall. Simultaneous contraction of the right and left middle pharyngeal constrictors acts like a sphincter and is important during swallowing.

The superior pharyngeal constrictor is located in the upper part of the oropharynx. Its origin is complex with four points of attachment: the pterygoid plate (of the sphenoid bone), pterygomandibular raphe (seam), inner side of the mandible, and posterolateral tongue. Its fibers course posteriorly to

Table 12.6 Muscles of the pharynx

Muscle	Origin	Insertion	Action	Innervation
Superior constrictor	Pterygomandibular raphe	Median raphe of pharyngeal aponeurosis	Pulls pharyngeal wall anteriorly, constricts pharyngeal diameter	Accessory (CN XI) and vagus (CN X) nerves
Middle constrictor	Horns of the hyoid	Median pharyngeal raphe	Narrows diameter of pharynx	Accessory (CN XI) and vagus (CN X) nerves
Inferior constrictor	Thyroid cartilage	Median pharyngeal raphe	Narrows the diameter of the pharynx	Accessory (CN XI) and vagus (CN X) nerves
Palatopharyngeus	Palatal aponeurosis and posterior margin of hard palate	Upper border of thyroid cartilage	Narrows the pharynx and lowers the soft palate	Accessory (CN XI) and vagus (CN X) nerves
Stylopharyngeus	Styloid process	Pharyngeal constrictors and posterior thyroid cartilage	Elevates and opens the pharynx	Accessory (CN XI) and vagus (CN X) nerves

insert into the median pharyngeal raphe. The most superior fibers of the superior constrictor muscle are horizontal and located at the level of the velum. Contraction reduces the cross-sectional area of the upper pharynx to achieve velopharyngeal closure. The paired superior pharyngeal constrictor muscles encircle the posterior and lateral walls of the upper pharynx; simultaneous contraction decreases the cross-sectional area of this part of the pharyngeal tube, similar to a sphincter.

The anterior fibers of the palatopharyngeus muscle originate from the anterior hard palate, and the posterior fibers arise from the midline of the soft palate posterior to the fibers of the levator veli palatini, attached to the palatal aponeurosis. Fibers from each muscle course laterally and inferiorly, forming the posterior faucial pillar and inserting into the posterior thyroid cartilage. This muscle intermingles with fibers of the stylopharyngeus and salpingopharyngeus muscles prior to insertion and assists in narrowing the pharyngeal cavity as well as lowering the soft palate.

The **stylopharyngeus muscle** extends between the styloid process of the temporal bone and the lateral wall of the pharynx near the juncture of the superior and middle pharyngeal constrictor muscles. Its fibers course inferiorly, anteriorly, and medially. When the stylopharyngeus contracts, it pulls the pharyngeal tube superiorly and draws the lateral wall of the pharynx laterally. When both the right and left stylopharyngeus muscles contract, the cross-sectional area of the pharyngeal tube increases, particularly in the oropharynx.

The Pharynx as an Articulator

The pharynx houses a complex array of muscles collectively referred to as the superior, middle, and inferior constrictors. During speech,

---

Box 12.6 Oral Cancer

Patients with oral cavity or oropharyngeal cancer often undergo surgery to remove the tumor. Although tissue is often taken from other parts of the body to provide tongue bulk and closure of the areas where the cancer was removed, structures of the oral cavity and oropharynx are significantly affected. These patients have difficulties with both speech and swallowing. Removal of tissue from the tongue and from the pharynx near the velopharyngeal port results in the most severe speech problems. Dental prostheses can be used to assist with speech and swallowing. For example, if one side of the tongue is removed, a palatal prosthesis can be made that lowers the palate on the side where the tongue was removed to assist the patient in making contact with the palate for palatal and alveolar consonants. If velopharyngeal port closure is impaired by the resection, a palatal obturator can be used to assist with closure of the velopharynx. In cases where a large amount of tissue is removed, particularly if the tongue is damaged, the patient may not be able to use speech to communicate. In these cases, rehabilitation should focus on working with the patient and family to identify augmentative and alternative methods of communication.

the constrictor muscles expand and contract to change the diameter and length of the pharynx to change the resonant properties of the vocal tract. The superior constrictor muscle primarily controls the size of the velopharyngeal port from the sides, which assists with velopharyngeal closure. The middle constrictor radiates from the hyoid bone to the pharyngeal wall and constricts pharyngeal diameter and retracts the hyoid bone. The inferior pharyngeal constrictor narrows the hypopharyngeal cavity during gestures in speech such as whispering.

Immobile Articulators

Teeth

As just described, the teeth are considered an immobile articulator, even though the lower teeth move during mandibular movement. The teeth are important for speech production because they serve as a point of contact for moveable articulators to produce speech sounds. The teeth are involved in production of linguadental speech sounds, /θ/, /ð/, as well as labiodental consonants /f/, /v/. As the names implies, linguadental sounds are produced by placing the tongue between the upper and lower teeth, and labiodental refers to a compression of the upper teeth onto the lower lip. In both cases, a movable articulator comes in contact with the immobile teeth to produce a speech sound.

Alveolar Ridge

The alveolar ridge is the bony part of the upper and lower gums where the tooth sockets reside. It is covered with a layer of mucous membrane. In terms of speech production, the maxillary alveolar arch is important for the production of alveolar sounds, where the tongue comes in contact with the alveolar ridge. These sounds include /t/, /d/, /s/, /z/, /l/, /n/. Some people may also produce /ɹ/ in this region.

Hard Palate

The hard palate is an immobile articulator, but it serves a role in the production of some speech sounds. For sounds such as /ʃ/, /ʒ/, /ʧ/, /ʤ/, the tip of the tongue approximates the anterior portion of the hard palate (e.g., the juncture of the hard palate and alveolar ridge). The /ɹ/ phoneme may also be produced in this region. In English, the only true palatal sound is /j/, where the blade of the tongue articulates with the hard palate.

■ Development of the Vocal Tract

The vocal tract, including the skeletal framework and soft tissue components of an infant, is clearly smaller than that of an adult, but the infant is not merely a small version of an adult. The infant vocal tract differs in relative sizes among the components of the vocal tract as well as their configuration. Proportional changes occur during development that have an impact on speech development. At birth, the skull is relatively large compared to the body of the newborn; however, the viscerocranium is small compared to that of an adult. In an infant, the face is about one-eighth the bulk of the cranium as opposed to about one-half in an adult (Zemlin 1998). After the first year of life, the viscerocranium grows at a more rapid rate than the neurocranium. A major feature of this development is the inferior and anterior growth of the face.

The neurocranium approximates adult size relatively early in childhood, at about 6 years of age (Melsen and Melsen 1982). The viscerocranium, on the other hand, continues to grow into adolescence and possibly adulthood (Kent and Vorperian 1995; Vorperian et al 2009). During this growth period, the anteroposterior depth of the hard palate nearly doubles, but lateral expansion is significantly less. Mandible growth is relatively steady until adulthood, with its length increasing to accommodate additional permanent teeth and the angle of the ramus and body becoming less obtuse (Zemlin 1998).

Soft tissue within the vocal tract also undergoes significant growth. The pharyngeal cavity of a newborn is approximately 4 cm in length and much shorter than the oral cavity (Crelin 1973). The pharynx almost triples in length, to approximately 12 cm, by adulthood. The junction between the pharyngeal and oral cavities is rounded in an infant rather than having the nearly right-angle orientation of an adult; this change occurs during puberty (Kent and Vorperian 1995).

The tongue of the newborn essentially fills the oral cavity (Crelin 1976). During the first year, the tongue begins to descend within the neck as the oral and pharyngeal cavities grow, and it continues to do so until about 5 years of age (Kent and Vorperian 1995). Growth of the tongue begins at about age 5 and continues through puberty. Growth of the tongue is similar to the growth pattern for the mandible (Kent and Vorperian 1995). The lips form a nearly round sphincter at birth but develop a more transverse elliptical sphincter in the adult. Reconfiguration of the lips occurs during the first

2 years of life (Burke 1980). As the lips grow, the thickness of the lower lip exceeds that of the upper lip. Rapid lip growth is reported between ages 10 and 17 years (Vig and Cohen 1979).

Growth of the vocal tract structures is accompanied by changes in various aspects of the nervous system. Changes include development and maturation of the regions of the brain, motor control, and other nervous system functions relevant for speech production. These changes in the nervous system include maturation in synaptic connections, axon diameters, dendrite branching, myelination of motor and sensory pathways, and establishment of neural networks (Netsell 1986; Paus et al 2001). Development of movement control for articulation is continuous and nonlinear during childhood (Netsell 1986). Some changes in movement control appear gradual, whereas others occur over shorter periods of time (Newell et al 2001). As an example, studies have shown slower rates of speech production and increased variability in children compared to adults (Smith et al 1983; Nittrouer 1993; Sturm and Seery 2007). Variability can be seen in velocity, timing, and general movement patterns during speech. The transition to more rapid and stable speech movements is gradual and may not be adultlike until around 12 to 14 years of age (Kent 1976; Smith and Zalaznik 2004; Walsh and Smith 2002). However, studies suggest short-term plasticity in school-age children using a repeated trials paradigm to demonstrate rapid improvements in performance (Walsh et al 2006). These data suggest improved coupling of the upper lip, lower lip, and mandible during later productions of an utterance within a single experimental session. This short-term plastic nature of speech

Table 12.7 American English vowels and diphthongs

Degree of Major Constriction	Place of Major Constriction		
	Front	**Central**	**Back**
High	i *heed* ɪ *hid*		u *who* ʊ *hood*
Mid	eɪ,e *hate* ɛ *head*	ɝ *bird*, ɚ *mother* ʌ *but*, ə *about*	oʊ,o *hoed* ɔ *caught*
Low	æ *had*		ɑ *hot*

Diphthongs: aɪ *dice*; aʊ *cow*; ɔɪ *boy*

production reveals a strong practice effect and suggests a high degree of flexibility in vocal tract coordination.

■ Articulation

Recall that eight primary articulators (five mobile and three immobile) produce changes in the shape of the vocal tract. With just these eight articulators, all sounds in American English can be produced. In American English, there are 26 letters of the alphabet, but approximately 44 speech sounds. To enable consistent scientific discussion of languages in which there are more speech sounds than alphabet letters, those for which there is no script, and those between which alphabets are used inconsistently, a special system called the International Phonetic Alphabet (IPA) was developed to represent each possible speech sound with a unique character. Some of the IPA symbols are ordinary alphabet letters, while others are new designs or modifications of existing letters. **Table 12.7** and **Table 12.8** provide a list of the

Table 12.8 American English consonants

Place of Production	Manner of Production							
	Stop/Plosive		Fricative		Affricate		Nasal	Semivowel
	U	**V**	**U**	**V**	**U**	**V**	**V**	**V**
Labial	p *pig*	b *big*					m *mice*	w *well*
Labiodental			f *face*	v *vase*				
Dental			θ *thin*	ð *then*				
Alveolar	t *tool*	d *duel*	s *sue*	z *zoo*			n *nice*	l *lake*
Palatal			ʃ *shoe*	ʒ *measure*	ʧ *cheap*	ʤ *jeep*		j *yellow*, ɹ *rake*
Velar	k *coat*	g *goat*					ŋ *sing*	
Glottal			h *how*					

U - unvoiced; V - voiced

American English vowels and consonants, respectively, with their corresponding IPA characters.

Vowels are described based on place of major constriction, which specifies the location within the vocal tract where the airway is maximally constricted during production, and the degree of that constriction. There are three locations coded for vowels: front, central, and back. The term "front" refers to constrictions between the tongue and alveolar process of the maxilla; "central" indicates a constriction between the tongue and the hard palate, or when no obvious constriction exists. The term "back" designates constrictions formed between the tongue and velum or between the tongue and posterior pharyngeal wall. The degree of constriction is coded as high, mid, or low, corresponding to the location of the highest point of the tongue surface. The vowels of American English are shown according to these categories in **Table 12.7**, with the IPA symbol for each followed by a common word that serves as an example, with the letters corresponding to the vowel sound italicized. A diphthong consists of two vowels produced within a single syllable. There are five diphthongs in American English; the three listed below the table are considered distinct **phonemes** (meaning they represent separate vowel categories of their own), while the other two are listed within the table because they are considered **allophones** (alternative ways of expressing another vowel category).

Consonants, unlike vowels, are produced with a substantially constricted or obstructed airway. Some are produced with voicing, and some are not. As shown in **Table 12.8**, consonants are coded along three dimensions: manner of production, place of production, and voicing. The manner of production refers to the way the structures within the vocal tract constrict the airway during production of a consonant. The manner of production includes five adjustments: stop or plosive, fricative, affricate, nasal, and semivowel. The place of production identifies where a consonant constriction or occlusion occurs along the vocal tract. Places of production include labial, labiodental, dental, alveolar, palatal, velar, and glottal, listed in order of position farther inward along the vocal tract. The voicing dimension for consonants is binary. That is, either the voice is on or off for consonant productions, so consonants are categorized as either voiced or unvoiced. In American English, there are no unvoiced nasal or semivowel consonants. Note that /j/ and /ɹ/ are both palatal semivowels, but for /j/ the body of the tongue is articulated to the palate, while for /ɹ/ the tip of the tongue is the movable articulator (strictly speaking). Moreover, /l/, unlike other alveolar consonants, is articulated with lateral margin relaxation, as discussed in the section on the tongue as an articulator.

Resonance

Resonance can be defined as the vibratory response of a body or air-filled cavity to a frequency imposed on it (Wood 1971). As discussed in the source-filter theory section that follows, the speech mechanism acts like a resonator. As the acoustic waveform generated by the vibration of the vocal folds travels through the vocal tract, it is shaped by the natural vibrating frequencies of the vocal tract structures.

Resonance, by definition, is a physical phenomenon; however, the term is also used to refer to the perceptual aspects of the speech signal as it varies under different resonating conditions. In other words, the term "resonance" is used to describe the perception of the relative amounts of sound emanating from the mouth and nose during speech production. This distinction in terminology was discussed in the section on the velum as an articulator. Speakers do not have speech patterns that are simply categorized as normal or abnormal with respect to resonance. Rather, resonance characteristics are on a continuum. Normal resonance is marked by some nasal resonance. A speaker may sound slightly more hypernasal than another, but both are considered to have normal resonance. If slightly more **nasality** is present, one might perceive vowels as being hypernasal. Hypernasality occurs when the oral and nasal cavities are abnormally coupled and the sound wave is diverted into the nasal airway. On the other hand, a speaker with too little nasal resonance on vowels might be considered hyponasal. Hyponasality is perceived when the nasal airway itself is partially blocked or the entrance to the nasal passages is partially occluded. The coupling of the oral and nasal cavities is controlled primarily by the velopharyngeal mechanism.

Source-Filter Theory

A widely accepted description of how the vocal tract shapes speech sounds is the source-filter theory of speech production. In general terms, this theory suggests that a primitive sound produced within the larynx is transformed, as it travels through the vocal tract, into the sound patterns a listener recognizes as speech. Although sound travels as a wave, it is often more revealing to specify the characteristics of a sound in terms of an amplitude spectrum. Much as a prism can separate white light into the colors of the rainbow, a spectrum shows how the energy in a sound wave is distributed from low to high frequency. In speech, the sound produced in the larynx

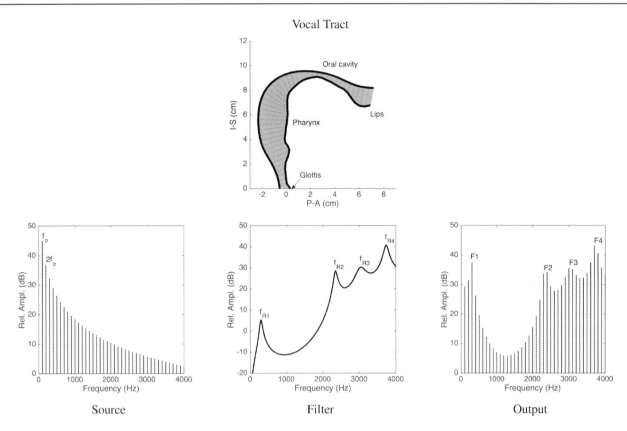

Fig. 12.46 Schematic representation of how the source (input) spectrum (left panel) and filter function (middle panel) are combined to produce a vocal tract output spectrum (right panel) for the vowel /i/. The upper center panel shows the vocal tract configuration corresponding to the filter function shown. The peaks in the output spectrum are the formants (F1, F2, F3) representing the first three resonance frequencies of the vocal tract (f_{R1}, f_{R2}, f_{R3}). Figure provided courtesy of Brad H. Story, Ph.D., University of Arizona. Reproduced with permission.

typically contains energy that is broadly spread across the spectrum with no distinct pattern. As it enters the vocal tract, multiple resonances come into play that impose a pattern on the incoming energy; by the time the sound exits the vocal tract at the lips, its spectrum has been reshaped into a series of precisely positioned peaks and valleys extending from low to high frequency. Each peak signifies a grouping of frequencies where the energy has been enhanced; these are called **formants** and are important acoustic cues used by listeners to perceive speech sounds.

The source-filter representation of the high front vowel /i/ is demonstrated in **Fig. 12.46**. The vocal tract shape is shown in the top middle panel and is configured so that the constriction is forward in the mouth, near the alveolar ridge just behind the front teeth; note that this representation is simply the airway shape and contains no anatomic structures. In the bottom left panel is a spectrum of a sound produced by vibration of the vocal folds (i.e., the "source"). The horizontal axis indicates frequency from low to high, whereas the vertical axis shows the amplitude (or energy). The leftmost

vertical line in the spectrum represents the vibrating frequency of the vocal folds, or fundamental frequency (f_o). The other vertical lines indicate the harmonics; recall that they are located at successively higher frequencies that are whole-number multiples of the fundamental frequency (as an example, the second harmonic is labeled as $2f_o$); note also that the amplitude of each successive harmonic decreases. Shown in the lower center panel is the filter, which depicts how the frequencies that are present in the source spectrum are enhanced or suppressed by passing through the vocal tract shape. Each peak in the filter represents an acoustic resonance of the vocal tract and is labeled as f_{R1}, f_{R2}, etc. The spectrum in the bottom right panel is the result of combining the source spectrum with the filter. You should appreciate that the fundamental frequency and harmonics produced by the source are still present, but the amplitude of the harmonics has changed based on the pattern imposed by the filter. Notice groupings of harmonics with higher amplitudes relative to other surrounding harmonics. These groupings are the formants and are labeled as F1, F2, etc. For the vowel /i/, we observe a peak for the first formant F1 at about 300 Hz and the second formant F2 at approximately 2,500 Hz.

The positions and movements of the individual articulators collectively determine the shape of the vocal tract and, thus, determine the pattern of acoustic resonances in the filter at any given time. When muscles are activated to move the articulators, the vocal tract shape changes. This change in vocal tract shape coincides with a change in the resonance or frequency response of the filter and ultimately results in a change of the formants. For example, when you move your tongue from the high front position for the /i/ vowel to a low back position for an /ɑ/ vowel, you change the shape of both your pharynx and your oral cavity, which shifts the formants from those present in **Fig. 12.46** to new locations along the frequency axis. The change in formant frequency is illustrated in **Fig. 12.47a**, where the change in vocal tract shape from /i/ to /ɑ/ is shown and is reflected acoustically as a change of the formant frequencies as time progresses, shown in **Fig. 12.47b**, called a wide-band spectrogram, where time is represented on the horizontal axis, frequency on the vertical axis, and amplitude is coded by color (yellow is high amplitude, blue is low). Simply, a spectrogram is a long sequence of instantaneous spectra like those in the right panel of **Fig. 12.46**, where each spectrum corresponds to a specific point in time. The highest-amplitude regions (yellow in this case) are displayed in the spectrogram as the wide bands of energy and represent the

formants. For purposes of analysis, the center of the formant bands can be "tracked" over time, as indicated by the thin black lines. Thus, precise movements of the articulators are the physiologic means by which speakers systematically produce a flow of speech sounds with distinctive characteristics. Consequently, spectrographic analysis of speech is a means of determining the characteristics of sound perceived by a listener, and it provides an indirect measure of articulator movement.

Consonants are also produced by a sound source combined with a filter. They are different from vowels in that the source is typically located near the point of primary constriction in the vocal tract rather than the larynx, and the filter consists of the portion of the vocal tract downstream of the constriction. For example, the fricative /s/, as in the word "see," is produced by moving the tongue tip to the alveolar ridge until only a small opening is left, through which air is forced. Airflow becomes turbulent or noisy as it exits the opening, creating a sound source near the teeth that is filtered by the short section of airway extending from this constriction to the lips. Stop consonants are produced by completely closing off the vocal tract (e.g., the stop /t/ is formed by pressing the tongue completely against the alveolar ridge) for a short time while pressure builds behind the constriction. When the constriction is released, the pressure causes air to flow rapidly and generates a burst of turbulence noise just downstream of the constriction that is filtered by the surrounding airspace. Consonants may

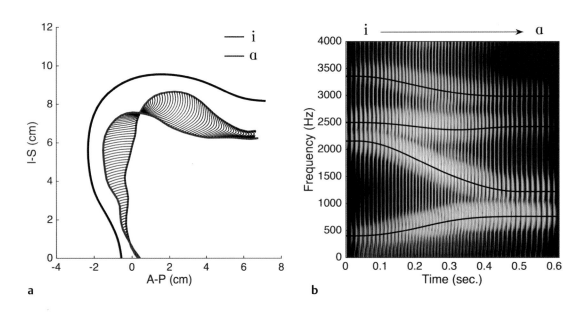

Fig. 12.47 **(a)** The change in vocal tract shape for the vowel-to-vowel sequence from /i/ (red line) to /ɑ/ (blue line). **(b)** The corresponding change in formant frequencies, shown as a wide-band spectrogram. The black lines in **(b)** indicate tracking of the formants for purposes of analysis. Figure provided courtesy of Brad H. Story, Ph.D., University of Arizona. Reproduced with permission.

also be produced while the vocal folds are vibrating, combining turbulence noise with the periodicity of laryngeal pulses; these are "voiced" consonants as compared with the "unvoiced" consonants produced in the absence of vocal fold vibration.

Just as the vocal tract shape is determined by the positions of the articulators, the overall size of the vocal tract (length and cross section) is determined by the size of the articulators. As a child grows from infancy to adulthood, the vocal tract undergoes continual restructuring with regard to the size of the larynx, pharynx, oral cavity, and nasal passages. In adulthood, there are also size differences between males and females as well as idiosyncratic differences from one person to the next. In general, the smaller the structure, the higher the frequencies produced. For the voice source, small vocal folds (e.g., children, adult females) produce high fundamental frequencies, whereas low fundamental frequencies are produced by large vocal folds (e.g., adult males). With regard to the vocal tract, a short length will have higher-frequency resonances (and formants) than a longer vocal tract. Adult males typically have lower formants than do adult females, who in turn have lower formants than children. During speech, an individual speaker may also dynamically lengthen or shorten the vocal tract by lip rounding and lip spreading or by raising and lowering the larynx. These maneuvers result in altered formants.

■ Measurement of Articulation and Resonance

The configuration of the vocal tract depends on the position of the speech articulators (tongue, lips, jaw, velum, and larynx). Furthermore, because the acoustics are continually changing during speech, it is the behavior of the speech articulators over time (e.g., changes of articulatory configuration and their acoustic consequences) that are of interest in the study of speech production. A number of different techniques have been used to investigate vocal tract structures during speech production. A brief description of some of these techniques follows.

Electromyography

Electromyography (EMG) is a technique used to measure muscle activity. Electrodes are placed on the skin (surface) or into muscles (intramuscular). EMG can be helpful to measure activity from multiple locations within a muscle, since activity can vary within a muscle belly. Surface electrodes are

noninvasive, but they detect a larger volume of muscle activity (e.g., all activity below the electrode), making it difficult to differentiate activity of one muscle from another. For example, a surface electrode placed on the submental surface will detect activity from the anterior belly of the digastric, the mylohyoid, and the geniohyoid, and it would be hard to distinguish which muscle was primarily responsible for the activity detected by the electrode. Intramuscular electrodes are more precise in the activity that they record, but they are invasive. EMG signals can be difficult to acquire because they can be sensitive to electromagnetic radiation in the environment, even that produced by the circuitry around fluorescent lights. Since EMG provides no information about the movement of structures, it is usually coupled with a technique that can provide this information.

Radiography

X-ray imaging is a powerful tool for studying the positions and movements of structures found within the vocal tract. Lateral X-ray images have long been used to provide a midsagittal view of the articulators in a still position. From these images, measures of the midline positions of the lips, mandible, tongue, velum, posterior pharyngeal wall, and hyoid bone in relation to each other can be made. One limitation of this technique is that images are obtained while a speaker sustains a single speech sound and thus are limited to vowels and to fricative and nasal consonants.

Cinefluoroscopy (or videofluoroscopy) is an X-ray technique that enables the study of structures in motion. This moving X-ray facilitates observation of the spatial and temporal coordination among the structures within the vocal tract as the speaker produces an utterance. Movement patterns can be seen for the lips, mandible, tongue, velum, posterior pharyngeal wall, and hyoid bone as well as other structures. Quantitative analysis is completed on a frame-by-frame basis and can be tedious and time-consuming; nonetheless, this technique is powerful for examining speech production behaviors, and a great deal of knowledge has been gained about both normal and abnormal (disordered) speech production.

Measurement of the outline of stationary and moving structures using cinefluoroscopy is very complex. One technique designed to simplify measurement involves attaching small metal markers at strategic locations on the structures of interest and using an X-ray beam to track their positions as a function of time. An example of where markers can be attached is shown in **Fig. 12.48.** The X-ray microbeam system, developed at the University of Tokyo (Kiritani et al 1975) and in the United States at the University of Wisconsin–Madison (Westbury 1991), was designed to track small pellets glued to structures in the oral cavity using an extremely thin X-ray beam to limit exposure to radiation by focusing the beam on the pellets, while the surrounding tissue receives only minimal radiation. This technique tracks the two-dimensional position of multiple pellets simultaneously. Research has shown that patterns of tongue movement with and without the pellets in position are not appreciably different, so the pellet-tracking protocol does not influence the usual behavior of the speaker (Weismer and Bunton 1999). An example of data obtained using the X-ray microbeam is shown in **Fig. 12.49**. The path, or "trajectory," of the pellet labeled T1 is shown in **Fig. 12.49a** for the utterance "eedah" (/idɑ/ in IPA) where the X and Y positions correspond to the front/back and high/low configurations of the tongue, respectively. These same X–Y positions are shown stretched out along time in the middle panel of **Fig. 12.49b**. The speed of the T1 pellet (derived from both the X and Y positions over time) is plotted in the bottom panel, and a spectrogram of the utterance is shown in the top panel. The minima in the speed plot indicate temporal boundaries of articulatory movements that can be related to phonetic segments. For example, during the time period between the first two dashed lines, the tongue tip moves rapidly superiorly and posteriorly away from its position for the initial /i/, and then

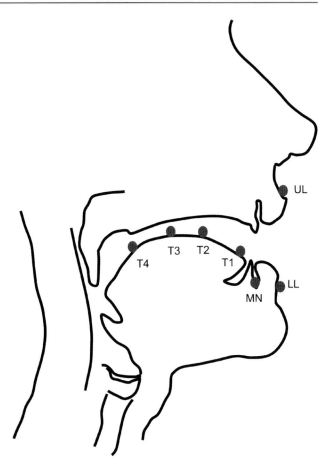

Fig. 12.48 Fleshpoint pellet positions used in X-ray microbeam studies of speech production. Figure provided courtesy of Brad H. Story, Ph.D., University of Arizona. Reproduced with permission.

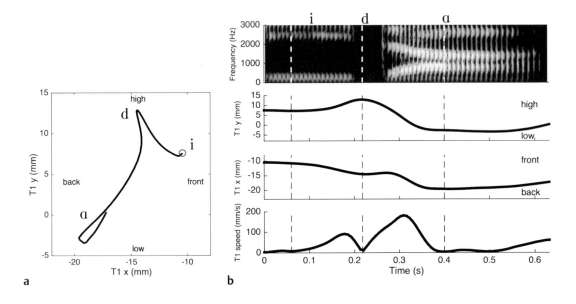

Fig. 12.49 X-ray microbeam data showing the tracking of a pellet attached at the tip of the tongue (T1). **(a)** Pellet moving in both the X- and Y- dimensions for the utterance /idɑ/. **(b)** Spectrogram for the same utterance (top); the X- and Y-dimensions shown individually and stretched out over time (middle); and speed of pellet movement (bottom). Figure provided courtesy of Brad H. Story, Ph.D., University of Arizona. Reproduced with permission.

its speed drops to nearly zero when it arrives at the desired point of constriction for the /d/ consonant. Movement of the tongue tip is initiated again, this time in an inferior direction, to release the /d/ and move toward the final /ɑ/ vowel. Studies using the X-ray microbeam have examined kinematic patterns of the oral structures in both individuals with normal speech production (Tasko and Westbury 2003) and individuals with neuromotor-based speech disorders (Weismer et al 2003; Weismer et al 2009).

Electromagnetic Sensing

Electromagnetic sensing, much like the X-ray microbeam, provides a means to track movement of points on the oral articulators (lips, tongue, and velum). Such sensing relies on detection and quantification of magnetic fields induced in receiving coils by generating coils. The data provide measures of the position of the receiving coil in one-, two-, or three-dimensional space. One such system is called an electromagnetic midsagittal articulometer (EMMA). EMMA uses a computer algorithm to calculate the distance between generating and receiving coils as the coils move through space over time. The EMMA system provides a useful means of understanding the speech mechanism, evaluating physiologic behaviors, and providing feedback that may be of value in the study of movement disorders affecting speech production. This technique is increasingly popular and appears to yield a more comprehensive understanding of normal speech production, abnormal speech production, and swallowing as well (Perkell et al 1992).

Electropalatography

Electropalatography (EPG) is a technique for sensing tongue contact with the palate. An acrylic mouthpiece shaped like the palate is made and fitted over the natural palate, and embedded electrodes sense tongue contact with the acrylic palate. Maps of tongue contact are then generated. EPG provides visual feedback during articulatory therapy and measures pre and post changes in therapy. However, there are some drawbacks. The acrylic palate likely alters normal articulatory movements. Also, posterior and alveolar contact are not well detected because of the distribution of the electrodes. It is important not to use this technique to train specific articulatory placements, because articulation is variable depending on the context of the target phoneme.

Camera Systems

Movements of the lips and jaw can be captured using a variety of camera systems. In most systems, markers are placed on the lips and jaw and are then tracked with a camera system. These systems have wide applicability, as they are also regularly used to track walking, balance, and other whole-body movements. Marker systems are noninvasive, but the markers must be kept in view of the cameras; thus, the tongue cannot be studied with marker-camera systems. These systems have been widely used to study the development of speech motor skills in children, largely because they are noninvasive and do not expose the speaker to radiation (Smith and Goffman 1998; Green et al 2002).

Ultrasound Imaging

Ultrasonic methods rely on the use of high-frequency sound waves to map the position and movements of the internal structures. A combined sound generator–sound receiver is placed on the outer surface of the skin. The ultrasonic waves are generated and directed inward through the body tissues. The waves propagate until they reach airspace. Ultrasonic waves do not travel well through air and are, therefore, reflected back through the same tissue and picked up by the sound receiver. The time it takes for ultrasonic energy to make the round trip provides a measure of whether the air-space boundary is moving toward or away from the receiver. The most widely imaged oral structure during speech production is the dorsal surface of the tongue (Stone 2005). When imaging the tongue, the receiver is positioned below the chin and oriented so that the sound beam can be swept to scan the interface between the airway and the surface of the tongue (Stone 1996).

As shown in **Fig. 12.50,** images of the surface of the tongue are most often obtained in midsagittal and coronal scans. Midsagittal scans are analogous to those observed in lateral X-ray images. Coronal scans provide views of the dorsum of the tongue that are at right angles to those provided by the midsagittal scans. This view makes it possible to look at behaviors such as tongue grooving that would be difficult to observe using a lateral image. Visualization of the tongue from these two perspectives provides a powerful research and clinical tool.

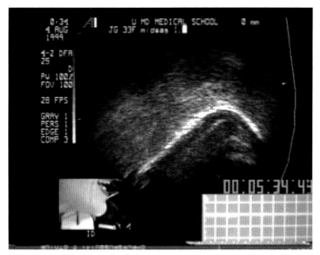

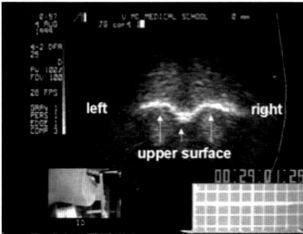

Fig. 12.50 Ultrasound images of the upper surface of the tongue shown in midsagittal and coronal scans. Images provided courtesy of Maureen Stone, Ph.D., University of Maryland Dental School, Baltimore, MD. Reproduced with permission.

Magnetic Resonance Imaging

Over the last two decades, a number of pioneering studies of vocal tract shapes have been reported using magnetic resonance imaging (MRI; Story et al 1996, 1998; Narayanan et al 1995). Midsagittal and three-dimensional images can be obtained for static speech sounds based on prolonged speech articulations. These static images enable detailed study of the airway shape during speech production. As an example, midsagittal images of /i/, /d/, and /ɑ/ obtained from a male speaker are shown in **Fig. 12.51**. These images were collected while the speaker was supine in an MRI scanner.

Recent improvements in temporal resolution have made it possible to examine the dynamics of vocal tract shaping during fluent speech using MRI. Although three-dimensional imaging is typically not possible, this method provides dynamic information for the entire vocal tract from the glottis to the lips in the midsagittal plane, which is not available with other methods for observing articulatory movements. Since image processing of the acquired data is automatic, the result can be observed immediately after recording, much like X-ray video but without any radiation exposure. Preliminary results suggest that this method has many possible applications to speech production research, such as the study of the articulatory coordination among multiple speech articulators.

Acoustic Observations

The acoustic signal recorded during speech production provides information on both sound generation and sound filtering, regardless of whether the

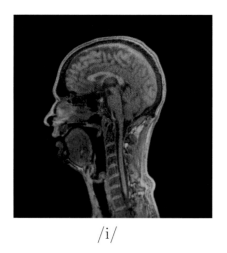

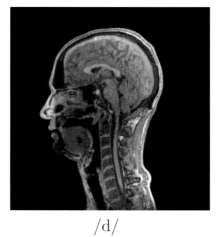

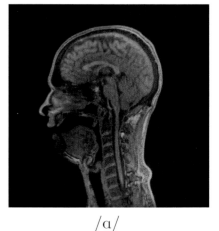

/i/   /d/   /ɑ/

Fig. 12.51 MRI views of the vocal tract taken in a midsagittal plane of an adult male speaker producing the sounds /i/, /d/, and /ɑ/. Images provided courtesy of Adam Baker, Ph.D., University of North Dakota, Grand Forks, ND. Reproduced with permission.

source is due to voicing, bursts, or turbulence. As discussed in the source-filter theory section, spectrograms provide information related to the possible positions and movements of the articulators across time during both vowel and consonant production. Most articulatory adjustments that make speech sounds distinct originate within the vocal tract. Understanding the relationship between speech physiology and speech acoustics is critically important for making logical inferences about the temporal and spatial coordination of underlying adjustments in both normal and abnormal speech production (Weismer 2006).

■ Coordinated Articulation

Speech is one of the most complex sequential motor tasks performed by humans. Early ideas about how speech is produced suggested that we simply linked basic movements into a series, like beads on a string. If the target word were "bead," the speaker would sequence the three separate sounds /b/, /i/, and /d/ to produce the word. Over the past few decades, however, research suggests that speech is not produced as a series of individual sounds but rather as a continuous blending of one sound into another, referred to as **coarticulation**. Coarticulation is accomplished by sequencing articulatory movements such that the characteristics of successive phonemes overlap in time. For example, the /ʃ/ sound in the word "shoe" is produced with rounded lips in anticipation of the following /u/ vowel, whereas there would be no rounding of the lips for the /ʃ/ produced in the word "she."

There are two basic sources of coarticulation. One is the biomechanical constraints of the speech articulators coupled with the fast rate at which speech is produced. In other words, because the articulators have mass, it takes time for them to be put into motion, change direction, or be brought to a stop. An example of this is the movement of the velopharyngeal port. Vowels produced near nasal sounds /m/, /n/, /ŋ/ tend to have more nasal resonance than vowels produced in a completely oral context. Nasal resonance is present because it takes more time to open and close the velum than is present between phonemes; the velum is lowered for some time before and after a nasal phoneme. A second source of coarticulation is a result of preparation for articulatory constraints of an upcoming phoneme. For example, lip rounding for an upcoming rounded vowel such as /u/ (as in "shoe") is present to some extent before and after that vowel, spanning up to 56% of the sentence (Goffman et al

2008). You may see lip rounding during the /s/ and /t/ in the word "suit" because of the rounded vowel at the syllable nucleus.

Researchers seek to better understand articulator control to produce speech. A major question is the nature of the goal (or target) of speech production. Is the goal based on a particular articulator achieving a desired position? Or is it the production of a particular acoustic or perceptual target? Depending on the point of view, explanations about how we produce speech vary. A second question concerns the basic unit of speech production. There are arguments for and against defining the smallest unit to be an individual phoneme, syllable, or even a whole word. How the smallest unit is defined will affect our understanding of how speech is coordinated.

Think for a moment about all of the muscles and structures you have learned about in this textbook. It should be easy to understand why speech production is so complex, in part because of the number of muscles and structures involved in speech production. The nervous system has to control and coordinate all of those structures very quickly to produce speech accurately. Controlling each of those muscles separately during speech production would be extremely difficult, and this pattern of activation is not thought to be practical. Some researchers propose that there are neuromuscular synergies within the articulators; for example, that the lips and jaw are controlled together to maintain a particular lip opening for a phoneme (Kelso et al 1984; Smith and Zelaznik 2004). Adults appear to use these organized and functional synergies to produce rapid sequences of speech sounds during connected speech production. Control and coordination in adults appears automatic, effortless, and usually error free. Young children, on the other hand, show greater variability in speech production, evidence that they have not fully developed neuromuscular synergies (Kent 1976; Smith and Zelaznik 2004; Walsh and Smith 2002). Reduced variability and more adultlike productions are present in young teens.

Theories and models of speech production must also include some form of feedback regarding the accuracy of production. There are three primary types of feedback that have been investigated: auditory (hearing your own production to determine how accurate your production was), somatosensory (perceiving how accurately your physical target was achieved during articulation), and feedback from external sources (such as a puzzled look on the face of a listener). Any comprehensive theory or model of speech production must clearly define the goal, units, and feedback as well as a mechanism

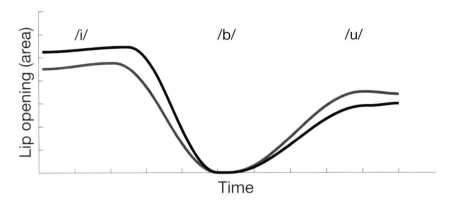

Fig. 12.52 Illustration of the interaction between motor equivalence and economy of effort in articulatory movements. The planned time course of the opening at the lips is shown by the black line and the actual trajectory is shown in red. When the lips are fully in contact for the /b/ in both the planned and actual trajectories, the area is zero. Figure provided courtesy of Brad H. Story, PhD, University of Arizona. Reproduced with permission.

for control and coordination across the articulators and the whole speech production system.

In building a theory or model, it is also important to characterize the various constraints under which speech production operates. One interesting characteristic of articulation is that a speaker can produce the same phoneme using a variety of articulatory movements. This phenomenon is known as **motor equivalence**. A good example of motor equivalence is the production of the /ɹ/ sound. The /ɹ/ sound can be produced with the tongue dorsum bunched or with the tongue tip retroflexed. Guenther et al (1999) demonstrated that speakers use different articulatory configurations for /ɹ/ in different phonetic contexts. They suggested that speakers are maintaining the same acoustic percept for /ɹ/ in a variety of phonetic contexts by using a range of articulatory configurations. Linked with the idea of motor equivalence is the idea of **economy of effort**. Economy of effort appears to be a characteristic of movement in general as well as a principle that guides speech movement planning. Speakers plan, in advance, the path that their articulators will travel to reach the target with the least amount of effort. The speaking context as well as rate of speech will influence the amount of articulatory movement produced and effort used (Lindblom 1996). In speaking situations that require a speaker to be clearer, we tend to articulate more distinctly, moving our articulators more (Lindblom 1996; Perkell et al 2002). On the other hand, in more casual speaking situations we may reduce the magnitude and speed of our articulatory movements (**Fig. 12.52**) with reduced effort. In this case, the acoustic characteristics may result in less clear speech, and the talker relies on context and familiarity of the listener to achieve the desired perceptual response. For example, imagine

your own speech when reading a book to a group of young children, compared to having a conversation with your friends. The expectations of the situation influence speech production.

One of the most common models of speech production referenced today is the Directions into Velocities of Articulation (DIVA) model (Guenther et al 1998; Callan et al 2000) (**Fig. 12.53**). DIVA is an extensive computational neural network model of speech motor skill acquisition and speech production. It has been used to simulate situations such as adaptation to articulatory perturbations, infant babbling and acquisition of speech, and stuttering. For example, in a simulation of speech acquisition, the model learns to control the movements of a computer-simulated vocal tract in order to produce speech sounds. The model's neural mappings are tuned during a babbling phase in which auditory feedback from self-generated speech sounds is used to learn the relationship between motor actions and their acoustic and somatosensory consequences. After learning, the model can produce arbitrary combinations of speech sounds, even in the presence of constraints on the articulators. This allows DIVA to be used to study a variety of speech disorders as well; for example, stuttering (Civier and Guenther 2005) or childhood apraxia of speech (Terband et al 2009).

According to the DIVA model, production of a phoneme or syllable starts with activation of a speech sound map cell (in left ventral premotor cortex) corresponding to the sound to be produced. This activation leads to production of the sound through two motor subsystems: a feedback control subsystem and a feedforward control subsystem. In the feedback control subsystem, signals from the premotor cortex travel to the auditory and somatosensory cortical areas through tuned

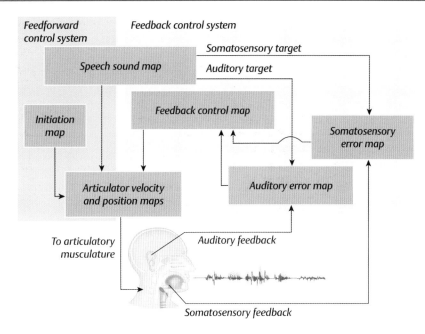

Fig. 12.53 Schematic of the DIVA model. Figure provided courtesy of Frank H. Guenther, Ph.D., Boston University. Reproduced with permission.

synapses that encode sensory expectations for the sound being produced. These expectations take the form of time-varying auditory and somatosensory target regions. The target regions are compared to the current auditory and somatosensory state, and any discrepancy between the target and the current state leads to a corrective command signal to the motor cortex. In the feedforward control subsystem, signals project from the premotor cortex to the primary motor cortex, both directly and via the cerebellum. These signals are tuned with practice by monitoring the commands from previous attempts to produce the sound, initially under feedback control. Feedforward- and feedback-based control signals are combined in the model's motor cortex to form the overall motor command.

Because the structure of DIVA is an appealing representation of the speech production process, it is occasionally used as a theoretical or conceptual model rather than an actual computational model capable of accepting input parameters and producing output. Complex speech production requires the control of many parameters simultaneously. DIVA provides unified explanations for a number of long-studied speech production phenomena, including motor equivalence, economy of effort, contextual variability, speaking rate effects, and coarticulation. Additionally, each block in the diagram corresponds to a hypothesized set of neurons in the human speech system and, thus, may facilitate further understanding of the neurophysiology of speech production.

■ References

Burke PH. Serial growth changes in the lips. *British Journal of Orthodontics, 7,* 17–30; 1980

Callan DE, Kent RD, Guenther FH, Vorperian HK. An auditory-feedback-based neural network model of speech production that is robust to developmental changes in the size and shape of the articulatory system. *Journal of Speech, Language, and Hearing Research, 43,* 721–736; 2000

Civier O, Guenther FH. Simulations of feedback and feedforward control in stuttering. In: Proceedings of the 7th Oxford Dysfluency Conference, St. Catherine's College, Oxford University; 29 June–2 July 2005.

Crelin ES. Functional Anatomy of the Newborn. Cambridge, MA: Yale University Press; 1973

Crelin ES. Development of the upper respiratory system. *Clinical Symposia, 28,* 1–30; 1976

Goffman L, Smith A, Heisler L, Ho M. The breadth of coarticulatory units in children and adults. *Journal of Speech, Language, and Hearing Research, 51,* 1424–1437; 2008

Green JR, Moore CA, Reilly KJ. The sequential development of jaw and lip control for speech. *Journal of Speech, Language, and Hearing Research, 45,* 66–79; 2002

Guenther FH, Hampson M, Johnson D. A theoretical investigation of reference frames for the planning of speech movements. *Psychological Review, 105,* 611–633; 1998

Guenther FH, Espy-Wilson CY, Boyce SE, Matthies ML, Zandipour M, Perkell JS. Articulatory tradeoffs reduce acoustic variability during American English /r/ production. *The Journal of the Acoustical Society of America, 105,* 2854–2865; 1999

Kelso JA, Tuller BV, Vatikiotis-Bateson E, Fowler CA. Functionally specific articulatory cooperation following jaw perturbations during speech: evidence for coordinative structures. *Journal of Experimental Psychology: Human Perception and Performance, 10,* 812–832; 1984

Kent RD. Anatomical and neuromuscular maturation of the speech mechanism: Evidence from acoustic studies. *Journal of Speech, Language, and Hearing Research, 19,* 421–447; 1976.

Kent RD, Vorperian HK. Development of the Craniofacial-Oral-Laryngeal Anatomy. San Diego, CA: Singular; 1995

Kier WM, Smith KK. Tongues, tentacles and trunks: the biomechanics of movement in muscular-hydrostats. *Zoological Journal of the Linnean Society, 83,* 307–324; 1985

Kiritani S, Itoh K, Fujimura O. Tongue-pellet tracking by a computer-controlled X-ray microbeam system. *The Journal of the Acoustical Society of America, 57,* 1516–1520; 1975

Lindblom B. Role of articulation in speech perception: clues from production. *The Journal of the Acoustical Society of America, 99,* 1683–1692; 1996

Melsen B, Melsen F. The postnatal development of the palatomaxillary region studied on human autopsy material. *American Journal of Orthodontics, 82,* 329–342; 1982

Moll KL. Velopharyngeal closure on vowels. *Journal of Speech, Language, and Hearing Research, 5,* 30–37; 1962.

Muller EM, Milenkovic PH, MacLeod GE. Perioral tissue mechanics during speech production. In: DeLisi C, Eisendfeld J, eds. Proceedings of the Second IMAC International Symposium on Biomedical Systems Modeling. Amsterdam, The Netherlands: North-Holland, 363–371; 1985

Narayanan SS, Alwan AA, and Haker K. An articulatory study of fricative consonants using magnetic resonance imaging. *The Journal of the Acoustical Society of America, 98,* 1325–1347; 1995

Netsell R. A Neurobiologic View of Speech Production and the Dysarthrias. San Diego, CA: College Hill Press; 1986

Newell KM, Liu Y-T, Mayer-Kress G. Time scales in motor learning and development. *Psychological Review, 108,* 57–82; 2001

Nittrouer S. The emergence of mature gestural patterns is not uniform: evidence from an acoustic study. *Journal of Speech, Language, and Hearing Research, 36,* 959–972; 1993

Paus T, Zijdenbos A, Worsley K, et al. Structural maturation of neural pathways in children and adolescents: in vivo study. *Science, 283,* 1908–1911; 1999

Perkell JS, Cohen MH, Svirsky MA, Matthies ML, Garabieta I, Jackson MT. Electromagnetic midsagittal articulometer systems for transducing speech articulatory movements. *The Journal of the Acoustical Society of America, 92,* 3078–3096; 1992

Perkell JS, Zandipour M, Matthies ML, & Lane H. (2002). Economy of effort in different speaking conditions. I. A preliminary study of intersubject differences and modeling issues. *The Journal of the Acoustical Society of America, 112*(4), 1627–1641

Smith A. The control of orofacial movements in speech. *Critical Reviews in Oral Biology and Medicine, 3,* 233–267; 1992

Smith A, Goffman L. Stability and patterning of speech movement sequences in children and adults. *Journal of Speech, Language, and Hearing Research, 41,* 18–30; 1998

Smith A, Zelaznik HN. Development of functional synergies for speech motor coordination in childhood and adolescence. *Developmental Psychobiology, 45,* 22–33; 2004

Smith BL, Sugarman MD, Long SH. Experimental manipulation of speaking rate for studying temporal variability in children's speech. *The Journal of the Acoustical Society of America, 74,* 744–749; 1983

Smith KK, Kier WM. Trunks, tongues, and tentacles: Moving with skeletons of muscle. *American Scientist, 77,* 28–35; 1989

Stone M. Instrumentation for the study of speech physiology. In: Lass NJ, ed., Principles of Experimental Phonetics. St. Louis, Mo: Mosby–Year Book, 495–524; 1996

Stone M. A guide to analysing tongue motion from ultrasound images. *Clinical Linguistics & Phonetics, 19,* 455–501; 2005

Story BH. A parametric model of the vocal tract area function for vowel and consonant simulation. *The Journal of the Acoustical Society of America, 117,* 3231–3254; 2005

Story BH, Titze IR, Hoffman EA. Vocal tract area functions from magnetic resonance imaging. *The Journal of the Acoustical Society of America, 100,* 537–554; 1996

Story BH, Titze IR, Hoffman EA. Vocal tract area functions for an adult female speaker based on volumetric imaging. *The Journal of the Acoustical Society of America, 104,* 471–487; 1998

Sturm JA, Seery CH. Speech and articulatory rates of school-age children in conversation and narrative contexts. *Language, Speech, and Hearing Services in Schools, 38,* 47–59; 2007

Tasko SM, Westbury JR. Defining and measuring speech movement events. *Journal of Speech, Language, and Hearing Research, 45,* 127–142; 2002

Terband H, Maassen B, Guenther FH, Brumberg J. Computational neural modeling of speech motor control in childhood apraxia of speech (CAS). *Journal of Speech, Language, and Hearing Research, 52,* 1595–1609; 2009

Vig PS, Cohen AM. Vertical growth of the lips: a serial cephalometric study. *American Journal of Orthodontics, 75,* 405–415; 1979

Vorperian HK, Wang S, Chung MK, et al. Anatomic development of the oral and pharyngeal portions of the vocal tract: an imaging study. *The Journal of the Acoustical Society of America, 125,* 1666–1678; 2009

Walsh B, Smith A. Articulatory movements in adolescents evidence for protracted development of speech motor control processes. *Journal of Speech, Language, and Hearing Research, 45,* 1119–1133; 2002

Walsh B, Smith A, Weber-Fox C. Short-term plasticity in children's speech motor systems. *Developmental Psychobiology, 48,* 660–674; 2006

Weismer G. Philosophy of research in motor speech disorders. *Clinical Linguistics & Phonetics, 20,* 315–349; 2006

Weismer G, Bunton K. Influences of pellet markers on speech production behavior: acoustical and perceptual measures. *The Journal of the Acoustical Society of America, 105,* 2882–2894; 1999

Weismer G, Yunusova Y, Bunton K. Measures to evaluate the effects of DBS on speech production. *Journal of Neurolinguistics, 25,* 74–94; 2012

Weismer G, Yunusova Y, Westbury JR. Interarticulator coordination in dysarthria: an X-ray microbeam study. *Journal of Speech, Language, and Hearing Research 46,* 1247–1261; 2003

Westbury JR. On coordinate systems and the representation of articulatory movements. *The Journal of the Acoustical Society of America, 95,* 2271–2273; 1994

Wood, K. Terminology and nomenclature. In: Travis LE, ed. Handbook of Speech Pathology and Audiology. New York: Appleton-Century-Crofts; 1971.

Zemlin W. Speech and Hearing Science: Anatomy & Physiology. Needham Heights, MA: Allyn & Bacon; 1998

■ **Suggested Readings**

Hoole P, Pouplier M. Interarticulatory coordination: speech sounds. In: Redford MA, ed. The Handbook of Speech Production. Hoboken, NJ: John Wiley & Sons, 133–157; 2015

Inouye JM, Perry JL, Lin KY, Blemker SS. A computational model quantifies the effect of anatomical variability on velopharyngeal function. *Journal of Speech, Language, and Hearing Research, 58,* 1119–1133; 2015

Kent RD, Kent JF, Rosenbek JC. Maximum performance tests of speech production. *Journal of Speech and Hearing Disorders, 52,* 367–387; 1987

Perkell JS. Five decades of research in speech motor control: What have we learned, and where should we go from here? *Journal of Speech, Language, and Hearing Research, 56,* S1857–S1874; 2013

Perry JL, Sutton BP, Kuehn DP, Gamage JK. Using MRI for assessing velopharyngeal structures and function. *The Cleft Palate–Craniofacial Journal, 51,* 476–485; 2014

Smith A. Development of neural control of orofacial movements for speech. In: Hardcastle WJ, Laver J, Gibbon FE, eds. The Handbook of Phonetic Sciences, 2nd ed. Chichester, UK: Wiley-Blackwell, 251–296; 2010

Stavness I, Nazari MA, Flynn C, et al. Coupled biomechanical modeling of the face, jaw, skull, tongue, and hyoid bone. In: Magnenat-Thalmann N, Ratib O, Choi HF, eds. 3D Multiscale Physiological Human. London, UK: Springer, 253–274; 2014

Tourville JA, Reilly KJ, Guenther FH. Neural mechanisms underlying auditory feedback control of speech. *Neuroimage, 39*, 1429–1443; 2008

Weismer G, Green JR. Speech production in motor speech disorders: lesions, models, and a research agenda. In: Redford MA, ed. The Handbook of Speech Production. Hoboken, NJ: John Wiley & Sons, 298–330; 2015

Yunusova, Y., Weismer G, Westbury JR, Lindstrom MJ. Articulatory movements during vowels in speakers with dysarthria and healthy controls. *Journal of Speech, Language, and Hearing Research, 51*, 596–611; 2008

■ Study Questions

1. Which of the following lists contain all paired bones?

A. Parietal, temporal, maxilla, zygomatic
B. Temporal, occipital, sphenoid, zygomatic
C. Mandible, maxilla, zygomatic, temporal
D. Parietal, temporal, palatine, frontal
E. Sphenoid, ethmoid, vomer, temporal

2. At one time a chewing tobacco company advertised the use of one of its products as "just a pinch between your cheek and gums." What is the name of the cavity or space in which the tobacco would be placed according to this ad (if you did decide to do such a thing)?

A. Glottis
B. Oral cavity
C. Buccal cavity
D. Mucosal space
E. Digastric cavity

3. The buccinator is best described as:

A. The deepest muscle of the face, principal muscle of the cheek, pulling mouth corners
B. Between the maxilla and the upper lip, raising the angle of the mouth up
C. An oval ring of muscle, located within the lips, puckering lips
D. Between the inner surface of the mandible and the hyoid bone, lowering mandible
E. Between the sides of the tongue and the midline of the soft palate, elevating the tongue

4. During a smile, which muscle would definitely *not* be contracted:

A. Levator anguli oris
B. Levator labii superioris
C. Zygomaticus major
D. Depressor anguli oris
E. Risorius

5. Which pair of muscles could be contracted to lower the mandible:

A. Digastric and palatoglossus
B. Temporalis and geniohyoid
C. Mylohyoid and geniohyoid
D. Masseter and internal pterygoid
E. Medial pterygoid and lateral pterygoid

6. The posterior faucial pillars are formed primarily by which muscle?

A. Palatoglossus
B. Palatopharyngeus
C. Hyoglossus
D. Faucial extensor posterioris
E. Styloglossus

7. The term "muscular hydrostat" means that the tongue:

A. Contains the only bones in the body that are filled with water
B. Is compressible, can increase or decrease in volume depending on which muscles contract
C. Provides its own skeletal support
D. Is incompressible, maintains a constant volume when muscles contract, and provides its own skeletal support
E. Utilizes muscle contraction to regulate the amount of saliva produced in the oral cavity

8. The muscles of the palate are *not* innervated by which of the following cranial nerves?

A. Trigeminal (CN V)
B. Facial (CN VII)
C. Vagus (CN X)
D. Accessory (CN XI)
E. Hypoglossal (CN XII)

9. If you wanted to move the tip of your tongue superiorly, you would contract the:

A. Transverse
B. Hyoglossus
C. Superior longitudinal
D. Inferior longitudinal
E. Anterior belly of the digastric

10. Which pair of intrinsic tongue muscles can work together to protrude the tongue?

A. Transverse and vertical
B. Superior longitudinal and transverse
C. Superior longitudinal and inferior longitudinal
D. Vertical and genioglossus
E. Transverse and genioglossus

11. Contraction of the transverse muscle of the tongue would have which effect:

A. Narrow and elongate the tongue
B. Elevate the tongue tip
C. Flatten and broaden the tongue
D. Pull the tongue superiorly and posteriorly
E. Lower the tongue tip

12. Which of the following muscles is most involved in elevating the velum?

A. Palatopharyngeus
B. Salpingopharyngeus
C. Levator veli palatini
D. Tensor veli palatini
E. Musculus uvulae

13. The function of the tensor veli palatini is best described as

A. Palatizing the tensor
B. Opening the eustachian tube and tensing the velum
C. Elevating the velum
D. Lowering the velum
E. Opening the nostril

14. If you wanted to depress the velum, you would contract the:

A. Stylopharyngeus
B. Palatoglossus
C. Nasalis
D. Musculus uvulae
E. All of the above

15. For normal production of the consonant /t/, what must be true about the state of the velopharyngeal port?

A. It must be elevated
B. It must be depressed
C. It must be closed
D. It must be open
E. It can be open or closed because the velopharyngeal port is not involved in production of /t/

16. Which muscle widens the cross section of the pharynx and elevates the pharynx

A. Stylopharyngeus
B. Thyroarytenoid
C. Levator pharyngeus
D. Buccinators
E. Middle constrictor

17. Secondary to some strange infection, a man lost the neural innervation to the posterior part of the genioglossus. Based on your knowledge of muscle activation and tongue position, production of which vowel will now become most problematic for this man:

A. /i/ as in "heat"
B. /æ/ as in "hat"
C. /u/ as in "hoot"
D. /ɑ/ as in "hot"
E. Vowel production would not be affected.

18. Which of the following sets of three consonants would all be produced with the same place of constriction in the vocal tract?

A. /n/, /d/, /t/
B. /m/, /d/, /b/
C. /n/, /g/, /k/
D. /n/, /m/, /b/
E. /s/, /t/, /k/

19. Production of the vowel /i/ as in "heat" can be described as having:

A. A high/front tongue position with the oral cavity more expanded than the pharynx
B. A high/front tongue position with the oral cavity more constricted than the pharynx
C. A low/front tongue position with the oral cavity more constricted than the pharynx
D. A low/back tongue position with the oral cavity more expanded than the pharynx
E. A low/back tongue position with the oral cavity more constricted than the pharynx

20. The term "coarticulation" refers to:

A. The ability to produce velar and alveolar consonants at the same time
B. The production of portions of multiple phonetic elements simultaneously
C. The ability of ventriloquists to produce a /b/ sound without bringing the lips together
D. A measurement technique in which the movement of an articulator is forced to coincide with the activity of a muscle
E. The ability of the jaw to move the tongue superiorly and inferiorly in the oral cavity

■ Answers to Study Questions

1. The correct answer is (A). There are two parietal bones, two temporal bones, two maxillae, and two zygomatic bones in the skull. (B) There is only one occipital and one sphenoid bone in the skull. (C) There is only one mandible in the skull. (D) There is only one sphenoid bone, one ethmoid bone, and one vomer in the skull.

2. The correct answer is (C). The word "buccal" refers to the cheek. (A) The glottis is the space between the vocal folds. (B) The oral cavity is the entire mouth cavity. (E) The digastric cavity, if it existed, would be associated with the digastric muscle below the oral floor.

3. The correct answer is (A). The buccinator pulls the mouth laterally and tenses the cheek. (B) This is the action for either the levator anguli oris or incisivus labii superioris. (C) This is the action for the orbicularis oris muscle. (D) This is the action for the mylohyoid muscle. (E) This is the action for the palatoglossal muscle.

4. The correct answer is (D). This muscle pulls the corners of the mouth inferiorly (as in frowning). (A) The levator anguli oris pulls the corner of the mouth superiorly. (B) The levator labii superioris pulls the upper lip superiorly. (C) The zygomaticus major raises the corners of the mouth. (E) The risorius pulls the corner of the mouth laterally.

5. The correct answer is (C). The mylohyoid and geniohyoid open the jaw and thus are important for jaw lowering. (A) The digastric opens the jaw; the palatoglossus raises the tongue body. (B) The temporalis closes (elevates) the jaw, and the geniohyoid opens (lowers) the jaw. (D) The masseter and medial pterygoid both close (elevate) the jaw. (E) The medial pterygoid closes (elevates) the jaw and the lateral pterygoid opens (lowers) the jaw.

6. The correct answer is (B). The palatopharyngeus, running from the palate to the pharynx, is housed in the posterior faucial pillar. (A) The palatoglossus runs in the anterior faucial pillar. (C) The hyoglossus runs from the hyoid bone to the tongue. (D) The faucial extensor posterioris is not a real muscle. (E) The styloglossus runs from the styloid process to the tongue.

7. The correct answer is (D). The tongue volume does not change when muscles contract. (A) The tongue is made almost entirely of muscle. (B) The tongue volume does not change during contraction. (C) While this is true, this is not the definition of a hydrostat. (E) The tongue being a muscular hydrostat does not have any effect on saliva production.

8. The correct answer is (B). (A) CN V innervates the tensor veli palatini. (C) CN X innervates the levator veli palatini, musculus uvulae, and palatopharyngeus. (D) CN XI innervates the levator veli palatini, musculus uvulae, and palatopharyngeus. (E) CN XII innervates the palatoglossal muscle.

9. The correct answer is (C). The superior longitudinal muscle elevates the tongue tip. (A) The transverse muscle narrows the tongue. (B) The hyoglossal muscle depresses the sides of the tongue. (D) The inferior longitudinal muscle depresses the tongue tip and aids in retraction. (E) The anterior belly of the digastric opens the jaw.

10. The correct answer is (A). (B) The superior longitudinal muscles helps in retraction of the tongue. (C) The superior and inferior longitudinal muscle assist in retraction. (D, E) The genioglossus retracts and protrudes the tongue.

11. The correct answer is (A). The transverse muscle narrows and elongates the tongue. (B) The superior longitudinal muscle elevates the tongue tip. (C) The vertical muscle flattens the tongue. (D) The superior longitudinal muscle assists in retraction. (E) The inferior longitudinal muscle lowers the tongue tip.

12. The correct answer is (C). (A) The palatopharyngeus serves to lower the velum. (B) The salpingopharyngeus muscle elevates the pharynx and larynx to aid in swallowing. (D) The tensor veli palatini opens the eustachian tube. (E) The musculus uvulae bunches the uvula during contraction.

13. The correct answer is (B). (A) The phrase "palatizing the tensor" has no meaning. (C) The levator veli palatini elevates the velum. (D) The palatoglossal muscle lowers the velum. (E) The nasalis muscle is responsible for flaring the nostrils.

14. The correct answer is (B). (A) The stylopharyngeus elevates and opens the pharynx. (C) The nasalis muscle is responsible for flaring the nostrils. (D) The musculus uvulae bunches the uvula upon contraction. (E) Only one muscle is correct.

15. The correct answer is (C). (A, B) Velar height is different in different contexts. (D, E) The plosive /t/ requires a buildup of oral pressure; therefore the VP cannot be open.

16. The correct answer is (A). (B) The thyroarytenoid muscle is an intrinsic muscle of the larynx. (C) The levator pharyngeus is not a single muscle, rather a group that has different action depending on the location. (D) The buccinator is a facial muscle. (E) The middle constrictor narrows the diameter of the pharynx.

17. The correct answer is (A). (B) Contraction of the posterior genioglossus pulls the tongue anteriorly to assist in protrusion. The vowel /æ/ is a low front vowel; therefore, the tongue needs to be flattened during production. (C) Contraction of the posterior genioglossus pulls the tongue anteriorly to assist in protrusion. The vowel /u/ requires elevation of the posterior tongue. (D) Contraction of the posterior genioglossus pulls the tongue anteriorly to assist in protrusion. The vowel /ɑ/ requires flattening of the posterior tongue. (E) Damage to any tongue musculature will affect both vowel and consonant production.

18. The correct answer is (A). (B) The place of articulation for /m/ and /b/ is bilabial, but that for /d/ is alveolar. (C) The place of articulation is alveolar for /n/ and velar for /k/ and /g/. (D) The place of articulation is bilabial for /m/ and /b/ but alveolar for /n/. (E) The place of articulation is alveolar for /s/ and /t/ but velar for /k/.

19. The correct answer is (B). (A) If the tongue were constricted in the front, the oral cavity size would decrease, not expand. (C, D, and E) The vowel /i/ is a high front vowel based on the location and degree of constriction.

20. The correct answer is (B). (A) Simultaneous production of velar and alveolar consonants is not common in speech production. (C) Ventriloquism is a challenge to learn, and when a ventriloquist learns to produce /b/ with a place of articulation within the vocal tract, this is an extreme example of motor equivalence, not coarticulation. (D) There are a variety of measurement techniques used to understand coarticulation. (E) The tongue cannot move superiorly and inferiorly at the same time.

13

Hearing

Jason Tait Sanchez and Tina M. Grieco-Calub

■ Chapter Summary

Hearing is the perception of sound. As one of the five sensory systems, it plays an important role in our everyday lives by providing us with the ability to monitor our environment and by supporting spoken communication. The study of anatomy and physiology of hearing is essential to the understanding of how sound is transduced to a neural signal that the brain can interpret and of how auditory pathologies compromise hearing. The purpose of this chapter is to provide an important foundation regarding the nature of sound and the anatomy and physiology of the human ear, including the peripheral and central auditory systems. Specifically, we will (1) introduce terminology related to sound, including a discussion of frequency, intensity, interaural cues, and sound transmission through different media, (2) describe the functional anatomy and physiology of the peripheral auditory system, including the outer ear, middle ear, and inner ear, as well as neural pathways that constitute the central auditory system, and (3) relate these concepts to the clinical management of hearing disorders.

■ Learning Objectives

- Describe the properties of sound
- Describe the transduction of sound through the peripheral auditory system
- Understand the functional neuroanatomy of the central auditory pathway

- Explain how the central auditory system encodes the properties of sound
- Describe the use of clinical hearing assessment procedures to understand disorders of the human auditory system

■ Putting It Into Practice

- The assessment and management of hearing require a basic understanding of how the peripheral auditory system transduces sound into a neural signal and how this neural signal is transmitted throughout the central auditory system.
- The study of the anatomy and physiology of the auditory system provides essential information about this transduction process, which is compromised in the presence of outer ear, middle ear, inner ear, and central auditory pathway pathologies.
- The processing of sound in the central auditory system involves a complex network of neural pathways that provide listeners with information to perceive both the content and the location of sounds in their environment.

■ Introduction

Hearing is the perception of **sound**. To hear, organisms have sensory systems that convert pressure waves into a signal that can be encoded by the central nervous system. In humans, that sensory system consists of the **peripheral auditory system**, referred to generally as the ear, and the **central auditory system**, which is composed of neural pathways that are responsible for encoding frequency, intensity, and temporal components of sound.

Hearing is the foundation for the development of a number of auditory and language skills. Hearing promotes (1) spoken language development (limited access to language in early childhood impairs behavioral, cognitive, and academic development); (2) communication and social/emotional well-being (individuals with hearing loss tend to withdraw from social interactions and can feel isolated); and (3) auditory skill development (the ability to localize sounds in space and distinguish target from nontarget sounds helps listeners monitor the safety of their environment and provides an advantage when attempting to understand speech in background noise). This chapter describes the general anatomy and physiology of the human auditory system. In addition, this chapter will provide (1) a description of the complexity of the auditory system; (2) an introduction to the methods used to measure auditory function; and (3) an overview of disorders that impair auditory function.

■ The Nature of Sound

Each sensory system has a physical stimulus to which it responds to exclusively: the eyes respond to light, the nose responds to odors, and the ears respond to vibrations in the media that surround us, perceived as sound. Sounds are all around us—we use them to communicate, enjoy them as music or a baby's laugh, and associate them with both happy and sad memories. The sounds that we encounter in our daily lives are often quite complex. Yet, broken down into its simplest form, sound is the byproduct of a vibrating or oscillating object, such as human vocal folds or strings on a guitar. As an object oscillates, it disturbs the air molecules immediately surrounding it. When those molecules are set into motion, they strike their neighboring molecules, causing them to oscillate as well, and so on. The end result is a cascade of vibrating molecules that emanate from the original vibrating source and travel to our ears.

To understand sound transmission better, consider the action of one air molecule that is adjacent to a drum's surface as illustrated in **Fig. 13.1a**. Suppose that, initially, the air molecule is motionless and is equidistant from its neighboring molecules. It remains so because of **inertia**, but as the drum is set into vibration, it physically pushes against the molecule, and the **force** of this action causes

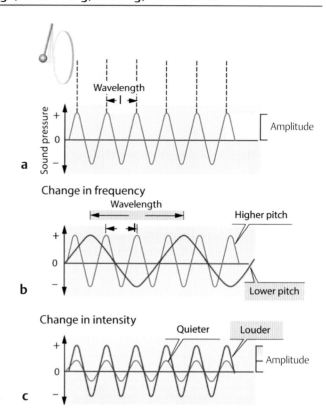

Fig. 13.1 Characteristics of sound. **(a)** Illustration of sound transmission from an object set into vibration. The vibrating drum sets adjacent air molecules into motion, which move toward other air molecules, creating areas of condensation (*blue shading*), and away from others, creating areas of rarefaction (*white shading*). The blue shading represents areas of peak sound pressure. As the approaching molecules collide and bounce away from each other, the rarefaction and compression areas move. **(b)** Faster vibrations result in a shorter wavelength and higher frequency. This results in higher pitch (*blue line*). Slower vibrations result in a longer wavelength and lower frequency. This results in lower pitch (*red line*). **(c)** Greater displacement of the drum results in greater displacement of molecules and the perception of a "louder" sound (*red line*).

the molecule to move away from the drum. As the molecule moves to the right, it moves *toward* its neighboring molecule, which creates a zone containing more molecules than usual, or **condensation**. In that same moment in time, the molecule moves *away* from the drum, which creates a zone containing fewer molecules than usual, or **rarefaction**. In the zone of condensation (i.e., molecules moving toward one another, *blue shading* in **Fig. 13.1a**), the molecule is more likely to collide with another air molecule. It and the molecule it struck are now moving away from each other, so where there had been condensation, there is now rarefaction (*white shading* in **Fig. 13.1a**), while there is new condensation out farther from the drum. The end result is a traveling pressure wave, whereby increases in sound pressure are observed during condensation and decreases in sound pressure are observed during rarefaction. In air near sea level, this pressure wave travels approximately 740 miles per hour (in contrast, light travels approximately 670 million miles per hour).

The fact that an air molecule set in motion bounces off other air molecules means that air is an elastic medium; the other air molecules act as a **restoring force**, which tends to reverse the direction of the molecule's movement toward its initial position. Inertia, however, keeps the molecule moving beyond its initial position until it bounces off yet another molecule; that is, the elastic forces redirect its motion again. Any physical system that includes both inertia and a restoring force tends to this to-and-fro variation, or **oscillation**; it tends to continue until **friction** (in this example, the result of collisions with adjacent molecules that are not head-on, so the molecules bounce up or down or from side to side rather than completely forward or backward) **damps** the oscillation. **Fig. 13.1b**, illustrates an oscillation pattern as a function of time in a plot known as a **waveform**. It shows the simplest form of oscillation, called **simple harmonic motion**, which yields a waveform called a **sine wave** or **sinusoid**. Sound waves that contain single sinusoids are **simple sounds** (such as might be heard from a flute or a tuning fork); sounds made up of multiple sine waves are called **complex sounds**. Sound waves that consist of elements that repeat at constant intervals over time, they are **periodic**. If the waveform does not repeat over time, it is **aperiodic**.

Sounds are typically characterized by their **frequency** and **intensity**. Frequency is the number of complete to-and-fro oscillations, or cycles, per second and is quantified in **hertz (Hz)**. A **cycle** is defined as one complete oscillation and is quantified in time (seconds). **Fig. 13.1b**, illustrates two sine waves that differ in frequency. Both are **pure tones** because they consist of a single frequency. The blue sine wave has a *higher* frequency because a greater number of cycles occur in the specified time window. Likewise, the red sine wave has a *lower* frequency because the completion of one cycle requires a longer duration of time. The perceptual correlate to frequency is **pitch**. For example, sounds containing high frequencies, like a bird chirping or a whistle blowing, are considered high-pitched sounds, and sounds containing low frequencies, like a fog horn or a large dog's bark, are considered low pitched sounds. Humans can detect sounds with frequencies between 20 and 20,000 Hz. Because sound travels at a constant speed through air at a given set of conditions, a related measure to frequency is **wavelength**, which is the distance in space between repeating elements of the wave. Because higher-frequency sounds generate a greater number of cycles, they have shorter wavelengths than lower-frequency sounds. Wavelength can be found by dividing the speed of sound by the frequency of the wave.

The frequency of the wave generated by an oscillating object depends on its physical properties as well as the forces (if any) acting upon it. An object in **free vibration** will oscillate at its **resonant** or **fundamental frequency**, which depends on the object's mass and stiffness. The equation for resonant frequency is:

$$f = [1/(2\pi)]\sqrt{(k/m)}$$

where f is the resonant frequency (Hz), k is the stiffness coefficient (newtons per meter) of the object, and m is the mass (kilograms) of the object. Objects that resonate at lower frequencies have more mass and less stiffness, whereas objects that resonate at higher frequencies have less mass and more stiffness. For additional reading on the physics of spring/mass systems, vibration, and frequency, see Gelfand (2007).

Objects can oscillate at frequencies other than their resonant frequency when external forces act upon them; this is known as **forced vibration**. As discussed in the following sections of this chapter, components of the human ear have their own resonant frequencies. They do, however, vibrate at other frequencies as well due to forced vibration caused by external forces.

Sound is also characterized by its **intensity**, or amplitude, which refers to the magnitude of the oscillation. The perceptual correlate of intensity is **loudness**. In **Fig. 13.1c**, intensity is illustrated on the vertical axis. Sounds with higher intensity ("louder") have waveforms with greater vertical displacement from zero. Sound pressure level (SPL) represents a conventional approach to quantifying the intensity of sound through air. Pressure (p) is defined as the amount of force (F) per area (A),

$$p = F/A$$

In the meter, kilogram, second (MKS) system of units, force is measured in newtons (N) and area is measured in square meters (m^2). Therefore, pressure is measured in newtons per square meter (N/m^2) or **pascals (Pa)**. The human range of hearing is from 0.00002 (i.e., 10^{-5}) to 200 (i.e., 10^2) Pa, or a range of 10^7 Pa. It turns out that intensity, being the amount of energy transferred by sound waves per unit time (i.e., power), is proportional to the square of the pressure variation:

$$I \propto p^2$$

where I is intensity and p is pressure. Thus, the dynamic intensity range of human hearing spans a scale of $(10^7)^2 = 10^{14}$. This wide range of intensities would be impractical to quantify on a linear scale. To solve this problem, a logarithmic scale is useful, as is usually the case with phenomena detected by the senses (see **Chapter 9, Sensory Systems**). The conventional logarithmic way to represent intensity is the **decibel (dB)**. A ratio of 10 to 1 in power (intensity) between two sounds corresponds to 10 dB (or one bel). A ratio of 10 to 1 in pressure corresponds to a ratio of $10^2 = 100$ to 1 in intensity, or 20 dB. For the purpose of measuring hearing sensitivity, the decibel is used to relate the sound pressure variation of a sound to a reference pressure, according to the following equation:

$$\text{dB SPL} = 20 \log_{10}(P_o/P_r)$$

where SPL stands for sound pressure level, P_o is the observed pressure, and P_r is the reference pressure. Because the decibel can be used to quantify the ratio of any two quantities that are on the same scale, the qualifier "SPL" is necessary to denote that this use is in reference to pressure. The reference pressure P_r is set equal to the minimum pressure change that humans can detect (0.00002 Pa). As previously discussed, the maximum pressure sensed by the human auditory system is 10^7 times this threshold level. Therefore, the dynamic range of human hearing corresponds to $20 \log (10^7) = 20 \times 7 = 140$ dB SPL.

When an object oscillates, the peak oscillation of air molecules (i.e., peak intensity level) occurs at the sound source. The pressure wave will propagate directly around and away from the source. As the pressure wave propagates, the same amount of force is distributed over a larger and larger area, making the pressure change less and less. As a result, sound pressure decreases as a function of the area, or the square of the distance, from the sound source. This is referred to as the **inverse square law**. For every doubling of the distance away from the sound source, the intensity drops by a factor of 4; the logarithm of 4 is about 0.6, so the change expressed in decibels is about $10 \times 0.6 = 6$ dB. For additional reading on the physics of intensity, pressure, and the decibel, see Gelfand (2007).

Up to this point, we have focused on sound in the **free field**. A sound pressure wave travels linearly until there is a change in medium (e.g., from air to water or a solid). These other media have vastly different **impedances** than air. Impedance refers to an object's opposition to the flow of energy. The **specific acoustic impedance (Z)** refers to a substance's opposition to the flow of sound pressure and is defined as the product of the substance's density (ρ) and acoustic velocity (V; how fast sound can travel within that substance). Note that both density and acoustic velocity of an object are influenced by temperature. The impedance match between two media

will determine the efficiency of sound transmission as the pressure wave travels from one medium to another. For example, let's consider the air–water interface. The specific acoustic impedances of air and water are approximately 420 Pa · s/m and 1.5 MPa · s/m, respectively, where Pa · s/m is pascal second per meter, or **rayl**. The impedances of air and water are mismatched by a factor of ~ 4000, which results in a large amount of sound reflection at the air–water interface. As the acoustic sound pressure wave reaches the water interface, most of it is reflected back into the air medium because the high impedance of the water limits transmission. The reflection coefficient of the air–water interface is over 0.999, meaning that less than 0.1% of sound can break the air–water impedance mismatch. The classic example of this phenomenon is attempting to communicate with someone who is submerged in a pool. The submerged individual is unable to hear a large majority of speech (the sound level is lowered by over 60 dB). In human hearing, we are also interested in sound transmission at the air–solid interface. Solids will vary in their impedance as a result of their material properties. Therefore, different solids have varying abilities to transmit sound. The most common example of this phenomenon is **reverberation**, or echoes, that one hears in a large room with hard surfaces. A sound that is generated in such a room is permitted to "bounce around," which is perceived as an echo until it damps out. As discussed later in this chapter, the human ear is specifically designed to overcome impedance mismatches as sound is transduced through the peripheral auditory system.

As sound approaches the ear, it interacts with the head. How the head influences the sound before it reaches each ear is highly dependent on the location of the sound source in space. First proposed by Lord Rayleigh (1907), the **duplex theory** of binaural hearing provides some explanation for the ability of humans to localize sounds produced along the horizontal plane. Sounds that originate directly on the midline (directly in front of or directly behind the head) reach the ears at the same time and at the same intensity. Sounds that are located to the right or left of midline reach the ears at different times and different intensities, referred to as **interaural timing differences (ITDs)** and **interaural level differences (ILDs)**, respectively. ITDs represent the timing difference between the arrival of sound (presented off of midline) at each ear. As illustrated in **Fig. 13.2a**, sound will reach the closer (left) ear before the farther (right) ear. This difference in the time of arrival is referred to as the lag, or ITD, and is quantified in microseconds (μs). A sound source located at 90° or 270° azimuth—representing the right and left ears, respectively, as you go around the head—generates a maximum ITD of ~ 700 μs in

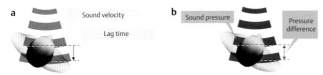

Fig. 13.2 The generation of interaural cues. **(a)** Sounds that originate from points in space that deviate horizontally from midline (0° and 180°) will arrive sooner at the near ear than at the far ear, resulting in an interaural timing difference, and **(b)** will be louder in the near ear than in the far ear, resulting in an interaural level difference.

adults. ITDs are more preserved by low-frequency sounds because low frequencies have longer wavelengths; therefore, differences in phase are more easily resolved by the auditory system. ILDs represent the intensity difference of sound at each ear. As illustrated in **Fig. 13.2b**, sound will reach the closer (left) ear at a higher intensity than the farther (right) ear. The **head shadow** contributes to the generation of ILDs because the head acts as an acoustic barrier as sound travels from one side of the head to the other. ILDs are more preserved in high-frequency sounds because the short wavelengths of high-frequency sounds are more susceptible to interference by the head. In addition to ITDs and ILDs, humans also have access to monaural cues, which are generated by the interaction between the sound and the **pinna**. Monaural cues are helpful in discerning the location of sound sources in the vertical plane. Humans use these auditory cues to locate sound sources in the environment and during segregation of speech from background noise.

■ Functional Anatomy of the Peripheral Auditory System

Bones Relevant to Hearing

The entirety of the auditory system is encased in the cranium, or skull, which is composed of four major bones: frontal, parietal, occipital, and temporal. The temporal bone houses the peripheral auditory system, including cranial nerves VII (facial) and VIII (vestibulocochlear) as well as the vascularization responsible for blood supply to the temporal bone structures (**Fig. 13.3**). The temporal bone contains four primary segments: the squamous, the tympanic, the mastoid, and the petrous, as well as the styloid process (**Fig. 13.4**). The four segments come together to create much of the peripheral auditory system, including components of the outer, middle, and inner ears. The squamous portion is the superior segment of the temporal bone. It serves as the lateral aspect of

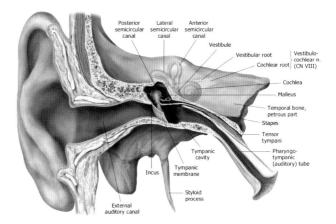

Fig. 13.3 The peripheral auditory system. Coronal section through right ear, anterior view. The tympanic membrane separates the outer ear (external auditory canal) from the middle ear (tympanic cavity). The stapes of the ossicular chain is in direct contact with the oval window (not labeled), which separates the middle ear from the vestibule of the inner ear.

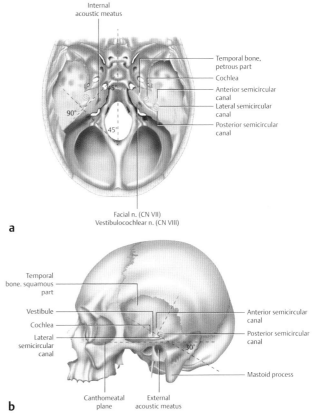

Fig. 13.4 **(a, b)** The temporal bone. The temporal bone contains four primary segments: the squamous, the tympanic, the mastoid, and the petrous. The tympanic portion provides structural support for the external auditory canal. The petrous portion of the temporal bone contains the middle and inner ear. The facial (CN VII) and vestibulocochlear (CN VIII) nerves pass through the internal auditory canal.

the middle cranial fossa, attaches the temporalis and masseter muscles, and contains sulci for the middle temporal and middle meningeal arteries. The tympanic portion is inferior to the squamous portion and provides structural support for the external auditory canal. The mastoid portion is the posterior segment of the temporal bone. Its lateral protrusion (the mastoid process) is located just posteriorly to the pinna of the ear and is an anatomic landmark used during hearing tests (**Box 13.1**). The mastoid portion of the temporal bone contains air cells, or air-filled spaces that communicate directly with the middle ear space via the **tympanic antrum**. The petrous portion of the temporal bone is the most medial aspect of the temporal bone and is one of the densest bones in the body. Internally, it contains cavities and canals that form the bony labyrinths of the cochlear and vestibular apparatuses. At the most medial point of the petrous portion (and therefore, the temporal bone), there is an opening known as the **internal auditory canal** (or **internal auditory meatus**), through which cranial nerves VII (facial nerve) and VIII (vestibulocochlear nerve) as well as

---

Box 13.1   Outer Ear, Aural Atresia, and Microtia

During embryonic development, the majority of head and neck structures arise from five branchial arches and their associated structures. The pinna of the outer ear emerges from the first and second branchial arches during the third and fourth weeks of gestation, and the external auditory canal emerges from the first branchial groove during the fourth and fifth weeks of gestation. The refinement of these structures continues throughout gestation: the pinna achieves adult-like structure (but not size) by the 20th week (~ fifth month) of gestation, and the external auditory canal is formed by the sixth month of gestation. Both the pinna and the canal continue to grow throughout the first decade of the child's life. For more detail about the embryology of the ear, see Northern and Downs (2014).

Any disruption that occurs during the development of the outer ear can result in a structural abnormality of the pinna, external auditory canal, or both. **Aural atresia** is the complete closure of the external auditory canal. It is differentiated from **stenosis**, which is a narrowing of the canal that continues to allow some sound transmission to the middle ear. Congenital aural atresia is present at birth and is often observed with other cranial and facial abnormalities. Aural atresia is associated with a number of genetic syndromes including Treacher Collins, Pierre Robin, CHARGE, and Goldenhar. It occurs in 1 of every 10,000 to 20,000 live births, and is more commonly observed unilaterally than bilaterally. Functionally, aural atresia results in a maximum conductive hearing loss (**Box 13.2**) because sound is prevented from directly stimulating the medial structures of the peripheral auditory system. It is important to note that middle ear abnormalities may also be present in individuals with aural atresia.

Aural atresia may or may not be observed with an abnormal pinna. **Microtia** is the technical term referring to a malformed or absent pinna. It occurs in 1 of every 20,000 births. Significant individual variability in the physical appearance of a microtic ear is common (**Box Fig. 13.1**). Although structural abnormalities of the pinna have a small impact on hearing function, they may be associated with other craniofacial abnormalities.

Microtia Grading System*

Grade 1	Grade 2	Grade 3	Grade 4
Small but almost normal	Some recognizable anatomy	Small rudiment of soft tissue	No external ear and no ear canal

*Marx Classification (1926)

Box Fig. 13.1   Photograph showing the grades of microtia. Photograph courtesy of Dr. Sheryl Lewin.

the blood supply to the peripheral auditory system pass.

The Outer Ear

The outer ear is considered the "sound collector." Due to its shape and location on the head, the outer ear structure captures and transmits sound to be processed by the more medial structures of the auditory system. Note, however, that the outer ear is not exclusive in its ability to funnel sound to the auditory system. Because the peripheral auditory system is encased in bone, any stimulus that can initiate bone conduction in the body has the potential to elicit an auditory percept (**Box 13.1** and **Box 13.2**).

The outer ear consists of the pinna and **external auditory canal** (ear canal, external auditory meatus) and terminates at the **tympanic membrane**. The pinna is the most lateral component of the auditory system. It is composed largely of cartilage, contains a number of folds and cavities, and is covered by skin. The ear lobe, which is the most inferior and most flexible part of the pinna, lacks

---

Box 13.2   Hearing Measurement

According to the World Health Organization (WHO; 2015), there are 360 million people with hearing loss. In children, hearing loss can interfere with the typical acquisition of spoken language, cognitive development, and academic achievement. In both children and adults, hearing loss can impact social relationships and lead to feelings of isolation and depression.

Audiologists use a battery of objective and subjective measures to quantify hearing sensitivity. The traditional hearing test includes hearing threshold estimation for octave frequencies between 250 and 8000 Hz in each ear. A **hearing threshold** is the lowest intensity that can be perceived by the listener on a specific number of trials. By convention, lower thresholds represent better hearing sensitivity. Using a calibrated **audiometer**, sounds are presented to the ear via **air conduction** or **bone conduction**. In air conduction, sounds are introduced to the ear through sound waves. Sound can originate from a loudspeaker or from headphones. Audiologists typically prefer to use headphones during hearing tests because they enable testing of each ear somewhat independently. Air-conducted sounds travel through the outer, middle, and inner ear before they are transduced into a neural signal at the junction of the inner hair cell and auditory nerve. The perception of sound, however, can also be elicited through direct stimulation of the hearing organ through bone conduction. Bone conduction occurs when a bone oscillator is placed on the head. The oscillator transduces sound into a vibratory signal, which is subsequently transmitted to the skull. Because the inner ear is encased in the petrous portion of the temporal bone, it can be stimulated from these vibrations. There can be some contribution from the outer and middle ear during bone conduction, but the major contribution is through direct stimulation of the inner ear structures (see Musiek and Baran [2007] for additional reading on the mechanisms of bone conduction). When considered together, air conduction and bone conduction thresholds can provide a general location of ear pathology.

Thresholds that are < 20 dB HL (15 dB HL for children) are considered to be normal. The dB HL (hearing level) scale is used in clinical audiometry to equate the average hearing threshold (in dB SPL) at each frequency. The use of dB HL is necessary because the human ear is not equally sensitive to all frequencies (see Durrant and Lovrinic [1995] for additional reading on the calculation of dB HL). A **sensorineural hearing loss** is defined as (1) air conduction thresholds that are > 20 dB HL; (2) bone conduction thresholds that are > 20 dB HL; and (3) air and bone conduction thresholds that are within 10 dB of each other. These findings indicate that sound travels equally well via air conduction and bone conduction, and therefore the source of the hearing loss is within the inner ear, auditory nerve (cochlear branch of the vestibulocochlear nerve, CN VIII), or central auditory system. A **conductive hearing loss** is defined as (1) air conduction thresholds that are > 20 dB HL; (2) bone conduction thresholds that are < 20 dB HL; and (3) air and bone conduction thresholds that differ by ≥ 15 dB. These findings indicate that sound is transmitted more efficiently via bone conduction (i.e., when it bypasses the outer and middle ear). A conductive hearing loss most often results from outer and middle ear pathology. There is one exception, referred to as "third window lesions," which represents abnormal sound transmission within the inner ear. Additional testing is necessary to differentiate the site of lesion in these cases. A **mixed hearing loss** is defined as (1) air conduction thresholds that are > 20 dB HL; (2) bone conduction thresholds that are > 20 dB HL; and (3) air and bone conduction thresholds that differ by ≥ 15 dB. These findings are suggestive of pathology impacting sound transmission in both air and bone conduction pathways. Mixed hearing loss results from pathology of the inner ear or auditory nerve as well as pathology within the outer and middle ears.

cartilage (**Fig. 13.5**). Although there is individual variability in size and position of the human pinna, it is fully developed in utero and contains a number of structural landmarks. The superior and posterior outer ridge of the pinna is the **helix**. Anterior to the helix is the **antihelix**. The bowl-like center of the pinna is the **concha**, which terminates at the opening of the ear canal. The most anterior landmark is the **tragus**. Between the concha and tragus is the opening to the ear canal. Inferior to the concha, the ear canal opening, and the tragus is the ear lobe. These anatomical structures aid in the collection and transmission of sound.

The ear canal is an air-filled tube that is opened on its lateral side and closed on its medial side as it terminates at the tympanic membrane (**Fig. 13.6**). The lateral one-third of the ear canal is composed of cartilage. The medial two-thirds of the ear canal is osseous and formed by the following structures: (1) the tympanic portion of the temporal bone, which forms the floor, anterior, and inferior-posterior walls; (2) the squamous portion of the temporal bone, which forms the roof and posterior walls; and (3) the condyle of the mandible bone, which forms the inferior-anterior wall and temporomandibular joint (Gelfand, 2009). In total, the ear canal is approximately 25 to 35 mm in length and is curved with two loose bends that form an **S** shape in adults. Although ear canal diameter varies significantly, it is ~ 0.75 cm in the normal adult. The ear canal is covered with tight-fitting epidermal lining that is continuous with the skin of the face and pinna laterally and forms the external layer of the tympanic membrane medially. The cartilaginous portion (lateral one-third) of the ear canal contains hair follicles and cerumen-producing

glands that are embedded in the external lining. Two types of glands are found in the ear canal: sebaceous glands and ceruminous glands. Sebaceous glands produce an oily substance called sebum that lubricates the epidermal lining of the ear canal. Ceruminous glands produce a waxlike substance that, when combined with sebum and dead epidermal cells, creates **cerumen** or earwax. The consistency of cerumen varies and can range from dry and flaky to wet and sticky.

The structure of the outer ear provides two mechanisms to protect the medial structures such as the tympanic membrane. First, its curvature provides protection from objects entering the ear that may cause structural damage. Second, the production and excretion of cerumen by the ear canal protects the ear from external particles and pathogens. Cerumen has some antibacterial and antifungal properties that make it difficult for pathogens to survive. Additionally, its "stickiness" captures particles before they enter the bony portion of the ear canal. The epidermal layer also has a natural process of migrating outward and carries cerumen with it, serving as a self-cleaning mechanism. Therefore, cerumen production is a healthy and normal process. In that regard, the use of cotton swabs to "clean out" the ear canal is counterproductive to the natural protective mechanisms of the outer ear. There are, however, conditions when cerumen is overproduced or becomes impacted, resulting in blockage of the ear canal. This becomes troublesome when the cerumen is pushed down into the bony portion of the ear canal, because this portion of the ear canal does not display the same epidermal migration processes as the cartilaginous portion.

The ear canal terminates at the tympanic membrane or eardrum, which is a drumlike, multilayered structure that divides the outer ear from the middle ear. It is fairly oval in shape

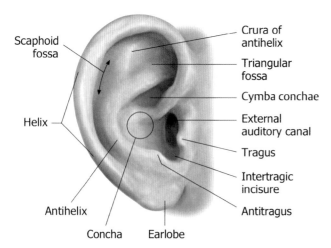

Fig. 13.5 Anatomic landmarks of the human pinna. Right auricle, right lateral view.

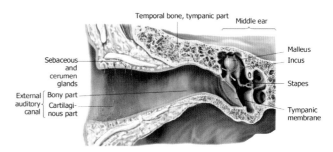

Fig. 13.6 Anatomic landmarks of the human external auditory canal and middle ear. Coronal section through right ear, anterior view. The outer third of the auditory canal is cartilaginous, and the inner two-thirds are osseous (tympanic part of temporal bone).

with an overall surface area of 85 mm² and is positioned at a 55° angle relative to the external ear canal. The tympanic membrane attaches to a small groove within the temporal bone called the tympanic sulcus. Although the tympanic membrane appears flat upon visual inspection, it is actually concave, with its maximum concavity (the **umbo**) located more medially than its outer rim. The structure comprises two subregions, which are separated by the posterior and anterior malleolar folds: the **pars tensa** and the **pars flaccida**. The pars tensa is the larger region, located inferiorly to the folds and approximately 55 mm² in surface area. The pars flaccida is the smaller region located superiorly to the folds (**Fig. 13.7**). Both regions are composed of two layers. The outer (lateral) layer is continuous with the epidermal lining of the external ear canal. The inner (medial) layer is continuous with the mucosal membrane of the middle ear. The pars tensa also contains a middle, collaginous layer that is composed of radial fibers and circular fibers. Radial fibers emanate outward from the center of the tympanic membrane, whereas the circular fibers make concentric circles that interconnect with the radial fibers. This dense, highly organized collection of collagen fibers not only provides support for the tympanic membrane but also facilitates the conversion of sound into mechanical motion. These fibers are very sparse and disorganized in the pars flaccida.

The tympanic membrane is a fairly translucent structure, which enables visualization of a number of landmarks during **otoscopy** (**Fig. 13.7**). The tympanic membrane connects the outer and middle ears through an attachment to the **malleus**

(hammer), which is the most lateral bone of the **ossicular chain** within the middle ear. The **manubrium** (or "handle") of the malleus is attached to the upper part of the tympanic membrane and is typically observed upon visual inspection. It is angled toward the 1 o'clock position in the right ear and toward the 11 o'clock position in the left ear. In cases of extreme middle ear pressure, the manubrium often appears to "pop out" into the ear canal. In very translucent tympanic membranes, other structures of the middle ear, such as the **oval** and **round windows**, can also be viewed. The **cone of light** is a reflection of the light used in otoscopy to visualize the tympanic membrane. The cone of light can be used to indicate which ear is being visualized. If the light angles to the lower right, it is the right ear. If the light angles to the lower left, it is the left ear.

The Middle Ear

The Tympanic Cavity

The middle ear is an air-filled cavity that houses the ossicular chain. A simplified model of the middle ear is that of a six-sided, hard-walled box that is lined with a mucosal membrane (**Fig. 13.8**). This large space is referred to as the tympanic cavity proper. There is also a small extension superiorly called the **epitympanic recess** (also called the epitympanum or attic). The lateral wall of the tympanic cavity is the tympanic membrane, which is the only wall that is membranous (i.e., not bone) and serves as the separation between the outer and middle ears.

The anterior wall of the tympanic cavity contains the opening of the **eustachian tube** and the carotid artery. The eustachian tube (also called the pharyngotympanic tube or auditory tube) connects the middle ear space with the nasopharynx. Approximately 35 mm in length, the eustachian tube is one-third osseous (proximal to middle ear) and two-thirds cartilaginous (near the nasopharynx). It is normally closed, and two muscles control its opening: the **tensor veli palatini** and the **levator veli palatini**. When opened, the eustachian tube equalizes middle ear pressure with atmospheric pressure. Abnormal eustachian tube function can result in middle ear pathology.

The medial wall of the tympanic cavity is the border between the middle ear and inner ear. Communication between these two parts of the peripheral auditory system occurs through the membranes located at the oval window and round window. Other landmarks on the medial wall

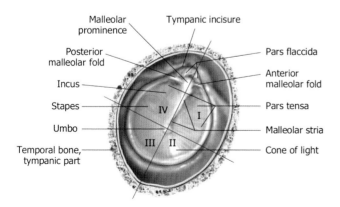

Fig. 13.7 Anatomic landmarks of the human tympanic membrane. Lateral view of the right tympanic membrane. The tympanic membrane is divided into four quadrants: anterosuperior (I), anteroinferior (II), posteroinferior (III), and posterosuperior (IV).

Box 13.3 Middle Ear Pathology

The balance of mass and stiffness within the middle ear space determines its efficiency to transmit sound between the outer ear and inner ear. This balance also determines the middle ear's resonant frequency, which is ~ 1200 Hz. A number of middle ear pathologies alter the mass and stiffness of the middle ear, resulting in differential changes in the resonant frequency. Thus, different middle ear pathologies alter sound transmission in a frequency-specific manner. Let's consider a few examples:

(a) Otitis media is an inflammation of the mucosal lining of the tympanic cavity of the middle ear. This inflammation is often the result of eustachian tube dysfunction, in which the eustachian tube is unable to equalize the pressure between the middle ear space and nasopharynx. Eustachian tube dysfunction results in a decrease in middle ear pressure, which disrupts the mucosal lining of the tympanic cavity. Otitis media may or may not present with effusion of fluid. Hearing loss is most often present in cases of otitis media with effusion (OME). Effusion can be sterile (serous OME) or infected (purulent OME). The extent to which OME affects sound transmission is dependent on the amount of fluid within the tympanic cavity and the location of the remaining air. If the fluid incompletely fills the tympanic cavity, there may be little to no change to hearing thresholds. Any reduction in sound transmission is typically isolated to low frequencies due to *increased stiffness* of the middle ear space resulting from eustachian tube dysfunction. The resulting hearing loss is a low-frequency conductive hearing loss. The accumulation of fluid within the tympanic cavity, however, adds both mass and stiffness to the system, resulting in a conductive hearing loss across the frequency range. It is important to note that the hearing loss associated with OME varies widely because of the differential effect on mass and stiffness of the middle ear system at each disease state. See Møller (2006) for additional reading on otitis media.

(b) Ossicular chain disarticulation (or **dislocation**) can result from trauma to the middle ear. These injuries are characterized by a break at any point of attachment within the contiguous ossicular chain. Incudostapedial joint discontinuities are the most common result of longitudinal temporal bone fractures. When the ossicular chain is disarticulated, there is a *decrease in stiffness* of the middle ear system. The system becomes mass-dominated, which results in a decrease in the transmission efficiency of high frequencies. The resulting hearing loss is a high-frequency conductive hearing loss, though flat configurations can also be observed.

(c) Otosclerosis, or otospongiosis, is a genetic metabolic disease of the temporal bone. It is characterized by abnormal bone remodeling in the tympanic cavity of the middle ear. Bone remodeling is a normal process by which bone renews itself. In otosclerosis, however, bone renewal becomes accelerated during the fourth or fifth decade of life, resulting in abnormal bone growth. The new bone is often highly vascularized and spongy. Early in the disease, a common lesion site is the stapes–oval window junction, whereby the stapes becomes fixed within the oval window. Stapes fixation results in an *increase in stiffness* of the middle ear system. In a stiffness-dominated system, transmission of low-frequency sounds is impaired. As the disease progresses, the additional bone adds mass to the system, which reduces the transmission of high-frequency sounds. As a result, patients with early-stage otosclerosis exhibit low-frequency conductive hearing loss, whereas patients with late-stage otosclerosis exhibit conductive hearing loss across the frequency range. Another hallmark of otosclerosis is a **Carhart notch**, which is a worsening of the *bone conduction* threshold at 2 kHz. This phenomenon is due to the pathology interfering with the ossicular chain's contribution to bone conduction (see Musiek and Baran [2007] for additional reading on bone conduction).

include the **promontory**, which is the first turn of the **cochlea** of the inner ear. The promontory is covered by the tympanic plexus, which is a network of fibers that innervate the mucous membranes of the middle ear, the eustachian tube, and the mastoid cells. Two prominences also protrude into the middle ear space on the medial wall: the prominence of the lateral (horizontal) semicircular canal of the vestibular system, and the prominence of the facial nerve canal. The prominence of the lateral semicircular canal is exploited during the clinical evaluation of vestibular function: clinicians stimulate the canal by irrigating the patient's ear canal with air or water.

The posterior wall of the tympanic cavity contains an opening, called the tympanic aditus (or the aditus to the mastoid antrum), which contains the entrance to the mastoid air cells via the tympanic antrum. The posterior wall also contains the **pyramidal eminence**, which is an extension off of the

Fig. 13.8 Schematic view of the tympanic cavity of the middle ear with anatomic landmarks. Right tympanic cavity; lateral view with the tympanic membrane (lateral wall) removed.

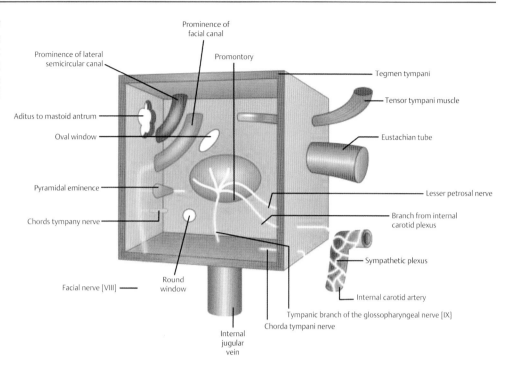

posterior wall from which the **stapedius muscle** arises. The superior wall of the tympanic cavity is called the tegmen tympani, which separates the middle ear space from the floor of the cranium. The inferior wall (floor) of the tympanic cavity consists of the tympanic plate of the temporal bone. The floor of the tympanic cavity separates the middle ear space from the jugular fossa, which is a canal in the temporal bone through which the jugular vein passes.

The Ossicular Chain

Suspended within the middle ear is the ossicular chain, which consists of three interconnected bones that link the tympanic membrane to the oval window of the inner ear. The three bones—the malleus, **incus**, and **stapes**—are the smallest bones in the human body (**Fig. 13.9**). As mentioned in the discussion of the external ear, the malleus is the most lateral bone. Its manubrium attaches firmly to the tympanic membrane and is visible during otoscopy. The malleus also has a head, neck, lateral process, and anterior process. The incus (anvil) is the middle bone and is characterized by a body, short limb, and long limb. The head and neck of the malleus articulate with the body of the incus at the **incudomallear joint**. At the tip of the long limb of the incus is a rounded projection called the lenticular process. The most medial aspect of the lenticular process

is covered with cartilage. The stapes (or stirrup, so called because of its structure), the smallest bone in the human body, is the most medial bone in the chain. It has a head, a neck, anterior crus, posterior crus, and a footplate. The head of the stapes articulates with the lenticular process of the incus at the **incudostapedial joint**. The purpose of the anterior crus and posterior crus is to connect the footplate to the neck of the stapes. The medial surface of the footplate of the stapes is covered by a thin layer of hyaline cartilage, which attaches to the bony wall of the oval window via

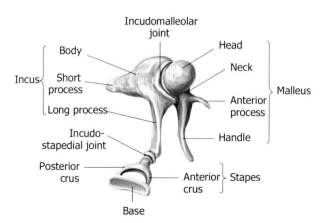

Fig. 13.9 Middle ear ossicles. Medial view of the ossicular chain in the left ear. The ossicular chain consists of three small bones that establish a mechanical linkage between the tympanic membrane and the oval window.

the **annular ligament** (Musiek and Baran 2007). The ossicular chain is suspended in the middle ear by ligaments, tendons, and muscles.

Muscles and Nerves in the Middle Ear

The major muscles of the peripheral auditory system are the stapedius muscle and the **tensor tympani muscle**; both are involved in the suspension of the ossicular chain in the middle ear space. The stapedius muscle is the smallest named muscle in the body. It is 1 mm in length, arises from the pyramidal eminence on the posterior wall of the middle ear, and attaches to the neck of the stapes. The stapedius muscle is innervated by the **stapedius nerve**, which branches from the main trunk of cranial nerve VII (facial nerve), which is located posterior to the middle ear as it traverses anteriorly to regions of the face. The tensor tympani muscle arises from the anterior wall of the middle ear and attaches to the neck of the malleus. It is innervated by the mandibular branch of the trigeminal nerve (CN V_3). In addition to providing structural support, the stapedius and tensor tympani muscles are involved in the **acoustic reflex**. The acoustic reflex is elicited by loud sounds, and its purpose is to increase the impedance of the middle ear system, therefore decreasing the transmission of acoustic energy.

The **chorda tympani**, which is a branch of the facial nerve (CN VII), has no relation to hearing; instead, it innervates taste buds. However, it passes through the middle ear space (behind the tympanic membrane), and therefore it may be compromised in cases of middle ear pathology.

The Inner Ear

The Labyrinths of the Inner Ear

The inner ear has two major divisions comprising the balance (vestibular division) and hearing (cochlear division) end organs. Both the vestibular and cochlear divisions of the inner ear, along with segments of the middle ear apparatus and the internal auditory canal, are located in the petrous portion of the temporal bone in a region appropriately called the (bony) labyrinth because of its numerous passages and canals: the cochlea for hearing and the semicircular canals of the vestibular system for balance (see **Chapters 9** and **15**). In both the cochlea and the vestibular system, the bony labyrinth is lined with elastic tissue called the membranous labyrinth. **Fig. 13.10** shows an anterior view of the inner ear with a portion of

the temporal bone removed to expose the orientation of the cochlea. The internal auditory canal provides the passageway for the vestibular and cochlear branches of the vestibulocochlear nerve (CN VIII, formerly called the auditory nerve) as well as the facial nerve (CN VII) into the lateral aspects of the lower brainstem.

The Bony Labyrinth of the Cochlea

The first, or basal, turn of the cochlea, which is located closest to the middle ear, is larger than the last, or apical, turn. Extending lateral from the central modiolus is the **osseous spiral lamina**, a double layer of thin bone that coils around the modiolus from base to apex of the cochlea. Small perforations in the osseous spiral lamina are referred to as the **habenula perforata**. These perforations in the bone allow the fibers of the cochlear branch of the vestibulocochlear nerve to exit the membanous labyritin of the cochlea. Once through, the nerve fibers spiral along a passage known as the **Rosenthal canal** and then project inside the internal auditory canal before terminating at the lower brainstem. The bony labyrinth in the cochlea (Latin for "snail shell") is a coil-shaped cavity (**Fig. 13.11**) that, in humans, consists of two and a half turns around a perforated central core known as the **modiolus**.

The Membranous Labyrinth of the Cochlea

Within the bony cochlea are three canals or ducts: the **scala vestibuli** (superior canal), **scala media** (middle canal, also known as the cochlear duct),

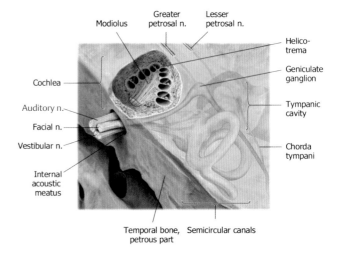

Fig. 13.10 Cochlea position in the temporal bone. A portion of the temporal bone removed to highlight orientation relative to the middle ear and vestibular structures. Cross section shows bony surrounding of the membranous labyrinth. See **Fig. 13.11** for more detail.

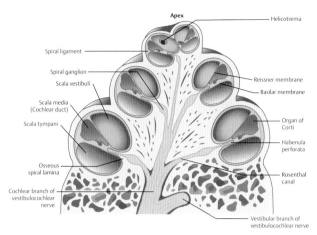

Fig. 13.11 The human cochlea. Anatomic landmarks of the membranous and bony labyrinths of the cochlea.

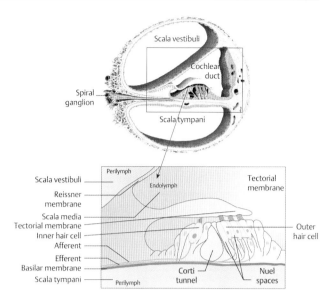

Fig. 13.12 The scala media and organ of Corti. Cross section of a single point along the membranous and bony cochlea. Red box (and arrow) highlights larger image below of the organ of Corti within the scala media (cochlear duct).

and the **scala tympani** (inferior canal) (**Fig. 13.11**). The scala media is separated from the scala vestibuli by the **Reissner membrane** and from the scala tympani by the **basilar membrane**. At the base of the cochlea, the oval window provides an opening from the middle ear to the scala vestibuli, while the round window provides an opening from the scala tympani to the middle ear. The stapes footplate is tightly coupled to the oval window by the annular ligament, while a thin membrane closes the round window. At the apex of the cochlea is a structure known as the **helicotrema**, which permits direct communication between the scala vestibuli and scala tympani.

The scala vestibuli and scala tympani are filled with a fluid known as **perilymph**. Perilymph's ionic content is similar to that of cerebrospinal fluid. It contains a high level of sodium ions and a low level of potassium ions in addition to chloride and calcium ions. The scala media is filled with a different fluid known as **endolymph**, whose ionic composition is unique for an extracellular space in that it contains a high level of potassium ions and a low level of sodium ions, which is typical of intracellular fluids. Fluid regulation of perilymph and endolymph plays an important role in the hydrodynamics of the membranous labyrinth. The regulation of perilymph and endolymph is primarily maintained by structures known as the **cochlear** and **vestibular aqueducts**, respectively. The cochlear aqueduct, which courses from the basal turn of the cochlea to the posterior aspect of the temporal bone, regulates the transfer of cerebrospinal fluid to the scala vestibuli and scala tympani. The vestibular aqueduct connects the posterior vestibule to the petrous portion of the temporal bone. Within the vestibular aqueduct

are the **endolymphatic sac** and **endolymphatic duct**, two structures thought to assist in regulating endolymph absorption.

The Cochlear Duct and the Organ of Corti

The cochlear duct (scala media) contains the **organ of Corti**, which is a network of sensory and supporting cells with interrupted space and fluid regions. In a cross section of the cochlea, one can view the three scalae (**Fig. 13.12**, top). The cochlear duct occupies the middle part of the labyrinth, and the organ of Corti sits upon the basilar membrane, the inferior boundary of the cochlear duct (**Fig. 13.12**, bottom). In humans, the basilar membrane is approximately 25 to 35 mm in length and courses along the entire distance of the cochlea, from base to apex. It is composed of extracellular matrix materials in which radially oriented tissue is securely embedded. The composition of embedded tissue is stiffer (~ 100 times as stiff) and narrower (~ 10 times as narrow) at the base than at the apex. This biophysical property permits better high-frequency tuning at the base and better low-frequency tuning at the apex. The **limbus** is a structure that makes up the medial edge of the organ of Corti (and the cochlear duct). It is attached to the osseous spiral lamina and contains numerous fibroblasts, capillaries, and filaments, the latter of which help make up the attachment point for the **tectorial**

Box 13.4   Otoacoustic Emissions (OAEs)

When OHCs change shape as their somatic motors operate, this motion itself produces sound waves that propagate in reverse direction even into the external auditory canal. A small and sensitive microphone can be placed in the auditory canal, and the emissions can be recorded. OAEs come in two primary varieties: spontaneous and evoked. Spontaneous emissions occur in the absence of external sound stimulation, while evoked emissions require a stimulus. The stimuli used for evoked emission are typically transient clicks and tones. OAEs are routinely tested in the clinical setting because they are noninvasive and easy to measure. They provide valuable information about the integrity of the inner ear and, more specifically, about OHC function. In addition, OAEs are utilized for newborn hearing screening programs that are designed to identify hearing loss in infants shortly after birth. All 50 states have implemented newborn hearing screening protocols within hospitals and birthing centers, and most OAE tests are performed prior to newborn discharge.

The primary types of OAEs measured in the clinic are transient and distortion product emissions (TEOAEs and DPOAE, respectively). DPOAEs are elicited by using two tones of similar frequencies. When the inner ear is stimulated using these two tones, a new set of tones, referred to as intermodulation distortion tones, is generated by the inner ear and can be recorded in the ear canal. The most prominent distortion products occur at two times the frequency of the first tone (F_1) minus the frequency of the second tone (F_2), or $2F_1 - F_2$. For example, if the frequency of tone 1 is 1,636 Hz and the frequency of tone 2 is 2,002 Hz, the inner ear distortion product will occur around $2 \times 1,636 - 1,200 = 3,272 - 2,002 = 1,270$ Hz. This provides frequency-specific information about the integrity of the OHC function of the inner ear. In fact, numerous reports have shown that lesions to inner hair cells (IHCs) have no effect on DPOAEs, further emphasizing that the frequency-specific loss of DPOAEs is intimately linked to the location of the damage along the organ of Corti.

---

membrane. The tectorial membrane defines the superior structure overlying the organ of Corti. It is a gelatinous matrix of embedded tissue consisting of ~ 95% water. A cluster of supporting cells known as **Hensen** and **Claudius cells** defines the lateral edge of the organ of Corti. The lateralmost wall of the cochlear duct itself contains the **stria vascularis** and the **spiral ligament**. The stria vascularis is important for endolymph production, as it consists of an intraepithelial network of capillaries and cell layers thought to secrete the high concentration of potassium ions found in endolymph. The spiral ligament provides structural support to both the Reissner membrane and the basilar membrane by anchoring them at the superior and inferior regions of the spiral ligament, respectively (**Fig. 13.12**, bottom).

Sensory and Supporting Cells of the Organ of Corti

The primary receptor structure of hearing is the organ of Corti. It contains two types of sensory cells known as **inner hair cells (IHCs)** and **outer hair cells (OHCs)** as well as numerous other nonsensory supporting cells (**Fig. 13.13**). The sensory hair cells occupy the superior upper half of the organ, while supporting cells are located medially, inferiorly, and laterally within the structure. IHCs and OHCs are separated from one another by supporting **pillar cells**. Pillar cells define the border of a triangular structure known as the **tunnel of Corti**: an open "tunnel" region that contains radially projecting afferent (i.e., toward the central nervous system, often called sensory) and efferent (i.e., away from the central nervous system, often called motor) nerve fibers. **Phalangeal cells** support IHCs, while each OHC is supported by a **Deiters cell**. Because of the inferior location of Deiters cells relative to each OHC body, adjacent regions between OHCs create openings known as the **space of Nuel**. Both the tunnel of Corti and the space of Nuel are filled with **cortilymph**, a fluid similar in its ionic content to perilymph—that is, it is high in sodium rather than potassium. Because of the tight junctions between sensory and supporting cells, cortilymph, in general, does not interact with the potassium-rich endolymph of the cochlear duct.

In humans, there is a single row of IHCs and three rows of OHCs that occupy the length of the cochlea, from base to apex. This arrangement allows for the initial establishment of a **tonotopic** organization of the cochlea, such that hair cells located at the basal end respond best to high frequencies and those located at the apical end respond best to low frequencies. It should be noted that the tonotopic organization of the cochlea arises as a result of the stiffness gradient along the basilar membrane (discussed in detail in the section on passive properties of basilar membrane macromechanics).

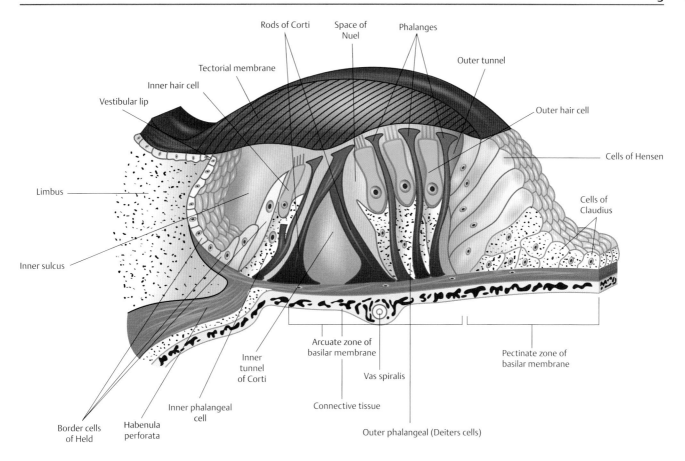

Fig. 13.13   The organ of Corti with anatomic landmarks.

There are approximately 3,500 IHCs and 13,500 OHCs per cochlea. The appearance of the IHC is "flask-shaped," with shorter cell bodies than OHCs, which are longer and cylindrical in shape (**Fig. 13.14**). In IHCs the nuclei are centrally located within the cell body, and organelles such

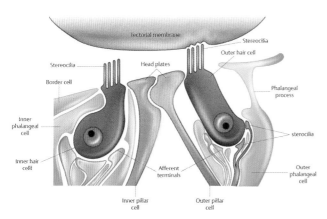

Fig. 13.14   Sensory and supporting cells of the organ of Corti with anatomic landmarks.

as mitochondria and lysosomes are dispersed throughout the cytoplasm. In OHCs the nuclei are located at the base of the cell body, while organelles are positioned mainly at the top and bottom of the cell body. At the basal pole of the IHC is a highly specialized structure known as the **ribbon synapse**. Important for extremely fast, precise, and sustained neurotransmitter release, this unique type of synapse plays an essential role in the perception of complex senses such as vision, balance, and hearing. As such, the ribbon synapse is found only in retinal photoreceptor cells, vestibular Type I hair cells, and IHCs of the cochlea. The function of these specialized structures will be discussed in greater detail in subsequent sections.

Projecting from the apex of hair cells are hair-like structures known as **stereocilia**. Three to four rows of stereocilia are arranged in a **U**-shaped pattern on IHCs, and three to five rows of stereocilia are arranged in a **W**- or **V**-shaped pattern on OHCs. Stereocilia are graded in length, with the shortest cilia located toward the medial side and the longest cilia positioned near the lateral edge of hair cells. IHC stereocilia do not come in contact with the tectorial membrane, whereas the tallest stereocilia of OHCs are embedded in the membrane. Also located at the top of hair cells is the **reticular lamina**, a dense structure that creates a tight junction around the base of stereocilia. Formed by the **cuticular plate** of hair cells along with the flattened phalangeal projections of adjacent supporting cells, the reticular lamina prevents endolymph from entering extracellular space surrounding the hair cells. Located near the upper portion of stereocilia are **tip links** and **crosslinks**, small filaments that connect to other stereocilia and open and close when the bundle is displaced toward the lateral or medial side of the cochlear duct, respectively. Later in this chapter, the opening and closing of the stereocilia by way of **mechanical transduction channels** will be discussed in more detail (see also **Chapter 9**). The small tip link and crosslink filaments help move the stereocilia in concert with one another when stimulated by hydromechanical vibrations. Their opening permits the entry of potassium-enriched endolymph from the cochlear duct into the hair cells, starting the sensory transduction process.

Inner and Outer Hair Cell Innervation

Both afferent and efferent nerve fibers innervate hair cells in the organ of Corti. Afferent fibers in the peripheral auditory system are axons of a type of bipolar neuron known as **spiral ganglion neuron**, whose cell bodies are located in the Rosenthal canal in the modiolus. Extending from the spiral ganglion cell body, the peripheral process (dendrite) of each neuron crosses the osseous spiral lamina, passes through the holes of the habenula perforata, and enters the organ of Corti to synapse onto IHCs and OHCs. In contrast to most dendrites, the peripheral process of a spiral ganglion neuron is myelinated, so it is sometimes referred to as the peripheral axon even though it carries action potentials toward the cell body rather than away. The central process (axon) traverses through the modiolus, exits the petrous portion of the temporal bone via the internal auditory canal, and travels in the vestibulocochlear nerve (approximately 22 to 26 mm long in humans) to enter the lower brainstem at the **cerebellopontine angle**.

There are two types of afferent spiral ganglion neurons: Type I and Type II. In humans, there are around 32,000 spiral ganglion neurons, of which the vast majority (~ 90 to 95%) are Type I, with Type II neurons making up the remaining 5 to 10%. Type I spiral ganglion neurons have large cell bodies, and their myelinated peripheral processes make restricted contact with individual IHCs. The peripheral process forms a small bouton ending located primarily on the base or basolateral side of the IHC. An individual IHC can receive as many as 10 to 20 spiral ganglion inputs (**Fig. 13.15**). Type II spiral ganglion neurons have small cell bodies with unmyelinated peripheral processes and connect exclusively to OHCs. An individual Type II afferent fiber can travel a great distance before forming bouton endings on the bases of multiple (~ 10) OHCs in one or more of the three rows (**Fig. 13.15**). Each OHC synapses with multiple Type II afferent fibers, but exact numbers are unknown.

Not only do hair cells transmit afferent signals to the central nervous system; they are also innervated by efferent axons from the brain. These efferent connections communicate largely with OHCs to extend the dynamic range of hair cell signaling and to protect the organ of Corti from acoustic overexposure. Efferent innervation to hair cells arises from neurons located in the **superior olivary complex (SOC)** of the brainstem. Efferent neurons send nerve fibers from both ipsilateral and contralateral locations within the SOC. Although exact numbers are not known, the number of efferent nerve fibers is considerably

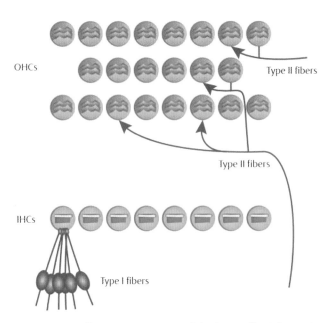

Fig. 13.15 Afferent innervation of the hair cells. Schematic drawing looking down on the top of outer (OHCs) and inner hair cells (IHCs). The tectorial membrane and stereocilia are removed to highlight afferent auditory nerve fiber innervation. Numerous type I auditory nerve afferent fibers innervate one IHC, while one type II auditory nerve afferent fiber innervates numerous OHCs.

less than that of afferent nerve fibers: approximately 500 total crossed and uncrossed fibers enter the cochlea from the brainstem. These efferent nerve fibers form part of the vestibulocochlear nerve and, together with cochlear hair cell innervation, constitute a system known as the **olivocochlear pathway**. Efferent nerve fibers enter the internal auditory canal, traverse the Rosenthal canal and the osseous spiral lamina, pass through the habenula perforata alongside afferent fibers, enter the organ of Corti, and synapse onto the bouton endings of Type I afferents (which synapse directly onto IHCs) or directly onto the base of OHCs, providing descending control of the organ of Corti (discussed in greater detail in subsequent sections).

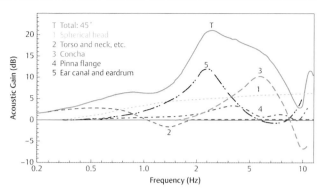

Fig. 13.16 Transfer function of the outer ear. The overall acoustic gain (T) at the level of the tympanic membrane from a sound source located at 45° (relative to the center-head position 0 at 0° horizontal azimuth) is shown. The contribution from individual body parts (1–5) is illustrated.

■ Physiology of the Peripheral Auditory System

The Outer Ear

The primary role of the outer ear is to funnel sound to the tympanic membrane. To accomplish this, the pinna and ear canal collect sound and transmit it to the tympanic membrane, which vibrates in response to the sound pressure wave. As discussed previously, the head influences sound as it reaches the outer ear. As sound reaches the ear, the cavernous structure of the pinna is exceptionally good at capturing and enhancing higher-frequency sounds, with a peak emphasis at ~ 5 kHz. This frequency range is also where monaural spectral cues are particularly strong. As sound passes through the ear canal, it is subjected to the canal's natural resonance. The ear canal is often thought of as a tube that is open on one end (lateral) and closed on the other end (medial, due to the tympanic membrane). Tubes with such a structure are known as quarter-wave resonators. Their resonant frequencies are determined by the equation

$$f = c/4L$$

where c = speed of sound and L is the length of the tube. The resonant frequency of the human adult ear canal is ~ 3 kHz. Note, however, that the resonant frequency of the ear canal is dependent on the length of the "tube." Therefore, the peak frequency in the transfer function may be lower than 3 kHz for larger-volume ear canals or higher than 3 kHz for smaller ear canal volumes. The combined effect of the head and outer ear on sound entering the auditory system can be determined by calculating the difference between the intensity of the sound at its source and the intensity of the sound

at the tympanic membrane (end of the ear canal). This difference is known as **head-related transfer function (HRTF)**, which typically shows a frequency emphasis between 2 and 7 kHz (**Fig. 13.16**). HRTFs help characterize how an ear receives sound and are dependent on the (1) location of the sound source; (2) size of the head; (3) size and location of the pinna; and (4) volume of the ear canal. HRTFs vary across individuals.

Tympanic Membrane: Transfer from Acoustic to Mechanical Energy

The tympanic membrane is the first point of energy transduction whereby sound (i.e., acoustic energy) is converted to a mechanical signal. As shown by Helmholtz in the 1800s and later confirmed by Bekesy in 1941, the tympanic membrane does not vibrate uniformly to all frequencies. For lower to mid frequencies, the tympanic membrane tends to vibrate like a disk, with maximum displacement in the inferior edge of the membrane. For higher frequencies, the tympanic membrane vibrates in a more segmented fashion, which likely facilitates the transmission of higher-frequency information by reducing the amount of membrane that needs to vibrate (as referenced in Musiek and Baran 2007; Pickles 2013).

The Middle Ear

Mechanical stimulation of the tympanic membrane forces vibration of the ossicular chain in the middle ear, which subsequently forces vibration of the oval window in the inner ear. Sound is maintained as mechanical energy throughout the middle ear.

The transduction of sound through the middle ear serves a pivotal role in our ability to hear because it solves the impedance mismatch between the air-filled ear canal and the fluid-filled cochlea that houses the organ of Corti. As discussed previously, sound traveling in air (low impedance) is largely reflected when it encounters water (high impedance). In the ear, the impedance mismatch between air (outer ear) and water (inner ear) would result in ~ 30 dB sound transmission loss without the impedance matching of the middle ear. Individuals with middle ear pathology experience hearing loss of similar magnitude (**Box 13.3**).

There are two primary ways in which impedance matching is accomplished: the area ratio and the lever ratio. The area ratio is between the area of the large tympanic membrane and that of the smaller oval window (which the footplate occupies). The area of the pars tensa is ~ 55 mm², and the size of the stapes footplate is ~ 3.2 mm². The differential area ratio is therefore 55/3.2 = 17:1. Recall that pressure is equal to force divided by area. To maintain the same force, a decrease in area will result in an increase in pressure. Using the formula for decibels referring to pressure,

$$dB = 20 \log P_o/P_r = 20 \log A_r/A_o$$
$$= 20 \log 17 = 24.6$$

Thus, the increase in pressure due to the differential area ratio accounts for an increase of ~ 25 dB at the oval window.

The lever ratio results from the manner by which the malleus, incus, and stapes are connected to form the ossicular chain. As a unit, the ossicular chain acts as a lever. By serving as the fulcrum of the lever, the short process of the incus divides the ossicular chain into a longer segment (malleus) and a shorter segment (long process of the incus). As the energy is transferred from the long segment to the short segment, there is a small increase in the force that is transferred to the oval window. The lever ratio of the long to short section is ~ 1.3:1, resulting in a ~ 2-dB gain at the oval window.

There has been some support in the literature for a third mechanism known as the buckling ratio. The theory posits that due to its concavity, the tympanic membrane has greater displacement during vibration, relative to the displacement of the manubrium. The shorter excursion of the manubrium results in an increase in force at the ossicular chain (Musiek and Baran 2007). The distance ratio between the tympanic membrane and manubrium is ~ 2:1, presumably resulting in a ~ 6-dB gain at the oval window. Together, these mechanisms generate ~ 33 dB gain, which compensates for the energy loss due to the impedance mismatch.

The ability of the middle ear to transmit sound is largely dependent on its **admittance** (the opposite of impedance). Normally, the middle ear has a resonant frequency of ~ 1200 Hz, the frequency at which it maximally responds. The transmission of lower frequencies is limited by the stiffness of the system (referred to as stiffness-dominated), and the transmission of higher frequencies is limited by the mass of the system (referred to as mass-dominated). As a result, the middle ear does not transmit frequencies equally well. As discussed in **Box 13.3**, changes in the middle ear's stiffness or mass are consequences of a number of middle ear pathologies. If the stiffness of the system increases, the resonant frequency of the middle ear becomes higher, and as a result, it is less effective at transmitting lower frequencies. Alternatively, if the middle ear system increases its mass, the resonant frequency becomes lower, resulting in reduced ability to transmit higher frequencies.

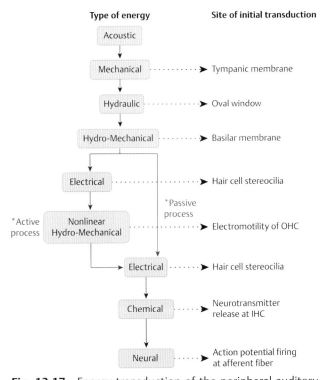

Fig. 13.17 Energy transduction of the peripheral auditory system. The system is simplified to include only the anatomic sites of energy transduction. The active process (red) represents activation of outer hair cells (OHC) during low-intensity stimulation. The passive process (blue) represents activation of inner hair cells during high-intensity stimulation.

The Cochlea of the Inner Ear

Cochlear Biophysiology

The common pathway that an acoustic signal takes from the pinna to the auditory nerve is depicted in **Fig. 13.17**. From this schematic, one can begin to appreciate that the peripheral auditory system is a remarkable feat of biological engineering designed for the specific function of hearing. This is especially true when we consider the biophysiology of the cochlea. Generally speaking, the function of the cochlea encompasses the change in vibratory and mechanical actions of the outer and middle ear into hydromechanical, chemical, and electrical impulses for the brain to interpret. Cochlear function, starting at the transduction site of the oval window, provides the necessary encoding of the frequency, intensity, and temporal components of sound and establishes the foundation for understanding behaviorally relevant communication signals.

Sensory encoding of sound begins in the cochlea. Pressure waves are delivered into the fluid-filled cochlea via the middle ear bones, setting the **cochlear partition** into motion. The cochlear partition consists of the basilar membrane, the organ of Corti, and the tectorial membrane (**Fig. 13.12**). As a result of this pressure wave and the mechanical properties of these structures, a relatively crude frequency analysis is performed by a vibratory pattern that occurs along the basilar membrane, a passive process known as the **traveling wave (Fig. 13.18a)**. In other words, the cochlea can "break down" a complex sound into its individual frequency components because of the mechanical properties of the cochlear partition. Because the basilar membrane is narrow and stiff at its base and wide and floppy at its apex, the traveling wave differentially stimulates specific regions along the basilar membrane. The traveling wave results in a vibratory pattern such that low-frequency sounds produce maximum displacement of the basilar membrane near the apical regions, while high-frequency sounds vibrate the basilar membrane maximally near basal regions (**Fig. 13.18b**).

Passive Properties of Basilar Membrane Macromechanics

Properties of basilar membrane movement originate with the mechanical stimulation of the stapes footplate and oval window of the scala vestibuli. This input is accommodated by the expansion of the round window of the scala tympani. When a compression sound wave is delivered to the cochlea,

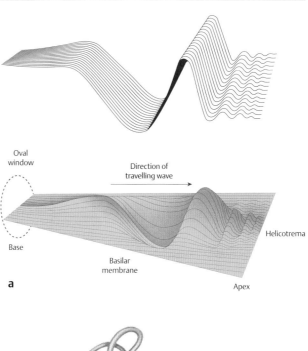

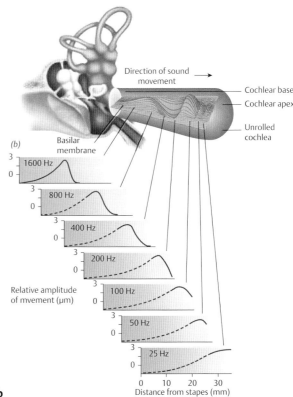

Fig. 13.18 The traveling wave. **(a)** Schematic of the traveling wave along the basilar membrane. The point of maximum vibration peaks close to the apical region, indicating a low-frequency input. **(b)** Uncoiled cochlea showing the direction of the traveling wave along the basilar membrane to seven different frequency inputs. For each subsequent frequency input (from 1,600 to 25 Hz), the peak of maximum vibration moves from base to apex, highlighting the tonotopic gradient of the cochlear partition.

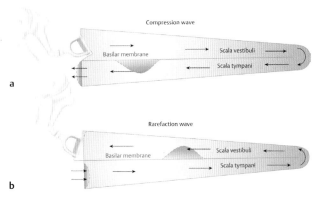

Fig. 13.19 Compression and rarefaction traveling waves. Uncoiled cochlea showing a compression and rarefaction traveling wave along the basilar membrane. **(a)** The compression wave pushes the stapes inward, causing an initial downward deflection of the basilar membrane (hyperpolarization, no excitation). **(b)** The rarefaction wave pulls the stapes outward, causing an initial upward deflection of the membrane (depolarization, excitation). Arrows indicate direction of fluid movement. See **Fig. 13.23** for more details on hair cell dynamics.

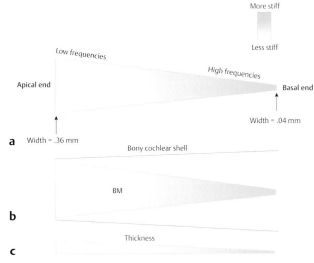

Fig. 13.20 Basilar membrane properties. **(a)** Schematic drawing looking down on the basilar membrane, highlighting its biophysical property differences between the apical and basal regions. **(b)** Relative dimensions of the basilar membrane in relation to the bony cochlear regions. **(c)** A side view showing the differences in thickness along the length of the basilar membrane from the apex to the base.

the stapes and oval window are pushed inward, the traveling wave moves from base to apex in the scala vestibuli and back in the scala tympani, and the round window is pushed outward (**Fig. 13.19a**). The opposite occurs when a rarefaction sound wave is presented. Here, the stapes and oval window are pushed outward while the round window adapts to this movement and pulls inward (**Fig. 13.19b**). The "push-pull" vibrations of the oval and round window set up a traveling wave in the cochlear fluids that propagates the length of the basilar membrane.

At the basal end of the basilar membrane, the traveling wave moves rapidly—approximately 328 feet per second, compared to about 10 feet per second in the apical region. The difference in traveling wave velocity is related to the biophysical characteristics of the basilar membrane that determine its stiffness and mass. For example, the basilar membrane is ~ 10 times as narrow and ~ 100 times as stiff at the base as at the apex, where it is wider, thicker, and more mobile (**Fig. 13.20**). As such, the basal region results in a high traveling wave velocity (stiffness dependent), and the apical region supports a low traveling wave velocity (mass loaded). This structural gradient confers a smooth shift of preferred vibration frequency along its length, with high frequencies maximally activating basal regions of the basilar membrane and low frequencies maximally activating apical areas (**Fig. 13.18**).

Another factor contributing to the macromechanics of basilar membrane movement and, thus, the traveling wave is its anatomic points of

attachment. The medial edge of the basilar membrane is attached to the osseous spiral lamina, which serves as a hinge for both the organ of Corti and the basilar membrane. The lateral portion of the basilar membrane is attached to the spiral ligament and is more elastic and mobile compared to the medial portion. This connectivity is present throughout the length of the basilar membrane and assists the cochlear partition in translating the frequency of vibration from a traveling pressure wave into a position of maximal displacement along its length.

The representation of frequency along the basilar membrane is accomplished by several primary principles known as the **place**, **temporal**, and **volley theories**. The place theory states that the encoding of a specific frequency is dependent on its *place* of maximum vibration along the basilar membrane (i.e., different frequencies produce traveling waves that reach their maximum deflections at different places). Because of the resonance characteristics of the basilar membrane, the traveling wave at high frequencies peaks at a place located near the basal region while the traveling wave at low frequencies peaks at a place near the apical region. One caveat to consider regarding the place theory is that the frequency tuning of the basilar membrane appears to be too broad, based on behavioral psychoacoustic measurements of frequency discrimination. That is, humans are able to discriminate very small changes in frequency, but the place theory suggests that the vibration pattern between two slightly different adjacent frequencies will not significantly differ. As such, an alternative temporal theory of frequency resolution was proposed, although not mutually exclusive with the place theory.

The temporal theory (also referred to as the frequency theory) states that the encoding of a specific frequency is dependent on the timing and rate of neuronal firing patterns (i.e., the rate at which an afferent Type I spiral ganglion nerve fiber can fire action potentials). In general, this theory claims that frequencies are encoded by the ability of neurons to fire action potentials at a rate that mimics the sound frequency. For example, if a sound has a frequency of 500 Hz, the traveling wave peaks at a *place* of maximum vibration that corresponds to a specific apical region of the basilar membrane as described in the preceding paragraph. At this specific apical location, the basilar membrane also vibrates 500 times per second and thus stimulates the adjoining Type I spiral ganglion nerve fibers at this same rate. However, because the range of human hearing extends to 20,000 Hz and afferent auditory nerve fibers cannot fire at this fast rate, the temporal theory has limitations to consider as well. In an effort to explain these caveats of frequency encoding on the basilar membrane, the volley theory was introduced.

The **volley theory** states that encoding of frequency is dependent on a population of neurons firing action potentials at a particular **phase** of the input frequency. An individual neuron does not need to fire at every phase of the frequency, so as long as it fires at the same phase for a given number of cycles (**Fig. 13.21**). When the combined firing of precisely timed action potentials is taken into consideration, higher frequencies can be encoded and represented by the population of neurons. However, as with the place and temporal theories, the volley theory also has caveats to consider. Because the ability of afferent Type I spiral ganglion neurons to fire synchronized phase-locked action potentials diminishes above 1,000 Hz, the volley theory cannot account for the higher-frequency range of human hearing.

As such, it is now generally agreed upon that hearing follows the rules of all three theories for frequency encoding. At frequencies below 1,000 Hz, the temporal and volley theories govern frequency encoding of the basilar membrane. Above 5,000 Hz, the place theory dominates. Between 1,000 and 5,000 Hz, all three principles work in concert. Encoding of sound frequency is determined by a specific region along the basilar membrane (place theory), and the rate of action potential firing

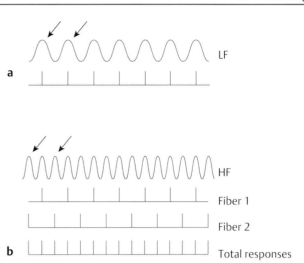

Fig. 13.21 The volley theory of hearing. **(a)** Principles of the volley theory represented by two sine waves. The arrows on both sine waves indicate the locations on the sine wave that the neuron may fire a phase-locked action potential. Vertical lines below the sine waves indicate a neural, phase-locked action potential response. The upper sine wave represents a low-frequency (LF) signal where an individual auditory nerve fiber fires phase-locked action potentials on every cycle. The lower sine wave is of a higher frequency (HF), and the individual nerve fibers (1 and 2) can lock onto only every other cycle. The summation (total response) of the firing of the two fibers captures the frequency of the high-frequency sine wave. **(b)** The higher the frequency (up to a certain point, see text), the greater the number of neurons needed to capture the input in their total response.

(temporal theory) by a population of neurons (volley theory).

Representation of sound intensity is also associated with maximal amplitude displacement of the traveling wave along the basilar membrane. High stimulus intensities result in larger traveling wave amplitudes, and low stimulus intensities yield smaller traveling wave amplitudes. Because of its biophysical characteristics (i.e., stiffness and mass), the passive properties of the basilar membrane establish a gradient of displacement that decreases from apex to base; displacement at its apical end is greater than at its basal end for the same intensity of stimulus. As the stimulus intensity increases, the shape of the traveling wave, or its **envelope**, becomes larger in amplitude and broader in width (**Fig. 13.22a**). A broad traveling wave at high stimulus intensities decreases frequency selectivity and tuning of the basilar membrane, while low-intensity stimuli result in sharper frequency selectivity. Large and broad displacements of the basilar membrane activate a greater number of hair cells and, thus, a larger proportion of afferent Type I spiral ganglion nerve fibers, resulting in greater loudness

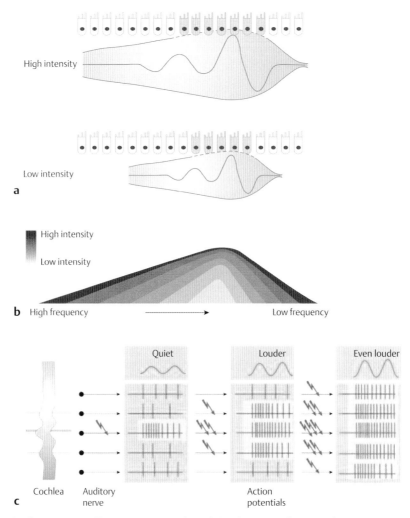

Fig. 13.22 Hair cell and afferent nerve fiber intensity coding. **(a)** Schematic showing the increase in the number of hair cells stimulated as the basilar membrane deflection increases with higher intensities. **(b)** Basilar membrane displacement with intensity increments. With higher intensities, the basilar membrane shows greater compression, less sharpness in tuning, and greater displacement along its length. **(c)** Increase in basilar membrane displacement as a result of higher intensities causes a greater firing rate and spread of auditory nerve afferent action potential excitation (going from quiet to louder and even louder intensities).

perception (**Fig. 13.22b, c**). However, despite the fact that the basilar membrane displacement is larger for high-intensity stimuli compared to low-intensity stimuli, there is progressively less change in displacement amplitude as a function of increasing intensity. In other words, a form of nonlinear compression of basilar membrane displacement exists for high intensity levels.

Active Transduction Properties of Hair Cell Micromechanics

The sensory receptors responsible for hydromechanical vibration transduction of the basilar membrane are the IHCs and OHCs of the organ of Corti. An important aspect of this sensory transduction process is the micromechanics of the hair cells themselves. As previously discussed, IHCs and OHCs contain stereocilia located on their apical surface. These **actin**-filled stereocilia contain mechanical transduction channels near the tips of the stereocilia bundles (**Fig. 13.14**). When stereocilia are deflected by movement of the basilar membrane, these channels alternately open, permitting movement of ions into the hair cells, and close, preventing such flow. Thus, IHCs and OHCs initiate the sensory transduction process of hearing by converting mechanical deflections of stereocilia bundles into electrochemical signals that are distributed throughout the rest of the auditory system.

How does sensory transduction work? In order to walk through the process of hair cell sensory transduction, it is necessary to start with the stereocilia bundles of the OHCs, which are the only stereocilia of the cochlear hair cells that make contact with the tectorial membrane. First, an acoustic compression pulse sets up a traveling wave that moves the basilar membrane downward. With this downward movement, the organ of Corti also moves downward and shears the tectorial membrane so that it pushes the stereocilia toward the limbus, or medially. Thus, downward movement of the basilar membrane drives the stereocilia bundles in the direction that causes the mechanical transduction channels to close, preventing the flow of potassium ions through the channel (**Fig. 13.23a, b**). If

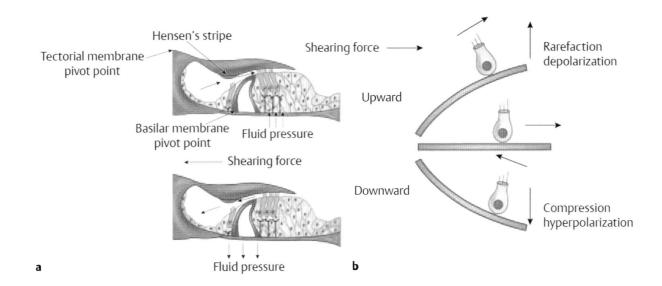

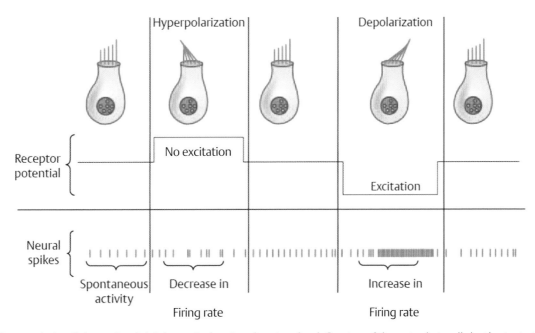

Fig. 13.23 Sensory hair cell dynamics. **(a)** Schematic drawing showing the deflection of the outer hair cells by the tectorial membrane for upward and downward movement of the basilar membrane. Upward movement (due to rarefaction) results in depolarization of the hair cell (excitation). Downward movement (due to compression) results in hyperpolarization (no excitation). **(b)** Image highlighting hair cell dynamics shown in (a), i.e., stereocilia deflection and basilar membrane movement. **(c)** Hair cell receptor potentials as a function of hyperpolarization and depolarization cause changes in afferent neural action potential firing rates.

no potassium ions flow into the hair cell, the cell is in a **hyperpolarized** state, and the attached vestibulocochlear nerve fiber fires fewer action potentials because of the decrease in neurotransmitter release from the IHCs (**Fig. 13.23c**). Second, when the basilar membrane is deflected upward as a result of an acoustic rarefaction pulse, the stereocilia of the OHCs are deflected in the opposite direction (toward the spiral ligament, or laterally). Thus, upward movement of the basilar membrane drives the stereocilia bundles in the direction that causes the mechanical transduction channels to open and **depolarize** the outer hair cell by an influx of potassium ions from the endolymphatic fluid (**Fig. 13.23**). This depolarization is critical for **electromotility** and the functioning of the **cochlear amplifier**, which is discussed in greater detail in following paragraphs.

Stereocilia deflection in IHCs is qualitatively different from that in outer hair cells. Because the IHC stereocilia bundles are not in contact with the tectorial membrane and, therefore, cannot shear against it, an alternative method of mechanical transduction must occur. The stereocilia of IHCs move, and mechanical transduction channels of IHCs open and close, as a result of the viscous drag that arises due to the traveling wave, basilar membrane movement, and OHC articulation with the tectorial membrane. In other words, fluid dynamics between the reticular lamina and the tectorial membrane cause the stereocilia of IHCs to move in the same direction. OHC movement drives this function. The opening of IHC mechanical transduction channels causes an unconventional form of depolarization (potassium-induced depolarization; see **Chapter 6**). This depolarization activates **voltage-gated calcium channels**, which triggers the release of the excitatory neurotransmitter **glutamate** via the ribbon synapse (**Fig. 13.24**). Glutamate is the primary excitatory neurotransmitter in the central nervous system, including the auditory pathway. When released from IHCs, glutamate binds to postsynaptic glutamate receptors known as **AMPA-type receptors** located on the peripheral processes (dendrites) of spiral ganglion neurons of the auditory nerve, initiating **saltatory conduction** of action potentials to central auditory nuclei in the brainstem.

The foregoing description of mechanoelectric transduction holds true for hair cells in all vertebrates. However, the classification into IHCs and OHCs and the differences between the two are remarkable and unique to mammals. IHCs are the primary sensory receptor, and as previously mentioned, they receive approximately 90 to 95% of afferent innervation. In contrast, OHCs receive

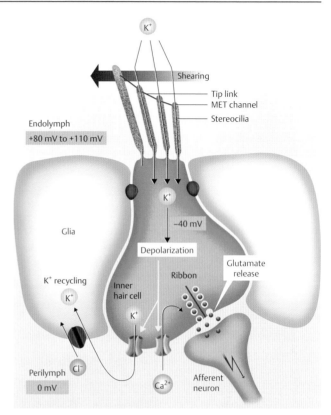

Fig. 13.24 Inner hair cell transduction. Shearing of stereocilia cause tip links to stretch and open mechanical transduction channels. Potassium (K$^+$) ions from the endolymph fluid move into the inner hair cell and cause depolarization. This opens voltage-gated calcium channels (Ca^{2+}), and Ca^{2+} influx in turn promotes the release of docked glutamate vesicles at the ribbon synapse. Released glutamate binds to receptors located on adjacent afferent vestibulocochlear nerve fibers. Excitation in the form of action potentials is generated and transmitted to the next-order auditory structure, located in the brainstem.

only around 5 to 10% of afferent contacts, suggesting a minor role in auditory transduction. Despite this dichotomy in afferent innervation, OHCs have highly specialized functions that contribute to what is known as the cochlear amplifier (**Fig. 13.25a**). The cochlear amplifier provides a form of positive feedback onto the basilar membrane upon OHC depolarization. Recall that as the basilar membrane moves upward, stereocilia deflect toward the spiral ligament, mechanical transduction channels open, potassium ions flow in, and depolarization occurs. Depolarized OHCs change shape because of molecules of a specialized protein known as **prestin** located within their cell body lateral walls. Prestin lengthens under membrane depolarization, which in turn lengthens the OHC, while prestin contraction leads to a decrease in OHC length. This ability to change OHC shape is referred to as the **somatic motor**.

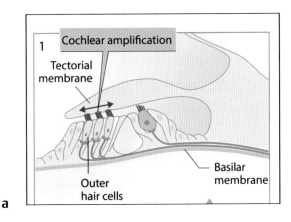

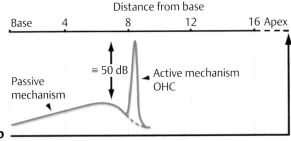

Fig. 13.25 Outer hair cell cochlear amplification. **(a)** Passive basilar membrane movement causes outer hair cells to vibrate optimally at their place of tonotopic tuning. This occurs best with low-intensity inputs in normal hearing individuals, providing amplification of the signal. **(b)** The amplification of the OHC provides positive feedback into the basilar membrane. This active mechanism provides ~ 50 dB of gain.

As OHCs contract and elongate following changes in membrane potential, they actively provide mechanical force onto the surrounding environment, a process termed electromotility. Electromotility is the driving force behind the cochlear amplifier, which is a mammalian evolution that increases sensitivity to incoming sounds. This increase in sensitivity can be as high as 100-fold in individuals with normal OHC function (providing ~ 50 dB of gain; **Fig. 13.25b**). By amplifying the signal, the cochlear amplifier produces a highly significant and spatially segregated enhancement of the basilar membrane vibratory amplitude. This enhancement provides narrowly tuned, frequency-specific information to afferent auditory nerve fibers via IHC activation. Accordingly, the relatively crude sensitivity and frequency selectivity of the basilar membrane that results from its passive biomechanical properties is substantially refined through OHC-driven cochlear amplification.

The cochlear amplifier is not always active during mechanoelectric transduction. For instance, cochlear amplification only occurs for low-intensity sounds and is diminished or lost for high-intensity signals, resulting in poorer frequency selectivity (**Fig. 13.22**). In addition, OHCs are more susceptible to damage than IHCs, and this damage reduces or eliminates the cochlear amplifier. Thus, damage to the OHCs broadens the frequency tuning selectivity and shifts the hearing threshold upward by 40 to 60 dB. Finally, contraction and elongation of OHCs is thought to be the mechanism underlying the generation of sound from the inner ear, known as otoacoustic emissions (OAEs), a clinically relevant by-product of the cochlear amplifier (**Box 13.4**).

Cochlear Electrophysiology

The precision of mechanoelectric transduction can be attributed, in part, to the electrical potential and ionic milieu in the endolymphatic space surrounding the apical surface of the hair cells, known as the **endocochlear potential** (EP). The EP is a positive electrical voltage (+80 to +100 mV), which can be recorded from the cochlear endolymphatic space. The EP is established between the endolymph and surrounding perilymph fluids. During the first week after hearing onset, the EP increases from 0 mV to +80 mV. The ramping-up of the electrical potential is complemented by the accumulation of high levels of potassium ions in the endolymphatic space, which further exaggerates the electrical gradient across the negative resting potential of the IHCs and OHCs (which is between –40 and –70 mV, respectively). The combination of high extracellular potassium ion concentrations and positive endocochlear potential work synergistically to effectively drive ionic currents through open mechanical transduction channels on the apical end of OHCs. This process generates large and rapid receptor potential changes that mediate neurotransmitter release at the synapse between the IHC and spiral ganglion fibers of auditory nerves. The endocochlear potential is established through the development of tight cellular junctions among epithelial cells, connective tissue, and supporting cells that completely partition the endolymph from the surrounding perilymph. These tightly bound networks also efficiently recycle potassium from the hair cell back into the endolymphatic space, where it can once again be used in mechanoelectric transduction.

In addition to the endocochlear potential, three other cochlear electrical potentials are associated with mechanoelectric transduction and hair cell depolarization: the **cochlear microphonic (CM)**, the **summating potential (SP)**, and the **compound action potential (cAP)**. The CM is an alternating current generated primarily by the OHCs and can be recorded by placing an electrode within the ear canal or on the tympanic membrane. When an acoustic signal of a given frequency is delivered to the ear, the CM generated by OHCs mirrors the waveform of the incoming signal. Thus, the CM reflects the flow of potassium ions into OHCs as a result of the opening and closing of stereocilia mechanical transduction channels. The SP is the extracellular direct current response generated largely by the IHCs as they move in conjunction with the basilar membrane. Again, a nearby placed electrode can record ionic flow into the IHC via the mechanical transduction channels. Although not technically a cochlear electrical potential, the cAP, is generated by the vestibulocochlear

nerve, represents the summed responses of the synchronous firing of phase-locked action potentials from the nerve fibers themselves and is discussed in greater detail in the following section (**Box 13.5**).

Afferent Neural Function

The cochlear division of the vestibulocochlear nerve, or auditory nerve, carries electrical impulses in the form of action potentials from the cochlea to the lower brainstem. The physiology of the auditory nerve accurately preserves encoded information

---

Box 13.5   Inner Ear Potentials

The inner ear and auditory nerve electrical potentials can be measured and recorded in response to sound by a test called **electrocochleography** (or ECochG). This procedure is used clinically to assess the cochlear microphonic (CM) and summating potential (SP) of hair cells as well as the compound action potential (cAP) of the vestibulocochlear nerve. The most common clinical applications of ECochG include objective identification and monitoring of **Ménière's disease**. In addition, ECochG is used to monitor the peripheral auditory system during surgery to the auditory periphery, to enhance the Wave I component of the **auditory brainstem response (ABR)**, and, more recently, in the diagnosis of **auditory neuropathy/dyssynchrony**.

Typically, a noninvasive electrode is placed in the ear canal or on the tympanic membrane of the "suspected" ear. This electrode is often referred to as an extratympanic (ET) electrode. Other electrodes are placed on the top of the head (or forehead) and on the opposite ear. The ET electrode has an advantage of not causing pain or discomfort to the patient, compared to transtympanic (TT) needle electrodes, which, as the name implies, must pass through the tympanic membrane, requiring sedation, anesthesia, and medical supervision. The TT needle electrode is placed on the promontory wall of the middle ear, between the oval and round windows. As a result, it provides a clearer, more robust electrical response with larger amplitudes than ET electrodes do because the TT electrode is placed nearer the voltage generators in the cochlea and vestibulocochlear nerve. Thus, the noninvasive ET electrode does not require sedation, anesthesia, or medical supervision, but the overall responses are smaller in magnitude.

The auditory signal used to generate the electrical potentials can be either clicks or tones. For clicks, the duration is usually 100 microseconds and the polar-

ity can be rarefaction, condensation, or alternating. For tones, the duration can be short or long and frequency specific. When tones are used, the CM is the alternating current voltage that mirrors the frequency of the tone. It is dominated by the outer hair cell and is proportional to the displacement of the basilar membrane. The SP is the stimulus-related potential of the cochlea and is often referred to as the direct current voltage response of the inner hair cells as they move in combination with the basilar membrane movement. Finally, the cAP represents the summed neural response of the synchronous action potential firing of vestibulocochlear nerve fibers. The cAP is the largest potential of the ECochG and is identical to Wave I of the ABR.

The clinical use of the ECochG is in the diagnosis of Ménière's disease. It is also used in differentiating between cochlear and retrocochlear deficits and in estimating hearing thresholds in difficult-to-test populations. The diagnosis of Ménière's disease is made when the SP is unusually large compared to the cAP, resulting in an SP/AP ratio that is more than 40% of the cAP. Although the criteria for abnormality are not universal, it is generally agreed upon that SPs larger than 40 to 50% of the cAP yield are highly specific for Ménière's disease. However, it should be noted that if the patient is asymptomatic at the time of testing, the SP/AP is, more often than not, normal.

In differentiating between cochlear and retrocochlear deficits, ECochG has proven useful, especially in individuals with auditory neuropathy/dyssynchrony, a relatively newly described disorder. Individuals with auditory neuropathy/dyssynchrony present with a wide range of symptoms, including mild to moderate hearing loss and severely impaired speech understanding in both quiet and noisy environments. One diagnostic indicator is the presence of the CM but abnormal or absent cAP, suggesting normal OHC function with abnormal vestibulocochlear nerve function.

from the IHC receptor potential, achieved in part by a specialized structure at the basal end of IHCs known as the ribbon synapse. As previously mentioned, the ribbon synapse is a type of synapse that can release multiple vesicle packets of the neurotransmitter glutamate. In addition to ideal localization of calcium channels, the ribbon synapse helps promote rapid glutamate release and sustained signal transmission upon activation of the IHC receptor potential.

Recall that the opening of the IHC mechanical transduction channels permits (1) potassium ion influx, (2) hair cell depolarization, (3) calcium channel activation, and (4) glutamate release through the ribbon synapse. Consequently, postsynaptic glutamate receptors located on the bouton endings of Type I afferent fibers (recall that these are the fibers that innervate IHCs) are activated. The glutamate receptor on the postsynaptic spiral ganglion fiber is an ion channel that, when glutamate binds to it, permits an inward flow of sodium ions into the afferent auditory nerve from the surrounding cortilymph. This conventional form of neuronal depolarization activated by the opening of sodium channels located on the afferent bouton generates an all-or-none action potential. The action potential rapidly propagates up the myelinated peripheral process (i.e., saltatory conduction) until it reaches the spiral ganglion cell body, from which it is further sent down along the central process (axon) to the **cochlear nucleus**, the first-order synapse in the central auditory system. The probability that an action potential will occur at any moment in time relative to the incoming sound is the basic foundation on which the central auditory system encodes and interprets sounds in the environment.

For all afferent auditory nerve fibers, there is a nonzero probability of action potential generation even in the absence of external stimulation (e.g., sound), referred to as **spontaneous action potential firing rate**. The overall range of spontaneous firing occurs between 0 and 100 action potentials per second (i.e., Hz) for all auditory nerve fibers. However, the distribution of spontaneous firing rates indicates two primary rates: low and high. Afferent auditory nerve fibers that have spontaneous firing rates between 0 and 2 Hz are called low-spontaneous-rate (low-SR) neurons. Auditory nerve fibers that exhibit firing rates between 60 and 70 Hz are termed high-spontaneous-rate (high-SR) neurons. Low and high spontaneous firing rates of auditory nerve fibers are the result of several factors. First, an individual IHC can spontaneously release different amounts of the neurotransmitter glutamate. Second, the location of the auditory nerve fiber synapse on an individual IHC differs; low-SR neurons terminate on the modiolar side of IHCs, while high-SR neurons terminate on the pillar side of IHCs. Finally,

the size of auditory nerve fibers also differs; low-SR fibers are thin, while high-SR fibers are thick.

What functional purpose might differences in spontaneous firing rates serve with respect to encoding sound? IHCs follow the waveform of a sound stimulus by hyperpolarizing and depolarizing their receptor potentials and thus, modulate the probability of generating an action potential by differentially releasing glutamate. Little to no glutamate is released when an IHC is hyperpolarized, and a sustained level of glutamate is released when the cell is depolarized. As such, the probability that an auditory nerve fiber will generate an action potential decreases and increases in a fashion that closely follows the IHC receptor potential described previously.

In order to encode sound information in this fashion, afferent auditory neurons must have a range of action potential firing *thresholds* for a given sound intensity. The intensity thresholds of afferent auditory neurons vary inversely with their spontaneous firing rate. Low-SR neurons have high intensity thresholds, while high-SR neurons have low intensity thresholds. The difference between spontaneous firing rate thresholds is significant: low-SR neurons have thresholds as much as 50 dB above their high-SR counterparts (**Fig. 13.26**).

Sound intensity is encoded at the auditory nerve not only by the total number of fibers involved (higher intensity = more fibers) but also by firing rate (higher intensity = greater firing rates) and the fiber-dependent threshold for action potential

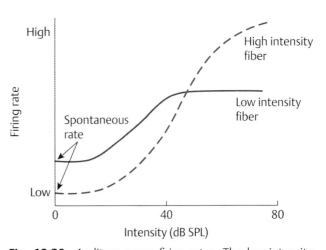

Fig. 13.26 Auditory nerve firing rates. The low-intensity fiber (higher spontaneous firing rate, solid line) begins to respond at low intensities at or near threshold and reaches saturation of firing at ~ 40 dB sound pressure level (SPL). The high-intensity fiber (lower spontaneous firing rate, dashed line) starts firing at mid-intensities and continues to respond at high SPLs. A wide intensity range is therefore coded by these two afferent auditory nerve fibers (~ 0–80 dB SPL).

activation (**Fig. 13.26**). Auditory nerve fibers with low spontaneous firing rates and high thresholds for action potential activation are better at encoding high-intensity sounds. Conversely, auditory nerve fibers with high spontaneous firing rates and low thresholds for action potential activation are best at encoding low-intensity sounds. Taken together, these auditory nerve properties are important for extending the dynamic range of sound intensity encoding.

How is sound frequency represented at the level of the afferent auditory nerve? The spatial organization and temporal characteristics of the cochlea are preserved throughout the auditory nerve. Frequency, therefore, is encoded by the auditory nerve based on the place, temporal, and volley principles established by the passive and active properties of basilar membrane mechanics. The one-dimensional tonotopic arrangement of the basilar membrane is preserved in tonotopic maps of preferred frequency within the auditory nerve. Afferent auditory nerve fibers that connect to hair cells running along the basilar membrane from base to apex, are graded in order to encode high to low frequencies, respectively, as delineated by the place theory. Because the cochlea is coil-shaped and the spiral ganglion curves with it, high-frequency auditory nerve fibers dominate the outer ring of the bundle, while low-frequency fibers are located in the central core.

This biophysical arrangement establishes that auditory nerve fibers are tuned tonotopically and have **characteristic frequencies** to which they best respond. Thus, the characteristic frequency of an individual auditory nerve fiber can be defined as the frequency to which the fiber best responds at the lowest possible sound intensity (i.e., threshold). The further away the stimulus frequency is from the nerve fiber's characteristic frequency, the greater the stimulus intensity must be in order for the nerve fiber to fire an action potential. This intensity/frequency relationship of auditory nerve fibers can be plotted as a **tuning curve**, which illustrates varying stimulus intensity as a function of changing frequencies above and below the characteristic frequency of the fiber (**Fig. 13.27**). The sharper the tuning curve, the better the frequency selectivity of the nerve fiber, the better the auditory "filter." Tuning curves are usually sharper for auditory nerve fibers located near the basal region of the cochlea (**Fig. 13.27a**), while fibers located more apically have slightly broader tuning curves (**Fig. 13.27b**). Interestingly, damage to OHCs results in decreased tuning curve sensitivity and sharpness regardless of position along the basilar membrane.

Temporal encoding of frequency by the auditory nerve is closely related to a phenomenon known as

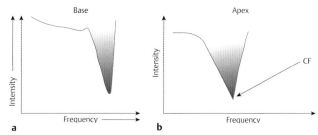

Fig. 13.27 Auditory tuning curves. **(a)** Schematic tuning curves of auditory nerve fibers recorded from the basal and apical regions along the basilar membrane in a normal cochlea (left and right, respectively). Although both neurons show sharp tuning at their respected characteristic frequencies (CF), the basal neuron is sharper in tuning and has a less pronounced "tail" of its tuning curve compared to the apically placed neuron. **(b)** Tuning curves of nerve fibers from the basal and apical regions of the basilar membrane in a cochlea containing damaged OHCs, showing loss of tuning curve sensitivity and sharpness.

phase locking. Simply put, phase locking reflects the neuron's ability to fire an action potential at a particular phase of the stimulus (**Fig. 13.22**). Thus, the firing rate of the auditory nerve fiber is closely related to the frequency of the stimulus (low frequency = low firing rate, high frequency = high firing rate). However, the relationship between phase locking and frequency encoding holds constant only for frequencies up to ~ 1,000 Hz, largely because the rate at which action potentials can be generated and propagate along afferent auditory nerve fibers is too slow to keep up with higher frequencies (albeit it is still faster than for most neurons in the central nervous system). As previously mentioned, the volley principle helps account for the encoding of higher frequencies at the level of the auditory nerve. For high-frequency sounds, an individual auditory nerve fiber may fire a phase-locked action potential every third or fourth cycle of the stimulus, while a subset of adjacent neurons may phase-lock to different cycles. In this way, a population of afferent auditory nerve fibers fire phase-locked action potentials at the same phase of different stimulus cycles. When summed together, they accurately represent the waveform of the sound and help maintain high-frequency encoding.

■ Functional Neuroanatomy of the Central Auditory System

The functional neuroanatomy linking the auditory periphery to the brain has at least seven essential processing stations: (1) sensory hair cells in the auditory periphery, which send chemical signals

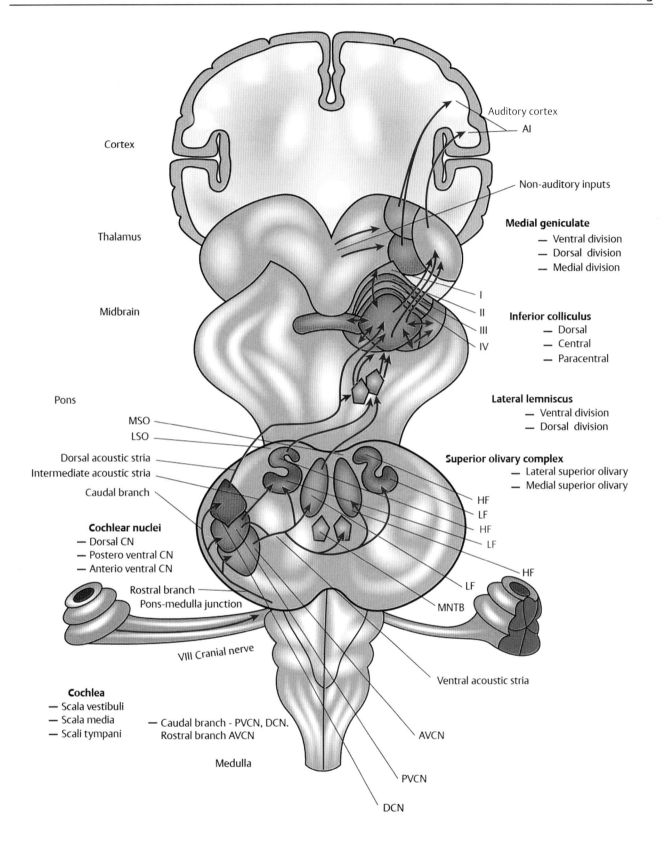

Fig. 13.28 The central auditory pathway. Schematic representation of the central ascending afferent auditory pathway. Major structures are the cochlear nucleus (CN) and the superior olivary nuclei (SOC), located in the pons region of the brainstem. The lateral lemniscus (LL) and the inferior colliculus (IC) are located in the midbrain of the brainstem. The medial geniculate body (MGB) is located in the thalamus, and the auditory areas are located on the cerebral cortex. Red lines indicate projections and inputs.

to the peripheral processes of spiral ganglion cells, (2) spiral ganglion neurons, which receive signals from the IHCs and OHCs and send signals along their central axon up the vestibulocochlear nerve to the brainstem, (3) the cochlear nucleus, a first-order auditory brainstem nucleus that is heavily innervated by cochlear nerve fibers, (4) the sound localization circuit, consisting of lower brainstem structures responsible for integrating time and intensity information used for binaural hearing, (5) the auditory **midbrain**, (6) the thalamic and cortical auditory regions, and (7) the efferent pathway, brainstem neurons whose efferent projections innervate IHCs, OHCs, and neurons of the cochlear nucleus (**Fig. 13.28**).

The Cochlear Nucleus

The central processes (axons) of spiral ganglion neurons, carried in the auditory nerve (cochlear branch of the vestibulocochlear nerve), terminate in the cochlear nucleus, the first major brainstem structure of the central auditory pathway. Located in the lateral-posterior region of the **pons**, between the **medulla oblongata** and **cerebellum** (a region referred to as the cerebellopontine angle), the cochlear nucleus is the first relay station of the ascending auditory pathway and is divided into three main divisions: the **anterior ventral cochlear nucleus (AVCN)**, **posterior ventral cochlear nucleus (PVCN)**, and **dorsal cochlear nucleus (DCN)**. Spiral ganglion axons bifurcate before reaching the cochlear nucleus. One branch terminates in the AVCN, the other in the PVCN or DCN (**Fig. 13.28**). Both branches project topographic inputs into each division of the cochlear nucleus and maintain a tonotopic organization. Low-frequency auditory nerve fibers project to the lateral regions, and high-frequency fibers project to the medial and dorsal regions of the AVCN, PVCN, and DCN. As such, auditory nerve fibers innervate different divisions of the cochlear nucleus, maintaining a tonotopic gradient and establishing the basis of parallel auditory processing, found throughout the central pathway.

Numerous cell types are found in the three divisions of the cochlear nucleus. Most notable, based in part on their cellular morphology and location in the cochlear nucleus divisions, are **spherical** and **globular bushy cells** of the AVCN; **multipolar**, **giant**, and **octopus cells** of the PVCN; and **granular** and **pyramidal cells** of the DCN. As one might expect, different cell types of the cochlear nucleus give rise to many different functional responses when activated by afferent auditory nerve fibers. Each of the different cell types either preserves or

modifies properties of the action potential firing pattern of the auditory nerve, such as the regularity, speed, or pattern of firing. In order to appreciate this preservation or modification of sensory information, the concept of **poststimulus time histograms (PSTHs)** is necessary. Generally speaking, PSTHs represent the action potential firing rate of cells over time. Different cell types within the cochlear nucleus yield different firing patterns that can be represented by the PSTH. For example, all afferent auditory nerve fibers have "primary-like" PSTHs, and bushy cells in the AVCN largely preserve this firing pattern (**Fig. 13.29**). Primary-like responses can be defined as action potential firing that lasts the entire duration of the stimulus, often being more robust at the onset of the signal but sustained throughout its time course. In contrast, octopus cells of the PVCN present with "onset-type" PSTHs and respond only at signal onset. Pyramidal cells of the DCN show "pauser" responses and respond at onset, followed by no response (e.g., pause) and then gradual buildup by the end of the signal. Regardless, the differences in PSTHs associated with the numerous cell types of the cochlear nucleus likely reflect variation in the structure and function of these cells as well as their tendency to preserve or modify the neural response pattern. In other words, specialized cells within the cochlear nucleus redefine the simple representation of the acoustic environment encoded by the auditory

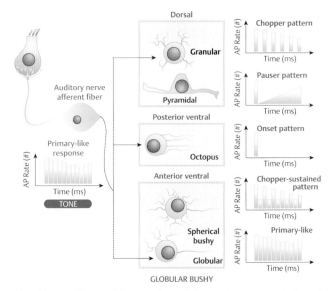

Fig. 13.29   The cochlear nucleus. Schematic representation of the different cell types and functional properties of the cochlear nucleus. *Left.* Input to the cochlear nucleus represented by a single inner hair cell and auditory nerve afferent fiber. Response of the auditory nerve to a sustained tone stimulus is considered to be "primary-like." The primary-like response pattern is changed, however, by the numerous cell types in the cochlear nucleus.

nerve by preserving and modifying the neural impulse pattern at the level of the cochlear nucleus.

Neural outputs represented by PSTHs from the cochlear nucleus travel along three primary routes to higher-order ascending auditory structures. AVCN fibers travel along the **ventral stria**, PVCN fibers along the **intermediate stria,** and DCN fibers along the **dorsal stria**. Fibers traveling along the ventral stria project both ipsilaterally and contralaterally to form what is known as the **trapezoid body**, a fiber tract that terminates in the SOC (**Fig. 13.28**). The intermediate stria contains ipsilateral and, largely, contralateral projections to the SOC, while the pyramidal cells of the DCN, which are thought to contribute to localization in elevation, bypass the SOC and project directly to the contralateral auditory midbrain. Together with the contralateral fibers from the ventral and intermediate striae, the dorsal projections combine to form the **lateral lemniscus**, a fiber tract that projects to the **inferior colliculus (IC)**, to be discussed in the following sections.

Lower Auditory Brainstem Sound Localization Circuit

The Superior Olivary Complex

Nerve fibers traveling from the cochlear nucleus project onto the superior olivary complex (SOC), the next major auditory structure, located in the pons region of the brainstem. As the name implies, the SOC consists of a complex of at least eleven subnuclei that make up the **periolivary group**, as well as three major nuclei, which are the most studied nuclei in the SOC. These major nuclei are the **medial superior olivary nucleus (MSO)**, the **lateral superior olivary nucleus (LSO)**, and **medial nucleus of the trapezoid body (MNTB)** (**Fig. 13.28**). The SOC is a binaural structure, indicating that it is the first major site of monaural convergence of auditory *time* and *intensity* information from the two ears. The complex comparisons of time and intensity information are the foundation for the key functions of the SOC. These include binaural computation used for auditory fusion, lateralization, and localization, as well as understanding speech in noise.

As previously mentioned, interaural time differences (ITDs) are used to localize low-frequency sounds (< 1,500 Hz) and interaural level differences (ILDs) are used to localize high-frequency sounds (> 2,000 Hz). However, the frequency ranges for ITDs and ILDs often overlap for the purpose of localization, as most "natural" sounds are composed of multiple low-and high-frequency components, strongly suggesting that the SOC utilizes both types of cues for binaural computation. Another limitation of the duplex theory is that it does not completely explain directional hearing for sound sources coming from directly in front of (i.e., 0° azimuth) or behind (i.e., 180° azimuth) the head, and it does not account for the use of the pinna cues in sound localization. Regardless of these limitations, the use of ITDs and ILDs is still the primary mechanism by which the SOC encodes binaural inputs.

The Medial Superior Olivary Nucleus

In humans, the MSO is the largest of the SOC nuclei and contains approximately 15,000 neurons. The primary type of neuron found in the MSO is a bipolar cell that has segregated dendrites that receive excitatory (i.e., glutamatergic) inputs from the right and left AVCN. Because the majority of MSO neurons (> 75%) receive excitatory inputs from both ears, they are referred to as excitatory/excitatory responders, or EE neurons. This function permits MSO neurons to encode disparities in the arrival time of action potential and computes ITDs, the foremost cue used to localize the azimuth of a low-frequency sound. For example, the time it takes for low-frequency sounds (< 1,500 Hz) to travel around the average adult human head is ~ 700 µs (dependent on the distance between the two ears and on the frequency of the sound). MSO bipolar neurons are able to encode time differences much smaller than this by responding optimally when excitatory inputs from the two ears arrive simultaneously at their segregated dendrites. This anatomical specialization (i.e., segregated dendrites that exclusively receive excitatory information from the two ears) makes MSO neurons **coincident detectors**. This enables individual MSO neurons to detect ITDs down to 10 µs, permitting sound source localization on the order of just a few degrees along the horizontal plane. Further refinement of ITD encoding is provided by the strong inhibitory inputs onto MSO cell bodies from the MNTB (described subsequently). Thus, the remaining 25% of MSO neurons respond to contralateral inhibitory projections and are referred to as excitatory/inhibitory responders, or EI neurons. The outputs of both types of MSO neurons (EE and EI) are sent via the ipsilateral lateral lemniscus to the IC for further binaural processing (**Fig. 13.28**).

The Lateral Superior Olive

The lateral superior olivary (LSO) nucleus has similar functions to the MSO but employs interaural level (intensity) differences (ILDs) instead of time disparities to encode sound source localization. The LSO receives excitatory, glutamatergic input from spherical bushy cells in the ipsilateral AVCN and strong inhibitory, **glycinergic** input from the MNTB. The MNTB is driven by excitatory input from globular bushy cells in the contralateral AVCN. Thus, the majority, if not all, of LSO neurons receive excitatory input from the ipsilateral ear and inhibitory input from the contralateral ear, making them EI responders. Projections from the cochlear nuclei are primarily from high-frequency (> 1,500 Hz) neurons, and the balance of excitation and inhibition is the foundation of ILD sensitivity and tuning. Frequencies greater than 1,500 Hz have wavelengths that are shorter than the distance between the two ears, producing a head shadow effect, and as such, the intensity or level difference provides the cue used for the localization of higher frequencies.

Fibers from the LSO project bilaterally to the inferior colliculus; ipsilateral projections are primarily inhibitory (glycinergic), while the contralateral projections are excitatory (glutamatergic). Additional projection targets include the dorsal and ventral nuclei of the lateral lemniscus (DNLL and VNLL). It should be noted that the inhibitory projections (which are primarily **GABAergic**) from the DNLL form a major source of GABA-mediated inhibition in the auditory brainstem and project bilaterally to the inferior colliculus and contralateral DNLL. These converging excitatory and inhibitory connections are thought to act synergistically to tune ILD sensitivity better in the midbrain.

The Medial Nucleus of the Trapezoid Body

The final primary nucleus of the major SOC group is the MNTB, located in the trapezoid region of the pons and consisting of principal neurons with round cell bodies. Each MNTB cell body receives a large, single excitatory input from the AVCN via a specialized synapse known as the **calyx of Held**. The calyx of Held is by far the largest synapse in the central auditory pathway (and the brain for that matter). Its function is related to rapid and reliable transmission of inhibitory information that it projects to the MSO and LSO. Because of the relatively large axon diameter of bushy cells from the AVCN and the even larger calyx synapse, MNTB principal neurons can send inhibitory (glycinergic) signals to the MSO and LSO in less than 200 µs following initial excitation within the cochlea. This < 200-µs time disparity is crucial for comparing binaural processing and establishes the balance between ipsilateral excitatory (via AVCN) and contralateral inhibitory (via MNTB) inputs used for ITD and ILD refinement.

The Upper Auditory Brainstem and Midbrain

The Lateral Lemniscus

As previously mentioned, the striae that originate from the cochlear nucleus formulate the most prominent fiber tract of the ascending central auditory pathway: the lateral lemniscus. Axon fibers from SOC neurons also contribute to the lateral lemniscus before terminating in the IC of the midbrain. Spanning a brainstem region that includes the upper pons and lower midbrain, the lateral lemniscus contains three nuclei: the **dorsal (DNLL)**, **intermediate (INLL)**, and **ventral (VNLL)** nuclei of the lateral lemniscus. The VNLL receives excitatory inputs from the contralateral SOC, while the DNLL receives inputs from both the ipsilateral and contralateral SOC, likely contributing to temporal processing (VNLL) and binaural hearing (DNLL), respectively. Little is known about the function of the INLL, where numerous neuronal cell types and complex PSTH response patterns are found. However, one known function of the lateral lemniscus is that it provides persistent GABAergic inhibitory inputs to the midbrain, shaping binaural response properties of IC neurons thought important for sound discrimination.

The Inferior Colliculus

The IC is the next auditory structure of the ascending pathway. Located in the midbrain and caudal to the visual system's superior colliculus, the IC is the major integration site of the lower brainstem nuclei, as all auditory inputs synapse in this nucleus. The IC contains three sections: the **central nucleus (ICC)**, **dorsal cortex**, and the **external** or **lateral shell**. Ascending inputs to the ICC include projections from the ipsilateral and contralateral CN, SOC, and DNLL. The VNLL sends only ipsilateral projections to the ICC. The dorsal cortex and the lateral shell receive numerous nonauditory inputs that are thought to regulate multimodal sensory perception, including the startle response and vestibuloocular reflex. Two primary neuronal cell types are found in the ICC: the **disk-shaped cells** and the **stellate cells**. Both cell types have numerous intrinsic functions that are related to their synaptic inputs. Axonal outputs of both cell types project ipsilaterally to the **medial geniculate body (MGB)** located in the **thalamus**. There are, however, projections to the contralateral MGB via the **commissure** of the IC, originating primarily from the dorsal and lateral IC regions.

The ICC is a laminar, or layered, structure, containing **isofrequency** sheets of tonotopically arranged inputs from the lateral lemniscus. Low-frequency inputs from the lateral lemniscus terminate in the dorsal-lateral isofrequency sheets, while high-frequency inputs terminate in the ventral-medial sheets. This configuration maintains a highly structured tonotopic arrangement. Although the ICC receives a great deal of lower auditory brainstem convergence, the isofrequency sheets appear to be highly segregated in function. For example, intensity-sensitive LSO cells (i.e., EI responders) terminate in ventral-medial sheets, whereas time-sensitive MSO cells (i.e., EE responders) terminate in dorsal lateral sheets.

Thus, functions of the IC are diverse, mainly due to the numerous auditory inputs it receives and its isofrequency tonotopic organization. In general, most ICC neurons have sharp tuning curves with varied dynamic ranges, indicating that ICC neurons sustain refined frequency selectivity coding strategies across multiple inputs and intensity changes. For example, some ICC neurons can code frequency bandwidths within tens of Hz across very narrow intensity changes (as little as 10 to 20 dB). These neurons are highly frequency-selective and have nonmonotonic intensity functions. Other ICC neurons can process multiple-frequency inputs that differ on the order of several magnitudes across broad intensity changes (as much as 60 to 80 dB). These neurons are **combination-sensitive** and have monotonic intensity functions. As one might predict with such diverse inputs from the lower auditory pathway, a single ICC neuron can possess any and all of the functions just mentioned. ICC neurons are also functionally well-tuned for long-duration signals, temporal encoding, phase locking, amplitude-modulated tones, and binaural processing. Like neurons within the SOC, many ICC neurons are responsive to binaural stimulation and show extreme sensitivity to disparities in interaural time and intensity cues from the two ears.

The Thalamic and Cortical Auditory Regions

The Medial Geniculate Body

The MGB is located in the thalamus and is the major set of relay nuclei for auditory projections originating in the IC. The MGB is divided into three divisions (ventral, medial, and dorsal regions), with the majority of inputs arising from the ipsilateral ICC and terminating at the ventral division. Thus, the ventral division of the MGB represents the "classic" ascending auditory pathway, while the medial and dorsal regions (which receive inputs from the dorsal cortex and external shell of the IC) form the "nonclassical" pathway.

Many different neuronal cell types are found in the MGB, including **thalamocortical relay cells** (principal cells) and **intrathalamic interneurons**. The ventral division contains large bushy cells and small stellate cells, while the medial and dorsal regions consist of varied stellate, bushy, **tufted**, and **elongated cells**. Because of the various cell types in the MGB and the complex innervation they receive from the IC, the functions of the nucleus are also diverse. In general, MGB cells from the ventral division present with "on," "off," "sustained," "late," and "suppressed" PSTHs, the latter of which is due to interneuron-induced inhibition. The primary function of the MGB is thought to be responsible for maintaining attention and direction to a sound source.

Basic auditory functionality in the MGB, such as intensity coding and binaural processing, however, is similar to that of ICC neurons. For example, intensity coding in the ventral division of the MGB is represented by neurons that have nonmonotonic and monotonic rate-level functions, with some neurons having dynamic ranges as high as 60 dB. Like some neurons in the ICC and SOC, neurons in the ventral division of the MGB are sensitive to interaural time (i.e., EE responders) and intensity differences (i.e., EI responders), implicating them in binaural processing. Therefore, damage to the ventral division of the MGB compromises these auditory functions. Temporal coding in the MGB, on the other hand, is different from that in all other lower auditory brainstem nuclei. In contrast to the SOC and ICC, the vast majority of neurons in the ventral division of the MGB (~ 90%) cannot phase-lock to signals above 250 Hz, with the remaining 10% able to encode only up to 1,000 Hz. Cumulatively, these features suggest that MGB neurons play a minimal role in temporal processing strategies.

MGB neurons send axonal projections to the auditory cortex and surrounding subcortical areas. The ventral division of the MGB projects via the **internal capsule** as part of fiber arrays, known as **acoustic radiations,** to the primary auditory cortex. The medial division projects via the **external capsule** to the **insula**, while the dorsal division courses through the internal capsule to secondary auditory regions of the cortex and the insula.

The Auditory Cortex and Subcortical Areas

The neural pathway connecting the MGB and auditory cortex is known as the thalamocortical pathway. Axonal fibers from the MGB course though this pathway via the internal capsule, a large white-matter tract connecting subcortical areas to the cortex. As such, the auditory cortex and subcortical areas receive input from the MGB via this route.

The auditory cortex and its surrounding subcortical areas are located deep in the superior portion of the temporal lobe, an area also referred to as the **transverse gyrus of Heschl**. Several other regions of this area have also been identified as key structures in processing auditory and "other" information. Aside from the **primary auditory cortex (A1)**, the **posterior auditory field (PAF)**, and the **anterior auditory field (AAF)**, other areas include the planum temporale, the inferior lobe, the angular gyrus, the submarginal gyrus, the superior temporal gyrus, and the insula. More recently, the primary auditory cortex is also referred to as the **core**, while the PAF, AAF, and all other surrounding regions make up the **belt** and **parabelt**. The belt is the area immediately surrounding the core; the parabelt sits adjacent to the lateral side of the belt.

Like all other cortical regions, the auditory cortex and subcortical areas have six layers that are defined by the neuronal cell types residing in each layer (designated by Roman numerals) (**Fig. 13.30a**). There are approximately 250,000 cells in

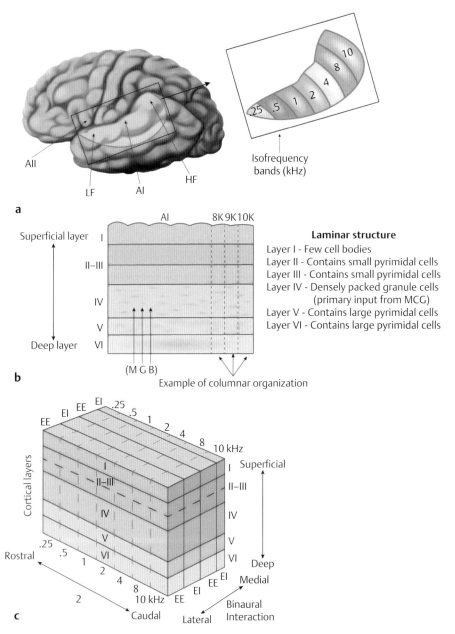

Fig. 13.30 The auditory cortex. **(a)** Laminar organization of the primary auditory cortex (AI). Each layer (I through VI) contains different cell types based on their structure and function, as well as place within the columnar organization of tonotopic tuning. **(b)** Schematic representation of the location and tonotopic tuning of the auditory cortical areas. **(c)** Columnar organization based on frequency of tonotopic tuning and binaural interactions from the lower auditory structures.

A1. The A1 region is tonotopically organized with low-frequency neurons located rostral-lateral and high-frequency neurons located caudal-medial (**Fig. 13.30b**). These tonotopic axes establish a columnar organization based on characteristic frequencies. In addition to this laminar and columnar organization, an organization based on binaural interactions also exists. EE and EI responders (i.e., neurons originating from the MSO and LSO, respectively) are interwoven within each column in a lateral-to-medial fashion (**Fig. 13.30c**). Communication between neurons within the core, belt, and parabelt regions as well as other nonauditory structures is accomplished via two primary pathways: the intrahemispheric and interhemispheric tracts.

The auditory cortex is composed of **gray matter**, which contains the cell bodies of the neurons, while subcortical auditory areas are composed of both gray and **white matter**, which consists of the myelin of the axons. The cortex contains both **sulci** (depressions or grooves) and **gyri** (the ridges or bulges), which together create the folded appearance of the brain. Within these folds and bulges, A1 neurons respond to sound, while neurons in the surrounding areas also respond to sound as well as receive input from other sensory modalities such as touch and vision. This interaction suggests that inputs to the auditory "brain" arise from other sensory pathways, providing a functionally complex interaction with our sensory world.

Of particular interest to human communication is the fact that the auditory cortex is highly involved in the perception of speech stimuli. In humans, speech stimuli create neural activity along the posterior temporal gyrus, and functional imaging studies have shown a greater "activity" preference for the left versus right hemisphere, consistent with studies suggesting a right-ear advantage for speech understanding. So how does the auditory brain encode sound? It involves a complex interaction between auditory cortical regions and the inputs they receive from lower auditory nuclei, as well as a balance of excitatory and inhibitory connections within the core structures themselves. For example, tuning curves (i.e., the relationship between frequency and intensity tuning) for auditory cortical neurons are sharp, often multipeaked, and increase in sharpness with more specific frequency tuning. These tuning curves are regulated by both excitatory and inhibitory connections; excitation drives the response, while inhibition shapes the sharpness of the curve, as blocking inhibitory inputs broadens the width of the tuning curve.

Encoding of sound intensity is represented by auditory cortical neurons in several different ways. Some neurons increase firing rate of action potentials as the intensity of sound increases, resulting in linear monotonic rate-level functions. Others decrease firing rate as stimulus intensity decreases, yielding nonmonotonic rate-level functions. The latter response is largely driven by strong inhibitory interconnections between neurons. Auditory cortical neurons also respond stronger (i.e., better) to signals that are modulated in the intensity (and frequency) domains (i.e., amplitude and frequency modulated) compared to steady-state tones.

Temporal processing by auditory cortical neurons is also diverse. Some neurons respond to periodicities only up to ~ 100 Hz, preferring slower changes in the modulation rate of a signal. Conversely, some neurons respond rapidly to click stimuli, with inter-stimulus intervals less than 1 ms, thus responding better to faster signal modulation. This accuracy in temporal precision by auditory cortical neurons is thought to assist in gap detection performance, as ablation of such neurons results in clear decrements in temporal, frequency, and intensity encoding. Localization and lateralization are also primary functions of auditory cortical neurons. Most neurons respond to changes in both interaural intensity and timing cues and utilize different excitatory and inhibitory properties to tune selectively to responses originating from the contralateral hemisphere.

The mechanisms that give rise to any sensory acuity, be it taste, smell, vision, balance or hearing, are often complex. The auditory system is one of the most complex and diverse sensory pathways of the nervous system. However, understanding the basic structure and normal function of the auditory system is an absolute prerequisite in order to truly appreciate and manage patients with hearing disorders.

■ Suggested Readings

Durrant JD, Lovrinic JH. Bases of Hearing Science. St. Louis, MO: Williams and Wilkins; 1995

Gelfand SA. Essentials of Audiology. New York, NY: Thieme; 2009

Kandel ER, Schwartz JH, Jessell TM, Siegelbaum SA, Hudspeth AJ. Principles of Neuroscience, 5th ed. New York, NY: McGraw-Hill; 2012

Møller AR. Hearing: Anatomy, Physiology, and Disorders of the Auditory System, 2nd ed. Amsterdam, The Netherlands: Elsevier; 2006

Musiek FE, Baran JA. The Auditory System: Anatomy, Physiology and Clinical Correlates. New York, NY: Pearson; 2007

Northern JL. Hearing Disorders, 3rd ed. Boston, MA: Allyn & Bacon; 1996

Northern JL, Downs MA. Hearing in Children, 6th ed. San Diego, CA: Plural; 2014

Pickles JO. An Introduction to the Physiology of Hearing, 4th ed. Leiden, The Netherlands: EJ Brill Academic; 2013

Sahley TL, Musiek FE. Basic Fundamentals of Hearing Science. San Diego, CA: Plural, 2015.

World Health Organization. Deafness and Hearing Loss Fact Sheet. Retrieved from www.who.int/mediacentre/factsheets/fs300/en/; 2015

Zemlin WR. Speech and Hearing Science: Anatomy and Physiology, 4th ed. Boston, MA: Allyn & Bacon; 1998

■ Study Questions

1. The auditory system utilizes many different types of chemicals, or neurotransmitters, to help convey synaptic activity from one neuron to the next. When released from the inner hair cell ribbon synapse, the excitatory neurotransmitter glutamate binds to what primary afferent postsynaptic spiral ganglion element to promote synaptic transmission?

A. AMPA-type receptors
B. GABA-type receptors
C. Glycine-type receptors
D. NMDA-type receptors
E. Nicotinic-type receptors

2. The ascending central auditory pathway contains at least six major "stations" before information reaches the primary and secondary auditory cortices. What ascending auditory structures receive information from both ears and are the first to be involved in binaural hearing?

A. Nuclei of the lateral lemniscus
B. Cochlear nucleus
C. Nuclei of the superior olivary complex
D. Inferior colliculus
E. Medial geniculate body

3. There are several major subdivisions of the inner ear. What portion of the inner ear is responsible for hearing?

A. The utricle
B. The semicircular canals
C. The saccule
D. The cochlea
E. The endolymphatic duct

4. Hearing loss can present itself with varying degrees (e.g., mild to profound) and different configurations (e.g., flat to sloping) and can affect one or more regions of the auditory pathway. If an individual presents with a pathophysiology of the vestibulocochlear nerve, what type of hearing loss might they have?

A. Conductive hearing loss
B. Neural hearing loss
C. Sensory hearing loss
D. Mixed hearing loss
E. Nonorganic hearing loss

5. The basilar membrane is approximately 25 to 35 mm in length and courses along the entire distance of the cochlea, from base to apex. It is composed of extracellular matrix materials in which radially oriented tissue is securely embedded. The composition of embedded tissue is stiffer (~ 100 times more stiff) and narrower (~ 10 times more narrow) at the base compared to the apex. This biophysical property helps permits what hearing specialization?

A. Tonotopic tuning of high-frequency sounds at the apex
B. Tonotopic tuning of low-frequency sounds at the base
C. Tonotopic tuning of mid-frequency sounds at the base
D. Tonotopic tuning of high-frequency sounds at the base and low-frequency sounds at the apex
E. Tonotopic tuning of low-frequency sounds at the base and high-frequency sounds at the apex

6. The bony labyrinth is filled with two fluids known as perilymph and endolymph. Perilymph's ionic content is similar to that of cerebrospinal fluid. It contains a high level of sodium ions and a low level of potassium ions, in addition to chloride and calcium ions. Perilymph is found in the scala vestibuli and scala tympani. Scala media is filled with endolymph, but what is its ionic composition similar to?

A. Intracellular fluid, with high potassium and low sodium levels
B. Extracellular fluid with high calcium levels
C. Extracellular fluid with high potassium and low chloride levels
D. Intracellular fluid with high sodium and low potassium levels
E. Intracellular fluid with high magnesium levels

7. Mechanical fluid displacement of the cochlea partition helps translate the frequency of vibration of the traveling pressure wave into a position of maximal neural response along a tonotopic map within the cochlear nuclei and higher. This representation of frequency is accomplished by which of the following sets of primary principles?

A. The space and null theories
B. The place and space theories
C. The temporal and frequency theories
D. The place, temporal, and volley theories
E. The space, volley, and null theories

8. Auditory nerve fibers are tonotopically tuned and have characteristic frequencies to which they best respond. Thus, the characteristic frequency of an individual auditory nerve fiber can be defined as the frequency to which the fiber best responds at the lowest possible sound intensity (i.e., threshold). The further away the stimulus frequency is from the nerve fiber's characteristic frequency, the greater the stimulus intensity must be in order for the nerve fiber to fire an action potential. This intensity/frequency relationship of auditory nerve fibers can be plotted as a graph known as what?

A. A volley firing plot
B. A tuning curve
C. A poststimulus time histogram
D. A phase-locking plot
E. An action potential graph

9. The neural outputs from the three divisions of the cochlear nucleus travel along three primary routes to higher-order ascending auditory structures. This helps maintain the tonotopic gradient and establishes the basis of parallel auditory processing found throughout the central pathway. What are the names of these three central pathways?

A. The spherical, globular, and multipolar pathways
B. The lateral lemniscus fiber tracts
C. The dorsal, ventral, and intermediate striae
D. The trapezoid body
E. The medial geniculate dorsal and ventral projections

10. The auditory cortex and its surrounding subcortical areas are located deep in the superior portion of the temporal lobe, an area also referred to as the transverse gyrus of Heschl. Several other regions of this area have also been identified as key structures in the processing of auditory and "other" information. Aside from the primary auditory cortex (A1), the posterior auditory field (PAF), and the anterior auditory field (AAF), other areas include the planum temporale, the inferior lobe, the angular gyrus, the submarginal gyrus, the superior temporal gyrus and the insula. More recently, the A1, PAF, and AAF have been referred to as what?

A. The core, belt, and parabelt regions
B. The primary, secondary, and tertiary regions
C. The major and nonmajor areas
D. The white and gray regions
E. The sulci and gyri areas

11. The conductive component of the peripheral auditory system refers to the:

A. Outer ear
B. Middle ear
C. Inner ear
D. A and B
E. A, B, and C

12. Which of the following is *not* a true statement about the stapedius muscle?

A. The stapedius attaches to the neck of the stapes.
B. The stapedius is involved in the acoustic reflex response.
C. The stapedius is innervated by the facial nerve.
D. The stapedius arises from the pyramidal eminence.
E. The stapedius is innervated by the trigeminal nerve.

13. Which of the following is *not* a true statement about the outer ear?

A. It collects sound waves and directs them toward the eardrum.
B. It protects the eardrum.
C. It converts sound into hydraulic energy.
D. It increases sound pressure exerted at the eardrum.
E. It is composed of the pinna and ear canal.

14. Which of the following is a property of outer hair cells?

A. There are three rows.
B. They are responsible for providing the sensory output of the cochlea.
C. There is a single row.
D. They are flask-shaped.
E. Their stereocilia are sheared by endolymph.

15. The eustachian tube acts to equalize pressure between the _____ and the _____.

A. Outer ear; middle ear
B. Inner ear; nasopharynx
C. Middle ear; mastoid
D. Outer ear; mastoid
E. Middle ear; nasopharynx

16. The intensity of sound is measured in which units?

A. Decibels (dB)
B. Hertz (Hz)
C. Ohms (Ω)
D. Amperes (A)
E. None of the above

17. Which of the following statements is *not* true about the impedance matching between the outer and inner ears by the middle ear?

A. The ossicular chain acts as a lever system.
B. The area over which the force is distributed decreases from the tympanic membrane to the oval window.
C. The air filling the middle ear amplifies the sound waves transmitted by the tympanic membrane.
D. The tympanic membrane buckles when it vibrates, increasing the force on the manubrium.
E. The impedance matching boosts the signal by ~ 30 dB.

18. Which of the following statements is true about interaural level differences (ILDs)?

A. They are generated when sounds arrive at each ear at different times.
B. They are better preserved at lower frequencies.
C. They occur when sound sources are located directly in front (0°) or behind (180°) the listener.
D. They are represented largely by neurons in the medial superior olivary nucleus.
E. They are influenced by the head shadow effect.

19. Which of the following pathologies does *not* create a conductive hearing loss?

A. Tumor on cranial nerve VIII
B. Otitis media
C. Cholesteatoma
D. Otosclerosis
E. Tympanic membrane perforation

20. Which of the following is true of sensorineural hearing loss?

A. It results in an air–bone gap of ≥ 15 dB on an audiogram.
B. It results from atresia of the ear canal.
C. It results from a pathology in the inner ear or along the auditory nerve.
D. It results from a hole in the tympanic membrane.
E. It can be diagnosed by air conduction audiometry alone.

21. Which of the following is true of cerumen?

A. It is produced by the sebaceous glands and ceruminous glands of the external ear canal.
B. It is a sign of a pathological condition.
C. It results from otitis media.
D. It is produced by the mastoid air cells.
E. It has no functional importance.

■ Answers to Study Questions

1. The correct answer is (A) because the only glutamate receptor known to be present on Type I afferent spiral ganglion neurons that is involved in sensory/synaptic transmission is the AMPA-type glutamate receptor. There is evidence that the NMDA-type glutamate receptor (D) is present extrasynaptically, but it is not directly involved in sensory transmission. The answer is not (B), (C), or (E) because the receptors neither bind glutamate nor are present at this synapse.

2. The correct answer is (C) because primary afferent inputs from the ipsilateral and contralateral cochlear nuclei, as well as the medial nuclei of the trapezoid body, terminate on neurons of the medial and lateral superior olivary nuclei, bilaterally. The answer is not (A), (D), or (E) because these nuclei are not the first to receive binaural inputs (they do, however, receive extensive binaural inputs from ipsi- and contralateral SOC neurons). The answer is not (B) because the cochlear nucleus is a monaural structure.

3. The correct answer is (D) because only the cochlea has the primary sensory organs for audition: the organ of Corti with its hair cells. The answer is not (A), (B), or (C) because these structures are involved exclusively in sense of balance, and the answer is not (E) because that structure is used to manage a fluid shared by both the hearing and balance systems.

4. The correct answer is (B) because the vestibulocochlear nerve, or cranial nerve VIII, is involved in balance and hearing. The cochlear branch of cranial nerve VIII sends sensory information from the inner hair cells of the cochlea to the lower brainstem by way of neural action potentials. Any damage to the nerve alone will result in neural deprivation and possible hearing impairments. The answer is not (A), (C), (D), or (E) because none of these types of hearing losses directly involves deficiency of the auditory nerve.

5. The correct answer is (D) because high-frequency sounds will peak toward the base because of its stiffness properties while low-frequency sounds will peak toward the apex because of its mass properties.

6. The correct answer is (A) because the concentration of potassium ions in endolymph is ~ 140 mM, while that of sodium ions is ~ 1 mM. This is very similar to intracellular concentration levels for both ions commonly found in neurons.

7. The correct answer is (D) because the place theory states that the encoding of a specific frequency is dependent on its *place* of maximum vibration along the basilar membrane; that is, different frequencies produce traveling waves that reach their maximum deflections at different places. The temporal theory states that the encoding of a specific frequency is dependent on the *timing* and *rate* of neuronal firing patterns; that is, the rate at which an afferent Type I spiral ganglion nerve fiber can fire action potentials, keeping up with the deflections of the basilar membrane. Finally, the volley theory states that the encoding of frequency is dependent on a population of neurons firing action potentials at a particular *phase* of the input frequency. All other options (A), (B), (C), (E) are fictional theories with respect to hearing.

8. The correct answer is (B) because a tuning curve is a graph that displays different stimulus intensities as a function of changing frequencies above and below the fiber's characteristic (or best) frequency. Options (A), (B), and (E) are fictional "graphs" with respect to hearing. Option (C) is not an answer because a poststimulus time histogram is a plot that represents the action potential firing rate of cells over time.

9. The correct answer is (C) because the neural outputs from AVCN fibers travel along the ventral stria, PVCN fibers along the intermediate stria, and DCN fibers along the dorsal stria. Option (A) is a fictional auditory tract (spherical, globular, and multipolar are types of neurons in the cochlear nucleus, not pathways) and thus not a correct answer. The other option choices are incorrect because although they are true auditory tracts, the trapezoid body (D) is only one pathway that consists of fibers from the ventral stria, the lateral lemniscus (B) is only one pathway that includes fibers from all three striae, while the medial geniculate dorsal and ventral projections (E) are not outputs from the cochlear nucleus.

10. The correct answer is (A) because the belt (consisting of more medial parts of the AAF and PAF) is the area immediately surrounding the core (or A1), and the parabelt (more lateral parts of the PAF and AAF) sits adjacent to the lateral side of the belt. The answer is not (B), (C), (D), or (E) because these are either fictional regions or unrelated to hearing function.

11. The correct answer is (D) because both the outer and middle ear contribute to conducting the sound waves to the inner ear. Abnormal function of either the outer or the middle ear can result in a conductive hearing loss. The answer is not (A) or (B) because neither is the complete conductive component. The answer is not (C) or (E) because the inner ear is the sensory, not the conductive, component of the peripheral auditory system.

12. The correct answer is (E) because a branch of the facial nerve (CN VII) innervates the stapedius muscle, whereas the trigeminal nerve (CN V) innervates the tensor tympani muscle. The answer is not (A), (B), (C), or (D) because all of those statements are true.

13. The correct answer is (C) because the motion of the stapes at the oval window converts sound into hydraulic energy; the stapes is driven by the ossicular chain connected to the tympanic membrane (eardrum), onto which the outer ear directs sound waves. The answer is not (A), (B), (D), or (E) because all of those statements are true.

14. The correct answer is (A) because there are three rows of outer hair cells and only one row of inner hair cells. The answer is not (B) because the synapses between the inner hair cells and the auditory nerve fibers provide the sensory output. The answer is not (C) or (D) because these are properties of inner hair cells. Outer hair cells are cylindrical. The answer is not (E) because the stereocilia of OHCs are sheared by the tectorial membrane.

15. The correct answer is (E) because the eustachian (auditory or pharyngotympanic) tube opens on the anterior (front) wall of the middle ear space and extends to the nasopharynx. The answer is not (A), (B), (C), or (D) because they are not consistent with known anatomy.

16. The correct answer is (A) because decibels are the units of the logarithmic system used to quantify the extremely large range of sound intensity. The answer is not (B) because the hertz is a unit of frequency. The answer is not (C) because ohms are units of electrical resistance. The answer is not (D) because amperes are units of electrical current. The answer is not (E) because the correct answer (A) is included in the option choices.

17. The correct answer is (C) because the air-filled tympanic cavity does not provide any additional force to sound as it travels through the middle ear. All of the other answer options, (A), (B), (D), and (E), are true statements.

18. The correct answer is (E) because the head acts as an acoustical blocker as sound travels from one side of the head to the other. The answer is not (A) or (B) because these are properties of interaural time differences (ITDs). The answer is not (C) because sounds that originate at 0° or 180° reach the ears at the same time and with the same intensity. Both ILDs and ITDs are useful for locating sound sources located off of midline. The answer is not (D) because ILDs are largely represented by neurons in the lateral superior olivary nucleus.

19. The correct answer is (A) because a tumor on cranial nerve VIII (often called an acoustic neuroma, but more accurately a vestibular schwannoma) results in a sensorineural hearing loss. The answer is not (B), (C), (D), or (E) because these pathologies all arise in the middle ear space and thus interfere with sound transmission to the oval window.

20. The correct answer is (C) because this is the only option choice to mention the sensory (inner ear) and neural (auditory nerve) elements of the hearing system. The answer is not (A), because an air–bone gap represents a conductive component to the hearing loss. The answer is not (B) or (D) because these conditions result in a conductive hearing loss. The answer is not (E), because a comparison between the air conduction and bone conduction scores needs to be made to approximate the site of the lesion.

21. The correct answer is (A) because cerumen is produced in the external ear canal to serve protective functions. Answer (B) is not correct because cerumen production is a normal function. The answer is not (C) because otitis media occurs in the middle ear, whereas cerumen is produced in the outer ear. The answer is not (D) because the mastoid air cells do not produce any substances. The answer is not (E) because cerumen has both cleaning and protective functions.

14

Swallowing

Michelle S. Troche and Alexandra E. Brandimore

■ Chapter Summary

Swallowing is a life-sustaining complex sensorimotor behavior that serves to transport food, liquid, and saliva from the oral cavity to the stomach for adequate nutrition and hydration. Additionally, normal swallowing is necessary in order to prevent airway compromise. Swallowing shares significant neuroanatomic and physiologic substrates with speech production. In fact, swallowing is a primary function for the subsystems you have learned about in this textbook (e.g., respiratory, laryngeal, and orofacial subsystems). Sensorimotor control of swallowing includes various neuroanatomic substrates: (1) sensory receptors in the oral, laryngeal, pharyngeal, and esophageal mucosa; (2) multiple cranial and spinal nerves that provide afferent and efferent information; (3) brainstem regions; (4) cortical regions; (5) subcortical regions including the motor control systems (e.g., basal ganglia and cerebellum); and, finally, (6) over 25 swallowing muscles. These neural processes control the swallowing sequence, which consists of four general phases: the oral-preparatory, oral, pharyngeal, and esophageal phases. Assessment and treatment of disorders of swallowing, or dysphagias, is an important part of the speech-language pathologist's scope of practice. The purpose of this chapter is to provide a solid understanding of the anatomic structures and complex physiologic processes involved in swallowing. Specifically, we will (1) provide a comprehensive overview of swallowing anatomy and physiology; (2) describe common etiologies, signs, symptoms, and consequences of dysphagia; and (3) discuss the role of the speech-language pathologist in the management of swallowing.

■ Learning Objectives

- Identify the anatomical structures involved in swallowing
- Describe the four phases of swallowing and the physiology associated with each phase
- Understand the sensorimotor control of swallowing, including peripheral and central nervous system components
- Identify normal variations in swallowing physiology based on bolus characteristics
- Evaluate the impact of dysphagia and identify some diseases that result in dysphagia

■ Putting It Into Practice

- The evaluation and management of swallowing function is an important part of the speech-language pathologist's scope of practice. During the assessment of swallowing function, the speech-language pathologist must distinguish normal variations in swallowing physiology from disordered swallowing.
- The assessment and management of dysphagia requires a comprehensive understanding of normal and disordered swallowing physiology. Understanding the neurophysiology of swallowing is essential for the development of therapeutic paradigms that are specific to a given pattern of dysfunction.
- Diverse diseases and disorders can result in dysphagia, and each alters the anatomy and physiology of swallowing in different ways.

The speech-language pathologist should determine the most appropriate method for the assessment of swallowing function in a given patient based on a complete understanding of anatomy and physiology and the advantages and disadvantages associated with each method.

■ Introduction

When you take a moment to think about all the things that we do in life that bring us enjoyment and satisfaction, many of them likely involve eating and drinking with family and friends. The processes that underlie eating and drinking are quite intricate and involve multiple systems working in a highly coordinated manner to ensure that the food and liquid we consume travels safely and efficiently into our esophagus and stomach without obstructing or entering the airway.

Several terms are used to describe the processes involved in transporting food and liquid safely from the mouth to the stomach during eating and drinking. Some of these terms overlap. **Swallowing** is a term used to refer to the entire process of bringing food to the oral cavity, maneuvering it, and propelling it into the pharynx and to the esophagus. **Deglutition** is commonly used synonymously with swallowing. Given that the two are so often used interchangeably, we will refer to this process as swallowing throughout this chapter. Dysfunction in the anatomy involved in swallowing or disorders of the brain regions involved in the control of swallow physiology can lead to dysphagia. **Dysphagia** is defined as difficulty in swallowing or disordered swallowing. This disorder often results in significant decrements to health and quality of life.

■ Biological Function of Swallowing, Chewing, and Feeding

Swallowing is a life-sustaining, complex sensorimotor behavior that transports food, liquid, and saliva from the oral cavity to the stomach. Swallowing enables us to maintain adequate nutrition and hydration. Additionally, normal swallowing is necessary in order to prevent airway compromise. In other words, if you swallow inappropriately, food can obstruct your airway, making it difficult to breathe, or liquid can enter the airway and descend into the lungs (**aspiration**), leading to an

infection called **aspiration pneumonia**. Both **airway obstruction** and respiratory infections such as aspiration pneumonia can be life-threatening. In fact, aspiration pneumonia secondary to deficits in airway protection is a leading cause of death in individuals with neurodegenerative disease.

Another process that has significant overlap with swallowing is feeding. **Feeding** is a term that is limited to the placement of food in the mouth and the oral stage of swallowing, including **mastication** or chewing. Dysfunction in feeding can also have significant consequences. One example is a newborn baby with a craniofacial anomaly who has trouble sucking. You have already learned that craniofacial anomalies can result in speech deficits, but they commonly result in feeding and swallowing problems as well. In this case, the child may be unable to achieve the nutritional status needed to thrive (**Box 14.2**). Mastication is part of feeding and swallowing. Mastication takes place during the oral-preparatory stage of swallowing. It serves as the beginning of digestion, when we cut or grind food into smaller particles and mix saliva with the food particles and liquid to form a **bolus** (a cohesive mass of food and liquid that should travel as a unit through the swallowing mechanism). Mastication is also the beginning of the enzymatic breakdown of the bolus. Therefore, disorders of mastication not only affect digestion but can also put patients at risk for airway obstruction if proper breakdown of the food and liquid has not occurred prior to swallowing.

■ Anatomy of Swallowing and Mastication

Overview

The functions of swallowing and mastication share significant neuroanatomic and physiologic substrates with speech production. Swallowing is a sensorimotor function relying highly on **afferent** information generated throughout the swallowing mechanism, which then shapes the **efferent** motor control of the swallowing sequence. In brief, the swallowing sequence consists of four general phases: the oral-preparatory, oral, pharyngeal, and esophageal phases. The successful completion of these phases requires a widely distributed neural network providing flexibility in the motor control of swallowing. In general, the sensorimotor control of swallowing includes various neuroanatomic substrates: (1) sensory receptors in

Box 14.1 Parkinson's Disease

Parkinson's disease (PD) is one of the most common neurodegenerative diseases in the elderly population (Box Fig. 14.1). Dr. James Parkinson first identified what he called the "shaking palsy" in 1817. Parkinson described a disease characterized by resting tremor, bradykinesia (slow movement), rigidity, and postural instability resulting in frequent falls. The motor deficits in PD result from dysfunction of the basal ganglia and depletion of the neurotransmitter dopamine. The basal ganglia are integral to motor programming (amplitude of motor movement) and sensorimotor integration (communication between the brainstem and cortex). Thus, all motor function, including swallowing and speaking, can be affected by PD.

Individuals with PD eventually develop dysphagia, or disordered swallowing. Interestingly, individuals with PD also present with concurrent cough dysfunction, or dystussia. Aspiration pneumonia is a leading cause of death in individuals with PD and in many other populations with neurologic conditions (Box Fig. 14.2). Thus, it is highly likely that the high incidence of aspiration-related lung infections in these

Box Fig. 14.2 Cough is an airway protective behavior that shares neurologic substrates with swallowing.

patients is not due to swallowing disorders alone but to a pervasive and degenerative disorder of airway protection (i.e., concurrent cough and swallowing dysfunction). Airway protection is functionally complex and includes a continuum of behaviors, with cough and swallowing at either end of the continuum. More specifically, effective swallowing prevents material from entering the airway, and effective coughing ejects the aspirate material from the airway when penetration and aspiration occur (Troche et al 2014a).

Cough and swallowing are sensorimotor behaviors that involve highly coordinated sequences of structural movements and also require reconfiguration of the ventilatory breathing pattern (Davenport et al 2011; Troche et al 2014a). Both functions can be triggered on command (voluntarily) or in response to a sensory stimulus (reflexively). Several studies describe the relationship between cough and swallowing in patients with PD and other neurologically impaired populations (Miles et al 2013; Troche et al 2014b). These studies highlight the need for both swallowing and cough dysfunction to be considered in the management of patients with PD and other neurodegenerative diseases in order to improve long-term health outcomes.

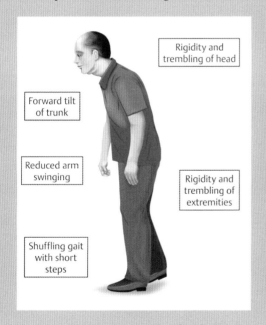

Box Fig. 14.1 Symptoms associated with PD.

Rigidity and trembling of head

Forward tilt of trunk

Reduced arm swinging

Rigidity and trembling of extremities

Shuffling gait with short steps

the oral, laryngeal, pharyngeal, and esophageal mucosa, (2) multiple cranial and spinal nerves that provide afferent and efferent information, (3) brainstem **central pattern generators** (CPGs), (4) cortical regions, (5) subcortical regions including the motor control systems (basal ganglia and cerebellum), and, finally, (6) over 25 swallowing muscles. The complex sensorimotor control of

swallowing will be discussed in much more detail later in this chapter. In this section, we will review the structures constituting the anatomic framework, the muscles that act on this framework, and the neural substrates controlling the successful transport of food and liquid from the oral cavity through the pharynx, past a closed laryngeal vestibule, and into the esophagus.

Box 14.2   Cleft Lip and Palate

Sucking is an important nutritive feeding strategy for infants. Effective sucking involves the generation of negative pressure within the oral cavity and simultaneous pressing of a nipple to stimulate milk flow from either the mother's breast or a bottle. To develop this negative pressure, the oral cavity must become what some researchers have referred to as a "closed box." This "closed box" must be appropriately sealed on all sides with coordinated muscular contraction of the lips (anterior wall), cheeks (lateral walls), palate (upper and posterior walls), and tongue (lower and posterior walls).

Infants born with craniofacial malformations such as cleft lip or palate are often confronted with severe feeding challenges. These challenges arise from the lack of an intact palate to seal off the oral and nasal cavities and from an inability to seal the lips. Thus, infants with cleft lip or palate cannot develop sufficient negative pressure to elicit milk from the feeding source (**Box Fig. 14.3**). Additionally, an infant with cleft lip or palate may have other dysphagia symptoms, including poor bolus formation and pre-swallow spill. In most infants with cleft lip and palate without concomitant syndromes, the cen-

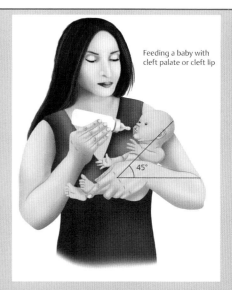

Box Fig. 14.4   Special feeding modifications must be made to compensate for dysphagia secondary to cleft lip or palate.

tral neural circuity is not damaged, and therefore, the challenges to feeding are purely anatomic (peripheral). Early intervention is critical in these infants to facilitate proper nutrition, weight gain, and parent/child bonding.

Assistive feeding bottles improve oral intake in infants with cleft lip or palate (**Box Fig. 14.4**). These devices enable the parent to control the delivery of milk directly into the oral cavity. Once the infant is old enough to undergo surgical modification, closure of the cleft lip and/or palate generally improves the child's ability to produce negative pressure and breastfeed naturally (Clarren et al 1987). Generally, four factors must be addressed: (1) temporary nutritive compensations to maintain oral intake and nutrition (e.g., Haberman Feeder [Athrodax Healthcare Ltd, Drybrook Park, UK] bottle, prostheses such as a Holt-type plate, enteral feeding), (2) peripheral modification of the cleft lip to ensure airtight closure of the lips around the mother's breast or bottle nipple, (3) surgical closure of the cleft in the palate to separate the nasal and oral cavities, and (4) improvement to the contact between the tongue and posterior palate.

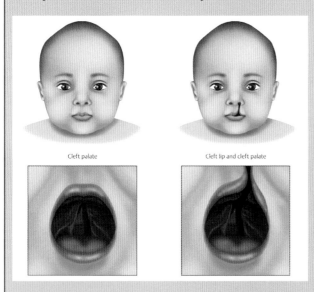

Cleft palate   Cleft lip and cleft palate

Box Fig. 14.3   Cleft lip and palate can result in dysphagia.

Anatomic Correlates

The process of swallowing begins in the oral cavity. The structures of the oral cavity involved in swallowing include the teeth, hard palate, soft palate, uvula, floor of mouth, tongue, faucial pillars (i.e., palatoglossal and palatopharyngeal arches), and mandible (**Fig. 14.1**). Sensory receptors in this region are among the first to provide afferent information to the brainstem about the material to be swallowed. This sensory information is provided to the brainstem via the trigeminal (CN V), facial (CN VII), glossopharyngeal (CN IX), and vagus (CN X) nerves. The muscle groups that act on the structures of the oral cavity during the process of swallowing are innervated by the trigeminal (CN V), facial (CN VII), vagus (CN X), and hypoglossal (CN XII) nerves.

The lips are the most anterior structure of the oral cavity. The lips are highly mobile structures containing several striated muscles, including the orbicularis oris. The orbicularis oris is involved in

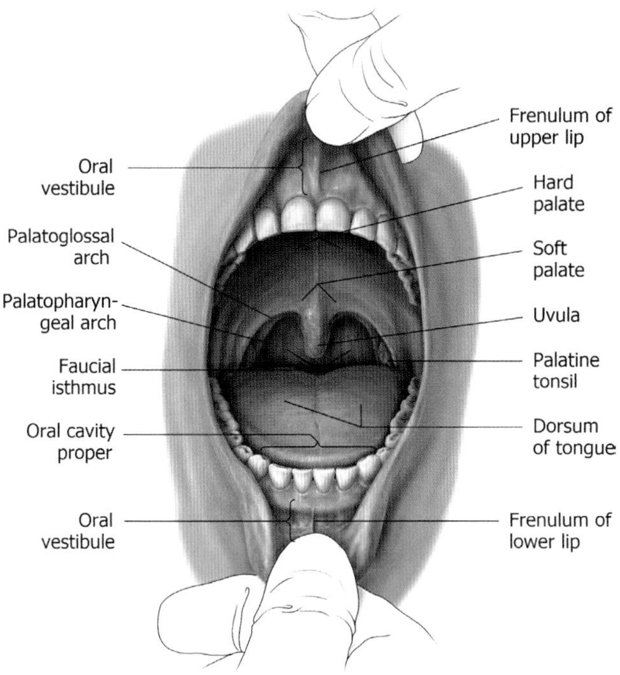
Oral vestibule
Palatoglossal arch
Palatopharyngeal arch
Faucial isthmus
Oral cavity proper
Oral vestibule
Frenulum of upper lip
Hard palate
Soft palate
Uvula
Palatine tonsil
Dorsum of tongue
Frenulum of lower lip

Fig. 14.1 Anterior view of structures in the oral cavity.

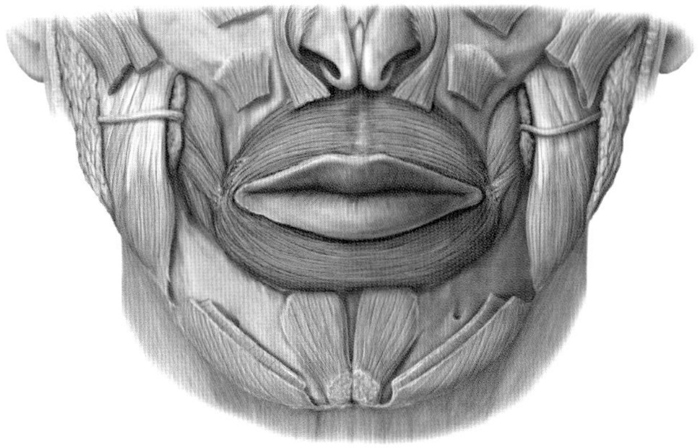

Fig. 14.2 Anterior view of the orbicularis oris.

lip rounding during speech and maintaining food in the oral cavity to avoid anterior labial leakage of the bolus (**Fig. 14.2**). Additionally, the lips contain several sensory receptors that judge texture and temperature of foods. This sensory information modifies the way a given food or liquid is swallowed. Both afferent and efferent information to and from the lips travels via the facial nerve (CN VII).

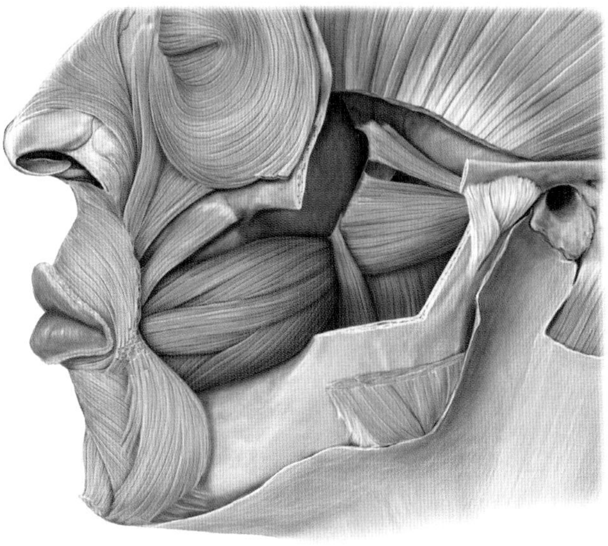

Fig. 14.3 Lateral view of the left buccinator muscle.

The cheeks are located lateral to the orbicularis oris and consist of several muscles that create the counterforce to the tongue for bolus control. The interior portion of the cheeks is formed by muscles controlling facial expression and mastication, primarily the buccinators, and is covered by a stratified squamous epithelium. When the buccinators contract, they tense the cheeks, thus maintaining the food between the molars (**Fig. 14.3**). They are also active during the process of sucking. These muscles are innervated by the trigeminal (CN V; sensory) and facial (CN VII; motor) nerves.

Just posterior to the lips and medial to the cheeks are the teeth, which are housed in the maxilla superiorly and the mandible inferiorly. The teeth are responsible for chewing and biting and are integral for bolus formation**.** The incisors serve to bite off food pieces, the canines to grasp and tear food, and the premolars and molars to grind food particles (**Fig. 14.4**). The teeth complete this function via the muscles of mastication, which move the mandible (**Fig. 14.5**). As discussed in **Chapter 12**, the mandible and the temporal bone articulate, creating the

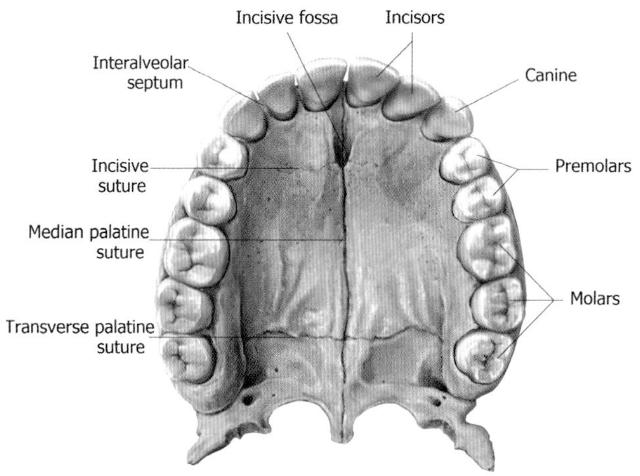
Incisive fossa
Incisors
Interalveolar septum
Canine
Incisive suture
Premolars
Median palatine suture
Molars
Transverse palatine suture

Fig. 14.4 Permanent maxillary teeth.

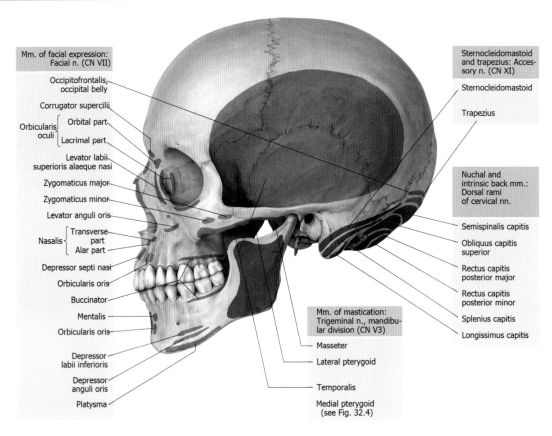

Mm. of facial expression:
Facial n. (CN VII)

Occipitofrontalis,
occipital belly

Corrugator supercilii

Orbicularis {   Orbital part
oculi {   Lacrimal part

Levator labii
superioris alaeque nasi

Zygomaticus major

Zygomaticus minor

Levator anguli oris

Nasalis { Transverse part
{ Alar part

Depressor septi nasi

Orbicularis oris

Buccinator

Mentalis

Orbicularis oris

Depressor
labii inferioris

Depressor
anguli oris

Platysma

Sternocleidomastoid
and trapezius: Acces-
sory n. (CN XI)

Sternocleidomastoid

Trapezius

Nuchal and
intrinsic back mm.:
Dorsal rami
of cervical nn.

Semispinalis capitis

Obliquus capitis
superior

Rectus capitis
posterior major

Rectus capitis
posterior minor

Splenius capitis

Longissimus capitis

Mm. of mastication:
Trigeminal n., mandibu-
lar division (CN V3)

Masseter

Lateral pterygoid

Temporalis

Medial pterygoid
(see Fig. 32.4)

Fig. 14.5   Lateral view of masticatory muscles; origins and insertions.

temporomandibular joint, around which movement of the mandible occurs. The various muscles of mastication produce movement around that joint. The masseter and medial pterygoid function to elevate the mandible (close the mouth) when contracted (**Fig. 14.6**). The temporalis muscle elevates and retracts the mandible (**Fig. 14.7**). Contraction of the lateral pterygoid depresses (opens) the mandible and produces rotary movement of the jaw during mastication (**Fig. 14.8**). These muscles are all innervated by the third (mandibular) division of the trigeminal nerve, cranial nerve (CN) V_3 (**Table 14.1**). Poor dentition or anatomic differences in mandibular structure can produce difficulty with mastication and bolus formation. The muscles of mastication also play an important role in posturing of the mandible

Pterygoid
process,
lateral plate

Medial
pterygoid
(superficial
head)

Medial
pterygoid
(deep head)

Mandibular
angle

Fig. 14.6   Lateral view of the medial pterygoid muscle.

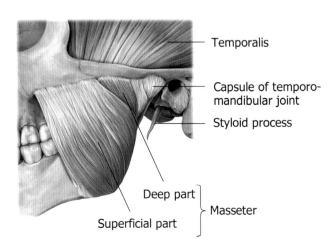

Temporalis

Capsule of temporo-
mandibular joint

Styloid process

Deep part
Superficial part   } Masseter

Fig. 14.7   Lateral view of the masseter and temporalis muscles.

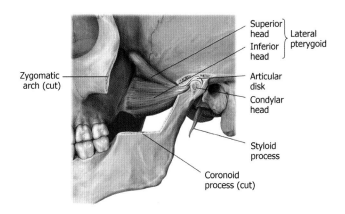

Fig. 14.8 Lateral view of the lateral pterygoid muscle.

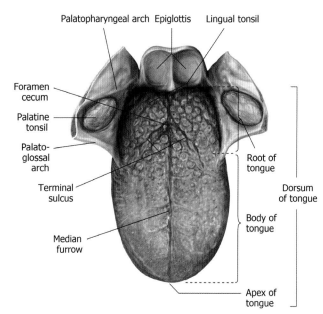

Fig. 14.9 Anatomy of the tongue.

during swallowing. The mandible must be elevated and the mouth basically closed in order to trigger a swallow. Try to swallow with your mouth open.

The tongue is one of the most important structures involved in swallowing (**Fig. 14.9**). It plays an integral role in the oral-preparatory, oral, and pharyngeal phases. The tongue is a complex structure made up of several muscles and is especially interesting because it functions as a **muscular hydrostat**. In a muscular hydrostat, the musculature itself creates both the movement and the support for the movement without a skeletal framework. More specifically,

the lingual muscles are integral for manipulation of the bolus in the oral cavity and propulsion of the bolus through the pharynx. The large number of lingual muscles, both intrinsic and extrinsic, that make up the tongue enable many gross and discrete movements that are essential for safe and efficient

Table 14.1 Muscles of mastication

Muscle		Origin	Insertion	Innervation	Action
Masseter		Superficial head: zygomatic arch (anterior two-thirds)	Mandibular angle (masseteric tuberosity)	Mandibular n. (CN V₃) via masseteric n.	Elevates (adducts) and protrudes mandible
		Deep part: zygomatic arch (posterior one-third)			
Temporalis		Temporal fossa (inferior temporal line)	Coronoid process of mandible (apex and medial surface)	Mandibular n. (CN V₃) via deep temporal nn.	*Vertical fibers:* elevate (adduct) mandible *Horizontal fibers:* retract (retrude) mandible *Unilateral:* lateral movement of mandible (chewing)
Lateral pterygoid	Superior head	Greater wing of sphenoid bone (infratemporal crest)	Temporomandibular joint (articular disk)	Mandibular n. (CN V₃) via lateral pterygoid n.	*Bilateral:* protrudes mandible (pulls articular disk forward) *Unilateral:* lateral movements of mandible (chewing)
	Inferior head	Lateral pterygoid plate (lateral surface)	Mandible (condylar process)		
Medial pterygoid	Superficial head	Maxilla (tuberosity)	Pterygoid tuberosity on medial surface of the mandibular angle	Mandibular n. (CN V₃) via medial pterygoid n.	Elevates (adducts) mandible
	Deep head	Medial surface of lateral pterygoid plate and pterygoid fossa			

Abbreviations: CN, cranial nerve; n., nerve; nn., nerves. *Source:*

swallowing. The intrinsic lingual muscles are important for maintaining appropriate lingual shape and tone (**Fig. 14.10**). The extrinsic lingual muscles function to modify the position of the tongue relative to other oral and pharyngeal structures (**Fig. 14.11**). These muscles are mainly innervated by the hypoglossal nerve (CN XII), but the palatoglossus muscle is innervated by the vagus (CN X) nerve. Therefore, given its important role in innervating the muscles necessary for bolus manipulation and propulsion, damage to the hypoglossal nerve can cause dysphagia (**Box 14.3**).

The tongue also has an essential role in providing sensory information about the bolus to the brainstem

---

Box 14.3   Unilateral Hypoglossal Nerve Lesion

The hypoglossal nerve (CN XII) provides motor innervation to all of the intrinsic and extrinsic lingual muscles (except for the palatoglossus, which is innervated by CN X). Peripheral damage to any portion of the hypoglossal nerve pathway can result in lingual muscle paresis (weakness) or paralysis. Lingual *paralysis*, in particular, has the potential of significantly impact to speech (causing dysarthria) and swallowing function. The causes of lingual paralysis are numerous and include vascular (e.g., cortical or brainstem stroke), neoplastic (i.e., tumor), inflammatory (e.g., multiple sclerosis), traumatic, and iatrogenic (i.e., tonsillectomy, tooth extraction) causes.

The hypoglossal nerve originates from the hypoglossal nucleus in the medulla (near the swallowing central pattern generator [CPG]). The hypoglossal nerve then exits the skull base via the hypoglossal canal in close proximity with the glossopharyngeal (CN IX), vagus (CN X), and accessory (CN XI) nerves and travels ipsilaterally to the lingual muscles. These nerves are medial to the internal jugular vein and lateral to the internal carotid artery. The hypoglossal nerve (CN XII) then descends vertically between the vessels until it reaches the angle of the mandible and ultimately to the lingual muscles themselves. Because of the proximity of the hypoglossal nerve to the glossopharyngeal (CN IX), vagus (CN X), and accessory (CN XI) nerves, peripheral nerve damage often results in additional damage to adjacent CNs and worse speech and swallowing deficits.

When evaluating a patient with unilateral lingual paresis or paralysis and dysphagia, it is important to differentiate among cortical, brainstem, and peripheral causes. To test the function of this nerve, ask the patient to protrude the tongue, move the tongue from side to side, and follow directional commands. A cortical lesion will likely cause a contralateral unilateral deficit to lingual function, whereas a lesion to the hypoglossal nucleus in the brainstem or the peripheral nerve will yield ipsilateral lingual weakness. In these cases, the patient may not be able to protrude the tongue or perform any coordinated tongue movements. With peripheral lesions, the tongue will deviate to the side of the lesion. The side of the tongue with adequate strength will overcompensate for the weak side and therefore bias towards the weak lingual muscles. Another way to think about it is that the tongue will point to the side of the weakness (**Box Fig. 14.5**).

Dysphagia in patients with lingual paralysis is generally characterized by oral phase deficits including poor bolus formation, inadequate mastication, food pocketing in the cheek, and delayed swallowing initiation, which can be viewed best during a clinical swallowing and videofluoroscopic evaluation. In general, hypoglossal nerve deficits tend to recover quite well over time, depending on the extent of injury. However, these deficits can be particularly troubling in the acute phase given the associated swallowing dysfunction. In the case of lingual paresis, treatment to improve tongue muscle strength and coordination through various exercise-based swallowing treatments is often used. Additionally, if the underlying pathophysiology is unclear or if additional speech/voice deficits are suspected, flexible nasoendoscopy should be performed to evaluate vocal fold movement, to determine whether the vagus nerve (CN X) is involved.

⚕ Clinical

Unilateral hypoglossal nerve palsy
Damage to the hypoglossal nerve causes paralysis of the genioglossus muscle on the affected side. The healthy (innervated) genioglossus on the unaffected side will therefore dominate. Upon protrusion, the tongue will deviate *toward* the paralyzed side.

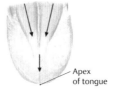

A Active protrusion with an intact hypoglossal nerve.

Apex of tongue

B Active protrusion with a unilateral hypoglossal nerve lesion.

Paralyzed genioglossus on affected side

Box Fig. 14.5 **(a)** Active normal tongue protrusion. **(b)** Active tongue protrusion with a unilateral hypoglossal nerve lesion.

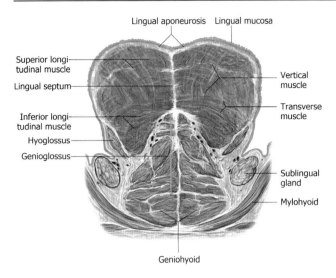

Fig. 14.10 Intrinsic muscles of the tongue. Coronal section, anterior view.

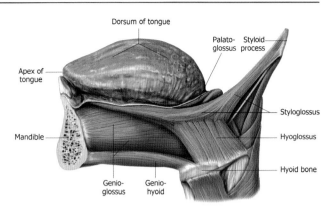

Fig. 14.11 Extrinsic muscles of the tongue.

control centers. This information comes from a high density of **mechanoreceptors** within and on the surface of the tongue. The tongue is covered with four different types of papillae that provide roughness for friction and contain taste buds. General sensory information from the anterior two-thirds of the tongue is carried to the brainstem via the lingual nerve, a branch of the trigeminal nerve (CN V). Taste from the anterior two-thirds of the tongue is transmitted to the brainstem via the facial nerve (CN VII). Taste and general sensory information from the posterior one-third of the tongue is carried to the brainstem by the glossopharyngeal nerve (CN IX) (**Fig. 14.12**).

Saliva production is essential for swallowing. Saliva serves to maintain oral moisture, reduce tooth decay, facilitate taste, destroy microorganisms, and assist in digestion. It also acts as a natural neutralizer of stomach acid that refluxes into the

esophagus. There are three main sets of salivary glands: the parotid glands, submandibular glands, and sublingual salivary glands. These glands are activated by the taste of the bolus and by movements of the orofacial structures during bolus preparation via the facial (CN VII) and glossopharyngeal (CN IX) nerves. The parotid gland is the largest of the glands and produces a thin and watery (serous) saliva, which makes up about 25% of saliva production. The parotid gland is located between the cheek and masseter muscle (**Fig. 14.13**). The submandibular gland, in the floor of the mouth, produces both serous and mucoidal (thick, viscous) saliva, which makes up 60% of saliva production. Lastly, the sublingual gland lies inferior to the tongue and produces

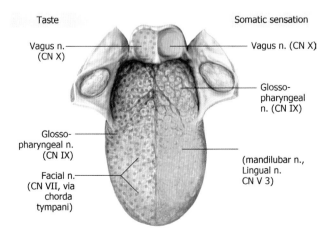

Fig. 14.12 Somatosensory and taste innervation of the tongue.

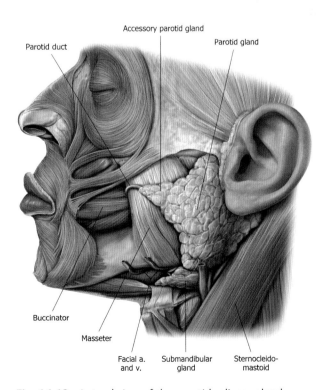

Fig. 14.13 Lateral view of the parotid salivary gland.

both serous and mucoidal saliva (**Fig. 14.14**). Saliva production can be disrupted in various conditions that affect the central nervous system and also diseases that influence peripheral receptors (**Box 14.4**).

After the bolus is prepared in the oral cavity, it travels into the pharynx on its way to the esophagus.

The pharynx is a fibromuscular tube extending from the base of the skull to the lower border of the cricoid cartilage, at which point the pharyngeal tube becomes the esophagus. The pharyngeal cavity is large and has several subdivisions. Most commonly, the pharynx is subdivided into the nasopharynx,

---

Box 14.4   Head and Neck Cancer

Cancer is the second leading cause of death in the United States. The term *head and neck (H&N) cancer* refers to a group of cancer types that occur in the oral cavity, pharynx, larynx, paranasal sinuses, nasal cavity, or salivary glands (**Box Fig. 14.6**). Medical advances have improved prevention, early detection, and treatment of cancer in general; however, a number of negative side effects are associated with the treatment of H&N cancer that require additional management and care. In fact, approximately 75% of patients treated for H&N cancer develop dysphagia after treatment.

Radiation therapy is often the primary treatment for individuals with H&N cancer. This treatment strategy utilizes localized high-energy X-rays to kill cancer cells, which in turn reduces the size of a tumor. Most often, radiation therapy is delivered once per day to the cancerous region for a specified period of time (approximately 2–6 weeks), followed by either surgical intervention (tumor resection/removal) or chemotherapy. Side effects from radiation significantly contribute to dysphagia in patients with H&N cancer and are common both during treatment (in the acute phase) and after treatment (latent long-term effects). Some of the most damaging side effects of radiation therapy to swallowing function are **xerostomia** and fibrosis.

Xerostomia, or chronic dry mouth, results from the destruction of salivary glands. Saliva production is essential for reducing oral bacteria, maintaining moisture in the oral cavity, preventing tooth and gum decay, and detecting taste in the variety of foods we eat. The inability to produce saliva can make it difficult to initiate a swallow, cause **odynophagia** (painful swallowing), increase the risk of infections such as candidiasis (caused by a fungus), impair taste perception, result in fewer swallowing events overall due to increased pain, and increase meal time duration (Logemann 1998).

Fibrosis occurs as a result of devascularization and damage to the peripheral nerves and muscle tissue in irradiated soft tissue regions. Patients with fibrosis may exhibit tissue that is hard or "woody." Thus, swallowing structures and tissue that have become fibrotic secondary to radiation therapy display significantly reduced range of motion. Reduced range of motion and strength of swallowing muscles has a particular impact on the anatomic structures involved in hyolaryngeal excursion (the lifting of the hyoid bone and larynx dur-

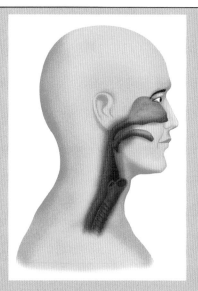

Box Fig. 14.6   Head and neck cancer regions that commonly receive radiation therapy.

ing swallowing, visible from the outside as the motion of the Adam's apple). Without adequate anterior and superior displacement of the hyolaryngeal complex, the epiglottis may not invert (increasing vallecular residue), and upper esophageal sphincter (UES) opening is reduced. As a result, patients with fibrotic H&N tissue and reduced hyolaryngeal excursion often have marked difficulty opening the UES to allow food/liquid to enter the esophagus. Consequently, food and liquid fill the pharyngeal cavity and piriform recesses and either overflow into the laryngeal vestibule, causing penetration and aspiration, or require expectoration.

Although both xerostomia and fibrosis can be observed acutely, the side effects of radiation can develop years after radiation therapy and sometimes years after cancer remission. It is important that patients with H&N cancer be managed as part of a multidisciplinary team throughout the treatment process. The speech-language pathologist serves to provide education, preventive exercises, timely evaluation of anatomic structures and physiology, and appropriate compensatory strategies to alleviate the negative side effects of treatment. It is important that patients maintain an adequate diet to prevent unintended weight loss. The efficacy of preventive swallowing exercises prior to and during radiation therapy warrants further study; however, it is clear that intervention throughout the continuum of care is necessary.

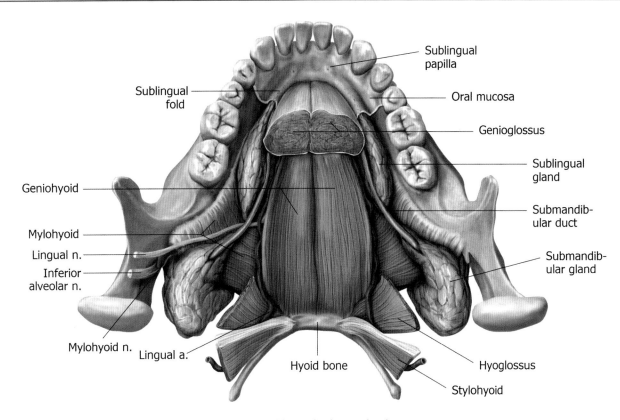

Fig. 14.14 Superior view of the submandibular and sublingual salivary glands.

oropharynx, and laryngopharynx (**Fig. 14.15**). The inferior portion of the pharynx is also referred to as the hypopharynx. The nasopharynx communicates with the nasal cavity to provide a passageway for air during breathing. During swallowing, this communication between the nasal and pharyngeal cavities is blocked in order to allow flow of the bolus from the oral cavity into the pharynx without entry into the nasal cavity. The velar muscles play a primary role in elevating the soft palate (velum) during the pharyngeal phase of swallowing and close off the nasal cavity in order to avoid nasal regurgitation of foods and liquids. The lack of velar closure can contribute to dysphagia; food or liquid can come out of the nose when eating. Among the most important velar muscles for swallowing is the levator veli palatini, which is innervated by the vagus (CN X) nerve.

The oropharynx is the portion of the pharynx immediately posterior to the oral cavity. It is a passageway for air during breathing, but it is also a passageway for food and liquid during swallowing. The anterior and posterior margins of the oropharynx are made up of the base of the tongue and the posterior pharyngeal wall. The oropharynx is also marked by the faucial pillars, which can be observed most posterolaterally in the oral cavity. The anterior faucial pillar on each side consists of the palatoglossus

muscle, and the posterior faucial pillar consists of the palatopharyngeus muscle. Sensory and motor information from the faucial pillars is carried to and from the brainstem via the vagus (CN X) nerve.

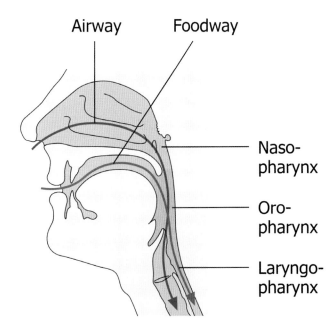

Fig. 14.15 Divisions of the pharynx.

The laryngopharynx is the portion of the pharynx nearest to the laryngeal region. The larynx and surrounding muscles play an important role in swallowing function. Swallowing interrupts the process of breathing. As you may recall from earlier chapters (particularly **Chapters 10** and **11**), the larynx is located superiorly to the trachea and must be open during breathing; however, during swallowing, the airway must be closed and the esophagus must be open. Given the very close proximity of the trachea and esophagus, it is critical that the larynx close quickly and completely during swallowing. If this closure does not happen, airway compromise and obstruction may occur. The floor of the mouth, tongue, hyoid bone, and larynx are all basically connected to one another by muscles and ligaments, creating intricate relationships among them. The floor of the mouth on either side is mainly composed of the mylohyoid muscle, geniohyoid muscle, and anterior belly of the digastric muscle. All three of these muscles are also known as suprahyoid muscles, with attachments to the mandible anteriorly and the hyoid bone posteriorly. The suprahyoid muscles mediate superior and anterior movement of the hyolaryngeal complex (hyoid bone and larynx), moving the larynx up and out of the way during swallowing. The intrinsic muscles of the larynx are responsible for adduction of the vocal folds during swallowing and include the lateral cricoarytenoid, interarytenoid, and thyroarytenoid muscles. Sensory and motor innervation of the laryngeal muscles is supplied by the vagus (CN X) nerve. Dysfunction that results in reduced range of motion or strength of the muscles of the hyolaryngeal complex can have significant consequences for airway protection (**Box 14.4**). A unique swallowing landmark in the laryngopharyngeal region is the **vallecula**. The valleculae are lateral spaces around the base of the tongue and epiglottis. These spaces often become receptacles for bolus material, especially in individuals with dysphagia (**Fig. 14.16**). Sensory innervation regarding taste from the epiglottis is provided by the vagus (CN X) nerve.

The muscular walls of the pharynx are composed of an outer layer made up of three circular muscles, known as pharyngeal constrictor muscles. They are intuitively named from superior to inferior: superior, middle, and inferior pharyngeal constrictor muscles. The inferior edges of the superior and middle pharyngeal constrictors approximate the next constrictor down. The inferior constrictor attaches to the lateral edges of the thyroid cartilage anteriorly. This attachment creates the piriform recess (commonly referred to as the piriform sinus) on either side of the thyroid cartilage (**Fig. 14.16**). The inferior edge of the inferior pharyngeal constrictor is thought to end in the cricopharyngeal muscle. The muscle fibers of the cricopharyngeal muscle attach to the posterolateral surface of the cricoid lamina (**Fig. 14.17**). These muscle fibers form part of the entrance to the esophagus, referred to as the upper esophageal

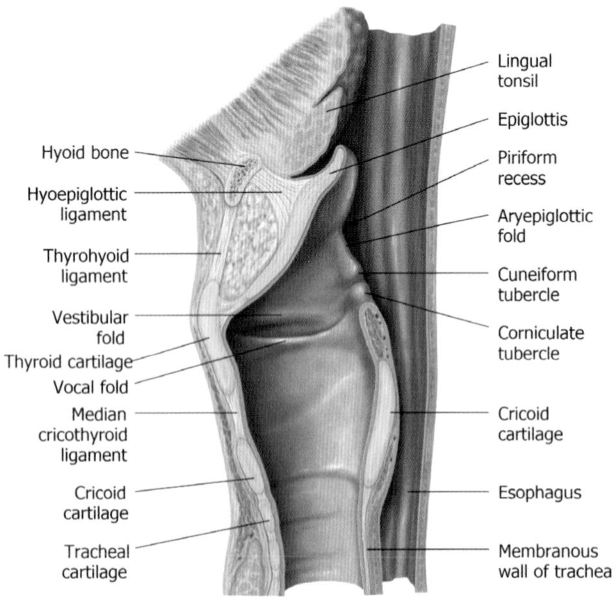

Fig. 14.16   Lateral anatomy of the laryngopharynx.

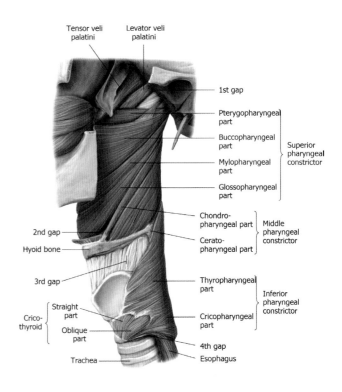

Fig. 14.17   Lateral view of the pharyngeal constrictor muscles.

sphincter (UES) or the pharyngoesophageal (PE) segment. At rest, the sphincter is closed by tonic contraction of the cricopharyngeal muscle, but when the muscle relaxes, it assists in the opening of the PE segment for swallowing. The motor innervation of the pharyngeal constrictor muscles comes from the vagus nerve (CN X) **(Table 14.2)**.

The esophagus is a long, collapsible tube connecting the pharynx to the stomach. This hollow muscular tube is approximately 25 centimeters in length and 2 centimeters in diameter. It is separated from the pharynx by the cricopharyngeal muscle and from the stomach by the lower esophageal sphincter (LES). The superior end of the esophagus is made up of striated muscle, the inferior two-thirds is made up of smooth muscle, and it courses inferiorly traversing past the heart, through the mediastinum and diaphragmatic hiatus, until it connects with the stomach (**Fig. 14.18**). This tube is lined with a protective, stratified, squamous epithelium that covers an inner layer of circular fibers and an outer layer of longitudinal fibers. Sensory innervation to the esophagus is provided by the vagus (CN X) nerve. The proximal esophagus, which includes the PE segment, receives motor innervation from the recurrent laryngeal nerve branch of the vagus nerve (CN X), which also innervates the intrinsic muscles of the larynx. Thus, the same peripheral nerve is responsible for simultaneous closing of the larynx and opening of the PE segment, thus facilitating safe passage of food and liquids into the esophagus. The distal region of the esophagus is mainly controlled by the **autonomic nervous system**.

■ Physiology

The Phases of Swallowing

Swallowing is a complex process, and in order for this process to be initiated and executed properly, a large series of neuromuscular systems and movements are involved. For simplicity's sake, the process of swallowing is most commonly divided into four phases: the oral-preparatory, oral, pharyngeal, and esophageal phases, as has been stated previously (Dodds et al 1990). However, it is important to note that these phases are merely a simplification of the process of swallowing and there is overlap between phases. That being said, the four phases are the traditional, and most often used, manner of describing swallowing. In this section, the physiology of swallowing will be discussed for each phase with reference to the anatomy introduced earlier in this chapter. The phases of swallowing are distinct in terms of their neural control. This control will be discussed in greater detail later in the chapter. In general, some of the phases of swallowing are under voluntary control, during which the process of swallowing can be paused and modulated in its entirety. Other phases are under involuntary control and mainly reflexive, but can be modified slightly.

Oral-Preparatory Phase

The oral-preparatory phase begins the swallowing process. The oral-preparatory phase also forms part of the feeding process, described at the beginning of this chapter. This phase is under voluntary control, with the goal of preparing the bolus to begin digestion and transport through

Table 14.2 Muscles of the pharynx

Muscles	Innervation	Action
Longitudinal muscles		
Salpingopharyngeus	Pharyngeal plexus–CN X	Elevates pharynx
Palatopharyngeus		Elevates pharynx and larynx
Stylopharyngeus	CN IX	Elevates pharynx
Circular muscles		
Superior constrictor	Pharyngeal plexus–CN X	Constricts pharynx
Middle constrictor		
Inferior constrictor	Pharyngeal plexus, superior laryngeal (external br.) recurrent laryngeal nn.–CN X	

Source:

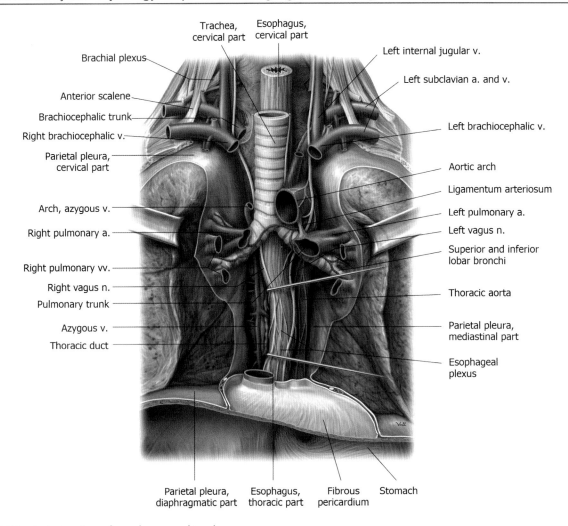

Fig. 14.18 Anterior view of esophagus and trachea.

the swallowing mechanism. In brief, during the oral-preparatory phase of swallowing the bolus is masticated (if necessary), mixed with saliva, and maneuvered in the oral cavity. In reality, the process of swallowing begins even prior to the food or liquid being placed in the oral cavity, during which time a person is receiving sensory information from visual and tactile sensory systems about the material which is about to enter the mouth. For example, when you see a piece of steak on your plate and decide to eat it, you know you are going to have to chew it. That information is already preparing the mechanism for the act of swallowing. This sensory feedback plus the sensory information regarding bolus viscosity, temperature, size, and other factors modify the oral-preparatory phase.

To begin, the mandible must depress and the lips open to allow the food or liquid to enter the oral cavity. Once the bolus has entered the oral cavity, the mandible is elevated and the lips are closed. Most anteriorly, the orbicularis oris is

the first sphincter of the swallowing mechanism (Leonard and Kendall 2013). The circular muscles of the lips help with puckering but are also essential for proper lip seal, which must be maintained to keep the bolus from falling out of the mouth. The buccinator muscles function to keep the bolus from pooling between the teeth and the cheeks (Bosma 1973).

Distinct differences are observed between the oral-preparatory phases of swallowing for liquids and for solids. When swallowing liquids, the tongue cups to receive and hold the bolus. At this point, the bolus is being held between the tongue and hard palate, while the anterior tongue flattens, the lateral tongue edges elevate, and the tongue tip is elevated behind the alveolar ridge. Individuals who demonstrate this pattern of oral preparation have been termed "tippers." In some rare cases, individuals hold the bolus on the floor of the mouth in front of the tongue. These individuals are referred to as "dippers" (only 20% of cases; Dodds et al 1990). The bolus is usually held in this position for about one second. The tongue also works in synchrony with the soft palate to maintain the bolus in the oral cavity and keep the bolus from escaping into the pharynx prematurely. The posterior portion of the tongue elevates secondary to contraction of the palatoglossus muscle against the soft palate, creating the second sphincter of the swallowing mechanism (Leonard and Kendall 2013).

In the case of solid foods, further oral preparation is required. Food must be mixed with saliva, and proper mastication must occur. The facial muscles play an important role by maintaining the bolus between the teeth for mastication. Mastication involves lateral movement of the mandible and tongue. Jaw movements are controlled by the masseter muscle, the temporalis muscle, and the medial and lateral pterygoid muscles. During and after chewing, the tongue maneuvers the food and helps to form a cohesive bolus to be transported in the next phase of swallowing: the oral phase. It is within normal variation for the soft palate to remain elevated during active chewing, resulting in initial presentation of the bolus head into the pharyngeal region. In general, the airway remains open and breathing continues during this phase of swallowing as long as the bolus has not passed into the pharynx.

The length of the oral-preparatory phase of swallowing varies greatly depending on whether a liquid or solid is being swallowed, whether the liquid is viscous or not, how hard the solid food is, how good or bad the food tastes, and even how distracted a person is. Marked individual variability in this phase of swallowing has been observed. For instance, some individuals take longer than others to savor food in the oral cavity prior to initiating the oral transport phase of swallowing. In some cases, the oral phase of swallowing may not be initiated if someone has decided they do not like the food or liquid they are consuming and decides to expectorate it.

Oral Phase

The oral phase of swallowing is also under voluntary control. The initiation of this phase of swallowing is marked by tongue movement that results in posterior transport of the bolus into the pharyngeal cavity. The oral phase begins when the tip of the tongue is placed at the alveolar ridge. Respiration ceases during this phase of swallowing to maintain adequate airway protection. If the individual is a "dipper" in the oral-preparatory phase, the bolus is transferred to the "tipper" position

prior to posterior movement of the bolus, followed by opening of the pharynx with elevation of the soft palate via contraction of the levator veli palatini, which breaks open the seal/sphincter described above in the oral-preparatory phase. Expansion of the posterior portion of the oral cavity creates a "chute" of sorts for transfer of material from the oral to the pharyngeal cavity. Depression of the tongue, allowing movement of the bolus, is controlled by contraction of the hyoglossus muscle and, to a lesser extent, the styloglossus muscle. The anterior portion of the tongue is then pressed against the alveolar ridge and the anterior part of the hard palate in rapid sequence, moving the bolus posteriorly on the dorsum of the tongue. This stripping action of the tongue is essential for the posterior movement of the bolus. At this point, contraction of the orbicularis oris and buccinators are essential to prevent escape of the bolus anteriorly or laterally. Soft palate elevation secondary to activation of the levator veli palatini allows the bolus to pass through the faucial pillars. This velar elevation is also essential for preventing leakage of the bolus or escape of air pressure into the nasopharynx. Toward the end of this phase, the hyoid bone begins to elevate in preparation for the pharyngeal phase of swallowing.

Pharyngeal Phase

The pharyngeal phase of swallowing is involuntary; therefore, once initiated, it cannot be reversed. However, evidence suggests that the pharyngeal phase of swallowing can be modulated by voluntary, cortical control. This phase is initiated about the time when the bolus head is passing any point between the anterior faucial pillars and the ramus of the mandible. During this phase of swallowing, the bolus passes from the pharynx into the esophagus, generally taking less than a second. The intricate relationship between respiration and swallowing is especially evident during this phase of swallowing. Both functions are life-sustaining, but a reconfiguration of the respiratory ventilatory cycle during swallowing is required to transport the bolus past the airway safely and efficiently. This relationship is described in detail subsequently when we discuss the sensorimotor control of swallowing.

The pharyngeal phase of swallowing is a complex sequence of events that occur in a rapid patterned sequence. The fundamental motor pattern has been described through electromyographic studies of the striated muscles involved in swallowing. The onset of the pharyngeal swallow is thought to begin with the contraction of the mylo-hyoid muscle. Concurrently, or rapidly following the contraction of the mylohyoid, the anterior digastric and the pterygoid muscles begin to contract, followed by the geniohyoid, stylohyoid, styloglossus, posterior tongue, superior constrictor, palatoglossus, and palatopharyngeus muscles. The middle and inferior constrictors then contract in an overlapping pattern ending when the wave of contraction reaches the UES (Doty and Bosma 1956; Miller 1982; Leonard and Kendall 2013).

This pattern of muscle activation can also be described in terms of the physiologic swallowing events that take place. To initiate the pharyngeal phase of swallowing, the soft palate is elevated (levator veli palatini) to close off the velopharyngeal port. This event tends to span the oral and pharyngeal phases of swallowing. At this point, the tongue acts like a piston, propelling the bolus posteriorly towards the pharynx, while the mandible remains in an elevated position. The pharyngeal constrictors are also essential in this phase of swallowing. The pharynx elevates and the pharyngeal constrictor muscles contract to create **peristaltic movement** of the bolus. The movements of the tongue and pharynx create the driving force to propel the bolus through the pharynx toward the pharyngoesophageal (PE) segment.

Simultaneously, the suprahyoid muscles contract, moving the hyolaryngeal complex superiorly and anteriorly. This motion serves to protect the larynx from penetration of the bolus into the airway, but it also opens or expands the hypopharynx. Additionally, this movement decreases the pressure at the PE segment, aiding in the opening of this sphincter (Doty and Bosma 1956; Kidder 1995). Several other protective mechanisms are triggered during this time including (1) inversion of the epiglottis, (2) adduction of the false vocal folds, and (3) adduction of the true vocal folds. Epiglottic inversion is mainly driven by elevation of the hyoid and larynx, paired with contraction of the thyrohyoid muscles and intrinsic laryngeal muscles to adduct the vocal folds.

The UES, also referred to above as the PE segment, is the final sphincter in the oropharyngeal swallowing system (Leonard and Kendall 2013). At rest, the sphincter is closed by the **tonic** contraction of the cricopharyngeus muscle. The sphincter opens when the cricopharyngeal muscle relaxes and is aided by hyolaryngeal excursion, which serves to expand the hypopharynx. Once the bolus has passed through the PE segment, the cricopharyngeus becomes active again to prevent stomach and esophageal contents from refluxing into the pharynx. The pharyngeal phase of swallowing is completed when the soft palate returns to its original position and the larynx reopens for respiration.

Esophageal Phase

The bolus is transported down the esophagus into the stomach during the esophageal phase of swallowing. The esophageal phase consists of a peristaltic wave of contraction that forces the bolus down the esophagus. Both gravity and the force with which the bolus arrives at the PE segment influences the speed and ease of bolus transport through the esophagus. During swallowing, lower esophageal sphincter tone is inhibited, which relaxes the sphincter to allow bolus passage into the stomach (Jean 2001). This phase of swallowing can last 8 to 20 seconds, depending on various bolus characteristics.

Summary

Swallowing consists of four stages: the oral-preparatory, oral, pharyngeal, and esophageal stages. In the oral-preparatory phase, the food, liquid, or saliva is formed into a cohesive bolus and made ready to be swallowed. During the oral phase, the bolus is moved posteriorly in the mouth to the oropharynx. To accomplish this movement, the tip of the tongue is elevated toward the superior alveolar ridge while the soft palate elevates to seal off the nasal cavity, and the posterior tongue depresses (Dodds et al 1990). The bolus is then propelled to the oropharynx as the tongue pushes the bolus posteriorly (Dodds et al 1990). The pharyngeal stage is also defined by a series of airway protective maneuvers including closure of the laryngeal complex, which involves three major events: (1) closure of the true vocal folds, (2) closure of the false vocal folds, and (3) inversion of the epiglottis. Simultaneously, the PE segment relaxes (opens), and the bolus is then delivered into the esophagus. Effective swallowing involves a rapid sequence of neuromuscular movements within a series of overlapping phases that create pressure gradients to ensure that a bolus is delivered safely and efficiently to the esophagus and, eventually, the stomach (**Fig. 14.19**). Therefore, changes in one phase of swallowing will result in changes to subsequent phases. This relationship becomes increasingly important when we think about dysphagia and its impact on swallowing physiology.

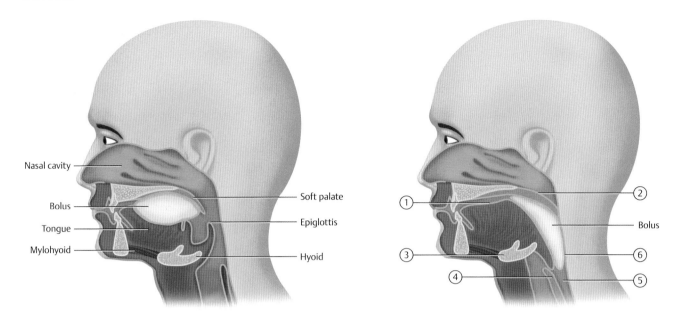

Nasal cavity

Bolus

Tongue

Mylohyoid

Soft palate

Epiglottis

Hyoid

Fig. 14.19 Schematic depicting the movement of a bolus through the oral and pharyngeal cavities during swallowing.

Respiratory–Swallowing Relationships

Swallowing and breathing serve distinct functions in humans but share anatomic and neural substrates. Healthy humans alternate between breathing and swallowing with apparent ease; however, these two life-sustaining mechanisms require intricate temporal coordination to maintain proper nutrition and to prevent aspiration (Shaw and Martino 2013). By way of review, air enters the human body through the nose or mouth and then flows through the pharynx, larynx, and abducted vocal folds into the trachea and lungs. Food, liquid, and secretions are moved from the oral cavity to the pharynx, bypassing a closed larynx with adducted vocal folds, through the PE segment, and into the esophagus. Swallowing in healthy individuals requires a reconfiguration of the normal ventilatory breathing pattern.

The respiratory system makes several accommodations before, during, and after the swallow to promote adequate airway protection. For example, a unique respiratory pattern exists that is most highly associated with safe swallowing, and also normal adaptations to lung volume made in response to varying bolus types and sizes. Researchers have found that the majority of healthy individuals exhale right before the initiation of the pharyngeal phase of swallowing, with a brief period of **apnea** during swallowing, and then exhale again when the swallow is complete (Martin et al 1994). The apneic period occurs secondary to brief closure of the vocal folds and upper airway and generally lasts between 0.5 and 1.5 seconds (Shaw and Martino 2013). The ending of the swallowing maneuver with exhalation has been theorized to provide additional protection from any residue pooling around the entrance to the airway (Matsuo and Palmer 2009). As you can imagine, if residue remained around the entrance of the airway after the swallow and one were to inhale, the likelihood of food or liquid penetrating the airway increases significantly.

Evidence suggests that sensory information from the upper airway influences lung volume and subglottal pressure during swallowing. Lung volume at swallow onset ranges from 50 to 55% vital capacity in healthy young adults, approximately 20% above functional residual capacity, and remains unchanged during completion of the swallow (Wheeler Hegland et al 2009). Additionally, lung volume initiation is higher for thin boluses than thick boluses (Wheeler Hegland et al 2009). These modifications to the respiratory system during swallowing are also thought to increase the safety and efficiency of the swallowing process by increasing the ability to generate expiratory airflow after a swallow as needed (i.e., cough). Pulmonary disease can disrupt these natural modifications of the respiratory system during swallowing, ultimately resulting in dysphagia (**Box 14.5**).

Box 14.5   Chronic Obstructive Pulmonary Disease

Chronic obstructive pulmonary disease (COPD), including emphysema and chronic bronchitis, is a progressive disease and the third leading cause of death in the United States (**Box Fig. 14.7**). In emphysema, the walls of the alveoli are damaged, which reduces gas exchange in the lungs. In chronic bronchitis, the mucosal lining of the airways becomes inflamed and irritated, resulting in thick mucus in the airway. Generally, people with COPD have both emphysema and chronic bronchitis but can also have asthma and/or cystic fibrosis (**Box Fig. 14.7**).

Respiratory symptoms of COPD include difficulty moving air in and out of the lungs, abnormalities in oxygen and carbon dioxide exchange, and lung hyperinflation characterized by failure to exhale sufficient amounts of carbon dioxide. The inability to adequately respire can cause significant anxiety and also impact swallowing function. COPD changes the pattern and coordination between breathing and swallowing. In most healthy individuals, the respiratory pattern during swallowing is exhalation prior to swallowing initiation, apnea during the pharyngeal phase, and then exhalation again. Patients with COPD tend to interrupt the normal apneic period during the pharyngeal phase with an inspiration secondary to "air hunger," thus increasing the risk of aspiration. Of concern, patients with COPD also exhibit ineffective or absent cough responses. In fact, one study reported silent aspiration in 42% of patients with COPD. Martin-Harris and colleagues (2015) found that retraining the respiratory–swallow pattern using visual biofeedback was effective for modifying the respiratory–swallow pattern in patients with head and neck cancer, some with concomitant COPD. Additionally, training improved laryngeal vestibule closure, tongue base retraction, and the amount of pharyngeal residue (Martin-Harris et al 2015). This finding is important, as it highlights the usefulness of treatment approaches targeted at the specific deficits underlying swallowing dysfunction.

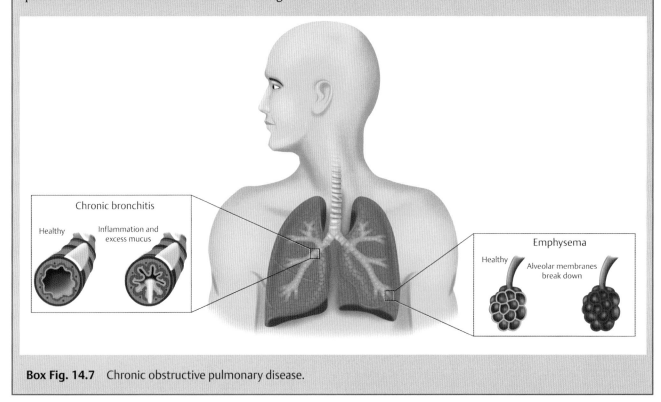

Box Fig. 14.7   Chronic obstructive pulmonary disease.

■ Variability in the Normal Swallowing Pattern

Swallowing is a motor act that requires significant sensory information for proper programming and execution. Much of the information that shapes the motor execution of the swallow comes from the bolus itself. Adaptability of a swallow is important given the variety of textures, tastes, sizes, and viscosities of foods and liquids that we regularly consume. Understanding the normal modifications of swallowing helps us to understand better the underlying neurophysiology and also provides targets for swallowing compensations in individuals with dysphagia. Therefore, it is important to understand the variations in bolus characteristics that impact swallowing biomechanics in healthy individuals.

Volume

Swallowing biomechanics must be modified in response to variations in bolus volume (size), and healthy individuals are able to do this with ease (Chi-Fishman and Sonies 2002). In healthy individuals, the normal volume of a bolus ranges from 10 to 25 mL depending on personal factors (e.g., sex, body size) and bolus delivery method (e.g., straw vs. cup). Small boluses (~ 3 mL) mostly result in systematic, gradual activation of the oral phase followed by the pharyngeal phase. In contrast, a large bolus (~ 10–30 mL) is usually associated with faster, simultaneous oral and pharyngeal phase muscle activity. Larger boluses also result in an earlier onset of tongue, velopharyngeal, laryngeal, hyoid, and PE segment activity; larger amplitude of hyoid movement and tongue contraction; greater velopharyngeal pressure; greater extent of pharyngeal wall and laryngeal muscle movements and longer duration of PE segment opening duration; and greater PE segment pressure generation.

As mentioned, a smaller bolus can improve bolus control as it moves from the oral cavity to the pharynx by the gradual activation of swallowing musculature. Thus, differences in bolus sizes can impact swallow safety. Increased frequency of laryngeal **penetration** and aspiration of thin liquids occurs as the size of a bolus increases (Bisch et al 1994; Daggett et al 2006). For example, Daggett and colleagues (2006) found that laryngeal penetration occurred more than twice as frequently with a 10-mL bolus compared to a 1-mL bolus. Therefore, based on the clinical manifestation of a patient's condition and dysphagia, speech-language pathologists may recommend reducing bolus volume to improve control and reduce the risk of airway compromise.

Viscosity

Bolus material is often characterized by **viscosity**, or thickness. Many different viscosities are consumed during normal meals, ranging from thin liquids (e.g., water) to thick consistencies (e.g., pudding) to mixed consistencies (e.g., cereal with milk, soups), and finally to solids (e.g., chicken or bread). Differences in bolus viscosity influence swallowing behavior. For example, a thin liquid bolus is generally held in the anterior oral cavity before being propelled to the pharynx all at once. In contrast, a chewed solid or a mixed consistency may be moved in stages to the pharynx, and held there, possibly in the valleculae, while the remaining bolus is masticated and formed in the oral cavity.

As the consistency of a bolus becomes thicker, greater tongue pressures are required to transport it from the oral cavity (Chi-Fishman and Sonies 2002; Steele and Van Lieshout 2009). Increased pressure results from greater muscular contraction of the tongue against the hard palate and from increased contact between the base of the tongue and the posterior pharyngeal wall. Paste boluses yield a greater duration and amplitude of infrahyoid and submental muscle activity compared to thin liquids. Increased muscular contraction during swallowing of thick consistencies has been associated with increased oral and pharyngeal phase duration times, increased apneic period durations, and greater PE segment opening extent compared to thin liquids. This increased "strength" of swallowing ensures that residue does not remain in the pharyngeal region after the swallow. In contrast, decreased bolus viscosity (i.e., thinner consistencies) results in earlier onset of the swallowing apneic period. The volume of air in the lungs prior to swallowing is greater for thin liquids compared to thick consistencies (Wheeler Hegland et al 2009). As mentioned earlier in this chapter, Wheeler Hegland and colleagues (2009) theorized that increased lung volume prior to swallowing thin liquids serves as a protective mechanism so that any penetrated, aspirated, or residual material can be removed from the airway with high airflow and/or effective coughs. Dietary modifications related to consistency are frequently used in the management of dysphagia. In some cases, patients may need thicker liquids to prevent aspiration, whereas in other cases patients may need softer solids or purees to increase ease of oral manipulation of the bolus.

Taste and Smell

Taste and smell are chemical senses that play an important role in the enjoyment and pleasure of eating and drinking and in modification of the swallowing motor response. The identification and experience of a specific flavor are considered to be a combination of taste, aroma, and chemical irritation of the tissues in the nasal and oral cavities. Five categories of taste have been identified: (1) sweet, (2) salty, (3) sour, (4) bitter, and (5) umami. Umami is the least discussed of the five tastes, but is generally described as savory. The ability to distinguish between different tastes is primarily accomplished by chemical stimulation of the taste bud receptors, known as papillae, located on the surface of the tongue, palate, and epiglottis. Between 5,000 and 10,000 taste buds are clustered throughout these regions.

The identification of different tastes can influence biomechanical aspects of swallowing behavior, including oropharyngeal swallowing pressures and muscular contraction. This finding is expected because peripheral taste receptors are linked neurologically to the nucleus of the solitary tract (part of the swallowing CPG) in the brainstem. Swallowing sweet, salty, and sour boluses results in greater lingual pressures compared to water boluses and greater overall activation of oropharyngeal swallowing musculature (Leow et al 2007). Additionally, sour boluses are associated with faster oral and pharyngeal phase initiations, reduced oral and pharyngeal bolus transit times, and increased swallowing effort and efficiency overall compared to other tastes (Logemann 1998). Cortical activation may increase with different bolus tastes as compared to water boluses because of the coactivation of sensory receptors for both taste and smell. Stimulation of the swallowing mechanism with boluses of various tastes improves swallowing biomechanics in some dysphagic populations.

Temperature

Very little consensus exists regarding the effects of bolus temperature on swallowing physiology. For example, Bisch et al (1994) reported that cold boluses delayed the initiation of pharyngeal muscular contraction and increased the duration of laryngeal elevation compared to room-temperature boluses in healthy individuals. In contrast, Selçuk and colleagues (2007) found that cold and hot boluses resulted in earlier initiation of the swallowing sequence and reduced pharyngeal transit times compared to room-temperature boluses. Matsubara and colleagues found that swallowing pressures did not differ in the velopharynx, mesopharynx, or hypopharynx with changes in bolus temperature in healthy individuals (Matsubara et al 2014).

Other studies of healthy adults have found that changes in bolus temperature impact esophageal function. For example, cold water slowed or abolished esophageal peristalsis, prolonged the contraction wave in the distal esophagus, and prolonged the relaxation of the lower esophageal sphincter in healthy adults. In contrast, hot water has been found to accelerate the response of the esophagus, evidenced by increased speed of peristaltic waves and a brief relaxation of the lower esophageal sphincter (Choi et al 2014). Additionally, researchers have found that cold water boluses result in significantly higher pressure at the PE segment compared to hot boluses (Matsubara et al 2014).

Despite limited evidence in healthy adults, modifications to bolus temperature are, at times, utilized clinically. There is evidence that pharyngeal transit times improve with cold boluses in patients with a history of stroke and other neurological conditions (Gatto et al 2013). Additionally, clinical anecdote suggests that the presentation of a cold or hot bolus increases patient awareness of the bolus, helping prompt the patient to modify the swallowing response voluntarily (Selçuk et al 2007).

■ Sensorimotor Control of Swallowing

From initiation to completion, swallowing is a patterned sensorimotor process controlled by both automatic and volitional control systems within a complex neural network (Hamdy et al 2001; Martin et al 2001). The brainstem, cortex, subcortical structures, and cerebellum are all involved in the production of a healthy, safe, and efficient swallow. Briefly, (1) receptors at the periphery detect the food and liquid to be swallowed and the sensory attributes of the bolus, (2) this information travels via sensory afferents that synapse in the brainstem on the CPG for swallowing, (3) a portion of this information also travels via the thalamus to the cortex for potential modulation of the behavior, (4) that information then descends to synapse again in the brainstem and (5) travels via efferents for execution of the swallowing behavior by the muscles of the respiratory, laryngeal, pharyngeal, velopharyngeal, and orofacial subsystems (**Fig. 14.20**). Further detail regarding this process is described in subsequent paragraphs.

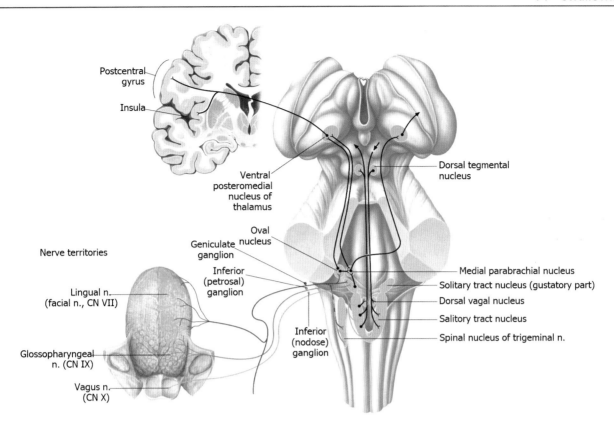

Fig. 14.20 Schematic of sensorimotor control of swallowing.

Afferents

Afferent information is critical to the generation of a normal swallow. Afferent activity is received by receptors located throughout the mucosal lining of the structures of the swallowing apparatus (oral, laryngeal, pharyngeal, and esophageal structures). The oral cavity, pharynx, and larynx contain some of the richest and most diverse sensory receptors in the human body (Mu and Sanders 2000), including both mechanoreceptors and **chemoreceptors**. Mechanoreceptors, also known as touch receptors, are sensitive to changes in pressure and muscular stretching or bending. Chemoreceptors are sensitive to chemical stimuli such as taste. In general, the afferent input from the receptors provides information related to (1) temperature, (2) taste, (3) changes in superficial and deep pressures within the aerodigestive tract, (4) muscular contraction and rate of change in muscular length, (5) surface deformation, and (6) noxious stimuli. Additionally, these receptors provide information about bolus size and texture. Additional sensory information from visual, auditory, and tactile-kinesthetic sensory systems can also affect swallowing physiology. For example, (1) visual appearance of food/bolus, (2) auditory cue from a clinician or caretaker, and (3) kinesthetic information from the hands as food is manipulated, cut, and so forth serve to modify swallowing performance in an efficient manner.

More specifically, the afferent receptors located throughout the lips, mandible, tongue, velum, pharynx, larynx, and esophagus are innervated by several cranial nerves that transmit sensory information to the brainstem. Specifically, the trigeminal (CN V), facial (CN VII), glossopharyngeal (CN IX), and vagus (CN X) nerves influence afferent sensation within the swallowing mechanism (Mu and Sanders 2000; Jean 2001). Not all of these cranial nerves participate equally during swallowing. For example, the trigeminal (CN V) and facial (CN VII) nerves are not directly involved in the initiation of swallowing, but they provide information about bolus shape and characteristics that can modify the swallow motor response. The trigeminal (CN V) nerve provides general sensory information from the muscles of mastication, lips, and tongue. The facial (CN VII) and glossopharyngeal (CN IX) nerves transfer sensory information related to taste from the tongue, and the vagus (CN X) nerve transfers taste information from the laryngeal region.

The initiation of swallowing is primarily controlled by stimulation of afferent fibers carried in the glossopharyngeal (CN IX) and vagus (CN X) nerves. The glossopharyngeal (CN IX) nerve provides sensory information from the posterior one-third of the tongue, tonsils, faucial pillars, epiglottis, walls of the posterior pharynx, inferior pharyngeal constrictor, and PE segment. The vagus (CN X) nerve has two primary branches that participate in swallowing, of which the superior laryngeal nerve provides sensory information to the brainstem. The internal branch of the superior laryngeal nerve (ISLN) is the only cranial nerve that can be directly stimulated to elicit a "pure" swallow. This phenomenon is related to the ISLN innervation of the laryngeal and pharyngeal mucosa, epiglottis, aryepiglottic folds, false and true vocal folds, cricoarytenoid joint, anterior wall of the laryngopharynx, and posterior pharyngeal wall (Mu and Sanders 2000; **Fig. 14.21**).

Brainstem

Afferent fibers of the cranial nerves involved in swallowing converge on the brainstem, mainly the nucleus of the solitary tract. Within the brainstem,

specifically on both sides of the medulla (bilaterally), a collection of neurons is responsible for the normal execution of a swallow. This group of neurons is commonly referred to as the swallowing central pattern generator (CPG). A CPG is a group of neurons that fire in a prescribed, rhythmic fashion to execute repetitive tasks. Within the brainstem, many CPGs facilitate various repetitive functions including walking, breathing, coughing, and swallowing so that little to no conscious awareness is required to complete the task. The swallow CPG is made up of two distinct groups of neurons: the dorsal swallow group in the rostrocaudal nucleus of the solitary tract and the ventral swallow group in the nucleus ambiguus (NA) (**Fig. 14.22**). Functionally, the swallowing CPG receives the afferent input from the cranial nerves (nucleus of the solitary tract) and allocates the appropriate neural drive to the nucleus ambiguus (motor component in the medulla) and surrounding reticular formation to activate various motor neurons and nerves that participate in swallowing (Jean 2001). What is unique about swallowing, and cough, for that matter, is that both are airway protective behaviors that require reconfiguration of the ventilatory respiratory cycle. Therefore, in many ways they disrupt the neurons that constitute the respiratory CPG. Strong evidence suggests that, although the swallowing and cough CPGs are unique entities, they share multifunctional neurons with the respiratory CPG. As a result, sensory information converges on the respiratory CPG in the brainstem, and then the appropriate airway protective behavior is elicited based on sensory information received. Based on sensory stimuli from the airway, an individual may, at times, initiate a swallow, at times initiate a cough, and at other times initiate a throat clear. Researchers have proposed something called the **behavioral control assembly** to explain this phenomenon better. The behavior control assembly is a pool of shared respiratory neurons that exert control over the various CPGs based on the received afferent stimuli. This hypothesis may explain why we are able to coordinate airway protective reflexes at the most basic level.

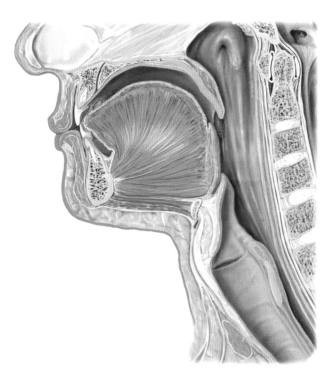

Fig. 14.21 Laryngopharyngeal regions receiving afferent information from the vagus nerve (CN X).

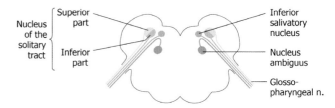

Fig. 14.22 Cross section of the medulla showing the nucleus ambiguus and nucleus of the solitary tract, which form the swallowing CPG.

Somatosensation and Volitional Control

Brainstem swallowing CPGs are capable of controlling swallowing independently. This enables us to swallow in our sleep. However, in awake and conscious humans, a large cortical network is involved that can tune, modulate, and modify swallowing behavior. More specifically, afferent sensory information received by the brainstem is simultaneously transmitted to the thalamus and then ultimately arrives at the cortex. The thalamus serves as a relay station by which sensory information from the periphery and brainstem is integrated and transmitted to higher cortical regions. This thalamic integration, or **gating**, is critical to filtering redundant sensory information from the periphery so that only necessary information is sent to the cortex. For most sensory information, the thalamus will filter out about half of the redundant stimuli, but this process appears to be different for swallowing. A study investigating the effects of paired pulsed air stimulations to the pharynx found that this sensory information is not gated out. Sensory gating is a mechanism controlled by the thalamus that controls the peripheral sensory information that is transmitted to the cortex. Reduced gating of air stimulation to the pharynx may reflect the biological need to react quickly and effectively with a swallow or cough in order to protect the airway adequately. The transfer of sensory information via the thalamus to the cortex allows for somatosensation of the stimuli and enables some level of volitional control to be exerted over the "reflexive swallow." This idea is supported by studies in which participants have identified an "urge to swallow" or have demonstrated differences in swallowing physiology in dual task conditions. Clinically, speech-language pathologists often ask patients to modify swallowing behaviorally, another indication of the volitional control of swallowing. Additionally, we are able to "swallow on command." In other words, the swallow can be initiated volitionally, or cortically.

The most advanced approach for evaluating the supramedullary regions involved in swallowing has been through the use of functional magnetic resonance imaging (fMRI). Using fMRI, researchers have identified a large cortical network involved in swallowing. This distributed cortical network is involved in sensorimotor integration, motor planning, and execution of the swallow. Many subcortical and cortical regions are involved in swallowing, including the premotor cortex, primary motor cortex, primary sensorimotor cortex, supplementary motor cortex, inferior frontal gyrus including the frontal operculum, and cingulate cortices (Humbert and Robbins 2007; Malandraki et al 2009). The insular cortex is also active during swallowing and is considered essential to sensorimotor integration between primary cortical and subcortical areas. Additionally, the role of the motor control circuits, namely the basal ganglia and cerebellum, cannot be excluded, as they are essential for proper coordination, sequencing, timing, learning, and memory of motion associated with swallowing. The diverse representation of swallowing along the neuroaxis makes it resilient to damage. In fact, destruction of several structures, including the frontal cortex, cerebellum, and pons, results in minimal changes to swallowing.

Efferent Motor Control

Swallowing requires the coordinated and patterned activation of a diverse set of muscle groups including oral, velopharyngeal, pharyngeal, laryngeal, and respiratory muscles. These efferent (motor) signals are transmitted via descending cranial nerves (V, VII, X, and XII) and spinal nerves (for respiration) away from the brainstem to the periphery (Jean 2001). The specific muscles involved in swallowing have been reviewed previously in this chapter. In general, the trigeminal nerve (CN V) innervates the muscles of mastication and floor-of-mouth muscles (**Fig. 14.23**); the

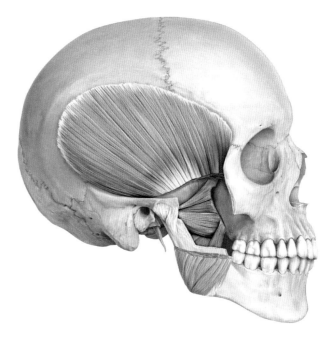

Fig. 14.23 Muscles innervated by the trigeminal nerve (CN V).

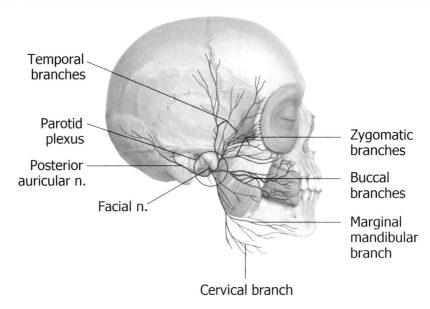

Fig. 14.24 Lateral view of the branches of the facial nerve (CN VII).

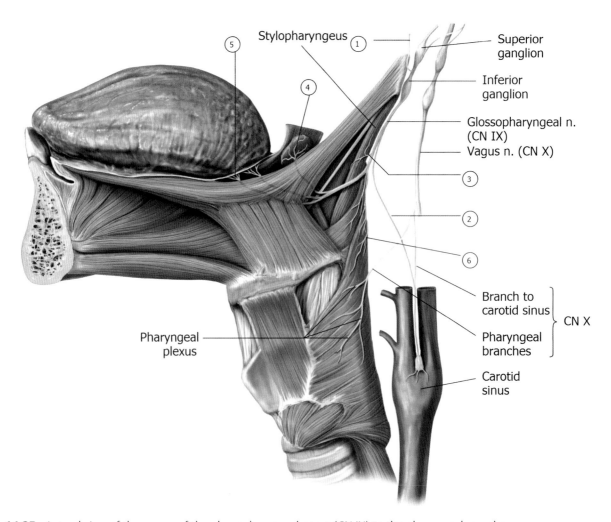

Fig. 14.25 Lateral view of the course of the glossopharyngeal nerve (CN IX) to the pharyngeal muscles.

facial nerve (CN VII) innervates the labial and buccinator muscles (**Fig. 14.24**); the glossopharyngeal nerve (CN IX) innervates the pharyngeal muscles (**Fig. 14.25**); the vagus nerve (CN X) innervates the palatal, laryngeal, pharyngeal, and esophageal muscles; and the hypoglossal nerve (CN XII) innervates the lingual muscles (**Fig. 14.26**). The collection of nerves involved in swallowing (V, VII, IX, X, and XII) constitute what is commonly known as the swallowing final common pathway (**Table 14.3**). Disruption of these nerve pathways can lead to significant swallowing problems because all cortical and subcortical information to the muscles is channeled through them.

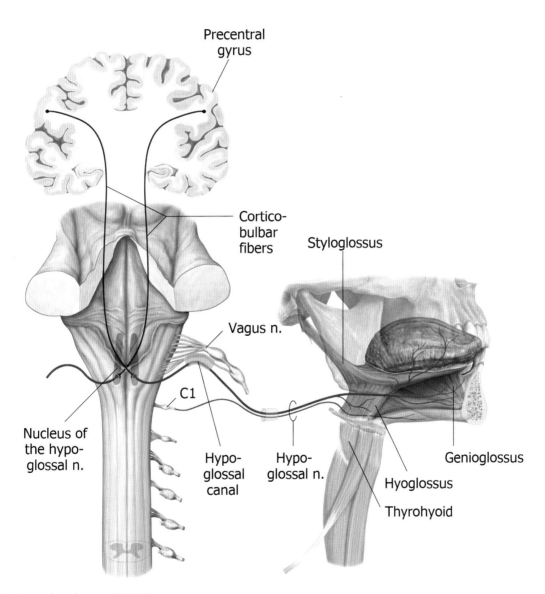

Fig. 14.26 Hypoglossal nerve (CN XII).

Table 14.3 Swallowing-specific cranial nerves and associated functions

	Course	Fibers	Nuclei	Function	Effects of nerve injury
Trigemi-nal nerve (CN V)	Exits from the middle cranial fossa *Maxillary division* (CN V$_2$): Enters pterygopalatine fossa through foramen rotundum *Mandibular division* (CN V$_3$): Passes through foramen ovale into infratemporal fossa	Somatic afferent	• Principal (pontine) sensory nucleus of the trigeminal nerve • Mesencephalic nucleus of the trigeminal nerve • Spinal nucleus of the trigeminal nerve	Innervates and provides sensation regarding pain, temperature, touch, and vibration to: • Facial skin (A) • Nasopharyngeal mucosa (B) • General sensation to the tongue (C) • Temporomandibular joint (D) • Proprioception to the jaw (A, D) • Soft and hard palate • Maxillary and mandibular teeth • Gums	• Sensory loss to the lips • Inadequate mastication • Some reduction in the extent of hyolaryngeal excursion
		Special visceral efferent	• Motor nucleus of the trigeminal nerve	Innervates: • Muscles of mastication—temporalis, masseter, medial and lateral pterygoids (D) • Oral floor muscles (mylohyoid, anterior digastric) • Tensor tympani • Tensor veli palatini	
		Visceral efferent pathway[a]	• Lingual nerve (CN V$_3$) conveys parasympathetic fibers from CN VII (via the chorda tympani) to the submandibular and sublingual glands • Auriculotemporal nerve (CN V$_3$) conveys parasympathetic fibers from CN IX to the parotid gland		
		Visceral afferent pathway[a]	• Gustatory (taste) fibers from CN VII (via chorda tympani) travel with the lingual nerve (CN V$_3$) to the anterior two-thirds of the tongue		
Facial nerve (CN VII)	Emerges in the cerebellopontine angle between the pons and olive; passes through the internal acoustic meatus into the temporal bone (petrous part), where it divides into: • Greater petrosal nerve • Stapedial nerve • Chorda tympani Certain special visceral efferent fibers pass through the stylomastoid foramen to the skull base, forming the intraparotid plexus	Special visceral afferent and efferent	• Facial nucleus	Sensory and motor innervation to: • Orbicularis oris and buccinators • Hard and soft palate • Stylohyoid • Digastric (posterior belly)	• Peripheral facial nerve injury: paralysis of muscles of facial expression on ipsilateral side of lesion • Associated disturbances of taste, xerostomia, hyperacusis, etc. • Reduction in bolus control during the oral-preparatory and oral phases of swallowing
		Visceral efferent (parasympathetic)[b]	• Superior salivatory nucleus	Synapse with neurons in the pterygopalatine or submandibular ganglion; innervate: • Small glands of nasal mucosa, hard and soft palate • Submandibular gland • Sublingual gland • Small salivary glands of tongue (dorsum)	
		Special visceral afferent[b]	• Nucleus of the solitary tract	Peripheral processes of fibers from geniculate ganglion form the chorda tympani (taste perception to the anterior two-thirds of tongue).	

Table 14.3 (*Continued*) Swallowing-specific cranial nerves and associated functions

	Course	Fibers	Nuclei	Function	Effects of nerve injury
Glossopharyngeal nerve (CN IX)	Emerges from the medulla oblongata; leaves cranial cavity through the jugular foramen	Visceral efferent (parasympathetic)	• Inferior salivatory nucleus	Parasympathetic presynaptic fibers are sent to the otic ganglion; postsynaptic fibers are distributed to: • Parotid gland (A) • Buccal gland • Labial gland	• Reduced taste perception • Impaired salivary production • Impaired pharyngeal constriction and pharyngeal peristalsis
		Special visceral efferent (branchiogenic)	• Nucleus ambiguus	Innervate: • Constrictor muscles of the pharynx (pharyngeal branches join with the vagus nerve to form the pharyngeal plexus) • Stylopharyngeus • Cricopharyngeal along with the vagus nerve	
		Special visceral afferent	• Nucleus of the solitary tract	• Receives general sensory information and taste perception from the posterior one-third of the tongue (via the inferior ganglion) (C) • Receives sensory information from faucial pillars, parotid gland, superior pharyngeal wall mucosa, and laryngeal mucosa	
		Somatic afferent	• Spinal nucleus of trigeminal nerve (CN V)	Peripheral processes of the intracranial superior ganglion or the extracranial inferior ganglion arise from the tongue, soft palate, pharyngeal mucosa, and tonsils (D, E)	
Vagus nerve (CN X)	Emerges from the medulla oblongata; leaves the cranial cavity through the jugular foramen; CN X has the most extensive distribution of all the cranial nerves (vagus = wandering, as in "vagabond"), consisting of cranial, cervical, thoracic, and abdominal parts	Special visceral efferent (branchiogenic)	• Nucleus ambiguus	Innervates: • Pharyngeal muscles including constrictors (via pharyngeal plexus with CN IX) • Muscles of the soft palate (levator veli palatini) • Laryngeal muscles (superior laryngeal nerve supplies the cricothyroid; recurrent laryngeal nerve supplies all other laryngeal muscles) • Palatoglossus	• Bilateral lesions can result in significant respiratory distress • Reduced laryngeal closure during the pharyngeal phase of swallowing • Reduced extent of hyolaryngeal elevation and excursion • Nasal regurgitation secondary to inadequate palatal elevation • Reduced extent and opening of the PE segment • Vallecular and piriform sinus residue secondary to impaired pharyngeal constriction
		Special visceral afferent	• Nucleus of the solitary tract (superior part)	Inferior (nodose) ganglion receives peripheral processes from: • Taste buds on the epiglottis and base of tongue (F)	
		Visceral afferent	• Nucleus of the solitary tract (inferior part)	Inferior ganglion receives peripheral processes from: • Mucosa of lower pharynx at its esophageal junction (cricopharyngeal muscle) (G) • Laryngeal mucosa above (superior laryngeal nerve) and below (recurrent laryngeal nerve) the vocal folds (G) • Pressure receptors in the aortic arch (B) • Tonsils • Soft palate • Valleculae • Posterolateral pharyngeal walls	

(Continued on page 510)

Table 14.3   (*Continued*) Swallowing-specific cranial nerves and associated functions

	Course	Fibers	Nuclei	Function	Effects of nerve injury
Hypo-glossal nerve (CN XII)	Emerges from the medulla ob-longata, leaves the cranial cavity through the hypo-glossal canal, and descends later-ally to the vagus nerve; CN XII enters the root of the tongue above the hyoid bone	Somatic efferent	• Nucleus of the hypoglossal nerve	Innervates: • All intrinsic and extrinsic muscles of the tongue (except palatoglossus, supplied by CN X)	• Flaccid paralysis: both nuclei injured; tongue cannot be protruded • Difficulty with bolus formation and propulsion • Pocketing of the bolus in the oral cavity
Respira-tory spinal nerves	Central control of respiration (including the respiratory CPG) occurs in the pons and medulla oblongata; spinal nerves originate in the vertebrae and extend to the muscles of respiration	Efferent	• C1–C8, T1–T12, L1–L2	Brainstem signals sent to the spi-nal cord where respiratory spinal nerves innervate respiratory muscles including: • Diaphragm (phrenic nerve [C3–C5]) • Intercostals (T1–T12) • Accessory inspiratory muscles • Expiratory muscles (T6–L2)	• Potential for marked respiratory distress • Mild injury may dirupt respiratory-swallow coordination and the effectiveness of cough production
		Afferent	• C1–C8, T1–T12, L1–L2	Spinal respiratory nerves receive afferent information from thoracic cavity and lung (chemoreceptors, baroreceptors, and mechanorecep-tors), which is then carried by CN IX and CN X to the brainstem respira-tory centers	

[a]Fibers of certain CNs adhere to division or branches of the trigeminal nerve, by which they travel to their destination.
[b]Grouped to form nervus intermedius, which aggregates with the visceral efferent fibers from the facial nerve nucleus

■ Disorders of Swallowing

Any disruption of the neurologic or peripheral con-trol of movements involving the muscles of the oral cavity, pharynx, larynx, esophagus, or respiratory system can result in dysphagia. These changes can occur throughout the lifespan, from infancy to adult-hood. A variety of diseases, disorders, and injuries can lead to dysphagia. More specifically, the causes of dysphagia can include, but are not limited to, tumors, trauma, surgical deformation, stroke, neu-rodegenerative diseases (e.g., Parkinson's disease, amyotrophic lateral sclerosis [**Box 14.6**], progressive supranuclear palsy), immune deficiency, pulmonary disease, premature birth, and craniofacial anoma-lies. Therefore, as you can imagine, dysphagia can manifest itself in many different ways. Any phase of swallowing can be disrupted, from minor changes in swallowing physiology to pervasive and severe swallowing disturbance. Regardless of the severity of swallowing deficits, the impact of dysphagia on a patient and their family cannot be ignored.

Dysphagia can lead to significant deterioration of health and quality of life. Of particular concern is the associated risk of aspiration, or ingestion of foreign particles into the airway, which can result in aspiration pneumonia, and thus, increased mor-bidity and mortality (Langmore et al 2002). Stud-ies suggest that 40% of adults aged 60 years and older have dysphagia. Additionally, pneumonia is the fifth leading cause of death in individuals 65 years or older and the third leading cause of death in individuals 85 years and older. In fact, aspiration pneumonia is often the leading cause of death in individuals with neurodegenerative diseases. In addition to aspiration pneumonia, the likelihood of malnutrition and dehydration also increases in individuals with airway compromise and dyspha-gia, given their inability to consume liquids and solids normally. Pediatric patients with dysphagia present a unique challenge in that dysphagia can lead to significant feeding challenges and **failure to thrive**, which can have long-term effects on overall health and well-being (**Box 14.7**).

Box 14.6 Amyotrophic Lateral Sclerosis

Amyotrophic lateral sclerosis (ALS), also known as Lou Gehrig's disease, is a rapidly progressive neuro-degenerative disease that results in widespread upper and lower motor neuron damage in the cerebral cortex, brainstem, and spinal cord. Upper motor neurons (UMNs) are nerve cells that originate in the cortical motor regions or brainstem and then carry efferent information to lower motor neurons in either the brainstem or the spinal cord. Lower motor neurons (LMNs) are nerve cells that originate in the cranial nerve motor nuclei of the brainstem or spinal cord and send signals to the neuromuscular junctions of the peripheral muscles (**Box Fig. 14.8**).

The clinical motor features of UMN deterioration include muscular spasticity with concomitant weakness, hyperreflexia, bradykinesia (slow movement), muscular spasms and cramps, and difficulty controlling the muscles of the face (Plowman 2015). The clinical motor features of LMN deterioration include muscular atrophy and weakness, hypotonia, fasciculations (uncontrolled rippling in the peripheral tissue), diminished reflexes, and bulbar palsy (i.e., disability of functions controlled in the medulla), which affects the strength and force of muscles innervated by the trigeminal (CN V), facial (CN VII), glossopharyngeal (CN IX), vagus (CN X), and hypoglossal (CN XII) nerves. Patients with ALS may present with any combination of both UMN and LMN symptoms. UMN and LMN damage to the efferent cranial nerve pathways involved in swallowing results in weakness or spasticity in the tongue, soft palate, pharynx, laryngeal, jaw, and facial muscles.

As a result of widespread motor system dysfunction, and especially bulbar symptoms, nearly all patients with ALS develop severe dysphagia, dysarthria (spastic and flaccid), and respiratory dysfunction. Dysphagia in patients with ALS is generally characterized by oropharyngeal dysfunction. Oral stage deficits include anterior labial leakage (weakness in orbicularis oris), inadequate mastication (reduced strength and force of masticatory muscles), inadequate bolus formation and transport (lingual atrophy, fasciculations, etc.), and marked oral residue (Plowman 2015). Pharyngeal stage deficits can include nasal regurgitation (inadequate contraction of levator veli palatini), vallecular and piriform sinus residue (reduced strength and force of pharyngeal constrictors), reduced hyolaryngeal excursion (spasticity), penetration and aspiration (weakness/spasticity of intrinsic laryngeal muscles), and reduced PE segment opening due to spasticity and reduced hyolaryngeal excursion. As mentioned earlier in this chapter, protection of the airway from food/liquid/saliva is dependent upon a continuum of behaviors including cough and swallowing (Troche et al 2014a). Of particular concern

is the severity of dysphagia in patients with ALS and the concomitant inability to voluntarily or reflexively produce an effective cough. Additionally, the marked respiratory dyscoordination and dysfunction secondary to deterioration of the spinal motor neurons only exacerbates the risk of airway compromise (disruption of the respiratory–swallow coordination pattern). Theses deficits are important to manage, as they frequently result in aspiration pneumonia, malnutrition, dehydration, choking, and even death.

Due to the insidious nature of ALS (average life expectancy is 2–5 years post symptom onset), early management and intervention by speech-language pathologists and other healthcare professionals is essential to maintain quality of life for these patients. One of the most common management strategies available to patients with severe dysphagia and ALS is placement of a percutaneous endoscopic gastrostomy (PEG) tube. A PEG tube is an alternative means of feeding in which patients have a tube placed in their stomach that provides all forms of nutrition and hydration, thus bypassing oral feeding. The placement of a PEG tube is not without risk, and if desired by the patient, it should be performed early in the disease process while respiratory function is adequate (i.e., forced vital capacity > 50% of predicted). Early education and counseling provided by speech-language pathologists is essential to assist patients with decision making regarding PEG tube placement and end of life issues.

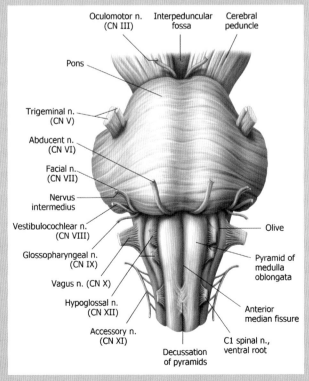

Box Fig. 14.8 Anterior view of the brainstem.

Box 14.7   Pierre Robin Sequence

Several congenital syndromes and sequences result in long-term, persistent dysphagia. **Pierre Robin sequence (PRS)** is a condition characterized by micrognathia (abnormally small mandible), glossoptosis (backward-positioned tongue), respiratory obstruction, and often cleft palate. PRS is considered a sequence and not a syndrome because the underdeveloped mandible begins a *sequence* of events leading to abnormal backward placement of the tongue and inadequate closure of the palatine bones in gestation, leading to formation of a cleft palate.

The anatomic changes associated with PRS often result in physiologic swallowing deficits, especially to the oral-preparatory and oral phases (**Box Fig. 14.9**). For example, micrognathia (class II malocclusion) can make it difficult to approximate the superior and inferior orbicularis oris and maintain a bolus in the oral cavity. The inability to close the first sphincter of swallowing has several negative consequences including anterior labial leakage, reduced pressure generation at the lips, and poor sucking-swallowing coordination. The posterior placement of the tongue and poor lingual movement also impact swallowing physiology. These lingual characteristics in PRS often result in inadequate bolus formation, difficulty propelling a bolus posteriorly in the oral cavity, and residue throughout the oropharyngeal mechanism due to reduced tongue stripping and pressure generation. The constellation of oral-preparatory and oral phase swallowing deficits in PRS likely contributes to the known pharyngeal phase deficits observed in these individuals. In particular, a lack of labial seal, inadequate bolus formation, and reduced pressure generation and speed of bolus delivery into the pharynx may contribute to asynchronous PE segment relaxation and frequent laryngeal penetration and aspiration. Dysphagia symptoms in PRS must be closely managed, as they can result in malnutrition, food refusal and aversions, failure to thrive (see following note), coughing and choking secondary to aspiration, and pulmonary infection (Monasterio et al 2004), thus increasing the morbidity and mortality in these individuals. Appropriate evaluation and treatment of infants with PRS should be completed by a multidisciplinary team that includes speech-language pathologists.

Note: Failure to thrive (FTT) can be caused by multiple medical causes (e.g., Down's syndrome, gastroenteritis, prematurity, thyroid deficiency, anemia, cerebral palsy, metabolic disorders) or environmental circumstances (e.g., abuse, neglect). Children diagnosed with FTT do not grow and develop normally compared to age-matched peers. For example, these children may weigh less or fail to gain weight at appropriate intervals. Children with FTT may also exhibit smaller head circumference, reduced height, poor social skills, and delayed developmental milestones (e.g., sitting, walking, puberty). Treatment for FTT depends on the underlying cause but can be improved with nutritional supplements, hormone/enzyme replacement, and/or counseling to address family dynamics and living conditions.

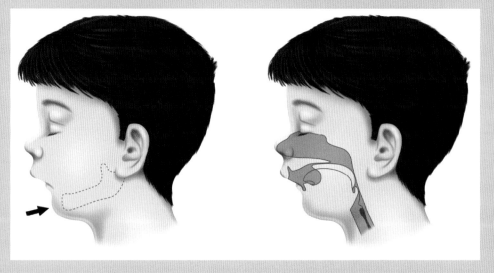

Box Fig. 14.9   Orofacial structural differences in the mandible associated with Pierre Robin sequence.

The deleterious effects of dysphagia on general health are relatively straightforward. However, often-ignored consequences of swallowing dysfunction can have a significant impact on quality of life. When swallowing is dysfunctional, a person's life and ability to engage in activities that are pleasurable can be greatly disrupted. In many cases individuals isolate themselves, stop participating in coffee dates or happy hours with friends, stop dining socially, or stop eating at the dining room table with family all together. All of these scenarios can greatly impact quality of life, leading to social isolation, depression, anxiety, and further physical decline. One factor that is also often ignored is the financial strain associated with special foods, supplemental nutrition, dysphagia therapy, and other aids to facilitate proper feeding and swallowing. Together these changes often result in familial stress, leading to decreases in quality of life for patients, loved ones, and caregivers as well.

■ Methods to Assess and Quantify Swallowing Function

Accurate evaluation of dysphagia is critical to the management, treatment, and quality of life for patients with dysphagia. Given the prevalence of "silent" aspiration and other deficits in swallowing that occur without patient awareness, visualization of the swallowing mechanism using appropriate instrumentation is important. For example, silent aspiration is so named because food and liquid enter the airway without inducing a cough response. Without proper identification and treatment of these conditions, the risk of respiratory infection and negative health complications related to dysphagia increases drastically. Many tools are used clinically and in research to evaluate swallow function. Several of these are presented in the following paragraphs.

Clinical Swallowing Evaluation

A variety of conditions that result in swallowing disorders (e.g., stroke, head and neck cancer surgery, intubation) are routinely observed in the acute inpatient healthcare setting. As a result, the evaluation and management of dysphagia in this setting often involves a multidisciplinary team of speech-language pathologists, nurses, dietitians, radiologists, oncologists, otolaryngologists, gastroenterologists, and neurologists. The speech-language pathologist is responsible for the evaluation

and behavioral management of oropharyngeal dysphagia. Most often, physicians make a request to the speech-language pathologist for a swallowing evaluation before allowing the patient to eat or drink after the medical event (surgery, trauma, etc.), or if swallowing deficits are suspected.

The clinical swallowing evaluation is a noninvasive approach to assess swallow function. A standard case history should be gathered with emphasis on diseases or disorders that may result in or modulate swallowing performance. The swallowing history should include information about the (1) method and schedule of feeding or eating, (2) diet, (3) onset and description of the problem, and (4) compensations that the patient might already be using to improve any swallowing difficulty. The clinical examination includes (1) assessment of the patient's overall condition, awareness, alertness, ability to follow directions, and cooperation; (2) posture and positioning; (3) breathing difficulties; and (4) potential for self-feeding. Direct physical examination includes a complete oral mechanism examination, assessing structure, sensation, reflexes, and volitional movement of the swallowing structures. Lastly, vocal quality, presence of signs of aspiration (cough, throat clear, change in oxygen saturations) during the swallowing of saliva, liquid, and solid trials are completed as appropriate based on the severity of the patient's condition. After the completion of the examination, impressions and recommendations are made regarding management. In many cases, an instrumental assessment of swallowing is needed to visualize the swallowing mechanism directly during eating and drinking.

Videofluoroscopy

Videofluoroscopy is often considered the "gold standard" for swallowing assessment. Videofluoroscopy provides a moving X-ray video of the swallowing mechanism while a patient swallows a variety of boluses mixed with barium sulfate. Barium sulfate is an insoluble, inert heavy metal salt that serves as contrast to enable easy visual observation of the bolus material as it moves from the oral cavity to the esophagus. The examination is generally performed in radiology. A radiologist or radiology technician typically operates the equipment, while the speech-language pathologist conducts the evaluation and provides an assortment of volumes of thin liquids, thickened liquids, pudding, soft solids, and possibly a barium tablet to the patient, depending on clinical presentation and symptoms. Delivery method of the boluses may also be varied by having the patient

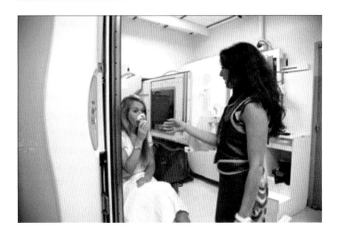

Fig. 14.27   Videofluoroscopic evaluation of swallowing.

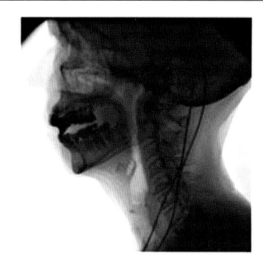

Fig. 14.28   Lateral still image from a videofluoroscopic evaluation of swallowing.

drink through a straw or from a cup to assess which mode is safest. This type of videofluorosopic evaluation of swallowing conducted by the speech-language pathologist is often referred to as the modified barium swallowing (MBS) evaluation (**Fig. 14.27**).

During the evaluation, the patient can be sitting or standing in the lateral or anterior viewing planes. The lateral view enables the visualization of mastication, bolus formation, timing and efficiency of bolus transport, velopharyngeal closure, residue (in the oral cavity, base of tongue, valleculae, piriform sinuses, etc.), extent of superior and anterior hyolaryngeal excursion, penetration or aspiration, epiglottic inversion, and PE segment opening extent and duration (**Fig. 14.28**). The anterior view provides information related to symmetry, timing, and efficiency of bolus flow through the oral, pharyngeal, and esophageal cavities. With respect to the esophagus, the speech-language pathologist can screen for esophageal disorders (e.g., reflux, dysmotility, and diverticulum); however, it is not the speech-language pathologist who diagnoses and treats these disorders.

Variability in measurement and description of the MBS findings is common between clinicians. Therefore, a number of assessment tools have been developed to help rate and quantify observations made from a videofluoroscopic evaluation. One of the most common assessment tools is the Penetration-Aspiration Scale (Rosenbek et al 1996). This scale rates the degree of laryngeal penetration and aspiration on an 8-point scale such that 1 indicates that contrast did not enter the airway, whereas 8 indicates that material entered the airway, passed below the vocal folds, and did not elicit a cough response to eject the material from the airway. The Modified Barium Swallow Impairment Profile (MBSImP) is an assessment tool that provides

a standardized method to quantify findings from the MBS (Martin-Harris et al 2008). The goal of the MBSImP is to provide a comprehensive, translatable description of the swallowing impairment from clinician to clinician and across healthcare facilities. The MBSImP examines 17 essential components of swallowing physiology and provides an objective profile of dysfunction that can be used to guide patient management.

As with any instrumentation technique, advantages and disadvantages of videofluoroscopy must be considered. The advantages of this technique include (1) noninvasiveness, (2) dynamic assessment of all phases of swallowing, (3) ability to assess patient response to swallowing modifications in real time, and (4) the ability to view the swallowing mechanism in two viewing planes. The disadvantages of using this technique include (1) short durations of radiation exposure, (2) the need to ingest barium, (3) indirect visualization of the structures of the swallowing mechanism, and (4) the need to coordinate equipment and scheduling with other departments in the hospital, which can be challenging in busy clinical settings.

Nasoendoscopy

Another common assessment tool for the visualization of swallowing physiology is flexible nasoendoscopy. This technique involves the use of a flexible endoscope inserted through the nasal cavity and nasopharynx into the laryngopharynx. This approach is most often referred to as a **flexible endoscopic evaluation of swallowing** (FEES) and is a portable technique that can be used at the bedside or in outpatient clinics. When the endoscope is positioned above the laryngopharynx, it allows visualization of the base of the tongue, laryngeal and pharyngeal mucosa, epiglottis, valleculae, vocal folds, glottis, piriform sinuses, and inlet to the esophagus. Placement of the endoscope in the nares allows the patient to speak and consume liquids and solids freely during the examination.

The image acquired by the endoscope is in color and allows visualization of the mucosa and laryngeal structures during swallowing. During a FEES evaluation, the speech-language pathologist first assesses for the presence of abnormalities in the swallowing structures (i.e. paralyses, growths, abnormal coloring of tissues). Swallowing function is then assessed by providing a variety of bolus types and volumes to the patient. This examination does not require a special type of contrast (such as barium sulfate in videofluoroscopy); however, food dye is generally added to all swallowed material to improve visualization of the bolus against the mostly pink tissues of the laryngopharynx. The speech-language pathologist evaluates the presence and amount of residue throughout the mechanism, whether or not the substance entered the laryngeal vestibule (penetration), and whether or not there is evidence that the substance traveled below the vocal folds into the glottis (aspiration). Due to the placement of the endoscope within the laryngopharynx, the actual pharyngeal phase of swallowing cannot be observed using this technique, because of the obstructed view caused by tongue and pharynx approximation during swallowing. The obstruction of the camera is called a "white out," and therefore airway compromise can be assessed only based on any evidence of the bolus that remains after a swallow is completed.

The advantages to FEES include (1) portability of the equipment for use at the bedside, (2) no radiation exposure or ingestion of barium, (3) direct visualization of laryngopharyngeal structures during swallowing, and (4) the ability of the speech-language pathologist to complete the examination independently without the need to coordinate with other specialties. The disadvantages of using FEES include (1) the lack of view of structures during the pharyngeal phase of swallowing and (2) the invasive nature of the exam, which can make it difficult for some patients to tolerate the procedure.

Electromyography

Electromyography (EMG) is a technique used to assess the activity and function of swallowing muscles. Two primary types of EMG are used to evaluate swallowing muscles: (1) needle EMG, where electrodes are inserted directly into the target muscle, and (2) surface EMG (sEMG), where electrodes are placed superficially on the skin either submentally (on the underside of the mandible), over the masseter, or on either side of the thyroid cartilage. Information from both of these EMG approaches enables clinicians and researchers to evaluate the duration and timing of swallowing events and intermittent and sustained activity of swallowing muscles throughout the duration of a swallow. This information is useful because reduced contraction of the swallowing musculature can increase the risk of aspiration and pneumonia. Surface EMG (sEMG) is most commonly used clinically for the evaluation and treatment of swallowing disorders.

During the evaluation of swallowing using sEMG, the patient sits comfortably and the targeted skin area is cleaned with alcohol. Surface electrodes are then placed on the target areas (submental, masseter, etc.). Patients are asked to complete various trials of voluntary dry or saliva swallows, single sips of water, large sips of water, and sequential sips of water. Swallowing function is evaluated based on the duration of muscular activity (in seconds), amplitude of the electrical signal (in microvolts or volts), and the number of swallows completed for each task. The findings from sEMG often serve as an impetus for further swallowing assessment and management. Clinicians also frequently use sEMG biofeedback as a therapeutic tool for patients with dysphagia. Thus, sEMG provides a useful means to evaluate and treat dysphagia; however, it does not provide a means to observe swallowing dysfunction directly. As a result, sEMG is generally used in combination with techniques that enable visualization of the bolus during swallowing (FEES or videofluoroscopy). In general, sEMG is considered a cost-effective, reliable, simple, and radiation-free diagnostic screening tool for dysphagia of various etiologies.

Manometry

Manometry is currently the most effective technique to assess oropharyngeal and esophageal swallowing pressures. As mentioned earlier in this chapter, completion of an oropharyngeal swallow involves a complex series of neuromuscular contractions to close air spaces throughout the oral cavity, nasopharynx, and glottis. Closure of these relatively long, asymmetrical cavities creates pressure gradients that serve to propel a bolus, in a timely fashion, from the oral cavity through the esophagus into the stomach. Oropharyngeal muscular contraction and closure of air cavities occurs in a systematic wave-like motion referred to as peristalsis. Thus, manometry provides important information about how well the oropharyngeal and esophageal muscles are performing peristalsis.

Traditional use of manometry involved the placement of a catheter with three sensors located near the PE segment. With advances in manometric technology, high-resolution manometry (HRM) catheters are now available with up to 36 circumferential sensors to capture changes in pressure throughout the entire length of the pharynx, PE segment, and esophagus. Manometric evaluation involves the insertion of a lubricated catheter through the nasal cavity into the pharynx and through the PE segment. Patients complete various volitional swallows of water and/or small solids during the evaluation. The output from this test provides information related to the magnitude of pressure generated during the pharyngeal peristaltic wave, the squeezing pressure of the PE segment during normal breathing, the magnitude of pressure drop as a bolus moves through the relaxed PE segment (Logemann 1998), and the magnitude of pressure generated during the esophageal peristaltic wave. Abnormal pressure generation may be indicative of impaired bolus control, PE segment dysfunction, esophageal strictures (narrowing), achalasia, esophageal cancer, or other esophageal dysfunction. Simultaneous videofluoroscopy with manometry can be performed to gain additional information about peristalsis and airway protection (Logemann 1998). Overall, researchers have found this technique to provide a reliable, sensitive, and direct way to evaluate esophageal dysfunction, but the equipment necessary to perform manometric evaluations can be expensive, often requires coordination with a gastroenterologist, and can be uncomfortable for patients.

Ultrasonography

Currently, **ultrasonography** is rarely used as an evaluative technique for the assessment of swallowing in the clinical management and treatment of patients with dysphagia. Ultrasonography involves the placement of a transducer directly on lubricated skin (usually submentally). The transducer generates and receives high-frequency sound waves that are sent through the tissue toward the airway and are then reflected back to the transducer once the sound waves contact air in the oropharyngeal cavity. This technique provides information related to lingual muscle thickness, lingual pressures against the hard palate, thickness of the masticatory muscles, and lateral pharyngeal wall movement. Reduced movement of the hyoid bone is associated with increased laryngeal airway compromise. A study by Tamura and colleagues (2012) found a relationship between lingual muscle thickness, identified by ultrasonography, and nutritional status in stroke patients. The authors suggested that use of this technique may be particularly helpful to identify dysphagia in patients with suspected sarcopenia (age-related muscle loss) and malnutrition (Tamura et al 2012). In summary, although ultrasonography does not provide direct information related to protection of the airway (penetration or aspiration), this technique can provide important information regarding swallowing dynamics in a reliable, inexpensive, and noninvasive manner. Generally, researchers recommend using ultrasonography in combination with other standardized evaluation techniques.

■ References and Suggested Readings

Bisch EM, Logemann JA, Rademaker AW, Kahrilas PJ, Lazarus CL. Pharyngeal effects of bolus volume, viscosity, and temperature in patients with dysphagia resulting from neurologic impairment and in normal subjects. *Journal of Speech and Hearing Research, 37,* 1041–1059; 1994

Bosma JF. Physiology of the mouth, pharynx, and esophagus. In: Paparella MM, Shumrick DA, eds. Otolaryngology. Vol 1: Basic Sciences and Related Disciplines, 1st ed. Philadelphia, PA: WB Saunders; 1973, 356–370

Chi-Fishman G, Sonies BC. Effects of systematic bolus viscosity and volume changes on hyoid movement kinematics. *Dysphagia, 17,* 278–287; 2002

Clarren SK, Anderson B, Wolf LS. Feeding infants with cleft lip, cleft palate, or cleft lip and palate. *Cleft Palate Journal, 24,* 244–249; 1987

Daggett A, Logemann J, Rademaker A, Pauloski B. Laryngeal penetration during deglutition in normal subjects of various ages. *Dysphagia, 21,* 270–274; 2006

Davenport PW, Bolser DC, Morris KF. Swallow remodeling of respiratory neural networks. *Head & Neck, 33* Suppl 1, S8–13; 2011

Dodds WJ, Stewart ET, Logemann JA. Physiology and radiology of the normal oral and pharyngeal phases of swallowing. *AJR American Journal of Roentgenology, 154,* 953–963; 1990

Doty RW, Bosma JF. An electromyographic analysis of reflex deglutition. *Journal of Neurophysiology, 19,* 44–60; 1956

Groher ME, Crary MA. Dysphagia: Clinical Management in Adults and Children, 1st ed. Maryland Heights, MO: Mosby Elsevier; 2010

Hamdy S, Aziz Q, Thompson DG, Rothwell JC. Physiology and pathophysiology of the swallowing area of human motor cortex. *Neural Plasticity, 8*, 91–97; 2001

Humbert IA, Robbins J. Normal swallowing and functional magnetic resonance imaging: a systematic review. *Dysphagia, 22*, 266–275; 2007

Jean A. Brain stem control of swallowing: neuronal network and cellular mechanisms. *Physiological Reviews, 81*, 929–969; 2001

Kidder TM. Esophago/pharyngo/laryngeal interrelationships: airway protection mechanisms. *Dysphagia, 10*, 228–231; 1995

Langmore SE, Skarupski KA, Park PS, Fries BE. Predictors of aspiration pneumonia in nursing home residents. *Dysphagia.* Fall 2002;17(4):298-307.

Leonard R, Kendall KA. Dysphagia Assessment and Treatment Planning: A Team Approach, 3rd ed. San Diego, CA: Plural Publishing; 2013

Leow LP, Huckabee ML, Sharma S, Tooley TP. The influence of taste on swallowing apnea, oral preparation time, and duration and amplitude of submental muscle contraction. *Chemical senses, 32*, 119–128; 2007

Logemann JA. Evaluation and Treatment of Swallowing Disorders. 2nd ed. Austin, TX: Pro-Ed Publishers; 1998

Malandraki GA, Sutton BP, Perlman AL, Karampinos DC, Conway C. Neural activation of swallowing and swallowing-related tasks in healthy young adults: an attempt to separate the components of deglutition. *Human Brain Mapping, 30*, 3209–3226; 2009

Martin BJ, Logemann JA, Shaker R, Dodds WJ. Coordination between respiration and swallowing: respiratory phase relationships and temporal integration. *Journal of Applied Physiology (1985), 76*, 714–723; 1994

Martin RE, Goodyear BG, Gati JS, Menon RS. Cerebral cortical representation of automatic and volitional swallowing in humans. *Journal of Neurophysiology, 85*, 938–950; 2001

Martin-Harris B, Brodsky MB, Michel Y, et al. MBS measurement tool for swallow impairment—MBSImP: establishing a standard. *Dysphagia, 23*, 392–405; 2008

Martin-Harris B, McFarland D, Hill EG, et al. Respiratory-swallow training in patients with head and neck cancer. *Archives of Physical Medicine and Rehabilitation, 96*, 885–893; 2015

Matsuo K, Palmer JB. Coordination of mastication, swallowing and breathing. *The Japanese Dental Science Review, 45*, 31–40; 2009

Miles A, Moore S, McFarlane M, Lee F, Allen J, Huckabee ML. Comparison of cough reflex test against instrumental assessment of aspiration. *Physiology & Behavior, 118*, 25–31; 2013

Miller AJ. Deglutition. *Physiological Reviews, 62*, 129–184; 1982

Monasterio FO, Molina F, Berlanga F, et al. Swallowing disorders in Pierre Robin sequence: its correction by distraction. *The Journal of Craniofacial Surgery, 15*, 934–941; 2004

Mu L, Sanders I. Sensory nerve supply of the human oro- and laryngopharynx: a preliminary study. *The Anatomical Record, 258*, 406–420; 2000

Plowman EK. Is there a role for exercise in the management of bulbar dysfunction in amyotrophic lateral sclerosis? *Journal of Speech, Language, and Hearing Research: JSLHR, 58*, 1151–1166; 2015

Rosenbek JC, Robbins JA, Roecker EB, Coyle JL, Wood JL. A penetration-aspiration scale. *Dysphagia, 11*, 93–98; 1996

Selçuk B, Uysal H, Aydogdu I, Akyuz M, Ertekin C. Effect of temperature on electrophysiological parameters of swallowing. *Journal of Rehabilitation Research and Development, 44*, 373–380; 2007

Shaw SM, Martino R. The normal swallow: muscular and neurophysiological control. *Otolaryngologic Clinics of North America, 46*, 937–956; 2013

Steele CM, Van Lieshout P. Tongue movements during water swallowing in healthy young and older adults. *Journal of Speech, Language, and Hearing Research: JSLHR, 52*, 1255–1267; 2009

Tamura F, Kikutani T, Tohara T, Yoshida M, Yaegaki K. Tongue thickness relates to nutritional status in the elderly. *Dysphagia, 27*, 556–561; 2012

Troche MS, Brandimore AE, Godoy J, Hegland KW. A framework for understanding shared substrates of airway protection. *Journal of Applied Oral Science, 22*, 251–260; 2014b

Troche MS, Brandimore AE, Okun MS, Davenport PW, Hegland KW. Decreased cough sensitivity and aspiration in Parkinson disease. *Chest, 146*, 1294–1299; 2014a

Wheeler Hegland KM, Huber JE, Pitts T, Sapienza CM. Lung volume during swallowing: single bolus swallows in healthy young adults. *Journal of Speech, Language, and Hearing Research, 52*, 178–187; 2009

■ Study Questions

1. Which of the following is *not* a muscle that contributes to hyolaryngeal elevation and excursion during swallowing?

A. Mylohyoid
B. Anterior digastric
C. Cricopharyngeus
D. Palatopharyngeus
E. Thyrohyoid

2. What cranial nerves are involved in the sensorimotor control of a swallow?

A. Trochlear, trigeminal, facial, vestibulocochlear, vagus, and hypoglossal
B. Trigeminal, facial, glossopharyngeal, vagus, and hypoglossal
C. Trochlear, facial, vestibulocochlear, glossopharyngeal, and vagus
D. Facial, glossopharyngeal, vagus, and hypoglossal
E. Trigeminal, facial, vestibulocochlear, glossopharyngeal, vagus, and hypoglossal

3. Which of the following is *not* true of videofluoroscopic swallowing (VFS) evaluations?

A. VFS involves exposure to radiation.
B. VFS allows for real-time assessment of penetration and aspiration.
C. VFS can assess both diet modifications and postural compensations.
D. VFS captures all phases of swallowing.
E. VFS provides the best visualization of the laryngopharyngeal mucosa.

4. Which of the following are *not* signs, symptoms, or consequences of dysphagia?

A. Malnutrition
B. Weight loss
C. Coughing and choking during meals
D. Aspiration pneumonia
E. All of the above are signs, symptoms, and consequences of dysphagia.

5. What muscle(s) innervated by the facial nerve (CN VII) are primarily responsible for maintaining an adequate labial seal during the oral phase of swallowing?

A. Orbicularis oris
B. Orbicularis oris and buccinators
C. Orbicularis oris and zygomatic
D. Risorius and buccinators
E. Risorius and zygomatic

6. During the pharyngeal phase of swallowing:

A. The vocal folds are abducted.
B. The epiglottis inverts.
C. The hyoid bone depresses.
D. The cricopharyngeal muscle is tonically contracted.
E. The velopharyngeal port is open.

7. The muscles of mastication are primarily innervated by CN_____, and are considered to be under_____ control.

A. V; voluntary
B. V; involuntary
C. VII; voluntary
D. VII; involuntary
E. X; voluntary

8. Which of the following are considered extrinsic muscles of the tongue?

A. Genioglossus, palatoglossus, stylopharyngeus
B. Genioglossus, stylopharyngeus, and inferior longitudinal
C. Palatoglossus, hyoglossus, and cricopharyngeus
D. Genioglossus, palatoglossus, hyoglossus, and styloglossus
E. Genioglossus, palatoglossus, hyoglossus, stylopharyngeus

9. Which of the following is *not* a technique that is used clinically to evaluate the structure and function of the swallowing mechanism?

A. Videofluoroscopy
B. Flexible fiber optic endoscopy
C. Magnetic resonance imaging
D. Ultrasonography
E. Manometry

10. Which of the following bolus characteristics can result in changes to muscular contraction during swallowing?

A. Volume
B. Viscosity
C. Taste
D. A and B
E. A, B, and C

11. Which of the following form part of the swallowing central pattern generator?

A. Bötzinger complex and surrounding reticular formation
B. Nucleus of the solitary tract and surrounding reticular formation
C. Nucleus ambiguus in the ventrolateral medulla
D. Dorsolateral pons and surrounding reticular formation
E. B and C

12. A patient presents to your clinic with a unilateral lingual paralysis. Which of the following would you expect to be the patient's most noticeable dysphagic symptom?

A. Penetration
B. Aspiration
C. Impaired PE segment opening extent and duration
D. Difficulty with bolus formation
E. Inadequate hyolaryngeal excursion

13. Which of the following are considered airway-protective behaviors?

A. Cough
B. Swallowing
C. Throat clearing
D. A and B
E. A, B, and C

14. Which of the following is *not* part of a bedside clinical swallowing evaluation administered by a speech-language pathologist:

A. Ocular motor testing
B. Oral mechanism exam
C. Cognitive-linguistic screening
D. Presentation of thin liquid, pudding, and cracker
E. Case history

15. Which of the following is *not* a cause of pediatric dysphagia?

A. Cleft lip and/or palate
B. Autism
C. Recurrent laryngeal nerve damage
D. GERD
E. Prolonged intubation

16. Which cranial nerve is primarily responsible for closure of the laryngeal vestibule during the pharyngeal phase of swallowing?

A. Trigeminal
B. Facial
C. Glossopharyngeal
D. Vagus
E. Hypoglossal

17. Radiation therapy associated with the treatment of head and neck cancer can result in which of the following symptoms that contribute to dysphagia?

A. Xerostomia
B. Odynophagia
C. Fibrosis
D. A and B
E. A, B, and C

18. The management of dysphagia in acute healthcare settings involves which of the following:

A. Nurses
B. Dietitians
C. Speech-language pathologists
D. All of the above
E. None of the above

19. Penetration is defined as the infiltration of swallowed material _____; aspiration is defined as the infiltration of swallowed material _____.

A. To or above the level of the vocal folds; below the level of the vocal folds
B. Above the level of the vocal folds; to the level of the vocal folds
C. Below the level of the vocal folds; to or above the level of the vocal folds
D. To the valleculae; to the piriform sinuses
E. To the piriform sinuses; to the valleculae

20. Which of the following *cannot* result in failure to thrive?

A. Difficulty latching on when breastfeeding
B. Glossoptosis
C. A retrognathic mandible
D. A and C
E. All of the above can result in failure to thrive.

■ Answers to Study Questions

1. The correct answer is (C). The mylohyoid (A), anterior digastric (B), palatopharyngeus (D), and thyrohyoid (E) all serve to elevate the larynx during swallowing. The cricopharyngeus muscle forms the upper esophageal sphincter, or PE segment, at the entrance to the esophagus. Hyolaryngeal elevation and excursion contribute to the relaxation and opening of the cricopharyngeus muscle when food approaches the entrance to the esophagus.

2. The correct answer is (B). The trigeminal (CN V), facial (CN VII), glossopharyngeal (CN IX), vagus (CN X), and hypoglossal (CN XII) nerves all contribute to completion of a swallow. The trochlear (CN IV) and vestibulocochlear (CN VIII) nerves do not directly participate in completion of a swallow.

3. The correct answer is (E). Fiber optic endoscopic evaluation of swallowing (FEES), not VFS, provides the best visualization of the laryngeal and pharyngeal mucosa. Answers (A), (B), (C), and (D) are all true of VFS evaluations.

4. The correct answer is (E). Dysphagia, or disordered swallowing, is associated with many negative health outcomes including malnutrition (A), weight loss (B), coughing and choking during meals (C), and aspiration pneumonia (D).

5. The correct answer is (A). The orbicularis oris encircles the mouth and is primarily responsible for preventing anterior labial leakage. The buccinators contribute to controlling the bolus in the oral cavity. The zygomatic and risorius muscles are more involved in facial expression.

6. The correct answer is (B). During the pharyngeal phase the vocal folds are *adducted* to prevent food and liquid from entering the airway (A). The epiglottis inverts to help protect the airway and direct food in the esophagus (B). The hyoid bone *elevates* (C), which assists in *relaxing* the cricopharyngeal muscle at the top of the esophagus (D). The velopharyngeal port is *closed* during the pharyngeal phase of swallowing.

7. The correct answer is (A). The masticatory muscles are innervated by the trigeminal nerve (CN V). Mastication occurs in the oral-preparatory and oral phases of swallowing and is considered to be under voluntary control.

8. The correct answer is (D). The extrinsic muscles of the tongue include genioglossus, palatoglossus, hyoglossus, and styloglossus. Stylopharyngeus is a pharyngeal muscle that contributes to pharyngeal constriction (A), (B), (E). The cricopharyngeal muscle (C) is tonically contracted at rest to keep the esophagus closed at all times except during swallowing.

9. The correct answer is (C). Functional magnetic resonance imaging is a useful technique to study the brain regions involved in swallowing function. However, this technique is not used clinically to evaluate swallowing structure and function in real time. All of the other techniques provide a means to directly evaluate swallowing structure and function in some manner in real time.

10. The correct answer is (E). Changes in bolus volume, viscosity, and taste have all been shown to result in changes in accommodations to swallowing physiology.

11. The correct answer is (E). The swallow CPG is made up of two distinct groups of neurons: the dorsal swallow group in the rostrocaudal nucleus of the solitary tract (B) and the ventral swallow group in the nucleus ambiguus (C).

12. The correct answer is (D). Unilateral lingual paralysis is a condition in which half of the tongue does not move appropriately. This type of deficit will most likely result in oral phase deficits. As a result of the lingual paralysis, the patient may have difficulty manipulating the food/liquid in the mouth and forming a bolus, may exhibit oral residue, and may have difficulty propelling the bolus posteriorly in the oral cavity.

13. The correct answer is (E). Protection of the airway involves a continuum of behaviors ranging from swallowing (preventing material from entering the airway) to cough (ejecting material from the airway). Thus, cough (A), swallowing (B), and throat clearing (C) are all behaviors that can help protect the airway from food and liquids.

14. The correct answer is (A). Ocular motor testing evaluates ocular alignment in many patients poststroke; however, it does not function as part of a bedside swallowing evaluation. During a bedside clinical swallowing evaluation, a speech-language pathologist will complete an oral mechanism exam (B); complete a cognitive-linguistic screening (C); present thin liquid, pudding, and cracker (C); and obtain a case history (D).

15. The correct answer is (B). Although autism can cause speech and language deficits, it does not generally result in pediatric dysphagia. All of the other conditions can result in temporary or persistent dysphagia.

16. The correct answer is (D). Closure, or adduction, of the vocal folds and laryngeal vestibule during the pharyngeal phase of swallowing is primarily controlled by the vagus nerve (CN X).

17. The correct answer is (E). Treatment of head and neck cancer with radiation therapy has many known side effects. These include xerostomia (dry mouth secondary to ablation of salivary glands; A), odynophagia (painful swallowing; B), and fibrosis (restricted movement of oropharyngeal structures; C).

18. The correct answer is (D). To provide optimal care for patients with dysphagia in the acute healthcare setting, a multidisciplinary approach is necessary. This requires the expertise of speech-language pathologists (C) to evaluate and treat signs and symptoms of dysphagia. Additionally, a dietitian (B) ensures the maintenance of adequate nutritive status, weight, and hydration, while a nurse (A) coordinates all aspects of patient care.

19. The correct answer is (A). Penetration is defined as the infiltration of swallowed material to or above the level of the vocal folds. Aspiration is defined by the infiltration of swallowed material below the level of the vocal folds into the trachea.

20. The correct answer is (E). Children considered to suffer from failure to thrive may have difficulty latching on when breastfeeding (A), glossoptosis (B), or a retrognathic mandible (C), resulting in the inability to increase weight to a healthy level.

15

Balance

Elizabeth Meztista Adams

■ Chapter Summary

Maintaining upright posture, perceiving movement when our head is in motion, and feeling at rest when we are not in motion are complex tasks accomplished through the involvement of multiple sensory systems (ears, eyes, the joints and skin, and connecting nerves) and the central nervous system. Each of the five main components of the balance system will be presented: the peripheral vestibular apparatus, the central vestibular nucleus complex, the vestibulo-ocular network, the vestibulospinal network, and the central vestibular nervous system. The anatomic structures of these systems and their function in the perception of motion and maintenance of balance will be presented. Knowledge of the anatomy and physiology of the balance system is critical in the assessment and management of patients reporting dizziness, imbalance, or unsteadiness related to a vestibular disorder.

■ Learning Objectives

- Understand the multiple sensory systems involved in the maintenance of balance including structures of the inner ear, visual system, and spinal system and that this sensory information is processed in multiple structures in the brain
- Define the role of each of the five sensory organs of the peripheral vestibular apparatus
- Describe the function of the central vestibular nucleus complex

- Understand the connections between the peripheral vestibular system and the visual system, the vestibulo-ocular network
- Understand the connections between the peripheral vestibular system and the proprioceptive system, the vestibulospinal network
- Explain the role of the vestibulocerebellum in the maintenance of balance and coordination of reflexive eye and postural movements
- Discuss the conscious perception of movement and spatial organization accomplished through processing of vestibular input by the thalamus and cortical areas of the brain

■ Putting It Into Practice

- To maintain balance and upright posture, information is gathered from multiple sensory systems (the peripheral vestibular apparatus, the visual system, and the somatosensory system) and integrated and processed by multiple structures of the central nervous system.
- Lesions at any level of the vestibular pathway can lead to symptoms of dizziness, imbalance, unsteadiness, or blurred vision when the head is in motion. Lesions in the peripheral vestibular organs may lead to additional auditory symptoms such as hearing loss, tinnitus, otalgia, and aural fullness, while lesions of the central vestibular nervous system may lead to more neurologically based symptoms such as difficulty coordinating

523

motor movements, swallowing, headache, slurred speech, and double vision.

- A test battery approach is employed to assess the balance system in individuals reporting difficulty with dizziness, imbalance, or unsteadiness. Tests in this battery include both behavioral, subjective measures and objective measures.
- Once a suspected site of lesion is determined, the disorder may be medically managed (i.e., with pharmacologic or surgical intervention), or may be nonmedically managed (i.e., with repositioning maneuvers and/or vestibular rehabilitation).

■ Introduction

The human body is amazing in its capacity to complete complex tasks efficiently and simultaneously. These tasks include respiration, digestion, circulation, processing sensory input (e.g., auditory, visual, proprioceptive inputs), and coordination of voluntary actions (e.g., walking and talking). All these tasks are mediated by electrical signals generated in the brain. The ability to maintain balance and feel at rest (as opposed to feeling dizzy) are other examples of these extraordinary activities. The feeling of stillness (quiescence) and the ability to keep our head and bodies upright may be something you take for granted, unless of course you have ever experienced unexpected dizziness or an imbalanced feeling.

Most people associate balance, or the abnormal feeling of dizziness, as being related only to the function of the structures of the inner ear. Five sensory organs of the inner ear sense head motion and position and send that information to the brain. However, these organs are only part of the complex balance system. Input from the visual and proprioceptive systems, along with information from the vestibular portion of the inner ears, is used to maintain balance and upright posture and to avoid feeling dizzy. This chapter includes a discussion of the connection between the inner ears and the visual and proprioceptive systems as well as a discussion of the centers of the brain responsible for conscious perception of head movement and for coordination of reflexive movements to aid with the maintenance of balance. If input from these sensory systems is not in agreement, sensations of dizziness, imbalance, or unsteadiness may occur. A battery of objective and subjective tests is commonly employed in patients with vestibular symptoms, and management of these patients is typically multidisciplinary (audiologists, physicians, physical therapists, etc.).

■ The Balance System

We tend to think of the balance system as simply the semicircular canals (SCCs). However, we employ input from multiple sensory systems to maintain our balance and upright posture and for conscious perception of movement and spatial orientation. This multisensory input includes information from the five vestibular end organs in each ear (three SCCs, the utricle, and the saccule), the visual system, and the proprioceptive system. Additionally, all of these sensory inputs are integrated and processed by higher brain centers so that movement, equilibrium, and spatial orientation can be consciously perceived (**Fig. 15.1**).

■ The Peripheral Vestibular Apparatus

Peripheral Vestibular Anatomy

Each inner ear contains five sensory organs that translate movement of the head into neural signals that can be sent along cranial nerve VIII (vestibulocochlear nerve, specifically its vestibular division)

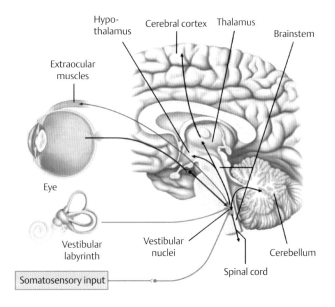

Fig. 15.1 The maintenance of balance and the perception of movement and spatial orientation are accomplished through the coordinated effort of multiple sensory systems. The vestibular sensory organs of the inner ear, the visual system, and the somatosensory/proprioceptive systems send information to the brain for integration and processing. As a result of this integrated information, conscious perception of movement and spatial orientation are achieved, and reflexive eye and postural movements are coordinated.

to the brain. Each structure in the peripheral vestibular apparatus is designed to sense and translate head movement in a specific three-dimensional plane. These structures are referred to by a number of names including the peripheral end organs, the sensory organs, the peripheral receptor apparatus, and the peripheral vestibular apparatus. No matter which name is used, the three SCCs (**anterior**, **posterior**, and **horizontal** SCCs) and two otolithic organs (**saccule** and **utricle**) are included. These sensory organs are encased in bone (the bony labyrinth), and within the bony labyrinth is a fluid-filled membrane (the membranous labyrinth). The anterior and posterior canals come together to form the **common crus**, a shared projection terminating at the vestibule. (The membranous labyrinth passages of the SCCs are also referred to as semicircular ducts; when that term is used, "semicircular canals" means the bony labyrinth specifically.) Between the bony labyrinth and membranous labyrinth is a fluid called **perilymph**. The composition of perilymph is very similar to that of cerebrospinal fluid, with a high concentration of sodium and low potassium concentration. Perilymph suspends and protects the membranous labyrinth within the bony labyrinth. The membranous labyrinth, on the other hand, is filled with **endolymph**. Endolymph contains higher amounts of potassium and lower amounts of sodium. Active infection (such as labyrinthitis) or active disease process (such as Ménière's disease) can lead to changes in the level or composition of endolymph, which may lead to balance disturbance and/or the perceived feeling of motion or **vertigo**. Vertigo is the sensation of movement or spinning in the absence of any movement.

The membranous labyrinth of the peripheral vestibular apparatus is continuous with the scala media within the cochlea, the hearing sensory organ (see **Chapter 13**). The two membranous structures are connected by the ductus reuniens, a small tube coursing from the saccule to the cochlear duct. Therefore, there are times when lesions related to fluid level in the peripheral vestibular system cause the patient to experience a loss of hearing, which can be temporary or permanent depending upon the exact nature of the lesion.

The SCCs constitute three of the five sensory organs of the vestibular system. The anterior, posterior, and horizontal SCCs are identified by their orientation and position in the skull (**Fig. 15.2**). The anterior canal is occasionally referred to as the *superior* canal, and the horizontal canal as the *lateral* canal. However, in this chapter, the canals will be referred to as anterior, posterior, and horizontal, as these names most accurately describe the position and orientation of each canal within the skull.

The SCCs contain the sensory cells responsible for transducing head movement into a neural impulse to be sent to the brain for processing.

The horizontal semicircular canal is oriented in the horizontal plane, and the anterior and posterior semicircular canals are vertically oriented in the skull. This orientation results in the horizontal SCCs being situated perpendicular to the anterior and posterior SCCs on the same side of the midline. The anterior SCC is oriented in the superior position relative to the vestibular labyrinth, and the posterior SCC is oriented in a posterior position, more dorsal, relative to the anterior canal. The anterior and posterior canals on the same side of the midline are positioned 90° from each other. The anterior canal on one side of the head is parallel to and in the same plane as the posterior canal on the other side of the midline (**Fig. 15.3**).

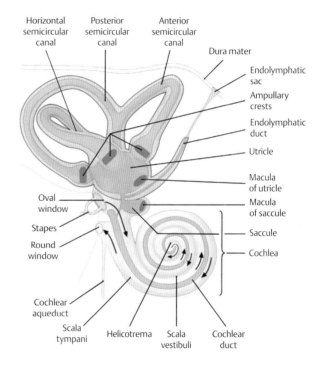

Fig. 15.2 The peripheral receptor apparatus includes five sensory organs: the anterior, posterior, and horizontal SCCs, the utricle, and the saccule. The anterior and posterior SCCs and saccule are vertically oriented, and the horizontal SCC and utricle are horizontally positioned in the skull. The sensory cells of each organ are noted in red; the sensory cells of the SCCs are contained within the ampulla, and the sensory cells of the utricle and saccule are noted as the "macula." Each of these sensory organs is contained within the membranous labyrinth (blue shaded area), which is filled with the fluid endolymph. The ductus reuniens connects the membranous labyrinth of the vestibular labyrinth with the cochlear duct of the cochlea. The membranous labyrinth is contained within the bony labyrinth, and the fluid perilymph fills the space between the bony and membranous labyrinths. The perilymph suspends and protects the membranous labyrinth and, thus, the sensory cells contained within.

Box 15.1   Clinical Correlation: Cochlear Hydrops and Ménière's Disease

The fluid contained within the membranous labyrinth of the peripheral vestibular system and the cochlear duct is endolymph. At times, the level of this fluid exceeds normal levels, due to either overproduction or underabsorption of endolymph. This fluid excess puts pressure on the sensory cells of the peripheral vestibular labyrinth as well as the sensory cells of the cochlea (**Box Fig. 15.1**). Increased endolymph is known as cochlear hydrops, and the condition can cause a number of symptoms in an otherwise healthy individual, including dizziness and hearing loss. The collection of symptoms associated with cochlear hydrops is called Ménière's disease, and possible causes include autoimmune disease, vascular insult, viral etiology, genetic predisposition, head injury, allergy-related, migraine, and endocrine system dysfunction.

Most often, Ménière's disease affects only one ear. However, the symptoms can be debilitating. The symptoms of Ménière's disease fluctuate as the level of endolymph fluctuates. When the level of endolymph is higher than normal, symptoms are present. When the fluid level returns to normal or near normal, the symptoms improve or resolve completely. During symptomatic times, individuals with Ménière's disease often experience a low-frequency sensorineural hearing loss and reduced ability to understand speech in the affected ear. The individual will report that their hearing is better on some days than others. Individuals with Ménière's disease also often report a low-pitched buzzing or humming sound called tinnitus. The sensation of aural fullness (the feeling that the middle ear is plugged or stopped up) is also common. Individuals may report feeling as if they have water or cotton stuck in their ear,

and attempts to perform the Valsalva maneuver are not effective at clearing the fullness. A few individuals with Ménière's disease even report otalgia (pain in the ear). The most debilitating symptom of Ménière's disease for most individuals is severe vertigo that accompanies cochlear hydrops. Vertigo may persist for days or weeks during an episode of cochlear hydrops, and the individual may experience nausea and vomiting.

Interestingly, some individuals experience some, but not all, of the symptoms associated with Ménière's disease. Therefore, Ménière's disease is at times categorized as cochlear in nature, sometimes as vestibular. If the individual experiences only cochlear symptoms, such as hearing loss, tinnitus, otalgia, and aural fullness, the disease is classified as cochlear Ménière's disease. If the individual experiences only the vestibular symptoms of vertigo, nausea, and vomiting, the disease is considered vestibular Ménière's disease.

In the early stages, Ménière's disease may be managed conservatively with dietary modifications. Restriction of sodium intake may improve symptoms, as sodium can lead to increased fluid retention in the body. Dietary modification may reduce symptoms in some individuals; however, the full effect may not be realized for weeks. Other dietary modifications include reduced caffeine intake, reduced nicotine use, and avoidance of certain foods such as wine, cheese, chocolate, and other foods related to migraine conditions, as Ménière's symptoms may be associated with migraine disorders. More aggressive treatments include the use of thiazide diuretics, which help rid the body of sodium and water, and antihistamines when an association between Ménière's and allergy symptoms is present. When dietary modification and pharmacologic treatments are not effective, streptomycin or gentamicin injections or surgical intervention may be indicated.

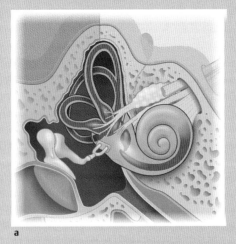
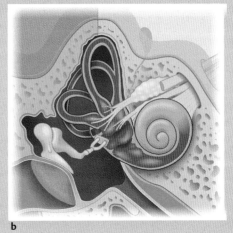

a   b

Box Fig. 15.1   (a) In the normal cochlea and vestibular labyrinth, the membranous labyrinth is filled with just the right amount of endolymph to fill the membrane without bulging. **(b)** Cochlear hydrops occurs when an excess of endolymph exists in the system, due to either overproduction or underabsorption of the fluid. In this case, the membranous labyrinth bulges like a squeezed, partially filled balloon, causing a number of symptoms including dizziness, hearing loss, aural fullness, and tinnitus.

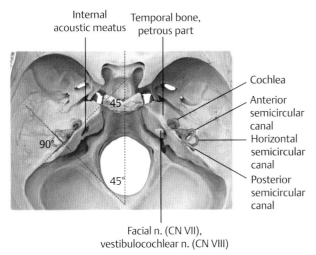

Internal acoustic meatus

Temporal bone, petrous part

Cochlea

Anterior semicircular canal

Horizontal semicircular canal

Posterior semicircular canal

Facial n. (CN VII),
vestibulocochlear n. (CN VIII)

Fig. 15.3   The position of the SCCs in the petrous portion of the temporal bone in the skull. The horizontal SCC is almost parallel to the plane of gravity, and the anterior and posterior SCCs are perpendicular to the horizontal SCC. The anterior and posterior canals are also oriented at a 90° angle from each other and, thus, at a 45° angle from the midline. The anterior canal on one side of the head is in a parallel plane to the posterior canal on the opposite side of the skull.

The otolithic organs—the utricle and saccule—also contain sensory cells, similar to those in the semicircular canals. These sensory cells transduce specific head movements into neural signals that are sent to the brain for processing. The utricles are oriented horizontally in the skull and, like the horizontal semicircular canals, are tilted slightly upward, approximately 30° relative to the

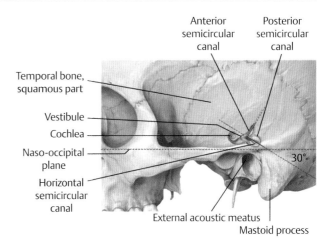

Anterior semicircular canal

Posterior semicircular canal

Temporal bone, squamous part

Vestibule

Cochlea

Naso-occipital plane

Horizontal semicircular canal

External acoustic meatus

Mastoid process

Fig. 15.4   The horizontal SCC is oriented at a 30° angle relative to the naso-occipital plane, and the anterior SCC is tilted 60° relative to the naso-occipital plane. During ambulation, the head is typically pitched downward approximately 30°, which positions the horizontal SCC parallel with the plane of gravity and the anterior SCC perpendicular to the plane of gravity, rendering both canals maximally sensitive to head movement.

naso-occipital plane (**Fig. 15.4**). The saccules are oriented vertically in the skull and are tilted 60° below the naso-occipital plane.

Neuroepithelium of the SCCs and Otolithic Organs

Contained within the SCCs and otolithic organs are the sensory cells necessary for head movement to be transduced into the neural impulse that

---

Box 15.2   Clinical Correlation: Responsiveness of Semicircular Canals and Otolithic Organs to Head Movement

Each SCC functions to transduce a specific angular excursion (rotation) of the head in the three dimensions of space (pitch, roll, and yaw). The horizontal SCC, oriented in the horizontal plane, responds to horizontal movements of the head. The vertical orientation of the anterior and posterior SCCs enables these canals to respond to vertical rotations of the head.

Complementing the function of the three SCCs are the two otolithic organs: the utricle and saccule. The otolithic organs are responsible for sensing acceleration in both the horizontal and vertical planes as well as certain head tilts (pitch and roll, specifically). Without otolithic organs, you would not be able to sense the acceleration of a moving car or vertical acceleration when riding in an elevator.

The utricle, oriented horizontally in the skull, is sensitive to acceleration in the horizontal plane, such as forward/backward and side-to-side movements. The horizontal SCCs are also oriented in the horizontal plane within the skull; however, the utricles and

horizontal SCCs do not sit completely horizontal in the skull. Both structures are tilted slightly upward, approximately 30° relative to the naso-occipital plane (**Fig. 15.4** in text). This slight tilt is functionally important because during walking or running, the head is pitched downward about 30°, which puts the line of sight a few meters in front of the feet. With the head tilted downward 30°, the horizontal SCCs and utricles are completely parallel with the ground and, thus, parallel to the plane of gravity and maximally sensitive to horizontal head movements.

The vertical orientation of the saccules cause these structures to be sensitive to movements in the vertical plane, specifically upward and downward. Recall that the anterior and posterior SCCs are also oriented vertically in the skull. These SCCs and the saccules are tilted at 60° below the naso-occipital plane, and with the head tilted downward 30° during ambulation, the vertical SCCs and saccules are completely perpendicular to the plane of gravity. This vertical positioning enables the vertical SCCs and saccules to be maximally sensitive to movements of the head in the vertical plane (**Fig. 15.4** in text).

is ultimately sent to the brain for processing. The neuroepithelium, a specialized layer of cells that sense external stimuli, of the peripheral end organs is made up of two main types of cells: supporting cells and sensory cells. Supporting cells cover the floor of the structure and are densely packed to support the sensory cells of the end organ, **hair cells**. Sensory cells of the peripheral vestibular apparatus are similar in structure and function to those of the hearing organ. These hair cells sense head rotation and acceleration and transduce these movements into a signal that can be transmitted by CN VIII to the brain for interpretation. These signals are ultimately perceived as a short-duration head movement, continuous head and body rotation, forward or backward whole body movement, or side-to-side movement of the body. These signals are also used by the brain to generate compensatory eye movements to maintain focused vision while the head is in motion, and to generate reflexive movements of the neck and limbs in order to maintain upright posture.

There are two types of *sensory* hair cells: type I and type II. Both type I and type II hair cells are innervated by both afferent and efferent nerve fibers, either directly or indirectly. Afferent nerve fibers transmit sensory information from the peripheral systems of the body to the brain. Efferent nerve fibers send neural information from the brain and spinal cord to the peripheral systems of the body, such as the muscles and sensory systems.

Type I hair cells are chalice-shaped and are innervated directly by afferent nerve fibers in a cuplike structure known as a nerve calyx. Type I hair cells are also innervated by efferent nerve fibers through synaptic bouton connections, an enlargement of the nerve ending with a buttonlike connection to the cell. Conversely, type II hair cells are cylindrical in shape and are innervated directly by both afferent and efferent nerve fibers with several bouton terminals (Sedó-Cabezón et al 2014; Soto and Vega 2010). The afferent and efferent connections to type I and type II hair cells can be seen in **Fig. 15.5**.

Each sensory hair cell is embedded with a bundle of 50 to 100 tiny microvilli or hairlike receptors called **stereocilia** and a single, longer **kinocilium** (Ciuman 2011) (**Fig. 15.5**). These stereocilia and kinocilia project from the **cuticular plate**, a firm layer of actin, on the apical surface of each hair cell. The bundle of stereocilia with the single kinocilium are arranged in descending height, such that the tallest stereocilia are closest to the kinocilium, and the stereocilia become shorter as the distance from the kinocilium increases (Ciuman 2011). The stereocilia and kinocilium of each hair cell are connected by tiny filaments that, along with the cuticular plate, function to maintain upright position of the hairlike receptors after they have been sheared, or bent.

The sensory hair cells of each SCC are housed in the **ampulla**, a swelling at the base of the SCC where it joins the vestibule. These sensory hair cells

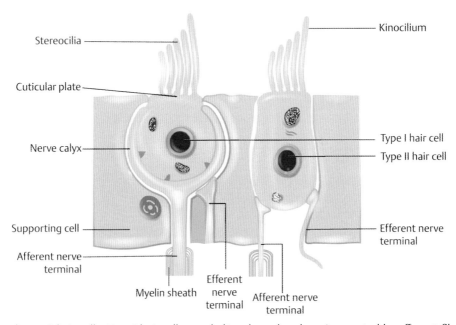

Fig. 15.5 Type I and type II hair cells. Type I hair cells are chalice-shaped and are innervated by afferent fibers in a nerve calyx wherein the nerve surrounds the hair cell. Efferent fibers connect to the type I hair cells through bouton connections with the afferent nerve fibers. Type II hair cells are cylindrical in shape and are innervated directly by afferent and efferent fibers through bouton connections. Embedded in the cuticular plate of each hair cell are a single kinocilium and 60 to 100 stereocilia, arranged in descending order of height.

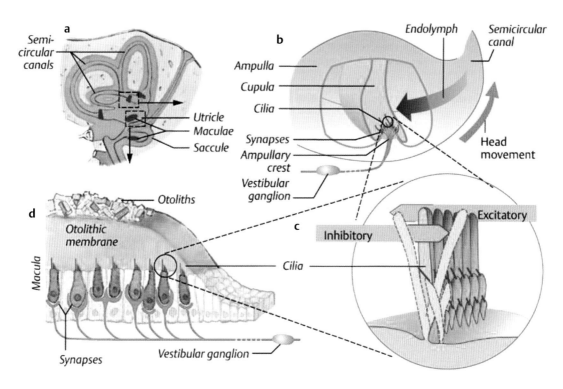

Fig. 15.6 Illustration of SCC and otolithic organ sensory cells. **(a)** Ampulla of SCCs and maculae of otolithic organs shown in their position in the vestibular labyrinth. **(b)** Cross section of the SCC ampulla, including the cupula, endolymph, kinocilia and stereocilia, and vestibular ganglion. Head movement results in movement of the endolymph in the direction opposite the head movement (shown with arrows). Movement of endolymph pushes against the cupula, which results in shearing (movement) of the kinocilia and stereocilia. **(c)** Cross section of the otolithic macula, including the otolithic membrane, otoliths, kinocilia and stereocilia, type I and type II hair cells, and vestibular ganglion. Linear acceleration (such as riding in an accelerating vehicle) and movements of the head relative to the plane of gravity result in movement of the otolithic membrane, which shears the kinocilia and stereocilia embedded within. **(d)** Illustration of the movement of the kinocilia and stereocilia with movement of the cupula (semicircular canals) or otolithic membrane (otolithic organs) in response to head movement/acceleration. Movement of the kinocilia and stereocilia toward the direction of the hair cell polarization (toward the kinocilium) results in an excitatory response. Movement of the kinocilia and stereocilia opposite the directional polarization (away from the kinocilium) results in an inhibitory response of the hair cell.

are supported by a mound of densely packed supporting cells, known as **cristae**. In the SCCs, type I hair cells are mostly clustered at the apex of the rounded cristae within the ampulla, and type II hair cells are more concentrated in the periphery of the cristae. The stereocilia and kinocilia of both type I and type II hair cells of the SCCs are embedded in a gelatinous membrane called the **cupula.** The cupula is affixed to the cristae on its inferior (bottom) surface and extends upward to the roof of the ampulla. A cross section of the SCC ampulla is shown in **Fig. 15.6**. Movement of the cupula ultimately moves and bends the stereocilia and kinocilia, leading to increased or decreased firing rate of CN VIII.

The sensory cells of the otolithic organs, the utricle and the saccule, are structurally similar to those found in the semicircular canals; however, some of the structures within otolithic organs are referred to by different terminology from that used

to describe the structures of SCC sensory cells. The otolithic organs contain type I and type II hair cells, from which multiple stereocilia and a single kinocilium project. Otolithic organs also contain cells that support these sensory hair cells. Recall that in the SCCs, these supporting cells are referred to as cristae. In the otolithic organs, the supporting cells are referred to as a **macula**.

The stereocilia and kinocilia of the otolithic organ hair cells are embedded in a gelatinous structure called the **otolithic membrane**, and atop the otolithic membrane lie calcium carbonate crystals, the **otoconia** (**Fig. 15.6**). Otoconia, or otoliths, are twice as dense as the endolymph contained within the organ. An electron microscope image of otoliths can be seen in **Fig. 15.7**. Because of their high density, otoconia are not displaced by slight movements of endolymph but are displaced by the force of gravity when head position is changed relative to gravitational pull. Therefore,

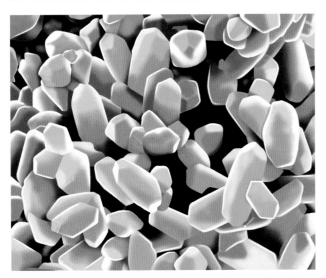

Fig. 15.7   Scanning electron microscope image of otoliths.

simple head movements do not result in movement of the otoconia, but forward and backward acceleration such as in a moving vehicle, or vertical acceleration such as that felt in a moving elevator, result in movement of the otoconia. Movement of the otoconia drags the otolithic membrane in the direction of the head movement, which ultimately causes the stereocilia and kinocilia embedded within to be sheared. The otoconia and otolithic membrane move when the head is tilted, with an initial acceleration, and with a change in the velocity of head movement. That movement can be processed and interpreted as head movement, but once movement of the otolithic membrane ceases, the feeling of movement also stops. The next time you are in a vehicle, pay attention to the feeling of movement you perceive when the vehicle begins to move from a stopped position. You will feel the initial acceleration, but once the vehicle reaches a constant speed, you no longer feel as if you are moving forward, although you clearly are. This sensation of being at rest, rather than moving with the car, occurs because once the vehicle is moving at a constant speed, the otolithic membrane returns to the resting position, which reduces the feeling of motion. If the otolithic membrane is at rest, the kinocilia and stereocilia are not being sheared, and there will be no perception of motion. The same will happen when the vehicle begins to decelerate.

Hair Cell Orientation

The position of the kinocilium and stereocilia on each hair cell dictates the directional orientation of the hair cell itself. This directional orientation is an important factor in sensing and transducing the exact direction of head movement into a neural impulse that can be interpreted by the brain. The kinocilia and stereocilia on the hair cells in each SCC are oriented in the same direction on one side of the head and with opposite orientation on the opposite side of the head (**Fig. 15.8**). Specifically, hair cells in the horizontal SCCs are oriented toward the utricle, with the kinocilia and longest stereocilia closest to the utricle. Hair cells in the anterior and posterior canals are oriented with the shortest stereocilia closest to the utricle. This arrangement is mirrored on both sides of the head (Tumarkin 1986). This anatomic orientation leads to functional physiologic orientation, which will be discussed later.

Hair cells of the otolithic organs are oriented in a different manner than the hair cells of the semicircular canals. Both otolithic organs, the utricle and the saccule, are bisected by the **striola** (**Fig. 15.9**), a curved indention in the macula (supporting cells) of the utricle and saccule, and hair cells of these otolithic organs are oriented relative to this depression. In the utricle, sensory hair cells are positioned toward the striola, with the kinocilium of each hair cell closest to the striola and the stereocilia in descending order from tallest to shortest moving away from the kinocilium. In the saccule, sensory hair cells are oriented away from the striola, such that the shortest stereocilia are closest to the striola with subsequently taller stereocilia and kinocilia positioned farther from the striola (**Fig. 15.8**). The macula of the saccule is hook-shaped; the macula of the utricle is kidney-shaped (Lindeman 1969).

Peripheral Vestibular Physiology

Any movement of the head causes movement of endolymph in the membranous labyrinth of the peripheral vestibular system. The exact direction of this head movement, as well as the orientation of the sensory hair cells in the vestibular labyrinth, causes hair cells within the semicircular canals and otolithic organs to respond in a specific manner. The response of hair cells to this head movement ultimately leads to increased or decreased firing rates on fibers of the vestibular division of CN VIII, the vestibulocochlear nerve, so that the signal that the head has moved can be sent to the brain.

Sensory hair cells of both the SCCs and the otolithic organs function in exactly the same manner, which incidentally is very similar to the function of the sensory cells of the cochlea. In SCCs, displacement of endolymph with head movement pushes the gelatinous cupula, which causes the kinocilia and stereocilia embedded in the cupula

Box 15.3 Clinical Correlation: Benign Paroxysmal Positional Vertigo

Benign paroxysmal positional vertigo (BPPV) occurs when otoconia from the utricle become dislodged and fall into one or more of the SCCs (**Box Fig. 15.2**). Any of the SCCs can be affected; however, it is the posterior SCC that is most often affected because of its position relative to gravity. In the SCC, the freed otoconia cause the fluid in the affected canal to move differently than the fluid in the unaffected corresponding canal on the other side of the head. Because the input to the vestibular system is asymmetrical, the individual experiences vertigo when the head is moved into certain positions, such as rolling over in bed. The name of the disease gives quite a bit of information about the symptoms it produces. "Benign" indicates that the disease is not life threatening. "Paroxysmal" indicates that the symptoms are distinct and episodic. The term "positional" indicates that the symptoms are typically induced by movement into a provoking position. Finally, "vertigo" indicates the hallmark of the disorder: a spinning sensation in the absence of actual movement. As many as half of BPPV cases are idiopathic, or without a known cause. Other possible causes of BPPV include viral etiology, spontaneous degeneration of the otolithic membrane, age-related changes in the otolithic membrane, weakened linking filaments between the otoconia, and head trauma.

The primary symptoms of BPPV are vertigo and nystagmus that are episodic and transient in nature. Individuals with BPPV frequently report distinct epi-sodes of dizziness that are typically of short duration (15 seconds to one minute). At times, the vertigo is severe enough to cause nausea and vomiting. Nystagmus (involuntary movement of the eyes) accompanies the vertigo. The direction of nystagmus is dependent on the specific SCC involvement; however, nystagmus is most often rotary in nature because the posterior SCC is most often affected. Individuals with BPPV may also report postural instability and an imbalanced feeling even between episodes.

BPPV is relatively easy to identify based on reported symptoms; however, the formal assessment used to identify BPPV is the Dix Hallpike maneuver. In this maneuver, the individual is moved into position with the head hanging slightly off of the examination table in an attempt to provoke the symptoms. The examiner observes for nystagmus and will inquire with the individual about any feelings of dizziness. Even when BPPV is strongly suspected, full vestibular assessment may be warranted to rule out any coexisting vestibular disorders. In as many as 50 to 70% of BPPV cases, the condition spontaneously resolves. However, the condition can be managed through otolith-repositioning maneuvers such as the Epley or Semont maneuvers, which were designed to move the otoconia from the SCC and back into the vestibule (**Box Fig. 15.3**). Pharmacologic intervention may be used at times to reduce the symptoms, but no pharmacologic interventions resolve BPPV.

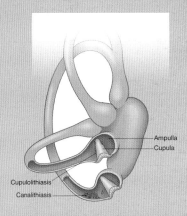

Box Fig. 15.2 BPPV occurs when otoconia from the utricle become displaced from their normal resting place atop the otolithic membrane and fall into one of the SCCs, most often the posterior SCC. The displaced otoconia cause the endolymph in the affected SCC to move differently than it moves in the the nonaffected corresponding canal on the opposite side of the head when the head is moved. This asymmetry in the input from the peripheral receptor apparatus to the central vestibular nervous system leads to the feeling of vertigo when the head is moved in certain positions.

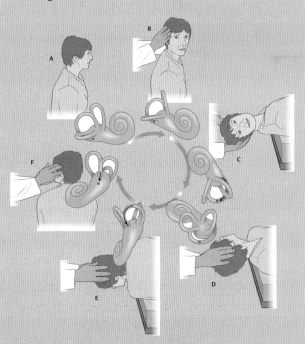

Box Fig. 15.3 The Epley maneuver for the treatment of BPPV. In the Epley maneuver, the individual is moved into various positions with the intent of moving the floating otoconia out of the affected SCC and back into the vestibule. Once the otoconia are moved out of the SCC, the vertiginous symptoms will resolve.

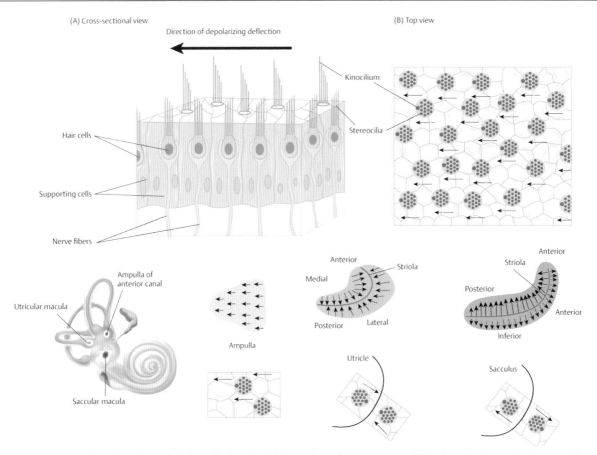

Fig. 15.8 Directional polarization of hair cells in the SCCs and otolithic organs. All hair cells in a single ampulla of an SCC are functionally polarized in the same direction. Hair cells of the utricles and saccules are arranged around the striola. In the utricles, the kinocilium and longest stereocilia are closest to the striola, and in the saccules, the kinocilium and longest stereocilia are oriented away from the striola. This arrangement enables functional polarization in one direction for one half of the organ and functional polarization in the other direction for the other half of the otolithic organ.

to move and bend, or shear (**Fig. 15.6**). In the otolithic organs, however, the kinocilia and stereocilia are not sheared simply with movement of the endolymph. The dense otoconia atop the otolithic membrane prevent shearing of the kinocilia and stereocilia with movement of the endolymph alone. Kinocilia and stereocilia of the otolithic organs are sheared only when the otoconia are displaced with enough force to drag the otolithic membrane across the kinocilia and stereocilia.

Because kinocilium and stereocilia are arranged such that the tallest stereocilia are closest to the single kinocilium on each hair cell, hair cells are considered to be directionally polarized. When stereocilia are sheared, or bent, with the kinocilium, an excitatory response is initiated, ultimately leading to increased firing rate of the corresponding fiber of CN VIII. Shearing of stereocilia away from or against kinocilium results in an inhibitory response, ultimately leading to decreased firing of the corresponding fiber of CN VIII (**Fig. 15.6**).

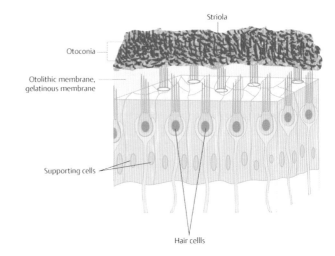

Fig. 15.9 Cross section of the otolithic (utricular) maculae. The striola is a curved indention in the macula and otolithic membrane that bisects each otolithic organ. The kinocilia and stereocilia of the otolithic organs are arranged around the striola so that with head movement, one half of each organ is stimulated and the other half of the organ is inhibited.

When the head moves, sensory hair cells in more than one SCC respond. Hair cells in one SCC respond in an excitatory manner, increasing firing on the canal's branch of CN VIII (the anterior, posterior, or lateral ampullary nerve). Conversely, hair cells in the other SCC respond in an inhibitory manner, decreasing firing on its ampullary nerve within CN VIII. This response pattern, wherein one SCC is excited and one SCC is inhibited, is considered a "push-pull" system. The response of the otolithic organs is also considered push-pull in nature, such that with movement of the otolithic membrane, one-half of the otolithic organ is excited and the other is inhibited.

The SCCs are grouped into **coplanar pairs**, which allows excitation of one SCC to be coupled with simultaneous inhibition of another associated SCC. The right and left horizontal SCCs are oriented in the same geometric plane and make up one of the three sets of coplanar SCC pairs. The right anterior and left posterior SCCs are in parallel geometric planes and are thus considered coplanar, as are the left anterior and right posterior SCCs. This arrangement of SCCs on opposite sides of the midline into coplanar pairs creates a push-pull system. With this arrangement, pairs of SCCs can work together in a functional, equal but opposite, fashion (**Fig. 15.10**).

This functional pairing is possible because of the orientation of the hair cells within the ampulla. Recall that hair cells of the horizontal semicircular canals are oriented with the kinocilia toward the utricle on both sides of the head, and the hair cells of the vertical canals are oriented with the kinocilia

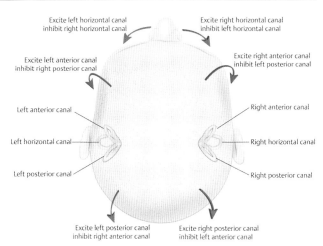

Fig. 15.10 A simplified illustration of head movements and subsequent SCC excitation and inhibition. The coplanar semicircular pairs include the right and left horizontal SCCs, and the anterior SCC on one side and the posterior SCC on the other. These canals work as a push-pull system such that when one canal of the pair is excited, the other canal in the coplanar pair will be inhibited. For example, with a simple rightward head turn, the right horizontal SCC (right lateral ampullary nerve) is excited and the left horizontal SCC (left lateral ampullary nerve) is inhibited.

away from the utricle on both sides. This hair cell arrangement creates a mirror image on either side of the head. Subsequently, when one SCC of the pair is stimulated, the other SCC in the pair is inhibited. For example, with a simple rightward head turn, the right horizontal SCC is excited, and the left

---

Box 15.4   Clinical Correlation: Vestibular Neuritis

With normal semicircular canal function, if one semicircular canal is excited, the other canal of its coplanar pair is inhibited. This arrangement leads to an equal but opposite response on both sides of the head, and the individual will perceive the head movement but will not feel dizziness. In an individual with a disordered vestibular labyrinth, at least one of these responses is reduced or possibly absent. Therefore, the response sent to the rest of the system is not symmetric, leading to vertiginous feelings.

One disorder that may lead to reduced output from one vestibular labyrinth is vestibular neuritis, also called vestibular neuronitis. Vestibular neuritis is a virally mediated infection that affects the vestibular division of CN VIII. Individuals often report having experienced a gastrointestinal or upper respiratory tract infection in close temporal proximity to the symptoms of vestibular neuritis, which include vertigo with accompanying nausea and imbalance. Auditory symptoms such as hearing loss, tinnitus, or otalgia are rare. In the early phase of the disorder, the vertigo is relatively constant. However, after a few days, the vertigo becomes less constant and more episodic. Specifically, individuals find that the vertigo is provoked by specific changes in head position relative to gravity.

Vestibular assessment of a patient with suspected vestibular neuritis should include an audiogram, vestibular evoked myogenic potential (VEMP), and videonystagmography (VNG) testing. Results should indicate normal hearing, or no change in hearing associated with the presence of vestibular neuritis, and vestibular hypofunction (reduced vestibular function) on the disordered side. The symptoms of vestibular neuritis can be medically managed through the use of antiemetics (antinausea medication) and vestibular suppressants, which reduce vertiginous symptoms. At times, antiviral medications may also be indicated. Recovery from vestibular neuritis can take weeks and may require vestibular rehabilitation to regain full functioning after the disorder has resolved.

horizontal SCC is inhibited (**Fig. 15.11**). Similarly, with a downward head tilt, both anterior SCCs are excited, and both posterior SCCs are inhibited. The opposite is true for an upward head tilt: the anterior SCCs are inhibited and the posterior SCCs are excited. These examples are simplistic; most head movements involve a more complex pattern of excitation and inhibition, as more than one set of coplanar SCCs respond.

The otolithic organs also function in a push-pull system, which is possible because of the orientation of the hair cells around the striola. In the utricle the kinocilia are oriented toward the striola, and in the saccule the kinocilia are oriented away from the striola, creating a mirror image of hair cell orientation around the striola within each otolithic organ. This arrangement of kinocilia and stereocilia generates a specific pattern of excitation and inhibition

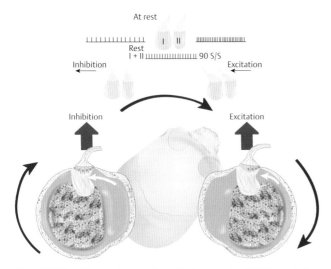

Fig. 15.11 The pattern of excitation and inhibition of the hair cells in the horizontal semicircular canal and the increased and decreased firing rate of the corresponding fibers of the vestibular division of CN VIII with a simple rightward head turn is shown. Because of the viscoelastic properties of endolymph, the rightward head rotation leads to the movement of endolymph in the direction opposite the head movement, toward the left in this example. The endolymph consequently pushes against the cupula within the ampulla, and the cupular movement results in shearing of the kinocilia and stereocilia embedded within. In the right horizontal SCC, the kinocilia and stereocilia are sheared toward the utricle (with the kinocilia), causing hair cell depolarization and ultimately an increase in firing rate on the right lateral ampullary nerve within CN VIII. This is an excitatory response. In the left horizontal SCC, the cupula is pushed away from the utricle and the stereocilia are sheared away from the kinocilia, causing the hair cell to be hyperpolarized and the neural firing rate (on the left lateral ampullary nerve) to decrease (an inhibitory response). The resting firing rate (without any head movement) is shown for reference, and the firing rates with the excitatory and inhibitory responses are also shown.

within each otolithic organ when the head is moved. With forward/backward acceleration, side-to-side acceleration, vertical acceleration, or head tilt, the otolithic organs on both sides of the head respond. However, approximately half of the hair cells within one otolithic organ are excited and the other half are inhibited (**Fig. 15.12**). In this way, the otolithic organs function in the same push-pull manner as SCCs. Because of the horizontal orientation of the utricle, this sensory organ is responsible for transducing head tilts, as well as forward and backward translations of the entire head (such as riding in a moving car), and side-to-side translations. Translations involve movement of the entire head in a forward/backward or side-to-side fashion, as opposed to rotational movement such as tilting the head or turning the head side-to-side. The vertical orientation of the saccule allows for sensing of pitch head tilts as well as vertical translations of the head (such as riding in an elevator).

Once the head moves and the endolymph displacement within the SCCs pushes the cupula and/or the otoconia pulls the otolithic membrane across the kinocilia and stereocilia, the stereocilia are sheared either toward or away from the kinocilia. Shearing of the stereocilia in the direction of the hair cell polarization opens potassium and calcium channels of the hair cell. Because endolymph is high in potassium (K^+) and is positively charged (+80 mV) relative to the hair cell, opening these channels allows potassium and calcium to flow into the cell, causing depolarization of the hair cell. Influx of these two ions results in release of the excitatory neurotransmitter, glutamate (Glu), the primary excitatory neurotransmitter released by the vestibular end organs (Sedó-Cabezón et al 2014; Soto et al 2013). **Fig. 15.13** illustrates the shearing of kinocilia and stereocilia, the influx of calcium (Ca^{++}) and potassium (K^+), and the subsequent release of glutamate (Glu). When the stereocilia are sheared away from the kinocilia, potassium and calcium channels are closed, causing hyperpolarization of the hair cell, and the release of glutamate is slowed. This inhibitory response leads to decreased firing on the saccular or utricular nerve within the vestibular portion of CN VIII.

Cranial Nerve VIII: The Vestibulocochlear Nerve

The release of neurotransmitters as a result of hair cell depolarization or hyperpolarization results in altered firing rate of the vestibular portion of CN VIII. The vestibulocochlear nerve has two main divisions: the cochlear branch, responsible for transmitting information from the cochlea, and the vestibular branch,

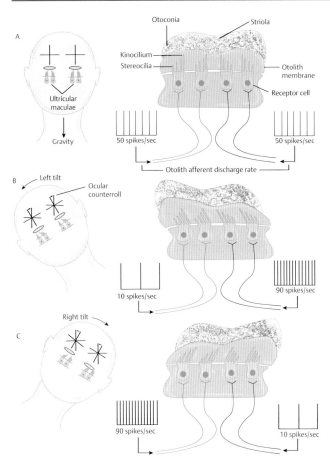

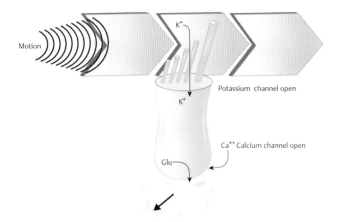

Fig. 15.13 With head movement, endolymph contained within the SCCs is displaced, leading to shearing of the kinocilia and stereocilia embedded in the sensory hair cells. When endolymph shears the stereocilia toward the kinocilium, potassium and calcium channels of the hair cell are opened, which allows potassium and calcium to flow into the hair cell. This influx leads to depolarization of the hair cell, causing the release of the excitatory neurotransmitter glutamate. The peripheral processes of CN VIII neurons contain receptors that absorb glutamate, which in turn leads to an increase in firing rate on the corresponding division of this nerve.

Fig. 15.12 The orientation and resting position of the kinocilia and stereocilia around the striola is shown for the utricle. In the utricle, the kinocilia and stereocilia are arranged around the striola such that on each side of the striola, the long kinocilium is closest to the striola and the shorter stereocilia are arranged in descending height from the kinocilium outward. This orientation of the kinocilia and stereocilia produces simultaneous excitation and inhibition of hair cells within the same utricle with appropriate head movements. For example, with a leftward head tilt, half of the stereocilia are sheared toward the kinocilium, and half of the stereocilia are sheared away from the kinocilium, which leads to depolarization of half of the hair cells and hyperpolarization of the other half. Therefore, the neural firing rate for fibers projecting into one half of the otolithic organ increases, while the neural firing rate for fibers projecting into the other half of the otolithic organ decreases. The response of the utricle for a rightward head tilt is also shown. Note the direction of shear and subsequent increased and decreased firing rates for separate portions of CN VIII.

responsible for transmitting information from the five sensory structures of the peripheral vestibular apparatus. The vestibular portion of CN VIII is further divided into superior and inferior branches, with each branch connecting to specific sensory structures of the vestibular labyrinth. The superior branch of the vestibular portion innervates the anterior and horizontal SCCs (the anterior and lateral ampullary nerves), the utricle (the utricular nerve), and the

"hook" portion of the saccule. The inferior branch of the vestibular portion innervates the posterior SCC (the posterior ampullary nerve) and the "shank" portion of the saccule (the saccular nerve; **Fig. 15.14**). These branches join to form the vestibular portion of CN VIII, which then joins with the cochlear portion of the nerve to form one nerve bundle that travels to the central structures of the auditory-vestibular pathway.

Interestingly, each of these branches of the vestibular portion of CN VIII fires continuously, even without stimulation. This response is likely due to a slow constant release of the excitatory neurotransmitter glutamate from the sensory hair cells, even when the cell is at rest. The resting firing rate of the vestibular portion of CN VIII is between 70 and 100 spikes per second, with an average of approximately 90 spikes per second. Displacement of the cupula or otolithic membrane as a result of head movement shears the kinocilia and stereocilia of the hair cells. If this shearing is in the direction of the hair cell polarization (i.e., with the kinocilia), the entire hair cell is depolarized and the neurotransmitter glutamate is released. This increase in the release of glutamate causes an increase in neural firing rate, thus an excitatory response. When stereocilia and kinocilia are sheared in the direction opposite of hair cell polarization, that is against the kinocilium, the hair cell is hyperpolarized and the release of glutamate is slowed significantly. Thus, nerve firing rate is decreased resulting in an inhibitory response.

Box 15.5   Clinical Correlation: Vestibular Schwannoma

Neoplasms can occur on cranial nerve VIII, the vestibulocochlear nerve. These tumors are typically slow growing and benign in that they do not erode into or replace brain tissue, so are therefore usually not life threatening. They have often been called acoustic neuromas, but most often, tumors on CN VIII arise from the vestibular division of the nerve and develop from Schwann cells (which produce myelin sheaths for peripheral nerve fibers), so they are most accurately termed vestibular schwannomas (**Box Fig. 15.4**). Vestibular schwannomas may result from the absence of a tumor suppressor gene, or they may be idiopathic in nature. Vestibular schwannomas may also develop as a result of neurofibromatosis type 2 (NF2), a disorder characterized by benign tumors on structures of the central nervous system. Most often, individuals with NF2 experience simultaneous or successive bilateral tumor growth affecting CN VIII. With the exception of individuals with NF2, most cases of vestibular schwannoma are unilateral.

Vestibular schwannomas are characterized by size. These tumors begin very small and are initially contained within the internal auditory canal. Larger growths tend to compress structures of the central nervous system, and symptoms therefore become more pronounced. Symptoms of vestibular schwannomas of small size include progressive hearing loss, speech comprehension difficulties, tinnitus, and dizziness. As the tumor grows, the brainstem, cerebellum, and other cranial nerves may be compressed, and individuals may experience all of the previously mentioned symptoms as well as facial weakness or numbness, difficulty swallowing, altered sense of taste, double vision, and headache. In rare instances, tumor growth may compress the brainstem and be fatal.

Initial treatment for vestibular schwannomas may be conservative and include monitoring the growth, with more aggressive treatment such as surgical removal during later stages. Surgical removal of the vestibular schwannoma typically leads to complete sacrifice of hearing and balance function. A third option is radiation therapy using Gamma Knife (Elekta, Stockholm, Sweden) technology. Gamma Knife radiation uses focused beams of radiation to retard the growth of the tumor, but does not destroy the tumor.

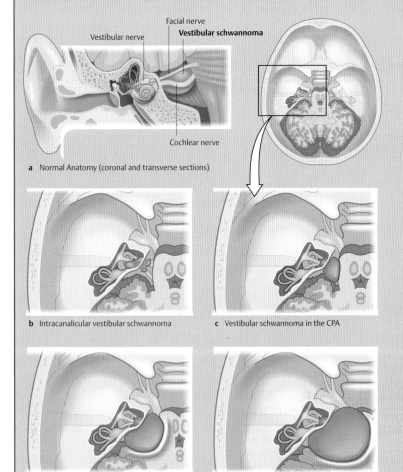

Facial nerve
Vestibular schwannoma
Vestibular nerve
Cochlear nerve

a   Normal Anatomy (coronal and transverse sections)

b   Intracanalicular vestibular schwannoma

c   Vestibular schwannoma in the CPA

d   Brainstem compressive stage

e   Final stage of vestibular schwannoma growth

Box Fig. 15.4   (a, b, c, d, e) Tumors of CN VIII are called vestibular schwannomas because they most often develop from Schwann cells of the vestibular branch of the nerve. When the tumor is smaller in size, it compresses the vestibulocochlear nerve, causing hearing loss, tinnitus, dizziness, and speech understanding difficulties to develop. As the tumor grows, it may begin to compress other surrounding structures such as the brainstem, facial nerve, and cerebellum, causing symptoms such as facial weakness or numbness, difficulty swallowing, headache, altered sense of taste, and double vision.

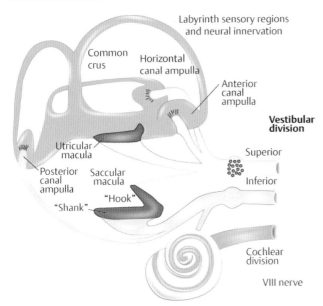

Fig. 15.14 Neural connections of CN VIII to the structures of the inner ear. CN VIII, the vestibulocochlear nerve, consists of a cochlear division and a vestibular division. The vestibular division is further subdivided into superior and inferior branches. The superior branch of CN VIII innervates the anterior SCC (anterior ampullary nerve), the horizontal SCC (the lateral ampullary nerve), the utricle (the utricular nerve), and the "hook" portion of the saccule. The inferior branch of CN VIII innervates the posterior SCC (posterior ampullary nerve) and the "shank" portion of the saccule (the saccular nerve).

Fig. 15.11 and **Fig. 15.12** illustrate the increase and decrease in firing rate of CN VIII for the SCCs and otolithic organs, respectively.

The increase or decrease in neural firing rate is transmitted along CN VIII to the central vestibular nervous system. At this point, the movement of the head has first produced fluid movement in the peripheral receptor apparatus, which has caused mechanical movement of the kinocilia and stereocilia, resulting in a neurochemical response. This neurochemical response leads to a change in the firing rate of CN VIII. Thus, head movement has been fully transduced into an electrical impulse that can be sent to the brain and other central nervous system structures for processing and interpretation.

■ The Central Vestibular Apparatus

Central Vestibular Nucleus Complex

The vestibulocochlear nerve originates in the brainstem as a cluster of nuclei called the **central vestibular nucleus complex** and projects to the

sensory organs of the peripheral vestibular system (the semicircular canals, the utricle, and the saccule). The central vestibular nucleus complex extends from the floor of the cerebellum through the brainstem, further connecting the structures of the peripheral receptor apparatus to higher structures in the brain. The central vestibular nucleus complex is not one structure but consists of two branches, one on each side of the brainstem, with four distinct nuclei on each side. These nuclei are the superior vestibular nucleus, the medial vestibular nucleus, the lateral vestibular nucleus, and the inferior vestibular nucleus (**Fig. 15.15**) (Barmack 2003). The central vestibular nucleus complex receives information from multiple sensory systems, integrates this information, and then distributes information to control reflexes in a number of systems of the body in response to vestibular input. This structure or set of structures plays a major role in our ability to maintain balance and upright posture.

The central vestibular nucleus complex is the first point of sensory integration for the maintenance of balance. This structure is responsible for the subconscious processing of peripheral vestibular, visual, and head/body movement information. In addition to the information received from the peripheral receptor apparatus about the movement and position of the head, the central vestibular nucleus complex receives visual input about the position of the head and body from the eyes. The central vestibular nucleus complex also receives information regarding

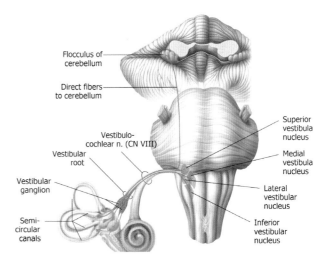

Fig. 15.15 Two sets of four nuclei (one set on each side of the brainstem) constitute the central vestibular nucleus complex within the brainstem. These nuclei are the superior, medial, lateral, and inferior vestibular nuclei. Neural signals from the peripheral vestibular apparatus are first sent along the vestibular division of CN VIII to the central vestibular nucleus complex for subconscious processing and integration with sensory input from the visual and somatosensory systems.

the reliability of the support (e.g., the ground) on which the individual is standing, the position of the body in space (e.g., lying down versus standing versus sitting), and the position of the body parts in relation to one another (e.g., having an arm extended over the head) from the proprioceptive and somato-sensory systems. Information regarding body posi-tion and the support surface reaches the central vestibular nucleus complex from the spinal system. The central vestibular nucleus complex integrates this multisensory information.

After receiving and processing information from multiple sensory systems, the central vestibular nucleus complex sends information to the visual system, cerebellum, spinal cord, thalamus, cortex, and reticular formation. Information sent to the visual system and cerebellum results in a set of reflexive eye movements that are equal in magnitude and opposite in direction of the movement of the head, the **vestibulo-ocular reflex**. Information sent to the spinal cord is used to generate **vestibulospinal reflexes**, which are postural reflexes to keep the body upright, the trunk centered over the hips, and the head centered over the trunk. The reticular formation is a structure within the brain involved with the regulation of cardiac function, breathing pattern, and state of arousal, as well as other functions. When postural changes are needed to prevent a fall as a result of loss of balance, cardiac function (blood flow) and breathing rate will increase in order to support the postural adjustment. A heightened state of arousal may also be needed to reduce the likelihood of the imminent fall. The signal from the central vestibular nucleus is also transmitted to higher centers of the brain, such as the thalamus and cortex, for conscious processing of motion and spatial orientation. **Fig. 15.16** outlines the connections between the central vestibular nuclei and the vestibular end organs, as well as the other sensory systems involved with the maintenance of balance.

If sensory information from the visual, proprioceptive, and vestibular systems is in agreement, balance is maintained and the individual will experience a feeling of quiescence or being still and at rest, rather than vertigo. If conflict exists between input from any of these sensory systems, the brain must choose which sensory information to rely upon, or the individual will experience a feeling of imbalance or true vertigo.

Vestibulo-Ocular Network

Reciprocal connections exist between the vestibular end organs and the visual system such that visual information is sent to the central vestibular nucleus complex to be integrated with vestibular input,

and the central vestibular nucleus complex sends information to the visual system to control reflexive eye movements in response to vestibular input. This series of reciprocal connections makes up the **vestibulo-ocular network**. The vestibulo-ocular network sends information to the vestibular system regarding the visual perception of head/body position, and to control eye movements in response to head movement (the vestibulo-ocular reflex). The vestibulo-ocular network also enables one to keep one's gaze fixed on an object when the head is moving.

Review of anatomy and physiology related to the ocular system is warranted in order to build

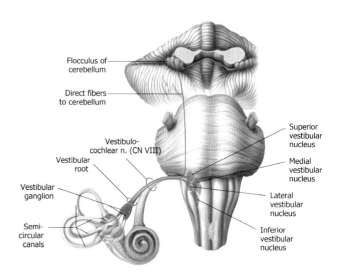

Fig. 15.16 Schematic illustrating the neural connections be-tween the central vestibular nuclei and three sensory systems, as well as between the central vestibular nucleus complex and the central nervous system structures that are responsible for maintenance of balance. Neural signals from the peripheral receptor apparatus are sent directly to the cerebellum and to the central vestibular nucleus complex. The central vestibular nucleus complex has reciprocal connections with the ocular and somatosensory systems, such that information is both sent to the central vestibular nucleus complex from these systems and sent from the central vestibular nucleus complex to these sensory systems. Visual and somatosensory input is sent to the central vestibular nucleus complex, where it is integrated with input from the peripheral vestibular apparatus. Once informa-tion from these three sensory systems is integrated, the central vestibular nucleus complex distributes information to the ocu-lar and somatosensory systems so that reflexive eye and pos-tural movements can be generated to maintain balance. The somatosensory (spinal) system, the peripheral receptor appa-ratus, and the ocular system are responsible for sensing infor-mation about the environment and the position of the head and body. The somatosensory and oculomotor systems are also responsible for reflexive movements in response to vestibular input. The central vestibular nucleus complex and the cerebel-lum are responsible for integration of these sensory inputs, and the thalamus and cortical areas are responsible for conscious perception of movement, balance, and spatial orientation.

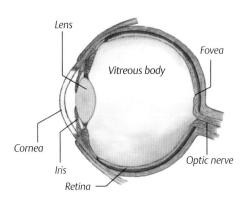

Fig. 15.17 Structures of the eye. The cornea is the clear covering on the eye. The iris is the pigmented part of the eye that dilates and constricts as the amount of ambient light changes. The lens functions to focus incoming light onto the retina, which contains the sensory cells of the eye. The point of highest visual acuity on the retina is the fovea. In order to view an object with the highest clarity, the eyeball must be oriented so that the image of interest is projected directly onto the fovea.

the connections between the vestibular and visual systems. The structure of the eye is shown in **Fig. 15.17**. Recall that the cornea is a clear covering on the surface of the eye, and the iris is the colored part of the eye that widens and constricts as the amount of light entering the eye changes. With more light, the iris constricts; with less light the iris dilates, or widens, to let in as much light as possible. The lens of the eye sits directly behind the iris and functions to focus incoming light on the retina. One of the most relevant structures of the eye related to the discussion of the vestibulo-ocular network is the **retina**, which contains the sensory cells (neuroepithelium) of the eye that capture incoming light and transduce it into a neural impulse that can be sent to the brain to be interpreted as a visual image. In the very center of the retina is the **fovea,** the region of the retina with the highest visual acuity. Images projected directly on the fovea are viewed with the highest resolution: and as the image moves farther from the fovea, image resolution declines and the image will be seen as more blurry. As you read this text (with normal or corrected vision), notice how the word you are currently reading is very clear, but the images in your periphery are blurred, even only slightly close to the word, and become more blurred the further in your periphery you attend. This phenomenon is why we look directly at what we want to see. When looking at something closely, we direct our gaze so that the image falls directly

on the fovea and is, therefore, seen with the greatest visual acuity.

The muscles of the eye (extraocular muscles) control reflexive eye movements that occur with input from the vestibular system. Each eye is equipped with six extraocular muscles (**Fig. 15.18**) that function to aim the eyeball. There are four rectus muscles (medial, lateral, superior, and inferior rectus muscles) and two oblique muscles (superior and inferior obliques). These extraocular muscles work in pairs to move the eye in specific directions such that when one muscle in the pair is contracted, the other muscle in the pair relaxes, creating a push-pull system. The medial and lateral rectus muscles function to move the eye horizontally; the superior and inferior rectus muscles function to move the eye vertically; and the superior and inferior obliques function to rotate the eye and, along with the rectus muscles, enable diagonal movement. All possible movements of the eye are shown in **Fig. 15.19**.

The six extraocular muscles of each eye are innervated by three cranial nerves. Cranial nerve III (oculomotor nerve) innervates the inferior rectus, medial rectus, and inferior oblique muscles on the ipsilateral side and the superior rectus muscle on the contralateral side. Cranial nerve IV (trochlear nerve) innervates the superior oblique muscle on the contralateral side. Cranial nerve VI (abducens nerve) innervates the ipsilateral lateral rectus muscle. This information is summarized in **Table 15.1**. Lesions in any of these three cranial nerves will lead to abnormal movements of the eye and may affect the ocular reflexes that occur in response to vestibular input.

These cranial nerves connect with the vestibular system via the **medial longitudinal fasciculus (MLF)**, a large nerve bundle with both ascending and descending tracts. The ascending tract of the MLF has projections that connect the central vestibular nucleus complex and the three cranial nerves that innervate the extraocular muscles: CN III, IV, and VI (Barmack 2003). This tract of the MLF carries most of the information between the central vestibular nuclei and the oculomotor nuclei, enabling the connection of the peripheral vestibular end organs (SCCs and otolithic organs) to the visual system. Therefore, this nerve fiber connection enables ocular reflexes to occur in response to vestibular input from head/body movement. The descending tract of the MLF connects the central vestibular nucleus complex to the spinal system.

Connections between peripheral vestibular structures and the ocular motor system allow compensatory eye movements when the head and/or body move. These compensatory eye movements are the first of three reflexes occurring in response to vestibular input: the vestibulo-ocular reflex previously mentioned. The vestibulo-ocular reflex is a collection of very-short-latency (~ 16 milliseconds) compensatory eye movements. The vestibulo-ocular reflex produces eye movements that are equal in magnitude and opposite in direction to the movement of the head, providing for stable gaze while the head is in motion. Without a functional

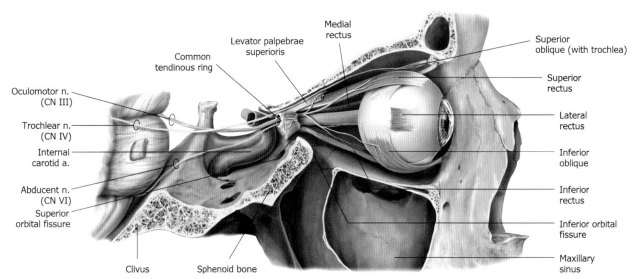

Fig. 15.18 Lateral view of the right eye showing the six extraocular muscles responsible for movement of the eye. These muscles work in functional pairs such that when one muscle in the pair is contracted, the other muscle of the pair is relaxed, serving to direct the eyeball. The functional pairs are the medial and lateral rectus muscles, the superior and inferior rectus muscles, and the superior and inferior oblique muscles. The insertion points for the superior, inferior, medial, and lateral rectus muscles enable the eye to move in the vertical (superior and inferior rectus) and horizontal planes (medial and lateral rectus muscles). The insertion points for the superior and inferior oblique muscles enable the eye to move diagonally and to rotate.

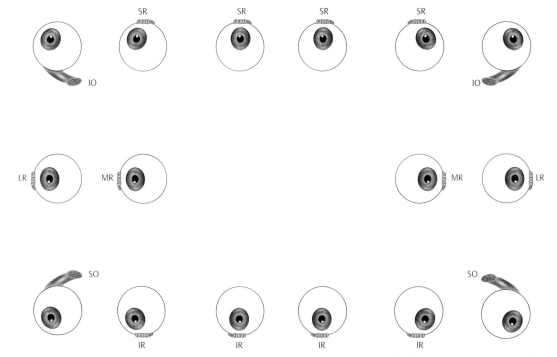

Fig. 15.19 All possible movements of the eye and the extraocular muscles responsible for each movement. Only the agonist (contracted muscle) of each functional pair is shown. For example, with a rightward gaze, the lateral rectus muscle of the right eye and the medial rectus muscle of the left eye are contracted, while the medial rectus of the right eye and lateral rectus of the left eye are relaxed.

Table 15.1   Innervation of and movements produced by the extraocular muscles

Extraocular muscle	Vertical eye movement	Horizontal eye movement	Rotary eye movement	Innervation
Superior rectus	Elevates	Adducts*	Rotates medially	CN III (oculomotor nerve)
Inferior rectus	Depresses	Adducts	Rotates laterally	CN III (oculomotor nerve)
Medial rectus	—	Adducts	—	CN III (oculomotor nerve)
Lateral rectus	—	Abducts**	—	CN VI (abducens nerve)
Superior oblique	Depresses	Abducts	Rotates medially	CN IV (trochlear nerve)
Inferior oblique	Elevates	Abducts	Rotates laterally	CN III (oculomotor nerve)

Data from Thieme Teaching Assistant, Table 35.3
*Adduct: To move toward the midline
**Abduct: To move away from the midline

vestibulo-ocular reflex, your vision would be blurred the entire time your head was in motion.

Neural signals generated in response to head movements in specific planes are sent to the central vestibular nucleus complex for integration with other sensory information, including information from the ocular system. The MLF then connects the central vestibular nuclei to the nuclei of the oculomotor, trochlear, and abducens nerves. These three cranial nerves innervate the ocular muscles and control their movement so that the muscles work in the functional pairs previously described. Head movement in the horizontal plane stimulates the horizontal SCCs and utricles, leading to compensatory eye movements in the horizontal plane (right- and leftward eye movements). Head movement in the vertical plane is transduced by the vertical SCCs (the anterior and posterior SCCs) and the saccules, which subsequently causes reflexive eye movements in the vertical plane (upward and downward eye movements). Stimulation of the vertical SCCs and utricles results in torsional (rotary) eye movements.

Stimulation of the Vestibulo-Ocular Reflex

A simple head turn toward the right will cause leftward compensatory eye movement. When the head is turned toward the right, the bony and membranous labyrinths of the SCCs are also accelerated toward the right. However, the viscoelastic properties of endolymph within the membranous labyrinth cause this fluid to lag behind. The endolymph ultimately moves in the opposite direction of the head movement. You can simulate this process using a simple bowl of water. If you turn the bowl of water in one direction, you can visualize how the water within lags behind slightly, and actually moves in the direction opposite that of the acceleration. Movement of the endolymph causes the cupula in each horizontal SCC to be deflected, causing excitation of the hair cells in the right horizontal SCC (depolarization) and inhibition of the hair cells in the left horizontal SCC (hyperpolarization). Depolarization of hair cells in the right horizontal SCC leads to increased firing rate of the lateral ampullary nerve within the vestibular portion of the right CN VIII, and hyperpolarization of the hair cells in the left horizontal SCC leads to decreased firing rate of lateral ampullary nerve within the vestibular portion of the left CN VIII. The signals then travel along the CN VIIIs to the central vestibular nucleus complex, where they are integrated with other sensory information. From the central vestibular nucleus complex, the signal crosses the midline and is sent to the contralateral CN VI (abducens nerve) nuclei, and then to the lateral rectus extraocular muscle and across the midline again to the CN III (oculomotor nerve) nuclei. From the CN III nucleus, the signal is sent to the ipsilateral medial rectus extraocular muscle. The excitatory reaction from the right horizontal SCC results in contraction of the lateral rectus muscle in the left eye and of the medial rectus muscle in the right eye. Additionally, the inhibitory response from the left SCC results in relaxation of the left medial rectus and right lateral rectus muscles. This pattern of contraction and relaxation of the extraocular muscles results in a leftward eye movement that is equal in magnitude and opposite in direction of the head turn (i.e., the vestibulo-ocular reflex). The vestibulo-ocular reflex is traced in **Fig. 15.20**.

If an individual was spinning and acceleration to the right continued, the eye would rotate to the left due to the vestibulo-ocular reflex but would reach maximal position in the orbit. Once the eye reaches the limit of the orbit, it recenters in a quick, jerking fashion mediated by the central nervous system. The result of this continuous acceleration to the right would be a slow drift of the eyes to the left, equal and

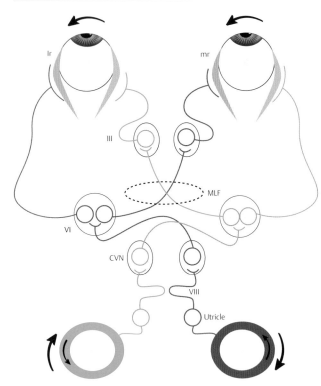

Fig. 15.20 Stimulation of the vestibulo-ocular reflex pathway by a simple rightward head turn. With rotation of the head toward the right, endolymph within the SCCs is displaced, which deflects the cupulas and shears the embedded kinocilia and stereocilia. Within the right horizontal SCC, the cupula is deflected toward the utricle, resulting in an excitatory response of the hair cells. The cupula of the left horizontal SCC is deflected away from the utricle, resulting in an inhibitory response. The excitatory response from the right horizontal SCC is sent via CN VIII to the central vestibular nucleus complex. From the central vestibular nucleus complex, the signal crosses the midline and is sent to the nuclei of CN VI (the abducens nerve). From CN VI nuclei, the excitatory signal is sent to the lateral rectus muscle of the left eye, triggering muscle contraction. The excitatory signal is also sent from CN VI nuclei back across the midline to the CN III nuclei and then to the medial rectus muscle of the right eye, which is subsequently contracted. The inhibitory signal from the left horizontal SCC can be traced similarly; however, the result is inhibition (relaxation) of the medial rectus muscle of the left eye and of the lateral rectus muscle of the right eye.

opposite relative to the head movement, with a quick jerk of the eyes back to the center of the orbit. This pattern of slow drift in the direction opposite from the head movement, with a quick jerking motion to recenter the eye is known as **nystagmus**. Nystagmus is an involuntary movement of the eyes consisting of two phases: a slow phase, most often mediated by the peripheral vestibular system, and a fast phase to recenter the eye, mediated by the central nervous system. Nystagmus can occur for a number of reasons and is often observed in individuals with lesions at some level of the vestibular pathway. You

can, however, cause temporary, nondamaging nystagmus by spinning around in place for 15 seconds or so. Once you cease spinning, have a friend observe your self-induced nystagmus. You can likely feel it, and your friend will see it if you keep your eyes open. Notice how the feeling of vertigo remains after you stopped spinning, and the nystagmus you experience should coincide with the vertiginous feeling. Nystagmus and vertigo should subside within a few seconds after you stop spinning.

Vestibulospinal Network

The visual system is not the only system that sends information to be integrated with vestibular input and responds when there is head and/or whole-body movement. One of the other systems that responds to head and/or body movement is the spinal network. This connection between the peripheral vestibular system and the spinal network is termed the vestibulospinal network. The **vestibulospinal network** connects the vestibular end organs to the spinal cord. Similar to the visual-vestibular connection (the vestibulo-ocular network), the connections within the vestibulospinal network are reciprocal, such that sensory input is received from the spinal cord to be integrated with vestibular input, and then the integrated information is sent back to the spinal cord to mediate postural reflexes.

Input to the vestibulospinal network comes from the somatosensory systems. These systems provide information about objects in the environment through touch and about the relative position of the parts of the body. The skin is the primary receptor for the somatosensory system, providing information about touch and pressure. Touch and pressure information from the feet when standing is sent to the brain to aid in our perception of where the body is located in space. When supine, the skin of the back, legs, arms, and back of the head provide the somatosensory information to perceive body position. The proprioceptive system is part of the somatosensory system, with the muscles, tendons, and joints functioning as proprioceptive receptors. These structures provide information regarding muscle tension and elongation so that the position of the limbs in space can be sensed without having to visualize where the limb is located. For example, if you were to extend your arm to the side and then close your eyes, it is your proprioceptive system that allows awareness that your arm is still extended, even though you cannot see it. Proprioceptive and somatosensory information about the position of the body and limbs is sent to the central vestibular nucleus complex and integrated with information about head and body movement from the peripheral end organs.

Once proprioceptive and somatosensory input is received by the central vestibular nucleus complex and integrated with information from the peripheral vestibular and visual systems, the vestibulospinal system sends information back to the spinal cord so that head movement, changes in axial musculature, and postural reflexes can be coordinated to maintain upright posture. Two major descending pathways connect the central vestibular nuclei to the spinal cord: the **lateral vestibulospinal tract** and the **medial vestibulospinal tract** (**Fig. 15.21**). These tracts mediate the remaining two of the three vestibular reflexes. Recall that the first vestibular reflex discussed was the vestibulo-ocular reflex, which is mediated by the vestibulo-ocular network and functions to control eye movements in response to vestibular input.

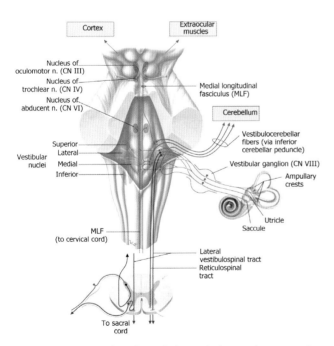

Fig. 15.21 Lateral and medial vestibulospinal tracts. The lateral vestibulospinal tract originates from the lateral and inferior vestibular nuclei and terminates in all levels of the spinal cord. This vestibulospinal tract mediates reflexive strategies to keep the center of gravity centered over the base of support in order to maintain upright posture. The medial vestibulospinal tract primarily originates from the medial vestibular nucleus and terminates in the cervical portion of the spinal cord and neck. The medial vestibulospinal tract mediates the vestibulocollic reflex, which functions to keep the head centered over the trunk.

Lateral Vestibulospinal Tract

The lateral vestibulospinal tract originates from neurons in the lateral and inferior vestibular nuclei and projects/terminates at all levels of the ipsilateral spinal cord. Actions of the lateral vestibulospinal tract are based upon information regarding head position received from the anterior and posterior SCCs and otolithic organs; the vestibulocerebellum; and proprioceptive and somatosensory information regarding body position from the spinal cord. The lateral vestibulospinal tract mediates postural reflexes below the neck to keep the trunk positioned over the **center of gravity** so that upright posture can be maintained. Four distinct **vestibulospinal reflexes** are mediated by the lateral vestibulospinal tract: the **ankle strategy**, the **hip strategy**, the **suspensory strategy**, and the **stepping strategy** (**Fig. 15.22**). The purpose of these strategies is to stabilize the body when the center of gravity has moved outside the base of support to help regain balance and prevent the individual from falling. The center of gravity is an imaginary point at which the mass of an object is equally balanced. The center of gravity in men and women has been found to be between approximately 54 and 58% of the individual's normal standing height, respectively, with the center of gravity only slightly higher in women compared to men (Croskey et al 1922). The exact center of gravity moves as an object changes shape or, in the case of the human, when we bend over, take a step, reach upward, or shift the body so that it is no longer in a straight vertical line as when standing. The **base of support** is defined as an outline of all ground contact points. In a standing position, the base of support is an imaginary oval-shaped outline around the feet. In a kneeling position, the base of support is the outline around the knees and feet. The optimal base of support in a standing position occurs when the feet are about shoulder width apart. This position provides the greatest stability. As the feet are moved closer together or are in tandem (heel to toe), the base of support, and therefore stability, is reduced.

The ankle strategy is used to correct small disturbances of balance and is accomplished through relatively small reflexive movements. With the ankle strategy, the leg muscles are contracted to keep the trunk aligned with the hips and knees, and the body moves on the ankle joints in a pendular motion. With slightly larger balance disturbances and in cases of reduced base of support, the hip strategy is used. As in the ankle strategy, the leg muscles are used to realign the trunk; however, the motions are completed on a larger scale. In addition to contractions of the leg muscles, the hips and head are moved in

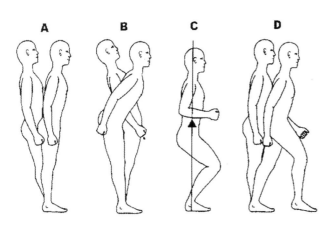

Fig. 15.22 The four vestibulospinal reflexes mediated by the lateral vestibulospinal tract are the ankle strategy, the hip strategy, the suspensory strategy, and the stepping strategy. **(a)** The ankle strategy is used for very small disturbances of balance. With this strategy, the leg muscles are contracted in order to keep the trunk aligned with the hips and knees. **(b)** For slightly larger disturbances of balance, the hip strategy is used. Using this strategy, the leg muscles are contracted and the hips and head are moved in opposite directions to redistribute the weight of the individual in order to maintain the center of gravity over the base of support. **(c)** The suspensory strategy is used when the base of support is reduced or the support surface is unreliable. With this strategy, stability can be increased by lowering the center of gravity, which is achieved through flexion of the knees, ankles, and hips. **(d)** The stepping strategy is used when the center of gravity has moved outside the base of support. With the stepping strategy, a corrective step, stumble, or hop is used to regain balance. This strategy is used when other reflexive movements are not sufficient to regain balance and/or upright posture.

opposite directions, wherein with forward movement of the head, the hips move back, and vice versa. This movement of the head and hips in opposing directions aids in redistributing weight to maintain a center of gravity within the base of support. Think of a gymnast on a balance beam and visualize the stance. The feet are in tandem, so the base of support is reduced. It is difficult to move on the balance beam while maintaining completely upright posture, which is part of gymnast training. Instead, the novice typically shifts her hips and head in opposite directions. The individual will also typically crouch down slightly, which brings us to discuss the suspensory strategy. These two strategies aid the person on

the balance beam with the maintenance of balance when the base of support has been reduced.

The suspensory strategy is used to lower the center of gravity, thereby increasing stability. Think of an action movie where the hero or heroine jumped onto a moving bus or train. Their feet were likely shoulder width apart or just slightly wider and they were probably crouched slightly. This crouched position is an example of the suspensory strategy. Using this strategy, the individual flexes at the knees, ankles, and hips, which lowers the center of gravity closer to the base of support. The last vestibulospinal reflex is the stepping strategy. The stepping strategy is used when very large corrections are needed, particularly in cases where the center of gravity has moved outside of the base of support and when other reflexive movements are unsuccessful in restoring balance. The stepping strategy typically involves a corrective step or stumble to regain upright posture. Each of the vestibulospinal reflexes may be reflexive or volitional. The stepping strategy is one example of a vestibulospinal reflex used quite often volitionally. During normal ambulation, the stepping strategy is used when the center of gravity is purposefully moved outside the base of support and a forward step (stepping strategy) is taken.

Medial Vestibulospinal Tract

The medial vestibulospinal tract primarily originates from the medial vestibular nucleus and terminates in the cervical portion of the spinal cord and neck. Actions of this tract are based upon input from the semicircular canals, utricles, and saccules, as well as the vestibulocerebellum and spinal cord. The medial vestibulospinal tract causes reflexive movements that function to keep the head centered over the body in response to vestibular stimulation. This reflex is known as the **vestibulocollic reflex**, or the head-righting reflex, because it functions to "right" the head when it becomes off-center relative to the position of the body. The vestibulocollic reflex is the third of three reflexive movements in response to vestibular input, causing the contraction and relaxation of muscles in the neck to stabilize the head when movement is sensed by the otolithic organs and semicircular canals. The vestibulocollic reflex causes head movement opposite in direction from a perceived falling motion.

In summary, the vestibulospinal network sends information about the position of the body in space to be integrated with information about head position sensed by the peripheral vestibular system and visual information about the head position sensed by the ocular system. All of this sensory information is integrated at the level of the central vestibular nucleus complex, from which information is sent to control postural reflexes to regain balance and maintain upright posture.

Central Vestibular Nervous System

In addition to receiving multisensory information and sending projections to the peripheral vestibular, ocular, and spinal systems, the central vestibular nucleus complex also sends ascending projections to the cerebellum, thalamus, and eventually two cortical areas. Connections between the peripheral vestibular apparatus and the thalamus and cortical areas make up the **vestibulothalamocortical network**. The vestibulothalamocortical network is responsible for further integration and processing of information from the vestibular, visual, and somatosensory systems to achieve conscious perception of balance and of the position and movement of the body in space.

The thalamus and two distinct cortical regions are the primary structures of this network. These connections are shown in **Fig. 15.1**.

In general, the thalamus is responsible for processing, modulating, and sending information to the cortex. The thalamus functions similarly in the vestibulothalamocortical network. The thalamus has two divisions, one on each side of midline, positioned at the top of the brainstem (**Fig. 15.23**). Neurons from the central vestibular nucleus complex project directly into these two parts of the thalamus, both ipsilaterally and contralaterally. Information received by the thalamus from the central vestibular nucleus complex maintains directional specificity that was encoded in the transduction process at the peripheral end organs (e.g., increased firing rate on the right lateral ampullary nerve and decreased firing rate on the left lateral ampullary nerve, indicating a rightward turn of the head). The thalamus also receives information from the visual and spinal systems, which is integrated with information from the peripheral vestibular system. Processing of this

---

Box 15.6 Clinical Correlation: Vestibular Evoked Myogenic Potentials

The vestibulocollic reflex is often measured in patients reporting difficulty with dizziness or imbalance using a test called the cervical vestibular evoked myogenic potential (cVEMP). In cVEMP, electrode sensors are placed on the patient and an intense acoustic stimulus is presented using insert earphones or a bone conduction oscillator. This loud acoustic stimulus is sensed by the saccule, which is not typically used for perception of acoustic stimuli in humans but has remnants as an acoustic receptor in lower animals and can still respond if a stimulus is intense enough. When the saccule receives this intense acoustic stimulus, the signal is sent via the inferior branch of CN VIII to the central vestibular nucleus complex, which then sends an inhibitory response to the ipsilateral sternocleidomastoid muscle in the neck. With this assessment, the function of the saccule, the inferior branch of CN VIII, the central vestibular nucleus complex, and the medial vestibulospinal tract is evaluated.

The patient is asked to contract the sternocleidomastoid muscle by lifting or turning the head. The measured response is the electrical potential caused by relaxation of this muscle, displayed as a waveform that can be analyzed for amplitude (size) and latency (time of the response following stimulation). Although an acoustic stimulus is used, structures of the *vestibular* system are being assessed through

an *evoked* response that is measured as a muscular ("*myogenic*") electric *potential*. Cervical VEMP can be used to determine whether specific pathologies of the peripheral or central vestibular pathways are present, including vestibular neuritis, Ménière's disease, superior canal dehiscence, and vestibular schwannoma, as well as neurologic pathologies such as multiple sclerosis and lesions of the brainstem.

Similarly, the vestibulo-ocular reflex is recorded during ocular vestibular evoked myogenic potential (oVEMP) protocols, which assess function of the utricle and superior branch of CN VIII. During oVEMP, electrodes are placed directly underneath the eyes and the individual is instructed to gaze upward while sitting or supine. The excitatory, myogenic precursors (the electrical activity generated in the eye muscles just before movement occurs) from the inferior oblique and inferior rectus muscles are measured. oVEMP is considered a "crossed" response, which occurs on the opposite side of midline from stimulation. For example, when assessing the right utricle and superior branch of CN VIII, the response from the left ocular muscles is observed. As with cVEMP, oVEMP is displayed as a waveform that is analyzed in terms of latency and amplitude of the response. Abnormal oVEMP results have been found in individuals with BPPV, vestibular neuritis affecting the superior portion of CN VIII, superior semicircular canal dehiscence, and Ménière's disease, as well as neurologic disorders such as multiple sclerosis.

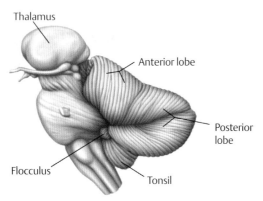

Fig. 15.23 Left lateral view of the brainstem, thalamus, and cerebellum. The thalamus is positioned at the top of the brainstem and has two divisions, one on each side of the midline. The thalamus receives vestibular input from the central vestibular nucleus complex, as well as input from the visual and somatosensory systems. The paraflocculus lobe (tonsil), anterior lobe, and posterior lobe of the cerebellum are also shown. The tonsil is involved with control of ocular and spinal reflexes in response to vestibular input, and the posterior lobe receives direct afferent and efferent projections from the central vestibular nuclei.

information enables cognitive distinction between active head movements (voluntary rotations) and passive head movements that occur when the entire body is moved, as well as the ability to distinguish different types of head rotations (Lopez and Blanke 2011). Multisensory processing at the level of the thalamus enables the conscious perception of movement and of the orientation of the body in space. Following thalamic processing, the integrated sensory information is then sent to the cortex for higher-level processing and interpretation.

Although no well-defined area of the cortex is thought to be the primary vestibular cortex, cortical areas 2v and 3a have been identified as the primary regions responsible for the perception of balance. Other regions of the brain, however, are also likely to contribute to the sense of balance, including the frontal lobe, parietal cortex, and hippocampus. Projections from the thalamus reach areas 2v and 3a on both sides of the brain (bilaterally). Cortical areas 2v and 3a are part of the **primary somatosensory cortex**, which is responsible for processing information from the somatosensory and proprioceptive systems such as touch, muscle tension, and joint pressure. Along with the input perceived by the peripheral vestibular apparatus and thalamus, area 2v receives information regarding pressure on the joints, as well as input from the visual system regarding the position of the head. Cortical area 2v uses this proprioceptive and visual input, along with input sensed by the peripheral end organs, for the conscious perception of movement. Area 3a receives input from the thalamus and peripheral receptor apparatus, as well as proprioceptive input regarding muscle elongation and contraction. This cortical area is responsible for volitional and reflexive motor control of the head and body when movement is perceived by the peripheral vestibular system, visual system, and proprioceptive systems. The result of the vestibulothalamocortical network is conscious perception of balance, the sense of gravity, the perception of the head and body in space, and sensation of movement

---

Box 15.7   Clinical Correlation: Lesion of the Cerebellum

Stroke can occur due to hemorrhage or due to restricted blood flow (ischemia) in a particular region of the brain. Hemorrhage or ischemia can cause permanent or transient damage to the brain, and symptoms during and following the event will vary based on the area of the brain that is affected. Symptoms of stroke are sudden in onset and include numbness or weakness of the face, arm, or leg; confusion; difficulty speaking; visual difficulty; and severe headache. When the stroke affects the cerebellum, central vestibular nucleus complex, or connections between the peripheral and central vestibular structures, vertigo, imbalance, and lack of coordination resulting in difficulty walking are common. Diplopia (double vision), nausea, and dysarthria (difficulty speaking or understanding speech) may also occur.

Although no treatments reverse permanent damage caused by stroke, therapies designed to minimize the damage caused during the stroke are available and stop the hemorrhage or dissolve the clot. However, these therapies must be administered acutely. Rehabilitation may be necessary poststroke to return the individual to a normal or near normal level of functioning.

Since the cerebellum has such an important role in the coordination of ocular motor and vestibulospinal reflexes, cerebellar involvement is likely to result in abnormal vestibulo-ocular and vestibulospinal reflexes. The vestibulo-ocular reflex may be present but delayed in latency (timing), may produce inaccurate movements, or may be completely absent. Additionally, the vestibulospinal reflex may be compromised, leading to impaired gait and postural instability.

(i.e., acceleration), as well as the motor planning involved in both reflexive and volitional movements.

The central vestibular nucleus complex and the peripheral vestibular apparatus also send projections to the cerebellum. The cerebellum is located dorsal to the brainstem and comprises a central midline structure called the vermis and two cerebellar hemispheres. The hemispheres of the cerebellum can be further divided into three lobes: the flocculonodular lobe, the anterior lobe, and the posterior lobe (**Fig. 15.24**). Because of the extensive connection to the vestibular system, the flocculonodular lobe, including the flocculus and nodulus, is also called the **vestibulocerebellum**. The vestibulocerebellum is one of the phylogenically oldest portions of the cerebellum and has also been referred to as the archicerebellum (Kheradmand and Zee 2011). Reciprocal connections exist between the peripheral vestibular system and the cerebellum, as between the peripheral vestibular system and visual and proprioceptive/somatosensory systems. Much of the input to the vestibulocerebellum is directly from projections of CN VIII, which directly connect the cerebellum to sensory cells of the peripheral vestibular system. The otolithic organs primarily connect with the uvula of the cerebellum, and neural fibers from the SCCs primarily project to the nodule (Barmack and Yakhnitsa 2011). Additionally, the posterior lobe of the cerebellum is connected to the central vestibular nuclei through both afferent and efferent projections (Gilman and Newman 2003). The paraflocculus (tonsil) has also been shown to be involved with ocular motor control and control of the limbs and axial musculature in response to vestibular input (Barmack 2003; **Fig. 15.24**).

The primary function of the vestibulocerebellum is coordination of both volitional (goal-oriented) and reflexive movements of the head, body, and eyes in response to vestibular input (Heck et al 2013). The majority of this coordination is subconscious; however, some evidence supports some cognitive control by the cerebellum. The vestibulocerebellum controls ocular movements that constitute the vestibulo-ocular reflex and can make adaptive changes to ocular movements that are occurring as a result of changes in head and body position. Interestingly, the vestibulocerebellum also contributes to ocular motor learning such that when retinal errors are made, the system can "learn" and adapt a new strategy to reduce the likelihood of repeating erroneous eye movement (Kheradmand and Zee 2011). Similarly, the vestibulocerebellum controls postural adjustments during vestibulospinal reflex actions and can learn to adapt when errors in reflexive postural adjustments occur (Pompeiano 2006).

Intact cerebellar function is imperative for proper function of the vestibulo-ocular reflex as well as the vestibulospinal reflexes. Lesions of the vestibulocerebellum can cause dizziness, disturbances of gait, imbalance, as well as abnormalities with the vestibulo-ocular reflex and vestibulocollic reflex (Shaikh et al 2011). Additionally, the vestibulocerebellum is crucial for adaptation following damage to the vestibular system. Damage to the vestibular system can cause significant dizziness and imbalance. Over time, the central system, through the vestibulocerebellum, can compensate and reduce the feelings of dizziness and imbalance experienced due to the damaged vestibular system. The cerebellum plays a crucial role in the coordination of postural reflexes and ocular motor movements in response to vestibular input.

■ Summary

The feeling of quiescence (being at rest), the maintenance of upright posture, and the ability to sense the position of the head and body in space are accomplished through the interaction of multiple sensory systems, including structures of the inner ear, the visual system, and the somatosensory system. The interconnections of these systems has been discussed in terms of the vestibulo-ocular and vestibulospinal systems. Specifically, these systems function to send sensory information to be integrated with information from the peripheral

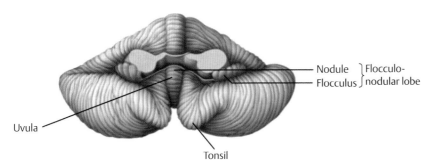

Fig. 15.24 Anterior view of the cerebellum showing the flocculonodular lobe (including the nodule and flocculus), the tonsil, and the uvula. The flocculonodular lobe has also been termed the vestibulocerebellum because of the extensive connection to the vestibular system. Neural fibers from the otolithic organs project to the uvula, and neural fibers from the SCCs primarily project to the nodule.

Uvula

Nodule ⎤ Flocculo-
Flocculus ⎦ nodular lobe

Tonsil

vestibular apparatus, which is accomplished at the level of the central vestibular nucleus complex. These systems receive this integrated information from the central vestibular nucleus so that reflexive eye and postural movements can be coordinated. These reflexive movements, and volitional eye and postural movements, are coordinated by multiple structures within the oldest portion of the

---

Box 15.8   Clinical Correlation: Migraine-Associated Vertigo

Migraines are a common and often debilitating condition that can be associated with vertigo or imbalance; however, migraine-associated symptoms of the auditory and vestibular systems vary widely across individuals. Migraines may be caused by a number of factors and may occur with or without the classic accompanying headache (Olesen 2004). Commonly reported symptoms of migraine include photophobia (sensitivity to light), decreased sound tolerance, nausea, decreased hearing sensitivity, tinnitus, and migraine-associated vertigo.

It can be difficult to diagnose migraine-associated vertigo with complete certainty due to marked variability in reported symptoms. Many individuals with migraine-associated vertigo do not experience classic migraine headaches with their vestibular symptoms. However, a history of migraine is a strong diagnostic indicator in individuals who experience vestibular deficits. Individuals may report true vertigo, imbalance, unsteadiness, or a combination of the three. Individuals may report vertiginous symptoms brought on by a change in position (i.e., positional). Others experience vertigo spontaneously (without cause); still others report experiencing both positional and spontaneous vertigo. Some individuals with migraine-associated vertigo report auditory symptoms such as loss of hearing sensitivity, tinnitus, otalgia, and aural fullness, which may be unilateral or bilateral. Interestingly, the loss of hearing sensitivity may be subjective and not measureable via standard hearing acuity testing audiogram (Johnson 1998).

Prevention is the most effective management strategy for migraine-associated vertigo. Prophylactic treatment can include dietary restrictions and lifestyle modification. Since migraines are often precipitated by certain foods and beverages, known triggers such as caffeine, chocolate, cheese, processed meats, and red wines should be avoided. Stress reduction, exercise, and enhanced sleeping patterns are also often recommended. Pharmacologic interventions may also be used in order to reduce the likelihood of developing migraine symptoms.

Box 15.9   Clinical Correlation: Vestibular Assessment

Assessment of vestibular system function and management of vestibular disorders are part of the defined scope of practice for audiologists. As such, audiologists must understand anatomy and physiology of the entire balance system, including the peripheral vestibular apparatus, vestibulo-ocular network, vestibulospinal network, vestibulocerebellum, and vestibulothalamocortical connections. Lesions at any point along the pathway can cause vertigo, nausea and emesis, imbalance and unsteadiness, as well as other conditions such as headaches and blurred vision. During vestibular assessment, a detailed case history is critical to determine which assessments should be performed. Frequently used assessments in the vestibular test battery include videonystagmography (VNG), passive and active rotational tests, vestibular evoked myogenic potentials (VEMP), electrocochleography (ECochG), auditory brainstem response (ABR), and posturography or the modified clinical test of sensory integration (mCTSIB). For example, VNG and mCTSIB enable evaluation of ocular motor movements and postural changes, respectively, in response to vestibular input. Others, such as ABR, ECochG, and VEMP, provide objective data regarding the function of specific structures within the vestibular system.

The results of the case history along with diagnostic audiometric (hearing test) and vestibular testing will be used to narrow down the suspected site of lesion. Based on all available information, the suspected site of lesion will be classified as a peripheral lesion, a lesion of the central vestibular pathway, lesions of both peripheral and central pathways, or lesions in other systems of the body unrelated to the peripheral or central vestibular systems. In most cases, the audiologist can also determine the specific site of lesion within each system, which would then be communicated to the referring physician in order to facilitate a management plan for the disorder. In some cases, medical management of symptoms through medications and/or surgical interventions is indicated. Individuals may also benefit from nonmedical management, such as repositioning maneuvers and a vestibular rehabilitation treatment program, to recover optimally from the vestibular disorder.

cerebellum, the vestibulocerebellum. Another central nervous system structure involved with maintenance of balance is the reticular formation in the brainstem. This structure functions to regulate respiration, heart rate, and state of arousal and responds accordingly when head and/or body movement is sensed by the peripheral receptor apparatus. Information about head and body position sensed by the peripheral vestibular system is also sent directly to the thalamus and cortex for processing. These structures further integrate and process this multisensory input to achieve conscious perception of movement and spatial orientation.

■ References

Barmack NH. Central vestibular system: vestibular nuclei and posterior cerebellum. *Brain Research Bulletin, 60,* 511–541; 2003

Barmack NH, Yakhnitsa V. Topsy turvy: functions of climbing and mossy fibers in the vestibulo-cerebellum. *The Neuroscientist, 17,* 221–236; 2011

Ciuman RR. Auditory and vestibular hair cell stereocilia: relationship between functionality and inner ear disease. *The Journal of Laryngology and Otology, 125,* 991–1003; 2011

Croskey MI, Dawson PM, Luessen AC, Marohn IE, Wright HE. The height of the center of gravity in man. *American Journal of Physiology, 61,* 171–185; 1922

Gilman S, Newman SW. Manter and Gatz's Essentials of Clinical Neuroanatomy and Neurophysiology, 10th ed. Philadelphia, PA: F.A. Davis Publishing Company; 2003

Heck DH, De Zeeuw CI, Jaeger D, Khodakhah K, Person AL. The neuronal code(s) of the cerebellum. *The Journal of Neuroscience, 33,* 17603–17609; 2013.

Johnson GD. Medical management of migraine-related dizziness and vertigo. *Laryngoscope, 108*(1), 1–28; 1998

Kheradmand A, Zee DS. Cerebellum and ocular motor control. *Frontiers in Neurology, 2,* article 53; 2011

Lindeman HH. Regional differences in structure of the vestibular sensory regions. *The Journal of Laryngology and Otology, 83,* 1–17; 1969

Lopez C, Blanke O. The thalamocortical vestibular system in animals and humans. *Brain Research Reviews, 67,* 119–146; 2011

Olesen J. The International Classification of Headache Disorders, 2nd edition. *Cephalalgia, 24*(1 Suppl):1–160; 2004

Pompeiano; 2006

Sedó-Cabezón L, Boadas-Vaello P, Soler-Martín C, Llorens J. Vestibular damage in chronic ototoxicity: a mini-review. *NeuroToxicology, 43,* 21–27; 2014

Shaikh AG, Marti S, Tarnutzer AA, et al. Ataxia telangiectasia: a "disease model" to understand the cerebellar control of vestibular reflexes. *Journal of Neurophysiology, 105,* 3034–3041; 2011

Soto E, Vega R. Neuropharmacology of vestibular system disorders. *Current Neuropharmacology, 8,* 26–40; 2010

Soto E, Vega R, Seseña E. Neuropharmacological basis of vestibular system disorder treatment. *Journal of Vestibular Research, 23,* 119–137; 2013

Tumarkin A. Stereocilia versus kinocilia Part II: the vestibular sensors. *The Journal of Laryngology and Otology, 100,* 1107–1114; 1986

■ Suggested Readings

Angelaki DE, Cullen KE. Vestibular system: the many facets of a multimodal sense. *Annual Review of Neuroscience, 31,* 125–150; 2008

Barmack NH. Central vestibular system: vestibular nuclei and posterior cerebellum. *Brain Research Bulletin, 60,* 511–541; 2003

Ciuman RR. Auditory and vestibular hair cell stereocilia: relationship between functionality and inner ear disease. *The Journal of Laryngology and Otology, 125,* 991–1003; 2011

Kheradmand A, Zee DS. Cerebellum and ocular motor control. *Frontiers in Neurology, 2,* article 53; 2011

Lopez C, Blanke O. The thalamocortical vestibular system in animals and humans. *Brain Research Reviews, 67,* 119–146; 2011

Sedó-Cabezón L, Boadas-Vaello P, Soler-Martín C, Llorens J. Vestibular damage in chronic ototoxicity: a mini-review. *NeuroToxicology, 43,* 21–27; 2014

■ Study Questions

1. Which of the following systems contribute to our ability to maintain balance and upright posture?

A.   The visual system
B.   The proprioceptive system
C.   The vestibular system
D.   The somatosensory system
E.   All of the above

2. The structures of the vestibular peripheral receptor apparatus do which of the following?

A.   Aid with the sense of hearing
B.   Transmit an electrical signal about head position to the brain
C.   Transduce head movements into a neural impulse
D.   Control reflexive eye movements
E.   Control reflexive postural changes

3. What type of fluid is found inside the membranous labyrinth of the peripheral vestibular apparatus?

A.   Blood
B.   Perilymph
C.   Cerebrospinal fluid
D.   Endolymph
E.   Saline

4. Which structure of the peripheral receptor apparatus allows for the perception of forward linear acceleration, as if you were riding in an accelerating car?

A.   Horizontal semicircular canal
B.   Anterior semicircular canal
C.   Posterior semicircular canal
D.   Saccule
E.   Utricle

5. Which semicircular canal(s) is/are responsible for transducing the angular head translation of pitch?

A.   Anterior
B.   Posterior
C.   Horizontal
D.   A and B
E.   B and C

6. At what angle do the utricles and horizontal semicircular canals sit relative to the naso-occipital plane?

A.   Not tilted at all but parallel with the naso-occipital plane
B.   Tilted 60° up
C.   Tilted 60° down
D.   Tilted 30° down
E.   Tilted 30° up

7. The neuroepithelium of the semicircular canals is contained within which of the following structures?

A.   Ampulla
B.   Cupula
C.   Otolithic membrane
D.   Otoconia
E.   Type I hair cells

8. Which of the following statements accurately describes the arrangement of kinocilia and stereocilia on the sensory hair cells?

A.   There are equal numbers of stereocilia and kinocilia on each hair cell.
B.   There is a single kinocilium with thousands of stereocilia on each hair cell.
C.   There is a single stereocilium with 50 to 100 kinocilia on each hair cell.
D.   There is a single kinocilium with 50 to 100 stereocilia on each hair cell.
E.   There is no way of knowing how many kinocilia and stereocilia are on each hair cell because they are too tiny to see.

9. Which of the following is necessary to stimulate the sensory hair cells of the otolithic organs?

A.   A force strong enough to move the otoconia and drag the otolithic membrane to shear the kinocilia and stereocilia
B.   Endolymph movement, which shears the kinocilia and stereocilia
C.   Perilymph movement, which shears the kinocilia and stereocilia
D.   Cupular movement
E.   Electric neural impulse

10. Which of the following statements is true regarding the orientation of the kinocilia and stereocilia on the hair cells in the semicircular canals?

A. The kinocilia and stereocilia are oriented toward the striola.
B. The kinocilia and stereocilia are oriented away from the striola.
C. The kinocilia and stereocilia are all oriented in the same direction within each semicircular canal.
D. The kinocilia and stereocilia are oriented in a haphazard manner within each semicircular canal.
E. There are no kinocilia or stereocilia contained within the semicircular canals.

11. What is the smallest possible number of semicircular canals that can be stimulated with an angular excursion of the head?

A. 5
B. 4
C. 3
D. 2
E. 1

12. The firing rate of the vestibulocochlear nerve increases in which of the following situations?

A. Kinocilia and stereocilia are sheared in the direction of the hair cell polarization.
B. Kinocilia and stereocilia are sheared in the direction opposite the hair cell polarization.
C. Glutamate rushes into the hair cell.
D. Calcium and potassium rush out of the hair cell.
E. Endolymph rushes out of the hair cell.

13. Which of the following statements accurately describes the function of the central vestibular nucleus complex?

A. Conscious perception of balance
B. Provide structural support of the brainstem
C. Connect the visual and proprioceptive/somatosensory systems
D. Conscious perception of spatial orientation
E. Receive, integrate, and distribute information from the visual, vestibular, and proprioceptive/somatosensory systems

14. Which of the following structures of the eye is used to view an object of interest with the greatest visual acuity?

A. Cornea
B. Iris
C. Fovea
D. Retina
E. Lens

15. Which of the following statements most accurately describes the function of the vestibulo-ocular network?

A. Connect the peripheral vestibular apparatus with the ocular motor system
B. Send visual information regarding the position of the head to the central vestibular nucleus complex
C. Receive information from the central vestibular nucleus that has been integrated with vestibular and proprioceptive/somatosensory information
D. Generate reflexive eye movements in response to input from the peripheral vestibular system
E. All of the above

16. The medial vestibulospinal tract is responsible for which of the following types of reflexive movements?

A. Changes in axial musculature
B. Reflexive movements of the neck
C. Flexing of the hips and ankles
D. Movement of the hips and head in opposite directions
E. Corrective step or stumble

17. Which of the following vestibulospinal reflexes is used when the center of gravity moves outside of the base of support?

A. Suspensory strategy
B. Stepping strategy
C. Hip strategy
D. Ankle strategy
E. Head-righting reflex

18. Which of the following statements accurately describes the function of the thalamus in the vestibulothalamocortical network?

A. It integrates information from the central vestibular nucleus complex, visual system, and proprioceptive/somatosensory systems for conscious perception of movement and the position of the body.
B. It performs subconscious processing of information from the peripheral receptor

apparatus, visual system, and proprioceptive/somatosensory systems.

C. It carries out the final processing stage of multisensory input for the maintenance of balance.

D. It performs motor planning of reflexive movements of the head and body in response to vestibular input.

E. It performs motor planning of volitional movements of the head and body in response to vestibular input.

19. Cortical areas 2v and 3a are responsible for which of the following tasks?

A. Subconscious processing of multisensory input for the maintenance of balance

B. Transduction of head movement into a neural impulse

C. Conscious perception of movement and the position of the head and body in space

D. Adaptation of reflexive movements when errors in movements are made

E. Coordination of reflexive eye and postural movements in response to vestibular input

20. Which of the following is *not* an accurate statement about the vestibulocerellum?

A. The vestibulocerebellum is responsible for coordination of visual and postural reflexes in response to vestibular input.

B. All areas of the cerebellum are used to some degree in the processing of vestibular information.

C. Fibers of CN VIII project directly into the vestibulocerebellum.

D. Most processing of information in the vestibulocerebellum is accomplished at subconscious levels.

E. The vestibulocerebellum will learn and adapt when erroneous reflexive eye and postural movements are made.

■ Answers to Study Questions

1. Answer (E) is correct. Input from the peripheral vestibular system regarding head movement is integrated with information about head position from the visual system as well as information about head and body position from the proprioceptive and somatosensory systems. This multisensory input is used to maintain balance and upright posture through reflexive eye and postural movements.

2. Answer (C) is correct. The structures of the peripheral receptor apparatus that function as sensory organs are the horizontal, anterior, and posterior SCCs, the utricles, and the saccules. The fluid inside the membranous labyrinth of these structures is displaced when the head is moved, ultimately generating a neural impulse that is sent to the brain by way of CN VIII.

The peripheral vestibular system is continuous with the organ of hearing, both of which are contained within the inner ear, but the peripheral vestibular apparatus does not aid with the sense of hearing (A). The five sensory structures of the peripheral receptor apparatus sense the position of the head that leads to the generation of an electrical impulse, but this signal is transmitted to the brain by the CN VIII, the vestibulocochlear nerve, not the periphal receptor structures (B). Lastly, while reflexive eye movements and postural movements are generated in response to the peripheral vestibular input, this is done by central nervous system structures, not the peripheral receptor apparatus (D), (E).

3. Answer (D) is the only correct choice. Endolymph is the fluid contained within the membranous labyrinth of the peripheral receptor apparatus. During head movement, the endolymph in the semicircular canals is displaced and pushed against the cupula, shearing the kinocilia and stereocilia. This process ultimately produces a signal regarding head movement, to be sent to the brain for processing.

Perilymph is found between the membranous and bony labyrinths (B). Perilymph is similar to cerebrospinal fluid in chemical composition, but cerebrospinal fluid is not found in the membranous labyrinth (C). Neither blood nor saline is normally found in the structures of the peripheral vestibular apparatus (D), (E).

4. Answer (E) is accurate because the otolithic organs respond to linear acceleration, and the utricle specifically responds to movements in the horizontal plane; therefore the utricle would respond during forward acceleration such as riding in an accelerating vehicle.

The saccule is responsible for the sensing of movement in the vertical plane, such as the vertical linear acceleration experienced in a moving elevator (D). The horizontal, anterior, and posterior SCCs are not sensitive to linear accelerations (A), (B), (C). Therefore, without the otolithic organs, linear acceleration would not be sensed.

5. Answer (D) is correct because the anterior and posterior semicircular canals are vertically oriented in the skull and therefore respond to rotations of the head in the vertical plane such as pitch.

Both sets of vertical canals respond during head rotations of pitch, not just one set, anterior (A) or posterior (B). The horizontal canals do not respond during head translations of pitch (C), (E).

6. Answer choice (E) is correct; the utricles and horizontal SCCs are oriented at a 30° angle relative to the naso-occipital plane. Additionally, the saccules and vertical SCCs sit 60° below the naso-occipital plane. These orientations are important because during ambulation, the head is typically pitched downward approximately 30° so that the eyes are easily focused on the ground in front of the individual. Equally important are the positions of the peripheral sensory organs. With the head pitched downward 30°, the utricles and horizontal SCCs sit completely horizontal and parallel with the force of gravity, and the saccules and vertical SCCs sit completely vertical, making all five peripheral sensory structures maximally sensitive to head movements (and thus potential loss of balance and fall!).

Answer (A) is incorrect because the utricles and horizontal canals are slightly tilted and do not sit exactly parallel with the naso-occipital plane. Answer choices (B), (C), and (D) incorrectly state the angle of the utricles and horizontal SCCs in the skull.

7. Answer A is accurate. The actual sensory cells, the hair cells, of the SCCs are located within the ampulla at the base of each SCC. Fluid movement in the ampulla pushes against the cupula, which shears the kinocilia and stereocilia atop the sensory hair cells.

The cupula is a gelatinous structure contained within the ampulla, in which the kinocilia and stereocilia of the neuroepithelium are embedded (B). The otolithic membrane is similar to the cupula in form, but it is located in the otolithic organs (C). The otoconia lie on top of the otolithic membrane and do not contain any sensory cells (D). Type I hair cells *are* the sensory cells of the neuroepithelium (E).

8. Answer (D) is correct. There are 50 to 100 stereocilia with a single longer kinocilium on each hair cell. These tiny hairlike receptors are arranged in ascending height, with the tallest stereocilia closest to the single kinocilium.

There are not equal numbers of stereocilia and kinocilia on each hair cell (A). Thousands of stereocilia would not physically fit on a single hair cell (B). There is a single kinocilium and many stereocilia on each hair cell (C). Finally, the number of kinocilia and stereocilia has been verified through histologic and electron microscope study (E).

9. Answer (A) is correct. The hair cells of the otolithic organs respond only when a strong force moves the otoconia, dragging the gelatinous otolithic membrane across the kinocilia and stereocilia of the utricle or saccule. Specifically, the otolithic organs respond when the position of the head is changed relative to the force of gravity.

The hair cells of the otolithic organs do not respond with simple endolymph movement (B). Perilymph is not contained within the otolithic organs (C). The cupula is located in the semicircular canals, not the otolithic organs (D). Lastly, the otolithic organs generate the electric neural impulse; they do not respond to it (E).

10. Answer (C) is correct because all hair cells within one SCC are polarized in the same direction. This is possible only because the kinocilia and stereocilia are oriented in the same direction on all hair cells within an SCC. The kinocilia and stereocilia of the same SCC on the opposite side of the head are arranged in a mirror image. This arrangement enables the canals to work in functional pairs (push-pull system).

The striola is found in the utricle and saccule, not the SCCs (A), (B). Answer choices (D) and (E) are simply incorrect.

11. Answer (D) is correct because with even the most simplistic movements of the head, such as right-to-left head rotation, at least two SCCs respond. The SCCs work in functional pairs such that when one canal in a pair (e.g., the left horizontal SCC) is excited, the other canal in the pair (e.g., the right horizontal SCC) is inhibited. This push-pull system ensures that an equal but opposite response is sent from both sides of the peripheral vestibular system so that the head movement is perceived accurately.

The SCCs function in pairs, so an odd number of responding canals is not possible (A), (C), (E). Although four canals could respond to head rotation, four is not the smallest number of responding canals possible (B).

12. Answer A is correct. The firing rate of CN VIII, the vestibulocochlear nerve, increases when the kinocilia and stereocilia are sheared in the direction of the hair cell polarization; that is, toward the kinocilium. This directional shearing depolarizes the hair cell and opens the calcium and potassium channels so that these two ions rush into the cell. The result is a neurochemical reaction causing the release of the excitatory neurotransmitter glutamate. Upon receiving the neurotransmitter glutamate, the firing rate of the nerve fiber on the vestibular portion of CN VIII that synapses on the hair cell is increased. This results in an excitatory response of the hair cell and vestibular portion of CN VIII.

Shearing of the kinocilia and stereocilia in the direction opposite the hair cell polarization (i.e., away from the kinocilium) would result in hair cell hyperpolarization, slowed influx of calcium and potassium, slowed release of glutamate, an inhibitory response that leads to a decreased firing rate of the vestibular portion of CN VIII. Glutamate travels out of the hair cell, not into it (C), and calcium and potassium rush into the hair cell, not out of it (D). Endolymph does not enter the hair cell (E).

13. Answer (E) is correct. The central vestibular nucleus complex receives information from the visual, vestibular, and proprioceptive/somatosensory systems and integrates this information. The central vestibular nucleus complex then distributes information so that reflexive eye and postural movements can be coordinated to aid in the maintenance of balance and upright posture.

The central vestibular nucleus complex processes this multisensory input at a subconscious level; conscious processing of both balance and spatial orientation occurs at the cortical level (A), (D). The central vestibular nucleus complex is a structure in the brainstem; however, the main function of the central vestibular nucleus complex is not structural support (B). Lastly, while the central vestibular nucleus complex does receive and integrate information from the visual and proprioceptive/somatosensory systems, the main function of the central vestibular nucleus complex is not connecting these two systems (C).

14. Answer (C) is correct. The retina contains the neuroepithelium of the eye and is therefore responsible for transducing the image of an object into a neural signal that can be processed and interpreted by the brain. The fovea is located in the center of the retina and is the region of the retina with the greatest visual acuity. When viewing an object of interest, an individual will look at the object so that the image is projected directly on the fovea.

Objects projected elsewhere on the retina, away from the fovea, are not viewed clearly (D). The cornea is the clear covering on the eye and mostly serves a protective and refractive function (A). The iris controls the amount of light entering the eye by dilating and constricting as the amount of ambient light changes (B). The lens functions to focus incoming light onto the retina (E).

15. Answer (E) is correct. The vestibulo-ocular network connects the peripheral receptor apparatus with the ocular motor system so that visual information can be received and integrated with vestibular input for accurate sensing of the head position in space. This integrated information is then distributed so that reflexive eye movements, the vestibulo-ocular reflex, can be generated to aid in the maintenance of balance and the feeling of being at rest.

Answers (A), (B), (C), and (D) are not accurate because none of these choices fully describes the scope of the vestibulo-ocular network function.

16. Answer (B) is correct. The medial vestibulospinal tract is one of the two vestibulospinal tracts of the vestibulospinal network. This tract begins in the central vestibular nucleus complex and terminates at the cervical spinal cord and in the neck. The medial vestibulospinal tract mediates reflexive movements to keep the head centered over the trunk. This reflex is called the vestibulocollic reflex, or the head-righting reflex.

Answers (A), (C), (D), and (E) relate to reflexive movements mediated by the lateral vestibulospinal tract. This tract of the vestibulospinal system also originates at the central vestibular nucleus complex; however, it terminates at all levels of the spinal cord. The lateral vestibulospinal tract mediates all postural reflexes below the neck, including the ankle, hip, suspensory, and stepping strategies.

17. Answer (B) is correct. When the center of gravity has moved outside the base of support, smaller postural adjustments are not likely to restore balance. In this case, the individual is likely to use the stepping strategy to take a corrective step or stumble. The stepping strategy is the last resort to keep the individual from falling when a loss of balance occurs.

The ankle strategy (D) is used with small disturbances of balance, and this strategy leads to contraction of the leg muscles so that the legs pivot on the ankles in a pendular motion; this strategy would not restore balance if the center of gravity moved outside of the base of support. Using the hip strategy (C), the head and hips are moved in opposite directions to redistribute weight; however, this strategy would not be sufficient to restore balance if the center of gravity moved outside the base of support. The suspensory strategy (A) involves lowering the center of gravity; however, if the center of gravity is outside the base of support, this strategy would not be useful. Lastly, the head-righting reflex (E) would serve to protect the head if a fall were to occur because the head would be moved opposite the direction of the fall. However, this reflexive movement would have no effect on the restoration of postural stability.

18. Answer (A) is correct. The thalamus receives and integrates information from the central vestibular nucleus complex, the visual system, and the proprioceptive/somatosensory systems. The processing that occurs at the level of the thalamus enables cognitive distinction between active head rotation (voluntary) and passive head rotation (which occurs when the whole body is moved). Processing at the level of the thalamus also enables distinction between specific types of head rotations.

Information from the peripheral end organs, visual system, and proprioceptive/somatosensory systems is integrated and subconsciously processed (B) at the level of the central vestibular nucleus complex, not the thalamus. The thalamus is not the final processing point of this multisensory input; from the thalamus the integrated signal is sent to two areas of the cortex for further processing (C). The thalamus is not responsible for motor planning of either reflexive (D) or volitional (E) movements in response to vestibular input.

19. Answer (C) is correct. Cortical areas 2v and 3a are responsible for the conscious perception of movement. 2v and 3a are also involved with the sensation of gravity and motor planning for both reflexive and goal-oriented movements of the eyes and body.

Subconscious processing of multisensory input first occurs at the level of the central vestibular nucleus complex, not the cortex (A). Cortical processing results in conscious perception. The transduction of head movement into a neural impulse occurs at the level of the peripheral end organs, not the cortex (B). Coordination of reflexive eye and postural movements occurs in the vestibulocerebellum (E), which is also responsible for motor learning and adaptation when erroneous movements are made (D).

20. Answer (B) is correct. The specific areas of the cerebellum that have been identified as contributing to ocular motor and musculoskeletal control are the flocculus and nodule of the vestibulocerebellum, as well as the paraflocculus (tonsil) and uvula.

The vestibulocerebellum is responsible for the coordination of visual and postural reflexes in response to vestibular input (answer A), and the vestibulocerebellum is capable of learning and adapting when errors are made in the reflexive movements it has coordinated (answer E). These visual reflexes are manifested as the vestibulo-ocular reflexes and the vestibulospinal reflexes. Fibers of CN VIII do project directly into the cerebellum (C). The cerebellum also receives fibers from the central vestibular nucleus complex. Processing at the level of the vestibulocerebellum is primarily on a subconscious level (D); however, it is possible that there is at least some conscious processing and control of the reflexive movements coordinated by the vestibulocerebellum.

Glossary

A

A bands Striations in myofibrils that contain the primary contractile proteins: actin and myosin

abducens nerve (CN VI) A small pure motor nerve that innervates the lateral rectus muscle of the eye; *see also* **oculomotor nerve (CN III)**, **trochlear nerve (CN IV)**

abduct To move a structure away from the midline

accessory nerve (CN XI) A motor nerve that innervates two muscles that control head and shoulder movements

acetylcholine (ACh) The neurotransmitter used for signaling a muscle to contract, also used in numerous locations in the central nervous system; *see also* **postsynaptic acetylcholine receptor (AChR)**

acetylcholinesterase (AChE) An enzyme located in the synaptic cleft that breaks down acetylcholine (ACh) into choline (which the presynaptic cell recycles) and acetate, regulating how much ACh is available to bind to postsynaptic receptors

achalasia Condition in which the smooth muscle of the esophagus does not relax, making it difficult for a bolus to flow through the esophagus

achromatopsia Loss of perception of color although retinal input into the visual system is normal, due to cortical damage at the juncture of the posterior temporal lobe and the occipital lobe

acoustic radiations A band of fibers that connect the medial geniculate body to auditory cortical areas

acoustic reflex Tightening of the stapedius and tensor tympani muscles in response to loud sounds, increasing the impedance of the ossicular chain to protect the inner ear

actin A protein that forms a thin filament that resembles two strings of pearls intertwined together, which is the location of the myosin contractile head binding site; together with myosin, actin provides contractile filaments of muscle cells and other sensory cells; it is also found in outer and inner hair cells

action potential A depolarization followed by a repolarization across the neuronal membrane that proceeds continuously along the axon without diminishment; typically represents the output information from the neuron; *see also* **all-or-none response**

action potential–initiating segment The site on a neuron where an action potential is initiated—typically, although not necessarily, the axon hillock

action tremor An involuntary rhythmic movement that is manifest when the individual attempts an action

active transport The transport of molecules in an energetically unfavorable direction across a membrane, coupled to the hydrolysis of ATP or other source of energy

adduct To move a structure toward the midline

adenoids Lymphoid tissue within the nasopharynx, also known as the pharyngeal tonsil

adenosine triphosphate (ATP) A nucleotide molecule containing the base adenine and the sugar ribose, with two more phosphate ions added; adding the second and especially the third phosphate group takes energy, and removing that group releases the energy to do useful work in the cell, such as muscle contraction or pumping ions across the cell membrane against a gradient

adherens junction A region of cell–cell adhesion at which the actin cytoskeleton is anchored to the plasma membrane

admittance Ability to transmit energy; the reciprocal of impedance

adult stem cells Undifferentiated cells found among differentiated cells in a tissue or organ

aerobic respiration Process of producing cellular energy involving oxygen

afferent Pertaining to conveying or carrying something (e.g., sensory information) toward something (e.g., the central nervous system)

affinity The strength of binding between a ligand such as a neurotransmitter or neuromodulator with its corresponding receptor; the tighter the binding, the greater the affinity of the receptor for the ligand

agonist (1) A chemical agent that binds to a receptor to replicate, to some degree, the action of the receptor's natural ligand such as a neurotransmitter; (2) A muscle whose contraction causes joint rotation in the intended direction. *See also* **antagonist**

air conduction Transmission of acoustic waves in air via the outer ear to the tympanic membrane

airway obstruction A blockage formed by foreign or endogenous material in the airway; it can be life-threatening.

akinesia   Loss of movement; for example, the loss of normal facial expressions in Parkinson's disease

ala (plural, alae)   A winglike projection

alkalemia   A condition in which the blood is too alkaline

all-or-none response   The principle that the electrical potential across the neuronal membrane must exceed a certain threshold before an action potential is generated; if there is an action potential at all, feedback mechanisms maintain the amplitude of the action potential over the whole length of the axon, so when the electrical potential across the neuronal membrane is less than the threshold, there is no action potential (none), but if the threshold is exceeded, the action potential is generated in its full strength (all)

allantois   Saclike structure that helps the embryo exchange gases and handle liquid waste

allele   One of the possible variations of a gene that an individual may possess, such as a single-base change or a variable number of nucleotide repeats

allophone   A member of a class of speech sounds that all represent one phoneme; which of the allophones is selected to represent the phoneme depends on particular conditions at the moment of production

alpha lower motor neuron (α-LMN)   A neuron in the brainstem or spinal cord whose axon synapses on a main extrafusal (outside the spindle) muscle fiber; *see also* **gamma lower motor neuron (γ-LMN)**

alveolar ducts   Branches of the respiratory bronchioles

alveolar macrophages   Cells that continually remove waste products from the alveolar wall

alveolar ridge   A ridge that forms the borders of the upper and lower jaws and contains the sockets of the teeth

alveolar sac   Group of alveoli that share a common opening into an alveolar duct

alveolar ventilation rate   The volume of air (per minute) actually involved in gas exchange within the respiratory zone

alveolus   Terminal of the airway and site of gas exchange between the respiratory and circulatory systems

amacrine cell   A cell involved in adjusting the output from bipolar cells in the retina by lateral inhibition; *see also* **horizontal cell**

amniotic cavity   The closed sac between the embryo and the amnion, containing amniotic fluid

amniotic membrane (amnion)   The membrane closest to the embryo, which fills with amniotic fluid and serves to protect the embryo

AMPA-type receptor   A type of glutamine receptor found on the synapses of the peripheral processes of Type I spiral ganglion neurons

amphipathic   Having both hydrophobic and hydrophilic regions within a molecule

amplitude   The level of acoustic power produced during vocal fold vibration; it corresponds to the perceptual quality of loudness and is measured in decibels (dB)

amplitude perturbation   Subtle change in amplitude of an oscillation from cycle to cycle; in a voice it is referred to as shimmer

ampulla   A swelling at the base of each semicircular canal, where the semicircular canal joins the vestibule, containing the hair cells of the semicircular canals that translate rotational accelerations of the head

amygdala   A nucleus within the limbic system (of each cerebral hemisphere) that lies deep within the anterior temporal lobe and is involved in regulating fear responses

anaerobic respiration   Cellular energy metabolism that occurs when oxygen is absent or scarce

anaphase   The shortest stage of mitosis, following metaphase and preceding telophase, during which chromosomes separate and the sister chromatids move to opposite poles of the cell

anatomic position   Standard posture, in which the full body is standing straight with the face directly forward, arms hanging down at the sides and palms facing forward, with fingers pointing straight down, knees facing forward, and feet slightly apart and pointed forward; used as a reference to describe a body part relative to another

anatomy   The study of the structure of a living organism

angle   A corner; a feature of the shape of a bone or other anatomic structure

angular gyrus   A gyrus that lies posterior to the supramarginal gyrus in the parietal lobe; it appears to have a central role in semantic processing (particularly understanding metaphors)

anion   An atom or molecule with more electrons than protons and therefore with a negative charge

ankle strategy   One of the four vestibulospinal reflexes, used for small disturbances of balance, in which the leg muscles are contracted to realign the trunk with the hips and knees; *see also* **hip strategy**, **stepping strategy**, **suspensory strategy**

annular ligament   Tissue that attaches the footplate of the stapes to the oval window

ansa cervicalis Branch of hypoglossal nerve that provides motor innervation to most of the infra-hyoid muscles

antagonist (1) A chemical agent that binds to a receptor to block the action of the receptor's natural ligand such as a neurotransmitter; (2) A muscle whose contraction causes joint rotation in the direction opposing the intended direction

anterior In front of, or before, another structure

anterior auditory field (AAF) A major subdivision of the primary auditory cortex

anterior cerebral artery (ACA) The blood vessel that supplies the frontal lobes, corpus callosum, and medial surfaces of the cerebral hemispheres

anterior commissure (in brain) Fiber bundle that connects the ventral frontal lobe and anterior temporal lobe across the hemispheres; (in larynx) The anterior point of attachment of vocal folds on the thyroid cartilage

anterior lingual primordia Cephalic pair of lingual primordia, located at the level of the first branchial arch; *see also* **root primordia**

anterior neuropore Rostral opening of the neural tube

anterior semicircular canal One of the three semicircular canals of the inner ear, oriented to the front (anterior) and top (superior) of the vestibular labyrinth and responsible for translating vertical head movements into neural impulses

anterior ventral cochlear nucleus (AVCN) One of three major divisions of the cochlear nucleus in the brainstem; *see also* **dorsal cochlear nucleus (DCN)**, **posterior ventral cochlear nucleus (PVCN)**

anterolateral system (ALS) A set of somatosensory pathways in the central nervous system that conveys information related to pain, temperature, crude touch, tickle, and itch from all parts of the body though the anterior and lateral spinothalamic tracts of the spinal cord

anticholinergic Blocking (antagonistic to) the effects of the neurotransmitter acetylcholine

antidromic action potential An action potential that travels in an axon toward the cell body from which the axon originated.

antihelix Cartilaginous ridge of the pinna, proximal to the helix

antrum Cavity in a body organ, especially a bone

aortic body A chemoreceptor within the aortic arch

aperiodic Not repeating at regular intervals of time; aperiodic sound waves are perceived as noise rather than tones; *see also* **harmonic frequency**

apex Tip

apnea Temporary cessation of breathing

apneustic center Part of the respiratory CPG, located within the lower pons; it assists in inspiration by exciting the dorsal respiratory group within the medulla

apraxia A disorder of movement typically not associated with weakness, sensory loss, or dysfunction of the basal ganglia or cerebellum; typically, the movements maintain a relatively normal appearance but are out of context, such as using a pen upside down

arachnoid barrier A tight junction on the arachnoid mater that separates the extracellular fluids from the cerebral cortex

arachnoid granulations Small protrusions of the arachnoid into the dura mater; also called arachnoid villi

arachnoid mater The middle layer of the meninges, containing a layer of cells that are bound tightly; the space below the arachnoid layers contains the major arterial vessels and the cerebrospinal fluid, which adds buoyancy to the brain.

arachnoid trabecula (plural, arachnoid trabeculae) A strengthening fiber that traverses the subarachnoid space and bears a passing resemblance to a spider web

arachnoid villus (plural, arachnoid villi) *See* **arachnoid granulation**

archicerebellum The flocculonodular lobe of the cerebellum, distinguished from the other regions by its anatomic connections to the vestibular system

archipallium The primitive cortex included in the rhinencephalon

articulate To join

articulation The act of moving different parts of the vocal tract to make different sounds

aryepiglottic folds The most superior aspect of the quadrangular membrane, connecting the arytenoid cartilages to the epiglottis and containing the cuneiform cartilages

aryepiglottic muscle Muscle fibers that are extensions of the oblique interarytenoid; its function is not well understood

arytenoid cartilages A pair of cartilages within the larynx to which the vocal folds attach; their rotation by the muscles of the larynx allows the vocal folds to be tensed, relaxed, or approximated (brought together)

aspiration Drawing of solid or liquid material such as food or saliva into the airway beneath the level of the vocal folds; see also **penetration**

aspiration pneumonia A lung infection resulting from food, saliva, liquids, or vomit entering into the lungs/airway

association The strength of the co-occurrence of allele and phenotype in sets of individuals; association in this context is defined for genetic studies

associational cortex Regions of the cerebral cortex other than those areas that directly receive information from the peripheral nervous system (for example, the auditory, somatosensory, and visual cortex) or directly project to effectors, such as muscles (for example, the motor and supplementary motor cortex); typically, there are various types of associational cortex depending on which primary cortex that the associational cortex projects to

astrocyte A type of glial cell that has numerous projections extending from its cell body that make contact with neurons but do not transmit information; instead, they provide metabolic support for neurons, create the blood–brain barrier, and may play important roles in neurotransmitter regulation

ataxia An abnormal movement in which the course or trajectory of the movement is abnormal; typically, it is irregular, in contrast to tremor, which is regular

atelectasis Partial or (rarely) total collapse of a lung

athetosis Continuous slow, sinuous movements caused by a hyperkinetic disorder

atmospheric pressure The pressure of the air outside the body; for inhalation to occur, the air pressure inside the lungs must be lower than atmospheric pressure

ATP *See* **adenosine triphosphate (ATP)**

attributable risk A measure of the public health impact of an exposure or characteristic (such as a gene); it is the rate of disease occurrence ("risk") in a group that carries a particular gene

audiometer A device used for measuring hearing sensitivity.

auditory brainstem response (ABR) Electrical signals generated by the cochlear branch of the vestibulocochlear nerve and the cochlear nuclei in the brainstem in response to an auditory stimulus; in individuals with normal hearing, the recording contains five to seven positive-going peaks, termed waves I–VII, that occur within the first 10–15 milliseconds after the onset of the auditory stimulus

auditory cortex *See* **primary auditory cortex**

auditory neuropathy/dyssynchrony A hearing disorder in which the outer hair cells of the cochlea are functionally normal, but sound information is not properly transmitted to the cochlear branch of the vestibulocochlear nerve and/or central auditory system

auditory nerve The vestibulocochlear nerve or its cochlear branch

auditory vesicle An invaginated structure consisting of epithelium surrounding a fluid-filled sac embedded in mesoderm, and that lies close to the early developing hindbrain and the developing vestibulocochlear-facial ganglion complex.

aural atresia Complete closure of the external auditory canal

auricle The external ear, formed of cartilage, which serves to focus sound pressure waves into the external auditory canal; also called pinna

auricular fold An elongated elevation that develops caudal to the three hillocks on the second arch and that arises during the sixth week of development

auricular hillocks Six small swellings that form from the first and second branchial arches during the sixth week of development at the hyoid-mandibular arch area and that give rise to the auricle

autocrine signaling Cell signaling in which molecules act on the same cells that produce them

autonomic nervous system (ANS) Part of the peripheral nervous system that delivers signals from the brain to regulate automatic or unconsciously directed bodily functions, such as heart rate, breathing, digestion, urination, and fight or flight responses

autoreceptor A receptor for a neurotransmitter that is located on the same presynaptic membrane from which the neurotransmitter is released; the neurotransmitter binding to the autoreceptor causes a change in further release of the neurotransmitter

autosomal recessive Of a heritable medical condition, manifesting only if both parents are carriers of the same mutation

autosome A chromosome that is not a sex chromosome; humans have 22 pairs of autosomes, numbered from the largest to the smallest, and receive one member of each pair from each parent

axial plane A horizontal plane that divides a region into superior and inferior parts; also called horizontal plane, transverse plane, or transaxial plane

axoaxonal synapse A synapse where an axon terminal contacts an axon of another neuron

axodendritic synapse A synapse where an axon terminal contacts a dendrite of another neuron

axon A long process (extension) of a nerve cell body (soma), also known as a nerve fiber, that conducts action potentials (the electrical nerve impulses) downstream (away from the cell body) to the terminal bouton and that makes synaptic contacts with other neurons, muscles, or glands; distinguished by the presence of voltage-gated ion channels that create positive and negative feedback necessary for action potential generation and conduction; *see also* **action potentials** and **soma**

axon collaterals   Minor branches of an axon

axon hillock   The junction of the axon and the soma of a neuron, typically a place where action potentials may be generated; *see also* **action potential–initiating segment**

axon terminal   The distal or terminal (end) structure of an axon that typically synapses on post-synaptic structures, such as another neuron or muscle fiber

axosomatic synapse   A type of synapse where an axon terminal contacts a soma of another neuron

α-LMN   *See* **alpha lower motor neuron**

B

babbling   Infant behavior that practices speech patterns before speech is developed

Babinski sign   A reflex typically seen in the presence of dysfunction of the corticospinal tract: when a painful stimulus such as scratching is applied to the lateral aspect of the plantar surface (sole) of the foot, the great toe extends and the other toes flex and flare

ballismus   Wild, flailing movements caused by a hyperkinetic disorder

bands   Alternating regions of dark and light that appear when chromosomes are stained

baroreceptor   Sensor within the blood vessels and kidneys that is able to detect changes in blood pressure

basal ganglia   A collection of deep (subcortical) gray matter nuclei that lie within the medial part of each cerebral hemisphere and appear to have a central role in the inhibition and release of action; they receive information from, and project to, wide regions of the nervous system including the supplementary motor area, motor cortex, and various motor-related structures in the brainstem, but they also function in emotion and cognitive function

base of support   an imaginary outline of all ground contact points; in a standing position, the base of support is an imaginary oval around the feet

basement membrane   A sheetlike extracellular matrix that supports epithelial cells and surrounds muscle cells, adipose cells, and peripheral nerves

basement membrane zone (BMZ)   A zone between the squamous epithelial layer and the superficial lamina propria in the vocal fold, containing fibrous proteins that connect the two layers

basilar artery   Blood vessel located at the base of the pons where the two vertebral arteries fuse

basilar membrane (BM)   The membrane that forms the floor dividing the scala media from the scala vestibuli in the cochlea and carries the organ of Corti; it varies from its base to its apex in thickness, stiffness, and width

beat interactions   Interactions between two oscillators (such as two different sound sources) that produce a third oscillation based on the differences in the frequencies of the initial two oscillators; for example, when a chord is played on a stringed instrument, such as a piano, additional pitches can be heard corresponding to the differences between the fundamental frequencies of the strings struck

behavioral control assembly   A hypothesized pool of neurons shared among the respiratory, swallowing, and cough central pattern generators, controlling them based on received afferent stimuli

belt   Secondary auditory cortical tissue that surrounds the primary auditory cortex or core

Bernoulli effect   Reduction in pressure in a more rapidly moving region of a flow of fluid

beta oscillation theory   A theory that the pathophysiology underlying Parkinson's disease is based on excessive oscillations in neuronal activities in the basal ganglia in the beta range (typically 15 to 30 Hz).

bifurcation   A relatively sudden change in the state of some system, typically one of two or more potential states; for example, consider a coin in the state of balancing on its edge until something else disturbs the coin and it falls flat in one of the two flat states—heads or tails; there has been a bifurcation from the upright state to either the heads or tails flat state

binocular visual zone   The central portion of the visual field created by the overlap of the left and right visual hemifields

bioenergetics   The process by which cells (such as muscle cells) use resources such as oxygen from air and molecules from food and liquid consumed to obtain energy and store it as ATP

bipolar neuron (bipolar cell)   A neuron that has a single dendrite extending in one direction from the soma and the axon extending in the opposite direction

blastocyst A structure formed about five days after fertilization that contains an inner cell mass, an outer layer of cells called the trophoblast, and an inner cavity called the blastocoele

blastomere A type of cell produced by cleavage (cell division) of the zygote after fertilization

blood–brain barrier Tight junctions formed by the endothelial cells in the blood vessels of the brain and glial end feet projections of astrocytes; the blood–brain barrier closely regulates diffusion of substances into and out of the central nervous system in order to maintain homeostasis of the extracellular environment

body stalk Connection of extraembryonic mesoderm between the chorion frondosum and the embryonic disc

bolus A cohesive mass of food and liquid that should travel together through the swallowing mechanism

bone The calcified supporting connective tissue forming the major portion of the skeleton of most vertebrates; in humans it is either compact bone or spongy bone

bone conduction Mechanical sound transmission through the skull that stimulates the inner ear directly

Boyle's law The principle that increases in volume of a gas produce decreases in pressure as temperature is held constant

brachium conjunctivum The output pathway from the deep cerebellar nuclei that is directed rostral to the red nucleus and thalamic nuclei

bradykinesia Abnormal slowness of movement, as might occur in Parkinson's disease

brainstem The caudal portion of the brain that is continuous with the spinal cord and contains the midbrain, pons, and medulla

branchial arches *See* **pharyngeal arches**

branchial grooves *See* **pharyngeal grooves**

branchial pouches *See* **pharyngeal pouches**

Broca aphasia A language disorder that is characterized by difficulty in generating grammatically connected speech, apparent in the patient's attempts at naming objects, reading aloud, and even writing; often with relative preservation of the ability to understand speech; generally caused by a stroke that creates a lesion in the Broca area and typically manifests with other symptoms, depending on the size of the lesion

Broca area A specific region within the inferior frontal gyrus of the frontal lobe that is responsible for speech planning and production

Brodmann areas A classification system for areas of the cerebral cortex based on distinctiveness of the cytoarchitecture or cellular stratification

bronchi Divisions of the air passage below the trachea, first left and right principal bronchi to direct air into the right and left lungs, then at a smaller scale to reach various regions within the lungs; reinforced with cartilages like the trachea

bronchiole Smaller-scale division of a bronchus without cartilage in its wall

buccal Of, or relating to, the cheek

buccinator Muscle that draws the lips laterally and tenses the cheek

bucconasal membrane A septum between the primitive nasal cavities and the future pharynx that disappears in the seventh week of development

buccopharyngeal membrane (oropharyngeal membrane) A septum between the primitive mouth and pharynx where the ectoderm and endoderm come into direct contact with each other

C

calcarine sulcus An indentation within the medial surface of the occipital lobe

calcium A chemical element (atomic number 20) that typically exists in the body as the divalent cation (an atom with a deficiency of two electrons, resulting in a positive charge of 2+).

calyx of Held A large synapse in the auditory brainstem connecting the globular bushy cells in the anterior ventral cochlear nucleus to the principal cells of the medial nuclei of the trapezoid body

cAMP *See* **cyclic adenosine monophosphate**

candidate gene A gene that is thought to influence a neurobiological process, cognitive ability, or disease susceptibility

canine A pointed tooth between the incisors and premolars

capillary basement membrane Membrane immediately outside the capillary wall; involved in gas exchange

capillary epithelium The wall of a capillary; involved in gas exchange.

capsule The mucopolysaccharide layer that lies outside the cell wall of bacteria

carbohydrates Molecules with the formula $(CH_2O)_n$, including simple sugars and polysaccharides

cardiac muscle Involuntary, striated muscle that is found in the walls and histologic foundation of the heart

Carhart notch A loss of sensitivity to bone-conducted stimuli at 2000 Hz, most often associated with otosclerosis

carotid body   A chemoreceptor within the carotid artery

carrier proteins   Proteins that selectively bind small molecules and transport them across a membrane

cartilage   Flexible, semirigid supportive connective tissue dominated by large amounts of the proteoglycan chondroitin sulfate in the extracellular matrix; cartilage is more flexible and compressible than bone and often serves as an early skeletal framework, becoming mineralized as the organism ages; principal types are elastic cartilage and hyaline cartilage

cartilaginous   Of, relating to, or composed of, cartilage

cartilaginous vocal fold   Part of the vocal fold closest to the vocal process of the arytenoid cartilage; *see also* **membranous vocal fold**

cation   An atom or molecule with fewer electrons than protons, and therefore with a positive charge

cauda equina   The most distal spinal nerves, into which the spinal cord divides

caudal   Toward the tail

caudate nucleus   A C-shaped component of the basal ganglia, having a large head portion in the frontal lobe that narrows into a body and tail sections as the nucleus curves posteriorly through the parietal lobe; the caudate nucleus wraps around the putamen, from which it is separated by the internal capsule

cell   The structural, functional, and biologic unit of all organisms

cell body   The part of a neuron that houses the nucleus and much of the metabolic machinery and excludes the branches formed by dendrites and axons; *see also* **soma**

cell culture   Removal of cells from an animal or plant and their subsequent growth in a favorable artificial environment

cell junction   Specialized region of connection between two cells or between a cell and the extracellular matrix

cell line   A perpetuating strain of cells in laboratory culture

cell surface receptors   Proteins that bind signaling molecules external to the cell with high affinity and, in response, produce one or more intracellular signals that alter the behavior of the target cell

cell wall   A rigid, porous structure forming an external layer that provides structural support to bacteria, fungi, and plant cells

cellular respiration   A series of metabolic processes that take place within a cell in which biochemical energy is harvested from an organic substance (e.g., glucose) and is stored in an energy carrier (ATP) for use in energy-requiring activities of the cell; respiration processes may use oxgen (aerobic respiration) or not (anaerobic respiration)

cellular transport   Movement of materials across cell membranes

cementum   The surface layer of the tooth root that is part of the periodontium and attaches to the alveolar bone via the periodontal ligament

center of gravity   An imaginary point at which the mass of an object is equally balanced

central auditory system   The part of the auditory system that processes information sent by the peripheral auditory system; includes the cochlear nucleus, superior olivary complex, lateral lemniscus, inferior colliculus, medial geniculate nucleus of the thalamus, acoustic radiations, and auditory cortex

central chemoreceptors   Medullary neurons that reside proximal to the respiratory control center; activated when the pH of nearby cerebrospinal fluid varies from the narrow range of normal values

central dogma   The principle that DNA is transcribed into RNA, which is then translated into proteins

central nervous system (CNS)   The division of the nervous system that consists of the brain and spinal cord; see also **peripheral nervous system**

central nucleus of the inferior colliculus (ICC)   Central or core region of the inferior colliculus

central pattern generator (CPG)   A grouping of neurons within the brainstem or spinal cord that fire in a prescribed, rhythmic fashion to produce a repetitive movement cycle

central   Pertaining to a core structure, generally of significant importance (e.g., brain and spinal cord of the central nervous system)

central sulcus   The sulcus that separates the frontal lobe from the parietal lobe and also the primary motor cortex from the primary sensory cortex; also called fissure of Rolando or rolandic fissure

central vestibular nucleus complex   *See* **vestibular nuclei**

centromedian nucleus   A nucleus within the thalamus that conveys information to the basal ganglia

centromere   The structure that joins two arms of the chromosome; responsible for tethering of chromosomes to the spindle during mitosis and meiosis

cephalic flexure   The first flexure, or bend, of the embryonic neural tube, which occurs in the region later to form the midbrain; it generally forms at the end of the third week or beginning of the fourth

cerebellar peduncles   The input and output pathways located on the dorsal aspect of the brainstem

cerebellopontine angle   Anatomic region where the peduncles of the cerebellum join the pons of the brainstem

cerebellum   A relatively large paired structure with left and right folded cortices, located in the posterior cranial fossa (back part of the brainpan in the skull) below the cerebral hemispheres and dorsal to the brainstem; the cerebellum is made up of the cerebellar cortex and cerebellar nuclei including the dentate, globose, emboliform, and fastigial nuclei; the cerebellum plays a major role in the coordination and control of movement and is essential for motor learning, but recent evidence suggests it also contributes to higher cognitive functions

cerebral aqueduct   Narrow channel that lies at the dorsal midbrain, connecting the third ventricle and the fourth ventricle

cerebral cortex   Folded, stratified gray matter that constitutes the superficial layer of the cerebrum; the cerebral cortex gives rise to consciousness, all higher-order cognitive functions, and integration of motor and sensory functions

cerebral hemispheres   Left and right paired divisions of the cerebrum that are made up of folded gray matter covering underlying white matter

cerebral peduncles   Large right and left columns of descending white matter in the ventral region of the midbrain, carrying motor signals to the brainstem, cerebellum, and spinal cord

cerebrospinal fluid (CSF)   Colorless body fluid secreted by choroid plexus cells in the ventricles of the brain, providing buoyancy, shock protection, and a closely regulated chemical environment to the brain

cerebrum   The largest portion of the brain in terms of surface area, weight, and volume; it includes the cerebral cortex and subcortex

cerumen   Earwax; waxy substance that is generated by sebaceous and ceruminous glands within the external auditory canal

cervical flexure   The flexure, or bend, of the embryonic brain that occurs at what will become the junction of the brain and the spinal cord

channel proteins   Proteins that form pores through a membrane through which a specific ion or molecule may pass

characteristic frequencies   Frequencies to which a neuron responds most strongly even at a minimal sound intensity level

chemoreceptor   A primary receptor responsible for detecting the presence of chemical agents and encoding information regarding smell or taste.

chest register   The register in which most speech is done, next above the pulse register; F_0 controlled mostly by the vocalis (contraction lowers F_0); speaker feels sensations primarily in the chest; see also **falsetto**, **head register**, **mixed register**

chiasmic groove   A narrow transverse groove that lies near the front of the superior surface of the body of the sphenoid bone, is continuous with the optic foramen, and houses the optic chiasm; also called optic groove

chloride   The monovalent anion (an atom with a single excess electron resulting in a charge of –1) from the element chlorine (atomic number 17)

choanae   Passages connecting the nasal cavities with the nasopharynx on either side of the posterior nasal septum; also called the posterior nasal apertures

cholinergic   Communicating by means of acetylcholine (ACh) as neurotransmitter

cholinergic/dopaminergic imbalance theory   A theory regarding the pathophysiology of the basal ganglia in movement disorders, formulated during the 1970s primarily from pharmacological observations, according to which relative excess of acetylcholine over dopamine in the striatum of the basal ganglia was thought to cause hypokinetic disorders such as Parkinson's disease, whereas relative deficiency of acetylcholine relative to dopamine was thought to cause hyperkinetic disorders such as Huntington's disease; pharmacological therapies were recommended to restore the balance

chondroglossus   Muscle often considered part of the hyoglossus that inserts more medially than the rest of the hyoglossus and depresses the tongue

chorda tympani   An important branch of the facial nerve that carries taste sensation to the gustatory nucleus in the brainstem but traverses the tympanic cavity

chorea   Quick, jerky movements at proximal joints, caused by a hyperkinetic disorder

chorion The outermost membrane surrounding an embryo, formed by extraembryonic mesoderm as well as the two layers of the trophoblast that surround the embryo, and containing chorionic villi

chorion frondosum The area on the surface of the blastocyst that exclusively retains chorionic villi

chorionic villi Processes that extend from the chorion and invade the endometrium to provide maximal area of contact to facilitate the transfer of substances such as nutrients and oxygen between maternal blood and fetal blood

choroid plexus A network of capillaries and ependymal cells in the cerebral ventricles that function in production of cerebrospinal fluid

chromosome A packaged and organized thread-like structure made of DNA and supporting proteins, located inside the nucleus of animal and plant cells; chromosomes may be autosomes or sex chromosomes

cingulate gyrus An arc-shaped structure extending across the medial surface of the frontal and parietal lobes

cingulate sulcus An arc-shaped cleft that separates the cingulate gyrus from the frontal and parietal lobe on the medial side

circle of Willis A circle of arteries located at the base of the brain, which receives blood from multiple arteries and distributes it to all parts of the brain; the circle provides redundant blood supply in case flow from one of the supplying arteries is impeded

cisternae Spaces containing fluid, such as the spaces occurring between the membranes of flattened sacs of the Golgi apparatus and the endoplasmic reticulum, as well as the spaces between the two membranes of the nuclear envelope

Claudius cell Columnar cell in the organ of Corti that provides support for outer hair cells

claustrum A small strip of gray matter seemingly separated from the cortex in the midst of rapid expansion

cleft A split or division in two

climbing fibers Axons that arise from cell bodies in the inferior olivary nucleus of the brainstem and that form a complex basket of connections onto the dendrites of the Purkinje neurons of the cerebellar cortex

closed phase The part of a cycle of vocal fold vibration when the folds are closed; *see also* **closing phase**, **opening phase**

closing phase The part of a cycle of vocal fold vibration when the folds are moving back toward the midline; *see also* **closed phase, opening phase**

CN See **cranial nerve**

coarticulation Production of sound as a continuous blend of one sound into another so that at any given moment, the articulatory characteristics of the preceding and following phonemes overlap

cochlea Bony cavity of the inner ear, coiled in a way that resembles the shape of a snail shell and including three parallel fluid-filled tubes or chambers, housing the primary sensory receptors for sound

cochlear amplifier The ability to amplify the neural signaling of auditory stimuli through the electromotility provided by the somatic motor

cochlear aqueduct Small space or opening between the jugular fossa and carotid canal that provides communication between the perilymphatic space and the subarachnoid space

cochlear microphonic (CM) A receptor potential generated by the outer hair cells; it is alternating current and follows the audio waveform

cochlear nuclei (CN) Ventral and dorsal nuclei in the lateral medulla oblongata, the principal target for afferents in the cochlear (auditory) branch of the vestibulocochlear nerve; project to the superior olivary complex

cochlear partition A region of the organ of Corti that contains the tectorial membrane and basilar membrane

codon A sequence of three bases in a messenger RNA molecule that code for a specific amino acid

coincident detectors Neurons in the brain that can encode information by detecting the occurrence of temporally close but spatially distributed input signals

collateral sulcus Indentation in the cerebral cortex that separates the posterior portion of the occipitotemporal gyrus and the parahippocampal gyrus

combination-sensitive Responsive to distinct frequency inputs at relatively low intensity levels; combination-sensitive neurons are responsible for spectral-temporal integration

commissure An anatomic structure that joins two paired structures; *see also* **anterior commissure**

common crus The portion of the anterior and posterior semicircular canals wherein the bony and membranous labyrinths of the two semicircular canals come together to form a shared projection that terminates at the vestibule

compact bone A type of osseous tissue consisting of closely packed osteons or haversian systems, which forms the extremely hard exterior of bones; *see also* **spongy bone**

complex sounds Sounds that are composed of multiple frequencies

complex spike A relatively long-duration action potential associated with multiple spikes in response to postsynaptic depolarization of the Purkinje neuron in response to action potentials arriving via the climbing fibers; the powerful response is thought to be the result of extensive synapses formed by the climbing fiber onto the Purkinje neuron soma

complex systems The dynamics, or changes in state over time, of systems with complex and large-scale structures (e.g., atmospheric systems that underlie weather); while often the result of clearly defined (determinate) processes, the complexity of the systems makes prediction difficult; for example, a great deal is understood about the motion of molecules, such as those that are involved in weather, but the size and complexity of weather systems make prediction of the weather difficult; many complex systems demonstrate "structure" or regularity (e.g., the swirl patterns in a whirlpool or the Great Red Spot of Jupiter); the phenomena of complex systems represent a challenge to current reductionist approaches, particularly in neuroscience, that initially attempt to understand simple or simplified systems and then build in complexity to achieve a complete understanding; complex systems theory suggests that in the evolution to increasing complexity, the dynamics of the system cease to be predictable by the underlying, slightly less complex systems

compliance The ability of a structure to undergo stretching or displacement

compound action potential (cAP) The combined electrical potentials resulting from activation of the cochlear branch of the vestibulocochlear nerve

concentration gradient The presence of different concentrations of a particular substance at different points in space; if possible, the substance tends to flow from regions of higher concentration to regions of lower concentration

concentric contraction Isotonic muscle activity that applies force as the muscle shortens in length; *see also* **eccentric contraction**

concha (plural, conchae) A body part that resembles a spiral shell; (1) part of the external ear; (2) nasal concha

concordant Of family members, displaying the same condition, or presence of the same trait

condensation The part of a sound wave where molecules are compressed together, where pressure is highest; *see also* **rarefaction**

conductive hearing loss A loss of hearing sensitivity due to pathology in the outer or middle ear

condylar process Prominence on the ramus of the mandibular bone that articulates with the temporal bone at the temporomandibular joint

cone One of the phototransducing cells of the retina that are responsible for vision during daylight and mediate color information; *see also* **rod**

cone of light The reflection of light observed in the anteroinferior quadrant of the tympanic membrane during otoscopy

confluence of sinuses Area where the superficial cerebral venous system and the deep cerebral venous system are joined

confluence The portion of the surface of a culture medium covered by cells, used as an estimate of the number of adherent cells

connective tissue Tissue that serves to hold in place, connect, and integrate the body's organs and systems

continuous cell line The descendants of a single cell type that can be serially propagated in culture indefinitely

continuous harmonic oscillator An oscillator that produces a smoothly varying periodic signal value, such as the varying air pressure around the plucked string of a guitar; *see also* **discrete oscillator**

contralateral On the opposite side; affecting the opposite side of the head or body

contraries A concept attributed to Aristotle that attempts to account for the diversity of phenomena by holding that a set of phenomena represent some mixture between the two (or more) extremes of the phenomena, for example, shades of gray as mixtures of black and white, or the dichotomization of neuronal influences into excitatory or inhibitory; however, the one-dimensional push-pull dynamics inherent in contraries is unlikely to provide a complete and satisfactory understanding, particularly in complex systems

conus elasticus *See* **cricothyroid ligament**

conus medullaris The termination of the spinal cord, from which the cauda equina extends

convergent glottis The condition during the opening phase of a vibration of the vocal folds, where the lower edges of the vocal folds are displaced wider than the upper edges; *see also* **divergent glottis**

coplanar pairs Pairing of semicircular canals such that when two semicircular canals within the same geometric plane respond to head movement, one canal is stimulated and the other is inhibited; also called functional pairs

copula A midline swelling that forms inferior to the tuberculum impar from the second and third branchial arches and gives rise to the epiglottis

copy number variation (CNV) Difference in the number of copies of a segment of DNA that is a departure from the usual two copies (one inherited from mother, the other from father)

core *See* **primary auditory cortex**

corniculate cartilages Two small conical nodules that articulate with the arytenoid cartilages and elongate from them posteriorly and medially; they form the posterior aspect of the laryngeal inlet

coronal plane A vertical plane that divides a region into anterior and posterior parts; also called frontal plane

coronoid process The anterior part of the upper end of the ramus of the mandible

corpus The main body or mass of a structure, such as the mandible or the hyoid bone

corpus callosum Band of nerve fibers located beneath the cortex at the longitudinal fissure, joining the two hemispheres of the brain and extending from the frontal lobe caudally to the occipital and temporal lobes

corpus striatum *See* **striatum**

corticobulbar tract The white matter between the brainstem and the cerebral cortex; its axons have their origin in the cortex, including the motor cortex and the supplementary motor area, and their terminals are located in the cranial nerve nuclei in the brainstem

corticospinal tract An important pathway for voluntary motor function, found in the white matter of the spinal cord; its axons have their origin in the cortex, and their terminals in the anterior horn of the spinal cord, where they synapse on lower motor neurons

cortilymph The fluid of the intracellular spaces of the organ of Corti, similar in ionic composition to perilymph

costal surface (of lungs) The surface of the lungs facing the inner surface of the rib cage

CPG See **central pattern generator**

cranial bones Bony structures that protect the brain

cranial nerve (CN) One of 12 paired nerves I–XII that emerge from the brain or brainstem rather than from the spinal cord; except for CN X the cranial nerves communicate with structures in the head and neck; from rostral to caudal they are the olfactory nerve (CN I), the optic nerve (CN II), the oculomotor nerve (CN III), the trochlear nerve (CN IV), the trigeminal nerve (CN V), the abducens nerve (CN VI), the facial nerve (CN VII), the vestibulocochlear nerve (CN VIII), the glossopharyngeal nerve (CN IX), the vagus nerve (CN X), the accessory nerve (CN XI), and the hypoglossal nerve (CN XII)

cremasteric reflex A reflex in which stroking the inner thigh of a man results in contraction of the cremaster muscle, which retracts the testicle; the cremasteric reflex is a superficial reflex that normally is present but can be lost with injury to the corticospinal tract

cricoarytenoid joint Articulations of the arytenoid cartilages with the cricoid

cricoarytenoid ligament Ligament running from the superior surface of the posterior cricoid lamina to the posterior and medial aspects of the base of the arytenoid cartilage

cricoid cartilage Ring-shaped cartilage in the larynx, set between the thyroid cartilage and the trachea

cricothyroid joint Joints where the inferior horns of the thyroid cartilage articulate with the lateral arches of the cricoid

cricothyroid ligament Sheet of connective tissue that connects the cricoid and thyroid cartilages, also called the conus elasticus, cricothyroid membrane, and cricovocal membrane; consists of the median and lateral cricothyroid ligaments

cricothyroid (CT) muscle Muscle that originates on the lateral arch of the cricoid and inserts on the inner surface of the thyroid lamina; contracting, it lengthens the vocal folds; two divisions (pars recta and pars obliqua) act together

cricotracheal membrane Ligament that connects the cricoid cartilage and the trachea

crista (1) A fold in the inner mitochondrial membrane extending into the matrix; (2) crista ampullaris; (3) crista galli

crista ampullaris The sensory organ of rotation, located in the ampulla of each semicircular canal of the inner ear; it senses angular acceleration and deceleration

crista galli Crest of the ethmoid bone

cross-bridge theory The theory that myosin heads attach themselves momentarily to the actin filament during contraction, forming cross-bridges

crosslink A chemical bond between different chains of atoms in a polymer or other complex molecule

cuneate fasciculus A bundle of axons in the dorsal column (more correctly, posterior funiculus) white matter of the spinal cord that houses primary afferent axons from the the upper trunk and upper extremities

cuneiform cartilages Paired cartilages that move with the arytenoids and are located within the aryepiglottic folds; they form the lateral aspect of the laryngeal inlet

cuneus gyrus Gyral structure that is superior to the calcarine sulcus of the occipital lobe; the cuneus gyrus is associated with processing spatial awareness and recognizing objects from memory

cupola *See* **cupula**

cupula A gelatinous domelike structure that crosses the lumen of the ampulla, in which stereocilia of semicircular canal hair cells are embedded; distortion of the cupula results in shearing of the stereocilia and depolarization/hyperpolarization of hair cells

cuticular plate A firm laminar structure in the organ of Corti to which the apical ends of the cochlear hair cells are attached and through which their stereocilia project

cycle *See* **vibratory cycle**

cyclic adenosine monophosphate (cAMP) A chemical agent derived from adenosine triphosphate (ATP) that often functions to convey information in many biochemical systems; for example, cAMP is the intermediary between the binding of some neurotransmitters and the subsequent changes in the electrical potential across the neuronal membrane

cyclic guanosine monophosphate (cGMP) A chemical similar to cyclic adenosine monophosphate (cAMP), but containing the base guanine rather than adenine; like cAMP, it conveys information within cells

cytokines Small protein molecules that affect cellular activity, used for signaling, especially in the immune system

cytoplasm The jellylike substance in a cell that contains the cytosol and organelles but not the nucleus

cytoskeleton A network of protein filaments that extends throughout the cytoplasm of eukaryotic cells, providing the structural framework of the cell and responsible for cell movement

cytosol In an intact cell, the liquid component of the cytoplasm surrounding the organelles and other insoluble cytoplasmic structures and where a wide variety of cell processes take place

cytotrophoblast A layer of cells that serves both to anchor the growing fetus to the maternal uterine tissue as well as to penetrate the maternal spiral arteries and route the blood flow through the placenta for the growing embryo to use

D

D$_1$ receptors A type of metabotropic postsynaptic receptor that binds dopamine or dopamine agonists, resulting in increased responsiveness to corticospinal action potentials

D$_2$ receptors A type of metabotropic postsynaptic receptor that binds dopamine or dopamine agonists and antagonists, resulting in decreased responsiveness to corticospinal action potentials

damp To remove energy from oscillation so that its amplitude decreases to zero

decerebrate posturing A reflex often producing long-duration contraction of the extensor muscles of the upper and lower extremities, typically seen in lesions of the brainstem between the inferior colliculus and the lateral vestibular nucleus

decibel (dB) Logarithmic unit of power or intensity of a wave form; a wave 10 dB higher than another has 10 times the power or $\sqrt{10}$ times the amplitude in pressure (of a sound wave) or in voltage or current (of an electromagnetic wave)

decomposition of movement Change in execution of movements that normally consist of complex simultaneous rotations about multiple joints, resulting in a smooth final trajectory of the limb, into a series of individually performed rotations, seen in some movement disorders, such as those associated with lesions of the cerebellar systems

decorticate posturing A reflex often producing long-duration contraction of the flexor muscles of the upper extremities and the extensor muscles of the lower extremities, typically seen in lesions of the cerebral cortex

deep Farther from the surface

deep brain stimulation (DBS) A revolutionary therapy for neurologic and psychiatric disorders involving the permanent implantation of stimulating electrodes in various brain regions

deep cerebellar nuclei Collections of neurons in the cerebellum beneath the cerebellar cortex (subcortical), including the dentate, globose, emboliform, and fastigial nuclei; the axonal output of the cerebellar system arises from these nuclei

deep cerebral vein Vein that drains the deep structures of the brain

deep lamina propria (DLP) The fourth layer in from the surface in the vocal fold, containing more collagen fibers than the intermediate lamina propria

deep tendon reflex A reflex in which a rapid stretch causes activation of muscle spindles, which is conducted by the axons of the muscle spindle receptors to synapse on the alpha lower motor neurons to result in a muscle contraction; the archetypical example is the knee or patellar reflex, in which striking the patellar tendon just below the kneecap (patella) with a rubber hammer, rapidly stretching the quadriceps muscle, sends action potentials from the muscle spindles to synapses on the α-LMNs controlling muscle fibers of the quadriceps muscle, resulting in a kicking out of the leg

deglutition   The entire process of bringing food to the oral cavity, maneuvering it in the oral cavity, and propelling it into the pharynx through the esophagus and into the stomach; the term is most often used synonymously with swallowing

degrees of freedom   The number of relevant variables in a system

dehydration   Condition in which there is not enough water in the body to maintain a healthy level of fluid in the body's tissues

Deiters cell   Modified support cell attached to the basilar membrane and inferior to outer hair cells

delayed-onset muscle soreness (DOMS)   Muscle tissue discomfort that is experienced about 24–48 hours after eccentric muscle exercise

dendrite   Part of the neuron, typically a branch-like projection extending from the cell body, usually shorter than an axon, that receives synaptic transmissions resulting in changes in the electrical potential across the local neuronal membrane; unlike action potentials, which occur typically in axons, the changes in electrical potentials in the dendrites dissipate over time and distance from the synaptic site

dendritic spines   Mushroom-shaped protrusions from the dendrite of a neuron that make synaptic contact with upstream neurons

dental lamina   Epithelium that extends into the mesoderm from the tooth germ; it begins developing during the sixth week of development

dental papilla   A condensation of odontoblasts that lies below the enamel organ

dentate nucleus   A deep cerebellar nucleus that receives inputs from the lateral zone of the neocerebellum and projects to the LMN via the rubrospinal and reticulospinal tracts; *see also* **emboliform nucleus, fastigial nucleus, globose nucleus**

dentin   Calcified tissue within the tooth that is usually covered by enamel on the crown and cementum on the root; it surrounds the entire pulp

deoxyribonucleic acid (DNA)   The double-helical nucleic acid that serves to store genetic information, consisting of nucleotides in which deoxyribose is the sugar and thymine is the base that pairs with adenine; *see also* **ribonucleic acid (RNA)**

depolarization   Decrease in the magnitude of the electrical potential across a cell membrane, such as the neuronal membrane (which is usually at a negative potential, so it is depolarized by positive charges entering the cell); *see also* **hyperpolarization**

depressor anguli oris   Muscle that pulls the corner of the mouth inferiorly and laterally

depressor labii inferioris   Muscle that pulls the lip inferiorly and laterally

dermatome   A specific zone or discrete area of the body innervated by a pair of spinal nerves or one spinal segment; formed from the most lateral portion of a somite, this area develops into the skin, fat, and connective tissue of the neck and trunk

desmosome   A region of contact between epithelial cells at which intermediate filaments are anchored to the plasma membrane

detraining effect   Weakening (over time) upon cessation of regular exercise

dexter (dextra, dextrum)   Located on the right-hand side of the body, as in the abbreviations used by audiologists (auris dextra, AD, right ear) and optometrists (oculus dexter, OD, right eye)

diaphragm   The primary muscle of inhalation, in the form of a sheet that divides the thoracic cavity from the abdomen

diencephalon   An embryologically defined subdivision of the brain that develops into the epithalamus, the thalamus, the hypothalamus, and the third ventricle; it is derived from the prosencephalon

diffusion   Passive movement of an atom, ion, or molecule through a medium, typically from a region of relatively high concentration to a region of lower concentration

digastric fossa   A depression on the internal surface of the mandible, where the anterior belly of the digastric muscle originates

digastric muscle   A muscle with two "bellies"; the anterior belly originates at the digastric fossa of the mandible, while the posterior belly originates at the mastoid process of the temporal bone; both join at the intermediate tendon, which is attached to the hyoid bone

diploid   Having both members of each pair of chromosomes; if the number of chromosome pairs is n, a diploid cell has $2n$ chromosomes; *see also* **haploid**

direct laryngoscopy   Viewing the larynx and vocal folds without mirror reflection through an endoscope; generally performed in an operating room; *see also* **indirect laryngoscopy**

direct pathway An anatomic pathway within the basal ganglia system in which connections from the striatum arrive at the globus pallidus internal segment directly; the anatomy of this pathway has been extrapolated into physiologic inferences related to the physiology and pathophysiology of the basal ganglia–thalamic–cortical system

disk-shaped cell Type of neuronal cell in the inferior colliculus

discrete oscillator An oscillator that produces a signal whose value does not vary smoothly, such as a flashing light that is either on or off for some period; *see also* **continuous harmonic oscillator**

distal Away from some reference point; located farther away from another structure or point; *see also* **proximal**

divergent glottis Condition during the closing phase of a vibration of the vocal folds, when the lower edges are closer together than the upper edges; *see also* **convergent glottis**

dizygotic (fraternal) twins Twins resulting from two separate eggs fertilized by two separate sperm

DNA *See* **deoxyribonucleic acid**

DNA sequencing The process of determining the exact order of the base pairs that make up chromosomes

dopamine A neurotransmitter

dopaminergic Communicating by means of dopamine as neurotransmitter

dorsal Toward the back (posterior) surface of the body or hand, or the upper side of the feet, the penis, or the thalamus, when in anatomic position; see also **ventral**

dorsal cochlear nucleus (DCN) One of three major divisions of the cochlear nucleus in the brainstem; *see also* **anterior ventral cochlear nucleus (AVCN)**, **posterior ventral cochlear nucleus (PVCN)**

dorsal-column medial lemniscal (DCML) pathway A somatosensory pathway in the central nervous system that conveys information related to touch and proprioception from all parts of the body through the spinal cord

dorsal-column system System that contains the fasciculus gracilis and fasciculus cuneatus and plays an important role in limb sensation

dorsal cortex Superior division of the inferior colliculus

dorsal nucleus of the lateral lemniscus (DNLL) Dorsal division of the lateral lemniscus

dorsal respiratory group Part of the medullary respiratory center; acts in cooperation with the pre-Bötzinger complex during inspiration

dorsal rhizotomy A surgical procedure that severs the afferent axons entering the spinal cord through the posterior root of a spinal nerve

dorsal root ganglion A collection of neurons that receive axons from receptors mediating deep sensations such as proprioception and vibration, and that send axons into the spinal cord through the posterior root of a spinal nerve

dorsal stria Fiber tract of axons that originate from the dorsal cochlear nucleus to the trapezoid body and form a portion of the lateral lemniscus tract

dorsum Upper surface of a horizontal body part

duplex theory The theory that humans are able to localize sounds by interaural timing differences and interaural level differences

dura mater The outermost, tough, leathery layer of the meninges, which forms a primary protective covering of the central nervous system

dysarthria A motor speech disorder that is associated with poor articulation

dysdiadochokinesia Inability to perform rapidly alternating movements

dyslexia Difficulty reading

dysmetric Inaccurate in distance, said of a bodily movement

dysosmia Distortions in the sense of smell

dysphagia Difficulty swallowing or disordered swallowing

dysphonia A perceptual sign or symptom of an underlying impairment in phonation; a deviation from the normal perceptual characteristics of voice production including pitch, loudness, quality, and variability (e.g., flexibility or intonation) that is appropriate for the speaker's age and sex

dyspnea Difficulty in breathing; the sense of breathlessness or "air hunger"

dystonia Abnormal sustained posture caused by a hyperkinetic disorder

dystussia Difficult or disordered cough

E

eccentric contraction Isotonic muscle activity that is characterized by muscle lengthening under tension and is used during muscle effort that requires a controlled descent against resistance (gravity); *see also* **concentric contraction**

economy of effort Planning of a series of bodily actions (such as speech) so that the moving structures reach their targets with the least amount of effort

ectoderm The outermost of the three primary germ layers, forming the epidermis; the nervous system; tooth enamel; the lining of the mouth, anus, and nostrils; sweat glands, hair, and nails

efferent Pertaining to conveying or carrying something (e.g., motor neural signals) outward or away (e.g., from the central nervous system)

efficacy The ability of a drug or other agent to produce the desired response

elastic cartilage A type of cartilage primarily consisting of elastin fibers rather than collagen, so it is less likely to harden or ossify with age; *see also* **hyaline cartilage**

elastic recoil Tendency of an elastic element (e.g., a lung or vocal fold) to snap back to its original position when displaced

electrocochleography (ECochG) Recording of the electrical signals emitted by the hair cells of the inner ear and the cochlear branch of the vestibulocochlear nerve; in normal-hearing individuals, the recording contains the cochlear microphonic (stimulus dependent), the summating potential, and the compound action potential

electromotility The capability for motion or movement of the outer hair cells in response to electrical stimulation

electromyography Detecting and recording the electrical potential generated by muscle cells when these cells are electrically or neurologically activated

electron microscopy Microscopy that uses an electron beam to form an image

elongated cell Neuronal cell type in the central auditory nervous system

emboliform nucleus One of the deep cerebellar nuclei that receives inputs from, the cortex of the paramidline of the neocerebellum and the archicerebellum and projects to the LMNs via the rubrospinal and reticulospinal tracts; *see also* **dentate nucleus**, **fastigial nucleus**, **globose nucleus**

embryonic stem cells Stem cells from early embryos

enamel Hard white substance covering the crown of a tooth

enamel organ Also known as the dental organ; a cellular aggregation above the dental papilla that functions in the formation of enamel, the initiation of dentin formation, the establishment of the shape of a tooth's crown, and the establishment of the dentogingival junction

endochondral ossification Process in which minerals accumulate in cartilage, making it more bonelike

endocochlear potential A positive voltage of +80 mV to +100 mV in the cochlear endolymphatic space relative to the perilymphatic fluid of the scalae vestibuli and tympani

endocrine signaling Cell–cell signaling in which endocrine cells secrete hormones that are carried by the circulation to distant target cells

endocytosis The uptake of extracellular material in vesicles formed from the plasma membrane

endoderm The innermost of the three primary germ layers; its cells develop into columnar epithelial cells that form the lining of multiple organ systems, including the gastrointestinal tract and respiratory tract

endolymph One of the two fluids in the inner ear, contained in the membranous labyrinth of the peripheral vestibular apparatus and in the cochlear duct (scala media), containing high concentrations of potassium and low concentrations of sodium ions

endolymphatic duct A small membranous canal connecting the saccule, the utricle, the semicircular ducts, and the cochlear duct to the endolymphatic sac

endolymphatic sac Structure of the inner ear that is connected to the the cochlear duct and the vestibular division of the membranous labyrinth; formed by an outpouching of the primitive membranous labyrinth around the fifth week of development; thought to regulate the production of endolymph

endophenotype Reliable fine-scale measure of components of particular disorders

endoplasmic reticulum An extensive network of membrane-enclosed tubules and sacs involved in protein sorting and processing as well as in lipid synthesis

endoscope Instrument used for viewing internal spaces of the body

endothelial cells Cells that form the inner lining of blood vessels

endothermic Able to regulate body temperature via internal (metabolic) means

enzyme Protein catalyst that speeds biochemical reactions

enzyme-linked receptors Transmembrane receptors that bind an extracellular ligand; the ligand binding causes enzymatic activity on the intracellular side

ependymal cell A type of glial cell (in the choroid plexus) that secretes cerebrospinal fluid

epiblast The outermost layer arising from the inner cell mass in the blastocyst

epidural hematoma Bleeding that occurs outside of the meninges (between the dura mater and the skull)

epigenetics The study of traits inherited by mechanisms other than the sequence of bases in DNA

epigenome The complete epigenetic state of a cell

epiglottis Leaf-shaped elastic cartilage that, during swallowing, covers the laryngeal vestibule and directs food toward the esophagus

epithalamus The dorsal segment of the diencephalon; its function includes regulation of the secretion of melatonin by the pineal body and regulation of motor pathways and emotions

epithelial basement membrane Membrane immediately outside the alveolar wall; involved in gas exchange

epithelial tissue Tissue that serves primarily as a covering or lining of body parts, protecting the body; it also functions in absorption, transport, and secretion

epitympanic recess Small cavity superior to the tympanic cavity proper

erythropoietin Hormone that increases production of hemoglobin-containing red blood cells within bone marrow, yielding increased total blood volume and, therefore, more O_2 to be delivered to tissues

estimated mean flow rate (EMFR) Prediction of airflow rate during phonation derived using the phonation quotient

ethmoidal air cells Multiple air-filled chambers in the ethmoid bone, located posterior to the nasal cavities between the eye sockets

eukaryotic cells Cells that have a nuclear envelope, cytoplasmic organelles, and a cytoskeleton; see also **prokaryotic cells**

eustachian tube A canal within the temporal bone with a cartilaginous extension that connects the middle ear space with the nasopharynx, allowing equalization of middle ear pressure with atmospheric pressure; the tensor veli palatini and levator veli palatini muscles open the eustachian tube; also called auditory tube or pharyngotympanic tube

excitation-contraction coupling The process in which neural excitation of the motor end plate leads to muscle fiber contraction

excitatory postsynaptic potential (EPSP) a change in the electrical potential across the neuronal membrane in a more positive direction, more accurately referred to as a depolarizing postsynaptic potential (DPSP)

exocytosis The process in which an intracellular vesicle (membrane-bound sphere) moves to the plasma membrane, where the vesicular membrane fuses with the plasma membrane, releasing the contents of the vesicle into the extracellular space; for example, exocytosis is involved in the release of a neurotransmitter stored in a vesicle into the synaptic cleft

exon Part of the sequence in a gene that is included in the code for the mature protein and that is separated from other exons in the gene by introns

expiration The process of exhaling

expiratory muscle strength training (EMST) Targeted, exercise-based conditioning of the muscles of expiration, primarily the abdominals and internal intercostals

expiratory reserve volume The volume of air that can be forcefully exhaled beyond what is exhaled during tidal breathing

extensor muscle Muscle that enlarges the angle between body parts

external auditory canal Also called the external auditory meatus; opening in the temporal bone of the skull where sound enters the ear

external branch of the superior laryngeal nerve (ESLN) Branch that provides motor innervation to the cricothyroid, inferior pharyngeal constrictor, and cricopharyngeus muscles

external capsule A series of white matter fiber tracts in the brain, separated from the internal capsule by the putamen and globus pallidus

external intercostal muscles Muscles that line the rib cage and are active during inspiration; upon contraction, they expand the rib cage

external (or lateral) shell A division of the inferior colliculus

exteroception Ability to sense stimuli that arise from outside the body

exteroreceptors Sensory organs that detect substances and conditions that exist outside of the body

extracellular matrix Secreted proteins and polysaccharides that fill spaces between cells and bind cells and tissues together

extradural space A space between the cranial bone and the dura mater

extraembryonic mesoderm Network of cells that gives rise to supporting structures for embryonic growth but does not contribute to formation of the embryo

extrapyramidal system Motor systems that are not directly related to the corticospinal tract, which descends via the medullary pyramids in the brainstem; axons of the extrapyramidal system originate in the basal ganglia, cerebellum, brainstem nuclei, and reticular formations

extrinsic laryngeal muscles Muscles that control and stabilize the position of the larynx as a whole during speech

F

facet A small, smooth area on cartilage or bone, usually forming part of a joint

facial nerve (CN VII) A mixed nerve that innervates all muscles of the upper and lower face and parts of the outer ear; it has a critical role in speech production

facilitated diffusion   The transport of molecules across a membrane by carrier or channel proteins

failure to thrive   Failure of a child to grow, gain weight, or develop normally compared to age-matched children

false vocal folds   *See* **ventricular folds**

falsetto   Register near the speaker's physologic maximum frequency, produced by maximum contraction of the cricothyroid with maximum relaxation of the vocalis; see also **chest register**, **head register**, **mixed register**, **pulse register**

fascia   Band or sheet of connective tissue, primarily collagen, that attaches, stabilizes, encloses, and separates muscles and other internal organs

fasciculus cuneatus   The lateral column in the caudal medulla and the posterior spinal cord conveying sensation from the arms to the brain

fasciculus gracilis   The medial column in the caudal medulla and the posterior spinal cord conveying sensation from the legs to the brain

fastigial nucleus   A deep cerebellar nucleus that receives inputs from, the cortex of the midline of the neocerebellum and the archicerebellum and projects to the brainstem and fastigiospinal tract; *see also* **dentate nucleus, emboliform nucleus, globose nucleus**

fastigiospinal tract   A pathway made up of axons that originate in the fastigial nucleus of the cerebellum and descend to synapse in the spinal cord, typically on motor neurons and interneurons

feeding   Placement of food in the mouth and the oral stage of swallowing, including mastication

fiberoptic endoscopic evaluation of swallowing (FEES)   A portable and instrumental swallowing evaluation technique that involves the use of a flexible fiber optic endoscope that is inserted through the nasal cavity and oropharynx into the laryngopharynx

fibrin   An insoluble protein found in blood clots

fibrinolysin   An enzyme that breaks down fibrin

fibroblast   Cell type found in connective tissue

fibrous   Consisting of, or characterized by, fibers

fight or flight response   A physiologic reaction to attack or threat

final common pathway   The alpha lower motor neuron that directly drives muscles, resulting in behavior; the alpha motor neuron expresses the combined influences of many pathways from the rest of the nervous system involved in motor control and, thus, is the effector in common for all these systems

finite cell line   Cell line that has a limited life span and goes through a limited number of cell generations

fissure   A large groove or depression within the cortical surface that typically separates cortical structures

fixation   A general term for the process of chemically preserving specimens at a moment in time; fixation prevents further deterioration, so that the specimen appears as close as possible to what it would be like in its original living state

flagellum   A microtubule-based projection of the plasma membrane that is responsible for cell movement

flexor muscle   Muscle that bends a body part at a joint

flocculonodular lobe   A caudally located lobe of the cerebellar cortex with direct inputs from the vestibular nuclei via the inferior cerebellar peduncle and connections to the spinal cord; involved in the control of balance, posture, and control of eye gaze; also known as the archicerebellum

flocculus   Small lobe located at the base of the cerebellum

flow separation vortices   Regions of airflow around regions of low pressure created during the closing phase of vibration of the vocal folds

foramen (plural, foramina)   An opening or short passage through a bone or other structure

foramen cecum   A depression in the dorsum of the tongue that is the most posterior point of the sulcus terminalis

foramen magnum   Large hole in the base of skull through which the spinal cord passes

foramen ovale   An oval opening in the greater wing of the sphenoid for passage of the mandibular branch of the trigeminal nerve

foramen rotundum   A circular hole in the sphenoid bone for passage of the maxillary branch of the trigeminal nerve

force   Transmission of motion to an object; the object accelerates at a rate proportional to the force and inversely proportional to the object's mass

forced vibration   Vibration of an object at a frequency that may or may not be its natural frequency, caused by the vibration of some other object; see also **free vibration**

formant   A frequency around which sound energy is concentrated by the oral/nasal cavity, prominent on a sound spectrogram

fornix   A large arch-shaped bundle of nerve fibers that posteriorly connects to the bottom of the splenium and anteriorly communicates with the hippocampus, carrying signals from the hippocampus to the mammillary bodies and then to the anterior nuclei of the thalamus

fossa (plural, fossae)   A shallow depression or hollow

fourth ventricle   Fluid-filled cavity in the brain that lies in the dorsal midline of the pons and medulla; see also **lateral ventricle**, **third ventricle**

fovea   A specialized and highly sensitive region of the retina that corresponds to the center of one's visual gaze

foveola   The centermost zone of the fovea, where the ganglion and bipolar cell layers are excluded to allow light to fall upon the photoreceptors (cones only) directly

free field   The sound field without any obstacles to sound pressure waves

free vibration   Vibration of an object at its natural frequency without a sustained external force; see also **forced vibration**

frequency   The rate of vibration, measured in cycles per second (Hz)

frequency perturbation   Subtle changes in the frequency of a vibration from cycle to cycle; in a voice it is referred to as jitter

friction   Resistance to movement of an object caused by contact with another object along a plane parallel with the motion

frons   Forehead

frontal bone   The bone that forms the anterior part of the skull and the upper part of the eye sockets

frontal lobe   The lobe located at the front or rostral portion of the brain, mostly responsible for volition, consciousness, action, and regulation of memory

frontal plane   A vertical plane that divides a region into anterior and posterior parts; also called coronal plane

frontal sinus   Air-filled chamber located above the eyes within the frontal (forehead) bone

frontalis   Muscle that raises the eyebrows and wrinkles the forehead

frontonasal prominence   A median bulge of ectoderm formed at about the third week of development from the ventral aspect of the forebrain

functional localization   The correlation between cerebral anatomy and behavior that contributes to prominent psychologic theories and neurologic examinations

functional residual capacity   Volume of air contained within the lungs at the end of tidal expiration

fundamental frequency   The lowest frequency produced by a vibrating object such as the vocal folds; usually determines the perceived pitch; measured in hertz (Hz) and symbolized by F_0; see also **aperiodic energy**, **harmonic frequency**

fundamental logical operator   In an information-processing system, the lowest-level operation that can be carried out on the smallest possible amount of information; in electronic computers the smallest amount of information is a number that is either zero or one or an answer that is either false or true, and a fundamental logical operator outputs such a value that depends on one or more inputs, such as NOT *a* (output true if the input is false and vice versa) or *a* NAND *b* (output true only if the inputs are all false, otherwise output false); more complicated operations are combinations of multiple fundamental logical operators (for example, all the logical operations can be performed by combining multiple NAND circuits); in a living nervous system the neuron is the fundamental logical operator

fusiform   Having muscle fibers oriented in a longitudinal fashion to the belly of the muscle; see also **pinnate**

G

G-protein   A protein within the cytoplasm that, when activated by a G-protein-coupled receptor, binds guanosine triphosphate (GTP), signaling a particular condition to which the cell's internal systems respond

G-protein-coupled receptor   Receptor characterized by seven membrane-spanning α helices; ligand binding causes a conformational change that activates a G-protein, thus transmitting the ligand's signal across the plasma membrane

GABA   See **gamma-aminobutyric acid**

GABAergic   Communicating by means of gamma-aminobutyric acid (GABA) as neurotransmitter

gamete   Cell that fuses with another gamete to produce a new individual during fertilization in organisms that sexually reproduce

gamma-aminobutyric acid (GABA)   A neurotransmitter that usually has a hyperpolarizing effect

gamma lower motor neuron (γ-LMN)   A motor neurons in the brainstem or spinal cord whose axon synapses on an intrafusal (inside the spindle) muscle fiber; see also **alpha lower motor neuron**

ganglia (singular, ganglion) Clusters of neuron cell bodies, typically peripheral nervous system structures, with the exception of the basal ganglia

gap junction A region where the plasma membranes of adjacent cells are brought close together and channels going through both membranes form a direct cytoplasmic connection between the cells

gastrulation A phase early in embryonic development during which the blastula is reorganized into a trilaminar gastrula; it is followed by organogenesis

gating The process, performed in the thalamus, of filtering redundant or unnecessary sensory information received at the brainstem out of the integrated signal transmitted to the cortex

gene A segment of DNA on the chromosome that makes a product, such as a protein; humans have 20,000 to 25,000 genes

genioglossus muscle Primary mover of the tongue, originating on the mandible and constituting most of the bulk of the tongue

geniohyoid muscle A paired muscle that originates at the inferior mental spine and inserts into the body of the hyoid bone and moves the hyoid bone and larynx forward and upward

genome The complete set of DNA in an organism

genome scan Examination of thousands (or millions) of markers throughout the genome for linkage or association

genotype The combination of alleles at a locus present in an individual

genu The anterior portion of the corpus callosum

giant cell Neuronal cell type in the posterior ventral cochlear nucleus

gingival line The line formed by the edge of the unattached gum tissue at the margin of the soft tissues beside the teeth

glia *See* **glial cells**

glial cell Nonneuronal cell of the central nervous system that provides support for the metabolic, electrical, or chemical functions of neurons; they include astrocytes, oligodendrocytes, ependymal cells, and microglia

glioblast Neuroglial progenitor cell, which has the capacity to differentiate into either neuroglial cells or neuroblasts

globose nucleus One of the deep cerebellar nuclei that receives inputs from the cortex of the paramidline of the neocerebellum and the archicerebellum and projects to the rubrospinal and reticulospinal tracts; *see also* **dentate nucleus**, **emboliform nucleus**, **globose nucleus**

globular bushy cell A type of neuron in the anterior ventral cochlear nucleus

globular process The most medial edge of the medial nasal process, which is projected posteriorly into the nasal cavity around the sixth week of development to form the nasal laminae

globus pallidus A structure in the basal ganglia that is closely connected to the putamen and is situated medial to it, having two subdivisions: GPe, the external (lateral) segment of the globus pallidus, close to the putamen, and GPi ("globus pallidus interna," though this phrase is grammatically incorrect), the internal (medial) segment of the globus pallidus, which connects to the thalamus and is the main output structure

globus pallidus interna rate theory The theory that increased neuronal activity in the internal segment of the globus pallidus prevents expression of movements, presumably those not intended, and reduced activity permits expression of intended movements; in Parkinson's disease, it is hypothesized that the firing rate of the globus pallidus internal segment neurons is increased, thereby preventing even intended movements, while in disorders manifesting involuntary movements, such as Huntington's disease, the neurons of the globus pallidus internal segment are said to be underactive

glossopharyngeal nerve (CN IX) A mixed cranial nerve that sends some somatic information to the CNS from the middle ear cavity and parts of the pharynx and visceral information from the carotid body and sinus

glossoptosis Abnormality that results in backward-positioning (or retraction) of the tongue

glottis The space between the vocal folds

glutamate A neurotransmitter in the brain that tends to have a depolarizing effect, increasing activation (or activity) of neurons the primary excitatory neurotransmitter of the peripheral vestibular system

glutamate receptors Transmembrane proteins to which glutamate can bind, involved in synaptic transmission

glycine An amino acid that acts as a neurotransmitter that usually has a hyperpolarizing effect, reducing the activity of neurons

glycinergic Using glycine as neurotransmitter

glycolysis A nonoxidative (no oxygen required) metabolic pathway that produces ATP from glucose molecules

glycosaminoglycan (GAG) Gel-forming polysaccharide of the extracellular matrix

Golgi apparatus Cytoplasmic organelle involved in the processing and sorting of proteins and lipids

Golgi tendon organ (GTO)   A sensor responsible for communicating to the CNS how much force is being produced by the muscle on a tendon

gracile fasciculus   A bundle of axons in the dorsal column (more correctly, posterior funiculus) white matter of the spinal cord that houses primary afferent axons from the lower limbs and lower trunk

graded potential   A change in electrical potential across a neuronal cell membrane that is caused by an event at a synapse, such as a neurotransmitter binding to its receptor, and that dissipates over time and distance from the synaptic site because of lack of positive feedback mechanisms maintaining the changes in the electrical potentials, in contrast to those mediating action potentials

granular cell   Neuronal cell type in the dorsal cochlear nucleus

granule cells   Interneurons found in the cerebellar cortex that receive mossy fiber inputs from the pontine nuclei; the neurons have an axon that ascends in the cortex and then branches to produce axons that run in parallel in opposite directions; thus, granule cells can affect a great number of Purkinje cells that align in the gyri of the cerebellar cortex

gray matter   Darker tissue of the brain and spinal cord, consisting mainly of nerve cell bodies and dendrites as well as unmyelinated axons, axon terminals (synapses), and glial cells; *see also* **white matter**

great cerebral vein   One of the deep cerebral veins; a large vein that extends from the internal cerebral veins and drains the cerebrum

greater cornu   Projection of the hyoid bone on either side; see also **lesser cornu**

ground substance   Gelatinous mixture of proteins other than collagen or elastin found outside cells, particularly in the superficial lamina propria of the vocal folds

gustation   The perception of taste

gyri (singular, gyrus)   A ridge or fold between two clefts (sulci) of the cerebral cortex of the brain

gyrus rectus   A straight gyral structure that is located medially to the olfactory sulcus

γLMN   *See* **gamma lower motor neuron**

H

habenula perforata   Small perforation in the osseous spiral lamina though which auditory nerve fibers traverse

hair cells (HC)   Mechanoreceptive cells with bundles of stereocilia on their top surfaces, found in the cochlea (where they are divided into outer and inner hair cells) and vestibular system; they produce graded receptor potential changes when stimulated by bending of stereocilia

haploid   Having only one member of each pair of chromosomes; if there are n pairs of chromosomes, such a cell would be said to have a haploid number n; *see also* **diploid**

harmonic frequency   An integer multiple of the fundamental frequency of a vibrating system, such as $2 \times F_0, 3 \times F_0, \ldots$; harmonics usually determine the quality of the perceived sound; see also **aperiodic energy**, **fundamental frequency**

harmonics-to-noise ratio   The ratio of the energy of periodic components in an acoustic signal to that of nonharmonic frequencies

hastening   A phenomenon associated with bradykinesia in patients with Parkinson's disease, in which patients asked to tap their fingers in sync with a metronome that is increasing its pace first maintain the same finger tapping rate and so fall behind the metronome until it reaches a certain frequency at which the patients increase their finger tapping rate ahead of the metronome and continue at that rate until they fall behind once again

head register   The register higher than chest register; speakers feel sensations mainly in the sinuses; F_0 is controlled primarily by the cricothyroid (contraction raises F_0); see also **falsetto**, **mixed register**, **pulse register**

head shadow   Blockage of sound waves by the head

head-related transfer function   The response of the ear as it receives a sound from a source in space

hearing threshold   The softest sound (lowest intensity) that can be perceived by a listener

Hebbian learning   A theory that posits that when two (or more) synaptic inputs (typically depolarizing) are repetitively active at the same time and same general vicinity, the postsynaptic neuron will become more likely to generate an action potential in response to the subsequent activations of the individual synaptic inputs, thus creating a form of learning

helicotrema   The most apical part of the cochlear labyrinth, where the scala tympani and scala vestibuli connect

helix   The superior and posterior outer ridge of the pinna

hemiballismus An involuntary movement characterized by forceful, often violent, sudden jerks of the muscle; this phenomenon particularly is associated with disorders of the subthalamic nucleus

hemidesmosome A region of contact between cells and the extracellular matrix at which intermediate filaments are attached to integrin

hemifield The portion of the visual field mediated by one retina

Henneman size principle The principle that normally, when one begins to exert a force that is progressively increased, the small motor units are recruited (activated) first, with larger units being recruited as the intended force increases; this is not the case in individuals with Parkinson's disease

Hensen cell One of the supporting columnar cells between the outer hair cells and Claudius cells in the organ of Corti

heparin An anticoagulant (substance used to prevent blood clots from forming) found in the lungs

Hering-Breuer inflation reflex Signal to the inspiratory control center within the medulla and pneumotaxic center within the pons, inhibiting inspiration and reducing respiratory rate

heritability The proportion of variation in the phenotype in the population that is due to genetic factors

hertz (Hz) Unit of frequency; one vibratory cycle per second

Heschl gyrus The main gyrus of the primary auditory cortex

hilum The lung root; a triangle-shaped depression in the medial (mediastinal) surface of each lung where the right or left bronchi enter the lung along with pulmonary blood vessels, nerves, and lymphatic vessels

hip strategy One of the four vestibulospinal reflexes in which the leg muscles are contracted and the hips and head are moved in opposite directions to rebalance weight distribution and regain balance; see also **ankle strategy**, **stepping strategy**, **suspensory strategy**

hippocampus A seahorse-shaped structure of the limbic system that lies medially within the temporal lobe of each hemisphere; the hippocampus is critical for the formation of new memories and it is thought to be the center of emotion

homeostasis Maintenance of the balance of conditions inside the body that is most conducive to health and life

homeostatic emotion Subjective, affective ("emotional") experiences related to temperature, itch, visceral distension (of bladder, stomach, rectum, or esophagus), muscle ache, hunger, thirst, breathlessness or dyspnea and sensual touch

homunculus The mapping of parts of the body to localized areas in the cerebral cortex; for example, the body parts are mapped to the primary motor cortex beginning with the head in the most lateral locations, then the hand, arm, trunk, and finally the lower extremities mapped to the medial surface of the hemisphere; the primary somatosensory cortex is similarly mapped

horizontal cell A cell involved in adjusting output of photoreceptors in the retina by lateral inhibition; see also **amacrine cell**

horizontal plane A plane that divides a region into superior and inferior parts; also called axial plane, transaxial plane, or transverse plane

horizontal semicircular canal One of the three semicircular canals of the inner ear, oriented in a semi-horizontal fashion, medial to the vestibular labyrinth; responsible for translating horizontal head rotation into neural impulses; see also **anterior semicircular canal**

Huntington's disease An autosomal dominant disorder associated with involuntary movements and cognitive and psychological problems; though there is widespread neuronal injury, the striatum appears to be involved the most

hyaline cartilage A type of cartilage that becomes harder with age; see also **elastic cartilage**

hydrocephalus Excess fluid in the ventricles of the brain

hydrophilic Soluble in water

hydrophobic Not soluble in water

hydrostasis The manner in which equal and opposing pressures generated by proximal liquids create a stable equilibrium

hydrostatic force Force generated by a fluid at rest, such as the surface tension force of pleural fluid that creates a stable relationship between the lungs and the thoracic cavity

hyoepiglottic ligament Ligament connecting the middle of the epiglottis to the hyoid bone

hyoglossus Muscle that originates at the hyoid bone and acts on the tongue

hyoid bone A **U**-shaped bone in the neck that supports the tongue and larynx

hyolaryngeal excursion Upward and forward movement of the larynx and hyoid bone caused by contraction of the geniohyoid muscle

hypercapnic hypoxia Condition of increased blood CO_2 (lowering blood pH) and reduced O_2

hyperdirect pathway An anatomic pathway within the basal ganglia system in which connections from the cerebral cortex are made to the subthalamic nucleus and from there to the globus pallidus internal segment; the anatomy of this pathway has been extrapolated into physiologic inferences related to the physiology and pathophysiology of the basal ganglia–thalamic–cortical system

hyperkinetic disorders Disorders of movement associated with involuntary movements excluding tremor

hypermetria Movements that take the limb beyond the intended target

hypernasal Having too much nasal resonance, as from inadequate closure of the velopharyngeal port

hyperplasia Increase in the number of cells

hyperpolarization Increase in the magnitude of the electrical potential across a cell membrane, such as the neuronal membrane (which is usually at a negative potential, so it is hyperpolarized by positive charges leaving or negative charges entering the cell); *see also* **depolarization**

hyperpolarizing A change in the electrical potential across the neuronal membrane in a more negative direction

hyperreflexia The phenomenon of exaggerated deep tendon reflexes

hypertonic solution Solution (e.g., extracellular fluid) with a higher solute concentration than another solution

hypertonus increased muscle tone defined as increased resistance to passive joint rotations

hypertrophy Muscle enlargement resulting from increase in cross-sectional area of muscle fibers rather than from increase in their number (which would be hyperplasia)

hypoblast The innermost layer arising from the inner cell mass in the blastocyst

hypoglossal nerve (CN XII) A pure motor nerve that innervates all of the tongue muscles and the geniohyoid and most infrahyoid muscles

hypokinetic disorders Disorders of movement associated with movements that are abnormally slow, such as those seen in Parkinson's disease

hypometria Movements that fall short of the intended target

hyponasal Having too little nasal resonance

hypophonic Having a voice volume typically less than would be normal

hypophysis *See* **pituitary gland**

hypothalamus A sugar cube-shaped structure located below the thalamus that forms the ventral aspect of the diencephalon, with multiple nuclei and specific white matter pathways; many of its various nuclei communicate with the pituitary gland; the hypothalamus is crucially involved in regulating homeostatic processes in the body

hypotonia Abnormally reduced resistance to passive joint rotation

hypotonic solution Solution (e.g., extracellular fluid) with a lower solute concentration than another solution

hypoxia Low concentrations of O_2 in the blood

I

ideational apraxia A type of apraxia most evident with tool use; for example, an affected individual may be able to name the tool and describe its function but be unable to demonstrate its use; *see also* **ideomotor apraxia**, **kinetic apraxia**

ideomotor apraxia A type of apraxia most evident when the subject is asked to imitate various actions, such as waving goodbye, or the use of an object; for example, an affected individual may be able to name a tool such as a hammer, describe its function, and even demonstrate the use of the actual tool but be unable to imitate the action of the tool; *see also* **ideational apraxia**, **kinetic apraxia**

IHC *See* **inner hair cell**

immediate energy system Anaerobic energy system that uses locally available energy stores to provide the primary energy pathway for muscle efforts that last less than 30 seconds

immunologic defense mechanisms Mechanisms for defending a bodily system that rely on the immune system's capability for recognizing specific pathogens

impedance The ability of an object to oppose the flow of energy through it in some form

incisivus labii inferioris Muscle that pulls the corner of the mouth inferiorly

incisivus labii superioris Muscle that elevates the corner of the mouth and draws it medially

incisor A narrow-edged tooth at the front of the mouth, adapted for cutting

incudomallear joint The joint connecting the malleus and incus in the middle ear

incudostapedial joint The joint connecting the incus and the stapes in the middle ear

incus Anvil; the middle bone of the ossicular chain within the middle ear, between the malleus and the stapes

indirect laryngoscopy Viewing of a reversed image of the larynx and vocal folds, as produced by a mirror introduced through the patient's mouth; *see also* **direct laryngoscopy**

indirect pathway An anatomic pathway within the basal ganglia system in which connections from the striatum arrive at the globus pallidus internal segment by way of the globus pallidus external segment and the subthalamic nucleus; the anatomy of this pathway has been extrapolated into physiologic inferences related to the physiology and pathophysiology of the basal ganglia–thalamic–cortical system

induced pluripotent stem cell A stem cell that has been created from an adult cell, such as a skin, liver, stomach, or other mature cell, through the introduction of genes that reprogram the cell and transform it into a cell that has all the characteristics of an embryonic stem cell

inertia The tendency of objects to either stay at rest or stay in motion

inertive reactance The effect of an inertial element, such as the mass of a column of air, on oscillations such as the acoustic waves produced by vocal fold vibration

inferior Below or under another structure

inferior cerebellar peduncle Pathway conveying information to and from the cerebellum that exits from the caudal portion of the cerebellum through the medulla of the brainstem

inferior colliculus (IC) The principal midbrain nucleus of the central auditory pathway, located on the tectum of the midbrain; this nucleus receives inputs from the superior olivary complex and the cochlear nuclei and is thought to create a 3D map of auditory space through integration of inputs from lower levels of the central auditory pathway; projects to the medial geniculate nucleus

inferior longitudinal muscle Paired intrinsic muscle of the tongue that depresses the tongue tip

inferior mental spine A small projection on the internal surface of the mandible

inferior olivary nucleus A collection of neuronal somas in the medulla of the brainstem that are a source of climbing fibers to the Purkinje neurons of the cerebellar cortex

inferior pharyngeal constrictor The lowest of the pharyngeal constrictor muscles; propels food into the esophagus

information Nonrandom changes in some state; it is not necessary that the state changes correspond to any given system of symbols (such as the sequence of letters *c*, *a*, *t*) but only that they be nonrandom, such as the activations of motor units to produce a nonrandom behavior, which are not symbolic but nonetheless contain information

infrahyoid muscle Muscle acting on the hyoid bone from below

infraorbital foramen Opening in the maxillary bone that allows passage of the infraorbital nerve, which is a branch of the maxillary branch of the trigeminal nerve

inhibitory postsynaptic potential (IPSP) a change in the electrical potential across the neuronal membrane in a more negative direction, more accurately referred to as a hyperpolarizing postsynaptic potential

inner cell mass The mass of cells inside the primordial embryo that ultimately gives rise to the embryo and forms or contributes to all of the extraembryonic membranes

inner hair cells (IHC) 3,000 to 4,000 cells forming a single row down the length of the organ of Corti, closest to the central axis of the cochlear spiral, sending 90% of afferent input to auditory nerve

insertion The more mobile point of attachment of a muscle

inspiration The process of taking air into the lung

inspiratory-expiratory muscle strength training (IMST-EMST) Combination of inspiratory and expiratory muscle strength training

inspiratory muscle strength training (IMST) Targeted, exercise-based conditioning of the muscles of inspiration, primarily the diaphragm and external intercostals

inspiratory reserve volume The volume of air that can be actively inhaled beyond that which is inhaled during tidal breathing

insula (insular cortex) Region of the cerebral cortex that is buried in the folds of the lateral fissure (lateral sulcus) beneath the frontal, temporal, and parietal lobes; thought to be involved in consciousness and to play a role in diverse functions linked to emotion or regulation of homeostasis

integral protein A protein embedded within the lipid bilayer of a cell membrane

integrin A transmembrane protein that mediates the adhesion of cells to the extracellular matrix

intensity With reference to sound, the magnitude of a sound pressure wave

interarytenoid (IA) muscle Muscle in two divisions (oblique and transverse) reaching from the base of one arytenoid cartilage to the apex of the other; contracting, it draws the arytenoids closer to each other and adducts the vocal folds

interaural level difference (ILD) The difference (in intensity) of sound between the left and right ear as it arrives from a sound source in space; also called interaural intensity difference (IID)

interaural timing difference (ITD) The difference in the timing of a sound between the left and right ear as it arrives from a sound source in space

intermaxillary suture The line of union of the two upper jaw bones

intermediate filament Cytoskeletal filament about 10 nm in diameter that provides mechanical strength to cells in tissues

intermediate lamina propria (ILP) The third layer in from the surface in the vocal fold, containing more elastin fibers than the superficial lamina propria but less stiff (containing less collagen) than the deep lamina propria

intermediate nucleus of the lateral lemniscus (DNLL) Intermediate division of the lateral lemniscus

intermediate stria A fiber tract of axons that originate from the posterior ventral cochlear nucleus and project to the trapezoid body and form a portion of the lateral lemniscal tract

internal auditory canal Canal within the petrous portion of the temporal bone through which the facial and vestibulocochlear nerves pass; also called internal auditory meatus

internal branch of the superior laryngeal nerve (ISLN) Main sensory nerve for mucous membranes of the epiglottis, tongue base, and upper larynx

internal capsule A white matter structure in the brain that carries information between the thalamus and the cortex, separated from the external capsule by the putamen and globus pallidus

internal carotid arteries The primary paired arteries for the cerebral hemispheres, located on each side of the head

internal cerebral vein One of the deep cerebral veins, located above the third ventricle; it is where the deep cerebral veins converge

internal respiration Gas exchange inside tissues; also called peripheral gas exchange

interneuron Neuron whose axon projects only a short distance to nearby neurons in the brain and spinal cord; the interneurons' dendrites and axons are confined to the local area, such as a specific organization in the cortex (e.g., a column), or in a collection of neurons (e.g., a nucleus); interneurons are thought to process information within the confines of the nucleus or column in the cortex

interoception Ability to sense stimuli that arise from within the body

interoreceptors Sensory organs that detect substances that exist inside of the body

interphase The resting phase of the cell cycle in which the cell spends the majority of its time; the cell prepares for mitosis by replicating its chromosomes during this time

interpositus nucleus Either the globose nucleus or the emboliform nucleus of the cerebellum

interthalamic adhesion A gray band that connects the two regions of the thalamus across the midline of the brain

interventricular foramen (plural, interventricular foramina) Narrow channel that connects the lateral ventricle and the third ventricle

intracellular receptors Receptors located in the cytoplasm that are activated by hydrophobic ligand molecules that can pass through the plasma membrane

intraembryonic mesoderm Mesoderm generated from epiblast cells migrating through the primitive streak; it becomes divided into paraxial mesoderm, intermediate mesoderm, and lateral plate mesoderm

intrafusal muscle fiber A muscle fiber within the muscle spindle, whose stretch activates receptors on the muscle. The intrafusal muscle fiber is innervated by axons from the gamma lower motor neuron, which affects the sensitivity of the spindle to detect stretch

intraglottal pressure differentials Differences in pressure between different regions of the glottis during the vibratory cycle of the vocal folds

intrathalamic interneuron Local neuron within the thalamus

intrinsic laryngeal muscles Muscles that move the vocal folds within the larynx

intron Part of the sequence in a gene that does not code for mature protein and that occurs between exons

inverse problem The situation in which a single phenomenon can be produced by any of multiple causes; the problem arises in that the specific cause among the many that could produce the phenomenon cannot be determined

inverse square law As a wave of sound or light propagates from its source, the same power is distributed over a larger area, so the intensity decreases in proportion to the area; that is, in proportion to the square of the distance

ion channel A protein structure that spans the neuronal membrane that contains a pore that can open or close so as to control the flow of a specific ion through the membrane

ionotropic directly causing changes in ion flux through channels in the postsynaptic cell membrane

ipsilateral Belonging to, or occurring on, the same side of the body

irritant receptors Sensors within the lungs that detect irritants

isofrequency A region within the auditory system defined by one frequency

isometric contraction Muscle activity that is characterized by tension being developed in the muscle tissue without any change in actual muscle length or joint angle

isotonic contraction Muscle activity that is characterized by shortening or lengthening of the muscle; it may be concentric or eccentric

isotonic solutions Two solutions having the same osmotic pressure across a semipermeable membrane

J

J-receptors Sensory nerve endings located within the alveolar walls, in juxtaposition to pulmonary capillaries, that detect fluid within the lung and accumulation of blood in the capillaries

jitter *See* **frequency perturbation**

joint Point at which two or more bones meet

jugum A connecting ridge or projection

just-noticeable difference (JND) The minimal difference in strength between a reference stimulus and a second stimulus whereby a difference can be detected

juxtacapillary receptors *see* **J-receptors**

juxtacrine signaling Contact-dependent signaling in which two adjacent cells must make physical contact in order to communicate

K

karyotype The organized profile of an individual's genome, characterized using form and numbers

kinesia paradoxica Paradoxical movement that appears normal in patients with bradykinesia and akinesia, such as those affected by Parkinson's disease

kinetic apraxia A type of apraxia where the individual is unable to perform an exact or precise movement, such as using a screwdriver to insert a small screw, but the inability is not associated with weakness, sensory loss, or evidence of involvement of the basal ganglia or cerebellum; *see also* **ideational apraxia, ideomotor apraxia**

kinocilium A special type of projection on the apex of hair cells in the inner ear

L

labeled-line principle of sensory systems The principle that perception is effectively localized and mapped by modality or class of sensation to specific components of the nervous system

labial Of, or relating to, the lips

lamina terminalis Sheet of tissue that stretches from the interventricular foramen to the recess at the base of the optic stalk; located along the median wall of the prosencephalon

large aspiny neurons interneurons of the striatum that typically utilize acetylcholine as neurotransmitter

laryngeal depressor Muscle originating below the larynx that pulls the larynx downward

laryngeal elevator Muscle originating above the larynx that pull the larynx upward

laryngeal prominence The central line where the two laminae of the thyroid cartilages have fused anteriorly; visible as "Adam's apple"

laryngeal ventricle The space between the ventricular fold (false vocal fold) and the vocal fold

laryngeal vestibule The upper part of the larynx above the vocal folds

laryngeal videostroboscopy Viewing of the larynx and vocal folds illuminated by a strobe light that flashes at a rate slightly less than the phonation frequency to show the periodic components of vocal fold vibration as if in slow motion

laryngologist An otolaryngologist who specializes in laryngeal impairments that cause voice and swallowing disorders, with special skills and training in diagnostic and therapeutic approaches to manage these disorders; most laryngologists complete a one-year fellowship in laryngology after completing a five-year residency in otolaryngology

laryngopharynx The lower part of the pharynx, posterior to the larynx; part of the alimentary system but not the respiratory system

laryngoscope Instrument used for viewing the larynx and vocal folds

laryngoscopy *See* **direct laryngoscopy**, **indirect laryngoscopy**, **laryngeal videostroboscopy**, **microlaryngoscopy**

laryngospasm Reflexive temporary stop in breathing when food or other substance reaches the vocal folds or the infraglottal region

larynx A cartilaginous structure, part of which is visible externally as "Adam's apple," which serves as a valve between the upper and lower respiratory tracts; location of the vocal folds

lateral To the side of another structure

lateral cricoarytenoid (LCA) muscle Muscle originating on the lateral arches of the cricoid cartilage and inserting on the muscular process of the arytenoid cartilage; contracting, it adducts the vocal folds; *see also* **posterior cricoarytenoid (PCA) muscle**

lateral cricothyroid ligament Thinner part of the cricothyroid ligament that connects the cricoid arch to the thyroid cartilage as well as to the vocal processes

lateral fissure (lateral sulcus) A prominent division between both the frontal and parietal lobes (superiorly) and the temporal lobe (inferiorly) of the brain; also called sylvian fissure

lateral geniculate nucleus (LGN) Nucleus of the thalamus receiving visual information from the optic tracts; it is retinotopically organized and consists of six layers that receive inputs from different classes of retinal ganglion cells

lateral inhibition A contrast enhancement mechanism whereby the activity of one receptive field is heightened through inhibition of adjacent receptive fields

lateral lemniscus A fiber tract that projects from the cochlear nucleus to the inferior colliculus (IC)

lateral lingual swellings Paired thickenings on the internal surface of the mandibular arch that develop in the fifth week of development to form the tongue

lateral nasal process The areas of the nasal process lateral to the nasal pits but medial to the nasolacrimal groove

lateral pterygoid Muscle originating on the sphenoid bone that opens and protrudes the jaw

lateral recess An extension of the fourth ventricle on each side at the cerebellar peduncles

lateral sulcus *See* **lateral fissure (lateral sulcus)**

lateral superior olivary nucleus (LSO) A specialized nucleus of the superior olivary complex involved in sound localization by comparing intensity differences between the two ears; *see also* **medial superior olivary nucleus (MSO)**

lateral thyrohyoid ligament Thickened lateral section of the thyrohyoid membrane, connecting to the greater thyroid horn

lateral ventricle One of a pair of fluid-filled cavities in the brain, with one in each hemisphere, are separated from the medial space of the brain by a thin membrane called the septum pellucidum; see also **fourth ventricle**, **third ventricle**

lateral vestibular nucleus A collection of neurons in the medulla of the brainstem that receive input from the vestibular apparatus in the inner ear

lateral vestibulospinal tract One of the two major descending pathways of the vestibulospinal network that originates at the central vestibular nucleus complex and terminates at all levels of the spinal cord; *see also* **medial vestibulospinal tract**

lateral zone of the cerebellum A region of the cerebellar cortex, involving but not limited to the neocerebellum, defined by reciprocal connections to the dentate nucleus

length-tension relationship Tension development in the muscle fiber that is relative to the degree to which actin and myosin filaments overlap at the start of muscle contraction

lesser cornu An upward projection on each side of the hyoid bone, located where the body and the greater cornu meet

levator anguli oris Muscle that elevates the corner of the mouth

levator labii superioris Muscle that elevates the upper lip and the angle of the mouth

levator labii superioris alaeque nasi Muscle with two bellies: one that opens the nostril and one that elevates the upper lip

levator veli palatini Principal muscle elevating the soft palate

levodopa A prodrug that, when administered, is metabolized to the neurotransmitter dopamine

ligament A band of fibrous tissue that connects bones or cartilages, serving to support and strengthen joints

ligand A substance that binds specifically and reversibly to another chemical entity to form a larger complex; binding of a ligand to a receptor often leads to a metabolic or structural change, such as opening or closing of an ion channel

ligand-gated ion channel A protein structure that spans the neuronal membrane and allows the flow of a specific positive or negative ion when it opens in response to the binding of a chemical, such as a neurotransmitter

light microscopy Microscopy in which the specimen is viewed under ordinary illumination

limb-kinetic apraxia Kinetic apraxia as it applies to the use of the limbs

limbic lobe The C-shaped lobe running from the medial surface of the cerebral cortex into the temporal lobe

limbic system A complex structure comprised of specific gray matter nuclei and white matter pathways within each lobe of each cerebral hemisphere that has a specific C-shape. The limbic system contributes to the regulation of emotion and memory formation; see also **amygdala**, **fornix**, **hippocampus**

limbus The border or margin of a structure

lingual Of, relating to, or facing the tongue

lingual gyrus Gyral structure that is inferior to the calcarine sulcus of the occipital lobe; involved in encoding complex images and recognizing written words

linkage Two markers are said to be linked on a chromosome when they segregate together more often than expected by chance

lipids Hydrophobic molecules that function as energy storage molecules, signaling molecules, and the major components of cell membranes

LMN *See* **lower motor neuron**

lobar bronchi Branches of the principal bronchi, in each lung, that extend into the individual lobes; the right lung contains three lobar bronchi and the left lung contains two

lobe An anatomic division of the cerebral cortex that is defined by specific landmarks

locus (plural, loci) A site of a specific gene or marker on a chromosome

longitudinal (hemispheric) fissure The long, deep cleft that divides the cerebrum into the right and left hemispheres

longitudinal tension Stretch of the vocal folds along their length

loudness The perceptual correlate of intensity of sound

lower motor neuron A motor neuron whose cell body is located in the anterior gray column of the spinal cord or a cranial nerve nucleus of the brainstem and whose axon synapses on muscle fibers

lower respiratory system The subdivision of the respiratory system consisting of the trachea, bronchi, and lungs (including all structures within the lungs)

lung buds Bilateral structures that form as lateral outgrowths at the caudal aspect of the laryngotracheal tube and that give rise to the bronchi of both lungs

lungs Paired conical organs of respiration

lysosome Cytoplasmic organelle containing enzymes that break down biologic polymers

lytic medication Medication that dissolves blood clots

M

macromolecule A large, complex molecule such as a nucleic acid, protein, or carbohydrate or lipid with relatively large molecular weight

macula A layer of specialized epithelium found in the otolithic organs, housing vestibular hair cells, innervated by the vestibular branch of the vestibulocochlear nerve (CN VIII) and sensitive to linear accelerations

macula flava Region at the anterior and posterior ends of the vocal folds, containing high concentrations of fibroblasts that produce the extracellular proteins that make up much of the folds

magnitude estimation A test in which participants use a numerical scale to estimate the magnitude of a stimulus

major gene effect The situation in which a single gene contributes substantially to the variance in a trait

malleus Hammer; the lateral bone of the tympanic membrane that transmits vibrations of the tympanic membrane to the incus

malnutrition Condition in which the body does not receive sufficient nutrients to maintain a healthy state

mammillary bodies A pair of pea-sized lumps, part of the hypothalamus, protruding anteriorly to the fornix

mandible The singular bone that makes up the lower jaw

mandibular branch (CN V₃) The most inferior branch of the trigeminal nerve, carrying all somatic innervation from the lower face, stretching from the lower lip around the jaw and chin to the upper neck; it also innervates the lower oral cavity, including the anterior two-thirds of the tongue, and provides jaw proprioception

mandibular foramen An opening on the medial surface of the ramus of the mandible

mandibular prominences Structures located caudal to the stomodeum/oral groove; they form from the first branchial arch

manometry Assessment of oropharyngeal and esophageal swallowing pressures by a catheter with sensors that detect pressure changes placed in the swallowing mechanism

manubrium A handle; the manubrium of the malleus attaches to the tympanic membrane; the superior end of the sword-shaped sternum is its manubrium

marker Naturally occurring variation in the DNA sequence that can be used to track the inheritance pattern of a particular chromosomal location in families or individuals

masklike facies A form of akinesia associated with a loss of the facial movements that convey affect, typically seen in individuals with Parkinson's disease

masseter Powerful muscle originating on the zygomatic arch that closes the mandible

mastication Chewing; part of feeding and swallowing

mastoid process A rounded conical prominence of the temporal bone behind the ear, to which neck muscles are attached

maxilla Paired bone forming the upper jaw

maxillary branch (CN V₂) The middle branch of the trigeminal nerve, mediating all somatic sensation in the intermediate face, from the lower half of the eyes down to the upper lip, and including the nasal cavity, upper teeth, and palate

maxillary prominences   Structures located superior and lateral to the stomodeum/oral groove; they form from the first branchial arch

maxillary sinuses   Air-filled chambers within the maxillary bones that are situated laterally to the nasal cavity

meatus   A passage or opening leading to the interior of a body

mechanical transduction channel   Mechanically gated ion channel that converts mechanical signals into chemical signals

mechanoreceptor   Primary receptor responsible for converting changes in pressure and muscular stretching or bending into information regarding touch, hearing, balance, and proprioception

medial   Located closer to the midline

medial compression   Force of the vocalis and cricothyroid muscles to hold the vocal folds together against airflow pressure

medial geniculate body (MGB)   Nucleus near the thalamus that receives auditory inputs from the inferior colliculus; the first location where neurons are activated by specific combinations of frequencies or are sensitive to specific time delays between the presentation of two frequencies

medial longitudinal fasciculus (MLF)   A large fiber bundle with two tracts; the ascending MLF connects the central vestibular nucleus complex to the three extraocular muscles, and the descending MLF connects the central vestibular nucleus complex to the medial vestibulospinal tract (VST)

medial nasal process   The segment of the nasal process between the two nasal pits

medial nucleus of the trapezoid body (MNTB)   Group of neurons associated with the trapezoid body and a primary structure within the superior olivary complex

medial pterygoid   Muscle originating on the sphenoid bone that closes the mandible; *see also* **lateral pterygoid**

medial superior olivary nucleus (MSO)   A specialized nucleus of the superior olivary complex involved in sound localization by comparing timing differences between the two ears; *see also* **lateral superior olivary nucleus (LSO)**

medial vestibulospinal tract   One of two tracts of the vestibulospinal network that originates in the central vestibular nucleus complex and terminates in the cervical spinal cord and neck; it functions to coordinate reflexive movements to keep the head centered over the body to maintain upright posture; *see also* **lateral vestibulospinal tract**

median cricothyroid ligament   Thicker center portion of the cricothyroid ligament, connecting the anterior arch of the cricoid to the posterior inferior undersurface of the thyroid cartilage

median fibrous septum   Vertical sheet of connective tissue that divides the tongue into left and right halves and serves as the origin for several tongue muscles

median laryngotracheal groove   Structure that appears on the floor of the foregut in the fourth week of development, deepens, and becomes the tubular lung bud

median sulcus   Groove or furrow along the midline of the dorsum of the tongue

median thyrohyoid ligament   Thickened middle portion of the thyrohyoid membrane

mediastinum   Membranous compartment containing the heart, blood vessels, esophagus, trachea, phrenic and cardiac nerves, thoracic duct, thymus, and numerous lymph nodes, dividing the thoracic cavity into two parts, each containing one lung

medium spiny neurons (MSNs)   Efferent neurons of the striatum of the basal ganglia typically using GABA as the neurotransmitter, comprising approximately 95% of the neurons in the striatum

medulla oblongata   The inferior part of the brainstem, between the pons and the spinal cord; often simply called the medulla

medullary respiratory center   Part of the respiratory CPG, located within the reticular formation

medulloblast   An undifferentiated cell of the embryonic neural tube that may develop into either astrocytes or oligodendrocytes

meiosis   A specialized type of cell division that produces haploid gametes by means of two meiotic divisions, meiosis I and meiosis II; *see also* **mitosis**

membrane potential   The electric potential that exists on the two sides of a membrane or across the wall of a cell

membranous vocal fold   Most of the length of the vocal fold except near the vocal process of the arytenoid

Ménière's disease   A disorder of the inner ear that causes spontaneous episodes of vertigo, or the sensation of spinning, along with fluctuating hearing loss, tinnitus, and the sensation of ear fullness

meninges   A collective term for the membranous tissues that cover the central nervous system: the dura mater, the arachnoid mater, and the pia mater

mental foramen   One of two holes located on the anterior surface of the mandible

mental protuberance   A midline swelling on the base of mandible on its anterior surface where the two sides of the mandible come together

mental symphysis   Union of the two halves of the mandible (lower jaw)

mental tubercle   A prominence on the inner border of either side of the mental protuberances of the mandible

mentalis   Muscle that depresses and protrudes the lower lip

mereological fallacy   The fallacy of ascribing the functions or operations of the whole to the part, such as ascribing to the globus pallidus internal segment the role of selecting movements to be executed when such actions actually represent the operations of the entire basal ganglia–thalamic–cortical system

mesencephalon   Midbrain; the superior part of the brainstem above the pons and medulla oblongata; develops from one of the three dilations of the neural tube, cephalad to the rhombencephalon but caudal to the prosencephalon

mesoderm   The middle layer of the three primary germ layers, which also lies outside of the embryo as extraembryonic mesoderm; intraembryonic mesoderm forms most of the connective tissues and muscles of the body

messenger RNA (mRNA)   A long single strand of ribonucleic acid, formed by transcription of exons, whose base sequence is to be translated into a protein by ribosomes

metabotropic   Causing a cascade of signals (G-coupled proteins) within the postsynaptic cell that ultimately modify the cell's response to signals

metaphase   The longest stage of mitosis, following prophase and preceding anaphase, during which the nuclear envelope fragments, the chromosomes attach to the microtubules of the mitotic spindle, and the microtubules align the chromosomes on the metaphase plate

metastable   A dynamical state of fragile stability such that the states can bifurcate to other states, for example when a coin is resting on its edge and falls flat on one face or the other

metencephalon   Part of the hindbrain that is located superior to the myelencephalon and inferior to the mesencephalon

method of concomitant variations   A logical method of induction according to which, if, when the magnitude of one variable changes, the magnitude of another variable also changes consistently, the two variables are considered to be related; either one causes the other or they are related by a common cause

method of difference   A logical method of induction, according to which, if two cases have all but one of a set of conditions in common and have all but one of a set of observed variables in common, the one variable they do not have in common is considered to be caused by the one condition they do not have in common

microfilament   Cytoskeletal filament composed of actin

microglia   A special type of phagocyte in the brain and spinal cord, thought to be involved primarily in inflammatory processes in the central nervous system as macrophages are in the rest of the body

microlaryngoscopy   Use of a microscope attachment with a laryngoscope to obtain an enlarged view of the larynx and vocal folds

microscope   An instrument used to obtain an enlarged image of small objects and reveal details of structure not otherwise distinguishable

microtia   The abnormal shape or absence of the pinna

microtubule   Cytoskeletal component formed by the polymerization of tubulin into rigid, hollow rods about 25 nm in diameter

midbrain   *See* **mesencephalon**

middle cerebellar peduncle   Communication pathway between the cerebellum and the pons of the brainstem

middle cerebral artery (MCA)   Blood vessel that supplies the lateral aspects of hemispheres and the basal ganglia

middle pharyngeal constrictor   Muscle originating on the hyoid bone, inserting on the occipital bone, and constricting the pharynx above the larynx during swallowing

midsagittal plane   A vertical plane that divides a region into equal left and right parts; also called median plane

minute ventilation   The volume of gas exchanged per minute of breathing

mitochondria   Cytoplasmic organelles responsible for synthesis of most of the ATP in eukaryotic cells by oxidative phosphorylation

mitosis   The usual type of cell division, which produces diploid daughter cells; the nuclei dissolve, the chromosomes separate from their duplicates, and the nuclei reform during prophase, metaphase, anaphase, and telophase, and the cytoplasm is divided into two new cells during cytokinesis; *see also* **meiosis**

mixed register   Phonation in the region of the boundary between chest and head registers, controlled by both the cricothyroid and vocalis muscles; used by skilled singers

modality   The general class and form of a sensory stimulus available to the nervous system; modalities include somatosensation, hearing, balance, vision, smell and taste

modiolus   The conical central axis of the cochlea

molar   A grinding tooth in the posterior of a mammal's mouth

monotone speech   Speech in which the rhythms of intonation and inflection are lost, typically seen in individuals with Parkinson's disease

monozygotic (identical) twins   Twins that develop from a single fertilized egg through its division into two genetically identical parts

morula   A round mass of about 12 to 16 cells present 3 to 4 days after fertilization

mosaic   Two or more genetically different cell types within a person developing from a single fertilized egg, instead of each cell being genetically identical

mossy fibers   Afferent neurons that carry signals to the cerebellar nuclei and cortex and that originate in the pontine nuclei of the brainstem

motor cortex   Region of the cerebral cortex comprising the precentral gyrus, also known as area 4; the source of axons that project to the lower motor neurons and interneurons of the brainstem and spinal cord and thus is involved in motor control

motor end plate   Terminal branch of a motor neuron that rests on the surface of the muscle fiber

motor equivalence   The ability of a speaker to produce the same phoneme using a variety of articulatory movements

motor unit (MU)   The smallest functional unit (fundamental logical operator) of motor control, which includes an alpha lower motor neuron, the neuromuscular junctions to which the neuron projects, and the muscle fibers the junctions affect; motor units vary in size depending on the number of muscle fibers within the unit; large motor units generate large forces, while small motor units generate less

MPTP   *See* **N-methyl-4-phenyl-1,2,3,6-tetrahydropyridine**

MU   *See* **motor unit**

mucociliary escalator   A line of defense against foreign bodies entering the lungs; consists of paired actions of secretion of mucus by the airway lining and upward propulsion of mucus by the ciliated epithelial tissue

multicellular   Having, or consisting of, many cells or more than one cell to perform all vital functions

multiple sclerosis   An adult-onset, progressive neurological disorder characterized by demyelination, plaques, and inflammation

multipolar neuron (multipolar cell)   Neuron that has multiple dendrites projecting from the soma; found in the posterior ventral cochlear nucleus and elsewhere; *see also* **bipolar cell**

muscle spindle   A sensory receptor within a muscle that detects changes in muscle length so as to regulate the speed of contraction and provide proprioceptive feedback to the central nervous system regarding how far and how fast the muscle fiber is moving; innervated by group Ia afferents

muscle tissue   Tissue that is capable of contracting and generating tension in response to stimulation, producing mechanical force

muscle tone   Resistance to passive joint rotation

muscular hydrostat   Biological structure in which the musculature itself creates both the movement of the structure and the support for the movement without a skeletal framework using fluid pressure without changing volume; the tongue is an example of a muscular hydrostat

muscular process   Posterolateral projection on the arytenoid cartilage, to which the muscles that rotate it are attached

muscularis muscle   The thyromuscularis muscle, a division of the thyroarytenoid; it acts to adduct the vocal folds

musculus uvulae   Muscle that shortens and thickens the palatine uvula

myelin   A fatty material, produced by glial cells, that forms an insulating layer around an axon and therefore promotes conduction of nerve transmission

myelin sheath   The covering of fatty tissue that protects and insulates axons in the central nervous system and peripheral nervous system, increasing the speed of action potential conduction

myelinated axon   An axon covered by a fatty layer called a myelin sheath

mylohyoid line   A thin line running horizontally across the inside of the mandible

mylohyoid muscle   Muscle originating on the mylohyoid line and inserts on the hyoid bone, forming the floor of the oral cavity

myoelastic-aerodynamic theory   Description of the vibration of vocal folds in terms of aerodynamic pressure variations and tissue elasticity and mass

myofibrils   Threadlike structures in a muscle fiber made up of serially arranged sarcomeres that contain the primary contractile proteins: actin and myosin

myogenesis   Muscle cell formation

myosin A thick filament contractile protein located in the sarcomere that slides alongside the thin filament, actin, in a corkscrew manner to produce force within the muscle

myospecificity The process through which muscle tissue becomes innervated

myotome Located immediately lateral to the sclerotome, the group of muscles that a single spinal nerve root innervates

N

nasal cavity A large, paired air-filled space above and behind the nose in the middle of the face

nasal concha One of three mucosa-lined bony projections from the nasal septum that divide the nasal cavity into superior, middle, and inferior nasal passages; the inferior nasal concha is a distinct bone, whereas the superior and middle conchae are part of the ethmoid bone; also called turbinate

nasal laminae Two plates formed from the globular process that fuse together to form the nasal septum

nasal pits Intermediate structures between nasal placodes and the olfactory epithelium of the nose; depressions on either side of the frontonasal process; they effectively divide the frontonasal process into a medial and two lateral nasal processes

nasal placodes Neural crest–derived ectodermal thickenings on either side of the frontonasal process; they give rise to the olfactory epithelium of the nose

nasal septum Structure in the midline of the nose that divides the two nasal cavities, made up of both cartilage and bone and covered by mucosa

nasality Quality of sound coming through the nose

nasolacrimal duct Passage that carries tears into the nasal cavity

nasopharynx The part of the pharynx posterior to the nasal cavity and superior to the oropharynx

negative resonance The condition in which periodic signals, such as sound waves, cancel each other out when combined; negative resonance is used in some noise-reduction headphones; see also **positive resonance**

negative symptom The lack of a phenomenon normally found, thought to reflect a loss of function; for example, the loss of strength with lesions of the upper motor neuron is thought to reflect a loss of the function of the upper motor neuron to drive movement

neocerebellum The posterior lobe of the cerebellum, with numerous connections to the pons

nerve A visible collection of numerous axons bound together within the peripheral nervous system

nervous tissue Tissue that is capable of sending and receiving information through electrochemical signals; consists of neurons and glial cells; also called neural tissue

neural folds Folds formed by the lateral margins of the neural plate, beginning just behind the rostral end of the embryonic disc, where they are continuous with one another, and from there extending inferiorly

neural groove The area between the neural folds, which deepens as the neural folds become elevated

neural plate Region located opposite the primitive streak in the embryo, consisting of thickened ectoderm

neural tissue *See* **nervous tissue**

neuraxis An imaginary line that is drawn through the middle of the central nervous system, from the bottom of the spinal cord through the front of the forebrain

neurocranium The part of the skull that surrounds the brain

neuroglia (neuroglial cells) *See* **glial cell**s

neuromere A region of intensified proliferation within the developing spinal cord, each of which supplies a defined segment of the body

neurometabolic imaging A type of imaging that utilizes changes in metabolism as the marker, such as functional magnetic resonance imaging (fMRI), which detects hemoglobin that has given up oxygen in metabolically active regions; in neuroscience, this change is thought to reflect neuronal activity, but this inference is not always valid

neuromodulator A chemical that binds to a receptor for another ligand that does not cause the same effect as occurs when the receptor's ligand binds to it but alter the receptor's response to the ligand; for example, benzodiazepine drugs bind to receptors for the neurotransmitter GABA and alter the affinity of the receptor for the GABA molecule; neuromodulators may persist and diffuse to many neurons simultaneously, thereby exerting a broader effect over many neurons

neuromuscular junction (NMJ) Juncture of a motor neuron axon with a muscle cell

neuron A specialized cell that conducts electrical or chemical signals entirely within the nervous system except for specific contacts with muscles and glands; also called nerve cell; a neuron typically includes a cell body or soma, dendrites, an axon, and terminal bouton

neuronal membrane The membrane (lipid bilayer) that contains the cytoplasm of a neuron; it contains various voltage-gated and ligand-gated ionic conductance channels and other specialized structures for the rapid integration of information from synapses and the transmission of action potentials over long distances along axons

neuroplasticity The concept that experience leads to changes in the neurophysiologic operations of neurons over time; typically, these sustained changes reflect anatomic or biochemical changes that do not require active reinforcement to sustain these changes; Hebbian learning is one conceptual form of neuroplasticity; actual instances include activity-dependent growth of dendritic spines, long-term potentiation (LTP), and long-term depression (LDP)

neurotransmitter A chemical released from the presynaptic terminal of a neuron into the synaptic cleft between the neuron's presynaptic membrane and the postsynaptic membrane of a target cell (another neuron or a gland or muscle cell); the neurotransmitter binds with a receptor on the postsynaptic membrane to effect a change in the behavior of the postsynaptic cell that depends on the postsynaptic receptor

nigrostriatal pathway The pathway consisting of axons whose origin lies in the substantia nigra and whose terminations reside in the striatum

N-methyl-4-phenyl-1,2,3,6-tetrahydropyridine (MPTP) A chemical that is converted to a toxin, MPP+, that can selectively destroy dopamine neurons; it is used to create an animal model of Parkinson's disease and has greatly enabled advances in understanding the pathoetiology and pathophysiology of this disease

nociception The encoding and processing of harmful or injurious stimuli that is consciously perceived as pain

nociceptor A primary sensory receptor that responds to a harmful or injurious stimulus and encodes it as pain

node of Ranvier A gap between two segments of myelin sheaths that contribute to the rapid conduction of action potentials, in which depolarization occurs only at the nodes of Ranvier; *see also* **saltatory conduction**

nodulus The anterior end of the inferior vermis in the cerebellum

nonlinear relationship A relationship between interacting agents in which the change in one agent is not a simple multiple of the change in the other; for example, a relationship described by $y = ax$, where a is a constant, is said to be linear, because doubling of x results in a doubling of y, but the relationship $y = x^a$ is not linear, because doubling of x does not lead to doubling of y; the interactions between neurons are nonlinear, which increases the likelihood that neuronal interactions will demonstrate complexity; *see also* **complex systems**

nonsense mutation A mutation that results in a truncated protein, as when a base pair change turns a codon for an amino acid into a "stop" codon, so the protein sequence is cut short

notochord An early-forming midline structure that transiently exists in the vertebrate embryo; it is required for signaling to, and patterning, the surrounding tissues; remnants of the notochord form the nucleus pulposus in the intervertebral disk

nuclear envelope The barrier separating the nucleus from the cytoplasm, composed of an inner and outer membrane, a nuclear lamina, and nuclear pore complexes

nucleic acids Macromolecules consisting of polymers of nucleotides, containing the genetic information important for all cellular functions and heredity: deoxyribonucleic acid (DNA) and ribonucleic acid (RNA)

nucleoid The portion of a prokaryotic cell where the genetic material is found

nucleolus The nuclear site of ribosomal RNA transcription, processing, and ribosome assembly

nucleotide The basic building block of nucleic acids (DNA and RNA), consisting of a combination of one of a small number of base molecules (adenine, cytosine, guanine, thymine, or uracil), a sugar molecule (ribose or deoxyribose), and a phosphate ion; the alternating sugars and phosphates form the strand, while the sequence of the bases attached to the sugars contain the information; when nucleotides are placed base to base, guanine pairs with cytosine while adenine pairs with thymine (DNA) or uracil (RNA), enabling transfer of information

nucleus In eukaryotic cells, the most prominent organelle, which contains the genetic material; in the central nervous system, a collection of neuronal cell bodies in a particular region with a particular function

nucleus ambiguus A collection of neurons in the medulla oblongata whose axons, carried in the vagus nerve, provide motor innervation to the pharynx and larynx

nucleus cuneatus A collection of neurons at the junction between the spinal cord and medulla that act as a relay between sensory neurons mediating proprioception and vibration in the upper part of the body to other structures in the brainstem, particularly the sensory relay nuclei in the thalamus

nucleus gracilis A collection of neurons at the junction between the spinal cord and medulla that act as a relay between sensory neurons mediating proprioception and sense of vibration in the lower part of the body to other structures in the brainstem, particularly the sensory relay nuclei in the thalamus

nucleus of the solitary tract (NST) A sensory nucleus in the medulla, target to several cranial nerve systems, including IX and X; the rostral portion of the NST is referred to as the gustatory nucleus and is the location for all afferent fibers carrying taste information

nystagmus Involuntary eye movements consisting of two phases: a slow drift of the eye (slow phase), which is often mediated by the peripheral vestibular system, and a quick recentering of the eye (fast phase), which is mediated by the central nervous system

O

occipital lobe The lobe located at the posterior end of the brain, which has primary responsibility for the reception and processing of visual information

occipitotemporal gyrus Gyral structure that is located on the ventromedial side of the brain and that extends from the occipital to the temporal lobe

occiput Most posterior portion of the skull

occlusal Of, or relating to, the portion of a tooth that comes in contact with a tooth in the other jaw

occlusion Blockage of a hollow vessel or organ; the contact between teeth in the upper and lower jaws

octopus cell A neuronal cell type in the posterior ventral cochlear nucleus

oculomotor nerve (CN III) A pure motor nerve that innervates four of the six extraocular muscles controlling eye movements (medial, superior, and inferior rectus and inferior oblique); *see also* **abducent nerve (CN VI)**, **trochlear nerve (CN IV)**

odorant A substance whose molecules are airborne and can be inhaled and stimulate olfactory receptors

odynophagia Painful swallowing

OHC *See* **outer hair cell**

olfaction The perception of odors; sense of smell

olfactory bulb A paired neural structure responsible for receiving odor information; it is the first area in which odor sensation enters the central nervous system

olfactory nerve (CN I) *See* **olfactory tract**

olfactory sulcus Indentation located in the midline of the frontal lobe on the ventral surface

olfactory tract The bundle of axons connecting the olfactory bulb to the orbitofrontal cortex, located within the olfactory sulcus; considered as the olfactory nerve (CN I), though it is actually an extension of the white matter of the brain

oligodendrocyte A type of glial cell that forms myelin in the central nervous system, in contrast to Schwann cells; similar in appearance to astrocytes, but with fewer protuberances, which project out to axons and spiral around them, creating myelin sheaths

oligogenic A trait influenced by a small, countable number of genes working together to contribute to a particular phenotype

olive Large, bulging, rounded structure in the ventral aspect of the medulla

olivocochlear pathway Part of the vestibulocochlear nerve that projects from the superior olivary complex to the cochlea

omohyoid muscle Laryngeal depressor muscle that originates on the clavicle and inserts on the hyoid bone; like the digastric, it has two bellies joined by a tendon

oogenesis The creation of an ovum (egg cell), the female form of gametogenesis, in which the primary oogonium divides meiotically (meiosis I) into a secondary oocyte and a polar body, and then the secondary oocyte divides meiotically (meiosis II) into a mature ovum and a second polar body

opening phase The part a cycle of vocal fold vibration when the folds are moving farther apart; *see also* **closed phase, closing phase**

ophthalmic branch (CN V₁) The superior branch of the trigeminal nerve, which innervates the upper face above the midline of the eyes up to the top of the forehead, carrying all forms of somatic sensation

optic canal Canal through the lesser wing of the sphenoid through which the optic nerve passes

optic chiasm X-shaped structure where the two optic nerves cross, located on the ventral surface of the brain

optic disc The region of the retina where all the axons from the retinal ganglion cells converge into the optic nerve; it contains no photoreceptors itself, so it forms the "blind spot"

optic nerve (CN II) A specialized cranial nerve (actually an extension of the brain) that conveys visual information from the retina

optic tract The collection of axons that convey visual information from the optic chiasm to the lateral geniculate nucleus and superior colliculus

optic radiations Massive bundle of axons conveying a complete mapping of the visual hemifield from the lateral geniculate nucleus to the primary visual cortex

oral cavity The region extending from the orifice of the mouth anteriorly, bounded laterally by the dental arches and posteriorly by the fauces

orbicularis oculi Muscle whose fibers run around the eye and closes the eyelids

orbicularis oris Muscle whose fibers run around the upper and lower lips, responsible for lip puckering and tight lip closure

orbitofrontal gyri Set of complex gyri on the ventral aspect of the frontal lobe that are located lateral to the olfactory sulcus

organ A collection of tissues joined in a structural unit to serve a common function

organ of Corti (OoC) Band of specialized epithelium running along the length of the basilar membrane and functioning as the site where acoustic stimuli in the form of hydraulic waves in the scala vestibuli are transduced into neural signals; also called the spiral organ

organelle A membrane-bound compartment or structure in a cell that performs a special function

orifice Opening

origin The less mobile point of attachment of a muscle

oropharynx The part of the pharynx posterior to the oral cavity, between the soft palate and hyoid bone

oscillation To-and-fro repeated changes in a physical system that has both inertia and a restoring force, such as air

oscillator phase changes Changes in the starting point of a periodic signal, such as a sine wave produced by an oscillator, independent of any change in frequency

osmosis Diffusion of a solvent (usually water molecules) through a semipermeable membrane from an area of low solute concentration to an area of high solute concentration

osseous spiral lamina A double layer of thin bone that coils around the modiolus from base to apex of the cochlea

ossicular chain The linkage consisting of three bones (malleus, incus, stapes) that transmit sound vibrations from the tympanic membrane to the cochlea

ossicular chain disarticulation or dislocation A fracture or dislocation within the ossicular chain, most often resulting from trauma to the temporal bone

otic placodes Sensory placodes that appear posterior to the second branchial arch during the fourth week of development

otitis media An inflammation of the mucosal lining of the tympanic cavity of the middle ear

otoacoustic emissions (OAEs) Sounds emitted by the outer hair cells in the cochlea as a result of the action of the somatic motor; they can be recorded using a microphone in the external auditory canal and indicate the condition of the inner ear

otoconia Small crystals of calcium carbonate in the saccule and utricle of the vestibular system that cause stimulation of the hair cells via their movement relative to cochlear fluid during acceleration

otolaryngologist Physician trained in the medical and surgical management and treatment of patients with diseases and disorders of the ear, nose, throat (ENT), and related structures of the head and neck

otolith organs The utricle and saccule, located at the base of the vestibular labyrinth, which provide information regarding linear acceleration as well as static position of the head relative to gravity

otolithic membrane A gelatinous membrane within the otolith organs, loaded with otoconia, in which the stereocilia and kinocilia of the otolithic organs are embedded

otosclerosis A genetic metabolic disease of the temporal bone characterized by abnormal bone remodeling in the tympanic cavity of the middle ear

otoscopy The visual examination of the external auditory canal and tympanic membrane with an otoscope

outer hair cell (OHC) A hair cell on the organ of Corti that is farther from the central axis of the cochlear spiral than the inner hair cells; there are approximately 12,000 OHCs arranged in three rows; they receive 5% of the innervation from the cochlear branch of the vestibulocochlear nerve; they can adjust their properties in response to efferent signals from the CNS, modifying the forces on the IHCs and altering their sensitivity

oval window Opening in the vestibule of the cochlea through which the stapes transmits sound vibrations to the fluid in the scala vestibuli; *see also* **round window**

overbite The overlapping of the lower teeth by the upper teeth

overjet The amount of horizontal protrusion of the upper teeth anterior to the lower teeth

overload principle The training principle that muscle must be worked at a level beyond what it is accustomed in order to realize strength gains; *see also* **reversibility principle**, **specificity principle**

ovum   Also called the egg; the female reproductive cell (gamete) in organisms that reproduce via sexual reproduction

oxidation   Chemical reaction in which there a molecule, atom, or ion loses electrons to an oxidizing agent (such as molecular oxygen), which is said to be reduced; loss of electrons increases the substance's oxidation state; *see also* **reduction**

oxidative phosphorylation   The aerobic (oxygen-requiring) energy pathway used by muscle tissue; an ATP-yielding system that is more efficient at delivering a larger number of ATP than anaerobic pathways

P

p arm   The short arm of a chromosome, (named from French *petit*)

palatal shelves   Palatine processes of the maxillae; structures that grow vertically initially from the maxillary prominences but elevate to a horizontal position between the seventh and eighth week of development and fuse in the midline to form the palate

palatine bone   Paired bone that forms the posterior fourth of the hard palate

palatoglossus   Muscle that forms the anterior faucial pillar and pulls the soft palate and tongue toward each other

palatopharyngeus   Muscle that forms the posterior faucial pillar and tenses and lowers the soft palate

paleocerebellum   Part of mostly the anterior lobe of the cerebellum that receives many spinocerebellar afferents

pallidotomy   A surgical procedure that involves the purposeful destruction of the globus pallidus internal segment to improve the symptoms and signs of a variety of movement disorders

parabelt   The most lateral subdivision of the auditory cortex, adjacent to the belt

parabrachial nuclei (PBN)   Lateral and medial brainstem nuclei located at the junction of the midbrain and the pons, receiving second-order neuron projections carrying taste information from the nuclei of the solitary tract in the medulla

paracrine signaling   Local cell–cell signaling in which a molecule released by one cell acts on a neighboring target cell

paradoxical vocal fold motion (PVFM)   Involuntary vocal fold adduction during inspiration

parafascicular nucleus   A nucleus within the thalamus that conveys information to the basal ganglia

parahippocampal gyrus   Gyral structure that is located at the medial aspect of the ventral temporal lobe and that overlies the hippocampus

parallel fibers   Axons arising from granule cells in the cerebellar cortex that synapse on Purkinje neurons

paranasal sinuses   Air-filled chambers within the bones of the skull and face

parasagittal plane   A vertical plane dividing a region into unequal left and right parts

parasympathetic system   Part of the autonomic nervous system that contains neurons in the brainstem and sacral spinal cord; the parasympathetic system restores homeostasis in the body; *see also* **sympathetic system**

paravermal zone of the cerebellum   A region of the cerebellar cortex, involving but not limited to the neocerebellum, defined by its reciprocal connections to the globose and emboliform deep cerebellar nuclei

parietal lobe   The lobe of the cerebral cortex located immediately posterior to the central sulcus and above the temporal lobe, responsible for reception of somatic sensory inputs and sensory-to-motor integration

parietal pleura   Membrane that lines the inner surface of the thoracic cavity (rib cage); see also **visceral pleura**

parieto-occipital sulcus   A deep cleft that can be seen in the medial aspect of the brain and that separates the occipital lobe from the parietal lobe

Parkinson's disease   The most common diagnosis that makes up the syndrome of parkinsonism; the symptoms include, but are not limited to, disorders of movement, such as bradykinesia and akinesia, increased muscle tone, and gait and postural abnormalities

pars flaccida   Small area of the superior part of the tympanic membrane

pars obliqua   One of the two divisions of the cricothyroid muscle

pars recta   One of the two divisions of the cricothyroid muscle

pars tensa   Large central area of the tympanic membrane that is primarily responsible for transducing acoustic to mechanical (vibratory) energy

pascal   Unit of pressure in the meter, kilogram, second system of units: one newton per square meter

Passavant ridge   A prominence on the posterior wall of the nasopharynx formed by constriction of the superior pharyngeal constrictor muscle

passive transport   The transport of molecules across a membrane in the energetically favorable direction

pathoetiology   Study of the mechanisms that cause disease, but not necessarily the mechanisms that cause the symptoms, signs, and disability of disease (the pathophysiology)

pathology   The scientific study of the structural and functional changes that affect an organism as a result of disease

pathophysiology   Study of the mechanisms that cause the symptoms and signs of a disease but not necessarily the mechanisms that cause the disease (pathoetiology)

pattern generator   Nucleus in the brainstem that causes repeating cascades of muscular activity

pedunculopontine nucleus   A collection of neurons in the mesencephalon of the brainstem with connections from the basal ganglia and projections to various brainstem structures; thought to be involved in motor functions such as gait and posture

penetrance   The probability that a person who has a mutation in a gene will show (express) the corresponding phenotype

penetration   Entry of solid or liquid matter material into the airway but not below the level of the vocal folds; *see also* **aspiration**

percept   A stimulus event as it is perceived through the central nervous system

perception   The process of interpreting information about sensed stimuli transmitted to the central nervous system; *see also* **sensation**

periaqueductal gray (PAG) matter   Region in the midbrain with connections to the limbic system and nuclei of spinal and cranial nerves

perilymph   One of the two fluids in the inner ear, located between the bony and membranous labyrinths of the peripheral vestibular apparatus and in the scala vestibuli and scala tympani of the cochlea; similar in ionic composition to cerebrospinal fluid (high sodium, low potassium); functions to suspend and protect the membranous labyrinth within the bony labyrinth and to transmit sound vibrations to the basilar membrane; *see also* **endolymph**

periodic   Repeating at regular intervals of time

periolivary group (or nuclei)   Subdivision of the superior olivary complex

peripheral auditory system   The part of the auditory system that receives sound wave energy and converts it to signals sent to the central auditory system; consists of the outer ear, middle ear, inner ear, and cochlear branch of the vestibulo-cochlear nerve

peripheral chemoreceptors   Structures located within blood vessels that detect changes in concentration of various chemicals vital to homeostasis, including O_2, CO_2, and blood glucose

peripheral gas exchange   *See* **internal respiration**

peripheral nervous system (PNS)   The division of the nervous system that consists of spinal nerves, cranial nerves, and autonomic/sensory ganglia; see also **central nervous system**

peripheral   Pertaining to structures located on the outer part or surface of another structure or body; toward the periphery

peripheral proteins   Proteins indirectly associated with cell membranes by protein–protein interactions

peristalsis (peristaltic movement)   Wavelike contraction that propagates movement down a tube (e.g., the esophagus or pharynx)

perisylvian region   Area of cerebral cortex around the sylvian fissure

permeability   The ability of a membrane to allow the passage of a particular atom, ion, or molecule.

perturbation   Subtle change in the behavior of a system over time; see also **amplitude perturbation**, **frequency perturbation**

pH   The negative logarithm of hydrogen ion concentration, expressing the relative acidity, or alkalinity, of an aqueous solution; pure water contains 10^{-7} mol/L H^+, so it has a pH of 7; lower values are more acidic, and higher values are more alkaline

pH buffer   A set of substances that maintains a solution such as the blood at a desired level of acidity or alkalinity

phalangeal cell   Support cell in the organ of Corti

phantosmia   Hallucination of smells

pharyngeal arches   A series of five paired swellings that surround the embryonic foregut from day 20 to day 35 of development

pharyngeal branch of the vagus nerve   Branch of the vagus nerve that provides motor innervation to muscles of the pharynx and the soft palate

pharyngeal cavity   The passageway between the posterior openings of the nasal passages and the esophagus

pharyngeal constrictors   The superior, middle, and inferior pharyngeal constrictor muscles

pharyngeal grooves   The ectodermally lined depressions between the pharyngeal arches

pharyngeal pouches   The endodermally lined depressions between the pharyngeal arches

pharyngeal raphe   The central line of the pharynx on the posterior wall, which serves as the origin and insertion of several pharyngeal constrictors

pharynx The throat; the space behind the oral and nasal cavities and between the oral cavity and the larynx and esophagus

phase A distinct point within the cycle of a vibration or oscillating signal

phase locking Performing some action, such as firing an action potential, at the same point in every successive cycle of a vibration or oscillating signal

phenotype The manifestation of particular physical or physiologic characteristics, associated with a genetic trait, that can be observed in cognition, behavior, anatomy, or physiology

philtrum The vertical groove between the base of the nose and the median vermilion ("Cupid's bow") of the upper lip.

phlegm Mucus secreted by the lining of the airway, forming a protective barrier between the wall of the airway and the air that passes through it; also serves to maintain moisture balance of airway epithelial tissues

phonation The physiologic process of vocal fold oscillation that results in the transformation of aerodynamic to acoustic energy

phonation periodicity *See* **periodicity**

phonation quotient (PQ) Vital capacity divided by maximum phonation time

phonation threshold pressure (PTP) The minimum amount of subglottal air pressure required to initiate vocal fold vibration

phonation volume Amount of air available for use for sustained vowel production

phoneme The smallest significant unit of sound production distinguished in a language

phospholipid bilayer The basic structure of biologic membranes, in which the hydrophobic tails of phospholipids are buried in the interior of the membrane and their polar head groups are exposed to the aqueous solution on either side

photoreceptor A primary receptor responsible for detecting photons of light and transmitting information regarding visual information

phrenic nerves Nerves that provide innervation to the diaphragm, derived from spinal nerves C3, C4, and C5

physiologic voice range The range of vocal F_0 that a person can produce, normally at least two octaves

physiology The scientific study of the functions of a living organism and its parts

pia mater The innermost layer of the meninges, which adheres closely to the cerebral cortex

Pierre Robin sequence A set of anomalies of the head and face, consisting of a small lower jaw (micrognathia), a tongue that is placed further back than normal (glossoptosis), and a cleft palate

pillar cell Support cell in the organ of Corti

pineal gland An endocrine gland found at the posterior portion of the thalamus; it regulates the daily rhythm of sleep and waking

pinna *See* **auricle**

pinnate Having muscle fibers oriented in a fan-shaped arrangement; *see also* **fusiform**

pitch The perception of frequency

pituitary gland Hypophysis; a pea-sized gland that hangs from the hypothalamus and regulates hormone production

place theory A theory of hearing that states that our perception of sound depends on where each component frequency produces vibrations along the basilar membrane

plane A flat or level surface

plasma membrane A phospholipid bilayer with associated proteins that surrounds the cell

platysma Broad muscle sheet that tenses the skin of the lower face and neck, pulls the corners of the mouth inferiorly, and assists with opening the mandible

pleiotropy Multiple phenotypes that are influenced by one gene or locus

pleural cavity Space between the visceral and parietal pleurae; normally contains pleural fluid

pleural fluid Fluid that fills the pleural cavities

pleural linkage Process by which the lungs are kept close to the inner chest wall by tension of pleural fluid

pleural membranes Tissue that lines the surface of the lungs (visceral pleura) and inner surface of the rib cage (parietal pleura)

pneumotaxic center Part of the respiratory CPG, located in the upper pons; inhibits inspiration, thereby reducing respiratory volume and rate

pneumothorax Lung collapse; commonly caused by a disruption in pleural linkage, admitting air into the pleural cavity

Poiseuille's law Equation that determines resistance to flow

polar body A small haploid cell without adequate cytoplasm to support a zygote if fertilized

polygenic A trait influenced by many genes, each with such a small effect that it cannot be easily identified using standard genetic methods

pons The middle subdivision of the brainstem between the mesencephalon and the medulla oblongata; named from the Latin word for bridge, after the transverse tracts that resemble a bridge across the ventral surface of the brainstem in this region

pontine flexure The flexure of the hindbrain at the junction between the metencephalon and the myelencephalon; it forms in the seventh week of development

pontine relay nuclei Groups of neuronal somas residing in the ventral region of the pons of the brainstem that are the source of mossy fiber afferents to the cerebellum

positive resonance The condition in which periodic signals, such as sound waves, reinforce each other when combined; used in radio receivers to amplify the signal from the desired station above the signals of all the other stations; *see also* **negative resonance**

positive symptom The occurrence of a phenomenon not normally found or not normally found in the degree at which it is observed; for example, the appearance of pathological reflexes or hyperreflexia of normally present reflexes with lesions of the upper motor neuron would be considered positive symptoms and signs

postcentral gyrus A prominent gyrus posterior to the central sulcus, containing the primary somatosensory cortex; *compare* **precentral gyrus**

posterior auditory field (PAF) A subdivision of the auditory cortex

posterior Behind or in back of another structure

posterior cerebral artery (PCA) Blood vessel that supplies the occipital lobe, the inferior surfaces of the hemispheres, the thalamus, the hypothalamus, the brainstem, and the cerebellum

posterior cricoarytenoid (PCA) muscle Muscle originating on the posterior lamina of the cricoid cartilage and terminating on the muscular process of the arytenoid; the only vocal fold abductor

posterior fossa The lower back (caudal) space within the skull beneath the tentorium cerebelli and above the foramen magnum

posterior neuropore Caudal opening of the neural tube

posterior root One of the two roots of a spinal nerve, in which afferent axons from the periphery enter the spinal cord

posterior semicircular canal One of the three semicircular canals of the inner ear, oriented posterior and superior to the vestibular labyrinth; along with the anterior semicircular canal, responsible for translating vertical head movements into neural impulses; *see also* **horizontal semicircular canal**

posterior ventral cochlear nucleus (PVCN) One of three major divisions of the cochlear nucleus in the brainstem; *see also* **anterior ventral cochlear nucleus (AVCN)**, **dorsal cochlear nucleus (DCN)**

posterolateral fissure Deep cleft that separates two adjoining cerebellar structures (the nodulus and flocculus) from the main body of the cerebellum

postural instability Decreased ability to respond reflexively to a force such as a push from the side so as to keep one's center of gravity over one's base of support, as seen in Parkinson's disease

postictal paralysis A form of paralysis that follows epileptic seizures; also known as Todd paralysis

poststimulus time histogram (PSTH) A graph representing a neuron's firing rate as a function of time, relative to an input stimulus

postsynaptic acetylcholine receptor (AChR) A protein molecule embedded in the postsynaptic cell membrane that binds to ACh that has traveled across the synaptic cleft

potassium A chemical element (atomic number 19) that typically exists in the body as the monovalent cationic form (an atom from which one electron has been removed, resulting in a charge of +1)

pre-Bötzinger complex (preBötC) Part of the respiratory center, in the ventrolateral medulla; it generates the regular rhythm of respiration in the form of regular and repetitive "bursts" of neuronal impulses, which stimulate the muscles of inspiration to contract

preoccipital notch An indentation in the inferior lateral side of the occipital lobe

precentral gyrus A large gyrus in the cerebral cortex anterior to the central sulcus, containing the primary motor cortex; *see also* **postcentral gyrus**

prechordal plate A thickened portion of endoderm that is in contact with ectoderm immediately rostral to the cephalic tip of the notochord

precuneus gyrus Gyral structure visible in the medial surface of the parietal lobe

premaxilla A pair of small cranial bones at the tip of the upper jaw in many animals, fused in humans with the maxilla to form part of the hard palate

premolar A tooth situated between the canine and molar teeth

premotor cortex Cortical region in the frontal lobe anterior to the primary motor cortex that is responsible for the planning of movements by both influencing the motor signals generated by the primary motor cortex directly and through a population of projection neurons that influence other motor functions

pressure Force per unit area acting perpendicular to a surface

prestin A protein in the outer hair cell membrane that lengthens when the membrane is depolarized, lengthening the cell, and shortens when the cell is hyperpolarized, constituting the somatic motor

primary afferent A sensory axon projecting from a peripheral sensory receptor to the spinal cord or brainstem

primary auditory cortex (A1) Cortical region in the posterior two-thirds of the superior temporal gyrus and extending into the lateral fissure; it is involved in the primary processing of auditory information, such as frequency, location, and loudness, performing basic and higher functions in hearing; it receives auditory input from the medial geniculate body and possesses a tonotopic representation originating in the basilar membrane and the cochlea; it is considered the core of the auditory system, surrounded by the belt; also called the Heschl gyrus or transverse gyrus

primary cell culture Maintenance of growth of cells dissociated from the parental tissue (using mechanical or enzymatic methods) in culture medium in suitable glass or plastic containers

primary fissure Large, deep cleft that separates the cerebellum into anterior and posterior lobes

primary motor cortex The cortex of the precentral gyrus that is associated with motor execution; somatotopically organized; its axons project to alpha lower motor neurons in the spinal cord via the corticospinal tract

primary palate The intermaxillary segment that arises from the fusion of the two medial nasal processes and the frontonasal process; the area anterior to the incisive foramen that includes the premaxilla and its overlying mucosa

primary somatosensory cortex The cortex of the postcentral gyrus, which participates in somatic sensation, such as touch or position; the central target for somatosensory neurons of the ventroposterolateral and ventroposteriomedial nuclei; somatotopically organized and segregated into separate regions mediating proprioceptive and tactile sensations, respectively

primary visual cortex (V1) The cortex above and below the calcarine sulcus in the occipital lobe that receives information from the retinas via the lateral geniculate nucleus; it is retinotopically organized into ocular dominance columns, orientation columns, and color-sensitive collections of neurons (blobs)

primitive streak A temporary structure that forms on the surface of the blastula; it gives rise to mesoderm, and its formation marks the beginning of gastrulation

proband The index case from whom other family members are identified

prodrug An inactive chemical compound that is chemically transformed into an active drug inside the body

projection neuron Neuron that has a long axon projecting far from the soma that sends signals to a distant target neuron, such as corticospinal neurons

prokaryotic cells Cells lacking a nuclear envelope, cytoplasmic organelles, and a cytoskeleton (primarily bacteria); *see also* **eukaryotic cells**

promontory Bony protrusion into the tympanic cavity formed by the first turn of the cochlea

prophase The first stage of mitosis, during which chromosomes condense and nucleoli disappear

proprioception Ability to identify how one's body is moving and positioned in space

prosencephalon The most cephalad of the dilations of the neural tube that forms the telencephalon and the diencephalon

prosopagnosia Inability to identify or recognize faces due to damage to the fusiform area of the inferior temporal gyrus

proteins Large, complex molecules made up of amino acids that define the function of a cell; each protein is a polypeptide with a unique amino acid sequence

proteome All the proteins in a cell

proximal Located closer to the center of a body; opposite of distal

psychometric function A means of defining normative measures for diagnostic purposes; achieved by plotting the detection level of a stimulus versus the intensity of the test stimulus

psychophysics The science of relating physical properties of a stimulus to humans' internal percepts

pulmonary artery Artery that directs oxygen-depleted blood directly from the right side of the heart into the lungs

pulmonary distention Stretching of blood vessels in the lung, enabling the lungs to accommodate more blood

pulmonary edema A dangerous condition where fluid accumulates within the lungs

pulmonary extraction   The process of removing drugs from the systemic circulation through the lungs

pulmonary irritant receptors   Sensory receptors in the lungs that detect the presence of irritants

pulmonary recruitment   The process of admitting blood into previously unperfused regions of the circulation in the lungs; prevents a "back loading" of blood that could produce dangerous increases in pulmonary arterial pressures

pulmonary stretch receptors   Sensory receptors in the lungs that detect stretching

pulmonary surfactant   Pulmonary fluid, which enhances the ability of the lungs to stretch and expand while simultaneously preventing lung collapse

pulse register   The lowest register of the voice, produced by complete relaxation of the cricothyroid with maximum contraction of the vocalis; individual vocal fold pulses can almost be heard; *see also* **chest register**, **falsetto**, **head register**, **mixed register**

pure tone   A sound containing a single frequency

Purkinje cell   The primary output neuron in the cerebellar cortex; characterized by a flasklike soma, an elaborate dendritic tree, and a single long axon

pursed-lip breathing   Technique used by patients experiencing dyspnea; narrowing the space through which the patient must exhale (by pursing the lips), thereby promoting positive air pressures back into the airways, holding the airways open and allowing more air to be exhaled prior to the next breath

putamen   A rounded mass of gray matter in the center of the cerebral hemisphere, part of the basal ganglia complex, lateral to the globus pallidus

pyramid   One of two prominent and large white matter bundles in the ventral aspect of the medulla, containing the corticobulbar and corticospinal tracts (pyramidal tracts)

pyramidal cell   A type of neuron found in the cerebral cortex (and in the dorsal cochlear nucleus) that has a triangular soma, a single large apical dendrite, multiple short basal dendrites, and a single long axon

pyramidal eminence   Bony projection from the posterior wall of the tympanic cavity where the stapedius muscle originates

pyramidal system   The system consisting of those structures whose efferent axons pass through the pyramids in the medulla of the brainstem; typically, they include fibers of the corticospinal and corticobulbar pathways

pyramidal tract   Pathways that mediate the pyramidal system

Q

q arm   The long arm of the chromosome, so called because the letter *q* follows the letter *p* (for *petit*) used for the short arm; *see also* **p arm**

quadrangular membrane   Ligament extending from the arytenoid cartilage to the epiglottis; its most inferior aspect forms the ventricular fold, while its most superior aspect forms the aryepiglottic fold

quarter-wave resonator   A tube that is open at one end and closed at the other; it resonates with sound waves four times its length

R

ramus (plural rami)   An arm or branch of a bone; branch of a nerve; branch of an artery

rapidly adapting (RA)   Of a sensory receptor, firing action potentials only at points of dynamic change during a stimulus event

rarefaction   The part of a sound pressure wave where molecules are spread apart, where pressure is lowest; *see also* **condensation**

rayl   Unit of specific acoustic impedance, equal to $1\ Pa \cdot s/m$

receptive field   The area (such as an anatomic zone of the body surface, a region of space, a range of frequencies) within which a stimulus will trigger a response (fire) in a given sensory receptor

receptor   Molecular structure within a cell or on the cell's surface characterized by selective binding of a specific substance and a specific physiologic effect that accompanies the binding

receptor potential   Graded electrical response to a stimulus occurring within a sensory receptor; can be depolarizing or hyperpolarizing

receptor segment   The input zone of a neuron that consists of the soma and dendrites; receptor segments receive input signals from other neurons

recurrent laryngeal nerve   Main motor nerve for intrinsic laryngeal muscles except the cricothyroid

red nucleus   A collection of neurons in the mesencephalon that have extensive connections from motor areas of the cerebral cortex as well as connections from the deep cerebellar nuclei; some efferents from the red nucleus innervate lower motor neurons (via the rubrospinal tract) and thus function in motor control

reduced preparation   An experimental method in which a component of a complex system is isolated from the other components in order to allow detailed analysis; for example, sections of the thalamus be removed and kept alive in chambers so that their "local" physiology can be studied independent of various inputs to the tissue

reduction Chemical reaction in which a molecule, atom, or ion gains electrons from a reducing agent, which is said to be oxidized; gaining electrons lowers the substance's oxidation state; *see also* **oxidation**

reflex A nerve pathway that connects muscle groups to others without involving the brain

refractory period A period of time, typically following the initiation of an action potential, during which the neuron is unable or unlikely to generate another action potential; there is an absolute refractory period in which an action potential cannot be generated at all under normal conditions because of the inactivation of voltage-gated sodium ion (Na^+) channels; there is also a relative refractory period, during which the threshold to generation of an action potential is increased but an action potential can still occur

Reinke space *See* **superficial lamina propria**

Reissner membrane A thin membrane in the cochlea that separates the scala vestibuli from the scala media

relaxation pressure curve A plot of changes in lung volumes and pressures that occur as a consequence of inhalation and exhalation

renin An enzyme that transforms angiotensinogen into angiotensin I

renin–angiotensin–aldosterone system (RAAS) Hormonal network responsible for regulating blood pressure

Renshaw cell A neuron in the spinal cord that receives direct depolarization input from an alpha lower motor neuron via an axon collateral but then has a hyperpolarizing effect on the same alpha lower motor neuron

residual volume The volume of air that remains in the lungs and cannot be exhaled

resolving power The ability of an optical instrument or type of film to separate or distinguish small or closely adjacent image elements

resonance Vibratory response of a body or air-filled cavity to a frequency imposed on it

resonant frequency The frequency at which an object vibrates freely, which is determined by its physical properties such as mass and stiffness

respiratory acidosis Dangerous reduction in blood pH that can lower the concentration of hemoglobin in the blood

respiratory bronchioles Branches of the terminal bronchioles

respiratory Of, or relating to, the bodily processes of respiration: the bodily exchange of carbon dioxide for oxygen that is accomplished by the muscles and organs of respiration, as well as the cellular processes of generating energy

resting tremor Abnormal tremor (as opposed to physiologic tremor) that manifests when the affected body part is at rest

restoring force The ability of an elastic medium to stop and reverse a body's motion; the presence of both inertia and a restoring force leads to oscillation

reticular formation A relatively amorphous collection of neuronal somas throughout the brainstem; various regions of the reticular formation, though not well defined visually, are thought to be involved in a variety of functions such as wakefulness; neurons in some regions in the reticular formation project to lower motor neurons and, thus, are involved in motor control

reticular lamina A thin extracellular layer that forms the ceiling of the sensory and supporting cells of the organ of Corti, through which the stereocilia of the hair cells protrude

reticular system A network of scattered gray matter nuclei in the central area of the brainstem that contributes to wakefulness

reticulospinal tract A tract that descends from the reticular formation in the brainstem and to lower moter neurons in the spinal cord and influences automatic posture- and gait-related movements

retina The neuroepithelium (sensory cells) of the eye, which changes the pattern of light that enters the eye into neural impulses that are sent to the brain to be interpreted as a visual image

retinotopy The mapping or organization of visual inputs from the retina through all components of the central visual pathway

reuptake The process in which a presynaptic cell reabsorbs neurotransmitter molecules it has released, recycling the neurotransmitter for future use

reverberation The prolongation of a sound

reversibility principle The training principle that metabolic, morphologic, and neurologic mechanisms suffer loss (downregulation) when a muscle is no longer worked at 70% of its maximum capacity; *see also* **overload principle**, **specificity principle**

rhinal sulcus Indentation that separates the anterior portion of the occipitotemporal gyrus and parahippocampal gyrus

rhinencephalon The part of the brain involved with olfaction; it includes the olfactory bulb, olfactory tract, anterior olfactory nucleus, anterior perforated substance, medial olfactory stria, lateral olfactory stria, parts of the amygdala, and prepiriform area

rhombencephalon   Hindbrain; the most caudal of neural tube dilations; it forms the medulla, pons, and cerebellum

ribbon synapse   A type of neuronal synapse characterized by unique mechanisms of multivesicular release and calcium channel positioning that promotes rapid neurotransmitter release and sustained signal transmission

ribonucleic acid (RNA)   A usually single-stranded nucleic acid, consisting of nucleotides in which ribose is the sugar and uracil is the base that pairs with adenine; RNA forms certain structures used in protein synthesis and also serves as the medium for translating informatin stored in DNA into protein molecules; *see also* **deoxyribonucleic acid (DNA)**, **messenger RNA (mRNA)**, **ribosomal RNA (rRNA)**, **transfer RNA (tRNA)**

ribosomal RNA (rRNA)   Ribonucleic acid molecules that make up part of the structure of a ribosome

ribosome   A structure composed of ribosomal RNA and proteins that is the site of RNA translation (protein synthesis)

rigidity   Resistance to passive joint rotations

risorius   A muscle that draws the angle of the mouth laterally

RNA   *See* **ribonucleic acid**

rod   One of the phototransducing cells of the retina that are responsible for vision in low light conditions and are exquisitely sensitive to light but cannot distinguish color; *see also* **cone**

root primordia   Caudal pair of lingual primordia, located at the level of the second branchial arch; *see also* **anterior lingual primordia**

Rosenthal canal   A section of the bony labyrinth of the inner ear where spiral ganglion cells converge

rostral   Toward the nose

rough endoplasmic reticulum   The region of the endoplasmic reticulum covered with ribosomes and involved in protein metabolism

round window   Opening in the cochlea through which sound waves exit the scala tympani

rubrospinal tract   A descending pathway from neuronal cell bodies in the red nucleus that project to neurons in the spinal cord, particularly interneurons and lower motor neurons

S

saccade   A rapid eye movement, such as when the eye jumps from looking at one object to looking at a different object

saccule   An otolithic organ in the vestibular labyrinth of the inner ear, vertically oriented and therefore responding to linear acceleration in the vertical plane and orientation of the head relative to gravity

sagittal plane   A vertical plane dividing a region into equal left and right parts

SAID principle   *See* **specific adaptation to imposed demand (SAID) principle**

saltatory conduction   The propagation of action potentials along myelinated axons from one node of Ranvier to the next node, increasing the conduction velocity of action potentials

sarcolemma   Muscle cell outer membrane

sarcomere   The smallest contractile unit of a muscle cell

sarcoplasmic reticulum (SR)   Organelle in the muscle cell that stores calcium needed for muscle contraction

scala media   The medial canal of the membranous labyrinth; also called the cochlear duct

scala tympani   The inferior canal of the membranous labyrinth

scala vestibuli   The superior canal of the membranous labyrinth

scanning electron microscopy (SEM)   Microscopy method in which electrons scattered from the surface of a specimen are analyzed to generate a three-dimensional image

scanning speech   Speech in which words are broken into separated syllables spoken with irregular or nonvarying stress

Schwann cell   A type of glial cell that forms a myelin sheath around an axon in the peripheral nervous system, in contrast to oligodendrocyte

sclerotome   An area formed from the most medial region of a somite, which gives rise to the individual vertebral bodies, the intervertebral disks, the ribs, and part of the occipital bone

second messenger   A substance whose metabolism is modified as a result of a ligand–receptor interaction; it functions as a signal transducer by regulating other intracellular processes

secondary palate   The portion of the palate that is posterior to the incisive foramen; it includes both the soft palate and part of the hard palate

segmental bronchi   Branches of the lobar bronchi that penetrate each of the lungs' ten bronchopulmonary segments

segmental   Operating entirely within a specific level of the spinal cord to control movement, such as lower motor neurons and interneurons, in contrast to suprasegmental motor control

self-oscillating system   A physical system in which a steady power input (e.g., airflow from the lungs) produces output that oscillates back and forth in some sense (e.g., vibrating vocal folds)

semicircular canals Three canals (horizontal, superior and posterior) located in the inner ear that provide sensory information related to rotational acceleration of the head

senescence Loss of a cell's power of division and growth

sensation The process by which sensory receptors detect stimulus events and convert the information about them into signals transmitted to the central nervous system; *see also* **perception**

sensorineural hearing loss A loss of hearing sensitivity due to pathology in the inner ear and/or the vestibulocochlear nerve

sensory physiology Study of the neural activity associated with a stimulus: how the stimulus is transduced and processed by specific neural regions or structures

sensory receptor A peripheral anatomical component that encodes and transduces external (real-world) stimulus energy into an electrochemical neural impulse

sensory system A neural system consisting of sensory receptors, neural pathways, and specific cortical areas dedicated to processing sensory information within a modality

sensory threshold The smallest magnitude input required to detect a stimulus event consciously

septum pellucidum Membrane that forms the medial wall of the lateral ventricles in each hemisphere

sex chromosome One of a pair of chromosomes that determine the sex of the individual; those of humans are called X and Y, where the individual normally has one X chromosome inherited from the mother and a chromosome inherited from the father that may be another X (in which case the individual is normally female) or a Y (in which case the individual is normally male); *see also* **autosome**

sexual reproduction Form of reproduction in which genetic information from two different parent organisms is combined to form the genome of the offspring; in the most common type, two gametes (a female's ovum and a male's sperm) fuse during fertilization to create a single-celled zygote that includes genetic material from both gametes

shimmer *See* **amplitude perturbation**

signal transduction A chain of reactions that transmits chemical signals from the cell surface to their intracellular targets

simple harmonic motion The simplest type of oscillation

simple sound Sound wave whose waveform consists of a single sinusoid

sine wave *See* **sinusoid**

sinister (sinistra, sinistrum) Located on the left-hand side of the body, as in the abbreviations used by audiologists (auris sinistra, AS, left ear) and optometrists (oculus sinister, OS, left eye)

sinus Cavity within a bone or other structure

sinusoid The curve illustrating the simplest type of periodic oscillations at a constant frequency; the plot of the height of a spot on the rim of a wheel that rotates at a constant rate, as a function of time; a single sinusoidal sound wave is heard as a pure tone

size principle The principle that the smallest and slowest motor units are ordinarily recruited first, followed by larger and faster motor units

skeletal muscle Voluntary muscle made up of elongated, multinucleated, transversely striated muscle fibers, having principally bony attachments

sliding filament theory The theory that muscle contraction is achieved by a sliding movement of the actin and myosin filaments past each other

slowly adapting (SA) Of a sensory receptor, beginning to fire action potentials at the onset of a stimulus event and continuing to fire them as long as the stimulus is present in the receptive field

SMA *See* **supplementary motor area**

smooth endoplasmic reticulum The major site of lipid synthesis in eukaryotic cells

smooth muscle Muscle tissue in which the contractile fibrils are not highly ordered, or striated; smooth muscle occurs in the gut and other internal organs and is not under voluntary control

sodium A chemical element (atomic number 11) that typically exists in the body as a monovalent cationic form (an atom from which one electron has been removed, resulting in a positive charge of +1)

sodium-potassium pump A protein structure found in the membranes of nearly all animal cells that transports potassium ions into the cell while simultaneously transporting sodium ions out of the cell to the extracellular fluid; in the neuronal membrane, it pumps out three sodium ions for every two potassium ions pumped in, making the membrane potential more negative; because it pumps against the concentration gradient and membrane potential, it requires energy in the form of ATP

solitary tract Compact nerve fiber bundle that travels through the posterolateral region of the medulla and conveys afferent information from stretch receptors and chemoreceptors in the walls of the cardiovascular, respiratory, and intestinal tracts

soma   The cell body of a neuron, including the nucleus and dendrites but not the axon; the soma is responsible for the production of proteins and neurotransmitters and integrates information received from other neurons via the dendrites

somatic motor fibers   Efferent fibers found in the spinal cord and brainstem that typically regulate action of skeletal muscles

somatic motor   The ability of outer hair cells to lengthen when depolarized and shorten when hyperpolarized, through the action of prestin

somatic nervous system (SNS)   Part of the peripheral nervous system that is responsible for voluntary movement and somatic sensation

somatic sensory fibers   Afferent fibers found in the spinal nerves and brainstem

somatotopy   The correspondence between the position of a receptor and the area of the cerebral cortex that enables systematic spatial organization of the body in the somatosensory system

somites   Bilaterally paired blocks of paraxial mesoderm that form along the axis of the neural tube. They give rise to the vertebrae of the spine, rib cage, skeletal muscle, cartilage, tendons, and dermal tissue

sound   The audible correlate of a vibration or oscillation of air

sound intensity   *See* **vocal intensity**

source-filter theory   Description of how the shape of the vocal tract (the filter) affects the sound waves produced by the vocal folds (the source)

space of Nuel   A fluid-filled region of the organ of Corti between outer hair cells

spasticity   A syndrome associated with hyperreflexia and hypertonus, typically due to lesions of the corticobulbar and corticospinal tracts

spatial summation   The additive effects of changes in electrical potentials of neuronal membranes consistent with synaptic effects that are in close proximity to each other on the neuronal membrane

specific acoustic impedance   The ability of a material to oppose the flow of energy by pressure waves

specific adaptation to imposed demand (SAID) principle   The principle that muscle tissue adapts in a specific manner to match the demands placed on it, also called the specificity principle; *see also* overload principle, reversibility principle

spectral acoustic analysis   Study of the distribution of energy by frequency in acoustic waves

speech   The oral expression of language through sound generated by the upper respiratory tract; speech utilizes voiced and unvoiced sounds, called phonemes, to represent thoughts and ideas in the form of words

sperm   Short for spermatozoon; the male germ cell consisting of a head, midpiece, and tail

spermatogenesis   The creation of spermatozoa; the male form of gametogenesis, in which the primary spermatocyte divides meiotically (meiosis I) into two secondary spermatocytes; each secondary spermatocyte divides into two spermatids by meiosis II

sphenoidal sinus   Air-filled chamber located within the sphenoid bone in the center of the skull

spherical bushy cell   A neuronal cell type in the anterior ventral cochlear nucleus

spinal cord   The portion of the central nervous system that extends from the brainstem down the vertebral column; the essential pathway for information flow between the brain and the limbs and trunk

spinocerebellum   The region of the cerebellum, particularly the archi- and paleocerebellum that has extensive afferents from and efferents to structures in the spinal cord

spinothalamic tracts   Tracts within the anterior and lateral funiculi of the white matter of the spinal cord carrying sensation information; the lateral spinothalamic tract is important for pain, temperature, tickle, and itch sensation, whereas the anterior spinothalamic tract is important for crude touch and pressure sensation

spiral ganglion neuron   One of the neurons around the cochlea that relay signals from the organ of Corti to the brain via the cochlear branch of the vestibulocochlear nerve

spiral ligament   A ligament located between the otic capsule wall and the stria vascularis; it covers the entire lateral wall of the scala media and extends inferiorly into the upper region of the scala tympani and provides support for the basilar membrane

spiral limbus   Thickening of the periosteum of the osseous spiral lamina on its upper plate, which ends in an external concavity, the sulcus spiralis internus

spiral organ   *See* **organ of Corti**

splenium   The posterior portion of the corpus callosum

spongioblast   A cell type formed from the primitive medullary epithelial cells

spongy bone The osseous tissue that fills the interior or cavity of bones with a latticework of small spicules or flat pieces of mineralized bars (trabeculae) and interstices containing bone marrow or fat; also called cancellous or trabecular bone; *see also* **compact bone**

spontaneous action potential firing rate Neural discharge activity that is present in the absence of an external stimulus

stapedius muscle A middle ear muscle that attaches to the neck of the stapes bone; the stapedius nerve innervates it

stapedius nerve An offshoot of the facial nerve that innervates the stapedius muscle

stapes Stirrup; the most medial bone of the ossicular chain, which transmits the motions of the incus to the cochlea through the oval window

stellate cell A neuronal cell type in the central auditory nervous system

stem cells Cells that have the ability to divide (self-replicate) for indefinite periods, often throughout the life of the organism, and give rise to more specialized cell types

stenosis The narrowing of a passage in the body (e.g., aorta, external auditory canal)

stepping strategy One of the four vestibulospinal reflexes, used when the center of gravity moves outside of the base of support and all other vestibulospinal reflexes have failed to regain balance; with the stepping strategy, the individual uses a corrective step or stumble to return the center of gravity to within the base of support; *see also* **ankle strategy**, **hip strategy**, **suspensory strategy**

stereocilia Stalklike projections arranged in bundles found on the top surfaces of hair cells; with their tip links, the location where hydromechanical energy is converted into electrochemical neural impulses

sternoclavicular ligament Ligament that joins fibers of the sternohyoid muscle to the clavicle

sternohyoid muscle Laryngeal depressor muscle that originates on the strernum and inserts on the hyoid bone

sternothyroid muscle Laryngeal depressor muscle that originates on the sternum and inserts on the thyroid cartilage

stochastic resonance A physical phenomenon in which a signal embedded in noise may be improved by adding more noise

straight sinus An area that receives blood from the great cerebral vein

stretch reflex A physical response to the extension of a muscle

stria vascularis A structure located on the lateral wall of the scala media that likely produces endolymph

striatum Subdivision of the basal ganglia comprising the caudate nucleus and the putamen, so called because of its striped appearance due to the layers of gray and white matter; the striatum is considered the input structure of the basal ganglia complex and is anatomically continuous with the thalamus

striola A curved indention of the macula (supporting cells) in the utricle and saccule that divides each otolithic organ into two sections

styloglossus muscle An extrinsic muscle of the tongue that originates at the styloid process, inserts into the inferior side of the tongue, and serves to pull the tongue superiorly and posteriorly

stylohyoid muscle A muscle originating on the styloid process of the temporal bone and inserting on the hyoid bone, serving to raise the hyoid and the larynx upward and rearward

styloid process A slender projection of bone from the temporal bone

stylopharyngeus muscle Muscle from the styloid process to the lateral wall of the pharynx that draws the pharynx up and the lateral pharyngeal wall laterally, increasing the cross-sectional area of the pharynx

subarachnoid space Space between the arachnoid mater and the pia mater; the subarachnoid space contains major arteries surrounded by cerebrospinal fluid

subculture A new cell culture made by transferring some or all cells from a previous culture to fresh growth medium

subdural hematoma *See* **subdural hemorrhage**

subdural hemorrhage Also called subdural hematoma; bleeding that takes place between the dura mater and the cerebral cortex

subdural space A space beneath the dura mater and occupied by the nonconnective tissue fibers called neurothelium

subglottal air pressure The partial pressure of exhaled air beneath a closed glottis

substantia nigra A large gray matter nucleus, located in the crus cerebri of the mesencephalon of the brainstem posterior to the pyramidal tract, that is responsible for producing the neurotransmitter dopamine; it plays an important role in reward, addiction, and movement

substantia nigra pars compacta The medial subdivision of the substantia nigra, containing neurons whose neurotransmitter is dopamine and that project to the striatum, among other targets; degeneration of the substantia nigra pars compacta is associated with idiopathic Parkinson's disease

substantia nigra pars reticulata The lateral subdivision of the substantia nigra, containing neurons that project to the thalamus, particularly the ventral anterior nucleus, and to brainstem structures thought to be related to control of eye movements

sulcus A grooves on the surface of the cerebral cortex

sulcus terminalis A groove on the dorsal surface of the tongue that originates in the foramen cecum and runs laterally and anteriorly on either side to the margin of the tongue; it marks the union of the anterior and posterior parts of the tongue

summating potential (SP) A sound-evoked potential arising from the inner (sensory) hair cells of the cochlea; it is direct current

superficial Closer to the surface

superficial abdominal reflex A reflex where stroking the skin over the abdomen causes a contraction of the rectus abdominis muscles, which can be observed as the umbilicus moving

superficial cerebral vein Vein that is located on the medial and lateral surface of the cerebral hemisphere and that courses along the sulci and drains the adjacent areas

superficial lamina propria (SLP) The second layer in from the surface in the vocal fold, the most pliable layer, with a gelatinous texture

superior Above or over another structure

superior cerebellar peduncle Pathway of afferents to and efferents from the deep cerebellar nuclei and the cerebellar cortex, that is rostral to the level of the deep cerebellar nuclei; targets include the red nucleus and the ventral intermediate thalamus

superior colliculus (SC) A nucleus found on the dorsal aspect (tectum) of the mesencephalon that receives visual information from the optic tracts and is active during reflexive turning or orienting of the eyes; also called the optic tectum, and usually described as the visual reflex center

superior laryngeal nerve (SLN) Branch of the vagus nerve that innervates the pharynx and larynx through its external and internal branches

superior longitudinal muscle Paired intrinsic muscle of the tongue that constitutes the upper layer and elevates the tip of the tongue

superior olivary complex (SOC) Medial and lateral nuclei in the brainstem that receives tonotopic inputs from the cochlear nuclei (low-frequency inputs project to the medial SOC, high-frequency inputs to the lateral SOC); the first point on the central auditory pathway where binaural inputs are combined; projects to the inferior colliculus

superior orbital fissure An opening in the sphenoid bone through which various nerves and vessels, including the nerves that control eye movement, pass into the orbit

superior pharyngeal constrictor Muscle with multiple origins from the pterygoid hamulus, the mandible, and the tongue, inserting on the occipital bone, which constricts the oropharynx during swallowing

superior sagittal sinus A large area located superiorly and dorsally to the brain where the blood and cerebrospinal fluid drain

superior temporal gyrus (STG) Gyrus immediately inferior to the lateral sulcus, home of the primary auditory cortex

supplementary motor area (SMA) A cortical region lying just anterior to the motor cortex predominantly over the medial convexity of the cerebral hemisphere; it receives inputs from the basal ganglia via the thalamus and projects to motor areas and to the brainstem and to the spinal cord via the corticobulbar and corticospinal pathways

suprahyoid aponeurosis Layer of connective tissue joining the intermediate tendon, and thus the digastric muscle, to the hyoid bone

suprahyoid muscle Muscle acting on the hyoid bone from above

supramarginal gyrus A gyrus curving around the end of the lateral sulcus, associated with recognition and generation of spoken language and written words

suprasegmental Of a neuronal system, originating outside of the specific level (segment) of the spinal cord that innervate the muscles and organs the neuronal system controls; structures of the suprasegmental motor control systems include the motor cortex, supplementary motor area, red nucleus, cerebellum, reticular formations, and basal ganglia

suspensory strategy One of the four vestibulospinal reflexes, used to lower the center of gravity and increase stability; when using the suspensory strategy, the individual flexes at the knees, ankles, and hips to lower the center of gravity and improve stability; *see also* **ankle strategy**, **hip strategy**, **stepping strategy**

suture Fibrous joint that occurs only in the skull

swallowing The entire process of bringing food to the oral cavity, maneuvering it in the oral cavity, and propelling it into the pharynx through to the esophagus

sympathetic system A division of the autonomic nervous system that contains neurons in the lateral gray column from the thoracic to lumbar spinal cord, as well as in the sympathetic trunks running along either side of the spine; the sympathetic system participates in the responses regulating reactions to stress and threats; *see also* **parasympathetic system**

synapse The structure that enables communication between an axon and the target cell to which the signal from the axon is to be delivered (such as a muscle cell or a dendrite of another neuron), consisting the presynaptic terminal (terminal bouton), the postsynaptic membrane, and the synaptic cleft between them; a signal is delivered by the release of neurotransmitter molecules from the presynaptic terminal into the synaptic cleft, which they cross to combine with receptors on the postsynaptic membrane

synaptic cleft Space in a synapse between the presynaptic membrane (e.g., axon terminal or motor end plate) and the postsynaptic membrane (e.g., dendrite of a nerve or muscle cell wall); neurotransmitters must cross the synaptic cleft to bind to their receptors

synaptic signaling Chemical signaling that travels between nerve cells through synapses

synaptogenesis The formation of a synapse such as the one that that connects the nerve and the muscle cell

synaptogenesis Creation of synapses between neurons

syncytiotrophoblast One of two cell layers of the chorionic villi that plays an important role in maternal–fetal gas exchange, nutrient exchange, and immunological and metabolic functions

synovial joint A joint that is surrounded by a fluid-filled membrane that lubricates the joint

syntax The structure of a communication, such as language, independent of the meaning (semantics)

s/z ratio The ratio of the maximum time a person can produce an unvoiced sound (/s/) to the maximum time the person can produce the voiced counterpart (/z/)

T

T cells White blood cells that destroy pathogens through a complex series of coordinated actions

tachycardia Rapid heartbeat

tastant A substance with water-soluble molecules that bind to and stimulate gustatory/taste receptors

taste buds Sensory receptors found primarily on the tongue and responsible for transducing taste information; taste buds are also found within regions of the mouth and pharynx

tectal ridge The equivalent of the premaxillary process, a set of bones fixed with the maxilla that later underlies the alveolar ridge

tectorial membrane (TM) A gelatinous layer that lies over the organ of Corti; outer hair cell stereocilia are embedded within this layer

tectospinal tract A pathway from the neuronal cell bodies in the tectum of the brainstem to terminations on neurons of the brainstem and spinal cord, thought to be involved in motor control

tectum The most dorsal layer of the most superior part of the brainstem (the mesencephalon), carrying the superior and inferior colliculi

telencephalon The embryologically defined subdivision of the prosencephalon that gives rise to both lobes of the cerebrum as well as the basal ganglia and limbic system

telophase The final stage of mitosis, during which the nuclear envelope forms around each group of chromosomes and the division of cytoplasm, or cytokinesis, begins

temporal fossa Depression on the side of the skull where soft tissue structures define the form of the head in the region of the temple

temporal lobe The lobe of the cerebrum located beneath the lateral sulcus, responsible for auditory input and processing and multiple aspects of speech recognition, language, and memory

temporal summation Additive effect of sequential postsynaptic potentials that are close together in time

temporal theory Theory that states that our perception of sound depends on the temporal patterns with which neurons respond to sound in the cochlea, so that the pitch of a pure tone would be determined by period of neuron firing patterns, either of single neurons or groups as described by the **volley theory**

temporalis Muscle originating on the temporal bone that closes the mandible

temporomandibular joint The hinge between the temporal bone of the skull and the lower jaw bone (mandible)

tendon Tough band of fibrous connective tissue that usually connects muscle to bone and is capable of withstanding tension

tensor tympani Muscle that increases the stiffness of the tympanic membrane

tensor veli palatini   Muscle that tightens the soft palate and opens the eustachian tube

terminal bouton   The endpoint structure of an axon that makes synaptic contact with downstream neurons; the terminal bouton is involved in the release of neurotransmitters that influence the response of the downstream neuron

terminal bronchioles   Branches of the segmental bronchi

terminal segment   Output zone of a neuron at the end of its axon, forming synapses; when an action potential reaches the terminal segment, neurotransmitters are released to complete neural communication

thalamocortical fibers   Third-order neurons that relay somatosensory signals from the thalamus to the cerebral cortex

thalamocortical relay cell   A neuronal cell type located in the thalamus

thalamus   A part of the diencephalon that is paired and symmetrical in the midline of the cerebrum, consisting of many gray matter nuclei that serve as the primary relay station of all afferent input (from cutaneous, visual, and auditory senses) to the cerebral cortex and as a processing region for complex actions; its medial surfaces constitute the upper part of the lateral walls of the third ventricle; the two halves of the thalamus are connected across the third ventricle by a band of gray matter called the interthalamic adhesion

thermoreceptor   A primary receptor responsible for detecting and encoding relative temperature information

third ventricle   Cavity of the ventricular system of the brain that is located in the midline of the diencephalon and is shared by both hemispheres; it communicates with the lateral ventricles through the interventricular foramen and with the fourth ventricle through the cerebral aqueduct

thoracentesis   Removal of fluid from the pleural cavity

thoracic cavity   Commonly referred to as the chest; bodily cavity encased by the ribs that contains the lungs and heart

thromboplastin   A substance produced by the lungs that promotes blood coagulation

three-mass model   The concept of the vocal fold as consisting of three elements (the lower edge, the upper edge, and the body), each having its own properties of elasticity and inertia

thyroarytenoid (TA) muscle   An intrinsic laryngeal muscle in two divisions; the thyrovocalis or vocalis tenses the vocal fold, whereas the thyromuscularis or muscularis acts on the muscular process of the arytenoid cartilage to adduct the vocal folds

thyroepiglottic ligament   Ligament connecting the inferior petiolus (stalk) of the epiglottis to the anterior wall of the thyroid cartilage

thyroepiglottic muscle   Muscle that may be considered as a third division of the thyroarytenoid, but it does not affect the vocal folds; widens the laryngeal vestibule

thyrohyoid membrane   Ligament connecting the thyroid cartilage to the hyoid bone

thyrohyoid muscle   Muscle that shortens the distance between the hyoid bone and the thyroid cartilage when contracting

thyroid cartilage   The superior cartilage component of the larynx

thyroid horns   Superior and inferior projections on the posterior margins of the thyroid cartilage

thyroid notch   Notch on the midline where the two thyroid laminae do not fuse

tidal volume   The volume of air that is repeatedly inhaled, then exhaled, during tidal breathing

tight junction   A continuous network of protein strands around the circumference of epithelial cells, sealing the space between cells and forming a barrier between the apical and basolateral domains

timbre   The attributes of a sound that give it a unique perceptual identity; pronounced "tamber"

tip links   Protein filaments connecting stereocilia together

tissue   An aggregate of cells in an organism that have similar structure and function

TMS   *See* **transcranial magnetic stimulation**

Todd paralysis   *See* **postictal paralysis**

tonic   Pertaining to slow and continuous action by a muscle fiber or nerve

tonotopy   Organization of acoustic signal processing in space by frequency in the auditory system

tooth buds   Groups of cells at the periphery of the dental lamina that appear around the seventh week of development

tooth germ   The structure consisting of the enamel organ and its contained dental papilla as well as the dental sac or follicle

total lung capacity (TLC)   The maximum volume of gas that the lungs are able to contain

trachea Windpipe; a tube reinforced by a series of cartilaginous rings that serves as a conduit for air passing in and out between the larynx and the lungs

tragus Most anterior landmark of the external ear

trait A distinguishing quality or characteristic of a specific part of a person

transaxial plane A horizontal plane that divides a region into superior and inferior parts; also called axial plane or transverse plane

transcranial magnetic stimulation (TMS) A method for causing or preventing depolarization of neurons in the central nervous system, typically over the cerebral cortex, cerebellum, and spinal cord, using a strong electromagnetic pulse generated outside the skull over the area to be affected; the advantage is that the skin and bones are less of a barrier to the magnetic flux than to electric flux

transcription The synthesis of an RNA molecule (message) from DNA in the cell nucleus

transfer RNA (tRNA) A molecule of ribonucleic acid folded into a form that presents three bases at one end to match a codon, while the other end is bonded to the specific amino acid the codon represents in order to bring the amino acid to the ribosome in the correct sequence

transglottal airflow Airflow between the vocal folds during a cycle of vibration

translation The synthesis of a protein from RNA in the cytoplasm

transmission electron microscopy (TEM) Microscopy method in which a beam of electrons is passed through a specimen stained with heavy metals

transmission segment Conducting zone of an axon, which propagates action potentials rapidly from the soma to the terminal segment

transverse gyrus (of Heschl) *See* **Heschl gyrus**

transverse muscles of the tongue Intrinsic muscles of the tongue that narrow the tongue when contracted

transverse palatine suture Union of the palatine processes of the maxillae with the horizontal plates of the palatine bones

transverse plane *See* **transaxial plane**

transverse tubules (T-tubules) Channels above the myofibrils that transport the action potential through the muscle fiber to facilitate muscle contraction

trapezoid body An area of transverse nerve fibers running over the posterior (deep) border of the pontine nuclei; formed by ascending auditory fibers that cross to the opposite side of the brainstem

traveling wave The movement of the cochlear partition in response to sound caused by fluid displacement as a result of movement of the stapes

trigeminal lemniscus An ascending axonal tract in the brainstem that conveys tactile and proprioceptive inputs from the head; fibers of the trigeminal lemniscus synapse onto neurons of the ventral posteromedial (VPM) nucleus of the thalamus

trigeminal nerve (CN V) A mixed nerve and the largest of the cranial nerves, having a large sensory root entering the brainstem and a much smaller motor root that exits the brainstem; it divides into the ophthalmic, maxillary, and mandibular branches

trigeminothalamic pathway A somatosensory pathway in the central nervous system that conveys information related to pain and temperature from the head; fibers of the trigeminothalamic pathway synapse onto neurons of the ventral posteromedial (VPM) nucleus of the thalamus

trochlear nerve (CN IV) A pure motor nerve that innervates the superior oblique muscle of the eye; *see also* **abducens nerve (CN VI)**, **oculomotor nerve (CN III)**

trophoblast Cells forming the outer layer of a blastocyst, which develop into a large part of the placenta

trophoblastic villi Fingerlike processes that extend out from the trophoblast into the endometrium and that grow into chorionic villi

tropomyosin A long, regulatory protein that wraps around the actin filament and covers the binding site for myosin

troponin A complex of three proteins located on the actin filament which regulates muscle contraction by controlling the interaction between actin and myosin

tuberculum impar A small elevation that forms between the lateral lingual swellings, thought to form the central part of the tongue immediately in front of the foramen cecum

tubulin A cytoskeletal protein that polymerizes to form microtubules

tufted cell A neuronal cell type in the central auditory nervous system

tuning curve A graph representing the intensity or other stimulus value needed to a sensory receptor fire action potentials against action potential frequency

tunnel of Corti A spiral passage within the organ of Corti

turbinate One of the nasal conchae

twitch The smallest contractile response of a muscle, resulting from a single action potential applied to a single motor unit

two-point discrimination A perceptual test that can assess the size, density, and distribution of receptive fields on the skin

tympanic membrane Eardrum; a translucent, drum head like, multilayer structure that separates the outer ear from the middle ear; it is responsible for transducing sound into a mechanical motion

type 2 alveolar cells Cells in the walls of alveoli that secrete alveolar fluid (pulmonary surfactant) to lower the surface tension of the alveolus, thereby preventing collapse

type 1 alveolar cells The cellular site of gas exchange in the walls of alveoli

U

ultrasonography Diagnostic imaging technique based on the application of ultrasound

umbo Point of maximum concavity of the tympanic membrane

uncus A protuberance at the rostral end of the parahippocampal gyrus

unicellular Having, or consisting of, a single cell

unipolar neuron Neuron that has only one projection from the soma, where the dendrite and axon are not separated

unmyelinated axon An axon that lacks a myelin sheath

upper motor neuron (UMN) A motor neuron whose soma resides in the motor area of the cerebral cortex or the supplementary motor area and whose axon projects to lower motor neurons in the brainstem and spinal cord

upper motor neuron syndrome A syndrome associated with lesions of the upper motor neuron or its axons in the corticobulbar and corticospinal tracts, with symptoms and signs including weakness or paralysis, emergence of pathological reflexes such as increased deep tendon reflexes and Babinski reflexes, and loss of superficial reflexes such as the abdominal and cremasteric reflexes

upper respiratory system The major subdivision of the respiratory system consisting of the larynx, pharynx, nasal cavities, and oral cavity

urge-to-cough (UTC) A conscious perception of the need to produce cough in response to stimulation

utricle An otolithic organ in the vestibular labyrinth of the inner ear, oriented in the horizontal plane and responsible for detecting linear acceleration in the horizontal plane, as well as head tilt relative to gravity

V

vagus nerve (CN X) A mixed cranial nerve that carries afferent and efferent information from the most diverse set of organs, including the larynx and pharynx; it serves as the primary motor innervation to the intrinsic laryngeal muscles and primary sensory innervation to tissues and structures of the larynx; its ten branches include the pharyngeal branch, the superior laryngeal nerve, and the recurrent laryngeal nerve

valleculae lateral recesses in the laryngopharynx, formed by the base of the tongue and epiglottis

Valsalva maneuver The process of inhaling, then tightly closing the vocal folds so as to trap a large volume of air within the lower respiratory tract, assisting with thoracic stabilization for tasks that put the thoracic and abdominal cavities under pressure

variable expressivity The ability of a genetic trait to present different degrees of severity and forms

vasoactive Able to alter vascular tone in blood vessels, dilating or constricting them, affecting blood pressure

velopharyngeal port Passage between the nasopharynx and the oropharynx

ventral Toward the front side of the body or hand, or the sole of the foot or the underside of the penis or the thalamus, when in anatomic position; *see also* **dorsal**

ventral intermediate nucleus of the thalamus The nucleus within the thalamus that relays information from the deep cerebellar nuclei to the motor cortex

ventral nucleus of the lateral lemniscus (VNLL) Ventral division of the lateral lemniscus

ventral respiratory group Part of the medullary respiratory center; acts in cooperation with the pre-Bötzinger complex during expiration

ventral stria Fiber tract of axons that originate from the anterior ventral cochlear nucleus to the trapezoid body and form a portion of the lateral lemniscus tract

ventral posterior (VP) nuclei Principal nucleus in the thalamus receiving vestibular information from the vestibular nuclei

ventral posterolateral (VPL) nucleus The nucleus in the thalamus that receives ascending cutaneous and proprioceptive inputs from second-order projections in the dorsal-column medial lemniscal (DCML) pathway

ventral posteromedial (VPM) nucleus The nucleus in the thalamus that receives ascending cutaneous and proprioceptive inputs from the head via the trigeminothalamic tract and trigeminal lemniscus

ventral thalamus pars oralis The nucleus within the thalamus that relays information from the basal ganglia to the supplementary motor area and to the motor cortex

ventricle Fluid-filled cavity within a bodily structure, such as the lateral, third, and fourth ventricles of the brain

ventricular folds Paired folds of tissue located above the vocal folds, formed by the inferior aspect of the quadrangular ligaments; also called false vocal folds and vestibular folds (because they are located in the laryngeal vestibule)

ventricular ligament Ligament running from the thyroid cartilage to the anterior surface of the arytenoid cartilage, covered by the ventricular fold

ventricular muscle Muscle fibers located along the length of the ventricular folds

ventricular system The interconnected cavities in the brain (the lateral, third, and fourth ventricles) that are filled with cerebrospinal fluid

vermal zone of the cerebellum Region of the cerebellum that is located in the midline and has reciprocal connections with the fastigial deep cerebellar nuclei; thought to be involved in control of posture and gait

vermis Flocculonodular lobe; a wormlike structure in the cerebellum

vertebral artery Major paired artery that is located in the neck and back, supplying the vertebral column and also contributing to the blood supply of the brain

vertebral-basilar artery Large paired blood vessels ascending from the vertebral column that fuse near the pontomedullary junction to form the single basilar artery; this artery is the primary blood supply for the brainstem, cerebellum and certain cerebral structures; *see also* **circle of Willis**

vertex Superior tip of the skull

vertical muscles of the tongue Intrinsic muscles of the tongue that flatten the tongue and withdraw it into the floor of the mouth

vertigo Sensation of movement or spinning; pathologic vertigo can be objective in nature, in which one feels as though the world is moving and spinning around one, or subjective in nature, wherein one feels as though one is spinning in the absence of actual head movement

vesicle Membrane-enclosed sac that transports a substance made in the cell, such as a protein or neurotransmitter, from the place it was made to the cell surface, where its membrane fuses with the cell membrane to release the substance into the extracellular environment

vestibular aqueduct The bony channel that encompasses the endolymphatic duct and contains endolymph

vestibular folds *See* **ventricular folds**

vestibular ligament *See* **ventricular ligament**

vestibular nuclei Four collections (superior, lateral, medial, and inferior) of neuronal cell bodies in the pons and medulla that receive sensory inputs from the vestibular apparatus in the inner ear that mediate balance and project to motor neurons via the vestibulospinal tracts; also called the central vestibular nucleus complex

vestibulo-ocular network (VON) A series of reciprocal connections between the peripheral vestibular apparatus and the visual system that functions to send visual information to the central vestibular nucleus complex and receive information from the central vestibular nucleus complex for control of reflexive eye movements in response to vestibular input

vestibulo-ocular reflex (VOR) A collection of compensatory eye movements that occur in response to head/body movement that are equal in magnitude and opposite in direction from the head movement that provoked them; they maintain eye gaze at a fixed target when the head or body is in motion

vestibulocerebellum Portion of the cerebellum responsible for processing input from the peripheral vestibular and visual systems for coordination of reflexive ocular and postural movements to maintain balance

vestibulocochlear nerve (CN VIII) Principal sensory nerve that originates from afferent terminals in the cochlea and the vestibular system and projects to both the cochlear and vestibular nuclei in the medulla to transmit auditory and balance-related input to these structures

vestibulospinal network (VSN) A network of connections between the peripheral vestibular apparatus and the spinal cord that functions to send proprioceptive information to the central vestibular nuclei and receive information from the central vestibular nucleus complex to coordinate reflexive head and body movements to maintain upright posture

vestibulospinal tracts The principal descending pathway (consisting of a lateral and a medial vestibulospinal tract) from neuronal cell bodies in the vestibular nuclei in the brainstem to synapses on motor systems of the trunk and lower limbs, functioning to maintain postural control and balance

vestibulothalamocortical network A network of connections between the central vestibular nucleus complex, the thalamus, and two regions of the cortex that enables further integration of vestibular, visual, and proprioceptive/somatosensory information to achieve conscious perception of balance and the position of the body in space

vibratory cycle One complete passage through the motions of a self-oscillating system from its starting point back to its starting point

videofluoroscopic evaluation of swallowing A radiographic swallowing evaluation technique that provides a moving X-ray video of the swallowing mechanism while a patient swallows a variety of boluses mixed with barium sulfate

visceral motor fibers Efferent fibers in the autonomic nervous system that regulate involuntary functions, such as heart rate, respiration, urination, digestion, and motor control of the vascular system and exocrine glands

visceral pleura Membrane that lines the outer surfaces of the lungs; *see also* **parietal pleura**

visceral sensory fibers Afferent fibers in the autonomic nervous system that carry information about involuntary functions, such as heart rate, respiration, urination, digestion, and status of the vascular system and exocrine glands

viscerocranium The part of the skull that comprises the facial skeleton

viscosity Thickness of a substance

visual field The total extent of the visual space that can be detected by both retinas; *see also* **hemifield**

vital capacity The maximum volume of air that can be passed in and out of the lungs

vocal folds A pair (left and right) of horizontally oriented and structurally stratified bands of connective tissue located within the larynx that function to close and open the airway for breathing and airway protection and modulate airflow through the glottis for voice production; sometimes called vocal cords; consist of epithelium and superficial lamina propria (vocal fold cover), intermediate and deep lamina propria (vocal ligament), and vocalis muscle (vocal fold body); *see also* **cartilaginous vocal fold**, **membranous vocal fold**

vocal fry Voice quality when F_0 is 70 Hz or less, described as a "creaky" voice

vocal intensity The average amplitude of vocal vibration; its perceptual correlate is loudness

vocal ligament The intermediate and deep lamina propria of the vocal fold, around the vocalis muscle

vocal process Anterior projection on the arytenoid cartilage, to which vocal folds attach

vocal tremor Effect of rhythmic muscle activity during phonation; perceived as a "shaky" voice

vocalis muscle (VM) The deepest layer of the vocal fold, which is also a division of the thyroarytenoid muscle; it tenses the vocal fold

voice Acoustic energy created when the vocal folds modulate airflow through the glottis

voice break Temporary failure of vocal folds to vibrate during the production of a voiced sound

voice quality The auditory-perceptual awareness of vocal acoustic features related to frequency (perceived as pitch), intensity (perceived as loudness), and timbre (e.g., breathiness, roughness)

voicing efficiency The amount of work needed to convert aerodynamic energy into acoustic energy

volley theory Theory that states that groups of neurons of the auditory system respond to a sound by firing action potentials slightly out of phase with one another so that, when combined, a greater frequency of sound can be encoded

voltage-gated ion channel A protein structure that spans the neuronal membrane and allows the flow of a specific positive or negative ion when it opens in response to the electric potential across the neuronal membrane

vomer Unpaired bone that forms the inferior part of the nasal septum

W

Waldeyer ring Arrangement of lymphoid tissue in multiple structures around the pharynx, including the pharyngeal, palatine, and lingual tonsils

waveform A curve illustrating oscillations of a sound or oscillating electrical signal

wavelength The distance in space between repeating elements of adjacent cycles of a periodic sound wave; calculated as the speed of sound divided by frequency of the wave

Wernicke aphasia A language disorder that is characterized by difficulty in comprehending one's own speech and the speech of others, caused by a stroke that produces a lesion in the posterior temporal lobe (Wernicke area); depending on the size of the lesion, there may be accompanying problems in reading and writing, repeating words, and naming objects; individuals symptomatically produce abundant but meaningless speech; *see also* **Broca aphasia**

Wernicke area   Area that is located posterior to the primary auditory cortex and that is responsible for speech perception

white matter   Substance in the brain and spinal cord characteristically consisting of myelinated axons and the glial cells that form myelin; *see also* **gray matter**

X

X chromosome   One of the two sex chromosomes in humans, found in both males and females

xerostomia   Chronic dry mouth

Y

Y chromosome   One of the two sex chromosomes in humans; the sex-determining chromosome found only in males

yolk sac   A membranous sac attached to an embryo, formed by cells of the hypoblast adjacent to the embryonic disc; it is situated on the ventral aspect of the embryo and is important in early embryonic blood supply; it is incorporated into the primordial gut during the fourth week of development

Z

Z-line   The juncture between two sarcomeres

zona pellucida   A thick glycoprotein layer that surrounds the ovum before implantation

zygomatic bone   Cheekbone, forming a bridge over the temporal fossa between the maxilla and the temporal bone

zygomaticus major   Muscle that draws the angle of the mouth superiorly and laterally

zygomaticus minor   Muscle that elevates the upper lip

zygote   Cell formed by fertilization between two gametes, the beginning of the offspring's existence, with a genome made up of a combination of the DNA in each gamete

Index

Note: an *f* indicates a figure; a *t*, a table.

A

AAF. *See* Anterior auditory field (AAF)
A-bands, 241
Abducens nerve, 162
Abduction, 360
ABR. *See* Auditory brainstem response (ABR)
ACA. *See* Anterior cerebral artery (ACA)
Accessory nerve, 162, 165
Acetylcholine (ACh), 193, 239
Acetylcholine (ACh) neurotransmitter, 238
ACh. *See* Acetylcholine (ACh)
Achilles tendon, 67*f*
AChRs. *See* Postsynaptic acetylcholine receptors (AChRs)
Acoustic analysis, 373*f*, 374*f*, 381–382
    amplitude perturbation, 382
    frequency perturbation, 382
    jitter, 382
    periodicity, 382
    physiologic voice, range, 382
    shimmer, 382
    sound intensity, 382
    spectral acoustic analyses, 382
    vocal intensity, 382
Acoustic observations, 432–433
Acoustic reflex, 454
Actin, 41, 241
Actin-filled stereocilia, 464
Action potential (AP), 58, 173, 176, 176*ff*, 178*t*, 193, 238, 264, 269, 269*f*
    depolarization, 176
    hyperpolarization, 176
Action potential-initiating segment, 178, 193
Action tremor, 218
Active cellular transport, 46–48
    endocytosis, 47, 48*f*
    exocytosis, 47, 48*f*
    membrane potential, 46
    sodium-potassium pump, 46–47, 48*f*
Active expiration, 321*f*
Active inspiration, 319–322, 320*f*, 321*f*
    active expiration, 321*f*
    alveolar ventilation rate, 321
    Boyle's law, 319, 320*f*
    expiratory reserve volume (ERV), 321
    inspiratory reserve volume (IRV), 321
    minute ventilation (MV), 321
    residual volume (RV), 321
    tidal volume, 321
    total lung capacity (TLC), 320
    vital capacity (VC), 321, 321*f*
Acute bronchitis, 339
Acute respiratory distress syndrome (ARDS), 340
Adduction, 360
Adenoids, 416, 416*f*
Adenosine triphosphate (ATP), 37, 175, 243, 312
Adherens junctions, 55
Adult stem cells, 61
Aerobic respiration, 43, 43*f*
    citric acid cycle, 43*f*
    electron transport chain, 43*f*
    glycolysis, 43–44, 43*f*
    pyruvate oxidation, 43*f*
Aerodynamic analysis, 380–381
    estimated mean flow rate, 380–381
    phonation quotient (PQ), 380
    phonation threshold pressure (PTP), 381
    phonation volume, 380

pressure, 381
    vital capacity (VC), 380
    voicing efficiency, 381
Afferent nerves, 140–141, 140*f*
Afferent neural functions, 468–470
    characteristic frequencies, 469
    cochlear nucleus, 469
    phase locking, 470
    spontaneous action potential firing rate, 469, 470*f*
    tuning curve, 470, 470*f*
Afferents, 484, 503
Affinity, 183
Age and gender differences in phonation acoustic energy characteristics, 377–379
    anatomy and physiology of larynx, 378–379
        cartilaginous vocal fold, 378
        membranous vocal fold, 378
    production of voice and voice quality, 378–379
Aging and coughing, 326
Aging and muscle adaptations, 257
Aging and respiration, 342
Agonists, 183
Air conduction, 449
Air conduction and filtration, 323–324, 323*f*
    mucociliary escalator, 323
    phlegm, 322
Airway protection, 324–328
    aging and coughing, 326
    cystic fibrosis, 324
    dystussia, 327
    homeostatic emotion, 325
    pulmonary infection, nontubercular mycobacteria (pNTM), 327
    urge-to-cough (UTC), 324, 324*f*, 325*f*
Alkalemia, 335
Akinesia, 207
Allantois, 107
Alleles, 80
Allophones, 426
All-or-none response, 193
Alpha lower motor neuron (α-LMN), 192, 237
ALS. *See* Anterolateral system (ALS)
Alveolar gas exchange, 316*f*
Alveolar process, 395, 396*f*
Alveolar ridge, 392, 424
Alveolar ventilation rate, 321
Alveoli, 316
Alzheimer's disease, 37, 184*t*
Amacrine cells, 281
American English consonants, 425*t*
American English vowels and diphthongs, 425*t*
Amnion, 107
Amniotic cavity, 107
Amniotic membrane, 107
AMPA-type receptors, 466
Amphipathic region, 36
Amplitude, 328
Amplitude perturbation, 382
Ampula, 296*f*, 297, 528–529, 529*f*
Amyotrophic lateral sclerosis, 184*t*, 511, 511*f*
Anaerobic respiration, 44
Anaphase, 105
Anatomically based theories, 208, 209*f*
Anatomic planes, 8
    anatomic position, anterior view, 8*f*
    axial plane, 8
    cardinal planes and axes, 10*f*

coronal plane, 8
    frontal plane, 8
    general terms, location and direction, 9
    horizontal plane, 8
    midsagittal plane, 8
    parasagittal plane, 8
    sagittal plane, 8
    transaxial plane, 8
    transverse plane, 8
Anatomic position, anterior view, 8*f*
Anatomy, 4
Angular acceleration by semicircular canals measurement, 297
    ampula, 296*f*, 297
    cupula, 297
Angular gyrus, 149
Anion, 173
Ankle strategy, 543, 544*f*
Ankyloglossia, 418
Annular ligament, 453
Anomic aphasia, 148–149
Ansa cervicalis, 368
Antagonists, 183
Anterior auditory field (AAF), 475
Anterior cerebral artery (ACA), 154
Anterior commissure, 150, 356
Anterior lingual primordia, 124
Anterior neuropore, 111
Anterior SCC, 525
Anterior ventral cochlear nucleus (AVCN), 472
Anterolateral system (ALS), 272, 278–279
Antidromic action potentials, 214
Antihelix, 450
Aortic body, 336
AP. *See* Action potential (AP)
Aperiodic energy, 374
Aperiodic sound waves, 445
Apex, 416
Aphasia, 147–149, 148*t*
    anomic aphasia, 148–149
    Broca's aphasia, 148
    conduction aphasia, 148
    global aphasia, 148–149
    Wernicke's aphasia, 148, 149
Apical membrane, 47, 47*f*
Apnea, 499
Apneustic center, 335
Arachnoid barrier, 155
Arachnoid granulations, 156–157
Arachnoid mater, 155
Arachnoid trabeculae, 155
Archicerebellum, 216
Archipallium, 115
ARDS. *See* Acute respiratory distress syndrome (ARDS)
Articulation and resonance, 391–441
    articulation, 425–429
        allophones, 426
        American English consonants, 425*t*
        American English vowels and dipthongs, 425*t*
        nasality, 426
        phonemes, 426
        resonance, 426
        source-filter theory, 426–429, 427*f*, 428*f*
    articulatory/resonance system anatomy, 392–393
        alveolar ridge, 392
        conchae, 392

laryngopharynx, 392
mandible, 392
meatuses, 392
nasal cavity, 392, 392f
nasopharynx, 392
oral cavity, 392, 392f
oropharynx, 392
pharyngeal cavity, 392
coordinated articulation, 433–435
coarticulation, 433
Directions into Velocities of Articulation
(DIVA) model, 434, 435f
economy of effort, 433, 433f
motor equivalence, 434
cranial bones, 397
frontal bone, 393f, 397
occipital bone, 393f, 398, 398f
parietal bones, 393f, 397–398
sphenoid bone, 398f, 399
temporal bone, 393f, 398–399, 398f
ethmoid bone, 399, 399f
facial muscles, 404–409, 404f, 405f, 406t
buccinator, 405, 406f
depressor anguli oris, 407, 407f
depressor labii inferioris, 406f, 407
frontalis muscle, 407, 408f
incisivus labii inferioris muscle, 407
incisivus labii superioris, 405
levator anguli oris, 407, 407f
levator labii superioris, 405, 406f
levator labii superioris aleque nasi, 404f,
405, 407
masseter muscle, 405
mentalis muscle, 407, 408f
orbicularis oculi, 407, 408f
orbicularis oris, 404, 404f
platysma muscle, 405, 405f, 407
risorius, 404–405, 405f
zygomaticus major, 407, 407f
zygomaticus minor, 407, 407f
immobile articulators, 424
alveolar ridge, 424
hard palate, 424
teeth, 424
innervation of articulatory structures,
403–404
jaw muscles, 409–412, 409t
geniohyoid, 409
infrahyoid muscle, 412f
mandible as articulator, 411–412
masseter, 409, 410f
masticatory muscle sling, 411f
medial pterygoid, 409, 410f
suprahyoid muscle, 412f
temporalis, 409, 410f
temporomandibular joint, 411, 413f
lacrimal bones, 393f, 397
lips as articulator, 409
mandible, 394, 394f, 395f
angle of the mandible, 394
condylar process, 394
coronoid process, 394
corpus, 394, 394f
lateral pterygoid muscle, 394
mental foramen, 394
mental protuberance, 394
mental symphysis, 394
ramus, 394
temporomandibular joint (TMJ), 394
maxillae, 395, 395f
alveolar process, 395, 396f
cleft, 395
infraorbital foramen, 395
intermaxillary suture, 395
medial portion, 395, 396f

premaxilla, 395, 397f
transverse palatine suture, 395
measurement, 429–433
acoustic observations, 432–433
camera systems, 431
electromagnetic sensing, 431
electromyography (EMG), 429
electropalatography, 431
magnetic resonance imaging, 432, 432f
radiography, 429–431, 430ff
ultrasound imaging, 431, 432f
nasal bones, 393f, 395
neurocranium and viscerocranium, bones,
393–394, 393ff
external auditory meatus, 393f, 394
foramen magnum, 394, 394f
frons, 394
mastoid process, 393f, 394
maxilla, 393
occiput, 394
orbit bones, 393f
palatine, 393
temporal fossae, 394
vertex, 394
vomer, 393
zygomatic arch, 393f, 394
zygomatic bones, 393
nose and nasal cavities, 399–401, 400ff
choane, 400
meatuses, 400
nasolacrimal duct, 401
orifices, 400
paranasal sinuses, 400–401, 401f
palatine bones and inferior nasal conchae,
396, 397f
pharynx muscles, 414f, 415f, 422–424, 423t
articulation, 423–424
inferior pharyngeal constrictor, 422
oral cancer, 423
pharyngeal raphe, 422
stylopharyngeus muscle, 423
teeth, 401–403, 401f
buccal surface, 402, 402f
canines, 401
cementum, 401
dental anomalies, 403
enamel, 401
gingival line, 401
labial surface, 402, 402f
lingual surface, 402, 402f
molars, 401
occlusal surface, 402, 402f
occlusion, 403, 403f
overbite, 403
overjet, 403
premolars, 401
primary vs. permanent, 402f
tongue, 416–422
ankyloglossia, 418
apex, 416
articulation, role in, 421–422
cerebral palsy, 417
chondroglossus, 421
dorsum, 416
extrinsic muscles, 419f, 420–421, 421t
foramen cecum, 417
genioglossus, 421
hyoglossus, 421
inferior longitudinal muscle, 420
inferior surface, 418f
intrinsic muscles, 419–420, 419ff, 420t
median fibrous septum, 417
median sulcus, 417
muscular hydrostat, 418
palatoglossus, 421

structures, 416f
superior longitudinal muscle, 420
transverse muscles of tongue, 420
vertical muscles of tongue, 420
Waldeyer ring, 417, 417f
velopharyngeal muscles, 412–416
adenoids, 416, 416f
hypernasal, 416
musculus uvulae, 413, 414f
palatoglossus muscle, 413
palatopharyngeus tenses, 414
Passavant ridge, 415–416
pharyngeal constrictors, 414f
pharyngeal musculature, 415f
soft palate muscles, 413t, 414f
velum as articulator, 414–415
vocal tract development, 424–425
vomer, 393f, 397
zygomatic bone, 393f, 397
Aryepiglottic muscle, 368
Arytenoid cartilages, 126, 357, 357f
Associated cortex, 218–219
ideational apraxia, 218
ideomotor apraxia, 218
kinetic apraxia, 218
limb-kinetic apraxia, 218
Associational cortex, 195
Asthma, 339
Astrocytes, 144, 174
Ataxia, 218
ATP. See Adenosine triphosphate (ATP)
ATP structure, 42f
Audiometer, 449
Auditory brainstem response, (ABR), 468
Auditory cortex, 295
Auditory cortex and subcortical areas, 475–477,
476f
anterior auditory field (AAF), 475
belt, 485
gray matter, 477
gyri, 477
parabelt, 475
posterior auditory field (PAF), 475
primary auditory cortex, 475
transverse gyrus of Heschl, 475
white matter, 477
Auditory cortical regions, 369
Auditory nerve and cochlear nuclei, 293
Auditory neuropathy/dyssynchrony, 468
Auditory-perceptual analysis, 379–380
Auditory system, 287–295
basilar membrane, 290–291, 290f
central auditory pathway structures, 292, 292f
auditory cortex, 295
auditory nerve and cochlear nuclei, 293
cochlear implants, 294
inferior colliculus, 292, 294
medial geniculate body (MGB), 292, 295
superior olivary complex, (SOC), 292
superior olivary complex and sound
localization, 293, 294f
cochlea, 289–290
scala media, 289
scala tympani, 289
scala vestibuli, 289
hair cells, 291–292
cochlear nuclei, 292, 292f
inner hair cells (IHCs), 291
kinocilium, 291
outer hair cells (OHCs), 291
stereocilia, 291
tip links, 292
organ of Corti (OoC), 289
presbycusis, 287
Aural atresia, 448

Autocrine cell signaling, 49–50, 50f
Autonomic nervous system (ANS), 19, 140f, 167, 496
Autoreceptor, 180
Autosomal dominant, 88t
Autosomal recessive, 88t
AVCN. See Anterior ventral cochlear nucleus (AVCN)
Axial plane, 8
Axoaxonal synapse, 142f, 143
Axodendritic synapse, 143
Axon collaterals, 217
Axon hillock, 178
Axons, 112, 141, 173
Axon terminal, 173
Axosomatic synapse, 143

B

Babbling, 369
Balance system, 523–555
    benign paroxysmal positional vertigo, 529, 529f
    central vestibular nervous system, 545–547
        cerebellum, 547, 547f
        primary somatosensory cortex, 546
        thalamus, 545, 546f
        vestibulocerebellum, 546
        vestibulothalamocortical network, 545
    central vestibular nucleus complex, 537–538, 537f
        vestibulo-ocular reflex, 538
        vestibulospinal reflexes, 538, 538f
    cochlear hydrops and Ménière disease, 526, 526f
    head movement and responsiveness of SCCs and otolithic organs, 527
    lateral vestibulospinal tract, 543–544, 543f
        ankle strategy, 543, 544f
        base of support, 543
        center of gravity, 543
        hip strategy, 543, 544f
        stepping strategy, 543, 544f
        suspensory strategy, 543, 544f
        vestibulospinal reflexes, 543
    lesions of the cerebellum, 546
    medial vestibulospinal tract, 544–545
        vestibulocollic reflex, 544
    migraine-associated vertigo, 548
    peripheral vestibular anatomy, 524–530, 524f
        ampula, 528–529, 529f
        anterior SCC, 525
        common crus, 525
        cristae, 529
        cuticular plate, 528
        endolymph, 525
        hair cell orientation, 530
        hair cells, 528, 528f, 531f
        horizontal SCC, 525, 527ff
        kinocilium, 528
        macula, 529
        neuroepithelium of SCCs and otolithic organs, 527, 529f
        otoconia, 529
        otolithic membrane, 529
        otoliths, 530f
        perilymph, 525
        peripheral receptor apparatus, 525f
        posterior SCC, 525
        saccule otolithic organ, 525
        stereocilia, 528
        utricle otolithic organ, 525
        vertigo, 525
    peripheral vestibular physiology, 530, 532–534
        coplanar pairs, 533, 533f

directional polarization, 532f
endolymph displacement, 535f
hair cell excitation and inhibition, 534f
kinocilia and stereocilia orientation and resting position, 535f
otolithic aculae, 532f
semicircular canals (SCCs), 524, 525f
vestibular assessment, 548
vestibular evoked myogenic potentials, 546
vestibular neuritis, 533
vestibular schwannoma, 536, 536f
vestibulocochlear nerve, 534–537
    firing rate, 534f, 535f
    neural connections, 537f
vestibulo-ocular network, 538–542
    extraocular muscles, 539, 540f, 541t
    eye movement possibilities, 540f
    fovea, 539
    medial longitudinal fasciculus (MLF), 540
    nystagmus, 542
    retina, 539
    stimulation of vestibulo-ocular reflex, 541, 542f
vestibulospinal network, 542–543, 543f
Ballismus, 207
Baroreceptors, 332
Basal ganglia (BGs), 139, 150, 147f, 192, 195f, 369
Basal ganglia-thalamic-cortical system, 202–215, 203f
    caudate nucleus, 203
    centromedian, 204
    D1 receptors, 205
    D2 receptors, 205
    direct pathway, 204
    dopaminergic neurons, 204
    gamma-aminobutyric acid (GABA), 204
    glutamate, 204
    hyperreflexia, 203
    indirect pathway, 204
    large aspiny neurons, 204
    medium spiny neurons (MSNs), 205
    mereological fallacy, 203
    parafascicular nuclei, 204
    putamen, 203
    sagittal plane reconstructions, 204f
    spasticity, 203
    striatum, 203
    substantia nigra pars compacta (SNc), 204
    substantia nigra pars reticulata (SNr), 203
Base, brain, 14f
Basement membrane, 54
Basement membrane zone (BMZ), 361
Base of support, 543
Basilar artery, 154
Basilar membrane, 290–291, 290f, 454–455
Basilar membrane macromechanics, passive properties, 461–464, 462ff
    place theory, 462
    temporal theory, 462
    traveling wave shape (envelope), 463, 464f
    volley theory, 462–463
Beat interactions, 224
Behavioral control assembly, 504
Belt, 475
Benign paroxysmal positional vertigo, 23, 529, 529f
    vestibular structure, inner ear, 23f
Bernoulli effect, 372
Beta oscillation theory, 210–211
BGs. See Basal ganglia (BGs)
Bifurcations, 213
Bilateral symmetry, 107, 107f
Binocular visual zone, 282–283
Bioenergetics, 244–247, 246f

glycolysis, 245
immediate energy system, 245
lactate, 247, 247f
oxidative phosphorylation, 246, 247f
Biomechanics of phonation, 371–373
    Bernoulli effect, 372
    convergent glottis, 372, 372f
    divergent glottis, 372, 372f
    elastic recoil, 372
    flow separation vortices, 372
    inertive reactance, 373
    intraglottal pressure differentials, 372
    medial compression, 371
    myoelastic-aerodynamic theory of phonation, 373
    three-mass model, 371, 371f
    transglottal airflow, 371, 371ff
    vocal folds nodules, 372
Bipolar neuron, 143, 143f
Blastocyst, 106, 107f
Blastomeres, 106
Blind spot, 282
Blood-brain barrier, 144, 157, 158f
    endothelial cells, 157
Blood pH and homeostasis, 334–335
    alkalemia, 335
    pH buffer, 334
Blood pressure, homeostasis and, 332
    baroreceptors, 332
    renin, 332
    renin-angiotensin-aldosterone system (RAAS), 332
Blood supply system, 154–155, 155ff
    anterior cerebral artery (ACA), 154
    basilar artery, 154
    cerebral artery distribution, 154f
    cerebral veins, 155f
    circle of Willis, 154f, 155
    confluence of sinuses, 155
    deep cerebral veins, 155
    dysarthria, 154
    dyslexia, 154
    great cerebral vein, 155
    internal carotid arteries, 154
    middle cerebral artery (MCA), 154
    posterior cerebral artery (PCA), 154
    straight sinus, 155
    superficial cerebral veins, 155
    superior sagittal sinus, 155
    vertebral arteries, 154
    vertebrobasilar and internal carotid branches, 154f
BMZ. See Basement membrane zone (BMZ)
Body stalk, 108
Body temperature regulation, 337, 337f
Bolus, 24
Bone, 10, 62–63, 63t, 64f
Bone conduction, 449
Bones of respiration, 317
Bones relevant to hearing, 447–448, 447ff
    internal auditory canal, 448
    internal auditory meatus, 448
    mastoid, 447
    petrous, 447
    squamous, 447
    temporal bone, 447
    tympanic, 447
    tympanic antrum, 448
Bony vertebral column, 16f
Boyle's law, 319, 320f
Brachium conjunctivum, 217
Bradykinesia, 207
Bradykinesia movement, 218
Brain and spinal cord, 138–140, 139f, 139t
    basal ganglia, 139

brainstem, 138, 139
  cerebellum, 138, 139*t*
  cerebral cortex, 139
  cerebral hemispheres, 138
  diencephalon, 138
  forebrain, 139*t*
  hindbrain, 139*t*
  limbic system, 139
  midbrain, 139*t*
  pituitary gland, 139
Brain development, 113–115, 113*f*
  archipallium, 115
  Broca area, 115
  cephalic flexure, 113
  cerebellum, 114
  cerebral aqueduct, 114
  cervical flexure, 113
  choroid plexus, 113
  claustrum, 115
  corpus callosum, 115
  corpus striatum, 115
  diencephalon, 113
  epithalamus, 114
  fornix, 115
  gray matter, 114–115
  hippocampus, 115
  hypothalamus, 114
  inferior colliculi, 114
  insular cortex, 115
  lamina terminalis, 115
  lateral fissure, 115
  mesencephalon, 113
  metencephalon, 114
  pons, 114
  pontine flexure, 113
  prosencephalon, 113
  rhinencephalon, 115
  rhombencephalon, 113
  sensory fibers, 113
  solitary tract, 113
  substantia negra, 114
  superior colliculi, 114
  telencephalon, 113
  thalamus, 114
  Wernicke area, 115
  white matter, 115
Brain stem, 138, 139, 161–163, 162*f*, 163*f*, 192, 195, 504
  medulla, 161–163
    abducens nerve, 162
    accessory nerve, 162
    facial nerve, 162
    fasciculus cuneatus, 162
    fasciculus gracilis, 162
    glossopharyngeal nerve, 162
    hypoglossal nerve, 162
    olive, 162
    pyramids, 162
    reticular system, 163
    vagus nerve, 162
    vestibulochlear nerve, 162
  midbrain, 161
    cerebral peduncles, 161
    corticospinal tracts, 161
    oculomotor nerve, 161
    substantia nigra, 161
    superior colliculi, 161
    trochlear nerve, 161
  pons, 161
    trigeminal nerve, 161
Brain structure functions hypotheses, 205–206
  contraries, 206
  inverse problem, 206
  method of concomitant variations, 206
  negative symptoms, 206

positive symptoms, 206
postictal paralysis, 206
Todd paralysis, 206
transcranial magnetic stimulation (TMS), 206
Branchial arches development, 116–118, 116*ff*
  branchial cleft anomalies, 117
  pharyngeal arches, 116–118, 116*f*, 118*t*
Branchial cleft anomalies, 117
Broca area, 115, 369
Broca's aphasia, 148
Brodmann areas, 6, 145–146, 146*f*, 199, 280
Bronchi, 313, 316*f*
Bronchial arches, 354
Bronchioles, 316
Buccal surface, 402, 402*f*
Buccinator muscle, 405, 406*f*, 487*f*
Bucconasal membrane, 120
Buccopharyngeal membrane, 109
Bushy cells, 475

C

Calcarine sulcus, 149–150
Calyx of Held, 474
Camera systems, 431
Canines, 401
cAP. *See* Compound action potential (cAP)
Capillary basement membrane, 322
Capillary epithelium, 322
Capsule, 33
Carbon dioxide transport from tissues to lungs, 322–323, 323*f*
  homeostasis, 322
Cardiac muscle, 19, 60, 61*f*
Cardiovascular system, 21
Carhart notch, 452
Carotid body, 336
Carrier proteins, 46
Cartilage, 10, 63, 64*t*
Cartilaginous joint, 18
Cartilaginous vocal fold, 378
Cation, 173
Cauda equina, 166
Caudal, 7
Caudate nucleus, 151, 203
Cell biology tools, 34
  electron microscopy, 34
  light microscopy, 34
  microscopes, 34
  relative sizes, logarithmic scale, 34*f*
Cell body, 193
Cell division, 86–87
  meiosis, 87, 87*f*
  mitosis, 86, 86*f*
Cell junctions, 55, 55*f*
Cell membrane structure, 174*f*
Cells, 32
  cytoplasm, 32
  definition, 32
  multicellular, 32
  plasma membrane, 32
  unicellular, 32
Cell signaling, 49–50
  autocrine, 49–50, 50*f*
  endocrine, 50, 50*f*
  gap junction, 49, 49*f*
  juxtacrine, 49, 49*f*
  neurotransmitters, 50
  paracine, 49, 49*f*
  synapse, 50
  synaptic, 50, 51*f*
Cell structure, 34–42
  cytoplasm, 39–41
    actin, 41
    cytoskeleton, 39, 40*f*
    cytosol, 39

dystrophin and Duchenne muscular dystrophy (DMD), 40
  intermediate filaments, 41, 41*f*
  microfilaments, 40, 41*f*
  microtubules, 40, 41*f*
  tubulin, 40
endomembrane system, 38–39
  cisternae, 39
  endoplasmic reticulum (ER), 38, 38*f*
  Golgi apparatus, 39, 39*f*
  lysosomes, 39
  rough ER, 38
  smooth ER, 38
extracellular matrix, 41–42, 41*f*
  fibroblasts, 42
  glycosaminoglycan (GAG), 42
  integrins, 42
mitochondria, 37–38
  adenosine triphosphate (ATP), 37
  Alzheimer's disease, 37
  cellular respiration, 37
  structure of, 38*f*
nucleus, 37, 37*f*
  nuclear envelope, 37
  nucleolus, 37
organelles, 34, 35*f*
plasma membrane, 35–37, 36*f*
  amphipathic region, 36
  hydrophilic heads, 35
  hydrophobic tails, 35
  inner ear hair cells, 35*f*
  integral proteins, 36
  peripheral proteins, 36, 36*f*
  phospholipid bilayer, 35
Cell surface receptors, 50
Cellular communication, 48–53
  Parkinson's disease and cell signaling, 53, 53*f*
  receptors, 48, 50–53
    cell surface receptors, 50
    enzyme, 51
    enzyme-linked receptors, 51, 52*f*
    G-protein-coupled receptors (GPCRs), 52, 52*f*
    intracellular receptors, 50–51, 51*f*
    ligand, 50
    second messengers, 52
    signal transduction, 51
  types of cell signaling, 49–50
    autocrine, 49–50, 50*f*
    endocrine, 50, 50*f*
    gap junction, 49, 49*f*
    juxtacrine, 49, 49*f*
    neurotransmitters, 50
    paracine, 49, 49*f*
    synapse, 50
    synaptic, 50, 51*f*
Cellular respiration, 37, 42–44
  aerobic respiration, 43, 43*f*
    citric acid cycle, 43*f*
    electron transport chain, 43*f*
    glycolysis, 43–44, 43*f*
    pyruvate oxidation, 43*f*
  anaerobic respiration, 44
  ATP structure, 42*f*
  during exercise, 44
  oxidation, 42
Cellular transport, 44–48
  active transport, 46–48
    endocytosis, 47, 48*f*
    exocytosis, 47, 48*f*
    membrane potential, 46
    sodium-potassium pump, 46–47, 48*f*
  passive transport
    carrier proteins, 46
    channel proteins, 46

diffusion, 45, 45f
  facilitated diffusion, 45–46, 45f
  hypertonic, 46
  hypotonic environment, 46
  isotonic environment, 46
  osmosis, 46, 46f
  in vocal folds, 47
    apical membrane, 47, 47f
    vocal fold surface fluid (VFSF), 47
Cell wall, 33
Cementum, 128, 401
Center of gravity, 543
Central auditory pathway structures, 292, 292f
  auditory cortex, 295
  auditory nerve and cochlear nuclei, 293
  cochlear implants, 294
  inferior colliculus, 292, 294
  medial geniculate body (MGB), 292, 295
  superior olivary complex, (SOC), 292
  superior olivary complex and sound localiza-
    tion, 293, 294f
Central auditory system, 444
Central auditory system functional neuroanat-
    omy, 470–477, 471f
  auditory cortex and subcortical areas,
      475–477, 476f
    anterior auditory field (AAF), 475
    belt, 485
    gray matter, 477
    gyri, 477
    parabelt, 475
    posterior auditory field (PAF), 475
    primary auditory cortex, 475
    transverse gyrus of Heschl, 475
    white matter, 477
  cochlear nucleus, 472–473, 472f
    anterior ventral cochlear nucleus (AVCN),
        472
    cerebellum, 472
    dorsal cochlear nucleus (DCN), 472
    dorsal stria, 472
    giant cells, PVCN, 472
    globular bushy cells, AVCN, 472
    inferior colliculus (IC), 473
    intermediate stria, 472
    lateral lemniscus, 473
    medulla oblongata, 472
    multipolar cells, PVCN, 472
    octopus cells, PVCN, 472
    pons, 472
    posterior ventral cochlear nucleus (PVCN),
        472
    poststimulus time histograms (PSTHs), 472
    pyramidal cells, DCN, 472
    spherical cells, AVCN, 472
    trapezoid body, 472
    ventral stria, 472
  inferior colliculus, 474–475
    central nucleus inferior colliculus, 474
    combination-sensitive neurons, 475
    commissure of the inferior colliculus, 474
    disk-shaped cells, 474
    dorsal cortex, 474
    external (lateral) shell, 474
    isofrequency sheets, 474
    medial geniculate body (MGB), 474
    stellate cells, 474
  lateral lemniscus, 474
    dorsal nuclei lateral lemniscus (DNLL), 474
    intermediate nucleus lateral lemniscus
        (INLL), 474
    ventral nucleus lateral lemniscus (VNLL),
        474
  lateral superior olive, 473–474
    GABAergic projections, 474

glycinergic input, 473
medial geniculate body, 475
  acoustic radiations, 475
  bushy cells, 475
  elongated cells, 475
  external capsule, 475
  insula, 475
  internal capsule, 475
  intrathalamic interneurons, 475
  thalamocortical relay cells, 475
  tufted cells, 475
medial nucleus of trapezoid body, 474
  calyx of Held, 474
medial superior olivary nucleus, 473
  coincident detectors, 473
superior olivary complex, 473
  lateral superior olivary nucleus (LSO), 473
  medial nucleus, trapezoid body (MNTB),
      473
  medial superior olivary nucleus (MSO), 473
  periolivary group, 473
Central chemoreceptors, 336
Central nervous system (CNS), 20–21, 264
  cerebellum, 20
  cerebrum, 20
  cranial nerves, 22f
  frontal lobe, 20
  gray matter, 20, 21f
  gyri, 20
  inferior surface, 21f
  left lateral surface, 21f
  occipital lobe, 20
  parietal lobe, 20
  peripheral nervous system, 21
  sulci, 20
  temporal lobe, 20
  white matter, 20, 21f
Central nucleus inferior colliculus, 474
Central olfactory pathway, 300–301
Central pattern generator (CPG), 335, 485, 504,
    504f
Central somatosensory pathways, 278–281
  anterolateral system (ALS), 278–279
  dorsal-column medial lemniscal (DCML)
      system, 278
  somatosensory cortex, 280
  trigemial lemniscus and trigeminothalamic
      tract, 278, 279f
Central sulcus, 146
Central vestibular nervous system, 545–547
  cerebellum, 547, 547f
  primary somatosensory cortex, 546
  thalamus, 545, 546f
  vestibulocerebellum, 546
  vestibulothalamocortical network, 545
Central vestibular nucleus complex, 537–538,
    537f
  vestibulo-ocular reflex, 538
  vestibulospinal reflexes, 538, 538f
Central vestibular pathway, 297–298, 298f
  flocculonodular lobe, 297
  lateral vestibulospinal tract, 298
  medial vestibulospinal tract, 298
  reticular formation, 298
  ventral posterior (VP) nuclei, 297
  vestibular nuclei, 297
  vestibulospinal tracts, 298
Central visual pathway, 286–288, 286f
  lateral geniculate nucleus (LGN), 286
  optic radiations, 286
  optic tract, 286
  primary visual cortex, 286
  retinotopy, 286
  superior colliculus (SC), 286
Centromedian, 204

Cephalic flexure, 113
Cerebellar disorders, 218
  action tremor, 218
  ataxia, 218
  bradykinesia movement, 218
  dymetric movement, 218
  dysdiadochokinesia, 218
  hypermetria, 218
  hypometria, 218
  hypotonia, 218
  scanning speech, 218
Cerebellar mutism, 153
Cerebellar penduncles, 159, 159f
Cerebellopontine angle, 458
Cerebellum, 20, 114, 138, 139t, 158–161, 158f,
    192, 195, 215–217, 370, 472, 547, 547f
  archicerebellum, 216
  axon collaterals, 217
  brachium conjunctivum, 217
  cerebellar penduncles, 159, 159f
  climbing fibers, 160, 217
  complex spike, 217
  dentate nuclei, 160, 216
  emboliform nuclei, 216
  fastigial nucleus, 160, 216
  flocculonodular lobe, 158
  flocculus, 158
  globose nuclei, 216
  granule cells, 160, 217
  inferior olivary nucleus, 217
  interpositus nucleus, 160, 216
  lateral zone, 216
  mossy fibers, 160, 217
  neocerebellum, 216
  nodulus, 158
  paleocerebellum, 216
  parallel fibers, 217
  paravermal zone, 216
  peduncles, 216, 216f
  pontine relay nuclei, 217
  posterior fossa, 216
  posterolateral fissure, 158
  primary fissure, 158
  Purkinje cell, 217, 217f
  spinocerebellum, 217
  tracts and functions, 159f
  vermal zone, 216
  vermis, 158
Cerebral aqueduct, 114, 156
Cerebral artery distribution, 154f
Cerebral cortex, 139, 145–150, 145f
  angular gyrus, 149
  anterior commissure, 150
  aphasia, 147–149
  Broca's area, 147
  Brodmann areas, 145–146, 146f
  calcarine sulcus, 149–150
  central sulcus, 146
  cingulate gyrus, 146f, 147
  collateral sulcus, 150
  corpus callosum, 146, 146f
  cuneus gyrus, 150
  fissures, 145
  fornix, 150
  frontal lobe, 146
  functional localization, 146
  genu, 150
  gyri, 145
  gyrus rectus, 150
  Heschl's gyrus, 149
  lateral fissure, 146, 146f
  lateral ventricle, 150
  limbic lobe, 147
  lingual gyrus, 150
  longitudinal fissure, 146, 146f

mammillary bodies, 150
occipital lobe, 147
occipitotemporal gyrus, 150
olfactory bulbs, 150
olfactory sulci, 150
olfactory tracts, 150
optic chiasm, 150
parahippocampal gyrus, 150
parietal lobe, 146
postcentral gyrus, 149
precentral gyrus, 147
premotor cortex, 147
preoccipital notch, 146–147
primary auditory cortex, 149
primary motor cortex, 147, 147f
primary somatosensory cortex, 149, 149f
primary visual cortex, 149–150
rhinal sulcus, 150
septum pellucidum, 150
splenium, 150
sulci, 145
superior temporal gyrus (STG), 147
supramarginal gyrus, 149
temporal lobe, 146
uncus, 150
Wernicke's area, 149
Cerebral hemispheres, 138
Cerebral palsy, 417
Cerebral peduncles, 161
Cerebral veins, 155f
Cerebrospinal fluid (CSF), 155
Cerebrospinal fluid circulation, 157f
Cerebrovascular system, 154–158
blood-brain barrier, 157, 158f
endothelial cells, 157
blood supply system, 154–155, 155ff
anterior cerebral artery (ACA), 154
basilar artery, 154
cerebral artery distribution, 154f
cerebral veins, 155f
circle of Willis, 154f, 155
confluence of sinuses, 155
deep cerebral veins, 155
dysarthria, 154
dyslexia, 154
great cerebral vein, 155
internal carotid arteries, 154
middle cerebral artery (MCA), 154
posterior cerebral artery (PCA), 154
straight sinus, 155
superficial cerebral veins, 155
superior sagittal sinus, 155
vertebral arteries, 154
vertebrobasilar and internal carotid
branches, 154f
meninges, 155
arachnoid barrier, 155
arachnoid mater, 155
arachnoid trabeculae, 155
cerebrospinal fluid (CSF), 155
dura mater, 155
epidural hematoma, 155
pia mater, 155
subarachnoid space, 155
subdural hemorrhage, 155, 156f
ventricular system, 156–157
arachnoid granulations, 156–157
cerebral aqueduct, 156
cerebrospinal fluid circulation, 157f
choroid plexus, 156, 157f
fourth ventricle, 156
interventricular foramina, 156
Cerebrum, 20
Cerumen, 450
Cervical flexure, 113

Cervical spine, 16
CF. See Cystic fibrosis (CF)
cGMP. See Cyclic guanosine monophosphate
(cGMP)
Channelopathies, 178
episodic ataxia type 2, 178
myasthenia gravis, 178
Channel proteins, 46
Chemoreceptors, 267, 503
Chest register, 377
Cheyne-Stokes respiration, 341
Chiari malformation, 26f
Chiasmic groove, 399
Choanae, 120, 400
Choanal atresia, 120
Cholinergic/dopaminergic imbalance theory,
208
Chondroglossus, 421
Chorda tympani, 454
Chorda tympani branch, 165
Chorea, 207
Chorion, 107
Chorion frondosum, 108
Chorionic villi, 108, 108f
Choroid plexus, 113, 156, 157f
Chromosomal abnormalities, 90–91, 94–98, 90t
cleft lip and palate, 97
Down syndrome, 94, 94f
fragile X syndrome, 96
parent-of-origin effects, 95, 95f
speech and language disorders, 98, 98f
Chromosomes, 78, 78f, 104
Chronic cough, 370
Chronic obstructive pulmonary disease (COPD),
339, 340, 500, 500f
Cingulate gyrus, 146f, 147
Circle of Willis, 154f, 155
Circuit-based model, 212, 212f
Circulatory system filtration, 329, 331
fibrin, 331
fibrinolysin, 331
heparin, 331
thromboplastin, 331
Cisternae, 39
Citric acid cycle, 43f
Claudius cells, 456
Claustrum, 115
Cleavage, 106, 107ff
blastocyst, 106, 107f
blastomeres, 106
inner cell mass, 106
morula, 106
trophoblast, 106
Cleft, 395
Cleft lip/palate, 25f, 97, 122, 396, 486, 486f
Climbing fibers, 160, 217
Clinical swallowing evaluation, 513
Closed phase, 371, 371f
CNS. See Central nervous system (CNS)
CNV. See Copy number variation (CNV)
Coarticulation, 433
Cochlea, 289–290, 451
scala media, 289
scala tympani, 289
scala vestibuli, 289
Cochlea position in temporal bone, 454f
Cochlear amplifier, 466, 467f
Cochlear aqueduct, 455
Cochlear electrophysiology, 467–468
cochlear microphonic (CM), 467
compound action potential (cAP), 467
endocochlear potential (EP), 467
summating potential (SP), 467
Cochlear hydrops and Ménière disease, 526,
526f

Cochlear implants, 294
Cochlear nuclei
Cochlear nucleus, 292, 292f, 469, 472–473, 472f
anterior ventral cochlear nucleus (AVCN), 472
cerebellum, 472
dorsal cochlear nucleus (DCN), 472
dorsal stria, 472
giant cells, PVCN, 472
globular bushy cells, AVCN, 472
inferior colliculus (IC), 473
intermediate stria, 472
lateral lemniscus, 473
medulla oblongata, 472
multipolar cells, PVCN, 472
octopus cells, PVCN, 472
pons, 472
posterior ventral cochlear nucleus (PVCN),
472
poststimulus time histograms (PSTHs), 472
pyramidal cells, DCN, 472
spherical cells, AVCN, 472
trapezoid body, 472
ventral stria, 472
Cochlear partition, 455f, 461
Codones, 83
Coincident detectors, 473
Collateral sulcus, 150
Combination-sensitive neurons, 475
Commissure of the inferior colliculus, 474
Common crus, 525
Compact bone, 63
Complex acoustic sound waves, 373
Complex sounds, 445
Complex spike, 217
Complex systems and network of oscillators
approach, 222–227
beat interactions, 224
continuous harmonic oscillators, 224
discrete oscillators, 224
kinesia paradoxica, 227
multiple neuron-like processing units, 224,
225f
necker cube, 223, 223f
neuronal action potentials, 223, 223f
nonlinear interactions, 222
oscillator phase changes, 224
resonance effect, 225, 225f, 226f
self-organization into attractor states, 223
systems oscillator theory, 224, 225f
Compound action potential (cAP), 467
Concentration gradient, 173, 175f
Concentric length, 249
Conchae, 392, 450
Condensation, 444
Conduction aphasia, 148
Conductive hearing loss, 449
Condylar process, 394
Cone of light, 451
Cones, 281
Confluence of sinuses, 155
Connective tissue, 55–57, 57f
Continuous and saltatory propagation of action
potentials, 179
Continuous harmonic oscillators, 224
Contralateral, 8
Contraries, 206
Conus elasticus, 358, 359f
Conus medullaris, 165
Convergent glottis, 372, 372f
Coordinated articulation, 433–435
coarticulation, 433
Directions into Velocities of Articulation
(DIVA) model, 434, 435f
economy of effort, 433, 433f
motor equivalence, 434

COPD. *See* Chronic obstructive pulmonary disease (COPD)
Coplanar pairs, 533, 533*f*
Copula, 124
Copy number variation (CNV), 90
Corniculate cartilages, 126, 357
Coronal plane, 8
Coronal section, 360, 361*f*
Coronoid process, 394
Corpus, 394, 394*f*
Corpus callosum, 115, 146, 146*f*
Corpus striatum, 115
Cortical innervation of facial nerve nuclei, 200
Corticospinal tracts, 161, 199*f*
Cortilymph, 456
Costal surface, 314
CPG. *See* Central pattern generator (CPG)
Cranial bones, 10, 13*f*
Cranial nerves, 22*f*, 145, 163–165, 163*f*, 164*tt*
   accessory nerve, 165
   chorda tympani branch, 165
   hypoglossal nerve, 165
   mandibular branch, 164
   maxillary branch, 164
   olfactory nerve, 163
   opthalmic branch, 164
   optic nerve, 163
   vagus nerve, 165
Cranial sutures, 15*f*
Cricoarytenoid ligament, 358
Cricoid cartilage, 356
Cricothyroid (CT) muscle, 366, 367*f*
Cricothyroid joints, 356, 356*t*
Cricothyroid ligament, 359, 359*f*
Cricotracheal membrane, 356
Crista galli, 399
Cross-bridge theory, 243, 243*f*
Cross links, 458
CSF. *See* Cerebrospinal fluid (CSF)
CT muscle. *See* Cricothyroid (CT) muscle
Cuneate fasciculi, 278
Cuneiform cartilages, 126, 357
Cuneus gyres, 150
Cupula, 297
Cutaneous mechanoreceptors, 273*f*, 274*t*
Cuticular plate, 458, 528
Cyclic guanosine monophosphate (cGMP), 285
Cystic fibrosis (CF), 324, 339
Cytokines, 329
Cytoplasm, 32, 39–41
   actin, 41
   cytoskeleton, 39, 40*f*
   cytosol, 39
   dystrophin and Duchenne muscular dystrophy (DMD), 40
   intermediate filaments, 41, 41*f*
   microfilaments, 40, 41*f*
   microtubules, 40, 41*f*
   tubulin, 40
Cytoskeleton, 39, 40*f*
Cytosol, 39
Cytotrophoblast, 108

D

Dampening, 445
dB. *See* Decibels (dB)
DBS. *See* Deep brain stimulation (DBS)
DCML pathway. *See* Dorsal-column medial lemniscal (DCML) pathway
DCML system. *See* Dorsal-column medial lemniscal (DCML) system
DCN. *See* Dorsal cochlear nucleus (DCN)
Deafness, genetics of, 76
   nonsyndromic hearing loss, 76
   syndromic hearing loss, 76

Decerebrate posturing, 221
Decibels (dB), 446
Decomposition of movement, 197
Decorticate posturing, 221
Deep brain stimulation (DBS), 185, 194, 196, 227
Deep cerebral veins, 155
Deep lamina propria (DLP), 361
Degrees of freedom, 221
Deiters cell, 456
Delayed onset muscle soreness (DOMS), 253
Dendrites, 58, 141, 173, 193
Dendritic spines, 143
Dental anomalies, 403
Dental lamina, 127
Dental papilla, 127
Dentate nucleus, 160, 216
Dentin, 128
Deoxyribonucleic acid (DNA), 74, 81–82, 81*f*
Depolarization, 176, 466
Depressor anguli oris, 407, 407*f*
Depressor labii inferioris, 406*f*, 407
Dermatomes, 111, 166, 277, 277*f*
Desmosomes, 55
Detraining adaptations, 256
Detraining effect, 330
Diaphragm, 23, 314, 317, 317*f*
Diencephalon, 113, 138, 152–153, 152*f*
Diffusion, 45, 45*f*, 175
Digastric fossa, 363
Digastric muscle, 364, 364*f*
Digestive system, 24
   bolus, 24
Diploid, 105
Directional polarization, 532*f*
Directions into Velocities of Articulation (DIVA) model, 434, 435*f*
Direct laryngoscopy, 382
Direct pathway, 204, 208
Discrete oscillators, 224
Disease, disorders, and injuries, effect on neurophysiology, 184–185, 185*t*
   Alzheimer disease, 184*t*
   amyotrophic lateral sclerosis, 184*t*
   epilepsy, 184*t*
   multiple sclerosis, 184*t*
   Parkinson's disease, 184*t*
   sensorineural hearing loss, 184*t*
   stroke, 184*t*
   traumatic brain injury, 184*t*
Disk-shaped cells, 474
Disordered speech, language, or swallowing effects, 342–343
Disorders, basal ganglia-thalamic cortical system, 207
   akinesia, 207
   ballismus, 207
   bradykinesia, 207
   chorea, 207
   dystonia, 207
   hastening, 207
   hemiballismus, 207
   Huntington disease, 207
   hyperkinetic disorders, 207
   hypokinetic disorders, 207
   kinesia paradoxica, 207
   levodopa, 207
   masklike facies, 207
   monotone speech, 207
   postural instability, 207
   resting tremor, 207
   rigidity, 207
Distal, 7
DIVA model. *See* Directions into Velocities of Articulation (DIVA) model
Divergent glottis, 372, 372*f*

DLP. *See* Deep lamina propria (DLP)
DMD. *See* Dystrophin and Duchenne muscular dystrophy (DMD)
DNA. *See* Deoxyribonucleic acid (DNA)
DOMS. *See* Delayed onset muscle soreness (DOMS)
D1 receptors, 205
Dopaminergic, 181
Dopaminergic neurons, 204
Dorsal, 7
Dorsal cochlear nucleus (DCN), 472
Dorsal column, 166
Dorsal-column medial lemniscal (DCML) pathway, 272
Dorsal-column medial lemniscal (DCML) system, 278, 278*t*
   cuneate fasciculi, 278
   gracile fasciculi, 278
   postcentral gyrus, 278
   thalamocortical fibers, 278
   ventral posteroateral (VPL) nucleus, 278
Dorsal cortex, 474
Dorsal nuclei lateral lemniscus (DNLL), 474
Dorsal respiratory groups, 335
Dorsal rhizotomy, 221
Dorsal root ganglia, 221
Dorsal stream, 287–288
Dorsal stria, 472
Dorsum, 416
Down syndrome, 94, 94*f*
Drugs, effect on neurophysiology, 180–184
   affinity, 183
   agonists, 183
   antagonists, 183
   efficacy, 183
   neuropharmacology, 183
D2 receptors, 205
Duplex theory, 446
Dura mater, 155
Dymetric movement, 218
Dynamic circuits, 213–214, 214*f*
Dysarthria, 154
Dysdiadochokinesia, 218
Dyslexia, 154
Dysosmias, 303
Dyspnea, 339
Dystonia, 207
Dystrophin and Duchenne muscular dystrophy (DMD), 40
Dystussia, 327

E

Early embryonic development, 105–111
   cleavage, 106, 107*ff*
      blastocyst, 106, 107*f*
      blastomeres, 106
      inner cell mass, 106
      morula, 106
      trophoblast, 106
   fertilization, 106, 106*f*
      diploid, 105
      gametes, 105
      gametogenesis, 105–106
      haploid, 105
      meiosis, 105
      oogenesis, 105, 105*f*
      ovum, 105
      polar body, 106
      sexual reproduction, 105
      sperm, 105
      spermatogenesis, 105, 105*f*
      X chromosome, 106
      Y chromosome, 106
      zona pellucida, 106
      zygote, 105

intraembryonic mesoderm division, 111
maternal/fetal communication establishment,
107–108, 108*f*
body stalk, 108
chorion frondosum, 108
chorionic villi, 108, 108*f*
cytotrophoblast, 108
extraembryonic mesoderm, 108, 108*f*
syncytiotrophoblast, 108
trophoblastic villi, 108
neural tube development, 109, 109*f*, 110*f*
neural fold, 109
neural grooves, 110
neural plate, 109
primitive streak and notochord, 108–109, 108*f*
buccopharyngeal membrane, 109
intraembryonic mesoderm, 108
prechordal plate, 109
somites formation, 109–111, 110*f*
dermatomes, 111
myotomes, 110
sclerotomes, 109
Eccentric length, 249
ECohG. *See* Electrocochleography (ECohG)
Economy of effort, 433, 433*f*
Efferent, 484
Efferent motor control for swallowing, 505–510
facial nerve, 508*t*
facial nerve branches, 506*f*
glossopharyngeal nerve, 506*f*, 509*t*
hypoglossal nerve, 507*f*, 510*t*
respiratory spinal nerves, 510*t*
trigeminal nerve, 508*t*
vagus nerve, 509*t*
Efferent nerves, 140*f*, 141
Efficacy, 183
Elastic recoil, 372
Electrocochleography (ECohG), 468
Electromagnetic sensing, 431
Electromotility, 466
Electromyography (EMG), 236, 429, 515
Electron microscopy, 34
Electron transport chain, 43*f*
Electropalatography, 431
Elongated cells, 475
Emboliform nuclei, 216
Embryology and development of speech and
hearing mechanism, 103–134
branchial arches development, 116–118, 116*ff*
branchial cleft anomalies, 117
pharyngeal arches, 116–118, 116*f*, 118*t*
early embryonic development, 105–111
cleavage, 106, 107*ff*
fertilization, 106, 106*f*
gametogenesis, 105–106
intraembryonic mesoderm division, 111
maternal/fetal communication establishment, 107–108, 108*f*
neural tube development, 109, 109*f*, 110*f*
primitive streak and notochord, 108–109,
108*f*
somites formation, 109–111, 110*f*
yolk sac development, 107
facial development, 118–120, 119*f*
choanal atresia, 120
frontonasal prominence, 119
globular process, 120
lateral nasal processes, 120
mandibular prominences, 120
maxillary prominences, 120
medial nasal processes, 120
nasal laminae, 120
nasal pits, 119*f*, 120
nasal placodes, 120
nasal septum, 120

larynx development, 126–127, 126*f*
arytenoid cartilages, 126
corniculate cartilages, 126
cuneiform cartilages, 126
laryngeal muscles, 126–127
T-shaped cleft, 126
lip and palate development, 120–124
bucconasal membrane, 120
choanae, 120
cleft palate, 122
facial and orofacial clefts, 121–122, 121*f*
lingual and labial ties, 124
palatal shelves, 120, 122–123, 123*f*
philtrum, 120
primary palate, 119*f*, 120
secondary palate, 120, 123*f*
tectal ridge, 123
mitosis and cell division, 104–105, 104*f*
anaphase, 105
chromosomes, 104
interphase, 104–105
metaphase, 105
prophase, 105
telophase, 105
nervous system development, 111–115
brain development, 113–115, 113*f*
neural folds fusion, 111–112
neural tube differentiation, 112
neural tube zones, 112
primitive medullary cells differentiation, 112
spinal cord development, 112–113
outer ear development, 128–130
auditory vesicle, 129
aural astresia, 128
auricle, 128
auricular fold, 129
auricular hillocks, 128, 129*f*
cristae ampullaris, 130
cupula, 130
endolymphatic sac, 129
kinocilia, 130
macula, 130
membranous labyrinth, 129, 130*f*
otic placodes, 129
otoconia, 130
saccule, 129
spiral limbus, 130
spiral organ, 130
utricle, 129
respiratory system development, 125–126
lung buds, 125
median laryngotracheal groove, 125
tracheobronchial tree, 125*f*
teeth development, 127–128, 127*f*
cementum, 128
dental lamina, 127
dental papilla, 127
dentin, 128
enamel organ, 128
tooth buds, 127
tooth germ, 128
tongue development, 124–125, 124*f*
anterior lingual primordia, 124
copula, 124
foramen cecum, 124
lateral lingual swellings, 124
root primordia, 124
sulcus terminalis, 124
tubercular impar, 124
Embryonic stem cells, 61
EMG. *See* Electromyography (EMG)
EMST. *See* Expiratory muscle strength training,
(EMST)
Enamel, 401
Enamel organ, 128

Endocochlear potential (EP), 182, 182*f*, 467
Endocrine cell signaling, 50, 50*f*
Endocytosis, 47, 48*f*
Endoderm, 107
Endolymph, 455, 525
Endolymphatic duct, 455
Endolymphatic sac, 455
Endolymph displacement, 535*f*
Endomembrane system, 38–39
cisternae, 39
endoplasmic reticulum (ER), 38, 38*f*
Golgi apparatus, 39, 39*f*
lysosomes, 39
rough ER, 38
smooth ER, 38
Endoplasmic reticulum (ER), 38, 38*f*
Endoscopic analysis, 382–384, 383*f*
direct laryngoscopy, 382
indirect laryngoscopy, 382, 383*f*
laryngeal videostroboscopy, 383, 383*f*
laryngoscopy, 382
microlaryngoscopy, 382
Endothelial cells, 157
Enzyme, 51
Enzyme-linked receptors, 51, 52*f*
EP. *See* Endocochlear potential (EP)
Ependymal cells, 174
Epiblast, 107
Epidural hematoma, 155
Epigenetics, 91, 98
Epiglottis, 357–358, 357*f*
Epilepsy, 184*t*
Episodic ataxia type 2, 178
Epithalamus, 114
Epithelial basement membrane, 322
Epithelial cells, 8
Epithelial tissue, 54–55, 54*tt*, 55*f*
adherens junctions, 55
basement membrane, 54
cell junctions, 55, 55*f*
desmosomes, 55
goblet cells, 55, 56*f*
hemidesmosomes, 55
smoking, effect on, 56
Epitympanic recess, 451
Epley maneuver, 531, 531*f*
ER. *See* Endoplasmic reticulum (ER)
ERV. *See* Expiratory reserve volume (ERV)
Erythropoietin, 333
Esophageal peristalsis, 60, 60*f*
Esophageal phase of swallowing, 498
oral phase of swallowing, 497
oral-preparatory phase of swallowing,
495–497
pharyngeal phase of swallowing, 497–498
Esophagus and trachea, 496*f*
Estimated mean flow rate, 380–381
Ethical, legal, and social issues of genetics, 75
Ethmoidal air cells, 312
Ethmoid bone, 399, 399*f*
Eustachian tube, 11, 451
Exercise adaptations, 255–256
Exercise and respiration, 44
Excitation-contraction coupling, 238–240
acetylcholine (ACh), 239
action potential (AP), 238
exocytosis, 239
motor end plates, 237*f*, 238
myelin sheath, 238
myofibrils, 239
network of channels in muscle cell, 239
neuromuscular junction, 240, 240*f*
postsynaptic acetylcholine receptors (AChRs),
239
presynaptic membrane, 239

sarcolemma, 239
   sarcoplasmic reticulum (SR), 239
   synaptic cleft, 238
   transverse tubules (T-tubules), 239
Exocytosis, 47, 48f, 239
Exons, 78
Expiration, 23
Expiratory muscle strength training, (EMST),
     329, 330
Expiratory reserve volume (ERV), 321
Extensor muscle, 168
External auditory canal, 449, 450f
External auditory meatus, 393f, 394
External capsule, 475
External intercostal muscles, 317, 318f
External (lateral) shell, 474
External muscles, 23
Exteroception, 272
Exteroceptors, 336
Extracellular matrix, 41–42, 41f
   fibroblasts, 42
   glycosaminoglycan (GAG), 42
   integrins, 42
Extraembryonic mesoderm, 108, 108f
Extraocular muscles, 539, 540f, 541t
Extrinsic muscles, tongue, 419f, 420–421, 421t,
     491
Eye movement possibilities, 540f

F

Facial and orofacial clefts, 121–122, 121f
Facial bones, 13f
Facial development, 118–120, 119f
   choanal atresia, 120
   frontonasal prominence, 119
   globular process, 120
   lateral nasal processes, 120
   mandibular prominences, 120
   maxillary prominences, 120
   medial nasal processes, 120
   nasal laminae, 120
   nasal pits, 119f, 120
   nasal placodes, 120
   nasal septum, 120
Facial muscles, 404–409, 404f, 405f, 406t
   buccinator, 405, 406f
   depressor anguli oris, 407, 407f
   depressor labii inferioris, 406f, 407
   frontalis muscle, 407, 408f
   incisivus labii inferioris muscle, 407
   incisivus labii superioris, 405
   levator anguli oris, 407, 407f
   levator labii superioris, 405, 406f
   levator labii superioris aleque nasi, 404f, 405,
     407
   masseter muscle, 405
   mentalis muscle, 407, 408f
   orbicularis oculi, 407, 408f
   orbicularis oris, 404, 404f
   platysma muscle, 405, 405f, 407
   risorius, 404–405, 405f
   zygomaticus major, 407, 407f
   zygomaticus minor, 407, 407f
Facial nerve branches, 506f
Facial nerves, 162, 368, 508–510t
Facilitated diffusion, 45–46, 45f
Failure to thrive, 510
Falsetto register, 375, 377
Fascia, 68
Fasciculus cuneatus, 162
Fasciculus gracilis, 162
Fastigial nucleus, 160, 216
Fatigue, 251–252
FEES. See Flexible endoscopic evaluation of
    swallowing (FEES)

Fertilization, 106, 106f
   zona pellucida, 106
Fibrin, 331
Fibrinolysin, 331
Fibroblasts, 42
Fibrosis, 492
Fibrous joints, 18
Fight or flight response, 141
Firing rate, 534f, 535f
Fissures, 145
Flagellum, 33
Flexible endoscopic evaluation of swallowing
    (FEES), 514–515
Flexor muscle, 168
Flocculonodular lobe, 158, 297
Flocculus, 158
Flow separation vortices, 372
Fontanelles, 14, 15f
Foramen cecum, 124, 417
Foramen magnum, 10, 394, 394f
Foramen ovale, 399
Foramen rotundum, 399
Foramina, 399
Force, 444
Forced vibration, 445
Forebrain, 139t
Fornix, 115, 150
Fourth ventricle, 156
Fovea, 281, 539
Foveola, 282
Fragile X syndrome, 96
Free arm movements, 201, 201f
Free field, 446
Free vibration, 445
Frequency, sound, 445
Frequency of muscle stimulation, 249
Frequency perturbation, 382
Friction, 445
Frons, 394
Frontalis muscle, 407, 408f
Frontal lobe, 20, 146
Frontal plane, 8
Frontal sinuses, 312
Frontonasal prominence, 119
Functional localization, 146
Fundamental frequency, 328, 373, 374–375,
    374f, 445
   falsetto register, 375
   hertz, 374
   pitch, 374
Fundamental logical operators, 172
Fusiform shape, 236, 236f

G

GABA. See Gamma-aminobutyric acid (GABA)
Gabaergic projections, 474
GAG. See Glycosaminoglycan (GAG)
Gametes, 105
Gametogenesis, 105–106
   diploid, 105
   gametes, 105
   haploid, 105
   meiosis, 105
   oogenesis, 105, 105f
   ovum, 105
   polar body, 106
   sexual reproduction, 105
   sperm, 105
   spermatogenesis, 105, 105f
   X chromosome, 106
   Y chromosome, 106
   zygote, 105
Gamma-aminobutyric acid (GABA), 204
Gamma lower motor neuron (γ-LMNs), 193
Gap junction cell signaling, 49, 49f

Gap junctions, 173
Gas exchange in tissue, 322
   capillary basement membrane, 322
   capillary epithelium, 322
   epithelial basement membrane, 322
   internal respiration, 322
   peripheral gas exchange, 322
Gastrulation, 107
Genes, 77
   chromosomes, 78, 78f
   exons, 78
   genome, 777
   nucleic acids, 78
   ribonucleic acid (RNA), 77–78
   transcription, 78, 79f
Genetic code, 85f
Genetic counseling, 74
Genetics, 73–102
   cell division, 86–88
     meiosis, 87, 87f, 88f
     mitosis, 86, 86f
   chromosomal abnormalities, 90–91, 94–98,
     90t
     cleft lip and palate, 97
     Down syndrome, 94, 94f
     fragile X syndrome, 96
     parent-of-origin effects, 95, 95f
     speech and language disorders, 98, 98f
   codones, 83
   copy number variation (CNV), 90
   deafness, genetics of, 76
     nonsyndromic hearing loss, 76
     syndromic hearing loss, 76
   deoxyribonucleic acid (DNA), 74, 81–82, 81f
   epigenetics, 91, 98
   ethical, legal, and social issues, 75
   genes, 77
     chromosomes, 78, 78f
     exons, 78
     genome, 777
     nucleic acids, 78
     ribonucleic acid (RNA), 77–78
     transcription, 78, 79f
   genetic counseling, 74
   KE family, 75
   Mendelian traits, 87–89
     autosomal dominant, 88t
     autosomal recessive, 88t
     mitochondrial, 88t
     X-linked dominant, 88t
     X-linked recessive, 88t
     Y-linked, 88t
   mitochondrial inheritance, 89
   multifactorial inheritance, 91, 92t
   nucleic acids, 79, 80f
     nucleotides, 79
   penetrance and expressivity, 89
     genotype, 89
     phenotype, 89
     variable expressivity, 89
   polymorphisms, 79–81, 81f
     alleles, 80
     genotypes, 80
     locus, 79
     markers, 81
   protein degradation, 85
   proteins, 82
     proteome, 82
     translation of mRNA, 81f, 82
   protein synthesis regulation, 84–85
     genetic code, 85f
     homeostasis, 84
     nucleotide base pairs, 85f
     ribosomal RNA (rRNA), 84
   recombination, 90, 91f

ribonucleic acid (RNA), 77–78, 81–82
  messenger RNA (mRNA), 82
  transcription, 82, 82f
ribosome, 83
technologies and diagnostic testing used in
  speech, language, swallowing, hearing,
  and balance disorders, 77, 77f
technologies for analysis of gene expression,
  84, 84f
traits, 74
transfer RNA (tRNA), 84
transcription, 82, 82f, 83, 83ff
translation of mRNA, 81f, 82, 83, 83ff
Genioglossus, 421
Geniohyoid muscle, 363, 363f
Genome, 79
Genotype, 80, 89
Genu, 150
Giant cells, PVCN, 472
Gingival line, 401
Glaucoma, 283
Glial cells, 58, 58f, 144, 172, 174, 172f, 175f
  astrocytes, 144, 174
  blood-brain barrier, 144
  ependymal cells, 174
  microglia, 144, 174
  oligodendrocytes, 144, 174
  Schwann cells, 144, 144f
Glioblasts, 112
Global aphasia, 148–149
Globose nuclei, 216
Globular bushy cells, AVCN, 472
Globular process, 120
Globus pallidus, 151
Globus pallidus internal segment (GPi) rate
  theory, 209–210, 210f
Glossopharyngeal nerve, 162, 506f, 509t
Glutamate, 204, 285, 466
Glycinergic input, 473
Glycolysis, 43–44, 43f, 245
Glycosaminoglycan (GAG), 42
Goblet cells, 55, 56f
Golgi apparatus, 39, 39f
Golgi tendon organ (GTO), 248–249
GPCRs. *See* G-protein-coupled receptors (GPCRs)
GPi rate theory. *See* Globus pallidus internal
  segment (GPi) rate theory
G-protein-coupled receptors (GPCRs), 52, 52f
Gracile fasciculi, 278
Graded potentials, 177, 178t
Granule cells, 160, 217
Gray matter, 20, 21f, 114–115, 144, 145f, 166,
  166f, 473
  dermatome, 166
  lower motor neurons, 166
Great cerebral vein, 155
Greater cornu, 358
Ground substance, 361
GTO. *See* Golgi tendon organ (GTO)
Gustatory system, 301
  dysosmias, 303
  gustatory pathways, 302f
  gustatory receptors and transduction,
  301–303, 302f
  nucleus of solitary tract (NST), 303
  parabrachial nuclei (PBN), 303
  phantosmias, 303
  taste buds, 301
  xerostomia, 302
Gyri, 20, 145, 199, 477
Gyrus rectus, 150

H

Habenula perforta, 454
Hair cell excitation and inhibition, 534f

Hair cell micromechanics active transduction,
  464–467, 465f, 466f, 467f
  actin-filled stereocilia, 464
  AMPA-type receptors, 466
  cochlear amplifier, 466, 467f
  depolarization, 466
  electromotility, 466
  glutamate, 466
  hyperpolarized state, 465
  prestin, 466
  saltatory conduction, 466
  somatic motor, 466
  voltage-gated calcium channels, 466
Hair cell orientation, 530
Hair cells, 291–292, 528, 528f, 531f
  cochlear nuclei, 292, 292f
  inner hair cells (IHCs), 291
  kinocilium, 291
  outer hair cells (OHCs), 291
  stereocilia, 291
  tip links, 292
Hair follicles, 274
Haploid, 105
Hard palate, 424
Harmonic frequencies, 373, 376
  idealized spectrum of sound, 373f
  normal and dysphonic sound, 374f
Hastening, 207
Head and neck cancers, 492, 492f
  fibrosis, 492
  odynophagia, 492
  xerostomia, 492
Head movement and responsiveness of SCCs and
  otolithic organs, 527
Head register, 377
Head-related transfer function (HRTF), 459, 459f
Head shadow, 447
Hearing, 443–482
  bones relevant to hearing, 447–448, 447ff
    internal auditory canal, 448
    internal auditory meatus, 448
    mastoid, 447
    petrous, 447
    squamous, 447
    temporal bone, 447
    tympanic, 447
    tympanic antrum, 448
  inner and outer hair cell innervation,
  458–459, 458f
    cerebellopontine angle, 458
    impedance matching, 459
    spiral ganglion neuron, 458
    superior olivary complex (SOC), 458
  inner ear bony cochlea labrinths, 454
    cochlea position in temporal bone, 454f
    habenula perforta, 454
    modiolus, 454
    osseous spiral lamina, 454
    Rosenthal canal, 454
  inner ear cochlear biophysiology, 460–461,
  460f
    olivocochlear pathway, 461
  inner ear cochlear duct and organ of Corti,
  455, 455ff
    Claudius cells, 456
    Hensen cells, 456
    limbus, 455
    otoacoustic emissions (OEAs), 456
    spiral ligament, 455f, 456
    stria vascularis, 456
    tectoral membrane, 455
  inner ear membranous cochlea labyrinth,
  454–455
    basilar membrane, 454–455
    cochlear aqueduct, 455

    endolymph, 455
    endolymphatic duct, 455
    endolymphatic sac, 455
    helicotrema, 455
    perilymph, 455
    Reisner membrane, 454
    scalia media, 454
    scala tympani, 454, 455f
    scala vestibuli, 454
    vestibular aqueduct, 455
  inner ear sensory and supporting cells of
  organ of Corti, 456–458, 457ff
    cortilymph, 456
    cross links, 458
    cuticular plate, 458
    Deiters cell, 456
    inner hair cells (IHCs), 456
    mechanical transduction channels, 458
    outer hair cells (OHCs), 456
    phalangeal cells, 456
    pillar cells, 456
    reticular lamina, 458
    ribbon synapse, 457
    space of Nuel, 456
    stereocilia, 457
    tip links, 458
    tonotopic organization, 456
    tunnel of Corti, 456
  measurement, 449
    air conduction, 449
    audiometer, 449
    bone conduction, 449
    conductive hearing loss, 449
    hearing threshold, 449
    mixed hearing loss, 450
    sensorineural hearing loss, 449
  middle ear muscles and nerves, 454
    acoustic reflex, 454
    chorda tympani, 454
    stapedius nerve, 454
    tensor tympani muscle, 454
  middle ear ossicular chain, 453, 453f
    annular ligament, 453
    incudomallear joint, 453
    incudostapedial joint, 453
    incus, 453
    stapes, 453
  middle ear pathology, 452
    Carhart notch, 452
    ossicular chain disarticulation, 452
    otitis media, 452
    otosclerosis, 452
  middle ear tympanic cavity, 451–453, 453f
    cochlea, 451
    epitympanic recess, 451
    eustachian tube, 451
    levator veli palatini, 451
    promontory, 451
    pyramidal eminence, 452
    stapedius muscle, 452
    tensor veli palatine, 451
  outer ear, 448–451
    antihelix, 450
    aural atresia, 448
    cerumen, 450
    concha, 450
    cone of light, 451
    external auditory canal, 449, 450f
    helix, 450
    malleus, 451
    manubrium, 451
    microtia, 448, 448f
    ossicular chain, 451
    otoscopy, 451
    oval window, 451

pars flaccida, 451
pars tensa, 451
pinna, 449, 450f
round window, 451
stenosis, 448
tragus, 450
tympanic membrane, 451f
umbo, 451
sound, 444–447, 444f
aperiodic sound waves, 445
central auditory system, 444
complex sounds, 445
condensation, 444
cycle, 445
dampening, 445
decibels (dB), 446
duplex theory, 446
force, 444
forced vibration, 445
free field, 446
free vibration, 445
frequency, 445
friction, 445
fundamental frequency, 445
head shadow, 447
hertz (Hz), 445
impedances, 446
inertia, 444
intensity, 445
interaural level differences (ILDs), 446
interaural timing differences, 446, 447f
inverse square law, 446
loudness, 445
oscillation, 445
pascals (Pa), 445
periodic sound waves, 445
peripheral auditory system, 444
pinna, 447
pitch, 445
rarefaction, 444
resonant frequency, 445
restoring force, 445
reverberation, 446
simple harmonic motion, 445
simple sounds, 445
sine wave, 445
sinusoid, 445
specific acoustic impedance (Z), 446
waveform, 445
wavelength, 445
Hearing threshold, 449
Heinneman size principle,11951
Helicotrema, 455
Helix, 450
Hemiballismus, 207
Hemidesmosomes, 55
Hemifield, 282
Hensen cells, 456
Heparin, 331
Hering-Breuer inflation reflex, 338
Hertz (Hz), 374, 445
Heschl's gyrus, 149
Hierarchical information-processing structure, 270
Higher-order sensory areas, 270
Hilum, 314
Hindbrain, 139t
Hippocampus, 115
Hip strategy, 543, 544f
Homeostasis, 84, 175, 322
blood pH and homeostasis, 334–335
alkalemia, 335
pH buffer, 334
blood pressure, homeostasis and, 332
baroreceptors, 332

renin, 332
renin-angiotensin-aldosterone system (RAAS), 332
blood reserves and homeostasis, 332–333
oxygen reserves and homeostasis, 333–334
erythropoietin, 333
hypoxia, 333
Homeostatic emotion, 325
Homunculus, 200, 200f, 280
Horizontal cells, 281
Horizontal plane, 8
Horizontal SCC, 525, 527ff
HRFT. See Head-related transfer function (HRTF)
Huntington's disease, 151, 207
Hyaline cartilage, 357
Hydrophilic heads, 35
Hydrophobic tails, 35
Hydrostasis, 315
Hydrostatic force, 315
Hyoglossus, 363, 421
Hyoid bone, 355, 355f, 356f
Hyolaryngeal excursion, 364
Hypercapnic hypoxia, 337
Hyperdirect pathway, 208
Hyperkinetic disorders, 207
Hypermetria, 218
Hypernasal, 416
Hyperpolarization, 176
Hyperpolarized state, 465
Hyperreflexia, 203
Hypertonic, 46
Hypertrophy, 330
Hyperventilation, 341
Hypoblast, 107, 108f
Hypoepiglottic ligament, 359, 359f
Hypoglossal nerve, 162, 165, 368, 507f, 510t
Hypokinetic disorders, 207
Hypometria, 218
Hypothalamus, 114, 152
Hypotonia, 218
Hypotonic environment, 46
Hypoventilation, 338
Hypoxia, 333
Hz. See Hertz (hZ)

I
IA muscle. See Interarytenoid (IA) muscle
IC. See Inferior colliculus (IC)
Idealized spectrum of sound, 373f
Ideational apraxia, 218
IHCs. See Inner hair cells (IHCs)
ILDs. See Interaural level differences (ILDs)
ILP. See Intermediate lamina propria (ILP)
Immediate energy system, 245
Immobile articulators, 424
alveolar ridge, 424
hard palate, 424
teeth, 424
Immunologic defense mechanisms, 329
Immunoprotection, 329
cytokines, 329
immunologic defense mechanisms, 329
T cells, 329
Impedance matching, 459
Impedances, 446
IMST. See Inspiratory muscle strength training, (IMST)
Incisivus labii inferioris muscle, 407
Incisivus labii superioris, 405
Incudomallear joint, 453
Incudostapedial joint, 453
Incus, 453
Indirect laryngoscopy, 382, 383f
Indirect pathway, 204
Induced pluripotent stem cells, 61

Inertia, 444
Inertive reactance, 373
Inferior colliculi, 114, 221, 292, 294
Inferior colliculus (IC), 473, 474–475
central nucleus inferior colliculus, 474
combination-sensitive neurons, 475
commissure of the inferior colliculus, 474
disk-shaped cells, 474
dorsal cortex, 474
external (lateral) shell, 474
isofrequency sheets, 474
medial geniculate body (MGB), 474
stellate cells, 474
Inferior longitudinal muscle, 420
Inferior mental spines, 363
Inferior olivary nucleus, 217
Inferior pharyngeal constrictor, 422
Inferior surface, 21f, 418f
Infrahyoid muscles, 362
Infraorbital foramen, 395
INLL. See Intermediate nucleus lateral lemniscus (INLL)
Inner and outer hair cell innervation, 458–459, 458f
cerebellopontine angle, 458
impedance matching, 459
spiral ganglion neuron, 458
superior olivary complex (SOC), 458
Inner cell mass, 106
Inner ear bony cochlea labyrinths, 454
cochlea position in temporal bone, 454f
habenula perforta, 454
modiolus, 454
osseous spiral lamina, 454
Rosenthal canal, 454
Inner ear cochlear biophysiology, 460–461, 460f
olivocochlear pathway, 461
Inner ear cochlear duct and organ of Corti, 455, 455ff
Claudius cells, 456
limbus, 455
Hensen cells, 456
otoacoustic emissions (OEAs), 456
stria vascularis, 456
spiral ligament, 455f, 456
tectoral membrane, 455
Inner ear hair cells (IHCs), 35f, 291, 456
Inner ear membranous cochlea labyrinth, 454–455
basilar membrane, 454–455
cochlear aqueduct, 455
endolymph, 455
endolymphatic duct, 455
endolymphatic sac, 455
helicotrema, 455
perilymph, 455
Reisner membrane, 454
scalia media, 454
scala tympani, 454, 455f
scala vestibuli, 454
vestibular aqueduct, 455
Inner ear potentials, 468
auditory brainstem response, (ABR), 468
auditory neuropathy/dyssynchrony, 468
electrocochleography (ECohG), 468
Ménière disease, 468
Inner ear sensory and supporting cells of organ of Corti, 456–458, 457ff
cortilymph, 456
cross links, 456
cuticular plate, 458
Deiters cell, 456
inner hair cells (IHCs), 456
mechanical transduction channels, 458
outer hair cells (OHCs), 456

phalangeal cells, 456
pillar cells, 456
reticular lamina, 458
ribbon synapse, 457
space of Nuel, 456
stereocilia, 457
tip links, 458
tonotopic organization, 456
tunnel of Corti, 456
Innervation of articulatory structures, 403–404
Insertion of muscle, 19
Inspiration, 23, 317
Inspiratory muscle strength training, (IMST),
329, 330
Inspiratory reserve volume (IRV), 321
Insula, 475
Insular cortex, 115
Integral proteins, 36
Integrins, 42
Intensity, 445
Interaural level differences (ILDs), 446
Interaural timing differences (ITDs), 446, 447f
Interarytenoid (IA) muscle (IA), 367, 367f
Intercostal muscles, 23
Intermaxillary suture, 395
Intermediate filaments, 41, 41f
Intermediate lamina propria (ILP), 361
Intermediate nucleus lateral lemniscus (INLL),
474
Intermediate stria, 472
Internal auditory canal, 448
Internal auditory meatus, 448
Internal capsule, 199, 475
Internal carotid arteries, 154
Internal respiration, 322
Interneurons, 144, 194
Interoception, 272
Interoceptors, 336
Interphase, 104–105
Interpositus nucleus, 160, 216
Interstitial lung disease, 341
Interthalamic adhesion, 151f, 152
Interventricular foramina, 156
Intracellular receptors, 50–51, 51f
Intraembryonic mesoderm, 108
Intraembryonic mesoderm division, 111
Intraglottal pressure differentials, 372
Intramuscular electromyographic (EMG)
activities, 214
Intramuscular EMG activities. See Intramuscular
electromyographic (EMG) activities
Intrathalamic interneurons, 475
Intrinsic muscles, tongue, 419–420, 419ff, 420t,
491f
Inverse problem, 206
Inverse square law, 446
Invertebral disks, 65f
Ion channels, 269
Ionotropic, 180
Ipsilateral, 8
Irritant receptors, 337
IRV. See Inspiratory reserve volume (IRV)
Isofrequency sheets, 474
Isometric activity, 249
Isometric muscle tension, 250f
Isotonic activity, 249
Isotonic environment, 46
ITDs. See Interaural timing differences (ITDs)

J
Jitter, 382
JNDs. Just-noticeable differences (JNDs)
Joints, 18–19, 64–65, 65f, 65t, 66f
cardiac muscle, 19
cartilaginous joint, 18

fibrous joints, 18
insertion of muscle, 19
invertebral disks, 65f
origin of muscle, 19
skeletal muscle, 19
skull sutures, 65f
traumatic brain injury and, 66f
smooth muscle, 19
synovial joint, 18, 66f
J-receptors. See Juxtacapillary receptors
(J-receptors)
Jugum, 399
Just-noticeable differences (JNDs), 266
Juxtacapillary receptors (J-receptors), 337
Juxtacrine cell signaling, 49, 49f

K
KE family, 75
Kinesia paradoxica, 207, 227
Kinetic apraxia, 218
Kinocilia and stereocilia orientation and resting
position, 535f
Kinocilium, 291, 528

L
Labeled-line principle of sensory systems, 265
Labial surface, 402, 402f
Labyrinthine artery, 26
Lacrimal bones, 393f, 397
Lactate, 247, 247f
Lamina terminalis, 115
Large aspiny neurons, 204
Laryngeal depressors, 362, 365t
Laryngeal elevators, 362, 363t
Laryngeal muscles, 126–127, 245, 245f
Laryngeal prominence, 356
Laryngeal vestibule, 352, 353f
Laryngeal videostroboscopy, 383, 383f
Laryngomalacia, 357
Laryngopharynx, 392, 494f
Laryngoscopy, 382
Laryngospasm, 370
Larynx. See Phonation and larynx
Larynx anatomy and physiology, 378–379
Larynx development, 126–127, 126f
arytenoid cartilages, 126
corniculate cartilages, 126
cuneiform cartilages, 126
laryngeal muscles, 126–127
T-shaped cleft, 126
Lateral, 7
Lateral cricoarytenoid (LCA) muscle, 367, 367f
Lateral fissure, 115, 146, 146f
Lateral geniculate nucleus (LGN), 286
Lateral inhibition, 268
Lateral lemniscus, 473, 474
dorsal nuclei lateral lemniscus (DNLL), 474
intermediate nucleus lateral lemniscus (INLL),
474
ventral nucleus lateral lemniscus (VNLL), 474
Lateral lingual swellings, 124
Lateral pterygoid muscle, 394, 489f
Lateral nasal processes, 120
Lateral superior olivary nucleus (LSO), 473
Lateral superior olive, 473–474
GABAergic projections, 474
glycinergic input, 473
Lateral thyrohoid ligament, 360
Lateral ventricle, 150
Lateral vestibular nucleus, 221
Lateral vestibulospinal tract, 298, 543–544, 543f
ankle strategy, 543, 544f
base of support, 543
center of gravity, 543
hip strategy, 543, 544f

stepping strategy, 543, 544f
suspensory strategy, 543, 544f
vestibulospinal reflexes, 543
Lateral zone, 216
LCA muscle. See Lateral cricoarytenoid (LCA)
muscle
Left lateral surface, 21f
Length-tension muscle relationship, 250–251
fatigue, 251–252
isometric muscle tension, 250f
load-velocity relationship, 251, 251f
muscle tension control, 251
shortening/lengthening velocity control, 251
Lesion and function correlation, 219–220, 220f
Lesions of the cerebellum, 546
Lesser cornu, 358
Levator anguli oris, 407, 407f
Levator labii superioris, 405, 406f
Levator labii superioris aleque nasi, 404f, 405,
407
Levator veli palatini, 368, 451
Levers in musculoskeletal system, 235f
Levodopa, 207
LGN. See Lateral geniculate nucleus (LGN)
Ligaments, 67–68, 67f
Ligand, 50
Ligand-gated ion channel, 178
Light microscopy, 34
Light transduction and retinal processing,
283–286
cyclic guanosine monophosphate (cGMP), 285
glutamate, 285
OFF bipolar cells, 285, 285f
ON bipolar cells, 285, 285f
phototransduction mechanism, 284f
rod and cone light wavelength sensitivities,
284f
second messenger system, 285
Limbic lobe, 147
Limbic system, 139, 153, 153f
Limb-kinetic apraxia, 218
Limbus, 455
Lingual and labial ties, 124
Lingual gyres, 150
Lingual surface, 402, 402f
Lip and palate development, 120–124
bucconasal membrane, 120
choanae, 120
cleft palate, 122
facial and orofacial clefts, 121–122, 121f
lingual and labial ties, 124
palatal shelves, 120, 122–123, 123f
philtrum, 120
primary palate, 119f, 120
secondary palate, 120, 123f
tectal ridge, 123
Lips as articulator, 409
Load-velocity relationship, 251, 251f
Lobes, 199
Lobar bronchi, 316
Locus, 79
Longitudinal fissure, 146, 146f
Loss of tissue compensation, 257
Loudness, 376, 445
Lower motor neurons, 166, 167
Lower respiratory system, 313–317, 312f
alveoli, 316
alveolar gas exchange, 316f
bones of respiration, 317
bronchi, 313, 316f
bronchioles, 316
costal surface, 314
diaphragm, 314, 317, 317f
external intercostal muscles, 317, 318f
hilum, 314

hydrostasis, 315
hydrostatic force, 315
inspiration, 317
lobar bronchi, 316
mediastinum, 314
phrenic nerves, 317
pleural cavity, 315, 315*f*
pleural linkage, 315
pneumothorax, 315–316, 315*f*
pulmonary artery and veins, 318, 318*f*
segmental bronchi, 316
trachea and bronchial tree, 313*ff*, 316*f*
LSO. *See* Lateral superior olivary nucleus (LSO)
Lumbar spine, 16
Lung buds, 125
Lung cancer, 340
Lungs, 312, 314*ff*
Lysosomes, 39

M

Macula, 296, 529
Macula flava, 362
Magnetic resonance imaging, 432, 432*f*
Magnitude estimation, 266
Malleus, 451
Mammillary bodies, 150
Mandible, 392, 394, 394*f*
    angle of the mandible, 394
    condylar process, 394
    coronoid process, 394
    corpus, 394, 394*f*
    lateral pterygoid muscle, 394
    mental foramen, 394
    mental protuberance, 394
    mental symphysis, 394
    ramus, 394
    temporomandibular joint (TMJ), 394
Mandibular branch, 164
Mandibular prominences, 120
Manometry, 515–516
Manubrium, 451
Markers, 81
Masklike facies, 207
Masseter and temporalis muscles, 488*f*
Masseter muscle, 405
Mastication, 487–490
    buccinator muscle, 487*f*
    lateral pterygoid muscle, 489*f*
    masseter and temporalis muscles, 488*f*
    mastication muscles, 489*t*
    masticatory muscles, 488*f*
    maxillary teeth, permanent, 487*f*
    medial pterygoid muscle, 488*f*
    oral cavity structures, 487*f*
    orbicularis oris, 487*f*
    temporomandibular joint, 488*f*
    tongue anatomy, 489*f*
    unilateral hypoglossal nerve lesion, 490, 490*f*
Mastoid, 447
Mastoid process, 364, 393*f*, 394
Maternal/fetal communication establishment,
        107–108, 108*f*
    body stalk, 108
    chorion frondosum, 108
    chorionic villi, 108, 108*f*
    cytotrophoblast, 108
    extraembryonic mesoderm, 108, 108*f*
    syncytiotrophoblast, 108
    trophoblastic villi, 108
Maxillae, 393, 395, 395*f*
    alveolar process, 395, 396*f*
    cleft, 395
    infraorbital foramen, 395
    intermaxillary suture, 395
    medial portion, 395, 396*f*

premaxilla, 395, 397*f*
    transverse palatine suture, 395
Maxillary branch, 164
Maxillary prominences, 120
Maxillary sinuses, 312
Maxillary teeth, permanent, 487*f*
MCA. *See* Middle cerebral artery (MCA)
Measurement of articulation, 429–434
    acoustic observations, 432–433
    camera systems, 431
    electromagnetic sensing, 431
    electromyography (EMG), 429
    electropalatography, 431
    magnetic resonance imaging, 432, 432*f*
    radiography, 429–431, 430*ff*
    ultrasound imaging, 431, 432*f*
Meatuses, 392, 400
Mechanical transduction channels, 458
Mechanoreceptors, 267, 503
Medial, 7
Medial compression, 371
Medial geniculate body (MGB), 292, 295, 473,
        475
    acoustic radiations, 475
    bushy cells, 475
    elongated cells, 475
    external capsule, 475
    insula, 475
    internal capsule, 475
    intrathalamic interneurons, 475
    thalamocortical relay cells, 475
    tufted cells, 475
Medial longitudinal fasciculus (MLF), 540
Medial nasal processes, 120
Medial nucleus of trapezoid body (MNTB), 473,
        474
    calyx of Held, 474
Medial portion, 395, 396*f*
Medial pterygoid muscle, 399, 488*f*
Medial superior olivary nucleus(MSO), 473
    coincident detectors, 473
Medial vestibulospinal tract, 298, 544–545
Median crichothyroid ligament, 359, 359*f*
Median fibrous septum, 417
Median laryngotracheal groove, 125
Median sulcus, 417
Median thyrohyoid ligament, 358
Mediastinum, 314
Medical root words, 5–7*t*
Medium spiny neurons (MSNs), 205
Medulla, 161–163
    abducens nerve, 162
    accessory nerve, 162
    facial nerve, 162
    fasciculus cuneatus, 162
    fasciculus gracilis, 162
    glossopharyngeal nerve, 162
    hypoglossal nerve, 162
    olive, 162
    pyramids, 162
    reticular system, 163
    vagus nerve, 162
    vestibulochlear nerve, 162
Medullary respiratory center, 335
Meiosis, 87, 87*f*, 105
Meissner corpuscle, 274
Membrane potential, 46
Membranous vocal fold, 378
Mendelian traits, 87–89
    autosomal dominant, 88*t*
    autosomal recessive, 88*t*
    mitochondrial, 88*t*
    X-linked dominant, 88*t*
    X-linked recessive, 88*t*
    Y-linked, 88*t*

Ménière disease, 468, 526, 526*f*
Meninges, 155
    arachnoid barrier, 155
    arachnoid mater, 155
    arachnoid trabeculae, 155
    cerebrospinal fluid (CSF), 155
    dura mater, 155
    epidural hematoma, 155
    pia mater, 155
    subarachnoid space, 155
    subdural hemorrhage, 155, 156*f*
Mental foramen, 394
Mentalis muscle, 407, 408*f*
Mental protuberance, 394
Mental symphysis, 394
Mereological fallacy, 203
Merkel disks, 274
Mesencephalon, 113
Mesoderm, 107
Messenger RNA (mRNA), 82
Metabotropic, 180
Metaphase, 105
Metencephalon, 114
Method of concomitant variations, 206
MGB. *See* Medial geniculate body (MGB)
Microfilaments, 40, 41*f*
Microglia, 144, 174
Microlaryngosocopy, 382
Microscopes, 34
Microtia, 448, 448*f*
Microtubules, 40, 41*f*
Midbrain, 139*t*, 161
    cerebral peduncles, 161
    corticospinal tracts, 161
    oculomotor nerve, 161
    substantia nigra, 161
    superior colliculi, 161
    trochlear nerve, 161
Middle cerebral artery (MCA), 154
Middle ear muscles and nerves, 454
    acoustic reflex, 454
    chorda tympani, 454
    stapedius nerve, 454
    tensor tympani muscle, 454
Middle ear ossicular chain, 453, 453*f*
    annular ligament, 453
    incudomallear joint, 453
    incudostapedial joint, 453
    incus, 453
    stapes, 453
Middle ear pathology, 452
    Carhart notch, 452
    ossicular chain disarticulation, 452
    otitis media, 452
    otosclerosis, 452
Middle ear peripheral auditory system physiol-
        ogy, 459–460
    cochlear partition, 455*f*, 461
    traveling wave, 461, 461*f*
Middle ear tympanic cavity, 451–453, 453*f*
    cochlea, 451
    epitympanic recess, 451
    eustachian tube, 451
    levator veli palatini, 451
    promontory, 451
    pyramidal eminence, 452
    stapedius muscle, 452
    tensor veli palatine, 451
Midsagittal plane, 8
Migraine-associated vertigo, 548
Migratory pathways of neural crest cells, 109*f*,
        111
Minute ventilation (MV), 321
Mitochondria, 37–38
    adenosine triphosphate (ATP), 37

Alzheimer's disease, 37
  cellular respiration, 37
  structure of, 38f
Mitochondrial inheritance, 88t, 89
Mitosis, 86, 86f
Mitosis and cell division, 104–105, 104f
  anaphase, 105
  chromosomes, 104
  interphase, 104–105
  metaphase, 105
  prophase, 105
  telophase, 105
Mixed hearing loss, 450
Mixed register, 377
MLF. See Medial longitudinal fasciculus (MLF)
Models, basal ganglia-thalamic cortical system,
      207–215
  anatomically based theories, 208, 209f
  antidromic action potentials, 214
  beta oscillation theory, 210–211
  bifurcations, 213
  cholinergic/dopaminergic imbalance theory,
      208
  circuit-based model, 212, 212f
  direct pathway, 208
  dynamic circuits, 213–214, 214f
  globus pallidus internal segment (GPi) rate
      theory, 209–210, 210f
  hyperdirect pathway, 208
  intramuscular electromyographic (EMG)
      activities, 214
  one-dimensional push-pull concept, 208
  Parkinson's and dopamine, 215
  physiologic and pathophysiologic models, 209
  polysynaptic nonlinear oscillators, 211, 211f
  stochastic resonance, 215
Modiolus, 454
Molars, 401
Monotone speech, 207
Morula, 106
Mossy fibers, 160, 217
Motor control hierarchy, 221–222
  decerebrate posturing, 221
  decorticate posturing, 221
  degrees of freedom, 221
  dorsal rhizotomy, 221
  dorsal root ganglia, 221
  inferior colliculi, 221
  lateral vestibular nucleus, 221
  one-dimensional conceptual approach, 222
  posterior (dorsal) roots, 221
  reduced preparations, 221
  Sherrington's reflexology, 222
Motor cortex, 192, 195
Motor end plates, 237f, 238
Motor equivalence, 434
Motor unit (MU), 192–194
  acetylcholine, 193
  action potential-initiating segment, 193
  action potentials, 193
  all-or-none response, 193
  cell body, 193
  dendrites, 193
  electrical activity generated by, 197
  interneurons, 194
  muscle spindle, 193
  Renshaw cell, 193
  segmental motor control, 194
Motor unit activation, 195–198
  decomposition of movement, 197
  deep brain stimulation (DBS), 196
  electrical activity generated by motor units,
      197
  Heinneman size principle, 195
  organization of information, 197–198

Parkinson's disease, 195
  subthalamic nucleus, 195
Motor unit and peripheral motor control,
      236–238, 249–250
  acetylcholine (ACh) neurotransmitter, 238
  alpha lower motor neuron, 237
  electromyography, 236
  frequency of stimulation, 249
  myogenesis, 237–238
  myospecificity, 237
  neuromuscular junctions (NJs), 237
  polysynaptic reflexes, 238f
  recruitment, 249
  size principle, 249
  synaptogenesis, 238
  tetanic contraction, 249
  twitch, 249, 250f
MRI. See Magnetic resonance imaging
mRNA. See Messenger RNA (mRNA)
MSNs. See Medium spiny neurons (MSNs)
MU. See Motor unit (MU)
Mucociliary escalator, 323
Multicellular, 32
Multiple neuron-like processing units, 224, 225f
Multiple sclerosis, 142, 143, 184t
Multipolar cells, PVCN, 472
Multipolar neuron, 143, 143f
Muscle adaptations, 254–257
  aging and muscle adaptations, 257
  detraining adaptations, 256
  exercise adaptations, 255–256
  loss of tissue compensation, 257
  overload principle, 254
  reversibility principle, 254
  specific adaptation to imposed demand (SAID)
      principle, 254
Muscle contraction types, 249
  concentric length, 249
  eccentric length, 249
  isometric activity, 249
  isotonic activity, 249
Muscle fiber types, 243–244, 244t
Muscle mechanics, 234–237
  fusiform shape, 236, 236f
  larynx, 245, 245f
  levers in musculoskeletal system, 235f
  pinnate arrangement, 236
  temporalis, 236, 237f
Muscle receptors, 247–249
  Golgi tendon organ (GTO), 248–249
  muscle spindles, 247–248, 248f
Muscle spindle, 193, 194, 194f, 247–248, 248f
Muscle strength training for respiration,
      330–331
  detraining effect, 330
  hypertrophy, 330
  inspiratory-expiratory muscle strength
      training (IMST-EMST), 330
  Poiseuille's law, 330
  pressure trainer, 331f
  resistive trainer, 330f
  synaptogenesis, 330
Muscle tension control, 251
Muscle tissue, 59–61
  cardiac muscle, 60, 61f
  esophageal peristalsis, 60, 60f
  skeletal muscle, 60, 60f
  smooth muscle, 59, 60f
Muscular dystrophy, 252
Muscular hydrostat, 418
Muscularis muscle, 366
Muscular system, 19
  cardiac muscle, 19
  insertion of muscle, 19
  origin of muscle, 19

  skeletal muscle, 19
  smooth muscle, 19
Musculoskeletal system, 62–68
  fascia, 68
  joints, 64–65, 65f, 65t, 66f
    invertebral disks, 65f
    skull sutures, 65f
    synovial joint, 66f
  ligaments, 67–68, 67f
  supportive connective tissues, 63–64
    bones, 62–63, 63t, 64f
    cartilage, 63, 64t
    compact bone, 63
    spongy bone, 63
  tendons, 66–67
    Achilles tendon, 67f
    omohyoid tendon, 67f
Musculus uvulae, 413, 414f
MV. See Minute ventilation (MV)
Myasthenia gravis, 178, 253
Myelin, 112, 143, 178
Myelinated axons, 143
Myelin sheath, 143, 238
Mylohyoid line, 363, 363f
Mylohyoid muscle, 363f, 364, 364f
Myoelastic-aerodynamic theory of phonation,
      373
Myogenesis, 237–238
Myosin, 241, 242f
Myospecificity, 237
Myotomes, 110

N

Nasal bones, 393f, 395
Nasal cavity, 392, 392f
Nasal conchae, 313
Nasality, 426
Nasal laminae, 120
Nasal pits, 119f, 120
Nasal placodes, 120
Nasal septum, 120, 312
Nasoendoscopy, 514–515
Nasolacrimal duct, 401
Nasopharynx, 392
Necker cube, 223, 223f
Necrotic tissue, 254
Negative symptoms, 206
Neocerebellum, 216
Nervous system, 19–22
  autonomic nervous system (ANS), 19
  central nervous system, 20–21
    cerebellum, 20
    cerebrum, 20
    cranial nerves, 22f
    frontal lobe, 20
    gray matter, 20, 21f
    gyri, 20
    inferior surface, 21f
    left lateral surface, 21f
    occipital lobe, 20
    parietal lobe, 20
    peripheral nervous system, 21
    sulci, 20
    temporal lobe, 20
    white matter, 20, 21f
  somatic nervous system (SNS), 19
Nervous system development, 111–115
  brain development, 113–115, 113f
    archipallium, 115
    Broca area, 115
    cephalic flexure, 113
    cerebellum, 114
    cerebral aqueduct, 114
    cervical flexure, 113
    choroid plexus, 113

claustrum, 115
corpus callosum, 115
corpus striatum, 115
diencephalon, 113
epithalamus, 114
fornix, 115
gray matter, 114–115
hippocampus, 115
hypothalamus, 114
inferior colliculi, 114
insular cortex, 115
lamina terminalis, 115
lateral fissure, 115
mesencephalon, 113
metencephalon, 114
pons, 114
pontine flexure, 113
prosencephalon, 113
rhinencephalon, 115
rhombencephalon, 113
sensory fibers, 113
solitary tract, 113
substantia negra, 114
superior colliculi, 114
telencephalon, 113
thalamus, 114
Wernicke area, 115
white matter, 115
neural folds fusion, 111–112
anterior neuropore, 111
migratory pathways of neural crest cells,
109f, 111
posterior neuropore, 109f, 111
neural tube differentiation, 112
neural tube zones, 112
primitive medullary cells differentiation, 112
axons, 112
glioblasts, 112
myelin, 112
oligodendrocytes, 112
spinal cord development, 112–113
Nervous tissue, 57–58
action potentials, 58
dendrites, 58
glial cells, 58, 58f
neurons, 58, 58f
Neural connections, 537f
Neural folds fusion, 111–112
anterior neuropore, 111
migratory pathways of neural crest cells, 109f,
111
posterior neuropore, 109f, 111
Neural tissue, 144–145
cranial nerves, 145
gray matter, 144, 145f
white matter, 144, 145f
Neural tube development, 109, 109f, 110f
neural fold, 109
neural grooves, 110
neural plate, 109
Neural tube differentiation, 112
Neural tube zones, 112
Neuroanatomy, 137–170, 137f
blood supply system, 154–155, 155ff
anterior cerebral artery (ACA), 154
basilar artery, 154
cerebral artery distribution, 154f
cerebral veins, 155f
circle of Willis, 154f, 155
confluence of sinuses, 155
deep cerebral veins, 155
dysarthria, 154
dyslexia, 154
great cerebral vein, 155
internal carotid arteries, 154

middle cerebral artery (MCA), 154
posterior cerebral artery (PCA), 154
straight sinus, 155
superficial cerebral veins, 155
superior sagittal sinus, 155
vertebral arteries, 154
vertebrobasilar and internal carotid
branches, 154f
brain and spinal cord, 138–140, 139f, 139t
basal ganglia, 139
brainstem, 138, 139
cerebellum, 138, 139t
cerebral cortex, 139
cerebral hemispheres, 138
diencephalon, 138
forebrain, 139t
hindbrain, 139t
limbic system, 139
midbrain, 139t
pituitary gland, 139
brain stem, 161–163, 162f
medulla, 161–163
midbrain, 161
pons, 161
cerebellum, 158–161, 158f
cerebellar penduncles, 159, 159f
climbing fibers, 160
dentate nucleus, 160
fastigial nucleus, 160
flocculonodular lobe, 158
flocculus, 158
granule cells, 160
interpositus nucleus, 160
mossy fibers, 160
nodulus, 158
posterolateral fissure, 158
primary fissure, 158
tracts and functions, 159f
vermis, 158
cerebral cortex, 145–150, 145f
angular gyrus, 149
anterior commissure, 150
aphasia, 147–149
Broca's area, 147
Brodmann areas, 145–146, 146f
calcarine sulcus, 149–150
central sulcus, 146
cingulate gyrus, 146f, 147
collateral sulcus, 150
corpus callosum, 146, 146f
cuneus gyrus, 150
fissures, 145
fornix, 150
frontal lobe, 146
functional localization, 146
genu, 150
gyri, 145
gyrus rectus, 150
Heschl's gyrus, 149
lateral fissure, 146, 146f
lateral ventricle, 150
limbic lobe, 147
lingual gyrus, 150
longitudinal fissure, 146, 146f
mammillary bodies, 150
occipital lobe, 147
occipitotemporal gyrus, 150
olfactory bulbs, 150
olfactory sulci, 150
olfactory tracts, 150
optic chiasm, 150
parahippocampal gyrus, 150
parietal lobe, 146
postcentral gyrus, 149
precentral gyrus, 147

premotor cortex, 147
preoccipital notch, 146–147
primary auditory cortex, 149
primary motor cortex, 147, 147f
primary somatosensory cortex, 149, 149f
primary visual cortex, 149–150
rhinal sulcus, 150
septum pellucidum, 150
splenium, 150
sulci, 145
superior temporal gyrus (STG), 147
supramarginal gyrus, 149
temporal lobe, 146
uncus, 150
Wernicke's area, 149
cerebrovascular system, 154–158
blood-brain barrier, 157, 158f
blood supply system, 154–155, 155ff
meninges, 155
ventricular system, 156–157
cranial nerves, 163–165, 163f, 164tt
accessory nerve, 165
chorda tympani branch, 165
hypoglossal nerve, 165
mandibular branch, 164
maxillary branch, 164
olfactory nerve, 163
opthalmic branch, 164
optic nerve, 163
vagus nerve, 165
glial cells, 144
astrocytes, 144
blood-brain barrier, 144
microglia, 144
oligodendrocytes, 144
Schwann cells, 144, 144f
meninges, 155, 156f
arachnoid barrier, 155
arachnoid mater, 155
arachnoid trabeculae, 155
cerebrospinal fluid (CSF), 155
dura mater, 155
epidural hematoma, 155
pia mater, 155
subarachnoid space, 155
subdural hemorrhage, 155, 156f
neural tissue, 144–145
cranial nerves, 145
gray matter, 144, 145f
white matter, 144, 145f
neurons, anatomy of, 141–143, 142f
axoaxonal synapse, 142f, 143
axodendritic synapse, 143
axon, 141
axosomatic synapse, 143
dendrites, 141
dendritic spines, 143
multiple sclerosis, 142, 143
myelin, 143
myelinated axons, 143
myelin sheath, 143
nodes of Ranvier, 143
soma, 139f, 141
structure, 141f
terminal boutons, 141
terminal segment, 141
transmission segment, 141
unmyelinated axons, 143
neurons, classification of, 143–144, 144f
bipolar neuron, 143, 143f
interneurons, 144
multipolar neuron, 143, 143f
projection neurons, 144
Purkinje cell, 143, 143f
pyramidal cell, 143, 143f

unipolar neuron, 143f, 144
peripheral nervous system (PNS), 140–141
    afferent nerves, 140–141, 140f
    autonomic nervous system, 140f
    efferent nerves, 140f, 141
    fight or flight response, 141
    parasympathetic system, 140f, 141
    somatic motor fibers, 141
    somatic nervous system, 141
    somatic sensory fibers, 141
    visceral motor fibers, 141
    visceral sensory fibers, 141
spinal cord, 165–168
    autonomic nervous system, 167
    cauda equina, 166
    conus medullaris, 165
    gray matter, 166
    lower motor neurons, 167
    reflexes, 168
    upper motor neurons, 167
    white matter, 166–167, 167f
subcortex, 150–153
    basal ganglia, 150, 151ff
    caudate nucleus, 151
    cerebellar mutism, 153
    diencephalon, 152–153, 152f
    globus pallidus, 151
    Huntington's disease, 151
    hypothalamus, 152
    interthalamic adhesion, 151f, 152
    limbic system, 153, 153f
    Parkinson's disease, 151, 152
    pineal gland, 152
    putamen, 150
    stratium, 151
    thalamus, 152
    third ventricle, 152
ventricular system, 156–157, 156f
    arachnoid granulations, 156–157
    cerebral aqueduct, 156
    cerebrospinal fluid circulation, 157f
    choroid plexus, 156, 157f
    fourth ventricle, 156
    interventricular foramina, 156
Neurocranium, 10, 13f
Neurocranium and viscerocranium, bones, 393, 393ff
    external auditory meatus, 393f, 394
    foramen magnum, 394, 394f
    frons, 394
    mastoid process, 393f, 394
    maxilla, 393
    occiput, 394
    orbit bones, 393f
    palatine, 393
    temporal fossae, 394
    vertex, 394
    vomer, 393
    zygomatic arch, 393f, 394
    zygomatic bones, 393
Neuroepithelium of SCCs and otolithic organs, 527, 529f
Neuromodulators, 180
Neuromuscular junction (NJs), 237, 240, 240f
Neuronal action potentials, 223, 223f
Neurons, 58, 58f, 172–173, 172f
    action potential, 173
    anion, 173
    axon, 173
    axon terminal, 173
    cation, 173
    cell membrane structure, 174f
    concentration gradient, 173, 175f
    dendrites, 173
    gap junctions, 173

ligand-gated ion channel
    neurotransmitters, 173
    permeability, 173
    soma, 173
    synapse, 173
    terminal bouton, 173
    voltage-gated ion channel, 173
Neurons, anatomy of, 141–143, 142f
    axoaxonal synapse, 142f, 143
    axodendritic synapse, 143
    axon, 141
    axosomatic synapse, 143
    dendrites, 141
    dendritic spines, 143
    multiple sclerosis, 142, 143
    myelin, 143
    myelinated axons, 143
    myelin sheath, 143
    nodes of Ranvier, 143
    soma, 139f, 141
    structure, 141f
    terminal boutons ,11417
    terminal segment, 141
    transmission segment, 141
    unmyelinated axons, 143
Neurons, classification of, 143–144, 144f
    bipolar neuron, 143, 143f
    interneurons, 144
    multipolar neuron, 143, 143f
    projection neurons, 144
    Purkinje cell, 143, 143f
    pyramidal cell, 143, 143f
    unipolar neuron, 143f, 144
Neuropharmacology, 183
Neurophysiology, 171–189
    action potential, 176, 176ff, 178t
        depolarization, 176
        hyperpolarization, 176
    deep brain stimulation, 185
    disease, disorders, and injuries, 184–185, 185t
        Alzheimer disease, 184t
        amyotrophic lateral sclerosis, 184t
        epilepsy, 184t
        multiple sclerosis, 184t
        Parkinson's disease, 184t
        sensorineural hearing loss, 184t
        stroke, 184t
        traumatic brain injury, 184t
    drugs, effect on, 180–184
        affinity, 183
        agonists, 183
        antagonists, 183
        efficacy, 183
        neuropharmacology, 183
    endocochlear potential, 182, 182f
    fundamental logical operators, 172
    glial cells, 172, 174, 172f, 175f
        astrocytes, 174
        ependymal cells, 174
        microglia, 174
        oligodendrocytes, 174
        Schwann cells, 174
    neurons, 172–173, 172f
        action potential, 173
        anion, 173
        axon, 173
        axon terminal, 173
        cation, 173
        cell membrane structure, 174f
        concentration gradient, 173, 175f
        dendrites, 173
        gap junctions, 173
        ligand-gated ion channel
        neurotransmitters, 173
        permeability, 173

        soma, 173
        synapse, 173
        terminal bouton, 173
        voltage-gated ion channel, 173
    neuroplasticity, 185–186
    neurotransmission, 179–182
        actions, 180
        multiple sclerosis, 179
        packing, docking, and release, 180
        types, 181, 182t
    postsynaptic potentials, 176–178
        channelopathies, 178
        graded potentials, 177, 178t
        spatial summation, 177
        temporal summation, 177
        tetrodotoxin, 177, 177f
    resting membrane potential, 174–175
        adenosine triphosphate (ATP), 175
        diffusion, 175
        homeostasis, 19
        sodium-potassium pump, 175
    saltatory conduction, 178–179
        action potential-initiating segment, 178
        axon hillock, 178
        continuous and saltatory propagation of action potentials, 179
        myelin, 178
        nodes of Ranvier, 178
Neuroplasticity, 185–186
Neurotransmission, 179–182
    actions, 180
        autoreceptor, 180
        ionotropic, 180
        metabotropic, 180
        neuromodulators, 180
    multiple sclerosis, 179
    packing, docking, and release, 180
        synaptic signal transmission, 180f
        vesicles, 180
    types, 181, 182t
        dopaminergic, 181
        noradrenergic, 181
Neurotransmitters, 50, 173
NJs. See Neuromuscular junctions (NJs)
Nociception, 276
Nociceptors, 267
Nodes of Ranvier, 143, 178
Nodulus, 158
Nonlinear interactions, 222
Nonsyndromic hearing loss, 76
Noradrenergic, 181
Normal and dysphonic sound, 374f
Nose and nasal cavities, 399–401, 400ff
    choanae, 400
    meatuses, 400
    nasolacrimal duct, 401
    orifices, 400
    paranasal sinuses, 400–401, 401f
NST. See Nucleus of solitary tract (NST)
Nuclear envelope, 37
Nucleic acids, 78, 79, 80f
    nucleotides, 79
Nucleoid, 33, 79
Nucleolus, 37
Nucleotide base pairs, 85f
Nucleus, 33, 37, 37f
    nuclear envelope, 37
    nucleolus, 37
Nucleus ambiguus, 368
Nucleus of solitary tract (NST), 303
Nystagmus, 542

O

Occipital lobe, 20, 147
Occipitotemporal gyrus, 150

Occiput, 394
Occlusion, 403, 403f
Occlusal surface, 402, 402f
Octopus cells, PVCN, 472
Oculomotor nerve, 161
Odynophagia, 492
OEAs. See Otoacoustic emissions (OEAs)
OFF bipolar cells, 285, 285f
OHCs. See Outer hair cells (OHCs)
Olfactory bulbs, 150
Olfactory nerve, 163
Olfactory sulci, 150
Olfactory system, 299
    central olfactory pathway, 300–301
    olfactory bulb, 299
    olfactory receptors and transduction mecha-
        nism, 299–300
    olfactory tract, 300
Olfactory tracts, 150
Oligodendrocytes, 112, 144, 174
Olive, 162
Olivocochlear pathway, 461
Omohyoid muscle, 364f, 365
Omohyoid tendon, 67f
ON bipolar cells, 285, 285f
One-dimensional conceptual approach, 222
One-dimensional push-pull concept, 208
OoC. See Organ of Corti (OoC)
Oogenesis, 105, 105f
Opening phase, 371
Opthalmic branch, 164
Optic canal, 399
Optic chiasm, 150
Optic disc, 281
Optic nerve, 163
Optic radiations, 286
Optic tract, 286
Oral cancer, 423
Oral cavity, 392, 392f
Oral cavity structures, 487f
Oral phase of swallowing, 497
Oral-preparatory phase of swallowing, 495–497
Orbicularis oculi, 407, 408f
Orbicularis oris, 404, 404f, 487f
Orbit bones, 393f
Organ of Corti (OoC), 289
Organs and organ systems, 61–62, 62t
Orifices, 400
Origin of muscle, 19
Orofacial region, 276–277
Oropharynx, 392
Oscillation, 445
Oscillator phase changes, 224
Osmosis, 46, 46f
Osseous spiral lamina, 454
Ossicular chain, 451
Ossicular chain disarticulation, 452
Otitis media, 11, 11f, 452
    eustachian tube, 11
Otoacoustic emissions (OEAs), 456
Otoconia, 296, 529
Otolithic membrane, 296, 529
Otolith organs, transduction of linear motion by,
        296–297, 296f
    macula, 296
    otoconia, 296
    otolithic membrane, 296
    saccule, 296
    utricle, 296
Otoliths, 530f
Otosclerosis, 452
Otoscopy, 451
Outer ear, 448–451
    antihelix, 450
    aural atresia, 448

cerumen, 450
concha, 450
cone of light, 451
external auditory canal, 449, 450f
helix, 450
malleus, 451
manubrium, 451
microtia, 448, 448f
ossicular chain, 451
otoscopy, 451
oval window, 451
pars flaccida, 451
pars tensa, 451
pinna, 449, 450f
round window, 451
stenosis, 448
tragus, 450
tympanic membrane, 451f
umbo, 451
Outer ear development, 128–130
    auditory vesicle, 129
    aural atresia, 128
    auricle, 128
    auricular fold, 129
    auricular hillocks, 128, 129f
    cristae ampullaris, 130
    cupula, 130
    endolymphatic sac, 129
    kinocilia, 130
    macula, 130
    membranous labyrinth, 129, 130f
    otic placodes, 129
    otoconia, 130
    saccule, 129
    spiral limbus, 130
    spiral organ, 130
    utricle, 129
Outer ear hair cells (OHCs), 291, 456
Outer ear peripheral auditory system physiol-
        ogy, 459
    head-related transfer function (HRTF), 459,
        459f
Oval window, 451
Overbite, 403
Overjet, 403
Overload principle, 254
Ovum, 105
Oxidation, 42
Oxidative phosphorylation, 246, 247f
Oxygen reserves and homeostasis, 333–334
    erythropoietin, 333
    hypoxia, 333

P

Pa. See Pascals (Pa)
Pacinian corpuscle (PC), 274
PAF. See Posterior auditory field (PAF)
PAG matter. See Periaqueductal gray (PAG)
        matter
Pain, 276
Palatal shelves, 120, 122–123, 123f
Palatine, 393
Palatine bones and inferior nasal conchae, 396,
        397f
Palatoglossus, 421
Palatoglossus muscle, 413
Palatopharyngeus tenses, 414
Paleocerebellum, 216
Parabelt, 475
Parabrachial nuclei (PBN), 303
Paracine cell signaling, 49, 49f
Paradoxical vocal fold motion (PVFM), 370
Parafascicular nuclei, 204
Parahippocampal gyrus, 150
Parallel fibers, 217

Paranasal sinuses, 312, 400–401, 401f
Parasagittal plane, 8
Parasympathetic system, 140f, 141
Paravermal zone, 216
Parent-of-origin effects, 95, 95f
Parietal lobe, 20, 146
Parkinson's disease, 151, 152, 184t, 195
    and cell signaling, 53, 53f
    and dopamine, 215
    and swallowing, 485, 485f
Parotid salivary gland, 491
Pars flaccida, 451
Pars obliqua, 366
Pars recta, 366
Pars tensa, 451
Pascals (Pa), 445
Passavant ridge, 415–416
Passive transport
    carrier proteins, 46
    channel proteins, 46
    diffusion, 45, 45f
    facilitated diffusion, 45–46, 45f
    hypertonic, 46
    hypotonic environment, 46
    isotonic environment, 46
    osmosis, 46, 46f
Pathology, 4
Pathophysiology, 192
Pattern generators, 370
PBN. See Parabrachial nuclei (PBN)
PC. See Pacinian corpuscle (PC)
PCA. See Posterior cerebral artery (PCA)
PD. See Parkinson disease (PD)
PE. See Pleural effusion (PE)
PE. See Pulmonary embolism (PE)
Peduncles, 216, 216f
Penetrance and expressivity, 89
    genotype, 89
    phenotype, 89
    variable expressivity, 89
Percept, 265
Perception, 264
Periaqueductal gray (PAG) matter, 369
Perilymph, 455, 525
Periodicity, 382
Periodic sound waves, 445
Periolivary group, 473
Peripheral auditory system physiology, 444,
        459–470
    afferent neural functions, 468–470
        characteristic frequencies, 469
        cochlear nucleus, 469
        phase locking, 470
        spontaneous action potential firing rate,
            469, 470f
        tuning curve, 470, 470f
    basilar membrane macromechanics, passive
        properties, 461–464, 462ff
        place theory, 462
        temporal theory, 462
        traveling wave shape (envelope), 463, 464f
        volley theory, 462–463
    cochlear electrophysiology, 467–468
        cochlear microphonic (CM), 467
        compound action potential (cAP), 467
        endocochlear potential (EP), 467
        summating potential (SP), 467
    hair cell micromechanics active transduction,
        464–467, 465f, 466f, 467f
        actin-filled stereocilia, 464
        AMPA-type receptors, 466
        cochlear amplifier, 466, 467f
        depolarization, 466
        electromotility, 466
        glutamate, 466

hyperpolarized state, 465
prestin, 466
saltatory conduction, 466
somatic motor, 466
voltage-gated calcium channels, 466
inner ear potentials, 468
auditory brainstem response, (ABR), 468
auditory neuropathy/dyssynchrony, 468
electrocochleography (ECohG), 468
Ménière disease, 468
middle ear, 459–460
cochlear partition, 455f, 461
traveling wave, 461, 461f
outer ear, 459
head-related transfer function (HRTF), 459, 459f
tympanic membrane, 459
Peripheral chemoreceptors, 336, 336f
Peripheral gas exchange, 322
Peripheral motor control, 233–261
bioenergetics, 244–247, 246f
glycolysis, 245
immediate energy system, 245
lactate, 247, 247f
oxidative phosphorylation, 246, 247f
excitation-contraction coupling, 238–240
acetylcholine (ACh), 239
action potential (AP), 238
exocytosis, 239
motor end plates, 237f, 238
myelin sheath, 238
myofibrils, 239
network of channels in muscle cell, 239
neuromuscular junction, 240, 240f
postsynaptic acetylcholine receptors (AChRs), 239
presynaptic membrane, 239
sarcolemma, 239
sarcoplasmic reticulum (SR), 239
synaptic cleft, 238
transverse tubules (T-tubules), 239
length-tension relationship, 250–251
fatigue, 251–252
isometric muscle tension, 250f
load-velocity relationship, 251, 251f
muscle tension control, 251
shortening/lengthening velocity control, 251
motor unit, 236–238, 249–250
acetylcholine (ACh) neurotransmitter, 238
alpha lower motor neuron, 237
electromyography, 236
frequency of stimulation, 249
myogenesis, 237–238
myospecificity, 237
neuromuscular junctions (NJs), 237
polysynaptic reflexes, 238f
recruitment, 249
size principle, 249
synaptogenesis, 238
tetanic contraction, 249
twitch, 249, 250f
muscle adaptations, 254–257
aging and muscle adaptations, 257
detraining adaptations, 256
exercise adaptations, 255–256
loss of tissue compensation, 257
overload principle, 254
reversibility principle, 254
specific adaptation to imposed demand (SAID) principle, 254
muscle contraction types, 249
concentric length, 249
eccentric length, 249
isometric activity, 249

isotonic activity, 249
muscle mechanics, 234–237
fusiform shape, 236, 236f
larynx, 245, 245f
levers in musculoskeletal system, 235f
pinnate arrangement, 236
temporalis, 236, 237f
muscle receptors, 247–249
Golgi tendon organ (GTO), 248–249
muscle spindles, 247–248, 248f
physical injury and overuse, 253–254
delayed onset muscle soreness (DOMS), 253
necrotic tissue, 254
skeletal muscle, 239, 241–244
A-bands, 241
actin, 241
adenosine triphosphate (ATP), 243
cross-bridge theory, 243, 243f
muscle fiber types, 243–244, 244t
myosin, 241, 242f
sarcomeres, 239, 242f, 243f
sliding filament theory, 243
striated muscle, 241f
structure, 241f
tropomyosin, 241, 242f
troponin, 241
Z-line, 241
skeletal muscle disease, 252–253
muscular dystrophy, 252
myasthenia gravis, 253
specific adaptation to imposed demand (SAID) principle, 234
Peripheral nervous system (PNS), 21, 140–141
afferent nerves, 140–141, 140f
autonomic nervous system, 140f
efferent nerves, 140f, 141
fight or flight response, 141
parasympathetic system, 140f, 141
somatic motor fibers, 141
somatic nervous system, 141
somatic sensory fibers, 141
visceral motor fibers, 141
visceral sensory fibers, 141
Peripheral neuropathy, 219
Peripheral proteins, 36, 36f
Peripheral receptor apparatus, 525f
Peripheral vestibular anatomy, 524–530, 524f
ampula, 528–529, 529f
anterior SCC, 525
common crus, 525
cristae, 529
cuticular plate, 528
endolymph, 525
hair cell orientation, 530
hair cells, 528, 528f, 531f
horizontal SCC, 525, 527ff
kinocilium, 528
macula, 529
neuroepithelium of SCCs and otolithic organs, 527, 529f
otoconia, 529
otolithic membrane, 529
otoliths, 530f
perilymph, 525
peripheral receptor apparatus, 525f
posterior SCC, 525
saccule otolithic organ, 525
stereocilia, 528
utricle otolithic organ, 525
vertigo, 525
Peripheral vestibular physiology, 530, 532–534
coplanar pairs, 533, 533f
directional polarization, 532f
endolymph displacement, 535f
hair cell excitation and inhibition, 534f

kinocilia and stereocilia orientation and resting position, 535f
otolithic aculae, 532f
Peristaltic movement, 498
Perisylvian regions, 370
Permeability, 173
Petrous, 447
pH, 312
Phalangeal cells, 456
Phantosmias, 303
pH buffer, 334
Pharmacokinetics, 332
prodrug, 332
pulmonary extraction, 332
Pharyngeal arches, 116–118, 116f, 118t, 354–355, 355f
Pharyngeal branch, 368
Pharyngeal cavity, 352, 392
Pharyngeal constrictor muscles, 414f, 494f
Pharyngeal musculature, 415f
Pharyngeal phase of swallowing, 497–498
Pharyngeal raphe, 422
Pharynx and swallowing, 493–496
autonomous nervous system, 496
esophagus and trachea, 496f
laryngopharynx, 494f
peristaltic movement, 498
pharyngeal constrictor muscles, 494f
pharynx divisions, 493f
pharynx muscles, 495t
tonic contraction, 498
Pharynx divisions, 493f
Pharynx muscles, 414f, 415f, 422–424, 423t, 495t
articulation, 423–424
inferior pharyngeal constrictor, 422
oral cancer, 423
pharyngeal raphe, 422
stylopharyngeus muscle, 423
Phase locking, 470
Phenotype, 89
Philtrum, 120
Phlegm, 322
Phonation acoustic energy characteristics, 373–379
age and gender differences, 377–379
anatomy and physiology of larynx, 378–379
cartilaginous vocal fold, 378
membranous vocal fold, 378
production of voice and voice quality, 378–379
aperiodic energy, 374
complex acoustic sound waves, 373
control of vocal intensity, 375
fundamental frequency, 373, 374–375, 374f
falsetto register, 375
hertz, 374
pitch, 374
harmonic frequencies, 373
idealized spectrum of sound, 373f
normal and dysphonic sound, 374f
vocal registers, 377
chest register, 377
falsetto register, 377
head register, 377
mixed register, 377
pulse register, 377
vocal fry, 377
voice quality, 375–377
harmonic frequencies, 376
loudness, 376
phonation periodicity, 376
timbre, 375
vocal tremor, 376–377
voice breaks, 376

Phonation and laryngeal function, 379–384
  acoustic analysis, 373f, 374f, 381–382
    amplitude perturbation, 382
    frequency perturbation, 382
    jitter, 382
    periodicity, 382
    physiologic voice, range, 382
    shimmer, 382
    sound intensity, 382
    spectral acoustic analyses, 382
    vocal intensity, 382
  aerodynamic analysis, 380–381
    estimated mean flow rate, 380–381
    phonation quotient (PQ), 380
    phonation threshold pressure (PTP), 381
    phonation volume, 380
    pressure, 381
    vital capacity (VC), 380
    voicing efficiency, 381
  auditory-perceptual analysis, 379–380
  endoscopic analysis, 382–384, 383f
    direct laryngoscopy, 382
    indirect laryngoscopy, 382, 383f
    laryngeal videostroboscopy, 383, 383f
    laryngoscopy, 382
    microlaryngosocopy, 382
Phonation and larynx, 351–370, 352f
  central neural supply, 369–370
    auditory cortical regions, 369
    babbling, 369
    basal ganglia (BGs), 369
    Broca area, 369
    cerebellum, 370
    chronic cough, 370
    direct pathway, 369
    laryngospasm, 370
    paradoxical vocal fold motion (PVFM), 370
    pattern generators, 370
    periaqueductal gray (PAG) matter, 369
    perisylvian regions, 370
    premotor cortex, 369
    pyramidal pathway, 369
    supplementary motor area, 369
    Wernicke area, 369
  extrinsic laryngeal muscles, 362–365
    digastric fossa, 363
    digastric muscle, 364, 364f
    geniohyoid muscle, 363, 363f
    hyoglossus, 363
    hyolaryngeal excursion, 364
    inferior mental spines, 363
    infrahyoid muscles, 362
    laryngeal depressors, 362, 365t
    laryngeal elevators, 362, 363t
    mastoid process, 364
    mylohyoid line, 363, 363f
    mylohyoid muscle, 363f, 364, 364f
    omohyoid muscle, 364f, 365
    sternoclavicular ligament, 364
    sternohyoid muscle, 364, 364f
    sternothyroid muscle, 364, 364f
    stylid process, 364, 364f
    stylohyoid muscle, 364, 364f
    suprahyoid aponeurosis, 364
    suprahyoid muscles, 362
    thyrohyoid muscle, 364f, 365
  intrinsic laryngeal muscles, 365–368, 365t
    aryepiglottic muscle, 368
    cricothyroid (CT) muscle, 366, 367f
    interarytenoid (IA) muscle (IA), 367, 367f
    lateral cricoarytenoid (LCA) muscle, 367, 367f
    muscularis muscle, 366
    pars obliqua, 366
    pars recta, 366

posterior cricoarytenoid (PCA) muscle, 367, 367f
    thyroarytenoid (TA) muscle, 366, 366f
    thyroepiglottic muscle, 367
    ventricular muscle, 368
  laryngeal development, 354–355, 355f
    bronchial arches, 354
    pharyngeal arches, 354–355, 355f
  laryngeal framework, 355–358
    anterior commissure, 356
    arytenoid cartilages, 357, 357f
    cartilages, 355t
    corniculate cartilages, 357
    cricoid cartilage, 356
    cricothyroid joints, 356, 356t
    cricotracheal membrane, 356
    cuneiform cartilages, 357
    epiglottis, 357–358, 357f
    greater cornu, 358
    hyaline cartilage, 357
    hyoid bone, 355, 355f, 356f
    laryngeal prominence, 356
    laryngeal vestibule, 352, 353f
    laryngomalacia, 357
    larynx, biologic functions, 352–354
    lesser cornu, 358
    pharyngeal cavity, 352
    thyroid cartilage, 355, 356f
    thyroid horns, 356
    thyroid notch, 356
    vallecula, 358
    vocal process, 357
  larynx membranes and ligaments, 358–360, 359t
    conus elasticus, 358, 359f
    cricoarytenoid ligament, 358
    cricothyroid ligament, 359, 359f
    hypoepiglottic ligament, 359, 359f
    lateral thyrohyoid ligament, 360
    median crichothyroid ligament, 359, 359f
    median thyrohyoid ligament, 358
    quadrangular membrane, 358
    respiratory epithelium, 360, 360f
    thyroepiglottic ligament, 360
    thyrohyoid membrane, 358
    vocal ligament, 358, 359f
  larynx, speech functions, 354
  peripheral neural supply, 368
    ansa cervicalis, 368
    facial cranial nerve, 368
    hypoglossal cranial nerve, 368
    levator veli palatini, 368
    nucleus ambiguus, 368
    pharyngeal branch, 368
    recurrent laryngeal nerve (RLN), 368
    superior laryngeal nerve, 368
    trigeminal cranial nerve, 38
    vagus nerve, 368
  vocal fold structure, 360–362
    abduction, 360
    adduction, 360
    basement membrane zone (BMZ), 361
    coronal section, 360, 361f
    deep lamina propria (DLP), 361
    ground substance, 361
    intermediate lamina propria (ILP), 361
    macula flava, 362
    phonation threshold pressure (PTP), 361
    Reinke space, 361
    superficial lamina propria (SLP), 361
    vocalis muscle (VM), 360, 361, 361f
    vocal ligament, 361
Phonation and respiratory system, 24
Phonation periodicity, 376
Phonation physiology, 370–373

biomechanics, 371–373
    Bernoulli effect, 372
    convergent glottis, 372, 372f
    divergent glottis, 372, 372f
    elastic recoil, 372
    flow separation vortices, 372
    inertive reactance, 373
    intraglottal pressure differentials, 372
    medial compression, 371
    myoelastic-aerodynamic theory of phonation, 373
    three-mass model, 371, 371f
    transglottal airflow, 371, 371ff
    vocal folds nodules, 372
  vibratory cycle, 370–371
    closed phase, 371, 371f
    opening phase, 371
    self-oscillating system, 370
Phonation quotient (PQ), 380
Phonation threshold pressure (PTP), 328, 361, 380
Phonemes, 426
Phospholipid bilayer, 35
Photoreceptors, 267
Phototransduction mechanism, 284f
Phrenic nerves, 317
Physical injury and overuse of muscles, 253–254
    delayed onset muscle soreness (DOMS), 253
    necrotic tissue, 254
Physiologic and pathophysiologic models, 209
Physiologic voice, range, 382
Physiology, 4
Pia mater, 155
Pierre Robin sequence (PRS), 512, 512f
Pillar cells, 456
Pineal gland, 152
Pinna, 447, 449, 450f
Pinnate arrangement, 236
Pitch, 374, 445
Pituitary gland, 139
Place theory, 462
Plasma membrane, 32, 35–37, 36f
    amphipathic region, 36
    hydrophilic heads, 35
    hydrophobic tails, 35
    inner ear hair cells, 35f
    integral proteins, 36
    peripheral proteins, 36, 36f
    phospholipid bilayer, 35
Platysma muscle, 405, 405f, 407
Pleural cavity, 315, 315f
Pleural effusion (PE), 341
Pleural linkage, 315
Pneumoconiosis, 340–341
Pneumonia, 340
Pneumotaxic center, 335–336
Pneumothorax, 341
PNS. See Peripheral nervous system (PNS)
pNTM. See Pulmonary infection, nontubercular mycobacteria (pNTM)
Poiseuille's law, 330
Polar body, 106
Polymorphisms, 79–81, 81f
    alleles, 80
    genotypes, 80
    locus, 79
    markers, 81
Polysynaptic nonlinear oscillators, 211, 211f
Polysynaptic reflexes, 238f
Pons, 114, 161, 472
    trigeminal nerve, 161
Pontine flexure, 113
Pontine relay nuclei, 217
Postcentral gyrus, 149, 278
Posterior auditory field (PAF), 475

Posterior cerebral artery (PCA), 154
Posterior cricoarytenoid (PCA) muscle, 367, 367f
Posterior (dorsal) roots, 221
Posterior fossa, 216
Posterior neuropore, 109f, 111
Posterior SCC, 525
Posterior ventral cochlear nucleus (PVCN), 472
Posterolateral fissure, 158
Postictal paralysis, 206
Poststimulus time histograms (PSTHs), 472
Postsynaptic acetylcholine receptors (AChRs),
        239
Postsynaptic potentials, 176–178
    channelopathies, 178
        graded potentials, 177, 178t
        spatial summation, 177
        temporal summation, 177
        tetrodotoxin, 177, 177f
Postural instability, 207
PQ. See Phonation quotient (PQ)
preBötC. See Pre-Bötzinger complex (preBötC)
Pre-Bötzinger complex (preBötC), 335
Precentral gyrus, 147
Prechordal plate, 109
Premaxilla, 395, 397f
Premolars, 401
Premotor cortex, 147, 369
Preoccipital notch, 146–147
Presbycusis, 287
Pressure, 381
Pressure trainer, 331f
Prestin, 466
Presynaptic membrane, 239
Primary afferent innervation zones, 276
Primary auditory cortex, 149, 475
Primary fissure, 158
Primary motor cortex, 147, 147f
Primary palate, 119f, 120
Primary sensory areas, 270
Primary somatosensory cortex, 149, 149f, 546
Primary visual cortex, 149–150, 286
Primary vs. permanent teeth, 402f
Primitive medullary cells differentiation, 112
    axons, 112
        glioblasts, 112
        myelin, 112
        oligodendrocytes, 112
Primitive streak, 107
Primitive streak and notochord, 108–109, 108f
    buccopharyngeal membrane, 109
    intraembryonic mesoderm, 108
    prechordal plate, 109
Prodrug, 332
Projection neurons, 144
Projections to α-LMNs, 198–199
Prokaryotes and eukaryotes, 32–34, 33f
    capsule, 33
    cell wall, 33
    comparison, 33t
    flagellum, 33
    nucleoid, 33
    nucleus, 33
    ribosomes, 33
Promontory, 451
Proprioception, 272, 275, 275f
Prosencephalon, 113
Protein degradation, 85
Proteins, 82
    proteome, 82
    translation of mRNA, 81f, 82
Protein synthesis regulation, 84–85
    genetic code, 85f
    homeostasis, 84
    nucleotide base pairs, 85f
    ribosomal RNA (rRNA), 84

Proteome, 82
Proximal, 7
PRS. See Pierre Robin sequence (PRS)
Pseudoathetosis, 219
PSTHs. See Poststimulus time histograms
        (PSTHs)
Psychophysics, 266
PTP. See Phonation threshold pressure (PTP)
Pulmonary artery and veins, 318, 318f
Pulmonary edema, 338, 340
Pulmonary embolism (PE), 341
Pulmonary extraction, 332
Pulmonary hypertension, 341
Pulmonary infection, nontubercular mycobacte-
        ria (pNTM), 327
Pulmonary stretch receptors, 337
Pulmonary surfactant, 338
Pulse register, 377
Purkinje cell, 143, 143f, 217, 217f
Putamen, 150, 203
PVCN. See Posterior ventral cochlear nucleus
        (PVCN)
PVFM. See Paradoxical vocal fold motion (PVFM)
Pyramidal cell, 143, 143f
Pyramidal cells, DCN, 472
Pyramidal eminence, 452
Pyramidal pathway, 369
Pyramids, 162
Pyruvate oxidation, 43f

Q
Quadrangular membrane, 358
Quantification of sensation and perception,
        265–266
    just-noticeable differences (JNDs), 266
    magnitude estimation, 266
    psychophysics, 266
    sensory threshold sensibility, 266

R
Radiography, 429–431, 430ff
Ramus, 394
Rapidly adapting (RA) receptors, 270
RA receptors. See Rapidly adapting (RA)
        receptors
Rarefaction, 444
Receptive field, 267, 267f
Receptor coding of intensity, 269
Receptors, 48, 50–53
    cell surface receptors, 50
    enzyme, 51
    enzyme-linked receptors, 51, 52f
    G-protein-coupled receptors (GPCRs), 52, 52f
    intracellular receptors, 50–51, 51f
    ligand, 50
    second messengers, 52
    signal transduction, 51
Recombination, 90, 91f
Recruitment, 249
Recurrent laryngeal nerve (RLN), 368
Reduced preparations, 221
Reflexes, 168
    extensor muscle, 168
    flexor muscle, 168
    stretch reflex, 168
Reinke space, 361
Reisner membrane, 454
Renin, 332
Renin-angiotensin-aldosterone system (RAAS),
        332
Renshaw cell, 193
Residual volume (RV), 321
Resistive trainer, 330f
Resonance. See Articulation and resonance
Resonance effect, 225, 225f, 226f

Resonant frequency, 445
Respiration, 311–350
    active inspiration, 319–322, 320f, 321f
        active expiration, 321f
        alveolar ventilation rate, 321
        Boyle's law, 319, 320f
        expiratory reserve volume (ERV), 321
        inspiratory reserve volume (IRV), 321
        minute ventilation (MV), 321
        residual volume (RV), 321
        tidal volume, 321
        total lung capacity (TLC), 320
        vital capacity (VC), 321, 321f
    adenosine triphosphate (ATP), 312
    air conduction and filtration, 323–324, 323f
        mucociliary escalator, 323
        phlegm, 322
    airway protection, 324–328
        aging and coughing, 326
        cystic fibrosis, 324
        dystussia, 327
        homeostatic emotion, 325
        pulmonary infection, nontubercular
                mycobacteria (pNTM), 327
        urge-to-cough (UTC), 324, 324f, 325f
    blood pH and homeostasis, 334–335
        alkalemia, 335
        pH buffer, 334
    blood pressure, homeostasis and, 332
        baroreceptors, 332
        renin, 332
        renin-angiotensin-aldosterone system
                (RAAS), 332
    blood reserves and homeostasis, 332–333
    carbon dioxide transport from tissues to
            lungs, 322–323, 323f
        homeostasis, 322
    circulatory system filtration, 329, 331
        fibrin, 331
        fibrinolysin, 331
        heparin, 331
        thromboplastin, 331
    gas exchange in tissue, 322
        capillary basement membrane, 322
        capillary epithelium, 322
        epithelial basement membrane, 322
        internal respiration, 322
        peripheral gas exchange, 322
    immunoprotection, 329
        cytokines, 329
        immunologic defense mechanisms, 329
        T cells, 329
    lower respiratory system, 313–317, 312f
        alveoli, 316
        alveolar gas exchange, 316f
        bones of respiration, 317
        bronchi, 313, 316f
        bronchioles, 316
        costal surface, 314
        diaphragm, 314, 317, 317f
        external intercostal muscles, 317, 318f
        hilum, 314
        hydrostatic force, 315
        hydrostasis, 315
        inspiration, 317
        lobar bronchi, 316
        mediastinum, 314
        phrenic nerves, 317
        pleural cavity, 315, 315f
        pleural linkage, 315
        pneumothorax, 315–316, 315f
        pulmonary artery and veins, 318, 318f
        segmental bronchi, 316
        trachea and bronchial tree, 313ff, 316f
    lungs, 312, 314, 314ff

muscle strength training for respiration, 330–331
  detraining effect, 330
  hypertrophy, 330
  inspiratory-expiratory muscle strength training (IMST-EMST), 330
  Poiseuille's law, 330
  pressure trainer, 331*f*
  resistive trainer, 330*f*
  synaptogenesis, 330
oxygen reserves and homeostasis, 333–334
  erythropoietin, 333
  hypoxia, 333
pH, 312
pharmacokinetics, 332
  prodrug, 332
  pulmonary extraction, 332
respiratory dysfunction, 338–341
  acute bronchitis, 339
  acute respiratory distress syndrome(ARDS), 340
  aging, 342
  asthma, 339
  Cheyne-Stokes respiration, 341
  chronic obstructive pulmonary disease (COPD), 339, 340
  cystic fibrosis (CF), 339
  disordered speech, language, or swallowing effects, 342–343
  dyspnea, 339
  hyperventilation, 341
  hypoventilation, 338
  interstitial lung disease, 341
  lung cancer, 340
  pleural effusion (PE), 341
  pneumoconiosis, 340–341
  pneumonia, 340
  pneumothorax, 341
  pulmonary edema, 340
  pulmonary embolism (PE), 341
  pulmonary hypertension, 341
  sleep apnea, 338
sensorineural control of respiration, 335–338, 336*f*, 337*f*
  aortic body, 336
  apneustic center, 335
  body temperature regulation, 337, 337*f*
  carotid body, 336
  central chemoreceptors, 336
  central pattern generator (CPG), 335
  dorsal respiratory groups, 335
  exteroceptors, 336
  Hering-Breuer inflation reflex, 338
  hypercapnic hypoxia, 337
  interoceptors, 336
  irritant receptors, 337
  juxtacapillary receptors (J-receptors), 337
  medullary respiratory center, 335
  peripheral chemoreceptors, 336, 336*f*
  pneumotaxic center, 335–336
  pre-Bötzinger complex (preBötC), 335
  pulmonary edema, 338
  pulmonary stretch receptors, 337
  pulmonary surfactant, 338
  reticular formation, 335
  tachycardia, 338
  ventral respiratory groups, 335
thermoregulation, 335
upper respiratory system, 312–313, 312*f*
  ethmoidal air cells, 312
  frontal sinuses, 312
  maxillary sinuses, 312
  nasal conchae, 313
  nasal septum, 312
  paranasal sinuses, 312

  sphenoidal sinuses, 312
  thoracic activity, 313
  Valsalva maneuver, 313
uptake and transformation of endogenous and exogenous substances, 332
  vasoactive, 332
venous and arterial systems connection, 335
vocal folds, 312
voicing and speech, 328–329
  amplitude, 328
  expiratory muscle strength training, (EMST), 329
  fundamental frequency, 328
  inspiratory muscle strength training, (IMST), 329
  phonation threshold pressure (PTP), 328
  subglottal air pressure, 328
Respiratory dysfunction, 338–341
  acute bronchitis, 339
  acute respiratory distress syndrome(ARDS), 340
  aging, 342
  asthma, 339
  Cheyne-Stokes respiration, 341
  chronic obstructive pulmonary disease (COPD), 339, 340
  cystic fibrosis (CF), 339
  disordered speech, language, or swallowing effects, 342–343
  dyspnea, 339
  hyperventilation, 341
  hypoventilation, 338
  interstitial lung disease, 341
  lung cancer, 340
  pleural effusion (PE), 341
  pneumoconiosis, 340–341
  pneumonia, 340
  pneumothorax, 341
  pulmonary edema, 340
  pulmonary embolism (PE), 341
  pulmonary hypertension, 341
  sleep apnea, 338
Respiratory epithelium, 360, 360*f*
Respiratory spinal nerves, 510*t*
Respiratory-swallowing relationships, 499
  apnea, 499
  chronic obstructive pulmonary disease (COPD), 500, 500*f*
Respiratory system, 23–24
  diaphragm, 23
  expiration, 23
  external muscles, 23
  inspiration, 23
  intercostal muscles, 23
  and phonation, 24
Respiratory system development, 125–126
  lung buds, 125
  median laryngotracheal groove, 125
  tracheobronchial tree, 125*f*
Resting membrane potential, 174–175
  adenosine triphosphate (ATP), 175
  diffusion, 175
  homeostasis, 19
  sodium-potassium pump, 175
Resting tremor, 207
Restoring force, 445
Reticular lamina, 458
Reticular formation, 298, 335
Reticular system, 163
Reticulospinal system, 167
Retina, 281–283, 539
  amacrine cells, 281
  binocular visual zone, 282–283
  blind spot, 282
  cones, 281

  fovea, 281
  foveola, 282
  glaucoma, 283
  hemifield, 282
  horizontal cells, 281
  optic disc, 281
  retinal layers, 281*f*
  rods, 281
  visual fields, 282*f*
Retinal layers, 281*f*
Retinotopy, 286
Reverberation, 446
Reversibility principle, 254
Rhinal sulcus, 150
Rhinencephalon, 115
Rhombencephalon, 113
Ribbon synapse, 457
Rib cage, 16
Ribonucleic acid (RNA), 77–78, 81–82
  messenger RNA (mRNA), 82
  transcription, 82, 82*f*
Ribosomal RNA (rRNA), 84
Ribosomes, 33
Rigidity, 207
Risorius, 404–405, 405*f*
RLN. *See* Recurrent laryngeal nerve (RLN)
RNA. *See* Ribonucleic acid (RNA)
Rod and cone light wavelength sensitivities, 284*f*
Rods, 281
Root primordia, 124
Rosenthal canal, 454
Rostral, 7
Rough ER, 38
Round window, 451
rRNA. *See* Ribosomal RNA (rRNA)
Ruffini endings, 274
RV. *See* Residual volume (RV)

S

Saccule, 296
Saccule otolithic organ, 525
Sacral spine, 16
Sagittal plane, 8
Sagittal plane reconstructions, 204*f*
SAID principle. *See* Specific adaptation to imposed demand (SAID) principle
Salivary glands, 491–493
  parotid salivary gland, 491
  submandibular and sublingual salivary glands, 493
Saltatory conduction, 178–179, 466
  action potential-initiating segment, 178
  axon hillock, 178
  continuous and saltatory propagation of action potentials, 179
  myelin, 178
  nodes of Ranvier, 178
Sarcolemma, 239
Sarcomeres, 239, 242*f*, 243*f*
Sarcoplasmic reticulum (SR), 239
SA receptors. *See* Slowly adapting (SA)
SC. *See* Superior colliculus (SC)
Scala media, 289, 455, 455*f*
Scala tympani, 289, 454, 455*f*
Scala vestibuli, 289, 454
Scanning speech, 218
SCCs. *See* Semicircular canals (SCCs)
Schwann cells, 144, 144*f*, 174
Sclerotomes, 109
Secondary palate, 120, 123*f*
Second messengers, 52
Second messenger system, 285
Segmental bronchi, 316
Segmental motor control, 194
Self-oscillating system, 370

Self-organization into attractor states, 223
Semicircular canals (SCCs), 524, 525*f*
Sensation loss, 219
    peripheral neuropathy, 219
    pseudoathetosis, 219
Sensation vs. perception, 264–265
    action potentials, 264
    central nervous system (CNS), 264
    labeled-line principle of sensory systems, 265
    percept, 265
    perception, 264
    sensory receptors, 264
Sensorimotor control of swallowing, 502–504, 503*f*
    afferents, 503
    behavioral control assembly, 504
    brainstem, 504
    central pattern generator (CPG), 504, 504*f*
    chemoreceptors, 503
    mechanoreceptors, 503
    vagus nerve, 504*f*
Sensorineural control of respiration, 335–338, 336*f*, 337*f*
    aortic body, 336
    apneustic center, 335
    body temperature regulation, 337, 337*f*
    carotid body, 336
    central chemoreceptors, 336
    central pattern generator (CPG), 335
    dorsal respiratory groups, 335
    exteroceptors, 336
    Hering-Breuer inflation reflex, 338
    hypercapnic hypoxia, 337
    interoceptors, 336
    irritant receptors, 337
    juxtacapillary receptors (J-receptors), 337
    medullary respiratory center, 335
    peripheral chemoreceptors, 336, 336*f*
    pneumotaxic center, 335–336
    pre-Bötzinger complex (preBötC), 335
    pulmonary edema, 338
    pulmonary stretch receptors, 337
    pulmonary surfactant, 338
    reticular formation, 335
    tachycardia, 338
    ventral respiratory groups, 335
Sensorineural hearing loss, 184*t*, 449
Sensory fibers, 113
Sensory receptors, 264
Sensory receptors, somatosensory system, 273–276
    pain, 276
    proprioception, 275, 275*f*
    temperature, 275–276
    touch, 273–274
Sensory systems, 263–307
    angular acceleration by semicircular canals measurement, 297
        ampula, 296*f*, 297
        cupula, 297
    anterolateral system (ALS), 278–279, 278*t*
        spinothalamic tract, 248
    auditory system, 287–295
        basilar membrane, 290–291, 290*f*
        central auditory pathways, 292–295
        cochlea, 289–290
        hair cells, 291–292
        organ of Corti, (OoC), 289
        presbycusis, 287
    central auditory pathway structures, 292, 292*f*
        auditory cortex, 295
        auditory nerve and cochlear nuclei, 293
        cochlear implants, 294
        inferior colliculus, 292, 294
        medial geniculate body (MGB), 292, 295

superior olivary complex, (SOC), 292
superior olivary complex and sound localization, 293, 294*f*
central somatosensory pathways, 278–281
    anterolateral system (ALS), 278–279
    dorsal-column medial lemniscal (DCML) system, 278
    somatosensory cortex, 280
    trigemial lemniscus and trigeminothalamic tract, 278, 279*f*
central vestibular pathway, 297–298, 298*f*
    flocculonodular lobe, 297
    lateral vestibulospinal tract, 298
    medial vestibulospinal tract, 298
    reticular formation, 298
    ventral posterior (VP) nuclei, 297
    vestibular nuclei, 297
    vestibulospinal tracts, 298
central visual pathway, 286–288, 286*f*
    lateral geniculate nucleus (LGN), 286
    optic radiations, 286
    optic tract, 286
    primary visual cortex, 286
    retinotopy, 286
    superior colliculus (SC), 286
chemical senses, 298–299
    central olfactory pathway, 300–301
    gustatory receptors and transduction, 301–303, 302*f*
    gustatory system, 301
    odorant molecules, 299
    olfactory receptors and transduction mechanism, 299–300
    olfactory system, 299
    tastant molecules, 299
dorsal-column medial lemniscal (DCML) system, 278, 278*t*
    cuneate fasciculi, 278
    gracile fasciculi, 278
    postcentral gyrus, 278
    thalamocortical fibers, 278
    ventral posterolateral (VPL) nucleus, 278
duration, 270, 270*f*
    rapidly adapting (RA) receptors, 270
    slowly adapting (SA) receptors, 270
gustatory system, 301
    dysosmias, 303
    gustatory pathways, 302*f*
    gustatory receptors and transduction, 301–303, 302*f*
    nucleus of solitary tract (NST), 303
    parabrachial nuclei (PBN), 303
    phantosmias, 303
    taste buds, 301
    xerostomia, 302
hair cells, 291–292
    cochlear nucei, 292, 292*f*
    inner hair cells (IHCs), 291
    kinocilium, 291
    outer hair cells (OHCs), 291
    stereocilia, 291
    tip links, 292
intensity, 269
    action potential, 269, 269*f*
    ion channels, 269
    receptor coding of intensity, 269
    receptor potential, 269, 269*f*
light transduction and retinal processing, 283–286
    cyclic guanosine monophosphate (cGMP), 285
    glutamate, 285
    OFF bipolar cells, 285, 285*f*
    ON bipolar cells, 285, 285*f*
    phototransduction mechanism, 284*f*

rod and cone light wavelength sensitivities, 284*f*
    second messenger system, 285
location, 267–268
    lateral inhibition, 268
    receptive field, 267, 267*f*
    two-point discrimination test, 268
modality, 267
    chemoreceptors, 267
    mechanoreceptors, 267
    nociceptors, 267
    photoreceptors, 267
    tuning curve, 267
olfactory system, 299
    central olfactory pathway, 300–301
    olfactory bulb, 299
    olfactory receptors and transduction mechanism, 299–300
    olfactory tract, 300
organization, 270–271
    hierarchical information-processing structure, 270
    higher-order sensory areas, 270
    primary sensory areas, 270
    regulation, 271
quantification of sensation and perception, 265–266
    just-noticeable differences (JNDs), 266
    magnitude estimation, 266
    psychophysics, 266
    sensory threshold sensibility, 266
retina, 281–283
    amacrine cells, 281
    binocular visual zone, 282–283
    blind spot, 282
    cones, 281
    fovea, 281
    foveola, 282
    glaucoma, 283
    hemifield, 282
    horizontal cells, 281
    optic disc, 281
    retinal layers, 281*f*
    rods, 281
    visual fields, 282*f*
sensation vs. perception, 264–265
    action potentials, 264
    central nervous system (CNS), 264
    labeled-line principle of sensory systems, 265
    percept, 265
    perception, 264
    sensory receptors, 264
sensory receptors, somatosensory system, 273–276
    pain, 276
    proprioception, 275, 275*f*
    temperature, 275–276
    touch, 273–274
somatosensory cortex, 280, 280*f*
    Brodman areas, 280
    homunculus, 280
somatosensory system, 271–278
    anterolateral system (ALS), 272
    dermatomes, 277, 277*f*
    dorsal-column medial lemniscal (DCML) pathway, 272
    exteroception, 272
    interoception, 272
    orofacial region, 276–277
    primary afferent innervation zones, 276
    proprioception, 272
    sensory receptors, somatosensory system, 273–276
    synesthesia, 271

trigeminal innervation zones, 277–278
trigeminal lemniscus, 272
trigeminothalamic pathway, 272
stimulus attributes related to perception, 267–270
  duration, 270, 270*f*
  intensity, 269
  location, 267–268
  modality, 267
touch, 273–274
  cutaneous mechanoreceptors, 273*f*, 274*t*
  hair follicles, 274
  Meissner corpuscle, 274
  Merkel disks, 274
  Pacinian (PC), 274
  Ruffini endings, 274
transduction of linear motion by otolith organs, 296–297, 296*f*
  macula, 296
  otoconia, 296
  otolithic membrane, 296
  saccule, 296
  utricle, 296
trigeminal lemniscus and trigeminothalamic tract, 278, 279*f*
  ventral posteromedial (VPM), 280
vestibular system, 295–298, 296*f*
  angular acceleration by semicircular canals measurement, 297
  central vestibular pathway, 297–298, 298*f*
  transduction of linear motion by otolith organs, 296–297
visual system, 281–288
  central visual pathway, 286–288, 286*f*
  dorsal stream, 287–288
  light transduction and retinal processing, 283–286
  retina, 281–283
  ventral stream, 288
Sensory threshold sensibility, 266
Septum pellucidum, 150
Sexual reproduction, 105
Sherrington's reflexology, 222
Shimmer, 382
Shortening/lengthening velocity control, 251
Signal transduction, 51
Simple harmonic motion, 445
Simple sounds, 445
Sine wave, 445
Sinusoid, 445
Size principle, 249
Skeletal and muscular system, 10–19
  extremities, 18, 18*f*
  joints, 18–19
    cartilaginous joint, 18
    fibrous joints, 18
    synovial joint, 18
  muscular system, 19
    cardiac muscle, 19
    insertion of muscle, 19
    origin of muscle, 19
    skeletal muscle, 19
    smooth muscle, 19
  skull, 10–14
    base, 14*f*
    cranial bones, 10, 13*f*
    cranial sutures, 15*f*
    facial bones, 13*f*
    fontanelles, 14, 15*f*
    foramen magnum, 10
    neurocranium, 10, 13*f*
    viscerocranium, 10, 13*f*
  torso, 16–18, 17*f*
    abdominal cavity, 17
    abdominopelvic cavity, 17

pelvic cavity, 17
rib cage, 16
thoracic cavity, 17
thoracic wall, 16, 17*f*
thorax, 16
vertebral column, 14–16
  bony vertebral column, 16*f*
  cervical spine, 16
  lumbar spine, 16
  sacral spine, 16
  thoracic spine, 16
Skeletal muscle, 60, 60*f*, 239, 241–244
  A-bands, 241
  actin, 241
  adenosine triphosphate (ATP), 243
  cross-bridge theory, 243, 243*f*
  muscle fiber types, 243–244, 244*t*
  myosin, 241, 242*f*
  sarcomeres, 239, 242*f*, 243*f*
  sliding filament theory, 243
  striated muscle, 241*f*
  structure, 241*f*
  tropomyosin, 241, 242*f*
  troponin, 241
  Z-line, 241
Skeletal muscle disease, 252–253
  muscular dystrophy, 252
  myasthenia gravis, 253
Skull, 10–15
  base, 14*f*
  cranial bones, 10, 13*f*
  cranial sutures, 15*f*
  facial bones, 13*f*
  fontanelles, 14, 15*f*
  foramen magnum, 10
  neurocranium, 10, 13*f*
  viscerocranium, 10, 13*f*
Skull sutures, 65*f*
Sleep apnea, 338
Sliding filament theory, 243
Slowly adapting (SA) receptors, 270
SLP. *See* Superficial lamina propria (SLP)
Smoking, effect on epithelial cells, 56
Smooth ER, 38
Smooth muscle, 19, 59, 60*f*
SNc. *See* Substantia nigra pars compacta (SNc)
SNr. *See* Substantia nigra pars reticulata (SNr)
SOC. *See* Superior olivary complex
Sodium-potassium pump, 46–47, 48*f*, 175
Soft palate muscles, 413*t*, 414*f*
Solitary tract, 113
Soma, 139*f*, 141, 173
Somatic motor, 466
Somatic motor fibers, 141
Somatic nervous system (SNS), 19
Somatic sensory fibers, 141
Somatosensation and volitional control of swallowing, 505
Somatosensory and taste innervation, tongue, 491
Somatosensory cortex, 280, 280*f*
  Brodman areas, 280
  homunculus, 280
Somatosensory system, 271–278
  anterolateral system (ALS), 272
  dermatomes, 277, 277*f*
  dorsal-column medial lemniscal (DCML) pathway, 272
  exteroception, 272
  interoception, 272
  orofacial region, 276–277
  primary afferent innervation zones, 276
  proprioception, 272
  sensory receptors, somatosensory system, 273–276

synesthesia, 271
trigeminal innervation zones, 277–278
trigeminal lemniscus, 272
trigeminothalamic pathway, 272
Somatotopy, 167
Somites formation, 109–111, 110*f*
  dermatomes, 111
  myotomes, 110
  sclerotomes, 109
Sound, 444–447, 444*f*
  aperiodic sound waves, 445
  central auditory system, 444
  complex sounds, 445
  condensation, 444
  cycle, 445
  dampening, 445
  decibels (dB), 446
  duplex theory, 446
  force, 444
  forced vibration, 445
  free field, 446
  free vibration, 445
  frequency, 445
  friction, 445
  fundamental frequency, 445
  head shadow, 447
  hertz (Hz), 445
  impedances, 446
  inertia, 444
  intensity, 445
  interaural level differences (ILDs), 446
  interaural timing differences, 446, 447*f*
  inverse square law, 446
  loudness, 445
  oscillation, 445
  pascals (Pa), 445
  periodic sound waves, 445
  peripheral auditory system, 444
  pinna, 447
  pitch, 445
  rarefaction, 444
  resonant frequency, 445
  restoring force, 445
  reverberation, 446
  simple harmonic motion, 445
  simple sounds, 445
  sine wave, 445
  sinusoid, 445
  specific acoustic impedance (Z), 446
  waveform, 445
  wavelength, 445
Sound intensity, 382
Source-filter theory, 426–429, 427*f*, 428*f*
SP. *See* Summating potential (SP)
Space of Nuel, 456
Spasticity, 203
Spatial summation, 177
Specific acoustic impedance (Z), 446
Specific adaptation to imposed demand (SAID) principle, 234, 254
Spectral acoustic analyses, 382
Speech and language disorders, 98, 98*f*
Speech systems, 24
Sperm, 105
Spermatogenesis, 105, 105*f*
Sphenoidal sinuses, 312
Sphenoid bone, 398*f*, 399
  chiasmic groove, 399
  crista galli, 399
  foramen ovale, 399
  foramen rotundum, 399
  foramina, 399
  jugum, 399
  medial pterygoid muscle, 399
  optic canal, 399

superior orbital fissure, 399
tensor veli palatini muscle, 399
Spherical cells, AVCN, 472
Spinal cord, 165–168
  autonomic nervous system, 167
  cauda equina, 166
  conus medullaris, 165
  gray matter, 166
    dermatome, 166
    lower motor neurons, 166
  lower motor neurons, 167
  reflexes, 168
    extensor muscle, 168
    flexor muscle, 168
    stretch reflex, 168
  upper motor neurons, 167
  white matter, 166–167, 167f
    dorsal column, 166
    reticulospinal system, 167
    somatotopy, 167
    spinothalamic tract, 166
    vestibulospinal tract, 167
Spinal cord development, 112–113
Spinocerebellum, 217
Spinothalamic tract, 166, 278
Spiral ganglion neuron, 458
Spiral ligament, 455f, 456
Splenium, 150
Spongy bone, 63
Spontaneous action potential firing rate, 469,
    470f
Squamous, 447
SR. See Sarcoplasmic reticulum (SR)
Stapedius muscle, 452
Stapedius nerve, 454
Stapes, 453
Stellate cells, 474
Stem cells, 61
  adult stem cells, 61
  embryonic stem cells, 61
  induced pluripotent stem cells, 61
Stenosis, 448
Stepping strategy, 543, 544f
Stereocilia, 291, 457, 528
Sternoclavicular ligament, 364
Sternothyroid muscle, 364, 364f
STG. See Superior temporal gyrus (STG)
Stimulus attributes related to perception,
    267–270
  duration, 270, 270f
    rapidly adapting (RA) receptors, 270
    slowly adapting (SA) receptors, 270
  intensity, 269
    action potential, 269, 269f
    ion channels, 269
    receptor coding of intensity, 269
  location, 267–268
    lateral inhibition, 268
    receptive field, 267, 267f
    two-point discrimination test, 268
  modality, 267
    chemoreceptors, 267
    mechanoreceptors, 267
    nociceptors, 267
    photoreceptors, 267
    tuning curve, 267
  touch, 273–274
    cutaneous mechanoreceptors, 273f, 274t
    hair follicles, 274
    Meissner corpuscle, 274
    Merkel disks, 274
    Pacinian (PC), 274
    Ruffini endings, 274
Stochastic resonance, 215
Straight sinus, 155

Stratium, 151, 203
Stretch reflex, 168
Striated muscle, 241f
Stria vascularis, 456
Stroke, 184t
Stylid process, 364, 364f
Stylohyoid muscle, 364, 364f, 423, 424
Subarachnoid space, 155
Subcortex, 150–153
  basal ganglia, 150, 151ff
  caudate nucleus, 151
  cerebellar mutism, 153
  diencephalon, 152–153, 152f
  globus pallidus, 151
  Huntington's disease, 151
  hypothalamus, 152
  interthalamic adhesion, 151f, 152
  limbic system, 153, 153f
  Parkinson's disease, 151, 152
  pineal gland, 152
  putamen, 150
  stratium, 151
  thalamus, 152
  third ventricle, 152
Subdural hemorrhage, 155, 156f
Subglottal air pressure, 328
Submandibular and sublingual salivary glands,
    493
Substantia nigra, 114, 161
Substantia nigra pars compacta (SNc), 204
Substantia nigra pars reticulata (SNr), 203
Subthalamic nucleus, 195
Sulci, 20, 145, 199
Sulcus terminalis, 124
Summating potential (SP), 467
Superficial cerebral veins, 155
Superficial lamina propria (SLP), 361
Superior colliculi (SC), 114, 161, 286
Superior laryngeal nerve, 368
Superior longitudinal muscle, 420
Superior olivary complex (SOC), 292, 458, 473
  lateral superior olivary nucleus (LSO), 473
  medial nucleus, trapezoid body (MNTB), 473
  medial superior olivary nucleus (MSO), 473
  periolivary group, 473
Superior olivary complex and sound localiza-
    tion, 293, 294f
Superior orbital fissure, 399
Superior sagittal sinus, 155
Superior temporal gyrus (STG), 147
Supplementary motor area, 369
Supportive connective tissues, 63–64
  bones, 62–63, 63t, 64f
  cartilage, 63, 64t
  compact bone, 63
  spongy bone, 63
Suprahyoid aponeurosis, 364
Suprahyoid muscles, 362
Suprasegmental motor control, 191–231
  alpha lower motor neuron (α-LMNs), 192
  anatomical system, 198–202, 198f
    Brodmann area, 6, 199
    cortical innervation of facial nerve nuclei,
        200
    corticospinal tract, 199f
    free arm movements, 201, 201f
    gyri, 199
    homunculus, 200, 200f
    internal capsule, 199
    lobes, 199
    motor cortex, 199–202
    projections to α-LMNs, 198–199
    sulci, 199
    upper motor neurons, (UMNs), 199
    ventral intermediate nucleus, 199

associated cortex, 218–219
  ideational apraxia, 218
  ideomotor apraxia, 218
  kinetic apraxia, 218
  limb-kinetic apraxia, 218
basal ganglia-thalamic-cortical system,
    202–215, 203f
  caudate nucleus, 203
  centromedian, 204
  D1 receptors, 205
  D2 receptors, 205
  direct pathway, 204
  dopaminergic neurons, 204
  gamma-aminobutyric acid (GABA), 204
  glutamate, 204
  hyperreflexia, 203
  indirect pathway, 204
  large aspiny neurons, 204
  medium spiny neurons (MSNs), 205
  mereological fallacy, 203
  parafascicular nuclei, 204
  putamen, 203
  sagittal plane reconstructions, 204f
  spasticity, 203
  striatum, 203
  substantia nigra pars compacta (SNc), 204
  substantia nigra pars reticulata (SNr), 203
brainstem, 192
brain structure functions hypotheses,
    205–206
  contraries, 206
  inverse problem, 206
  method of concomitant variations, 206
  negative symptoms, 206
  positive symptoms, 4
  postictal paralysis, 206
  Todd paralysis, 206
  transcranial magnetic stimulation (TMS), 206
cerebellar disorders, 218
  action tremor, 218
  ataxia, 218
  bradykinesia movement, 218
  dymetric movement, 218
  dysdiadochokinesia, 218
  hypermetria, 218
  hypometria, 218
  hypotonia, 218
  scanning speech, 218
cerebellum, 192, 215–217
  archicerebellum, 216
  axon collaterals, 217
  brachium conjunctivum, 217
  climbing fibers, 217
  complex spike, 217
  dentate nuclei, 216
  emboliform nuclei, 216
  fastigal nuclei, 216
  globose nuclei, 216
  granule cells, 217
  inferior olivary nucleus, 217
  interpositus nuclei, 216
  lateral zone, 216
  mossy fibers, 217
  neocerebellum, 216
  paleocerebellum, 216
  parallel fibers, 217
  paravermal zone, 216
  peduncles, 216, 216f
  pontine relay nuclei, 217
  posterior fossa, 216
  Purkinje cell, 217, 217f
  spinocerebellum, 217
  vermal zone, 216
complex systems and network of oscillators
    approach, 222–227

beat interactions, 224
continuous harmonic oscillators, 224
discrete oscillators, 224
kinesia paradoxica, 227
multiple neuron-like processing units, 224, 225f
necker cube, 223, 223f
neuronal action potentials, 223, 223f
nonlinear interactions, 222
oscillator phase changes, 224
resonance effect, 225, 225f, 226f
self-organization into attractor states, 223
systems oscillator theory, 224, 225f
correlation, lesion and function, 219–220, 220f
deep brain stimulation, limb vs. speech, 194
disorders, basal ganglia-thalamic cortical
system, 207
akinesia, 207
ballismus, 207
bradykinesia, 207
chorea, 207
dystonia, 207
hastening, 207
hemiballismus, 207
Huntington disease, 207
hyperkinetic disorders, 207
hypokinetic disorders, 207
kinesia paradoxica, 207
levodopa, 207
masklike facies, 207
monotone speech, 207
postural instability, 207
resting tremor, 207
rigidity, 207
gamma lower motor neuron (γ-LMNs), 193
models, basal ganglia-thalamic cortical
system, 207–215
anatomically based theories, 208, 209f
antidromic action potentials, 214
beta oscillation theory, 210–211
bifurcations, 213
cholinergic/dopaminergic imbalance theory, 208
circuit-based model, 212, 212f
direct pathway, 208
dynamic circuits, 213–214, 214f
globus pallidus internal segment (GPi) rate
theory, 209–210, 210f
hyperdirect pathway, 208
intramuscular electromyographic (EMG)
activities, 214
one-dimensional push-pull concept, 208
Parkinson's and dopamine, 215
physiologic and pathophysiologic models, 209
polysynaptic nonlinear oscillators, 211, 211f
stochastic resonance, 215
pallidotomy, 209
motor control hierarchy, 221–222
decerebrate posturing, 221
decorticate posturing, 221
degrees of freedom, 221
dorsal rhizotomy, 221
dorsal root ganglia, 221
inferior colliculi, 221
lateral vestibular nucleus, 221
one-dimensional conceptual approach, 222
posterior (dorsal) roots, 221
reduced preparations, 221
Sherrington's reflexology, 222
motor cortex, 192
motor unit (MU), 192
acetylcholine, 193
action potential-initiating segment, 193

action potentials, 193
all-or-none response, 193
cell body, 193
dendrites, 193
interneurons, 194
muscle spindle, 193
Renshaw cell, 193
segmental motor control, 194
motor unit activation, 195–198
decomposition of movement, 197
deep brain stimulation (DBS), 196
electrical activity generated by motor units, 197
Heinneman size principle, 195
organization of information, 197–198
Parkinson's disease, 195
subthalamic nucleus, 195
muscle spindle, 194, 194f
pathophysiology, 192
sensation loss, 219
peripheral neuropathy, 219
pseudoathetosis, 219
suprasegmental control, 192
suprasegmental structures, 195, 195t
associational cortex, 195
basil ganglia, 195
brainstem, 195
cerebellum, 195
motor cortex, 195
Suspensory strategy, 543, 544f
Swallowing, 483–521
anatomy of swallowing, 484–495
afferent, 484
buccinator muscle, 487f
central pattern generators (CPGs), 485
cleft lip and palate, 486, 486f
efferent, 484
esophagus and trachea, 496f
extrinsic muscles, tongue, 491
intrinsic muscles, tongue, 491f
laryngopharynx, 494f
lateral pterygoid muscle, 489f
medial pterygoid muscle, 488f
masseter and temporalis muscles, 488f
mastication muscles, 489t
masticatory muscles, 488f
maxillary teeth, permanent, 487f
oral cavity structures, 487f
orbicularis oris, 487f
Parkinson disease (PD), 485, 485f
parotid salivary gland, 491
pharyngeal constrictor muscles, 494f
pharynx divisions, 493f
pharynx muscles, 495t
somatosensory and taste innervation,
tongue, 491
submandibular and sublingual salivary
glands, 493
temporomandibular joint, 488f
tongue anatomy, 489f
unilateral hypoglossal nerve lesion, 490, 490f
assessment methods, 513–516
clinical swallowing evaluation, 513
electromyography (EMG), 515
flexible endoscopic evaluation of swallowing (FEES), 514–515
manometry, 515–516
nasoendoscopy, 514–515
ultrasonography, 516
videofluoroscopy, 513–514, 514ff
biological function, 484
airway obstruction, 484
aspiration, 484
aspiration pneumonia, 484

bolus, 484
deglutition, 484
dysphagia, 484
feeding, 484
mastication, 484
disorders, 510–513
amyotrophic lateral sclerosis, 511, 511f
failure to thrive, 510
Pierre Robin sequence (PRS), 512, 512f
efferent motor control, 505–510
facial nerve, 508t
facial nerve branches, 506f
glossopharyngeal nerve, 506f, 509t
hypoglossal nerve, 507f, 510t
respiratory spinal nerves, 510t
trigeminal nerve, 508t
vagus nerve, 509t
head and neck cancers, 492, 492f
fibrosis, 492
odynophagia, 492
xerostomia, 492
phases, 495–499, 499f
esophageal phase, 498
oral phase, 497
oral-preparatory phase, 495–497
pharyngeal phase, 497–498
respiratory-swallowing relationships, 499
apnea, 499
chronic obstructive pulmonary disease
(COPD), 500, 500f
sensorimotor control of swallowing, 502–504,
503f
afferents, 503
behavioral control assembly, 504
brainstem, 504
central pattern generator (CPG), 504, 504f
chemoreceptors, 503
mechanoreceptors, 503
vagus nerve, 504f
somatosensation and volitional control, 505
variability in pattern, 500–502
taste and smell, 501–502
temperature, 502
viscosity, 501
volume, 501
Synapse, 50, 173
Synaptic cell signaling, 50, 51f
Synaptic cleft, 238
Synaptic signal transmission, 180f
Synaptogenesis, 238, 330
Syncytiotrophoblast, 108
Syndromic hearing loss, 76
Synesthesia, 271
Synovial joint, 18, 66f
Systems oscillator theory, 224, 225f

T

Tachycardia, 338
TA muscle. See Thyroarytenoid (TA) muscle
Taste and smell and swallowing, 501–502
Taste buds, 301
T cells, 329
Technologies and diagnostic testing used in
speech, language, swallowing, hearing,
and balance disorders, 77, 77f
Technologies for analysis of gene expression,
84, 84f
Tectal ridge, 123
Tectoral membrane, 455
Teeth, 401–403, 401f
buccal surface, 402, 402f
canines, 401
cementum, 401
dental anomalies, 403
enamel, 401

gingival line, 401
  labial surface, 402, 402*f*
  lingual surface, 402, 402*f*
  molars, 401
  occlusal surface, 402, 402*f*
  occlusion, 403, 403*f*
  overbite, 403
  overjet, 403
  premolars, 401
  primary vs. permanent, 402*f*
Teeth development, 127–128, 127*f*
  cementum, 128
  dental lamina, 127
  dental papilla, 127
  dentin, 128
  enamel organ, 128
  tooth buds, 127
  tooth germ, 128
Telencephalon, 113
Telophase, 105
Temperature, 275–276
Temperature and swallowing, 502
Temporal bone, 447
Temporal fossae, 394
Temporalis, 236, 237*f*
Temporal lobe, 20, 146
Temporal summation, 177
Temporal theory, 462
Temporomandibular joint (TMJ), 394, 488*f*
Tendons, 66–67
  Achilles tendon, 67*f*
  omohyoid tendon, 67*f*
Tensor tympani muscle, 454
Tensor veli palatini muscle, 399, 451
Terminal boutons, 141, 173
Terminal segment, 141
Terms of orientation, 4–10
  anatomic planes, 8–10
    anatomic position, anterior view, 8*f*
    axial plane, 8
    cardinal planes and axes, 10*f*
    coronal plane, 8
    frontal plane, 8
    general terms, location and direction, 9
    horizontal plane, 8
    midsagittal plane, 8
    parasagittal plane, 8
    sagittal plane, 8
    transaxial plane, 8
    transverse plane, 8
  caudal, 7
  contralateral, 8
  deep, 7
  distal, 7
  dorsal, 7
  ipsilateral, 8
  lateral, 7
  location and direction, 9*t*
  medial, 7
  medical root words, 5–7*t*
  proximal, 7
  rostral, 7
  superficial, 7
  ventral, 7
Tetanic contraction, 249
Tetrodotoxin, 177, 177*f*
Thalamocortical fibers, 278
Thalamocortical relay cells, 475
Thalamus, 114, 152, 545, 546*f*
Thermoregulation, 335
Third ventricle, 152
Thoracic activity, 313
Thoracic spine, 16
Thoracic wall, 16, 17*f*
Thorax, 16

Three-mass model, 371, 371*f*
Thromboplastin, 331
Thyrohyoid membrane, 358
Thyrohyoid muscle, 364*f*, 365
Thyroid cartilage, 355, 356*f*
Thyroid horns, 356
Thyroid notch, 356
Tidal volume, 321
Timbre, 375
Tip links, 292, 458
Tissues, 54–61
  connective tissue, 55–57, 57*f*, 57*tt*
  epithelial tissue, 54, 54*tt*, 55*f*
    adherens junctions, 55
    basement membrane, 54
    cell junctions, 55, 55*f*
    desmosomes, 55
    goblet cells, 55, 56*f*
    hemidesmosomes, 55
    smoking, effect on, 56
  muscle tissue, 59–61
    cardiac muscle, 60, 61*f*
    esophageal peristalsis, 60, 60*f*
    skeletal muscle, 60, 60*f*
    smooth muscle, 59, 60*f*
  nervous tissue, 57–58
    action potentials, 58
    dendrites, 58
    glial cells, 58, 58*f*
    neurons, 58, 58*f*
Tissues and systems, 8–9
  bone, 10
  cartilage, 10
  epithelial cells, 8
TLC. *See* Total lung capacity (TLC)
TMJ. *See* Temporomandibular joint (TMJ)
TMS. *See* Transcranial magnetic stimulation (TMS)
Todd paralysis, 206
Tongue anatomy, 489*f*
Tongue and articulation, 416–422
  ankyloglossia, 418
  apex, 416
  articulation, role in, 421–422
  cerebral palsy, 417
  chondroglossus, 421
  dorsum, 416
  extrinsic muscles, 419*f*, 420–421, 421*t*
  foramen cecum, 417
  genioglossus, 421
  hyoglossus, 421
  inferior longitudinal muscle, 420
  inferior surface, 418*f*
  intrinsic muscles, 419–420, 419*ff*, 420*t*
  median fibrous septum, 417
  median sulcus, 417
  muscular hydrostat, 418
  palatoglossus, 421
  structures, 416*f*
  superior longitudinal muscle, 420
  transverse muscles of tongue, 420
  vertical muscles of tongue, 420
  Waldeyer ring, 417, 417*f*
Tongue and swallowing, 491
  extrinsic muscles, tongue, 491
  intrinsic muscles, tongue, 491*f*
  somatosensory and taste innervation, tongue, 491
Tongue development, 124–125, 124*f*
  anterior lingual primordia, 124
  copula, 124
  foramen cecum, 124
  lateral lingual swellings, 124
  root primordia, 124
  sulcus terminalis, 124

  tubercular impar, 124
Tonic contraction, 498
Tonotopic organization, 456
Tooth buds, 127
Tooth germ, 128
Torso, 16–18, 17*f*
  rib cage, 16
  thoracic wall, 16, 17*f*
  thorax, 16
Total lung capacity (TLC), 320
Touch, 273–274
  cutaneous mechanoreceptors, 273*f*, 274*t*
  hair follicles, 274
  Meissner corpuscle, 274
  Merkel disks, 274
  Pacinian (PC), 274
  Ruffini endings, 274
Trachea, 12
Trachea and bronchial tree, 313*ff*, 316*f*
Tracheobronchial tree, 125*f*
Tracheoesophageal fistulas, 12, 12*f*
Tragus, 450
Traits, 74
Transaxial plane, 8
Transcranial magnetic stimulation (TMS), 206
Transcription, 78, 79*f*, 82, 82*f*, 83, 83*ff*
Transfer RNA (tRNA), 84
Transglottal airflow, 371, 371*ff*
Translation of mRNA, 81*f*, 82, 83, 83*ff*
Transmission segment, 141
Transverse gyrus of Heschl, 475
Transverse muscles of tongue, 420
Transverse palatine suture, 395
Transverse plane, 8
Transverse tubules (T-tubules), 239
Trapezoid body, 472
Traumatic brain injury, 184*t*
Traumatic brain injury skull sutures, 66*f*
Traveling wave, 461, 461*f*
Traveling wave shape (envelope), 463, 464*f*
Trigeminal innervation zones, 277–278
Trigeminal lemniscus, 272
Trigeminal lemniscus and trigeminothalamic tract, 278, 279*f*
  ventral posteromedial (VPM), 280
Trigeminal nerve, 161, 368, 508*t*
Trigeminothalamic pathway, 272
tRNA. *See* Transfer RNA (tRNA), 84
Trochlear nerve, 161
Trophoblast, 106
Trophoblastic villi, 108
Tropomyosin, 241, 242*f*
Troponin, 241
T-shaped cleft, 126
T-tubules. *See* Transverse tubules (T-tubules)
Tubercular impar, 124
Tubulin, 40
Tufted cells, 475
Tuning curve, 267, 470, 470*f*
Tunnel of Corti, 456
Twitch, 249, 250*f*
Two-point discrimination test, 268
Tympanic segment of temporal bone, 447
Tympanic antrum, 448
Tympanic membrane, 451*f*, 459

U

Ultrasonography, 516
Ultrasound imaging, 431, 432*f*
Umbo, 451
UMNs. *See* Upper motor neurons (UMNs)
Uncus, 150
Unicellular, 32
Unilateral hypoglossal nerve lesion, 490, 490*f*
Unipolar neuron, 143*f*, 144

Unmyelinated axons, 143
Upper motor neurons UMNs), 167, 199
Upper respiratory system, 312–313, 312f
　ethmoidal air cells, 312
　frontal sinuses, 312
　maxillary sinuses, 312
　nasal conchae, 313
　nasal septum, 312
　paranasal sinuses, 312
　sphenoidal sinuses, 312
　thoracic activity, 313
　Valsalva maneuver, 313
Uptake and transformation of endogenous and
　　exogenous substances, 332
　vasoactive, 332
Urge-to-cough (UTC), 324, 324f, 325f
UTC. See Urge-to-cough (UTC)
Utricle, 296
Utricle otolithic organ, 525

V

Vagus nerve, 162, 165, 368, 504f, 509t
Vallecula, 358
Valsalva maneuver, 313
Variable expressivity, 89
Vasoactive, 332
VC. See Vital capacity (VC)
Velopharyngeal muscles and articulation,
　　412–416
　adenoids, 416, 416f
　hypernasal, 416
　musculus uvulae, 413, 414f
　palatoglossus muscle, 413
　palatopharyngeus tenses, 414
　Passavant ridge, 415–416
　pharyngeal constrictors, 414f
　pharyngeal musculature, 415f
　soft palate muscles, 413t, 414f
　velum as articulator, 414–415
Velum as articulator, 414–415
Venous and arterial systems connection, 335
Ventral, 7
Ventral intermediate nucleus, 199
Ventral nucleus lateral lemniscus (VNLL), 474
Ventral posterior (VP) nuclei, 297
Ventral posterolateral (VPL) nucleus, 278
Ventral posteromedial (VPM), 280
Ventral respiratory groups, 335
Ventral stream, 288
Ventral stria, 472
Ventricular muscle, 368
Ventricular system, 156–157
　arachnoid granulations, 156–157
　cerebral aqueduct, 156
　cerebrospinal fluid circulation, 157f
　choroid plexus, 156, 157f
　fourth ventricle, 156
　interventricular foramina, 156
Vermal zone, 216
Vermis, 158
Vertebral arteries, 154
Vertebral column, 14–16
　abdominal cavity, 17
　abdominopelvic cavity, 17
　bony vertebral column, 16f
　cervical spine, 16
　lumbar spine, 16
　pelvic cavity, 17
　sacral spine, 16
　thoracic cavity, 17
　thoracic spine, 16
Vertebrobasilar and internal carotid branches,
　　154f
Vertex, 394
Vertical muscles of tongue, 420

Vertigo, 525
Vesicles, 180
Vestibular aqueduct, 455
Vestibular assessment, 548
Vestibular nuclei, 297
Vestibular schwannoma, 536, 536f
Vestibular structure, inner ear, 23f
Vestibulocerebellum, 546
Vestibulocochlear nerve, 162, 534–537
　firing rate, 534f, 535f
　neural connections, 537f
Vestibulocollic reflex, 544
Vestibulo-ocular network, 538–542
　extraocular muscles, 539, 540f, 541t
　eye movement possibilities, 540f
　fovea, 539
　medial longitudinal fasciculus (MLF), 540
　nystagmus, 542
　retina, 539
　stimulation of vestibulo-ocular reflex, 541,
　　542f
Vestibulo-ocular reflex, 538
Vestibulo-ocular reflex stimulation, 541, 542f
Vestibulospinal network, 542–543, 543f
Vestibulospinal reflexes, 538, 538f, 543
Vestibulospinal tract, 167, 298
Vestibulothalamocortical network, 545
VFSF. See Vocal fold surface fluid (VFSF)
Vibratory cycle in phonation, 370–371
　closed phase, 371, 371f
　opening phase, 371
　self-oscillating system, 370
Videofluoroscopy, 513–514, 514ff
Visceral motor fibers, 141
Visceral sensory fibers, 141
Viscerocranium, 10, 13f
Viscosity and swallowing, 501
Visual fields, 282f
Visual system, 281–288
　central visual pathway, 286–288, 286f
　　lateral geniculate nucleus (LGN), 286
　　optic radiations, 286
　　optic tract, 286
　　primary visual cortex, 286
　　retinotopy, 286
　　superior colliculus (SC), 286
　dorsal stream, 287–288
　light transduction and retinal processing,
　　283–286
　　cyclic guanosine monophosphate (cGMP),
　　　285
　　glutamate, 285
　　OFF bipolar cells, 285, 285f
　　ON bipolar cells, 285, 285f
　　phototransduction mechanism, 284f
　　rod and cone light wavelength sensitivities,
　　　284f
　　second messenger system, 285
　retina, 281–283
　　amacrine cells, 281
　　binocular visual zone, 282–283
　　blind spot, 282
　　cones, 281
　　fovea, 281
　　foveola, 282
　　glaucoma, 283
　　hemifield, 282
　　horizontal cells, 281
　　optic disc, 281
　　retinal layers, 281f
　　rods, 281
　　visual fields, 282f
　ventral stream, 288
Vital capacity (VC), 321, 321f, 380
VM. See Vocalis muscle (VM)

VNLL. See Ventral nucleus lateral lemniscus (VNLL)
Vocal folds, 312
Vocal folds cellular transport, 47, 47f
　apical membrane, 47, 47f
　vocal fold surface fluid (VFSF), 47
Vocal folds nodules, 372
Vocal fold structure, 360–362
　abduction, 360
　adduction, 360
　basement membrane zone (BMZ), 361
　coronal section, 360, 361f
　deep lamina propria (DLP), 361
　ground substance, 361
　intermediate lamina propria (ILP), 361
　macula flava, 362
　phonation threshold pressure (PTP), 361
　Reinke space, 361
　superficial lamina propria (SLP), 361
　vocal ligament, 361
　vocalis muscle (VM), 360, 361, 361f
Vocal fold surface fluid (VFSF), 47
Vocal fry, 377
Vocal intensity, 382
Vocal intensity, control of, 375
Vocalis muscle (VM), 360, 361, 361f
Vocal ligament, 358, 359f, 361
Vocal process, 357
Vocal registers, 377
　chest register, 377
　falsetto register, 377
　head register, 377
　mixed register, 377
　pulse register, 377
　vocal fry, 377
Vocal tract development, 424–425
Vocal tremor, 376–377
Voice and voice quality production, 378–379
Voice breaks, 376
Voicing and speech, 328–329
　amplitude, 328
　expiratory muscle strength training, (EMST),
　　329
　fundamental frequency, 328
　inspiratory muscle strength training, (IMST),
　　329
　phonation threshold pressure (PTP), 328
　subglottal air pressure, 328
Voicing efficiency, 381
Volley theory, 462–463
Voltage-gated calcium channels, 466
Volume and swallowing, 501
Voltage-gated ion channel, 173
Vomer, 393, 393f, 397
VPL nucleus. See Ventral posterolateral (VPL)
　　nucleus
VPM. See Ventral posteromedial (VPM)
VP nuclei. See Ventral posterior (VP) nuclei

W

Waldeyer ring, 417, 417f
Waveform, 445
Wavelength, 445
Wernicke area, 115, 149, 369
Wernicke's aphasia, 148, 149
White matter, 20, 21f, 115, 144, 145f, 166–167,
　　167f, 477
　dorsal column, 166
　reticulospinal system, 167
　somatotopy, 167
　spinothalamic tract, 166
　vestibulospinal tract, 167

X

X chromosome, 106
Xerostomia, 302, 492

X-linked dominant, 88*t*
X-linked recessive, 88*t*

Y

Y chromosome, 106
Y-linked traits, 88*t*
Yolk sac development, 107
   allantois, 107
   amnion, 107
   amniotic cavity, 107
   amniotic membrane, 107
   bilateral symmetry, 107, 107*f*
   chorion, 107
   endoderm, 107
   epiblast, 107
   extraembryonic mesoderm, 107
   gastrulation, 107
   hypoblast, 107, 108*f*
   mesoderm, 107
   primitive streak, 107

Z

Z. *See* Specific acoustic impedance (Z)
Z-line, 241
Zona pellucida, 106
Zygomatic arch, 393*f*, 394
Zygomatic bone, 393, 393*f*, 397
Zygomaticus major, 407, 407*f*
Zygomaticus minor, 407, 407*f*
Zygote, 105

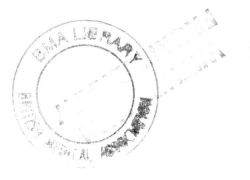